ESSENTIAL
REPRODUCTIVE
MEDICINE

NOTICE

Medicine is an ever-changing science. As new research and clinical experience broaden our knowledge, changes in treatment and drug therapy are required. The editors and the publisher of this work have checked with sources believed to be reliable in their efforts to provide information that is complete and generally in accord with the standards accepted at the time of publication. However, in view of the possibility of human error or changes in medical sciences, neither the editors nor the publisher nor any other party who has been involved in the preparation or publication of this work warrants that the information contained herein is in every respect accurate or complete, and they are not responsible for any errors or omissions or for the results obtained from use of the information. Readers are encouraged to confirm the information contained herein with other sources. For example and in particular, readers are advised to check the product information sheet included in the package of each drug they plan to administer to be certain that the information contained in this book is accurate and that changes have not been made in the recommended dose or in the contraindications for administration. This recommendation is of particular importance in connection with new or infrequently used drugs.

ESSENTIAL REPRODUCTIVE MEDICINE

BRUCE R. CARR, MD

Director
Division of Reproductive Endocrinology
Department of Obstetrics & Gynecology
University of Texas Southwestern Medical Center
Dallas, TX

RICHARD E. BLACKWELL, PhD, MD

Professor
Division of Reproductive Biology & Endocrinology
Department of Obstetrics & Gynecology
University of Alabama at Birmingham
Birmingham, AL

RICARDO AZZIZ, MD, MPH, MBA

Chair
Department of Obstetrics & Gynecology
Cedars-Sinai Medical Center
Professor
Department of Obstetrics & Gynecology and Gynecology
David Geffen School of Medicine at UCLA
Los Angeles, CA

McGraw-Hill

MEDICAL PUBLISHING DIVISION

New York   Chicago   San Francisco   Lisbon   London   Madrid   Mexico City
Milan   New Delhi   San Juan   Seoul   Singapore   Sydney   Toronto

Essential Reproductive Medicine

Copyright © 2005 by The **McGraw-Hill Companies,** Inc. All rights reserved. Printed in the United States of America. Except as permitted under the United States copyright Act of 1976, no part of this publication may be reproduced or distributed in any form or by any means, or stored in a data base or retrieval system, without the prior written permission of the publisher.

1 2 3 4 5 6 7 8 9 0   DOC DOC   0 9 8 7 6 5 4

ISBN 0-07-140993-9

This book was set in Garamond by ATLIS Graphics.
The editors were Andrea Seils, Michelle Watt, and Regina Y. Brown.
The production supervisor was Catherine Saggese.
The cover designer was Aimee Nordin.
The indexer was Robert Swanson.
RR Donnelley was printer and binder.

This book is printed on acid-free paper.

Library of Congress Cataloging-in-Publication Data

Essential reproductive medicine / edited by Bruce R. Carr, Richard E.
  Blackwell, Ricardo Azziz.
      p. ; cm.
   Includes bibliographical references and index.
   ISBN 0-07-140993-9
    1. Endocrine gynecology.   2. Human reproduction—Endocrine
aspects.   3. Infertility—Treatment.   4. Generative organs—Diseases.
I. Carr, Bruce R.   II. Blackwell, Richard E.   III. Azziz, Ricardo.
  [DNLM: 1. Endocrine Diseases—Handbooks.   2. Contraception—
Handbooks.   3. Infertility—Handbooks.   4. Menopause—Handbooks.
WK 140 E78 2005]
RG159.E85 2005
618.2—dc22
                                                    2003071023

Contents

SECTION 1

Fundamentals of Reproductive Medicine / 1

SECTION 2

Disorders of the Endocrine System / 171

SECTION 3

Infertility / 359

SECTION 4

Contraception / 631

SECTION 5

Menopause / 663

Contributors

SANJAY K. AGARWAL, MD

Department of Obstetrics & Gynecology
University of California, San Diego
San Diego, CA
(Chapters 15 and 21)

DAVID F. ARCHER, MD

Professor of Obstetrics and Gynecology
Director, CONRAD Clinical Research Center
Eastern Virginia Medical School
Norfolk, VA
(Chapter 31)

AYDIN ARICI, MD

Professor and Director
Division of Reproductive Endocrinology & Infertility
Department of Obstetrics & Gynecology
Yale University School of Medicine
New Haven, CT
(Chapter 20)

RICARDO AZZIZ, MD, MPH, MBA

Chair,
Department of Obstetrics & Gynecology
Cedars-Sinai Medical Center
and Professor, Departments of Obstetrics and Gynecology,
    and Medicine
David Geffen School of Medicine at UCLA
Los Angeles, CA
(Chapters 13, 15, and 21)

RICHARD BLACKWELL, MD, PhD

Professor and Acting Director
Division of Reproductive Biology & Endocrinology
Department of Obstetrics & Gynecology
University of Alabama at Birmingham
Birmingham, AL
(Chapters 2, 10, 17, and 32)

KAREN D. BRADSHAW, MD

Professor
Obstetrics & Gynecology
University of Texas Southwestern Medical Center
(Chapter 9)

GLENN D. BRAUNSTEIN, MD

Chairman, Department of Medicine
Cedars-Sinai Medical Center
The James R. Klinenberg, MD Chair in Medicine
Professor of Medicine, David Geffen School of Medicine
    at UCLA
Los Angeles, CA
(Chapter 29)

GREGORY A. BRENT, MD

Professor of Medicine and Physiology
David Geffen School of Medicine at UCLA
Chief, Endocrinology and Diabetes Division
VA Greater Los Angeles Healthcare System
Los Angeles, CA
(Chapter 12)

SERDAR E. BULUN, MD

Professor and Distinguished Friends of Prentice
Physician, Department of Obstetrics and Gynecology
Head
Section of Reproductive Biology Research
Northwestern University
Feinberg School of Medicine
Chicago, IL
(Chapter 1)

WENDY Y. CHANG, MD

Fellow
Division of Reproductive Endocrinology and
    Infertility
Department of Obstetrics and Gynecology
David Geffen School of Medicine at UCLA, and
    Cedars-Sinai Medical Center
Los Angeles, CA
(Chapter 15)

BRUCE CARR, MD

Director
Division of Reproductive Endocrinology
Department of Obstetrics & Gynecology
University of Texas Southwestern Medical Center
Dallas, TX
(Chapters 4, 9, and 30)

SEJAL DHARIA, MD

Instructor/Fellow
Division of Reproductive Endocrinology and
 Infertility
Department of Obstetrics and Gynecology
University of Alabama at Birmingham
Birmingham, AL
(Chapter 17)

SABRINA GILL, MD

Division of Endocrinology
St. Paul's Hospital
Vancouver, Canada
(Chapter 3)

BARBARA A. GOWER, PhD

Associate Professor
Division of Physiology and Metabolism
Department of Nutrition Sciences
University of Alabama at Birmingham
Birmingham, AL
(Chapter 14)

JANET E. HALL, MD

Reproductive Endocrine Unit,
Department of Medicine
Massachusetts General Hospital and Harvard
 Medical School
Boston, MA
(Chapter 3)

ROBERT HEYMANN, MD

Fellow
Division of Endocrinology
David Geffen School of Medicine at UCLA
VA Greater Los Angeles Healthcare System
Los Angeles, CA

PETER N. KOLETTIS, MD

Associate Professor
Division of Urology
University of Alabama at Birmingham
Birmingham, AL
(Chapter 16)

ASHIM KUMAR, MD

Fellow
Division of Reproductive Endocrinology and Infertility
Department of Obstetrics & Gynecology
David Geffen School of Medicine at UCLA, and
 Cedars-Sinai Medical Center
Los Angeles, CA
(Chapter 21)

WILLIAM H. KUTTEH, MD, PhD, HCLD

Professor
Obstetrics & Gynecology
Director, Reproductive Endocrinology and Infertility
Director, Reproductive Immunology
University of Tennessee, Memphis
Memphis, TN
(Chapter 24)

LAWRENCE C. LAYMAN, MD

Professor
Chief, Section of Reproductive
 Endocrinology Information & Genetics
Department of Obstetrics & Gynecology
Medical College of Georgia
Augusta, GA
(Chapter 5)

JUERGEN LIEBERMAN, MD

University of Würzburg
Department of Obstetrics & Gynecology
Shady Grove Fertility RSC
Rockville, MD
(Chapter 23)

JOHN MAHAN, MT, MA

Laboratory Manager
OB/GYN Research & Diagnostic Laboratory
Department of Obstetrics & Gynecology
University of Alabama at Birmingham
Birmingham, AL

NEAL G. MAHUTTE, MD

Assistant Professor
Reproductive Endocrinology & Infertility
Department of Obstetrics & Gynecology
Yale University School of Medicine
New Haven, CT
(Chapter 20)

DEBORAH MANZI-SMITH, MD

Advanced Reproductive Medicine
University of Colorado Health Sciences Center
Denver, CO
(Chapter 18)

DAVID R. MELDRUM, MD

Scientific Director
Reproductive Partners
Medical Group, Inc.
Redondo Beach, CA
(Chapter 22)

NORA R. MILLER, MD

Fellow, Division of Reproductive Endocrinology
    and Infertility
Department of Obstetrics, Gynecology, & Women's
    Health
Albert Einstein College of Medicine
Bronx, NY

LYNNETTE K. NIEMAN, MD

Senior Investigator
Pediatric and Reproductive Endocrinology Branch
National Institute of Child Health and Human
    Development
Bethesda, MD
(Chapter 11)

YINKA OYELESE, MD

Division of Maternal Fetal Medicine
Department of Obstetrics, Gynecology, and Reproductive
    Sciences
UMDNJ-Robert Wood Johnson Medical School
Camden, NJ
(Chapter 19)

C. RICHARD PARKER, JR. PHD

Professor of Obstetrics & Gynecology
University of Alabama at Birmingham
Birmingham, AL
(Chapter 6)

RICHARD H. REINDOLLAR, MD

Beth Israel Deaconess Medical Center
Boston, MA
(Chapter 8)

DAVID A. RYLEY

Beth Israel Deaconess Medical Center
Boston, MA
(Chapter 8)

NANETTE SANTORO, MD

Professor
Albert Einstein College of Medicine
Department of Obstetrics, Gynecology, & Women's
    Health
Division of Reproductive Endocrinology and
    Infertility
Bronx, NY
(Chapter 28)

WILLIAM D. SCHLAFF, MD

Advanced Reproductive Medicine
University of Colorado Health Sciences Center
Denver, CO
(Chapter 18)

DALE W. STOVALL, MD

Professor and Director,
Division of Reproductive Endocrinology
    and Assisted Reproduction Program
Department of Obstetrics and Gynecology
Virginia Commonwealth University Medical Center
Richmond, VA
(Chapter 25)

HUGH S. TAYLOR, MD

Associate Professor
Director of Research in Reproductive Endocrinology
    and Infertility
Division of Reproductive Endocrinology and Infertility
Department of Obstetrics, Gynecology, and Reproductive
    Sciences
Yale University School of Medicine
New Haven, CT
(Chapter 7)

LORNA TIMMRECK, MD

Shady Grove Fertility
Rockville, MD
(Chapter 8)

MICHAEL J. TUCKER, PHD, FIBIOL, HCLD

Georgia Reproductive Specialists
Atlanta, GA
(Chapter 23)

CRAIG A. WINKEL, MD, MBA

Department of Obstetrics & Gynecology
Georgetown University School of Medicine
Washington, DC
(Chapter 19)

ELLEN E. WILSON, MD

Clinical Assistant Professor
UT Southwestern Medical Center at Dallas
Dept of Obstetrics & Gynecology
Division of Reproductive Endocrinology & Infertility
Dallas, TX
(Chapter 30)

Preface

Reproductive medicine has continued its relentless growth since the birth of the first child by *in vitro* fertilization in the late 1970's. We now have available new generations of dopamine agonists for the treatment of pituitary tumors and hyperprolactinemic syndromes, highly purified urinary and recombinant gonadotropins for ovulation induction, gonadotropin releasing hormone antagonists, significant advancement in the use of transvaginal ultrasonography, and an exploding new technology in the field of minimally invasive surgery. Accompanying these advances has been a steady improvement in the pregnancy rate with assisted reproductive technology and the introduction of intracytoplasmic sperm injection for the treatment of male infertility and preimplantation genetic studies.

In addition to these scientific changes there has been a redirection of the specialty of obstetrics and gynecology and reproductive medicine. Gynecologists now deal with the general area of women's medicine and are assuming a greater role in the diagnosis and treatment of diseases of the breast. These new roles are assumed in an environment of changing health care delivery, managed care. The new health care is delivered through the use of algorithms that are based on evidence-based medicine and cost-effective analysis. The outcomes of these treatments are subjected to rigorous statistical analysis.

It is the purpose of this book to furnish the practicing obstetrician/gynecologist with a sound scientific basis for diagnosing and managing contemporary reproductive endocrine and infertility problems. The book utilizes the strength of numerous clinicians and scientists from many institutions including our own, The University of Texas Southwestern Medical Center at Dallas, the David Griffin School of Medicine at UCLA and the University of Alabama Medical School at Birmingham to achieve this goal.

Dedication and Acknowledgment

This book is dedicated to our mentors, Dr. Paul C. MacDonald (Dr. Bruce Carr), Dr. Roger Guillemin (Richard Blackwell) and Nestor J Azziz (Ricardo Azziz). The excellent scientific research and teaching done in laboratories such as theirs forms the foundation for this *Essential Reproductive Medicine*. We would also like to thank our respective wives, Phyllis Carr, Kathryn Blackwell, and Cynthia Azziz for their support during the preparation of this book.

Finally, the publication of this book would not have been possible without the help of our associates who contributed to it and the administrative staff who helped prepare it. We wish to express our thanks to Janice Fain (Dr. Carr's administrative assistant), Murrill Lynch (Dr. Blackwell's administrative associate), and Lois Dollar (Dr. Azziz's administrative assistant).

SECTION I

Fundamentals of Reproductive Medicine

CHAPTER 1

Hormone Action

Serdar E. Bulun

This chapter provides general information regarding mechanisms of action of hormones. It is not our intention to provide a complete database of the known signaling pathways; rather we have attempted to familiarize the reproductive endocrinologist with the molecular mechanisms that are responsible for the hormone action that is directly related to reproductive function. Common abbreviations used in this chapter are denoted in Table 1-1.

The term "hormone" applies to a chemical substance that, after being produced in one part of the body, enters the circulation and is carried to distant organs and tissues to modify their structure and function. From the turn of the century until some 40 years ago, the pursuit of endocrinology was confined to determining the chemical nature and properties of the various compounds that could justifiably be termed hormones and estimating their levels in

the blood and other body fluids. During that period, almost nothing was known about their mechanisms of action. It was only with the development of techniques to radiolabel molecules to very high specific activities that it became apparent that the first step in the series of events that led to a cellular response was the binding of an excitatory substance to a receptor. This event, which was found to occur with high specificity and affinity, served therefore as the initial point of contact between the regulatory ligand and the responsive cell. Indeed, the presence of cellular receptors specific for a particular ligand determines the capacity of a cell to respond to that particular hormone.

Over the past four decades, enormous progress has been made in the characterization of a large number of receptors and also of the second messenger systems to which they are coupled, due in large part to the widespread

▶ **TABLE 1-1:** LIST OF ABBREVIATIONS USED IN CHAPTER 1

ANP	Atrial natriuretic peptide	MLCK	Myosin light chain kinase
BNP	Brain natriuretic peptide	N-CoR	Nuclear receptor corepressor
CBP	CREB-binding protein	NFκβ	Nuclear factor kappa beta
CREB	Cyclic AMP response element binding protein	NO	Nitric oxide
		PDGF	Platelet-derived growth factor
CSF-I	Colony stimulating factor-I	PEPCK	Phosphoenol pyruvate carboxy kinase
DAX-1	Dosage-sensitive sex adrenal hypoplasia congenita critical region in the X chromosome, gene 1	PIP$_2$	Phosphatidylinositol 4,5-biphosphate
		PLCγ	Phospholipase-Cγ
DAG	Diacylglycerol	RAR	Retinoic acid receptor
EGF	Epidermal growth factor	RXR	Retinoid-X receptor
FADD	Fas-activating death domain	SCR-1	Steroid receptor coactivator-1
FGF	Fibroblast growth factor	SF-1	Steroidogenic factor-1
G protein	GTP-binding protein	Sgk	Serum/glucocorticoid-activated protein kinases
GRB-2	Grab-2		
HAT	Histone acetyltransferase	SH2	Src-homology-2
HER-2	Human epidermal growth factor receptor-2	SMAD	Sma mothers against decapentaplegic
ICE	IL-Iβ converting enzyme	SMRT	Silencing mediator for retinoid and thyroid hormone receptors
IGF-I	Insulin-like growth factor-I		
Iκβ	Inhibitor kappa beta	SOS	Son of sevenless (Guanine nucleotide exchange factor)
IL-1β	Interleukin 1β		
IP$_3$	Inositol-1,4,1-triphosphate	STAT	Signal transducer and activator of transcription
IRS	Insulin receptor substrate		
Jak	Janus kinase	TFIIA	Transcriptional initiation factor-IIA
LIF	Leukemia inhibitory factor		
LXR	Liver-X-receptor	TNF	Tumor necrosis factor
MAPKK	Mitogen-activated protein kinase kinase	TRADD	TNF-α-receptor-activating death domain

deployment of the tools of molecular and cellular cloning. In general, it can be considered that hormone receptors fall into two categories: those present on the cell surface, which in general interact with hormones that are water soluble such as peptide and protein hormones, as well as prostaglandins, catecholamines and other neurotransmitters (Table 1-2). On the other hand, lipophilic hormones such as steroids, as well as thyroid hormones, retinoic acid, and 1,25 dihydroxyvitamin D3 interact with receptors primarily localized within the nucleus (Table 1-1). To interact with nuclear receptors, therefore, these compounds presumably have to diffuse freely through the lipophilic plasma membrane, cytoplasm and nuclear membrane to interact with their receptors.

Many of these substances do not fall into the strict definition of the term *endocrine* in that they are not necessarily produced at a site distal to the target cell. On the contrary, many regulatory substances are produced and secreted by cells proximal to the target cell, e.g. neurotransmitters. The term *paracrine* has been coined to define such factors. It also is recognized that some regulatory substances interact with receptors on the surface of the same cells that produce them. Such factors are known as *autocrine* agents. And, finally, it now appears that there are intracellular receptors that interact

► **TABLE 1-2:** CLASSIFICATION OF RECEPTORS

Cell-surface receptors
G protein–coupled receptors (e.g., receptors for epinephrine, norepinephrine, LH, hCG, FSH, TSH)
Receptor kinases
    Receptor tyrosine kinases (e.g., receptors for insulin, IGF-1, EGF, FGF)
    Receptor serine/threonine kinases (e.g., receptors for TGF-β activin, inhibin)
Cytokine receptors (e.g., receptors for GH, prolactin, cytokines)
Receptor guanylate cyclases (e.g., receptors for ANP, NO)
Ligand-gated ion channels (e.g., muscarinic receptor for acetylcholine, receptor for GABA)

Hormone-activated transcription factors (nuclear receptors)
Steroid hormone receptors
    Estrogen receptors (e.g., ERα and ERβ, receptors for estradiol)
    Progesterone receptors (e.g., PR-A and PR-B, receptors for progesterone)
    Androgen receptor (receptor for testosterone and DHT)
    Glucocorticoid receptor (receptor for cortisol)
    Mineralocorticoid receptor (receptor for aldosterone)
Thyroid hormone receptors (e.g., TRα and TRβ, receptors for T_3)
Receptors for vitamins
    Vitamin D receptor (VDR, receptor for 1, 25-(OH)$_2$-vitamin D_3)
    Retinoic acid receptors (RARα, RARβ, RARδ; receptors for all-trans-retinoic acid)
    Retinoid X receptors (RXRα, RXRβ, RXRδ; receptors for 9-cis-retinoic acid)
Receptors for metabolic products and environmental toxins
    Liver-X receptors (LXRα and LXRβ, receptors for oxysterols)
    Peroxisome proliferator–activated receptors (PRARα, PRARβ, PRARδ; receptors for fatty acids
        and troglitazones)
    Sterol and xenobiotic receptor (SXR).
Orphan receptors (putative ligands are not known; e.g., SF-1, DAX-1, COUP-TF).

with ligands present within the same cell and never leave that cell. The term *intracrine* has been introduced to define this type of ligand-receptor interaction.

A receptor recognizes one particular ligand among all other molecules in the environment of the cell. Binding of this hormone or ligand to its receptor gives rise to transmission of a signal that results in a biological response. Hormones are normally present in the circulation and tissues in very low concentrations. Thus, a hormone must bind to a receptor much more avidly in comparison with other molecules in the environment in order to initiate a signal. This is referred to as "affinity." The hormone must also bind to a receptor with high specificity to produce a predictable biological outcome.

The affinity of a hormone-receptor interaction is defined in terms of the "equilibrium dissociation constant (K_d)." In a system in which there is a single class of binding sites with no interactions among receptors, the K_d is defined as the concentration of hormone required for binding to 50 percent of the receptor sites at equilibrium. The affinity can also be expressed in terms of the "equilibrium association constant (K_a)," the reciprocal of the K_d.

Analogues of hormones that bind to receptors and elicit the same biologic response as the naturally occurring hormone are termed "agonists." Molecules that bind to receptors but fail to elicit the normal biologic response are termed "competitive antagonists" because they occupy the receptors and prevent the binding of the biologically active molecules. Molecules that bind to receptors, but are less biologically active than the native hormone, are termed "partial agonists." The term "partial antagonist" also applies because partial agonists bind to receptors and prevent the binding of the fully biologically active native hormone. A large number of therapeutic agents fall into the category of hormone agonists, antagonists or partial agonist-antagonists.

The receptors have two principal functions: (*i*) to bind a hormone and (*ii*) to activate an intracellular signaling cascade upon hormone binding. Based on these properties and the location of a receptor in a cell, there are two broad categories of receptors: 1) cell-surface receptors and 2) nuclear receptors (Table 1-1). The first group of receptors interacts with hormones that do not enter cells. In this case, hormone-receptor interaction generates a signal via second messengers. GTP binding (G) protein-coupled receptors and receptor tyrosine kinases represent some of the major superfamilies in this category of cell-surface receptors (Table 1-1). The second category of receptors is activated by ligands that can enter the cells readily and include receptors for steroid and thyroid hormones.

▶ G PROTEIN-COUPLED RECEPTORS

These receptors contain seven transmembrane α helices connected by 3 intracellular loops and 3 extracellular loops with an extracellular amino terminus and an intracellular carboxyl terminus (Fig. 1-1). The ligands of these receptors include protein and peptide hormones, prostaglandins, catecholamines, and other neurotransmitters. Such receptors are integral membrane proteins that traverse the plasma membrane. As indicated earlier, the function of a receptor is to interact with its regulatory ligand. In the case of plasma membrane receptors, this interaction results in the transduction, followed by the amplification, of a signal. This signal generally takes the form of a second messenger molecule, such as cyclic adenosine monophosphate (cAMP) or inositol triphosphate, or calcium ions.

G-protein-coupled receptors represent a large superfamily of receptors, which includes the β- and α-adrenergic receptors, muscarinic cholinergic receptors, and receptors for prostaglandins, gonadotropins, thyrotropin (TSH), corticotropin (ACTH), gonadotropin releasing

---

Figure 1-1 The G protein-coupled receptor (GPCR) superfamily: diversity in ligand binding and structure. Each panel depicts various members of the GPCR superfamily in cartoon form. The seven membrane-spanning α helices are shown as cylinders with the extracellular amino terminus and three extracellular loops above and the intracellular carboxyl terminus and three intracellular loops below. The superfamily can be divided into three subfamilies on the basis of amino acid sequence conservation within the transmembrane helices. Family 1 includes (*A*) the opsins, in which light (*jagged arrow*) causes isomerization of retinal covalently bound within the pocket created by the transmembrane helices (*bar*); (*B*) monoamine receptors, in which agonists (*arrow*) bind noncovalently within the pocket created by the transmembrane helices (*bar*); (*C*) receptors for peptides such as vasopressin, in which agonist binding (*arrow*) may involve parts of the extracellular amino terminus and loops as well as the transmembrane helices (*bar*); and (*D*) glycoprotein hormone receptors, in which agonists (*oval*) bind to the large extracellular amino terminus, thereby activating the receptor through as yet undefined interactions with the extracellular loops or transmembrane helices (*arrow*). Family 2 includes receptors for peptide hormones such as parathyroid hormone (PTH) and secretin. Agonists (*arrows*) may bind to residues in the extracellular amino terminus and loops as well as transmembrane helices (*bar*). Family 3 includes the extracellular Ca^{2+} sensing receptor and metabotropic glutamate receptors. Agonists (*sphere*) bind in a cleft of the Venus flytrap-like domain in the large extracellular amino terminus, thereby activating the receptor through as yet undefined interactions with the extracellular loops or transmembrane helices (*arrow*).

FAMILY 1

A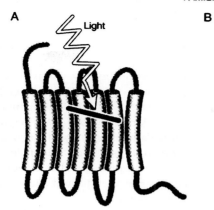

Light

B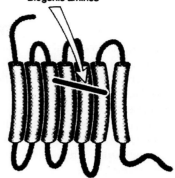

Biogenic amines

C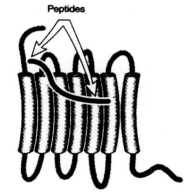

Peptides

D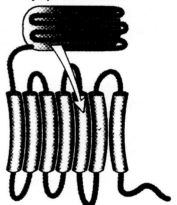

Glycoprotein hormones

FAMILY 2

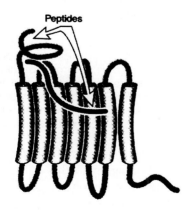

Peptides

FAMILY 3

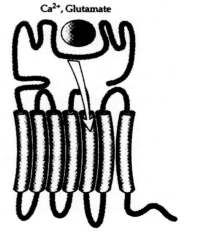

Ca^{2+}, Glutamate

hormone (GnRH), angiotensin II, serotonin, and substance P, as well as the receptor mediating the response of the retinal rod cells to light, namely, rhodopsin[1] (Fig. 1-1). These receptors are characterized by having seven transmembrane domains; signal transduction is mediated by a second group of receptor interacting proteins known as guanine nucleotide-binding or G proteins (discussed below).

We will emphasize the receptors for glycoprotein hormones and associated signaling pathways in the following section, because hormone receptors of particular interest to the reproductive endocrinologist, namely, FSH and LH/hCG receptors belong to this family. The associated signaling pathways in ovarian cells typically involve activation of adenylate cyclase, cAMP, PKA and subsequent binding of certain transcription factors (CREB/ATF, SF-1, C/EBPs) to the steroidogenic genes.

Receptors For Glycoproteins

This subgroup of the G protein-coupled superfamily of receptors interacts with large hydrophilic molecules as ligands, namely, the glycoprotein hormones, human chorionic gonadotropin (hCG), luteinizing hormone (LH), follicle-stimulating hormone (FSH), and TSH[1]. The extracellular N-terminal region of these receptors is extremely long and maintains the conformation of the ligand-binding site by forming disulfide bridges (Fig. 1-1). The LH receptor, which mediates the actions of LH and hCG, is a transmembrane polypeptide. The C-terminal half of the protein contains seven hydrophobic regions, each of sufficient length to span the plasma membrane, and therefore traverses the plasma membrane seven times (Fig. 1-1). The cytoplasmic loop between the fifth and sixth transmembrane domains is especially large and is involved in interaction with G proteins[2]. The binding of LH or hCG to LH receptors promotes interaction of the receptors with the stimulatory

guanine nucleotide-binding protein of adenylate cyclase (G_s). Interaction of the LH receptor with G_s promotes the activation of adenylate cyclase that gives rise to formation of cAMP (see below). There also is evidence for activation of phospholipase C by LH receptor.

We should point out here that the receptor for the decapeptide, GnRH, also has seven transmembrane domains but does not belong to the family of glycoprotein hormone receptors. In contrast to glycoprotein hormone receptors, the extracellular domain of the GnRH receptor, is much smaller. The mechanism of signal transduction by this receptor gives rise to an increase in the levels of cytosolic free calcium ion. Calcium appears to be the intracellular mediator of GnRH action on LH release, which involves calmodulin[3].

Signal Transduction Mechanisms Utilized by the G Protein-Coupled Glycoprotein Hormone Receptors

The second messenger hypothesis of hormone action was proposed in the early 1960s when it was discovered that the activation of glycogen phosphorylase by epinephrine and glucagon in liver slices was mediated by the formation of a heat-stable compound, identified as cAMP. Cyclic AMP is formed from Mg^{++} adenosine triphosphate (ATP) by a membrane-associated enzyme, adenylate cyclase[1]. According to this concept, the hormone, or first messenger, carries information from its site of production to the target cell where it binds to specific receptors on the cell surface. This results in the activation of a membrane-bound enzyme or effector (e.g., adenylate cyclase), which generates a soluble intracellular second messenger (e.g., cAMP), which then transmits the information to the cellular machinery, resulting in a biologic response. Following this seminal observation, a number of other effector/second messenger systems have been discovered that mediate the actions of a variety of hormones on cellular metabolism and function[1].

Hormone-Sensitive Adenylate Cyclase

The hormone-sensitive adenylate cyclase system has at least three components: the receptor (R), a form of guanine nucleotide-binding regulatory protein (G_s or G_i), and the catalytic component (C), namely adenylate cyclase itself, which enzymatically converts $Mg^{++} \cdot ATP$ to cAMP (Fig. 1-2). The guanine nucleotide-binding regulatory protein, G_s, mediates the actions of hormones that stimulate adenylate cyclase activity, whereas G_i mediates the actions of those hormones that inhibit adenylate cyclase. A number of different types of hormone receptors on a single cell can interact with the same pool of regulatory and catalytic components, and these combined interactions result in either a net stimulation or inhibition of adenylate cyclase activity. G_s and G_i are heterotrimers comprised of a unique α-subunit ($α_s$ or $α_i$) and identical β- and γ-subunits. Numerous different

α-subunit proteins have now been characterized, as well as several β- and γ-subunits.

Receptor-Mediated Stimulation of Adenylate Cyclase

The proposed mechanism for the hormonal activation of adenylate cyclase is presented in Figure 1-3[1]. As discussed above, G_s has three subunits, $α_s$, β, and γ. In the inactive state, the guanine nucleotide bound to the α-subunit of G_s is guanosine diphosphate (GDP). The binding of hormone (H) to receptor (R) is believed to promote the formation of the ternary complex, $H \cdot R \cdot G$, which facilitates the dissociation of GDP and the binding of GTP to the G_sα-subunit. The binding of GTP to G_sα results in the dissociation of $α_s$ from the βγ-subunits. The G_sα·GTP then associates with the catalytic subunit (C) of the adenylate cyclase to form the active holoenzyme (G_sα·GTP·C). The activated catalytic subunit then converts $Mg^{++} \cdot ATP$ to cAMP. The activated G_sα contains a GTPase activity, which rapidly catalyzes the

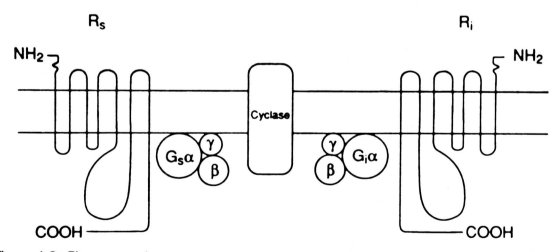

Figure 1-2 Plasma membrane components of hormone-sensitive adenylate cyclase. Hormone-sensitive adenylate cyclase is composed of the following integral proteins of the plasma membrane: receptors for either stimulatory (R_s) or inhibitory (R_i) hormones, the guanine nucleotide-binding regulatory proteins G_s or G_i, and the catalytic component (cyclase). G_s is comprised of a unique α-subunit, $M_r \cong 45,000$, and β and γ subunits, $M_r \cong 35,000$ and $10,000$, respectively. G_i has a unique α-subunit, $M_r = 41,000$, and β- and γ-subunits that appear to be similar to those of G_s.

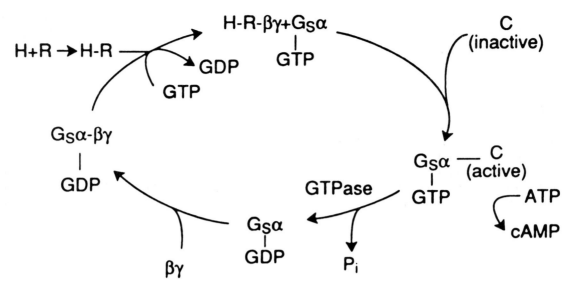

Figure 1-3 Proposed mechanism for the hormonal activation of adenylate cyclase. G_s is composed of three subunits, α_s, β, and γ (depicted here as $G_s\alpha$ and $\beta\gamma$). In the absence of the binding of a stimulatory hormone to its receptor, the guanine nucleotide GDP is bound to $G_s\alpha$, and adenylate cyclase is in the inactive state. The binding of hormone to receptor facilitates the dissociation of GDP and the association of GTP with the α-subunit of G_s. This, in turn, results in the dissociation of $G_s\alpha$ from the $\beta\gamma$ subunits and its association with the catalytic component (C), resulting in adenylate cyclase activation. The activated $G_s\alpha$ has GTPase activity, which hydrolyzes the bound GTP to GDP, resulting in a return of adenylate cyclase to an inactive state. Cholera toxin, which inhibits the GTPase activity, causes a persistent activation of adenylate cyclase.

hydrolysis of GTP to GDP and terminates the cycle of adenylate cyclase activation. Substitution of a nonhydrolyzable analogue of GTP, e.g., GTPγS, or inhibition of the GTPase activity can result in permanent activation of G proteins. For example, cholera toxin, produced by the bacterial organism *Vibrio cholera,* binds to gangliosides (complex glycolipids) on the cell surface and penetrates the cell membrane. Once within the cell membrane, the toxin catalyzes the adenosine diphosphate (ADP) ribosylation of $G_s\alpha$, which results in inhibition of the GTPase activity (Fig. 1-3), causing a persistent activation of adenylate cyclase. In intestinal mucosal cells, the binding of cholera toxin and subsequent activation of adenylate cyclase results in the stimulation of ion (primarily Cl^-) and water secretion across the intestinal brush border, causing massive diarrhea. A mutation in the $G_s\alpha$ gene may also give rise to the inhibition of its

GTPase activity and ligand-independent stimulation of multiple endocrine glands including gonads. Such is the case in McCune-Albright syndrome, in which a postzygotic mutation becomes manifest as autonomous activation of $G_s\alpha$ in the ovaries, testes, parathyroids, adrenals and melanocytes of the skin.

Receptor-Mediated Inhibition of Adenylate Cyclase

A number of hormones inhibit adenylate cyclase activity. These include catecholamines that bind to α_2-adrenergic receptors, muscarinic-cholinergic agonists, and opioids. These hormones bind to cell surface receptors that interact with the inhibitory guanine nucleotide-binding regulatory protein, G_i. Like $G_s\alpha$, $G_i\alpha$ contains a guanine nucleotide-binding site. The binding of these hormones to their receptors promotes the exchange of GTP for GDP on $G_i\alpha$.

This results in the dissociation of α_i from $\beta\gamma$. The inhibition of adenylate cyclase activity appears to be mediated primarily by the interaction of the free $\beta\gamma$-subunits of G_i with the α-subunit of G_s, reducing the concentration of free $G_s\alpha$. Islet-activating protein, one of the toxins of *Bordetella pertussis,* prevents the dissociation of G_i, which results in adenylate cyclase activation, because less free $\beta\gamma$ is available to interact with $G_s\alpha$. Thus, cholera toxin activates adenylate cyclase by promoting the dissociation of G_s, whereas islet-activating protein activates adenylate cyclase by inhibiting the dissociation of G_i. However, there are several examples, including one form of adenylate cyclase, in which the $\beta\gamma$ dimer can also interact directly with an effector molecule to mediate signal transduction.

Structure of Adenylate Cyclase

The structure of adenylate cyclase has been deduced on the basis of the sequence of cDNA clones (Fig. 1-4)[4]. The cyclase is a large transmembrane glycoprotein comprised of two similar regions, each of which has six transmembrane domains, separated by a long (~42 kDa) cytoplasmic loop. Both the N- and the C-termini are intracellular, and the N-terminal

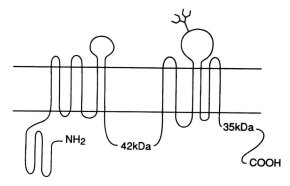

Figure 1-4 Structure of adenylate cyclase deduced from sequencing of the cDNA. The cyclase can be considered to be composed of two halves; each of which has six transmembrane domains, separated by a long cytoplasmic loop. Both the N- and C-termini are intracellular. The extracellular domain is glycosylated.

portions of each region are quite homologous to each other, as well as to sequences present in guanylate cyclases. Interestingly, the cyclase bears some topological homology to the multiple drug resistance (MDR) gene product, as well as the cystic fibrosis gene product, both of which are channel proteins.

Regulation of Cellular Function by Cyclic AMP

The major mechanism by which cAMP regulates cellular function is through its binding to cAMP-dependent protein kinase (protein kinase A). The cAMP-dependent protein kinase holoenzyme is comprised of a regulatory subunit (R) dimer and two catalytic subunits (C). The R subunit is a cAMP-binding protein, while the C subunit, when free of R, expresses protein kinase activity. Each molecule of R dimer binds four molecules of cAMP. The binding of cAMP to R causes dissociation of the inactive holoenzyme to yield two active catalytic subunits (Fig. 1-5). The active free catalytic subunits can now catalyze the phosphorylation of cellular proteins. Protein kinase A catalyzes the transfer of a phosphate from ATP to the hydroxyl groups of serine and, to a lesser extent, threonine residues on cellular proteins. The phosphorylation of enzymes may result in increases or decreases in activity. For example, phosphorylation of hormone-sensitive lipase, cholesteryl esterase, or glycogen phosphorylase results in enzyme activation. On the other hand, phosphorylation of glycogen synthase causes a decrease in enzyme activity[5]. The specific responses of various cell types to an increase in cAMP and the activation of protein kinase A is determined by the cellular phenotype and, therefore, by the enzymes and substrates available for regulation. Thus, a

$$R_2C_2 + 4cAMP \rightarrow R_2{\cdot}4cAMP + 2C$$
(inactive)   (active)

Figure 1-5 Mechanism of protein kinase A activation. Abbreviations: R, regulatory subunit; C, catalytic subunit.

major response of a liver cell to an increase in cAMP is the formation of glucose through glycogenolysis and gluconeogenesis. In a fat cell, on the other hand, the primary response to an increase in cAMP is lipolysis of the triglycerides stored in the lipid droplets, giving rise to free fatty acids and glycerol.

In addition to regulating the catalytic activity of enzymes, cAMP also regulates the transcription of specific genes in eukaryotic cells. An effect of cAMP at the level of gene transcription has been found for a number of eukaryotic genes, including steroidogenic P450s such as aromatase, 17α-hydroxylase, 21-hydroxylase and cholesterol side chain cleavage enzyme. The mechanism by which this occurs in many genes has been uncovered with the discovery of the cAMP-response element binding protein (CREB), which mediates the action of cyclic AMP to regulate specific genes. CREB is a member of a large family of DNA-binding proteins, the activating transcription factors (ATF proteins), which bind to a common palindromic DNA sequence TGACGTCA. These proteins serve a role as transcription factors and belong to the group of *trans*-acting regulatory proteins that possess an amino acid motif known as a leucine zipper, *i.e.,* a sequence of some five leucines, each separated by seven other amino acids. This zipper-like motif effects dimerization of the protein. CREB interacts with the TGACGTCA sequence, referred to as the cAMP response element (CRE), a *cis*-acting enhancer element in a number of a cAMP-stimulated genes, such as vasoactive intestinal peptide (VIP), somatostatin, and PEPCK. CREB also binds to DNA sequences that are similar to the CRE as is found in the aromatase P450 gene, resulting in an activation of transcription. CREB is activated by phosphorylation via cAMP-dependent protein kinase A at a specific serine residue.

Other Second Messenger Systems that Interact with G Protein-Coupled Receptors: Phospholipid Turnover and Inositol Triphosphate

Hormones that act through cAMP- and adenylate cyclase-mediated mechanisms include ACTH, glucagon, and the pituitary glycoprotein hormones, LH, FSH, and TSH. The glycoprotein hormone of human placental origin, hCG, which is highly homologous to LH and binds to LH receptors, also increases cAMP formation. Other hormones, such as a_1-adrenergic agonists, angiotensin II, and some hypothalamic releasing hormones, act through mechanisms independent of cAMP. Certain hormones may act through a cAMP-mediated mechanism in one tissue and by a cAMP-independent mechanism in another. For example, vasopressin binds to a specific subset of receptors (V_2) on cells of the kidney collecting tubules and loop of Henle to promote sodium and water reabsorption. These actions of vasopressin are mediated by increased cAMP formation and cAMP-dependent protein kinase activation. On the other hand, in the liver vasopressin acts through another subset of receptors (V_1) to enhance glycogenolysis, and this effect is mediated by a cAMP-independent pathway. The catecholamines, epinephrine and norepinephrine, bind to several subsets of receptors present in different relative amounts in various tissues. Binding of catecholamines to β-adrenergic receptors activates adenylate cyclase and increases cAMP formation. Interaction of catecholamines with α_2-adrenergic receptors, on the other hand, inhibits adenylate cyclase, while binding to α_1-adrenergic receptors increases inositol phospholipid turnover with a resulting increase in the levels of free cytosolic calcium ion and an activation of protein kinase C.

In addition to catecholamines acting through α_1-adrenergic receptors, a number of other regulatory ligands cause increased phospholipid turnover, protein kinase C activation, and increased cytosolic free calcium[6]. Hormone-receptor interactions that result in the formation of these second messengers include the binding of vasopressin to V_1 receptors and angiotensin II to G protein-coupled receptors on liver cells. The binding of hormone to receptor results in the rapid activation of a plasma membrane-associated phospholipase. Although enzymes with phospholipase C activity have received the most attention in this regard, phospholipases A and D may also have regulatory functions in certain second messenger systems, particularly those in which metabolites of arachidonic acid are involved. The phospholipase C in question catalyzes the hydrolysis of a specific inositol phospholipid within the plasma membrane, namely, phosphatidylinositol 4,5-biphosphate (PIP_2), to form the second messengers diacylglycerol (DAG) and inositol 1,4,5-triphosphate (IP_3). The hormonal activation of the specific phospholipase C is mediated by the interaction of the receptor with a specific G protein (Gq)[7]. At least three different phospholipase C (PLC) proteins have been characterized, namely, PLC-β, -γ, and -δ. The particular isoform involved in interaction with this family of receptors is PLC-β[8]. The hydrolysis of PIP_2 to form IP_3 is specifically associated with an increase in the levels of free cytosolic calcium ion and the subsequent physiological response. Furthermore, incubation of permeabilized cells with IP_3 results in a profound increase in the release of calcium ion from intracellular stores, primarily the endoplasmic reticulum. A receptor for IP_3 present on the endoplasmic reticulum has been cloned and characterized. In addition to mediating IP_3-stimulated Ca^{++} influx to the cytosol from the endoplasmic reticulum, this receptor also may act in conjunction with dihydropyridine-gated calcium channels to facilitate Ca^{++} influx from outside the cell. Once formed, IP_3 is rapidly hydrolyzed to IP_2, IP, and inositol by the actions of specific phosphomonoesterases. The action of the esterase that hydrolyzes IP to inositol is inhibited by lithium ion.

Calcium as a Second Messenger

The levels of free calcium ion in the cytoplasm are normally quite low ($\approx 10^{-7}$ mol/L) compared to the levels of calcium ion in the extracellular fluid ($\approx 10^{-3}$ mol/L). Within the cell, calcium is stored in relatively high concentrations in the mitochondria and endoplasmic reticulum (sarcoplasmic reticulum of muscle cells). An increase in the levels of free cytosolic calcium ion can have a variety of effects on the cell, including changes in cell motility,

contraction of muscle cells, increased release of secretory proteins, and activation of a number of regulatory enzymes. Calcium ion exerts most of these effects in cells by binding to specific calcium binding proteins, such as *calmodulin*. The binding of calcium results in the activation of calmodulin, enabling it to bind to various enzymes or effector molecules, causing a change in their activities.

Two enzymes activated by the calcium-calmodulin complex are phosphorylase kinase and myosin light-chain kinase (MLCK), in smooth muscle. Phosphorylase kinase has four subunits, α, β, γ, and δ. The δ-subunit is calmodulin and the γ-subunit is the catalytic component of the enzyme. The α- and β-subunits are phosphorylated by cAMP-dependent protein kinase. Phosphorylase kinase is an example of an enzyme activated by an increase either in intracellular calcium ion (*e.g.*, in response to angiotensin II) or cAMP (in response to glucagon). This provides an example of a system in which the actions of cAMP and calcium occur in the same direction. There are also examples in which the actions of calcium and cAMP are opposed. In smooth muscle, MLCK is activated by Ca^{++}-calmodulin, following the increase in cytosolic Ca^{++} triggered by muscarinic cholinergic activation. This results in phosphorylation of myosin light chains and activation of the contraction mechanism. On the other hand, increased cAMP levels resulting from β-adrenergic activation cause phosphorylation of MLCK via protein kinase A. This causes a decrease in the affinity of MLCK for Ca++-calmodulin and decreased kinase activity, with the result that relaxation ensues.

Binding of GnRH to its G protein-coupled receptor on the surface of the gonadotroph also gives rise to an increase in the levels of free cytosolic calcium ion. This activates the formation and secretion of FSH and LH from pituitary gonadotrophs.

Role of Protein Kinase C

The other product of the hydrolysis of inositol phospholipids, diacylglycerol, also serves as a second messenger by acting within the cell membrane to activate protein kinase C[9]. Protein kinase C is a phospholipid- and calcium-dependent enzyme that catalyzes the phosphorylation of serine and threonine residues on a number of cellular proteins. Diacylglycerol dramatically increases the affinity of the enzyme for calcium ion and therefore promotes an increase in enzyme activity at resting levels of intracellular calcium. The diacylglycerol-mediated hormonal activation of protein kinase C can be mimicked by incubating cells with tumor-promoting phorbol esters, which interact with the enzyme at the same site as diacylglycerol. Because phorbol esters are not rapidly degraded, these agents cause long-term activation of protein kinase C.

In addition to phosphorylating serine and threonine residues on enzyme proteins, protein kinase C, like protein kinase A, is capable of mediating the regulation of expression of specific genes. Just as the action of protein kinase A to regulate gene expression is mediated by a transcription factor, namely, CREB, so the action of protein kinase C is mediated by a transcription factor known as AP-1. This is a heterodimer of two related proteins containing leucine-zipper motifs, namely, c-fos and c-jun, both of which are recognized proto-oncogenes. AP-1 binds to a regulatory element on responsive genes that differs from the CRE by a single nucleotide, namely, TGAC/GTCA. A family of protein kinase C isoforms exists, and the roles for the various family members are currently being investigated.

▶ RECEPTOR TYROSINE KINASES

This large group of cell surface receptors is characterized by having an extracellular domain with a ligand binding site, a single transmembrane domain and a cytoplasmic tail that contains a protein tyrosine kinase domain, *i.e.,* the ability to phosphorylate tyrosyl residues in specific proteins. There are at least 16 families of receptor thyrosine kinases (Fig. 1-6). Some of the well-defined families that fall into this

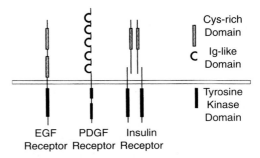

Figure 1-6 Receptor tyrosine kinases. This diagram illustrates 3 of the 16 families of receptor tyrosine kinases[41,42]. All receptor tyrosine kinases possess an extracellular domain containing the ligand-binding site, a single transmembrane domain, and an intracellular domain containing the tyrosine kinase domain. Several structural motifs (i.e., cysteine-rich domain, immunoglobulin-like domain, tyrosine kinase domain) in these receptor tyrosine kinases are indicated on the right side of the figure. Cys, cysteine; EGF, epidermal growth factor; Ig, immunoglobin; PDGF, platelet-derived growth factor.

category include: (1) the EGF, HER-2, v-*erb*B family; (2) the family that includes receptors for PDGF, c-fms/CSF-I, and the product of the c-kit protooncogene and (3) the insulin, IGF-I receptor family. The three families are indicated diagrammatically in Fig. 1-6.

The EGF Receptor Family

The EGF receptor is comprised of a single polypeptide chain of 1186 amino acids. The protein can be divided into three domains: an N-terminal domain of 621 amino acids that contains the EGF binding site; a membrane-spanning domain of 26 hydrophobic amino acids; and a C-terminal cytoplasmic domain of 542 amino acids that shares sequence homology with other tyrosine-specific protein kinases. The tyrosine kinase activity of the receptor is stimulated upon binding of EGF and is believed to mediate most of its actions[10]. The N-terminal region contains many cysteine residues, which are clustered into two regions that may form an EGF-binding cleft. The EGF receptor is found to be overproduced in a number of tumor cell lines, suggesting that overexpression of the EGF receptor gene may contribute to the phenotype of cellular transformation. It also is of interest that the cytoplasmic portion of the EGF receptor, which encodes the tyrosine kinase, has a very high degree of sequence homology with one of the transforming proteins of the avian erythroblastosis virus, the v-*erb*-B oncogene product[11]. The v-*erb*-B gene product induces cellular transformation because of the constitutive expression of the tyrosine kinase domain in the absence of expression of the regulatory EGF-binding domain. Another member of this family is HER-2, a transmembrane protein homologous to the EGF receptor and the *neu* oncogene. Amplification of HER-2 occurs in many adenocarcinomas and is overexpressed in breast tumor tissues of nearly 30 percent of women with breast malignancies. A natural ligand for this receptor has not yet been identified, although ligands for other family members, namely HER-3 and HER-4, are known, e.g., heregulin.

The essential role of HER-2 in the HER signaling network led to the development of anti-HER2 monoclonal antibodies for cancer therapy[12,13]. In particular, the recombinant humanized anti-HER2 monoclonal antibody, inhibits the growth of breast cancer cells overexpressing HER-2 and is widely used for the treatment of women with HER-2-over-expressing breast carcinomas[14]. The efforts are under way to produce substances that target HER-2[14].

The Insulin Receptor Family

The polypeptide hormone, insulin, exerts a variety of metabolic and growth-promoting effects on its target cells that are initiated by its interaction with specific plasma membrane receptors. The insulin receptor is a high-molecular-weight glycoprotein that exhibits insulin-dependent tyrosine-specific protein kinase activity (Fig. 1-7). The receptor exists in the plasma membrane as a tetramer consisting of two disulfide-linked heterodimers $\alpha\beta()2$.[15] The α- and β-subunits of the insulin receptor are synthesized as part of a single 180-kDa precursor polypeptide chain, which is subsequently proteolytically cleaved and inserted into the plasma membrane. The α-subunit can be chemically cross-linked to radio-labeled insulin and contains the hormone-binding site of the receptor. The β-subunits exhibit insulin-dependent tyrosine kinase activity and contain the membrane-spanning domain. The α-subunit of the receptor does not contain a hydrophobic membrane-spanning sequence and is localized exclusively on the outer face of the plasma membrane. Like the N-terminal extracellular domain of the EGF receptor, the α-chain is rich in cysteine residues (Figs. 1-6 and 1-7).

The receptor for IGF-I is quite similar in primary structure and organization to the insulin receptor. The only regions of significant divergence are in the extracellular cysteine-rich region, believed responsible for ligand binding, and in the C-terminus downstream of the tyrosine kinase. The highest homology is in the tyrosine kinase domain, although the IGF-I receptor has a nine amino acid insertion in the kinase domain as compared to the insulin receptor.

The receptor initially characterized as the IGF-II receptor was originally isolated as one of the mannose-6-phosphate receptors. This molecule has a single transmembrane-spanning region and a large extracellular domain, some 2200 amino acids with 15 repeating segments, each containing multiple cysteines. There is a relatively short (164 amino acids) cytoplasmic domain lacking homology to tyrosine kinases. There is evidence to suggest that the role of this receptor is to clear these molecules from the extracellular space rather than serve a second messenger role. It is likely that the biological actions of IGF-II are mediated by its binding to the IGF-I receptor, since the affinity

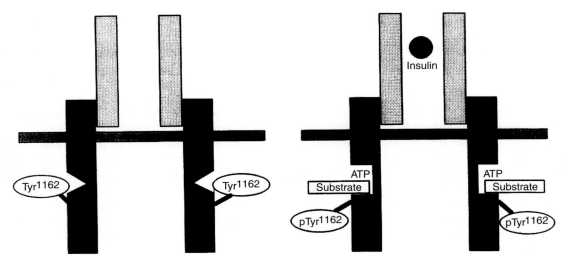

Figure 1-7 Phosphorylation of tyrosine residues in the activation loop leads to activation of the insulin receptor tyrosine kinase. The extracellular α-subunits were shown by shaded rectangles, whereas transmembrane solid black rectangles represent β-subunits. A hypothetical mechanism for ligand-stimulated activation of the insulin receptor tyrosine kinase is illustrated. The model is based on the three-dimensional structure of the isolated insulin receptor tyrosine kinase as determined by x-ray crystallography[43–45]. In the inactive insulin receptor kinase (*left*), Tyr1162 blocks the active site so that substrates cannot bind. In contrast, when the tyrosine residues in the activation loop (including Tyr1162) become phosphorylated (*right*), Tyr1162 moves out of the way, and there is a conformational change that allows binding of adenosine triphosphate (ATP) and protein substrate so that the kinase reaction can proceed. *(Reproduced, with permission, from Spiegel A, Carter-Su C and Taylor S. Mechanism of action of hormones that act at the cell surface, in: Larson PR, Kronenberg HM, eds.* William's Textbook of Endocrinology, *10th ed. Philadelphia, Pa., WB. Saunders, 2003; pp 45–64.)*

of IGF-II for IGF-I receptor is only about two-fold less than that for IGF-I, whereas the affinity for insulin is 100-fold less.[16]

The PDGF and CSF-I Receptor Family

The proteins belonging to this family are all receptors that once again contain a single transmembrane-spanning domain and tyrosine kinase domains in their cytosolic tail (see Fig. 1-6). The extracellular portions of these receptors have 5 immunoglobulin-like domains with a pattern of cysteines distinct from those of the EGF receptor and insulin receptor families. In addition, their tyrosine kinase domains contain 70 to 100 amino acid insertions compared to the tyrosine kinase domains of the EGF receptor and insulin receptor families, and are consequently divided into two segments. The ligands, PDGF and CSF-I, are both disulfide-linked dimeric molecules. PDGF specifically stimulates the proliferation of mesenchymal cells by acting early in the transition from the quiescent state to G_1. It is released from plate-lets when they adhere to injured vessels. However, it is also probably produced by endothelial cells and macrophages. The macrophage growth factor, CSF-I, stimulates hemopoietic precursor cells to form colonies containing mononuclear phagocytes. It selectively binds to hemopoietic precursor cells and promotes their differentiation.

The FGF Receptor Family

Another receptor thyrosine kinase family is that which binds FGF, including acidic and basic FGFs, VEGF, and the int-2 gene product. This group of hormones appears to be important in angiogenesis and wound-healing, as well as the maintenance of neuronal cell viability. The receptor is a 91-kDa protein with a single trans-membrane region. The extracellular portion has three immunoglobulin-like domains found in the PDGF receptor family. The FGF receptor differs from other tyrosine kinase receptors in that the distance between the transmembrane region and the start of the tyrosine kinase domain is longer, some 87 amino acids instead of the 50 amino acids in other receptors of this type. Similar to the PDGF receptor family, the tyrosine kinase domain of the FGF receptor is split by an insert of some 14 amino acids.

Signal Transduction by the Tyrosine Kinase Family of Cell Surface Receptors

A considerable body of evidence exists to support the view that most, if not all, of the actions of this group of receptors are a consequence of the tyrosine kinase activity stimulated upon binding of the ligand. Many of these ligands have growth-promoting activities on their target cells; frequently, overexpression of the receptors can result in the development of a transformed phenotype. Mutations of these receptors, which result in constitutive activation of the tyrosine kinase, also can frequently lead to transformation. An important question that arises then is the nature of the protein substrates for the tyrosine kinase activities of these receptors.

It is now appreciated that these receptors interact to form homo- or heterodimers. In the case of insulin receptors, these exist as tetramers of two disulfide-linked heterodimers. In this way, transphosphorylation of specific tyrosines on the cognate receptor is mediated by the tyrosine kinase of its partner. This gives rise to phosphorylation of thyrosine residues on insulin receptor substrates (IRSs) including IRS-1 and IRS-2. These phosphorylated tyrosines, together with the adjacent amino acid sequences, comprise recognition sequences for adaptor proteins, which mediate the signal transduction cascade (Fig. 1-8). Once such adaptor protein is GRB-2. In common with other adaptor proteins, GRB-2 has a region known as a Src-homology-2 (SH2) domain which recognizes a phosphotyrosine sequence on IRSs and binds to this region. GRB-2 then recruits another protein, SOS, by means of another Src-homology region (SH3), which recognizes a proline-rich region in SOS. SOS, which also is known as guanine nucleotide releasing factor, activates GTP-binding to ras by releasing GDP, and this initiates a phosphorylation cascade involving kinases of the MAPKKK, MAPKK, MAPK families[17]. In this case, MAPKKK is raf, but other possible cascades also have been recognized. Ultimately, the MAPK components activate transcription factors such as members of the Ets family and AP-1 which results in expression of selected genes.

Another enzyme that appears to be activated by the insulin receptor is phosphatidylinositol-3-kinase (PI-3-kinase), which in addition to its catalytic subunit has a regulatory subunit containing SH2 domains (Fig. 1-8). Activation of PI-3-kinase leads to subsequent activation of a variety of signaling molecules including PKC, Akt (PKB) and Sgk (Fig. 1-8).

In conclusion, it is now evident that the tyrosine kinase family of cell surface receptors can activate in overlapping as well as parallel fashions various second messenger systems that are activated by cell surface receptors that interact with G proteins. Clearly, some of these interactions are additive or synergistic, whereas others are opposing. However, the net result is the integrated control of cellular homeostasis, function, and growth.

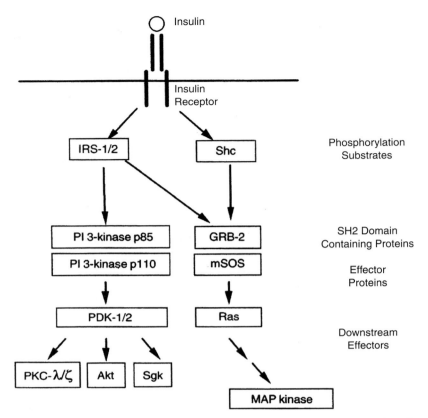

Figure 1-8 Simplified model of signaling pathways downstream from the insulin receptor. Insulin binds to the insulin receptor, thereby activating the receptor tyrosine kinase to phosphorylate tyrosine residues on insulin receptor substrates (IRSs) including IRS-1 and IRS-2[46]. Consequently, phosphotyrosine residues in IRS molecules bind to Src homology 2 (SH2) domains in molecules such as growth factor receptor-binding protein 2 (Grb-2) and the p85 regulatory subunit of phosphatidylinositol (PI)-3-kinase. These SH2 domain-containing proteins initiate two distinct branches of the signaling pathway. Activation of PI-3-kinase leads to activation of phosphoinositide-dependent kinases (PDKs) 1 and 2, which activates multiple protein kinases including Akt/protein kinase B, atypical protein kinase C (PKC) isoforms, and serum/glucocorticoid-activated protein kinases (Sgk)[47]. Grb-2 interacts with m-SOS, a guanine nucleotide exchange factor that activates Ras[48]. Activation of Ras triggers a cascade of protein kinases leading to the activation of mitogen-activated protein (MAP) kinase. *(Reproduced, with permission, from Spiegel A, Carter-Su C and Taylor S. Mechanism of action of hormones that act at the cell surface. in: Larson PR, Kronenberg HM, eds.* William's Textbook of Endocrinology, 10th ed. *Philadelphia, Pa., WB. Saunders, 2003; pp 45–64.)*

Receptor Serine/Threonine Kinases (TGFβ, Activin, Inhibin, MIS)

Receptors for this family of ligands have a unique signal transducing mechanism. The cytoplasmic domains of these receptors contain a serine/threonine kinase. Binding of ligand results in heterodimerization of R1 and R2 receptor isoforms and transphosphorylation. Although many of the downstream events are still unclear, the signal appears to be trans-duced by a series of proteins known as SMADs which upon activation tanslocate to the nucleus where they may activate transcription.

▶ CYTOKINE RECEPTORS

Members of the cytokine receptor family lack obvious kinase homology regions in their cytoplasmic domains. In this case, tyrosine kinase activity resides in a protein that associates with the cytokine receptor. As in the case of tyrosine kinases, ligand binding to the cytokine receptor activates the associated kinase.

The ligands that bind to members of the cytokine receptor family have diverse functions. An important group of ligands for cytokine receptors include GH that is critical for normal stature, prolactin that is essential for lactation, and leptin that regulates the appetite and rate of metabolism. Other ligands of cytokine receptors regulate hematopoiesis and immune response. These ligands include erythropoietin, the majority of interleukins and interferons. The genetic defects in some of these receptors were identified as the etiologies of the human disease: mutations of GH receptor give rise to dwarfism, and mutations of the leptin receptor are associated with severe obesity.

In the case of the class I cytokines, namely interleukin 6 (IL-6), IL-11, leukemia inhibitory factor (LIF) and oncostatin M, the receptor complex contains homo- or heterodimers of a transmembrane component, gp130, which binds a member of the soluble tyrosine kinase family, the Janus family of tyrosine kinases (Jaks).[18] Upon dimerization of gp130 with another subunit that is specific for a particular cytokine, the Jak protein is phosphorylated and in turn, catalyzes the phosphorylation of the transcription factor STAT, which has been recruited to a phosphotyrosine recognition site on gp130 via an SH2 domain (Fig. 1-9). These SH2 domains now recognize the newly phosphorylated tyrosine of another STAT protein, resulting in formation of a STAT homodimer. The STAT homodimer translocates to the nucleus where it binds to a DNA sequence element on responsive genes such as interferon-_ activating sequence, resulting in activation of transcription[18] (Fig. 1-9). Similar mechanisms operate to mediate signal transduction from GH and prolactin, except that different members of the Jak and STAT families are employed.

A direct clinical application of molecular genetics research related to signaling pathways is the discovery of a Janus tyrosine kinase inhibitor currently used in the treatment of leukemia. Imatinib mesylate is a protein tyrosine kinase inhibitor that blocks the Bcr-Abl tyrosine kinase, the constitutively active tyrosine kinase created by fusion of genes on the abnormal Philadelphia chromosome in chronic myeloid leukemia (CML). This tyrosine kinase inhibitor is effectively used to treat CML.[19]

Receptors with Death Domain (TNF, FAS)

These factors, together with IL-1β, are capable of initiating apoptosis in a variety of cell types.[20] However, TNF also has powerful anti-lipotropic activity and is capable of reversing the adipocyte differentiation process. Unlike Fas and IL-1β, TNF also can activate the transcription factor NFκB. These trimeric ligands bind to receptors, which also are trimeric. FAS receptor seems to transduce uniquely the apoptotic pathway. These receptors have no intrinsic kinase activities; however, each contains a sequence known as a death domain, which permits recruitment of the death domain-containing proteins, namely TRADD in the case of the TNF receptor type 1 (p 60), and FADD in the case of the FAS receptor. TRADD initiates a series of events leading to activation of NFκB. This involves phosphorylation of the NFκB inhibitory partner, IKB, leading to its dissociation and activation of NFκB. FADD initiates a cascade of events leading to apoptosis and cell death, which involves activation of ICE-related proteases. TRADD also initiates a similar sequence of events, but does so by first

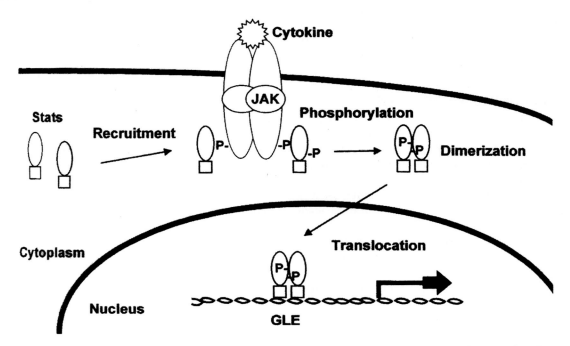

Figure 1-9 Cytokines activate signal transducers and activators of trascription (STATs). STAT proteins are latent cytoplasmic transcription factors. STATs bind, through their Src homology 2 (SH2) domains, to one or more phosphorylated tyrosines in activated receptor-JAK complexes. Once bound, they themselves are tyrosyl phosphorylated, presumably by the receptor-associated JAKs. STATs then dissociate from the receptor-JAK complexes, homodimerize or heterodimerize with other STAT proteins, move to the nucleus, and bind to gamma interferon-activated sequence-like elements (GLEs) in the promoters of cytokine-responsive genes. *(Reproduced, with permission, from Spiegel A, Carter-Su C and Taylor S. Mechanism of action of hormones that act at the cell surface. in: Larson PR, Kronenberg HM, eds. William's Textbook of Endocrinology, 10th ed. Philadelphia, Pa., WB. Saunders, 2003; pp 45–64.)*

interacting with FADD. Many of the actions of TNF at the cellular level can be mimicked by ceramide, indicating that sphingomyelinase activity is involved.

▶ THE GUANYLATE CYCLASE RECEPTOR FAMILY

Shortly after the discovery of cAMP, another cyclic nucleotide, namely cyclic guanosine monophosphate (cGMP), also was discovered. Considerable excitement was generated for several years over the possibility that these two cyclic nucleotides might work in opposite fashions to regulate cell metabolism, the so-called Yin-Yang hypothesis. With the failure of

efforts to confirm consistent cellular responses to cGMP, however, interest in this molecule as a potential second messenger waned. However, investigations into the role of cGMP have intensified with the recent characterization of several proteins containing guanylate cyclase activity and the clear involvement of this cyclic nucleotide in a number of cell regulatory mechanisms.

Soluble Guanylate Cyclases

The first guanylate cyclase to be characterized was found to be soluble and present in the cytoplasm. This protein is now recognized to be activated by exogenous nitrovasodilators such as nitroglycerine and azide. This soluble guanylate cyclase mediates the rapid vasodilatory effects of nitroglycerine on cardiac vasculature. These nitrovasodilators, as well as a number of endogenous activators of the enzyme, such as acetylcholine, histidine, and endothelin, give rise to a common second messenger signal, namely, the formation of the molecule nitric oxide (NO). NO activates soluble guanylate cyclase, which is a heterodimer of subunits of 82 and 70 kDa, each of which has a heme group that binds the NO, as well as a catalytic site. This activation, in turn, leads to increased levels of cGMP. Endogenous nitric oxide is formed from the side chain of the amino acid, arginine, via the activity of the enzyme nitric oxide synthase, which requires calcium and ATP. Several forms of this enzyme exist, which are activated by the endogenous stimulators of this pathway such as acetylcholine, histidine, and endothelin.

Membrane-Bound Guanylate Cyclases

In addition to the soluble guanylate cyclase, there are a number of transmembrane receptors that contain guanylate cyclase activity. These receptors bind such ligands as atrial natriuretic peptide (ANP) and related proteins such as brain natriuretic peptide (BNP) through their extracellular domains and mediate induction of guanylate cyclase activity. ANP an BNP induce natriuresis, diuresis, and vasodilation partially or entirely through the increased production of the second messenger, cGMP.[21] The ANP and BNP receptors are ~130 kDa proteins that have at least four distinct domains; namely, ligand binding, transmembrane, kinase-like, and guanylate cyclase catalytic domains. The kinase-like domain appears necessary for ANP stimulation of guanylate cyclase activity. The guanylate cyclase catalytic domain has sequence similarity to domains found in both the α- and β-subunits of the soluble guanylate cyclase and to the intracellular N-terminal region of adenylate cyclase. In addition to these transmembrane guanylate cyclases, there is another type of guanylate cyclase protein present in retinal rod cells, which is responsible for synthesis of the cGMP involved in transduction of the rhodopsin-mediated light-induced signal. This guanylate cyclase is attached to structural elements within the cell.

One question that arises then is, how does cGMP work in these systems? In the case of the retinal rod cells, there is a cGMP-gated ion channel that allows sodium and calcium ions to enter the cell in the presence of cGMP. Activation of cGMP phosphodiesterase by GTP-bound transducin in response to the light signal results in closure of the channel, thus preventing the uptake of sodium and calcium ions. This results in hyperpolarization of the plasma membrane, which is transmitted to the synaptic terminal at the other end of the cell and conveyed to neurons of the retina. In other cell types, cGMP actions may include activation of a cGMP-dependent phosphodiesterase which, in turn, lowers cAMP levels, and activation of cGMP-dependent protein kinases. Thus, cGMP may indeed oppose some effects of cAMP at various times.

▶ HORMONE SENSITIVITY AND CELL-SURFACE RECEPTORS

Fluctuations in hormone secretion and blood/tissue levels of a hormone represent important determinations of hormone action. An equally important determinant is the sensitivity of a target cell to a given concentration of a hormone. For example, changes in concentration of cellular receptors for a specific hormone can markedly alter the sensitivity of the target cell to that hormone; a decrease in the concentration of receptors can decrease sensitivity to the hormone, whereas an increase in receptor concentration can increase the sensitivity of the target cell for the hormone. It is apparent that the concentration of cellular receptors for a specific hormone can vary considerably with the physiological state. Most commonly, an increase in the level of a specific hormone will cause a decrease in the available number of its cellular receptors. This decrease in available receptors can be due either to a sequestration of receptors away from the cell surface or an actual disappearance or loss of receptors from the cell. This hormonally induced negative regulation of receptors is termed *homologous downregulation* or *desensitization*[22]. Studies of the downregulation of receptors for insulin and EGF by the homologous hormones indicate that downregulation is caused, at least in part, by a clustering of hormone-receptor complexes in coated pits on the cell surface, internalization within coated vesicles, and degradation by lysosomal enzymes. Coated pits and coated vesicles are so named because they contain a protein, clathrin, that forms a "coat" on their cytoplasmic surfaces. There is little doubt that receptor internalization provides an important homeostatic mechanism that serves to protect the organism from the potential toxic effects of hormone excess.

Desensitization is defined as a decrease in the responsiveness of a cell to a constant level of hormone or factor upon prolonged exposure. Homologous desensitization can also result from a hormone-induced alteration in the receptor, which uncouples it from some component of the signal transduction pathway. Another form of desensitization, *heterologous desensitization,* occurs when incubation with one agonist reduces the responsiveness of a cell to a number of other agonists that act through different receptors. This phenomenon is most commonly observed with receptors that act through the adenylate cyclase system. Heterologous desensitization reflects a broad pattern of refractoriness that has a slower onset than homologous desensitization.

▶ NUCLEAR RECEPTORS

Members of the nuclear receptor superfamily are ligand-dependent transcription factors that regulate the expression of target genes via binding to specific cis-acting (hormone-response) elements (Fig. 1-10). The superfamily consists of receptors for steroid hormones (estrogens, progestins, androgens, and corticosteroids), sterol derivatives (1,25 dihydroxyvitamin D_3), and nonsteroids (retinoids and thyroid hormone). It also includes a growing number of structurally related proteins for which ligands have yet to be identified, referred to as "orphan receptors" (see Table 1-2).

Classical steroid hormone receptors comprise an important group, but small component of the nuclear receptor superfamily. Steroids travel in the circulation predominantly bound to several classes of serum proteins. Estrogens and androgens are transported in the circulation bound to testosterone binding globulin (TeBG), which binds estradiol and testosterone with relatively high affinity ($K_d \approx 10^{-9}$ mol/L). These steroids also are weakly bound to serum albumin. Glucocorticoids and progesterone are bound in the circulation to corticosteroid binding globulin (CBG), also referred to as transcortin (Fig. 1-10). Presumably, steroids can freely diffuse across the plasma membranes of all cells but are sequestered only within cells that contain specific intracellular receptors. The steroid binds to its receptor with an affinity ($K_d \approx 10^{-10}$ mol/L) that is at least ten-fold greater than the affinity with which it binds to the serum globulins.

Steroid hormone receptors and other nuclear receptors are synthesized in the cytosol. Entry of nuclear receptors into the nucleus requires the nuclear localization signal, located near the border of C and D domains (Fig. 1-11). Owing to this nuclear translocation signal, most nuclear receptors reside in the nucleus in the presence or absence of a ligand. One exception is the glucocorticoid receptor that is found in the cytoplasm. Binding of hormone transforms the glucocorticoid receptor into an active form by mediating the dissociation of heat shock proteins and allowing the dimerization of receptor proteins. The activated receptor is now able to bind the hormone responsive element in genomic DNA as a homodimer and stimulate, or in some

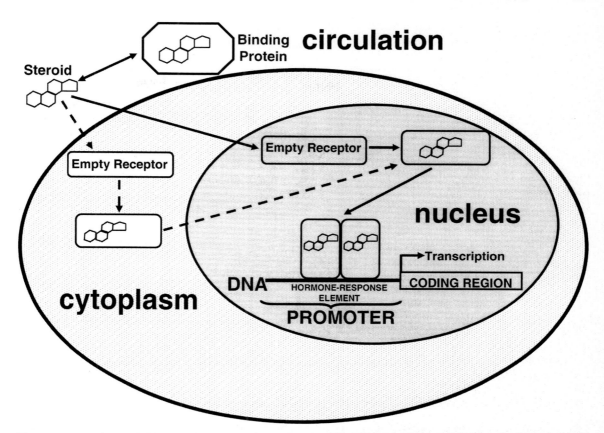

Figure 1-10 A model for steroid hormone action. Biologically active steroids in the circulation are bound to blood proteins. A very small fraction of the circulating steroid is free. The unbound steroid can diffuse into the cytoplasm and nucleus freely. The steroid hormone binds to transcription factors termed "steroid receptors" in the target cell. Steroid receptors are primarily located in the nucleus. Binding of a steroid to its specific receptor activates this receptor. The receptors that contain steroids bind as dimers to specific DNA sequences in the promoters of specific genes. These specific DNA sequences are termed "hormone-response elements." Binding of a dimer of activated steroid receptors to a gene promoter usually initiates transcription, which eventually gives rise to protein synthesis.

cases repress, the expression of target genes (see Fig. 1-10).

The second group within the superfamily are the nonsteroidal, ligand-activated receptors, which consists of the receptors for thyroid hormone, retinoic acid (RAR) and 1,25 dihydroxyvitamin D_3. These receptors are located in the nucleus in their free or bound state, and are bound to their hormone response elements as homo- or heterodimers with another member of the family, the retinoid-X-receptor (RXR) with the absence or presence of ligand: In the absence of ligand, these receptors act as silencers of the genes with which they interact. Ligand binding, however, dramatically alters the activity of these receptors from transcriptional silencers to transcriptional enhancers.

Orphan receptors comprise the largest component of the nuclear receptor superfamily. These receptors can bind as monomers or as heterodimers to defined DNA motifs and may

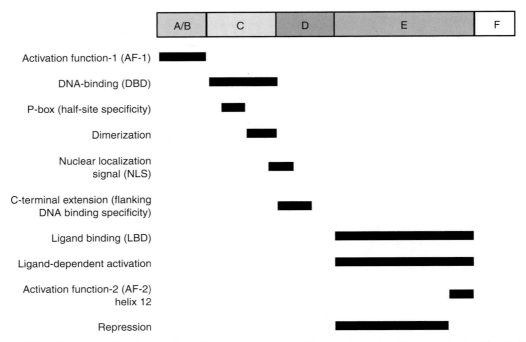

Figure 1-11 Domain structure of nuclear receptors. *(Reproduced, with permission from Lazar MA. Mechanism of action of hormones that act on nuclear receptors: in: Larson PR, Kronenberg HM, eds. William's Textbook of Endocrinology, 10th ed. Philadelphia, Pa., WB. Saunders, 2003; pp 35–44.)*

be constitutively active. Two of the orphan receptors are of particular importance for reproduction: Steroidogenic factor-1 (SF-1, also known as Ad4 binding protein) and DAX-1 [DSS (dosage-sensitive sex) - AHC (adrenal hypoplasia congenita) critical region in the X chromosome, gene-1). SF-1 was originally described by two separate groups for its role in the regulation of the 11-hydroxylase and 21-hydroxylase genes[23,24]. Knockout of the SF-1 gene in mice results in the failure of gonadal and adrenal development, as well as impaired ventromedial hypothalamic nucleus development and gonadotropin secretion. DAX-1 is another orphan receptor. Mutagenesis of the DAX-1 gene has been reported to be responsible for X-linked AHC and hypogonadotropic hypogonadism[25]. SF-1, immediately followed by DAX-1 is expressed in mouse embryos at very early developmental stages in the hypothalamus, pituitary, adrenals and gonads suggesting vital

roles for both factors in the development of these tissues. DAX-1 also is one of the candidate determining factors of gonadal sex.

Receptor Structure

Amino acid sequence analysis indicates that the nuclear receptors share common structural motifs, thus suggesting that they are evolutionarily linked[26]. These domains are referred to as A to F, and each domain accomplishes a particular function. All nuclear receptor proteins have the same general structure, as well as a high degree of homology in their hormone (ligand) and DNA binding regions (see Fig. 1-11). In each case, the ligand binding domain (LBD or E) is localized at the carboxy terminus of the molecule. Within the central portion of the protein lies the DNA binding domain (DBD or C), which contains two repeated units enriched in the amino acids Cys,

Lys, and Arg. Each of these units is folded into a finger-like structure with a zinc ion at its center. These DNA binding "fingers" have the capacity to insert into a half-turn of DNA. The hydrophilic region (D), which varies in length and sequence among the different receptors, may serve as a hinge between the ligand and DNA binding domains. The carboxy terminal regions of the members of the steroid/thyroid receptor gene family all have a high degree of sequence homology with the v-*erb*-A protein of the oncogenic avian erythroblastosis virus. This is the viral counterpart of c-*erb*-A, which encodes the thyroid hormone receptor[27].

High-affinity binding of a lipophilic ligand that can traverse cell membranes is a shared characteristic of many nuclear receptors. The C-terminal ligand-binding domain (LBD) is localized in regions D and E (see Fig. 1-11) mediates this function of the nuclear receptor. This region also has other functions such as transcriptional regulation (also known as activation function-2 or AF-2). The major structural change induced by ligand binding is an internal folding of the most C-terminal helix (H12), which forms a cap on the ligand binding pocket. And this configurational change in H12, in turn, plays important roles in the recruitment of coregulators and thus transcriptional activation and repression in response to specific ligands with pure or mixed agonist or antagonist properties. These observations partially explain the mechanism of action of tissue-selective partial agonism/antagonism (e.g., selective estrogen response modulators or SERMs, see below).

Of potential importance is the finding that most nuclear receptors are phosphoproteins that can be phosphorylated upon hormone binding. These receptors are substrates for protein kinases, such as protein kinase A. For example, in the case of the progesterone receptor, inhibition of protein kinase A can block progesterone action. It is likely, therefore, that phosphorylation plays an important role in modulating the action of nuclear receptors[28].

Target Gene Recognition by Nuclear Receptors

The steroid receptors directly link extracellular signals to transcriptional responses and comprise, in fact, a family of ligand-modulated transcription factors that regulate homeostasis, reproduction, development, and differentiation. Understanding of their mode of action, therefore, requires knowledge of the *cis*-acting (hormone-response) elements of the regulated genes, *i.e.*, the linear sequence of bases that constitutes a regulatory element on the gene with which these ligand-modulated transcription factors interact. These receptors can be divided into several groups depending upon the sequences of the response elements with which they interact (Fig. 1-12). One large group comprises the glucocorticoid, mineralocorticoid, progesterone, and androgen receptors, which all bind as homodimers to the same double-stranded idealized inverted repeat of a six nucleotide sequence (half-site) with a three nucleotide spacer, namely, AGAACAnnnTGTTCT. Members of another broad group, which comprises receptors for thyroid hormones, retinoids, and 1,25-dihydroxyvitamin D_3, usually bind as heterodimers with RXR to a double-stranded direct hexameric repeat of the sequence AGGTCA separated by a spacer of 1-5 nucleotides ($AGGTCAn_{1-5}AGGTCA$). Binding specificity is determined by the number of nucleotides in the spacer (see Fig. 1-12). On the other hand, the estrogen receptor binds to an inverted repeat of a half-site identical to that recognized by the thyroid/retinoid/vitamin D3 receptor subfamily; however, in the case of the estrogen receptor, this is an inverted repeat with a 3 nucleotide spacer, namely AGGTCAnnnTGACCT[29].

As noted earlier, most nuclear receptors bind inverted or direct repeats of their hormone response elements in promoters as dimers. Steroid receptors including ER, function primarily as homodimers, which preferentially bind inverted (palindromic) repeats (Fig. 1-12). The major dimerization domain in steroid receptors is within

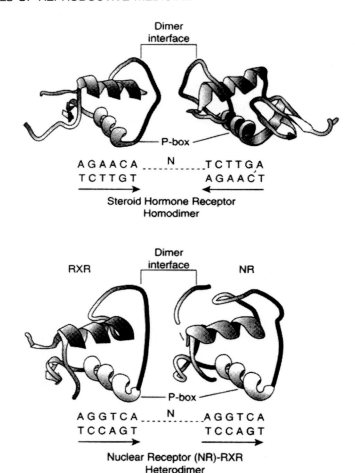

Figure 1-12 Structural basis of nuclear receptor (NR) DNA binding specificity. Ribbon diagrams of receptor DNA-binding domains (DBDs) are shown. *A,* Steroid hormone receptor binding as homodimer to inverted repeat (*arrows*) of AGAACA half-site. *B,* RXR-NR heterodimer binding to direct repeat of AGGTCA. The position of the P-box, the region of the DBD that makes direct contact with DNA, is shown. N, number of base pairs between the two half-sites; RXR, retinoid X receptor. *(Reproduced, with permission from Lazar MA. Mechanism of action of hormones that act on nuclear receptors: in: Larson PR, Kronenberg HM, eds. William's Textbook of Endocrinology, 10th ed. Philadelphia, Pa., WB. Saunders, 2003; pp 35–44.)*

the C-domain (see Fig. 1-11). Most other receptors including thyroid hormone receptor, retionic acid receptor, vitamin D_3 receptor and LXR bind to DNA as heterodimers with RXR.

The fact that the glucocorticoid, androgen, mineralocorticoid and progesterone receptors interact with the same response element implies that specificity of transcription of a target gene, in response to a particular hormone, is governed by whether or not the required hormone receptor is present within that particular cell type. In the case of the thyroid/retinoid/vitamin D_3 receptors, binding specificity is determined, in part by the number of nucleotides in the spacer between direct repeats of the half-site.

Regulation of Transcription of Specific Genes by Nuclear Receptors: Roles of Co-Regulators

Nuclear receptors may activate or repress the transcription of specific genes in the presence or absence of ligands. Ligand-dependent activation of a gene is the best studied function of nuclear receptors and their ligands. Upon binding of a ligand to the LBD, the receptor binds to a hormone response element (HRE) in the gene promoter via its DBD. Transcriptional activation is then mediated primarily by the LBD region, which also mediates an activation function known as AF-2. Activation of transcription requires the assembly of a large multimeric complex that eventually includes RNA polymerase II. A number of basal transcription factors bind to RNA polymerase II and comprise the complex of general transcription factors (GTFs, Fig. 1-13).

The nuclear receptor-ligand complex recruits cofactor proteins, named coregulators. In the case of transcriptional activation, corepressors are recruited, and these adaptor molecules possibly provide the positive physical interaction between the ligand-bound nuclear receptor and the general transcription factors. Coactivators increase the rate of transcription by their DNA unwinding activity and histone acetyl transferase (HAT) activity. For example, SRC-1 (belonGs to the p160 family) and CBP/p300 are recruited by ligand-bound steroid receptors to enhance transcription (Fig. 1-13).

The unliganded nuclear receptors also bind to DNA, and on this occasion, inhibit promoter activity. The unliganded nuclear receptor recruits negatively acting coregulators, named, corepressors to the target promoter. Two well-studied corepressors are N-CoR and SMRT. The corepressors may recruit histone deacetylases (HDACs), thereby reversing acetylation of DNA-bound histones (Fig. 1-13).

Binding of certain ligands to certain nuclear receptors may also give rise to ligand-dependent recruitment of corepressors and inhibition of gene transcription. In this case, ligand-bound receptors recruit corepressors and HDAC to the promoter region and suppress transcription (see Fig. 1-13).

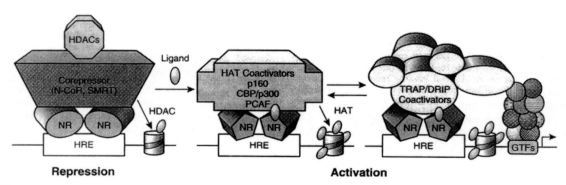

Repression   **Activation**

Figure 1-13 Coactivators and corepressors in transcriptional regulation by nuclear receptors. CBP, CREB-binding protein; DRIP, Dreceptor-interacting protein; HRE, hormone response element; HAT, histone acetyltransferase; HDAC, histone deacetylase; N-CoR, nuclear receptor corepressor; NR, nuclear receptor; PCAF, p300/CBP-associated factor; SMRT, silencing mediator of retinoid and thyroid receptors; TRAP, thyroid hormone receptor-associated protein. *(Reproduced, with permission from Lazar MA. Mechanism of action of hormones that act on nuclear receptors: in: Larson PR, Kronenberg HM, eds.* William's Textbook of Endocrinology, 10th ed. *Philadelphia, Pa., WB. Saunders; 2003; pp 35–44.)*

Tissue-Selective Agonist vs. Antagonist Activity of a Ligand

Certain ligands act as agonists in some tissues but as antagonists in others. This is best exemplified by the introduction of selective estrogen response modulators (SERMs) widely used in the treatment of breast cancer[30]. One such compound, tamoxifen, acts as an agonist in the bone and endometrium but as an antagonist in the breast cancer tissue, which led to its widespread use to treat breast cancer (Fig. 1-13).

The following factors may determine whether a compound will act as an agonist or antagonist in a given tissue: (*i*) nuclear receptor levels and their phosphorylation states, (*ii*) ligand levels, (*iii*) structure of the ligand, (*iv*) the types and levels of coactivators vs. corepressors, and (*v*) the complement of target genes that are expressible and available to hormone regulation in that particular tissue.

Thus, when a ligand (e.g., SERM) reaches a specific tissue and interacts with ERs, the conformation of ERs change (Fig. 1-14). This conformational change gives rise to recruitment of a coactivator or a corepressor based on the availability of these regulatory factors in this particular tissue[30]. The coactivator binding gives rise to an agonist-effect, whereas corepressor binding renders this compound an antagonist (Fig. 1-14).

It is hypothesized that estradiol induces specific conformational changes in the ER in the breast, bone and endometrium leading to coregulator recruitment that is favorable for growth. Thus, estradiol acts as an agonist in all 3 tissues. Tamoxifen, on the other hand, is an agonist in the bone and endometrium, possibly because it leads to recruitment of coregulators to the ER, which favor growth in these tissues (see Fig. 1-14). Tamoxifen, however, acts as an antagonist in the breast, possibly, because it is successful in recruiting coregulators to the ER-based transcriptional complexes giving rise to a gene expression profile that favors suppression of growth. We should emphasize that this is a rather simplistic model and there may be additional levels of complexity responsible for tissue-selective nuclear receptor ligands.

▶ ENDOCRINE DISORDERS DUE TO DEFECTS IN SIGNAL TRANSDUCTION

Most of the genetic defects that result in endocrine disorders have been localized to the hormone receptors (Table 1-3). The following are some examples that are relevant to the reproductive endocrinologist: Mutations in the LH receptor gene giving rise to inactivation [[2557]] or autonomous activation of the LH receptor have recently been described[31,32]. A homozygous inactivating mutation (recessive) in the sixth transmembrane domain of the LH receptor has been found to give rise to Leydig cell hypoplasia with deficient testosterone formation in 46,XY fetuses[31]. This results in male pseudohermaphroditism. Activating heterozygous mutations (dominant) in the sixth transmembrane domain and third cytosolic loop of the LH receptor, on the other hand, become manifest as male-limited precocious puberty (testotoxicosis), which is characterized by increased testosterone synthesis in the absence of testicular stimulation by LH[32]. The female members of these families that carry this mutation are phenotypically normal.

The overproduction of endogenous hCG during pregnancy has been associated with spontaneous ovarian hyperstimulation syndrome. Yet the syndrome has also been observed in women with normal levels of hCG. Two recent reports described recurrent gestational spontaneous ovarian hyperstimulation syndrome in women with heterozygous mutations in the FSH receptor[33,34]. The mutant FSH receptors responded to hCG.

Clinical manifestations of $G_s\alpha$ defects are extremely diverse. Mutations that give rise to autonomous activation of $G_s\alpha$ are manifest as the McCune-Albright syndrome. In this disorder, the mutant $G_s\alpha$ associated with LH, FSH,

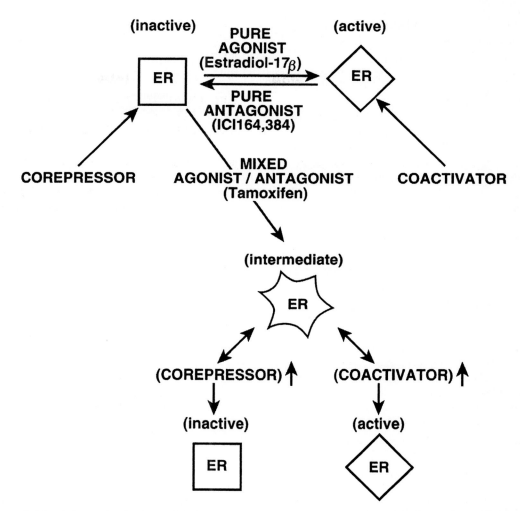

Figure 1-14 A hypothetical model that explains the mixed agonistic/antagonistic properties of the SERM, tamoxifen. This figure indicates that receptor conformation is dependent on which ligand binds to the receptor (ER). The ER conformation induced by pure agonist (e.g., estradiol-17β can make it interact with coactivators, whereas conformation induced by pure antagonists (e.g., ICl164,384) results in interaction with corepressors. For mixed agonists/antagonists (e.g., tamoxifen), the conformation varies depending on the relative ratio of coactivator and corepressor within the cell. When the intracellular corepressor is high (e.g., breast tissue), ER will be inactivated. In contrast, when the intracellular coactivator is high (e.g., endometrial tissue), the ER will shift to bind to the coactivator, resulting in an active receptor. *(Reproduced, with permission from Bulun SE and Simpson ER. Estrogen action, breast. in: Knobil E and Neill J, eds.* Encyclopedia of Reproduction, *Academic Press, San Diego, CA., 1999: Volume 2, pp 71–79.)*

▶ **TABLE 1-3:** ENDOCRINOPATHIES IN HUMANS DUE TO GENE DEFECTS IN SIGNAL TRANSDUCTION

Mutated Gene	Inheritance	Result	Phenotype
LH receptor[31]	Autosomal recessive	Inactivation	Leydig cell hypoplasia (Male pseudohermaphroditism)
LH receptor[32]	Autosomal dominant	Activation	Testotoxicosis (Familial male-limited precocious puberty)
FSH receptor[33,34]	Autosomal dominant	Activation	Spontaneous ovarian hyperstimulation syndrome during pregnancy
TSH receptor	Autosomal dominant	Activation	Non-autoimmune autosomal dominant hyperthyroidism
$G_s\alpha$	Postzygotic mutation	Activation	McCune-Albright syndrome (Male and female precocious puberty and other endocrine hyperfunction)
$G_s\alpha$[15]	Postzygotic mutation	Temperature-sensitive activation/ inactivation	Testotoxicosis and PTH-resistant (pseudo)hypoparathyroidism
$G_s\alpha$	Postzygotic mutation	Inactivation	Pseudohypoparathyroidism
Estrogen receptor[36]	Autosomal recessive	Inactivation	Estrogen resistance (Tall stature, continued linear growth and osteoporosis in adult men)
Androgen receptor	X-linked recessive	Inactivation	Androgen resistance (Male pseudohermaphroditism)
Glucocorticoid receptor[37]	Autosomal recessive	Inactivation	Glucocorticoid resistance (Androgen excess in women)
Vitamin D receptor	Autosomal recessive	Inactivation	Vitamin D resistance (Rickets)
Thyroid hormone receptor[38]	Autosomal dominant	Inactivation	Thyroid hormone resistance

melanocyte stimulating hormone (MSH), ACTH, TSH and PTH receptors causes activation the signaling cascade in an uncontrolled fashion. The mutant $G_s\alpha$ has decreased GTPase activity, leading to constitutive adenylate cyclase activation. This, in turn, gives rise to isosexual precocity in boys and girls, discoloration of the skin, adrenal and thyroid hyperfunction, and cystic bone lesions. On the other hand, certain forms of pseudohypoparathyroidism have been associated with inactivating mutations in the $G_s\alpha$. Most of these patients show hypocalcemia and a characteristic phenotype referred to as Albright's hereditary osteodystrophy, which comprises short stature, skeletal abnormalities, and subcutaneous calcifications. Affected individuals also show resistance to hormones other

than PTH. A temperature-sensitive activating mutation in the $G_s\alpha$ in two unrelated boys intriguingly gave rise to a paradoxical combination of textoxicosis and pseudohypoparathyroidism type Ia, a condition marked by resistance to PTH and TSH[35]. While the $G_s\alpha$ protein with this mutation is quite stable at testicular temperature giving rise to autonomous testosterone secretion, it is rapidly degraded at 37°C, explaining the PTH and TSH resistance caused by loss of $G_s\alpha$ activity.

Defects in androgen receptors give rise to varying degrees of androgen resistance, which is the most common form of male pseudohermaphroditism. An estrogen receptor defect that is associated with extremely tall stature, continued linear growth during the adult life and osteoporosis in a 28-year-old man has recently been described[36]. This case report demonstrated the crucial role of estrogen action in men in closure of epiphyses and maintenance of bone mass. Glucocorticoid receptor defects may be manifest in boys as isosexual precocity due to elevated adrenal androgen precursors that are partially converted to testosterone in the periphery. In women, glucocorticoid resistance gives rise to androgen excess by the same mechanism[37]. Anovulation and hirsutism of pubertal onset are common presenting symptoms of glucocorticoid resistance in women. Among the other members of the nuclear receptor superfamily, mutant vitamin D receptors are detected in cases of vitamin D-dependent rickets (Type II) and mutations in the thyroid hormone receptor-β are associated with symptoms of hypothyroidism but elevated levels of free T_3 and free T_4[38].

Various mutations in hormone receptors are also demonstrated in certain neoplasias. Constitutively active forms of mutated estrogen receptors in breast cancer or androgen receptors in prostate cancer are some examples. Somatic mutations in the TSH gene is associated with hyperfunctioning thyroid adenomas.

Finally, no gene defects in the insulin receptor have been demonstrated to date in the most common form of insulin resistance, which is non-insulin-dependent diabetes mellitus associated with obesity. However, in a limited number of women with extremely severe insulin resistance, ovarian hyperthecosis and acanthosis nigricans, mutations in the insulin receptor were found, most of which interfere with its tyrosine kinase activity. In the much more common form of the polycystic ovary syndrome (PCOS) with milder insulin resistance, however, mutations of receptors could not be demonstrated. In these relatively common conditions that are associated with mild insulin resistance, namely, obesity and PCOS, decreased receptor number on target cells or postreceptor defects (e.g., excessive serine phosphorylation of the insulin receptor) are likely mechanisms for insulin resistance[39,40].

KEY POINTS

1. Hormone action takes place through a variety of signal transduction pathways, activation of which give rise to alterations in gene expression in a cell-, hormone-, receptor-, signaling cascade-, and target gene-specific manner.

2. There is a wide variety of hormone receptors located in the cell membrane, cytoplasm or nucleus.

3. Glycoprotein hormones (FSH, LH, hCG, TSH) act via binding to specific seven-transmembrane-domain G-protein coupled receptors in the cell membrane giving rise to formation of intracellular cAMP. Other hormones interact with other specific G-protein-coupled receptors to cause alterations in phospholipid turnover and intracellular calcium concentrations.

4. Insulin, IGFs, EGF, FGF, PDGF, and a number of other growth factors act via a large family of cell membrane receptors that exhibit ligand-dependent tyrosine kinase activity, i.e., phosphorylation of tyrosine residues on cytoplasmic proteins that interact with these receptors.

5. Members of the TGFβ receptor family (receptors for TGFβs, activins, inhibins, MIS) also reside in the cell membrane and function via phosphorylation of serines and threonines in other proteins that interact with the receptor.

6. Receptors for cytokines and prolactin comprise another distinct family, which reside in the cell membrane and phosphorylate tyrosine residues on cytoplasmic signaling molecules.

7. Serial phosphorylations of dephosphorylations of a cascade of proteins in the cytoplasm and nucleus comprise a common and critical mechanism for signal transduction associated with many receptors.

8. Activation of a signal transduction pathway may give rise to binding of transcription factors to specific genes and alter the rate of transcription, may modify protein synthesis via post-transcriptional mechanisms or may modify protein function via post-translational mechanisms.

9. Nuclear receptors for estrogen, progesterone, cortisol, thyroid hormone, vitamin D and a number of other substances function as ligand-activated transcription factors. The hormone-nuclear receptor complex directly binds to a gene promoter to alter the rate of transcription.

10. Certain abnormalities in receptors and signaling pathways give rise to specific endocrine disorders that affect reproductive function.

11. Targeting receptors or specific elements of signal transduction by pharmaceutical compounds led to development of novel treatments of human disease.

REFERENCES

1. Gilman AG. G proteins and dual control of adenylate cyclase. *Cell* 1984;36:577.
2. Ascoli M, Fanelli F, Segaloff DL. The lutropin/choriogonadotropin receptor, a 2002 perspective. *Endocr Rev* 2002;23:141.
3. McArdle CA, Franklin J, Green L, et al. The gonadotropin-releasing hormone receptor: signalling, cycling and desensitisation. *Arch Physiol Biochem* 2002; 110:113.
4. Krupinski J, Coussen F, Bakalyar HA, et al. Adenylyl cyclase amino-acid sequence: possible channel- or transporter-like structure. *Science* 1989;244:1558.
5. Cohen P. The role of protein phosphorylation in neural and hormonal control of cellular activity. *Nature* 1982;296:613.
6. Berridge MJ. The molecular basis of communication within the cell. *Sci Am* 1985; 253:142.
7. Smrcka AV, Hepler JR, Brown KO, et al. Regulation of polyphosphoinositide-specific phospholipase C activity by purified Gq. *Science* 1991;251:804.
8. Rhee SG, Suh PG, Ryu SH, et al. Studies of inositol phospholipid-specific phospholipase C. *Science* 1989;244:546.
9. Kikkawa U, Kishimoto A, Nishizuka Y. The protein kinase C family: Heterogeneity and its implications. *Ann NY Acad Sci* 1989;58:31.
10. Ullrich A, Coussens L, Hayflick JS. Human epidermal growth factor receptor cDNA sequence and aberrant expression of the amplified gene in A431 epidermoid carcinoma cells. *Nature* 1984;309:418.
11. Downward J, Yarden Y, Mayes E. Close similarity of epidermal growth factor receptor and v-erb-B oncogene protein sequences. *Nature* 1984;307:521.
12. Baselga J, Norton L, Albanell J, et al. Recombinant humanized anti-HER2 antibody (Herceptin) enhances the antitumor activity of paclitaxel and doxorubicin against HER2/ neu overexpressing human breast cancer xenografts. *Cancer Res* 1998;58: 2825.
13. Albanell J, Codony J, Rovira A, et al. Mechanism of action of anti-HER2 monoclonal antibodies: scientific update on trastuzumab and 2C4. *Adv Exp Med Biol* 2003;532:253.
14. Murali R, Liu Q, Cheng X, et al. Antibody like peptidomimetics as large scale immunodetection probes. *Cell Mol Biol* (Noisy-le-grand) 2003; 49:209.
15. Ebina Y, Ellis L, Jarnagin K. The human insulin receptor cDNA: The structural basis for hormone-activated transmembrane signalling. *Cell* 1985; 40:747.
16. Czech MP. Signal transmission by the insulin-like growth factors. *Cell* 1989;59:235.
17. Canman CE, Kastan MB. Three paths to stress relief. *Nature* 1996;384:213.
18. Zhao Y NJ, Bulun SE, Mendelson CR, et al. Aromatase P450 gene expression in human adipose tissue: Role of a Jak/STAT pathway in regulation of the adipose-specific promoter. *J Biol Chem* 1995;270:16449.
19. Kurzrock R, Kantarjian HM, Druker BJ, et al. Philadelphia chromosome-positive leukemias: from basic mechanisms to molecular therapeutics. *Ann Intern Med* 2003; 138:819.
20. Nagata S. Apoptosis by death factor. *Cell* 1997; 88:355.
21. Yamaguchi M, Rutledge LJ, Garbers DL. The primary structure of the rat guanylyl cyclase A/atrial natriuretic peptide receptor gene. *J Biol Chem* 1990;265:20414.

22. Sibley DR, Lefkowitz RJ. Molecular mechanisms of receptor desensitization using the α-adrenergic receptor-coupled adenylate cyclase system as a model. *Nature* 1985;317:124.

23. Morohashi K, Honda S, Inomata Y, et al. A common trans-acting factor, Ad4-binding protein, to the promoters of steroidogenic P450s. *J Biol Chem* 1992;267:17913.

24. Lala DS, Rice DA, Parker KL. Steroidogenic factor I, a key regulator of steroidogenic enzyme expression, is the mouse homolog of Sushitaraza-factor I. *Mol Endocrinol* 1992;6:1249

25. Muscatelli F, Strom TM, Walker AP, et al. Mutations in the DAX-1 gene give rise to both X-linked adrenal hypoplasia congenita and hypogonadotropic hypogonadism. *Nature* 1994; 372:672.

26. Green S, Chambon P. A superfamily of potentially oncogenic hormone receptors. *Nature* 1986;324:615.

27. Weinberger C, Thompson CC, Ong ES. The c-erb-A gene encodes a thyroid hormone receptor. *Nature* 1986; 324:641.

28. Denner LA, Schrader WT, O'Malley BW, et al. Hormonal regulation and identification of chicken progesterone receptor phosphorylation sites. *J Biol Chem* 1990; 265:16548.

29. Forman BM, Samuels HH. Interactions among a subfamily of nuclear hormone receptors: The regulatory zipper model. *Mol Endocrinol* 1990; 4:1293.

30. Bulun S, Simpson E. Estrogen action, breast. in: Knobil E NJ, ed. Vol. 2. San Diego: Academic Press, Inc., 1999; p 71.

31. Laue LL, Shao-Ming W, Kudo M, et al. Compound heterozygous mutations of the luteinizing hormone receptor gene in leydig cell hypoplasia. *Mol Endocrinol* 1996; 10:987.

32. Kawate N, Kletter GB, Wilson BE, et al. Identification of constitutively activating mutation of the luteinising hormone receptor in a family with male limited gonadotrophin independent precocious puberty (testotoxicosis). 1995; 32:553.

33. Vasseur C, Rodien P, Beau I, et al. A chorionic gonadotropin-sensitive mutation in the follicle-stimulating hormone receptor as a cause of familial gestational spontaneous ovarian hyperstimulation syndrome. *N Engl J Med* 2003; 349:753.

34. Smits G, Olatunbosun O, Delbaere A, et al. Ovarian hyperstimulation syndrome due to a mutation in the follicle-stimulating hormone receptor. *N Engl J Med* 2003;349:760.

35. Iiri T, Herzmark P, Nakamoto JM, et al. Rapid GDP release from G_s alpha in patients with gain and loss of endocrine function. *Nature* 1994; 371:164.

36. Smith EP, Boyd J, Frank GR, et al. Estrogen resistance caused by a mutation in the estrogen-receptor gene in a man. *N Engl J Med* 1994;331: 1056.

37. Stratakis CA, Karl M, Schulte HM, et al. Glucocorticosteroid resistance in humans. Elucidation of the molecular mechanisms and implications for pathophysiology. *Ann NY Acad Sci* 1994;746:362.

38. DeRoux N, Misrahi M, Braunder R, et al. Four families with loss of function mutations of the thyrotropin receptor. *J Clin Endocrinol Metab* 1996;81:4229.

39. Dunaif A. Insulin resistance and the polycystic ovary syndrome: mechanism and implications for pathogenesis. *Endocr Rev* 1997;18:774.

40. Venkatesan AM, Dunaif A, Corbould A. Insulin resistance in polycystic ovary syndrome: progress and paradoxes. *Recent Prog Horm Res* 2001;56:295.

41. Hunter T. The Croonian Lecture 1997. The phosphorylation of proteins on tyrosine: its role in cell growth and disease. *Philos Trans R Soc Lond B Biol Sci* 1998;353:583.

42. Hanks SK, Hunter T. Protein kinases 6. The eukaryotic protein kinase superfamily: kinase (catalytic) domain structure and classification. *Faseb J* 1995;9:576.

43. Hubbard SR. Crystal structure of the activated insulin receptor tyrosine kinase in complex with peptide substrate and ATP analog. *EMBO J* 1997;16:5572.

44. Hubbard SR, Mohammadi M, Schlessinger J. Autoregulatory mechanisms in protein-tyrosine kinases. *J Biol Chem* 1998;273:11987.

45. Ullrich A, Schlessinger J. Signal transduction by receptors with tyrosine kinase activity. *Cell* 1990; 61:203.

46. Yenush L, White MF. The IRS-signaling system during insulin and cytokine action. *Bioessays* 1997;19:491.

47. Belham C, Wu S, Avruch J. Intracellular signalling: PDK1-a kinase at the hub of things. *Curr Biol* 1999;9:R93.

48. Avruch J, Khokhlatchev A, Kyriakis JM, et al. Ras activation of the Raf kinase: tyrosine kinase recruitment of the MAP kinase cascade. *Recent Prog Horm Res* 2001;56:127.

CHAPTER 2

Laboratory Assessment of Reproductive Hormones

RICHARD E. BLACKWELL AND JOHN MAHAN

In the past, endocrinopathies were diagnosed by clinical phenotype. Today, these disorders are diagnosed much earlier, and accurate measurement of reproductive hormones, which in the past were unmeasurable, today forms the backbone of modern reproductive endocrinology. It should be recalled that the reproductive hormones were not isolated and purified until the early 1940s and 1950s. In 1849, testes from castrated roosters were implanted in the intestines, which prevented the occurrence of the usual side effects of castration. This is considered to be the first bioassay. In the early 1900s, the estrus cycle of rodents was described using changes in vaginal cornification. Progesterone was isolated and purified in 1929, luteinizing hormone (LH) was discovered in 1941, and follicle-stimulating hormone (FSH) was discovered in 1950. The evaluation of all these hormones depended on complex bioassays frequently involving changes in various reproductive organ weights or identification of ovulation. It should be remembered that the standards we use today in various assays ultimately are still referenced to these early bioassays.

As hormone chemistry became more advanced, a number of 24-hour urinary assays were developed, including the Porter, Silber, and Zimmerman reactions for 17-ketosteroids, 17-ketogenic steroids, and 17-hydroxycorticosteroids. These were complex and cumbersome assays that formed the basis of endocrine evaluation in the 1960s and 1970s.

The original radioimmunoassay can be traced to Berson and colleagues[1] in 1956. This group was the first to demonstrate that patients who had been treated with insulin developed nonprecipitated antibodies capable of binding ^{131}I-labeled insulin. Further, this group showed that nonlabeled insulin could compete and displace the labeled hormone from binding sites on the antibody. Subsequently, two members of this group described the first radioimmunoassay for insulin.[2] The assay employed hematoelectrophoresis to separate the antibody-bound insulin from the unbound hormone. Concomitantly, Grodsky and Forsham[3] 1960 described a similar method for the assay of ^{131}I-labeled insulin. They used salt fractionation to separate their product instead of electrophoresis.

The next major contribution to the field was made by Hales and Randle[4] in 1963, who developed a radioimmunoassay method involving the separation of antibody-antigen complex from free-antigen complex from free antigen by precipitation with anti-gamma-globulin serum. This assay was based on the findings of

Skom and Talmadge (1958), who first showed that antiserum could cause precipitation of antigen-antibody complexes. The Hales-Randle method has been named the *double-antibody method;* it is more efficient that older types of assays.

In 1963, Herbert and colleagues[5] devised a method by which antigen-antibody complex could be separated from unbound material using dextran-coated charcoal. This assay makes use of the phenomenon that charcoal-dextran mixtures almost instantly absorb free antigen but will not bind the antigen-antibody complex. This type of separation is more rapid than conventional precipitation methods and makes use of ^{131}I-labeled hormone prepared using the method of Hunter and Greenwood.[6]

During the same period, Utiger and colleagues[7] expanded the use of radioimmunoassay by developing an assay for human growth hormone (GH). Later, Greenwood and colleagues[8] introduced a now classic method for the iodination of human GH that yields materials with specific activity of 200 to 500 mC/mg. This method involves oxidation of carrier-free sodium iodine with chloramine T, substitution of the reaction product onto the phenyl ring of tyrosine and the imidazole ring of histidine, and reduction of the nonreactive material after 1 min to prevent excess hormone damage. The method was described by Hughes in 1957. Subsequently, Meyer and Knobil[9] developed an assay based on separation by charcoal for the measurement of human and simian GH.

The first radioimmunoassay to be developed for the measurement of a gonadotropin made use of antibodies to human chorionic gonadotropin (anti-hCG antibody was shown to bind both hCG and human LH).[10–12] One of these assays[11] was new to the field of radioimmunoassay. Catt showed that antibodies could be coupled to diazotized polystyrene disks. This eliminated the need for separating the antibody-antigen complex by precipitation or absorption. Later, Catt and colleagues[11] were able to absorb the antibody directly onto unsaturated polystyrene at a basic pH. Faiman and Ryan[13] were the first to develop an antiserum to a pituitary gonadotropin (human LH). Subsequently, radioimmunoassays were developed for rat LH.[14–18]

The development of radioimmunoassay methods for the measurement of FSH, as with LH, began with clinical studies in mind. In 1967 and 1968, several groups announced the development of radioimmunoassays for various types of human FSH.[19,20] All these methods are based on double-antibody techniques.

The first radioimmunoassay for prolactin was developed to quantitate the hormone in ovine and bovine plasma because human material was not available. Aria and Lee in 1967 were the first to announce an assay for ovine prolactin based on double-antibody technology. They were followed by numerous other investigators during 1968 and 1969.

▶ THEORY OF RADIOIMMUNOASSAY

Radioimmunoassay is based on the ability of an unlabeled hormone to inhibit the binding of a labeled hormone to specific antibodies. The inhibition is thought to be a simple competition, as represented by the equations labeled antigen + antibody = labeled complex and unlabeled antigen + antibody = unlabeled complex. Therefore, the number of molecules of labeled hormone that are part of the antigen-antibody complex is inversely proportional to the amount of unlabeled hormone. This is somewhat of a naive concept, and as our knowledge becomes more sophisticated, we may find that the mechanism is more complex (Figs. 2-1 and 2-2).

The radioimmunoassay traditionally has been carried out at either 4°C or 37°C in phosphate-buffered saline at pH 7 or 8 or in a barbital buffer at pH 8 or 9. The reaction time varies from 2 to 24 h depending on the affinity of the antibody for the antigen and the de-

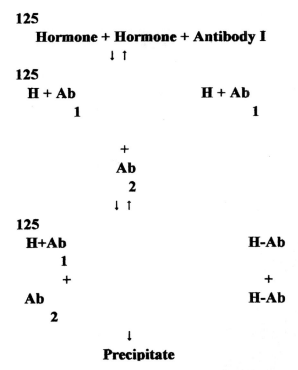

Figure 2-1 Antigen-antibody reaction in RIA.

gree of sensitivity desired. It should be noted that automated machinery and improved preparation of antibodies have shortened this incubation time markedly. Following completion of antigen-antibody formation, the complex is sep-

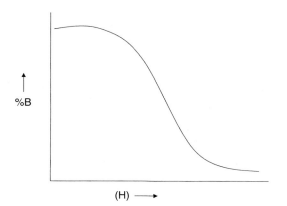

Figure 2-2 Binding curve showing relationship of free to bound unlabeled hormone.

arated from unattached elements by one of three methods described earlier; i.e., precipitation with anti-gamma-globulin, absorption with dextran-coated charcoal, or escalation of the reaction medium, leaving the antigen-antibody complex bound to polystyrene. The radioactivity of the complex is measured by conventional methods.

▶ PRODUCTION OF ANTISERUM

The antiserum that is used in radioimmunoassays has been produced in several species of animals including rabbit, chicken, guinea pig, duck, goat, and sheep. The rabbit is the most widely used species for first-antibody production, and the sheep is the most widely used for second-antibody production where needed.

Many methods of immunization exist, the most common involving injection of antigen into the footpad intradermally or into the regional lymph nodes or spleen. Because of the short life of antigens in the host organism, it is necessary to present the material with a carrier substance, the most popular carrier being the oil kill tubercle bacteria mixture Freund's adjuvant.[21] Other carriers that have found wide use are albumin, ferritin, methylated bovine serum albumin, charcoal, and Sephadex. Obviously, the choice of carrier determines the site of inoculation.[22]

The immunization usually consists of an initial exposure of the animal to the antigen, followed by secondary exposure at 15- and 30-day intervals. The serum antibody titer should rise rapidly after several injections, but if it does not, the animal should be discarded.

Serum samples are obtained by several methods: cardiac puncture, puncture of the marginal ear vein, or puncture of the central ear artery. The alternative method of choice when using rabbits is bleeding by tiny puncture in the marginal vein by vacuum (Hoppe et al., 1969). This may be done with or without pretreatment of the ear with xylene to

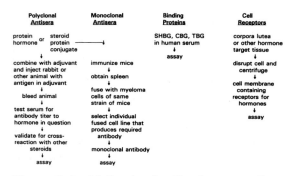

Polyclonal Antisera	Monoclonal Antisera	Binding Proteins	Cell Receptors
protein or steroid hormone protein conjugate		SHBG, CBG, TBG in human serum ↓ assay	corpora lutea or other hormone target tissue ↓
combine with adjuvant and inject rabbit or other animal with antigen in adjuvant ↓	immunize mice ↓ obtain spleen ↓		disrupt cell and centrifuge ↓
bleed animal ↓	fuse with myeloma cells of same strain of mice ↓		cell membrane containing receptors for hormones ↓
test serum for antibody titer to hormone in question ↓	select individual fused cell line that produces required antibody ↓		assay
validate for cross-reaction with other steroids ↓	monoclonal antibody ↓		
assay	assay		

Figure 2-3 Methods of antibody preparation.

produce local vasodilatation. When bleeding sheep, we prefer using puncture to the external jugular vein with a blood collection kit and removal of samples by vacuum (Abbovac blood collection set, 36 in).

Once the serum has been separated from whole blood, complement should be destroyed by incubation of the serum at 57°C for 30 min. Before freezing or storage, one may add sodium azide or Merthiolate to prevent bacterial or fungal growth.

A second method of obtaining antibodies involves monoclonal technology. This has been described by Chard.[23] Mice are immunized as in the production of polyclonal antiserum. The antibody spleen cells of these mice are fused in vitro with myeloma cells from the same strain of mice. This results in a cell line that

produces antibody. One can then select individually fused cells that produce exactly the antibody desired, and the lines can produce antibodies indefinitely (immortalized cell lines). The advantage of a monoclonal antibody includes production of high-grade antibodies that are more predictable and are more consistent than polyclonal screens. Further, large quantities of antibodies can be produced. The technology is expensive, and sophisticated facilities are needed to produce monoclonal antibodies (Figs. 2-3 and 2-4).

▶ PREPARATION OF IODINATED HORMONES

As mentioned earlier, the method generally used for iodination of protein hormones is that of Greenwood and Hunter.[8] The original Greenwood method used iodine-131 as the label. However, this has the disadvantage of a short half-life, and therefore, very frequent iodination

(A) Iodination of a peptide or protein hormone or large protein such as an antibody

(B) Iodination of a steroid hormone (progesterone-11-α-hemisuccinate tyrosine methyl ester)

(C) Tritiated I, 2,6,7-^{3}H- progesterone

Figure 2-5 Preparation of labeled hormones.

human LH, FSH, HCG ⇓	steroids ⇓
foreign proteins in non-human species ⇓	not antigenic in any species ⇓
immunize non-human species ⇓	complex with large proteins, i.e., bovine serum albumin, human serum albumin, etc. ⇓
obtain antigenic reaction ⇓	immunize foreign species ⇓
harvest antisera	obtain antigenic reaction ⇓
	harvest antisera

Figure 2-4 Steps in assay of proteins & steroids using RIA.

is necessary. We prefer to use iodine-125 in this method because the isotope has an appreciably longer half-life. This variation was introduced by Wilde and colleagues in 1967. Both iodine-131 and iodine-125 emit hard gamma rays; therefore, the emission can be measured with ease. The procedure yields labeled hormone with a specific activity of 100 to 250 mC/mg (Fig. 2-5).

▶ CRITERIA FOR VALID RADIOIMMUNOASSAYS

The criteria for good radioimmunoassays are not too different from those generally applied to bioassays. They must be specific, sensitive, reliable, and repeatable and should be as simple as possible. In addition, the assay should not be affected by the medium being assayed (blood or serum). These criteria have been reviewed by Midgley and colleagues,[16] and thus only a few comments will be made here.

Specificity is the most important consideration in developing a radioimmunoassay. In the case of FSH, specificity is a major problem because most anti-FSH serum reacts with thyroid-stimulating hormone (TSH) or LH to some degree. This is due to the structural similarity of the three molecules, notably the α chain. Most of the antibodies contained in a particular serum sample may be directed toward the common chain; therefore, serum cannot be rendered specific. However, if the converse is true, one may absorb the serum with unwanted antigens to eliminate the population of interfering antibodies.

Cross-reaction is sometimes a problem in developing radioimmunoassays for prolactin. Prolactin and GHs are similar in proximal structure, and it should be noted that nonspecific antiprolactin serum usually can be rendered specific by absorption.

When using radioimmunoassays to measure hormone in plasma, it is of the utmost importance to determine the nonspecific effect that plasma may be having on the measurement. In many cases plasma will have no specific effect; in others it may produce gross overestimation of hormone concentrations or lead to false-positive results in the experiment. The same test should be applied to assays used to measure hormones in vitro, i.e., Eagle's medium or Krebs' or Ringer's bicarbonate buffer.

The sensitivity of radioimmunoassays is determined on the basis of the number of picograms or nanograms that can be measured in 1 mL of fluid as based on a particular reference preparation. Therefore, the reported degree of sensitivity of a system is directly proportional to the standard used in the assay. Based on this information, there are some comments that we must make about various radioimmunoassays: Adrenocorticotropic hormone (ACTH) assays tend to be sensitive in the midpicogram range, whereas LH, GH, and prolactin assays can be measured in a few nanograms. Most FSH assays are sensitive and show a minimum sensitivity of 1 to 25 ng/mL.

The reliability of repeatability of a radioimmunoassay can only be ascertained by a working knowledge of the characteristics of the particular assay system under a well-defined set of conditions. This is done by comparison of values obtained by multiple assays of various samples.

▶ NONLABELED RADIOIMMUNOASSAYS

A considerable amount of discussion has been devoted to radioimmunoassay because of its historical importance and because it represents the basic principles involved in hormone assays. Most of the assays used in automated instruments today are of the nonradiolabeled type. In fact, many laboratories today are isotope-free. All assays use certain basic principles and components: the hormone to be measured, the antibody-binding protein or receptor, the label or tracer, and the means of separating free from bound antibody. These assays all operate at the basic principle of mass action described previously. Nonradiolabeled tracers may be colorimetric, fluorescent, bioluminescent, or chemoluminescent. Some of these agents, it should be noted, pose potential health risks and should be handled as biohazards.

▶ REFERENCE PREPARATIONS

Reference preparations generally are produced by the World Health Organization (WHO) or by the National Institutes of Health (NIH). Purification of these various hormone standards in their day was considered a massive science public work project involving many collaborating and competing laboratories. Obviously, the basic source of these hormones was human tissue obtained at autopsy. Because of supply limits, commercial preparations have been prepared by various manufacturers and are calibrated against either WHO or NIH material. Therefore, one must be clear when a standard is being used in reporting data and when comparing data with those of other investigators. For instance, over 20 standards have been prepared for the measurement of LH, FSH, prolactin, and hCG.[24]

▶ HORMONAL ASSAYS

A few points need to be made about commonly used specific assays. The hCG assay is one of the most widely used assays in reproductive endocrinology. The standard β-chain assay is not the same as a free-β-subunit-only measurement. The β subunit measures the whole hCG molecule plus any circulating free β subunit. There remains a slight possibility of LH cross-reacting in today's hCG assays, and it is felt that measurements of levels below 5 mIU/mL may not be accurate.

The assays for FSH and LH are well established and may be of either the radioisotope or nonradioactive type. There are many reliable standards, but there may not be agreement be-

tween bioassay and immunologic activity of a particular preparation. The prolactin assay likewise is fairly reliable, but it should be remembered that prolactin follows a diurnal variation. Therefore, early-morning levels may be elevated. A recent work by our group has shown that breast examination does not increase prolactin level, nor does the intake of foods high in tyrosine, tryptophan, or arginine, reported stimulators of prolactin secretion, a misconception that existed for many years.[25] The TSH assay is well established, and the high-sensitivity assays are extremely reliable for the diagnosis of both hyper- and hypothyroidism.

The measurement of 17β-estradiol poses a significant problem. Contemporary assays used for infertility measure free 17β-estradiol, but it should be remembered most estradiol is bound to sex hormone–binding globulin (SHBG) or albumin and may or may not be biologically active in these bound forms. Further, there is very little estradiol circulating in free form, and many of the assays operate at the limit of their accuracy. Finally, there is often great variability between estradiol levels obtained in one system versus those in the other.[26]

The measurement of androgens poses a special problem, particularly the measurement of testosterone. The best technology uses a solvent extraction followed by determination of SHBG capacity and, finally, determination of the level of free circulating testosterone. Further, it should be remembered that in developing antibodies to steroids it is necessary to couple these agents with various carriers such as methylated serum albumin to increased antigenicity.[27] In addition, steroids are tritiated, not labeled with radioactive iodine, and therefore do not emit gamma but beta radiation and must be counted in a scintillation counter.[28]

▶ QUALITY CONTROL

The laboratory, being another form of business, has certain licensing and certification requirements. First, the laboratory must be licensed by the state in which it practices because, after all, this is a form of medical practice. Further, the laboratory falls under a number of federal guidelines. STARK II (Omnibus Budget Reconciliation Act of 1993) requirements become exceedingly important when multiple individual physicians invest in a peripheral laboratory, and there are stringent penalties, both civil and criminal, for referral abuse. The Federal Clinical Laboratory Improvement Act of 1988 (CLIA) helps to ensure the delivery of accurate and reliable data. There are various levels of CLIA certification, and most reproductive endocrine practices would fall under CLIA level III, laboratories that perform complex functions.

Quality control lies at the very heart of laboratory certification and accreditation. Requirements include the following: Procedure manuals need to be stringently maintained and updated. Records need to be maintained on such things as refrigerator and freezer temperatures used to store samples; there needs to be daily temperature records for these devices. Instruments such as pipettes need to be calibrated at least quarterly. Accuracy of RPM gauges needs to be confirmed every 6 months. In general, scintillation and gamma counters, spectrophotometers, and so on all need to be calibrated each day of use. The laboratory must have a flawless archiving system, and the licensing agency must be able to track every sample from its entry into the laboratory to the reporting of data output. Records usually are maintained on file for at least 2 years. Samples frequently are discarded after 24 hours.

Comprehensive quality control involves three processes: (1) a validation recording of assay characteristics, (2) internal quality control samples for each assay, and (3) participation in some external certifying program. An example would be the College of American Pathology Proficiency Program. A set of samples is sent quarterly for assay under normal laboratory conditions, and the laboratory performance is graded by comparison with other laboratories using the same diagnostic kits.

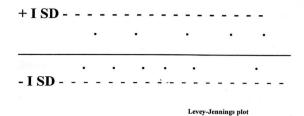

Figure 2-6 Levey-Jennings plot evaluation multiple assays.

Assay *precision* is the term that defines the reproducibility of measuring a given quantity of hormone in medium. Precision is measured using the coefficient of variation (CV) both within and between assays. CV is basically a standard deviation expressing the percentage of the mean of repeated measurements of the same sample. Values should be less than 10 percent for both within- and between-assay variation, and the CVs are used to compare it over an extended time period. The measurement can be plotted on a Levey-Jennings plot, which furnishes a picture of performance over time (Fig. 2-6). In addition to the coefficiency of variation, internal quality control samples should be used for every assay (see Fig. 2-3). Two such samples should come from a high and a low pool. They can be obtained commercially or prepared internally, and they are generally aliquotted and frozen and can be used over a year's time.

▶ CLIA CERTIFICATION

The Clinical Laboratory Improvement Act (CLIA) was passed by Congress in 1967 to improve laboratory practices. It targeted the operation and maintenance of instrumentation and the proficiency of laboratory personnel. In 1988, CLIA was amended (CLIA 88), and the final rule was effective September 1, 1992. All laboratory tests performed in the United States fall under CLIA guidelines, including those performed in physicians' office laboratories (POLs).

CLIA 88 very specifically delineates who may do testing and what quality control procedures must be followed when doing such testing. Quality control procedures are based on the complexity of the methodology and the instrumentation being used to do the test. There are three levels of complexity: waved, moderate and high complexity. Laboratories may perform only waved tests or a combination of all three categories.

To receive a certificate, laboratories must supply the Health Care Financing Administration (HCFA) with certain information and pay a fee. This is accomplished by contacting the laboratory accrediting agency, typically the Department of Public Health in the state where the laboratory is located. The initial step is to complete HCFA Form 116 describing the type of testing performed, test volume, and so on. This form becomes a certificate of application that is evaluated by HCFA. This form is available on federal Web sites.

Depending on the complexity (degree of difficulty) of testing, laboratories will receive either (1) a certificate and waiver that permits the laboratory to perform only tests identified as waived, (2) a certificate to perform microscopy, or (3) an interim registration certificate the allows the laboratory to perform waved tests and tests of moderate and high complexity. Once the laboratory is judged by HCFA to be in compliance, a permanent certificate of compliance can be issued.

CLIA 88 categorizes all tests according to complexity or difficulty in performing these tests. The Food and Drug Administration (FDA) categorizes all test systems and methodologies based on knowledge, skill, and background necessary to perform an individual test. The most recent information on test complexity may be obtained from HCFA's Web site. Each test category has requirements for personnel, quality control, quality assurance, proficiency of testing, and so on. In addition, each category's requirements depend to some degree on the accrediting agency.

▶ INSPECTION BY PROFESSIONAL ORGANIZATIONS

Laboratories voluntarily choosing to be accredited by an organization such as the Joint Commission on Accreditation of Health Care Organizations (JCAHO), the College of American Pathologists (CAP), or the Commission on Office Laboratory Accreditation (COLA) will receive a certification from the organization instead of HCFA once the laboratory is inspected and found to meet the organization's standards. Laboratories that wish to be accredited by this mechanism must begin by applying for a registration certificate. On the certificate the laboratory indicates that it wishes to be accredited by one of those organizations.

The CAP accreditation program has provided the longest-standing continuously offered inspection program. The inspections are unique in that they are conducted by trained teams of peers. Inspections tend to focus on the laboratory director and clearly hold him or her responsible for the quality of all aspects of laboratory operation. A separate checklist for all areas of testing is updated, clarified, and improved continuously. CAP also recognizes advances or changes in technology. Regulations and the many checklists fit large pathology-directed laboratories as well as different testing sites. The CAP program is often looked to nationally by regulators, states, and professional organizations to provide cutting-edge thinking about the laboratory issues of the day.

If a laboratory is not examined by one of the accrediting agencies, it will be inspected by a CLIA inspector. The CLIA inspector is either an employee of the health department in the state the laboratory is located or a federal government employee. The inspection will be based on the CLIA 88 regulations. If the laboratory chooses to be accredited by JACHO, CAP, COLA, or another organization, it must meet the specific requirements of that organization, and the inspector and inspections will be chosen by the specific organization. The inspector or inspectors will use the organization's standard or checklist. If the laboratory is located in a state with CLIA-exempt status (Washington, Oregon, or New York), it will need to meet the requirements of that state, and the inspector will be a state employee.

A feature of the CLIA 88 regulations is that up to 5 percent of all laboratories may be selected randomly for reinspection by a federal CLIA inspector. This is actually a quality-controlled check on the inspection process. While HCFA has not reinspected 5 percent of the laboratories each year, a summary inspection is occurring. It is part of the process, and for the laboratory chosen, it should pose no problem as long as it is meeting the standards specified by its accrediting organization.

► AUTOMATED EQUIPMENT

Automated chemoluminescence assay analyzers have continued to evolve over the years with improvements in assay sensitivity and instrument automation. Many of the improvements can be attributed to advanced chemoluminescence detector techniques and better systems design. Immunoassay forms of chemoluminescence detection techniques have been accepted increasingly as the platforms for immunoassay automation. Moreover, signals can be amplified manyfold if coupled with an enzyme label such as horseradish peroxidase or alkaline phosphatase. The combination of chemoluminescence detection of the enzyme amplification has produced some of the most sensitive assays available today.

The demand for increasing productivity and decreasing cost in managed-care settings have generated considerable interest in laboratory automation. Managed care has a profound effect on the operation, management, and infrastructure of a clinical laboratory. Automation of radioimmunoassays has been at the forefront of the changes taking place in clinical laboratories. Automated chemoluminescence assays

clearly offer unparalleled advantages. Simplicity in assay format has made it easier to adapt to automated systems, and low detection limits have made sensitive automated assays an achievable goal. With improvements in systems design and automated technology, many features of automated chemistry analyzers are found in automated chemoluminescence immunoassay analyzers such as random access, bar coding of specimens, extensive menus, primary tube sampling, onboard dilution, and reflux testing.

Several major chemoluminescence systems available currently on the market: Access by Beckman Coulter, Inc.; the ACS Sentor by Circon Diagnostics; Immulyte and Immulyte 2000 by Diagnostics Products Corp.; Victrose, ECI, by Johnson & Johnson Clinical Diagnostics; Elecys 10/10 and 20/10 by Roache Diagnostic Systems; the Architect I 2000 by Abbott Diagnostics; and Advantage by Nichols Diagnostics are fully automated analyzer systems. In general, this means that such instruments are capable of hands-off operation as a result of bar-code reading, primary tube sampling, incubation, autodilution, reflux testing, and online data transfer.

► TEST MENUS

Expanded test menus now provide the opportunity for laboratories to offer complete panels of automated tests similar to the chemistry analyzers such as the thyroid profile. Profiles projected include those for hepatitis, reproductive endocrine/infertility, anemia, oncology, congenital disorders, calcium, and bone metabolism. Competition among vendors is so intense that menus are constantly being updated and improved.

Ultrasensitive chemoluminescence detection systems have been accepted increasingly as the platform for immunoassay automation. In the future, requirements for increased sensitivity and specificity will continue to be the driving force for further improvements in automated immunoassay analyzers that will stretch current technologies and spawn new ones.

Laboratory automation offers many advantages: decreased operating cost, decreased labor cost, increased productivity, decreased sample size, and increased volume capacity with increased proficiency. The only disadvantage of the latest technology is the increased upfront cost. The purchase of any instrument and associated maintenance cost should not exceed the cost to lease the instrument based on a reagent rental or cost per reportable basis. The determination of whether to obtain instrumentation via capital equipment purchase or lease based on various types of reagent rental agreement depends on many factors. In most cases, it is more cost-effective for the laboratory to purchase reagents on a cost per reportable basis than to purchase instruments if maintenance is the responsibility of the manufacturer. In addition, membership in any large buying organization also will influence this decision. In most cases, manufacturers have the largest profit margin on reagents, not on instruments. This is one circumstance where comparative shopping and careful negotiation are a must. In addition, you should consider the type of maintenance agreements available. While most vendors offer a wide variety of options, including same-day and weekend service, the amount of downtime you are willing to accept will increase or decrease cost, but this is usually about 10 percent of the analyzer cost per year.

Finally, it is important to realize that selection of new automated instrumentation for any laboratory will be successful only if all parties—laboratory director, laboratory supervisor, and operators—are in agreement. In addition, this teamwork must carry over into the operational phase of the decision, in which the instrument is selected and placed in operation. It is particularly important that the laboratory work with selective vendors to ensure optimal operation in selecting instruments and cooperation with the vendor.

▶ INFORMATICS, LIS SYSTEM

The laboratory information system (LIS) has become an indispensable tool to laboratories for follow-up of patients and the entire team of health care providers. An effective information flow means expedited patient registration and order entry, instant access to electronic medical records, rapid turnaround of test results, point of care, expert systems, and a host of other automated applications. Patient satisfaction skyrockets, errors are reduced, safety is increased, and the clinical workflow is accelerated.

The LIS should be used as a primary vehicle for communication between the laboratory and other medical staff. A single phone call to a laboratory for a result has a dramatic and additive financial effect. Advanced LISs automate communications in a variety of ways. The ability to fax results directly from the LIS to multiple locations not only is a timesaver for laboratories, but it also significantly improves communication to the medical staff. Most of today's advanced LISs provide remote printing as a communications option. This option connects the LIS directly to a specific printer via the computer network and through a phone connection.

Newer LISs also have the capacity to securely communicate results over the Internet. This is particularly important in terms of the new Health Insurance Portability and Accountability Act (HIPAA) regulations. Physicians and other medical staff access these data using the Internet through assessment of specific medical portals such as Bednexus or Web MD. Using these portals, the physician has access to past and present patient results in real time. Some systems also can be linked to hospital LIS programs, giving inpatient access as well.

Advanced LISs provide physicians, and ultimately their patients, with the benefits of better communication. They also provide managers with the tools and time to manage their laboratories effectively, improving quality and cost-effectiveness. The laboratory and software sophistication employed by these systems continue to improve and allow for capabilities that did not exist until recently.

► SUMMARY

Protein and hormone assays can be carried out using today's automated instrumentation for nonisotopic assays. The manner in which these assays are carried out is regulated by CLIA 88, and external validation of assay accuracy can be furnished by participation in the CAP Proficiency Program. All these improvements allow for accurate measurement of hormonal assays and efficient and accurate patient care.

KEY POINTS

1. Monoclonal antibodies are produced from spleen cells fused with myeloma cells.

2. Criteria for radioimunoassays include specificity, sensitivity, reliability, repeatability, and simplicity.

3. Components of assays include hormone-antibody tracer and a means of separation.

4. Difficult hormones to measure include 17β-estradiol, DHEAS, and testosterone.

5. Laboratory operations are regulated by STARK II and CLIA 88.

6. Assay precision should be less than 10 percent within and between assays.

7. Advantages of automated systems include simplicity and increased sensitivity.

REFERENCES

1. Berson SA, Yalow RS, Bauman A, et al. Insulin-^{131}I metabolism in human subjects: Demonstration of insulin binding globulin in the circulation of insulin treated subjects. *J Clin Invest* 1956;35:170.

2. Yalow RS, Berson SA. Immunoassay of endogenous plasma insulin in man. *J Clin Invest* 1980;39:1157.

3. Grodsky GM, Forsham PH. An immunochemical assay of total extractable insulin in man. *J Clin Invest* 1960;39:1070.

4. Hales CN, Randle PJ. Immunoassay of insulin with insulin-antibody precipitate. *Biochem J* 1963;88:137.

5. Herbert V, Kam-Seng L, Gottlieb CW, et al. Coated charcoal immunoassay of insulin. *J Clin Endocrinol* 1965;25:1375.

6. Hunter WM, Greenwood FC. Preparation of iodine-131-labeled human growth hormone of high specific activity. *Nature* 1962;194:495.

7. Utiger RD, Parker ML, Daughady WH. Studies on human growth hormone: A radioimmunoassay for human growth hormone. *J Clin Invest* 1962;41:254.

8. Greenwood FC, Hunter FM, Glover JS. The preparation of I-131-labeled human growth hormone. *Biochem J* 1963;89:114.

9. Meyer V, Knobil E. Growth hormone secretion in the unanesthetized rhesus monkey in response to noxious stimuli. *Endocrinology* 1967;80:16371.

10. Midgley AR Jr. Radioimmunoassay: A method for human chorionic gonadotropin and human luteinizing hormone. *Endocrinology* 1966;79:10.

11. Catt KJ, Niall HD, Tregear GW. Solid-phase radioimmunoassay. *Nature* 1967;213:825.

12. Catt KJ, Niall HD, Amenomori Y, et al. Disc solid-phase radioimmunoassay of human luteinizing hormone. *J Clin Endocrinology* 1968; 28:121.

13. Faiman C, Ryan RJ. Radioimmunoassay for human follicle stimulating hormone. *J Clin Endocrinol Metab* 1967;27:444.

14. Parlow AF. Bioassay of pituitary luteinizing hormone by depletion of ovarian ascorbic acid, in Albert A (ed), *Human Pituitary Gonadotropins.* Springfield, IL: Charles C Thomas, 1961, p 300.

15. Amoss MS, Guillemin R. Solid-phase radioimmunoassay of ovine, bovine and murine luteinizing hormone. in Rosenberg E (ed), *Gonadotropins 1968*. Los Altos, CA: Geron-X, 1968, p 313.

16. Midgley AR Jr, Gay VL, Caligaris CS, et al. Radioimmunologic studies of rat LH, in Rosemberg E (ed), *Gonadotropins*. Los Altos, CA: Geron-X, 1968, p 307.

17. Niswender GD, Midgley AR Jr, Reichert LE Jr. Radioimmunologic studies with murine, bovine, ovine and porcine luteinizing hormone, in

Rosemberg E (ed), *Gonadotropins 1968*. Los Altos, CA: Geron-X, 1968, p 299.

18. Monroe SE, Parlow AF, Midgley AB Jr. Radioimmunoassay for rat luteinizing hormone. *Endocrinology* 1968;83:1004.

19. Aono T, Taymor ML. Radioimmunoassay for follicle-stimulating hormone (FSH) with ^{125}I-labeled FSH. *Am J Obstet Gynecol* 1968;100:110.

20. Aono T, Goldstein DP, Taymor ML, et al. A radioimmunoassay method for human pituitary luteinizing hormone (LH) and human chorionic gonadotropic (hCG) using ^{125}I-labeled LH. *Am J Obstet Gynecol* 1967;98:996.

21. Freund J. Effect of paraffin oil and mycobacteria on antibody formation sensitization. *Am J Clin Pathol* 1951;21:645.

22. Saxana BB, Gandy H, Peterson R. Radioimmunoassay of FSH and LH in body fluids, in Rosemberg E (ed), *Gonadotropins 1968*. Los Altos, CA: Geron-X, 1968, p 339.

23. Chard T. *An Introduction to Radioimmunoassay and Related Technology*. New York: Elsevier, 1983.

24. Bauthman DR, Berryman I, Burger H, et al. An international collaborative study of 691004, a reference preparation of human pituitary FSH and LH. *J Clin Endocrinol* 1973;36:647.

25. Hammond KR, Steinkampf MP, Boots LR, Blackwell RE. Effect of routine breast examination on serum prolactin levels. *Fertil Steril* 1996;65:869.

26. Thomas CMG, Van der Berg RT, Segers MFG. Measurement of serum estradiol comparison of three "direct" radioimmunoassays and the effect of organic solvent extraction. *Clin Chem* 1987;33:1946.

27. Erlanger BF, Borek F, Beiser SM, et al. Steroid protein conjugates. I. Preparation and characterization of conjugates of bovine serum albumin with testosterone and with cortisol. *Biol Chem* 1989;228:713.

28. Wheeler MJ, Shaikh M, Jennings RD. An evaluation of 13 commercial kits for the measurement of testosterone in serum and plasma. *Am Clin Biochem* 1986;23:303.

CHAPTER 3

Neuroendocrinology

SABRINA GILL AND JANET E. HALL

The neuroendocrine axis regulates and integrates neural and hormonal information and translates these signals to physiologic actions that have an impact on the synthesis and secretion of different hormonal systems. The hypothalamic-pituitary-gonadal (HPG) system is composed of: the gonadotropin-releasing hormone (GnRH)-producing neurons in the hypothalamus, the gonadotropes in the pituitary that secrete luteinizing hormone (LH) and follicle-stimulating hormone (FSH), and the ovary that responds to gonadotropin secretion with follicular development ovulation and secretion of gonadal steroids and peptides that modulate the hypothalamic and pituitary components of the reproductive axis (Fig. 3-1).

► ANATOMY

The hypothalamus is a phylogenetically old component of the central nervous system (CNS). Weighing approximately 10 g, it is located ventral to the ventral thalamus, caudal to the lamina terminals, rostral to the mamillary complex, and lateral to the third ventricle. The hypothalamus is comprised of three components: lateral, medial, and periventricular zones, each zone consisting of three groups of nuclei: anterior, tuberal, and posterior. In the anterior and tuberal hypothalamus are located the ma-

jority of the hypothalamic hormone-producing neurons. The median eminence, a prominence in the infundibular stalk extending from the hypothalamus to the anterior lobe of the pituitary, contains axons of the hypophysiotropic neurons responsible for control of hormonal secretion from the anterior pituitary. The hypothalamic pituitary portal system serves as the prime route of communication between the pituitary and hypothalamus.

The adult pituitary gland consists of the anterior and posterior lobes and is connected to the median eminence by the infundibular stalk and pars tuberalis. The main cell types within the anterior pituitary include the somatomammotropes that secrete growth hormone (GH) and prolactin, the corticotropes that secrete adrenocorticotropic hormone (ACTH); the thyrotropes that secrete thyroid-stimulating hormone (TSH), and the gonadotropes that secrete luteinizing hormone (LH) and follicle-stimulating hormone (FSH). Both thyrotropes and gonadotropes also secrete glycoprotein free α subunit. In addition to the trophic hormones secreted by the pituitary, activin, inhibin, and follistatin are also present within the pituitary and are critical to the autocrine/paracrine regulation of FSH. The posterior pituitary is composed of glial tissue and axonal termini and secretes antidiuretic hormone (ADH) and oxytocin. While hypothalamus–anterior pituitary

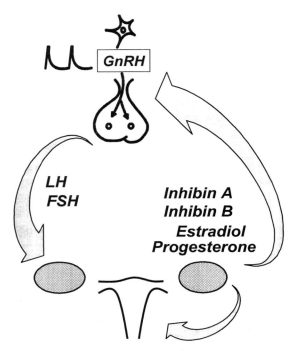

Figure 3-1 The hypothalamic, pituitary, and gonadal components of the reproductive axis are integrated through hormonal feedback.

gland communication is primarily vascular, hypothalamus-posterior pituitary interaction is neuronal.

▶ GnRH STRUCTURE

GnRH is a decapeptide isolated independently by two groups in the early 1970s led by Schally[1-3] and Guillemin.[4] The linear sequence of mammalian GnRH is pyro-Glu^1-His^2-Trp^3-Ser^4-Tyr^5-Gly^6-Leu^7-Arg^8-Pro^9-Gly^{10} amide. The half-life of the molecule is less than 10 minutes. Amino acid changes can extend the half-life to hours and days. Amino acid substitutions also can change the biologic activity of the molecule from an agonist to an antagonist.

There is now evidence that mammals, including humans, simultaneously express more that one molecular form of GnRH (for review, see ref. 5). GnRH II is widely expressed both within and outside the brain and works through

its own receptor. It is a potent stimulator of LH and FSH in both in vitro and in vivo animal models. While there is evidence that GnRH II may play a role in reproductive behavior in lower animal species, its role in the human is unknown. GnRH III has a similar hypothalamic distribution to that of GnRH in human brain, as indicated by immunohistochemistry, and may act through the GnRH receptor. Although there is some evidence in several animal species that GnRH III may have preferential FSH-releasing properties,[6] a GnRH III consensus sequence has not been found in the human genome,[5] and its role in the human is unclear.

▶ GENES THAT CONTROL GnRH

The GnRH gene is located at 8p21-8p11.2.[7] However, to date, mutations in this gene have not been found to be the cause of GnRH deficiency in humans. Recent evidence indicates that mutations in the gene encoding GPR54 are associated with hypogonadotropic hypogonadism, pubertal delay, and sexual infantilism that can be corrected by administration of exogenous GnRH.[8] Deletions in X-linked genes such as the KAL gene and DAX gene (dosage-sensitive sex-reversal AHC critical region on human X chromosome gene 1) may present with hypogonadotropic hypogonadism in conjunction with anosmia and renal agenesis or adrenal insufficiency, respectively.[9]

▶ GnRH RECEPTOR

The GnRH receptor (GnRHR) is a 327- to 328-amino-acid protein with seven transmembrane domains characteristic of a G protein-coupled receptor and an extracellular N terminus but no intracellular C terminus (Fig. 3-2). Studies elucidating GnRHR gene structure and signal transduction have been conducted using the αT3-1 cell line derived from a pituitary tumor in transgenic mice.[10] The GnRHR is coupled to G proteins of the G_q/G_{11} family, leading to production of inositol phosphates and increases

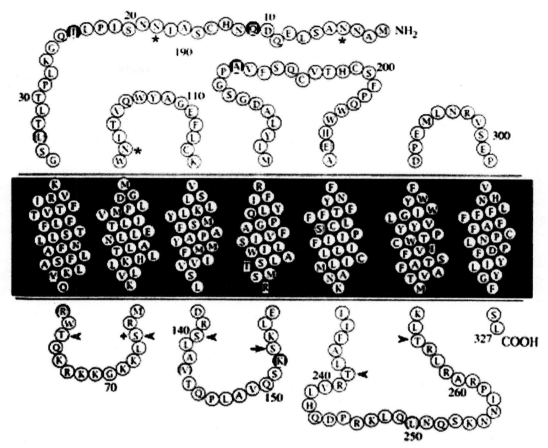

Figure 3-2 Model of the rat GnRHR. *(Reproduced with permission from Kaiser UB, et al. Iso-lation and characterization of cDNAs encoding the rat pituita gonadotropin-releasing hormone receptor. Biophys Res Commun 1992;189:1645–1652.)*

in intracellular calcium levels and resulting in activation of phospholipase C and protein kinase C.[10,11] The mitogen-activated protein kinase pathway also has been shown to be activated by GnRH and may be important in control of α-subunit gene expression by GnRH.[10,12] Activation of adenyl cyclase isoenzymes raises cAMP levels and intracellular calcium levels.[13] With continuous hormonal stimulation, gonadotropin receptors undergo desensitization, caused by phosphorylation and conformational changes of the receptor and uncoupling from the G proteins, in conjunction with internalization of the receptor and decreased receptor synthesis.[13]

The GnRHR is expressed on gonadotropes that comprise approximately 10 percent of all anterior pituitary cells.[10] Mutations affecting GnRHR structure, receptor binding of GnRH, or signal transduction may result in variable features of hypogonadotropic hypogonadism.[9]

► PITUITARY GONADOTROPINS

The gonadotropins, LH and FSH, hCG and TSH are non-covalently-linked dimers of glycoprotein subunits: the common glycoprotein α subunit and distinct hormone-specific β subunits that allow differential actions and functions. The α subunit consists of 92 amino acid residues with disulfide linkages encoded by a single gene on chromosome 6q12.21. The β subunits are specific for each hormone but have homology between LH and TSH and LH-hCG. These subunit genes are located on different chromosomes, with the genes for LH/hCGβ located on chromosome 19q12.32, FSHβ located on chromosome 11p13, and TSHβ located on chromosome 1p13.[13]

Gonadotropin receptors belong to the family of G protein–coupled receptors and have a large extracellular hormone-binding domain at the N terminus. LH and hCG bind to the same LH receptor, whereas FSH and TSH receptors are distinct. The amino acid sequence encoded by exons 2 through 9 confers hormone specificity[14] and coupling to Gs proteins.

LH and FSH are heterogeneous compounds with different isoforms that result from variations in their carbohydrate side chains. Both GnRH and gonadal steroids alter the isoform composition of stored and secreted LH and FSH. Basic isoforms are observed during normal menstrual cycles,[15] whereas more acidic isoforms are observed in postmenopausal women and men.[16] Although basic isoforms are more bioactive in in vitro assays, they have been shown to be less bioactive in vivo due to more rapid clearance from the circulation.[15,17]

▶ ONTOGENY OF THE REPRODUCTIVE AXIS

In the developing embryo, GnRH is found in neurons that originate in the olfactory placode and extend across the nasal septum through the nervus terminalis into the forebrain.[18,19] Fetal cells in the olfactory area respond to sex steroids and odorant stimuli to secrete GnRH in a time-dependent manner.[20] By embryonic day 14, GnRH cells migrate from the olfactory bulb along the olfactory tract into the mediobasal hypothalamus in the preoptic area and arcuate nucleus. Various factors and signals guide GnRH neuronal migration, including a neuronal cell adhesion molecule.[18] These hypothalamic neurons then proceed to send projections to the pituitary via the median eminence. The association of GnRH neurons with the olfactory system is best demonstrated by the high frequency of anosmia in patients with GnRH deficiency (Kallmann syndrome).[21]

GnRH neurons have been found in the fetal hypothalamus by 9 to 10 weeks of gestation and are detected in the portal system by 16 weeks, although human embryonic brain extracts[22] suggest that GnRH may be present as early as 4 to 5 weeks of gestation. Gonadotropins are detected in the pituitary at approximately 10 weeks and are measurable in peripheral blood by 12 weeks, peaking at midgestation in response to pulsatile GnRH release and decreasing in the third trimester due to gonadal negative feedback at the pituitary.[22,23]

During the gestational and neonatal periods, the HPG axis is transiently active in a gender-specific pattern.[24,25] Sexual dimorphism of gonadotropin secretion begins in utero, extending from infancy to 7 years of age, with both LH and FSH levels peaking earlier in females and remaining higher during gestation and neonatal periods than in males.[26,27] The capacity for gonadal steroid secretion during gestation occurs earlier in males compared with females, potentially accounting for this variability in gonadotropin secretion. Placental steroids, primarily hCG, bind to LH receptors at the testes early in gestation, stimulating androgen secretion.[28] Gonadal peptides, such as inhibin α and β subunits, are also detected at midgestation in the human male testes.[29] Thus testosterone secreted by the testes at 10 weeks of gestation results in negative feedback at the pituitary, inhibiting gonadotropin secretion.[30] In the female fetus, FSH receptors have not been detected until the ninth month of gestation,[31] consistent with the observed lack of inhibin secretion by the ovary at this time[29] and resulting in increased FSH secretion by the pituitary.

Postpartum, the loss of placental and gonadal steroids eliminates the negative feedback of sex steroids. This results in activation of the HPG axis at 1 to 2 weeks of age with an increase in LH and FSH secretion (albeit at lower amplitudes and duration than that at puberty) and stimulation of gonadal steroids.[24,25] Parturition triggers an LH surge in males that stimulates a transitory rise in testosterone levels for approximately 12 hours, after which the levels decline to those seen in females.[32] Gonadotropin levels eventually decline by 6 months, followed by decreases in testosterone. Inhibin B exceeds adult levels during early infancy and exhibits a more gradual decline.[33–35] In girls, the postparturition rise in FSH levels is significantly greater than that of LH levels and persists for 1 to 2 years.[33–35] Inhibin B levels decline by 12 months, while inhibin A levels remain immeasurable throughout.[32,36]

Following this initial HPG activity, the reproductive axis undergoes a quiescent hypogonadal period until puberty. The mechanisms involved in the reversible inhibition of the GnRH pulse generator during childhood remain unclear but seem to affect inhibition of GnRH secretion instead of synthesis.[37,38] Various factors that may be involved in modulating GnRH secretion include opioids,[38] neurotransmitters such as glutamate and aspartate,[39] and leptin.[40]

With the onset of puberty, the HPG axis undergoes a sleep-entrained reactivation characterized by increased GnRH pulse amplitude and resulting in increased nocturnal augmentation of LH secretion without any significant changes in pulse frequency.[41] In response to hypothalamic-pituitary stimulation, gonadal steroid and peptide secretion increases initially during the night and subsequently during the day as puberty progresses.[41]

▶ GnRH PULSE DYNAMICS

Neuroendocrine regulation of hormones involves a complex integrated network of feedback mechanisms between the hypothalamus, pituitary, and target organs (see Fig. 3-1). Understanding the physiology of GnRH secretion has been a challenge given the limited access to the hypophyseal-portal system. Since direct sampling of GnRH is not feasible in the human and peripheral blood measurements of GnRH do not accurately reflect GnRH secretion due to its rapid half-life of 2 to 4 minutes,[42] different approaches and probes have been used. There is ample evidence from studies in animal models that LH pulses in peripheral blood directly mirror pulses of GnRH in the pituitary portal circulation. In human studies, frequent blood sampling with measurement of LH and free α subunit in both normal and disease models and pharmacologic probes such as GnRH antagonists have been used to evaluate the physiology of GnRH secretion. Traditionally, LH has been used as a surrogate marker of GnRH pulse generator activity,[43,44] although glycoprotein free α subunit (FAS) has been shown to be a superior marker of GnRH secretion[45,46] in some settings due to its faster clearance. The ablation-replacement model of administration of GnRH to patients with hypogonadotropic hypogonadism and the use of probes such as GnRH antagonists that can provide a semiquantitative estimate of endogenous GnRH secretion have provided further insights into the physiology of GnRH secretion in the human.[45,47,48]

In the healthy young male, pulses of LH are secreted at approximately every 120 minutes, with a mild increase in frequency during the night.[49] During a single pulse of LH, levels can vary between 4.7 and 18.4 IU/mL, as seen in one series.[49] Conversely, the frequency of pulsatile GnRH and the amplitude of pulsatile LH secretion vary dramatically in women across the ovulatory cycle secondary to changing gonadal feedback (Fig. 3-3). The menstrual cycle is divided into two stages, follicular and luteal, linked by the midcycle surge (MCS). In the early follicular phase, LH pulse frequency increases from one pulse every 4 h (in the late luteal phase) to a pulse of every 90 minutes. During

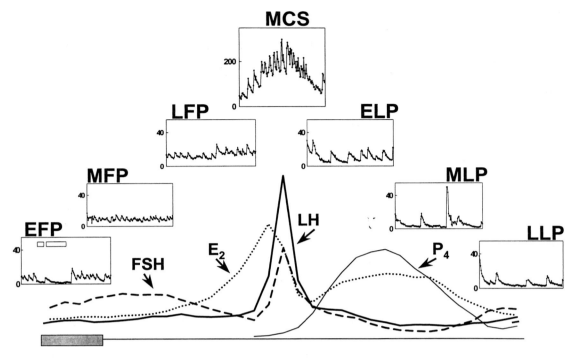

Figure 3-3 The pattern of LH (shown in boxes, IU/L) secretion changes across the normal menstrual cycle from the early, middle, and late follicular phases (EFP, MFP, LFP) through the midcycle surge (MCS) to the early, middle, and late luteal phases (ELP, MLP, LLP) reflecting changes in the frequency of GnRH secretion and the pituitary response to GnRH. Gonadotropin secretion stimulates follicular development, ovulation, and formation of the corpus luteum, resulting in secretion of estradiol (E_2) and progesterone (P_4). *(Reproduced with permission from Hall JE, Martin KA, Taylor AE. Body weight and gonadotropin secretion in normal women and women with reproductive abnormalities. In: Hansel W, Bray GA, Ryan DH, eds. Pennington Center Nutrition Series: Vol 6 Nutrition and Reproduction. Louisiana State University Press, Baton Rouge, 1998, pp. 378–393.*

the midfollicular phase, LH pulse frequency increases to one pulse per hour, and this frequency is maintained through the MCS. After the midcycle LH surge and ovulation, the GnRH pulse generator slows down to one LH pulse every 90 min, followed by a progressive decline in the LH pulse frequency during the luteal phase to pulses every 4 h in response to rising progesterone levels.[50–52] Although secretion of most gonadal steroids is apulsatile, both estrogen and progesterone concentrations can fluctuate dramatically in the mid (MLP) and late luteal phases (LLP) from 2.3 to 40.1 ng/mL in response to pulsatile secretion of LH.[53]

▶ MODULATION OF GnRH SECRETION

While there is now evidence that GnRH neurons are intrinsically pulsatile, various factors influence the coordinated pulsatile secretion of GnRH. GnRH release is stimulated by neurotransmitters such as nitroprusside, norepinephrine, and glutamic acid via nitric oxide (NO) pathways that increase guanylate cyclase. Increased production of cGMP mediates alterations in intracellular calcium and increases prostaglandin E_2 activity. These changes promote cAMP release, activating protein kinase A and leading to the exocytosis of GnRH secretory granules.[54] Opioid peptides appear to be involved in the negative-feedback effects of gonadal steroids on the brain but likely work through indirect mechanisms,[55] possibly through increasing gamma-aminobutyric acid (GABA) and cholinergic activity. Dopamine may stimulate hypothalamic GnRH release.[56] Neuropeptide Y stimulates GnRH secretion and is altered by the gonadal hormone milieu.[57] GABA suppresses GnRH release by inhibiting NO-driven GnRH release.

Leptin is a 167-amino-acid secreted peptide that is the product of the *ob* located on chromosome 6 and is expressed primarily in adipose tissue.[58] In *ob/ob* mice with phenotypic features of obesity, infertility, hyperinsulinemia, and impaired thyroid function,[59] diet restriction does not restore fertility, but leptin does,[60] suggesting a role for leptin in reproduction. Leptin receptors have been located on the gonadotrope cell surface and in the hypothalamus, and leptin stimulates the release of LH and FSH. Leptin increases GnRH pulse amplitude in female rats either directly or mediated by cocaine and amphetamine-regulated peptide (CART).[61] It also may work through inhibition of neuropeptide Y secretion,[62] which increases noradrenergic generated release of NO and activates GnRH release. Leptin also has been shown to accelerate the onset of puberty.[62] However, there is still lack of consensus on the exact role of leptin on puberty and reproduction, and studies are needed to elucidate this relationship.

▶ CONTROL OF GONADOTROPIN SECRETION BY GnRH

GnRH stimulates GnRHRs on anterior pituitary gonadotrophs, resulting in activation of heterodimeric GTP-binding (G) proteins, generation of inositol phosphates (IPs), influx of calcium into the cells, activation of protein kinase C (PKC) with generation of cAMP, and activation of mitogen-activated protein kinases. These steps are part of the cascade of events that re-

sult in synthesis and ultimate secretion of LH and FSH. Cell lines transfected with human FAS, LHβ, or FSHβ genes have been used to evaluate gonadotropin synthesis and release.[63] The effect of GnRH at its receptor occurs both directly and through increasing GnRHR numbers. The latter is accomplished at a posttranscriptional level through increasing mRNA translational efficiency.

LH is secreted through a regulated pathway, whereas most of the FSH is released constitutively, consistent with the observation that FSH secretion is more tightly coupled to FSH biosynthesis and that the magnitude of FSH secretion in response to secretagogues is generally smaller than that of LH.[10]

The pulsatile nature of the GnRH signal is critical to normal gonadotropin secretion. Varying GnRH pulse frequencies and amplitudes have an impact on the number of GnRHRs on gonadotropes, thereby influencing the magnitude of stimulation of gonadotropin subunit promoter activity.[64] Different GnRH pulse frequencies also differentially regulate LH and FSH synthesis and secretion. At low GnRH pulse frequencies (every 2 h), GnRHR concentrations on gonadotrope cell surfaces are low, with activation of a single signal-transduction pathway stimulating expression of α subunit, LHβ, and FSHβ. At higher GnRH pulse frequencies (every 30 min), GnRHR concentrations increase, resulting in greater activation of the signal-transduction pathway and stimulation of α and LHβ genes. In contrast, higher GnRH pulse frequencies stimulate a second signal-transduction pathway that specifically inhibits FSHβ gene expression, and the net result is preferential α and LHβ gene expression.[65]

Pioneering animal studies by Knobil and colleagues[43] demonstrated the absolute requirement for a pulsatile or phasic GnRH signal to stimulate gonadotropin secretion and the paradoxical desensitization of the gonadotrope that occurs with continuous GnRH stimulation. Sustained exposure or exposure to high concentrations of GnRH results in a decreased response to GnRH. This feature has permitted the therapeutic use of GnRH agonists for decreasing gonadotropin stimulation of gonadal steroid secretion in the treatment of precocious puberty, endometriosis, and prostate and breast cancers. The mechanism of gonadotrope desensitization is not completely understood but appears to involve both receptor and postreceptor mechanisms. Studies in αT3-1 pituitary cell lines suggest that unlike desensitization associated with other G protein receptors, the desensitization of GnRH signaling is primarily a postreceptor phenomenon.

Studies in the rat and sheep also have suggested that there may be a separate hypothalamic releasing factor that preferentially controls secretion of FSH. In the rat, GnRH III appears to selectively stimulate FSH secretion, and studies in rat hemipituitaries have demonstrated binding of biotinylated GnRH III to 80 percent of FSH gonadotropes and 50 percent of LH gonadotropes at low concentrations (10^{-9} M).[66] A second GnRH receptor (GnRH-IIR) has been reported in the human genome. This receptor is a G protein–coupled transmembrane receptor having a C-terminal cytoplasmic tail, unlike GnRHR, and resembles type II receptors of amphibians and fish rather than humans.[67]

▶ GONADAL FEEDBACK EFFECTS

Gonadal hormones exert negative and positive feedback actions either directly at the pituitary or indirectly through alterations in hypothalamic GnRH secretion. Estrogen, progesterone, and testosterone receptors are members of the nuclear receptor family that modulate transcription by DNA regulatory sequences. Nuclear receptors for estrogen, androgen, and progesterone have been detected in the brains of several species.[68] In their inactive state, gonadal hormone receptors are associated with corepressor molecules. Binding of gonadal hormones causes a conformational change in the receptor and leads to interaction with coactivator molecules that activate the transcriptional activity of genes that contain the specific receptor-binding enhancer DNA sequences.[69,70]

Two estrogen receptors (ERs) have been identified with distinct gene and chromosomal derivations. ERα and ERβ have equal affinity for estrogen but are unique in their terminal domains and have distinct transcriptional activities and distribution. ER localization can be challenging, and there are discrepancies between different species.[71] ERα is expressed in mammary glands, uterus, testis, pituitary, liver, kidney, heart, and skeletal muscle, whereas ERβ is seen predominantly in the prostate and ovary but is also present in the pituitary and brain. Within tissue types, there may be a different expression pattern for the ERs. For example, in the ovary, ERβ is localized to the granulosa cells, whereas ERα is detected in the thecal cells.[72] In the pituitary there is a significantly greater population of ERα compared with ERβ,[71] consistent with findings from studies in ER knockout rodent models that have demonstrated a greater role for ERα in the negative regulation of transcription of the gonadotropin subunit genes.[71] The inhibitory and stimulatory effects of estrogen involve modulation of direct neurochemical and neuronal pathways to influence GnRH neurons, with hyperpolarization of the GnRH neurons and GABA release to induce a negative-feedback effect on GnRH secretion and release of stimulatory neurotransmitters and inhibition of GABA to induce a positive-feedback effect in lower animal species.[73]

In women there is ample evidence supporting the negative-feedback effects of estradiol on gonadotropin secretion. In humans, studies have supported increased expression of GnRH mRNA in estrogen-deficient postmenopausal and young oophorectomized women.[74,75] Recent studies indicate that the hypothalamus is a major site of estrogen negative feedback in women. While some studies have suggested that the frequency of GnRH secretion is decreased, others have found no change. However, the overall quantity of GnRH is decreased, suggesting that there also may be a negative-feedback effect on GnRH pulse amplitude.[76] Estradiol has been shown to result in a dose- and time-dependent reduction in GnRHR number, noted within 24 hours of exposure and maximal after 4 to 5 d.[79]

Progesterone has been associated with slowing of the GnRH pulse generator in the luteal phase,[53,77] with a marked decrease in mean levels of LH and FSH seen in post-menopausal women.[76,78] Thus progesterone has predominately a hypothalamic site of negative feedback on the neuroendocrine components of the reproductive axis. Activin A increases GnRHR in a time- and dose-dependent fashion within 24 h of exposure and has been shown to modulate the responsiveness of GnRH activity at the pituitary by modulating the expression of GnRHRs.[80] Follistatin, on the other hand, inhibits the impact of activin on the GnRHR gene.[10]

In addition to the negative-feedback effects on gonadotropins in women, estrogen also exerts a positive-feedback effect on the development of the preovulatory LH surge. In lower animal species, an increase in GnRH is critical to development of the preovulatory gonadotropin surge. However, although it is critical that pulsatile stimulation of the gonadotrope continues, there is no evidence that an increase in GnRH is required to generate a normal surge in women.[81] There is no increase in GnRH pulse frequency at the onset of the surge in normal women,[82] and there is an overall decrease in the quantity of GnRH secreted.[83] This suggests that in women the changes that occur at the pituitary in response to increasing concentrations of estrogen (increased GnRHR number and postreceptor amplification of the GnRH signal) are of paramount importance in generating the normal midcycle LH surge.

In the rat,[84] sheep,[85] and humans,[86] progesterone and progesterone receptors may play a role in facilitating increased gonadotropin se-

cretion and possibly mediate a decrease in ER levels in the anterior pituitary, thereby counteracting the negative-feedback effects of estradiol.[87] This collective estrogen and progesterone effect on inducing the LH surge may suggest an estradiol-stimulated (via ERβ) increase in progesterone receptors in the hypothalamus and anterior pituitary gland.

In males, testosterone and estradiol have a negative-feedback effect on gonadotropin secretion, as demonstrated by both animal[88] and human studies.[89] To differentiate the feedback effects of estrogen and testosterone at the pituitary and hypothalamus, studies in patients with hypogonadotropic hypogonadism and in normal men treated with aromatase inhibitors elegantly demonstrate a significant increase in gonadotropin secretion and LH pulse amplitude, supporting the pituitary site of action for estradiol negative feedback and enhanced pituitary sensitivity to GnRH.[90] Greater suppression of gonadotropins observed in normal compared with GnRH-deficient men and increased LH pulse frequency with estradiol suppression indicate an additional hypothalamic effect.[90] Furthermore, the increase in LH pulse frequency with aromatase inhibitor–induced estrogen suppression despite a rise in testosterone levels suggests that estradiol has a greater negative-feedback effect compared with testosterone.[90,91] While the testosterone negative-feedback effects on LH are mediated directly via androgen receptors and indirectly by aromatization to estradiol, testosterone negative-feedback effects on FSH appear to be mediated primarily by estradiol[92] via ERα and ERβ receptors.[93]

With castration in the male, FSHβ, LHβ, and α subunit significantly increase, However, administration of testosterone suppresses expression of LHβ and α subunit to a much greater degree than that of FSHβ. Similar effects are seen in women, in whom oophorectomy is associated with a marked increase in FSH and LH, and gonadal steroids are much more effective at suppressing LH than FSH. Taken together, these data provide evidence for control of FSH by nonsteroidal gonadal feedback.

▶ GONADAL PEPTIDE FEEDBACK

Inhibin is a dimeric protein composed of a glycosylated α-subunit disulfide linked to β subunits βA and βB. The two subunits, βA and βB, are linked to the α subunit to form inhibin A and B, respectively. Inhibin selectively suppresses expression of FSHβ but not LHβ or glycoprotein α subunit.[94] Inhibin is secreted by the Sertoli cells of the testis and the granulosa and, to a lesser extent, the theca cells of the ovary. Inhibin B is the physiologically predominant inhibin in males as a marker of Sertoli cell function. It is stimulated by FSH and has a significant negative-feedback effect on FSH.[92,95,96] In women, inhibin A is a marker of the mature follicle and corpus luteum. It may contribute to suppression of FSH during the luteal phase, and its decline is associated with the rise of FSH that occurs during the luteal-follicular transition. However, its secretion is paralleled by estradiol, which also inhibits FSH secretion, and thus the relative role of estradiol and inhibin A in FSH control during the luteal-follicular transition is still under investigation. Inhibin B increases with administration of FSH in the early follicular phase in association with an increase in the number of granulosa cells. It appears to be constitutively secreted by granulosa cells and is a marker of granulosa cell number. A decrease in inhibin B is associated with the early increases in FSH that are a part of normal reproductive aging, well before changes in estradiol occur. Inhibin B also may play a role in the normal decrease in FSH that is critical to monofollicular development in the normal menstrual cycle.[97,98]

Activin is a dimer composed of two β subunits, comprising activin A (βAβA), activin B (βBβB), and activin AB (βAβB), all of which selectively stimulate GnRH-independent FSH secretion.[99] Follistatin is a gonadal protein that binds and inactivates activin, thereby inhibiting FSH biosynthesis and secretion.

▶ FEEDBACK DURING THE MENSTRUAL CYCLE

In women, dynamic hormonal changes in GnRH pulse frequency and gonadal function occur across the ovulatory menstrual cycle (see Fig. 3-3). FSH levels rise threefold in the early follicular phase in response to release of the negative-feedback effect of gonadal steroids (estradiol and progesterone) and peptides (inhibin A) and the increase in GnRH pulse frequency during the luteal-follicular transition.[50] FSH stimulates a new cohort of follicles, one of which eventually will become dominant. Rising levels of estradiol and inhibin B inhibit FSH, which reaches its nadir by the late follicular phase. During the midcycle surge and early luteal phase, FSH increases along with LH in response to the positive feedback of gonadal steroids but falls to very low levels by the midluteal phase and remains low until luteolysis. LH levels rise during the follicular phase and peak at the midcycle surge, increasing ten-fold within hours of a substantial increase in estradiol levels. LH levels subsequently decrease and reach a nadir by the late luteal phase. Estradiol levels increase with folliculogenesis during the follicular phase until peak levels are reached prior to ovulation, with subsequent negative feedback on the pituitary and hypothalamus. Estradiol concentrations continue to rise until they reach a peak approximately 1 day prior to ovulation, exerting a positive-feedback effect on gonadotropin secretion to elicit the midcycle surge. Ovulation occurs within 36 h of the LH peak, and estradiol levels decline rapidly in the luteal phase. Progesterone secretion begins with luteinization of the theca-granulosa cells after ovulation, reaching peak concentrations in the midluteal phase and declining in the late luteal phase to a nadir in the luteal-follicular transition.

▶ CONCLUSIONS

Normal reproductive function requires integration of the hypothalamus, pituitary, and gonad. Increased understanding of the components of this complex system provides an ever-greater sophistication in our understanding of both the physiology of reproduction and the disorders that result in abnormalities in reproductive function.

KEY POINTS

1. GnRH secretion from the hypothalamus dictates reproductive function; characteristic changes occur throughout the life cycle.

2. In reproductive-age women, the frequency of pulsatile GnRH secretion is every 90 min during the early follicular phase; this increases to every 60 min in the mid-follicular phase, maintains this frequency through the midcycle surge; and declines during the luteal phase. Pulsatile GnRH controls gonadotropin secretion, follicular development, and gonadal steroid secretion; GnRH and the pituitary response to GnRH are modified by secretion of gonadal steroids and peptides.

3. In men, GnRH pulse frequency is maintained every 2 h.

4. LH secretion has an impact on ovarian theca cell function in women and testicular Leydig cell function in men. FSH secretion stimulates ovarian follicular development in women and spermatogenesis in men.

5. Neuroendocrine regulation of reproduction is achieved by both positive- and negative-feedback effects at the hypothalamus and pituitary by various factors, including gonadal steroids and inhibin, leptin, opioids, and other hormonal and neurotransmitter systems.

REFERENCES

1. Baba Y, Matsuo H, Schally AV. Structure of the porcine LH- and FSH-releasing hormone: II. Confirmation of the proposed structure by conventional sequential analyses. *Biochem Biophys Res Commun* 1971;44:459–463.

2. Matsuo H, Baba Y, Nair RM, et al. Structure of the porcine LH- and FSH-releasing hormone: I. The proposed amino acid sequence. *Biochem Biophys Res Commun* 1971;43:1334–1339.

3. Schally AV, Arimura A, Baba Y, et al. Isolation and properties of the FSH and LH-releasing hormone. *Biochem Biophys Res Commun* 1971;43:393–399.

4. Guillemin R. Chemistry and physiology of hypothalamic releasing factors for gonadotrophins. *Int J Fertil* 1967;12:359–367.

5. Neill J. GnRH and GnRH receptor genes in the human genome. *Endocrinology* 2002;143:737–743.

6. McCann SM, Karanth S, Mastronardi CA, et al. Control of gonadotropin secretion by follicle-stimulating hormone–releasing factor, luteinizing hormone–releasing hormone, and leptin. *Arch Med Res* 2001;32:476–485.

7. Seminara SB, Hayes FJ, Crowley WF Jr. Gonadotropin-releasing hormone deficiency in the human (idiopathic hypogonadotropic hypogonadism and Kallmann's syndrome): Pathophysiological and genetic considerations. *Endocr Rev* 1998;19:521–539.

8. Seminara S, Messager S, Chatzidaki E, et al. The GPR54 gene as a regulator of puberty. *N Engl J Med* 2003;349:1614–1627.

9. Seminara SB, Oliveira LM, Beranova M, et al. Genetics of hypogonadotropic hypogonadism. *J Endocrinol Invest* 2000;23:560–565.

10. Kaiser UB, Conn PM, Chin WW. Studies of gonadotropin-releasing hormone (GnRH) action using GnRH receptor–expressing pituitary cell lines. *Endocr Rev* 1997;18:46–70

11. Stojilkovic S, Reinhart J, Catt K. Gonadotropin-releasing hormone receptors: Structure and signal transduction pathways. *Endocr Rev* 1994;15:462–499.

12. Roberson M, Misra-Press A, Laurance M, et al. A role for mitogen-activated protein kinase in mediating activation of the glycoprotein hormone α-subunit promoter by gonadotropin-releasing hormone. *Mol Cell Biol* 1995;15:3531–3539.

13. Themmen A, Huhtaniemi I. Mutations of gonadotropins and gonadotropin receptors: Elucidating the physiology and pathophysiology of pituitary-gonadal function. *Endocr Rev* 2000;21:551–583.

14. Baraun T, Schofield P, Strengel R. Amino-terminal leucine-rich repeats in gonadotropin recptors determine hormone selectivity. *EMBO J* 1991;10:1885–1890.

15. Wide L, Bakos O. More basic forms of both human follicle-stimulating hormone and luteinizing hormone in serum at midcycle compared with the follicular or luteal phase. *J Clin Endocrinol Metab* 1993;76:885–889.

16. Wide L, Wide M. Higher plasma disappearance rate in the mouse for pituitary follicle-stimulating hormone of young women compared to that of men and elderly women. *J Clin Endocrinol Metab* 1984;58:426–429.

17. Mulders J, Derksen M, Swolfs A, Maris F. Prediction of the in vivo biological activity of human recombinant follicle stimulating hormone using quantitative isoelectric focusing. *Biologicals* 1997;25:269–281.

18. Schwanzel-Fukuda M, Jorgenson K, Bergen H, et al. Biology of normal luteinizing hormone–releasing hormone neurons during and after their migration from olfactory placode. *Endocr Rev* 1992;13:623–634.

19. Schwanzel-Fukuda M, Pfaff D. Origin of luteinizing hormone–releasing hormone neurons. *Nature* 1989;998:161–164.

20. Barni T, Maggi M, Fantoni G, et al. Sex steroids and odorants modulate gonadotropin-releasing hormone secretion in primary cultures of human olfactory cells. *J Clin Endocrinol Metab* 1999;84:4266–4273.

21. Spratt DI, Carr DB, Merriam GR, et al. The spectrum of abnormal patterns of gonadotropin-releasing hormone secretion in men with idiopathic hypogonadotropic hypogonadism: Clinical and laboratory correlations. *J Clin Endocrinol Metab* 1987;64:283–291.

22. Grumbach M, Kaplan S. The neuroendocrinology of human puberty: An ontogenetic perspective, in Grumbach M, Sizonenko P, Aubert M (eds), *Control of the Onset of Puberty.* Baltimore: Williams & Wilkins, 1990;1–68.

23. Kaplan S, Grumbach M. The ontogenesis of human foetal hormones: II. Luteinizing hormone (LH) and follicle stimulating hormones. *Acta Endocrinol* 1976;81:808–829.

24. Grumbach M. The neuroendocrinology of human puberty revisited. *Horm Res* 2002;57:2–14.

25. Ojeda S, Andrews W, Advis J, White S. Recent advances in the endocrinology of puberty. *Endocr Rev* 1980;1:228–257.

26. Waldhauser F, Weibenbacher G, Frisch H, Pollak A. Pulsatile secretion of gonadotropins in early infancy. *Eur J Pediatr* 1981;137:71–74.

27. Wierman M, Crowley WF. Neuroendocrine control of the onset of puberty, in Falkner F, Tanner J (eds), *Human Growth: A Comprehensive Treatise,* Vol 2. New York: Plenum Press, 1986;225–241.

28. Axelrod L, Neer R, Kliman B. Hypogonadism in a male with immunologically active, biologically inactive luteinizing hormone: An exception ot a venerable rule. *J Clin Endocrinol Metab* 1979;48:279–287.

29. Rabinovici J, Goldsmith PC, Roberts VJ, et al. Localization and secretion of inhibin/activin subunits in the human and subhuman primate fetal gonads. *J Clin Endocrinol Metab* 1991;73:1141–1149.

30. Resko J, Ellinwood W. Negative-feedback regulation of gonadotropin secretion by androgens in fetal rhesus macaques. *Biol Reprod* 1985;33:346–352.

31. Huhtaniemi I, Yamamoto M, Ranta T, et al. Follicle-stimulating hormone receptors appear earlier in the primate fetal testis than in the ovary. *J Clin Endocrinol Metab* 1987;65:1210–1214.

32. Winter JS, Hughes IA, Reyes FI, Faiman C. Pituitary-gonadal relations in infancy: 2. Patterns of serum gonadal steroid concentrations in man from birth to two years of age. *J Clin Endocrinol Metab* 1976;42:679–686.

33. Winter JS, Faiman C, Hobson WC, et al. Pituitary-gonadal relations in infancy: I. Patterns of serum gonadotropin concentrations from birth to four years of age in man and chimpanzee. *J Clin Endocrinol Metab* 1975;40:545–551.

34. Faiman C, Winter JS. Sex differences in gonadotrophin concentrations in infancy. *Nature* 1971;232:130–131.

35. Burger H, Yamada Y, Bangah M, et al. Serum

gonadotropin, sex steroid, and immunoreactive inhibin levels in the first two years of life. *J Clin Endocrinol Metab* 1991;72:682–686.

36. Chellakooty M, Schmidt I, Haavisto A, et al. Inhibin A, inhibin B, follicle-stimulating hormone, luteinizing hormone, estradiol and sex-hormone binding globulin levels in 473 healthy infant girls. *J Clin Endocrinol Metab* 2003;88:3515–3520.

37. Plant T, Shahab M. Neuroendocrine mechanisms that delay and initiate puberty in higher primates. *Physiol Behav* 2002;77:717–722.

38. Wiemann M, Clifton D, Steiner R. Pubertal changes in gonadotropin-releasing hormone and proopiomelanocortin gene expression in the brain of the male rat. *Endocrinology* 1989;124:1760–1767.

39. Mahachoklertwattana P, Sanchez J, Kaplan S, Grumbach M. *N*-Methyl-D-aspartate (NMDA) receptors mediate the release of gonadotropin-releasing hormone (GnRH) by NMDA in a hypothalamic GnRH neuronal cell line (GT1-1). *Endocrinology* 1994;134:1023–1030.

40. Mantzoros C, Flier JS, Rogol AD. A longitudinal assessment of hormonal and physical alterations during normal puberty in boys: V. Rising leptin levels may signal the onset of puberty. *J Clin Endocrinol Metab* 1997;82:1066–1070.

41. Boyar R, Rosenfeld R, Kapen S, et al. Human puberty: Simultaneous augmented secretion of luteinizing hormone and testosterone during sleep. *J Clin Invest* 1974;54:609–618.

42. Pimstone G, Epstein S, Hamilton S, et al. Metabolic clearance and plasm half-disappearance time of exogenous gonadotropin-releasing hormone in normal subjects and in patients with liver disease and chronic renal failure. *J Clin Endocrinol Metab* 1977;44:1169–1173.

43. Belchetz P, Plant T, Nakai Y, et al. Hypophysial responses to continuous and intermittent delivery of hypothalamic gonadotropin-releasing hormone. *Science* 1978;202:631–633.

44. Clarke I, Cummins J. The temporal relationship between gonadotropin-releasing hormone (GnRH) and luteinizing hormone (LH) secretion in ovariectomized ewes. *Endocrinology* 1982;111:1737–1739.

45. Crowley WF Jr, Filicori M, Spratt DI, Santoro NF. The physiology of gonadotropin-releasing hormone (GnRH) secretion in men and women. *Recent Prog Horm Res* 1985;41:473–531.

46. Whitcomb RW, O'Dea LS, Finkelstein JS, et al. Utility of free alpha-subunit as an alternative neuroendocrine marker of gonadotropin-releasing hormone (GnRH) stimulation of the gonadotroph in the human: Evidence from normal and GnRH-deficient men. *J Clin Endocrinol Metab* 1990;70:1654–1661.

47. Hall JE, Whitcomb RW, Rivier JE, et al. Differential regulation of luteinizing hormone, follicle-stimulating hormone, and free alpha-subunit secretion from the gonadotrope by gonadotropin-releasing hormone (GnRH): Evidence from the use of two GnRH antagonists. *J Clin Endocrinol Metab* 1990;70:328–335.

48. Hall JE, Brodie TD, Badger TM, et al. Evidence of differential control of FSH and LH secretion by gonadotropin-releasing hormone (GnRH) from the use of a GnRH antagonist. *J Clin Endocrinol Metab* 1988;67:524–531.

49. Spratt DI, O'Dea LS, Schoenfeld D, et al. Neuroendocrine-gonadal axis in men: Frequent sampling of LH, FSH, and testosterone. *Am J Physiol* 1988;254:E658–E666.

50. Hall JE, Schoenfeld DA, Martin KA, Crowley WF Jr. Hypothalamic gonadotropin-releasing hormone secretion and follicle-stimulating hormone dynamics during the luteal-follicular transition. *J Clin Endocrinol Metab* 1992;74:600–607.

51. Filicori M, Flamigni C, Vizziello G, et al. Hypothalamic control of gonadotropin secretion in the human menstrual cycle. *Prog Clin Biol Res* 1986;225:55–74.

52. Filicori M, Santoro N, Merriam GR, Crowley WF Jr. Characterization of the physiological pattern of episodic gonadotropin secretion throughout the human menstrual cycle. *J Clin Endocrinol Metab* 1986;62:1136–1144.

53. Filicori M, Butler JP, Crowley WF Jr. Neuroendocrine regulation of the corpus luteum in the human: Evidence for pulsatile progesterone secretion. *J Clin Invest* 1984;73:1638–1647.

54. McCann SM, Kimura M, Walczewska A, et al. Hypothalamic control of FSH and LH by FSH-RF, LHRH, cytokines, leptin and nitric oxide. *Neuroimmunomodulation* 1998;5:193–202.

55. Kaur G, Kaur G. Role of cholinergic and GABAergic neurotransmission in the opioids-mediated

GnRH release mechanism of EBP-primed OVX rats. *Mol Cell Biochem* 2001;219:13–19.

56. Nazian S, Landon C, Muffly K, Cameron D. Opioid inhibition of adrenergic and dopaminergic but not serotonergic stimulation of luteinizing hormone–releasing hormone release from immortalized hypothalamic neurons. *Mol Cell Neurosci* 1994;5:642–648.

57. Woller M, McDonald J, Reboussin D, Terasawa E. Neuropeptide Y is a neuromodulator of pulsatile luteinizing hormone–releasing hormone release in the gonadectomized rhesus monkeys. *Endocrinology* 1992;130:2333–2342.

58. Zhang Y, Proenca R, Maffei M, et al. Positional cloning of the mouse obese gene and its human homologue. *Nature* 1994;372:425–432.

59. Dubuc P. The development of obesity, hyperinsulinemia and hyperglycemia in *ob/ob* mice. *Metabolism* 1976;25:1567–1574.

60. Chehab F, Lim M, Lu R. Correction of the sterility defect in homozygous obese female mice by teatment with the human recombinant leptin. *Nature Genet* 1996;12:318–320.

61. Parent A, Lebrethon M, Gerard A, et al. Leptin effects on pulsatile gonadotropin-releasing hormone secretion from the adult rat hypothalamus and interaction with cocaine- and amphetamine-regulated transcript peptide and neuropeptide Y. *Regul Pept* 2000;92:17–24.

62. Chehab F, Mounzih K, Lu R, Lim M. Early onset of reproductive function in normal female mice treated with leptin. *Science* 1997;275: 88–90.

63. Muyan M, Ryzmkiewicz D, Boime I. Secretion of lutropin and follitropin from transfected GH3 cells: Evidence for separate secretory pathways. *Mol Endocrinol* 1994;8:1789–1797.

64. Katt J, Duncan J, Herbon L, et al. The frequency of gonadotropin-releasing hormone stimulation determines the number of pituitary gonadotropin-releasing hormone receptors. *Endocrinology* 1985;116:2113–2115.

65. Kaiser UB, Sabbagh E, Katzenellenbogen R, et al. A mechanism for the differential regulation of gonadotropin subunit gene expression by gonadotropin-releasing hormone. *Proc Natl Acad Sci USA* 1995;92:12280–12284.

66. Childs G, Miller B, Chico D, et al. Preferential expression of receptors for lamprey gonadotropin-releasing hormone III by FSH cells: Support for its function as an FSH-RF.

83rd Annual Meeting of the Endocrine Society, Denver, CO, June 20–23, 2001.

67. Neill J, Duck L, Sellers J, Musgrove L. A gonadotropin-releasing hormone receptor specific for GnRH II in primates. *Biochem Biophys Res Commun* 2001;282:1012–1018.

68. Kawata M. Roles of steroid hormones and their receptors in structural organization in the nervous system. *Neurosci Res* 1995;24:1–46.

69. Klinge C. Estrogen receptor interaction with estrogen response elements. *Nucl Acids Res* 2001;29:2905–2919.

70. McKenna N, O'Malley B. Combinatorial control of gene expression by nuclear receptors and coregulators. *Cell* 2002;108:465–474.

71. Couse J, Korach K. Estrogen receptro null mice: What have we learned and where will they lead us? *Endocr Rev* 1999;20:358–417.

72. Schomberg D, Couse J, Mukerjee A, et al. Targeted disruption of the estrogen receptor-alpha gene in female mice: Characterization of ovarian responses and phenoype in the adult. *Endocrinology* 1999;340:2733–2744.

73. Herbison A. Multimodal influence of estrogen upon gonadotropin-releasing hormone neurons. *Endocr Rev* 1998;19:302–330.

74. Rance N, Uswandi S. Gonadotropin-releasing hormone gene expression is increased in the medial basal hypothalamus of postmenopausal women. *J Clin Endocrinol Metab* 1996;81: 3540–3546.

75. Abel T, Rance N. Stereologic study of the hypothalamic infundibular nucleus in young and older women. *J Comp Neurol* 2000;424: 679–688.

76. Gill S, Lavoie HB, Bo-Abbas Y, Hall JE. Negative-feedback effects of gonadal steroids are preserved with aging in postmenopausal women. *J Clin Endocrinol Metab* 2002;87: 2297–2302.

77. Soules M, Steiner R, Clifton D, et al. Progesterone modulation of pulsatile luteinizing hormone secretion in normal women. *J Clin Endocrinol Metab* 1984;58:378–383.

78. Cagnacci A, Melis G, Paoletti A, et al. Influence of oestradiol and progesterone on pulsatile LH secretion in postmenopausal women. *Clin Endocrinol (Oxf)* 1989;31:541–550.

79. McArdle C, Schomerus E, Groner I, Poch A. Estradiol regulates gonadotropin-releasing hormone receptor number, growth and inositol

phosphate production in aT3-1 cells. *Mol Cell Endocrinol* 1992;87:95–103.

80. Fernandez-Vazquez G, Kaiser UB, Albarracin C, Chin WW. Transcriptional activation of the gonadotropin-releasing hormone receptor gene by activin A. *Mol Endocrinol* 1996;5:356–366.

81. Karsch F, Dierschke D, Weick R, et al. Positive and negative feedback control by estrogen of luteinizing hormone secretion in the rhesus monkey. *Endocrinology* 1973;92:799–804.

82. Adams JM, Taylor AE, Schoenfeld DA, et al. The midcycle gonadotropin surge in normal women occurs in the face of an unchanging gonadotropin-releasing hormone pulse frequency. *J Clin Endocrinol Metab* 1994;79:858–864.

83. Hall J, Taylor A, Martin K, et al. Decreased release of gonadotropin-releasing hormone during the prevoulatory midcycle luteinizing hormone surge in normal women. *Proc Natl Acad Sci USA* 1994;91:6894–6898.

84. Leadem C, Kalra S. Stimulation with estrogen and progesterone of luteinizing hormone (LH)–releasing hormone release from perifused adult female rat hypothalami: correlation with the LH surge. *Endocrinology* 1984;114:51–56.

85. Clarke I. Variable patterns of gonadotropin-releasing hormone secretion during the estrogen-induced luteinizing hormone surge in ovariectomized ewes. *Endocrinology* 1993;133:1624–1632.

86. Kolp L, Pavlou S, Urban R, et al. Abrogation by a potent gonadotropin-releasing hormone antagonist of the estrogen/progesterone-stimulated surge-like release of luteinizing hormone and follicle-stimulating hormone in post-menopausal women. *J Clin Endocrinol Metab* 1992;75:993–997.

87. Mahesh V, Brann D. Regulation of the preovulatory gonadotropin surge by endogenous steroids. *Steroids* 1998;63:616–629.

88. Gharib S, Wierman M, Shupnik M, Chin W. Molecular biology of the pituitary gonadotropins. *Endocr Rev* 1990;11:177–199.

89. Quigley C, de Bellis A, Marschke K, et al. Androgen receptor defects: Historical, clinical and molecular perspectives. *Endocr Rev* 1995;16:271–321.

90. Hayes FJ, Seminara SB, Decruz S, et al. Aromatase inhibition in the human male reveals a hypothalamic site of estrogen feedback. *J Clin Endocrinol Metab* 2000;85:3027–3035.

91. Finkelstein JS, O'Dea LS, Whitcomb RW, Crowley WF Jr. Sex steroid control of gonadotropin secretion in the human male: II. Effects of estradiol administration in normal and gonadotropin-releasing hormone–deficient men. *J Clin Endocrinol Metab* 1991;73:621–628.

92. Hayes FJ, DeCruz S, Seminara SB, et al. Differential regulation of gonadotropin secretion by testosterone in the human male: Absence of a negative-feedback effect of testosterone on follicle-stimulating hormone secretion. *J Clin Endocrinol Metab* 2001;86:53–58.

93. Couse J, Hewitt S, Bunch D, et al. Postnatal sex reversal of the ovaries in mice lacking estrogen receptors α and β. *Science* 1999;286:2328–2331.

94. Carroll RS, Corrigan AZ, Gharib SD, et al. Inhibin, activin, and follistatin: Regulation of follicle-stimulating hormone messenger ribonucleic acid levels. *Mol Endocrinol* 1989;3:1969–1976.

95. Anawalt B, Bebb R, Matsumoto A, et al. Serum inhibin B levels reflect Sertoli cell function in normal men and men with testicular dysfunction. *J Clin Endocrinol Metab* 1996;81:3341–3345.

96. Seminara SB, Boepple PA, Nachtigall LB, et al. Inhibin B in males with gonadotropin-releasing hormone (GnRH) deficiency: Changes in serum concentration after shortterm physiologic GnRH replacement—A clinical research center study. *J Clin Endocrinol Metab* 1996;81:3692–3696.

97. Welt CK, Smith ZA, Pauler DK, Hall JE. Differential regulation of inhibin A and inhibin B by luteinizing hormone, follicle-stimulating hormone, and stage of follicle development. *J Clin Endocrinol Metab* 2001;86:2531–2537.

98. Welt CK, Adams JM, Sluss PM, Hall JE. Inhibin A and inhibin B responses to gonadotropin withdrawal depends on stage of follicle development. *J Clin Endocrinol Metab* 1999;84:2163–2169.

99. Carroll RS, Kowash PM, Lofgren JA, et al. In vivo regulation of FSH synthesis by inhibin and activin. *Endocrinology* 1991;129:3299–3304.

CHAPTER 4

The Ovary and the Normal Menstrual Cycle

Bruce R. Carr

► THE OVARY

The ovaries serve as the source of ova and the hormones that regulate female sexual function. The rapid growth of a single follicle that will become dominant and eventually ovulate and the consistent regularity of this process for an average of 38 years are truly remarkable phenomena. The development of predictable, regular, cyclic, and spontaneous ovulatory menstrual cycles is regulated by complex interactions of the hypothalamic-pituitary axis, the ovaries, and the genital tract. The cyclic *nature* of the female reproductive process depends on the ability of the ovary to change in both structure and function. The complex compartmentalization in the ovary that allows follicular growth is regulated by gonadotropins, steroid hormones, and local factors produced within the ovary. Estrogens and progestins, the principal steroid hormones secreted by the ovary, promote growth and differentiation of the uterus, fallopian tubes, and vagina, as well as other signs of sexual maturation. Alteration in this complex process can result in disorders of the ovary, as well as the development of sexual precocity, disorders of the menstrual cycle, androgen excess, and infertility. As a consequence of aging, the majority of remaining follicles undergo atresia such that by age 50 few follicles remain. Estrogen levels then decline, resulting in atrophy and regression of secondary sexual characteristics and the onset of menopause.

► FETAL OVARY

The development of the gonads takes place early in fetal life. While sexual differences between fetuses are not seen until development of the gonads, the genetic sex is determined at conception. The bipotential gonadal anlagen, which give rise to either the ovary or testis, can be identified in human embryos within 1 month of the conception.[1] Three principal cell types play key roles in the developing ovary: (1) coelomic epithelial cells, which are derived from the gonadal ridge and later differentiate into the granulosa cells, (2) mesenchymal cells of the gonadal ridge, which give rise to the ovarian stroma, and (3) primordial germ cells, which arise from the endoderm of the yolk sac and differentiate into ova.

During the third week of gestation, the primordial germ cells arise in the yolk sac at the caudal end of the ovary. During the sixth week, the primordial germ cells migrate into the underlying mesenchyme and become incorporated into the primary sex cords. Primordial cell migration can be traced by cytochemical techniques due to their high alkaline phosphatase activity. The mechanisms that control the ameboid movement of primordial cells to the gonadal ridge are still being investigated; however, chemotactic substances secreted by the gonadal anlagen are thought to play a role in regulating the migratory process.[2] During migration, the continued replication of the germ cells acts to amplify the original number of cells from the yolk sac. In the human embryo, approximately 1000 germ cells are present at 5 weeks, and by 8 weeks, they may be increased to 600,000 cells.[3]

The sex of the migrating primordial cells often can be predicted by the status of the sex chromatin. Specifically in female germ cells, one X chromosome is inactivated during migration to the gonadal ridge. As proposed by Lyon,[4] a dose compensation by X chromosome inactivation prevents aneuploidy. Two X chromosomes are required for normal development of the ovary. In individuals with a 45, X karyotype, initial ovarian development occurs with primordial germ cells appearing in the gonad, but follicular development is reduced and the rate of atresia is accelerated so that only a fibrous streak remains at the time of birth.[5]

Histologic recognition of the ovary cannot be made until 10 to 11 weeks of fetal life, whereas the fetal testis is distinguishable somewhat earlier. After the primordial cells reach the fetal gonad, they continue to proliferate by successive mitotic division (Fig. 4-1). The ovary

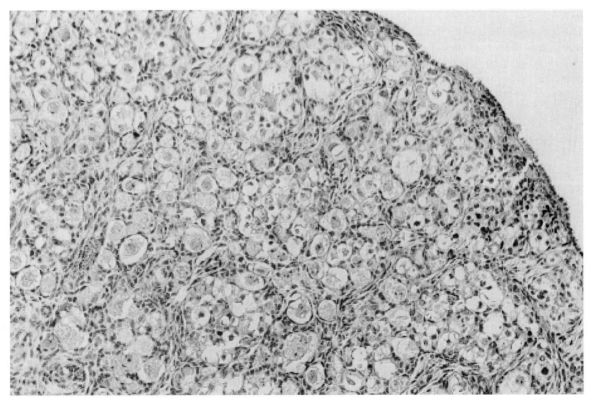

Figure 4-1 Histologic section of an ovary from a 16-week human fetus. *(Reproduced, with permission, from Carr BR. Disorders of the ovary and female reproductive tract. In: Wilson JD, Foster DW, eds. William's Textbook endocrinology, 8th ed. Phihldelphia, Pa., W. B. Saunders, 1992:733-798)*

will contain a finite number of germ cells, a maximal number of 6 to 7 million oogonia being reached by the twentieth week of gestation.[3] Follicular maturation continues following midgestation with follicular programming through the antral stage and ending in atresia. Most of the germ cells are lost in utero so that only 1 million remain at birth.[6] The process of follicular maturation and atresia continues throughout adult life.

Recent evidence suggests the ovary may be capable of postnatal germ cell development but the clinical relevance in humans remains unclear.[6a] During early fetal development, the ovary is in close proximity to the mesonephros (a primordial functioning kidney). The mesnephros influences both testicular and ovarian differentiation and is required for completion of ovarian development.[7] The ovarian-mesonephros association is retained during early ovarian differentiation, with the meso-nephros tissue regressing slowly. In the human, the ovary is invaded by mesonephric cells that form the ovarian medulla and force the germ cells to occupy the ovarian cortex. The oogonia continue to undergo mitosis until they enter meiosis, after which they are converted to primary oocytes, which begins as early as the twelfth week of gestation.[8] The primary oocytes initiate meiosis, but meiosis is arrested at the diplotene or resting stage of the first meiotic division and remains there until the onset of ovulation at puberty, when the first meiotic phase is completed (Fig. 4-2).

The second meiotic phase will be initiated following fertilization by spermatozoa. The arrest in meiosis appears to be controlled by substances produced locally in the ovary, namely, *meiosis-preventing substance* (MPS), also known as *oocyte-maturation inhibitor* (OMI).[9] After the primary oocyte arrests at the diplotene stage of meiosis, it becomes surrounded by a layer of primitive granulosa cells, giving rise to the primordial follicle, the morphologic marker of fetal ovarian differentiation. A basement membrane is formed that separates the primordial follicle from the sur-

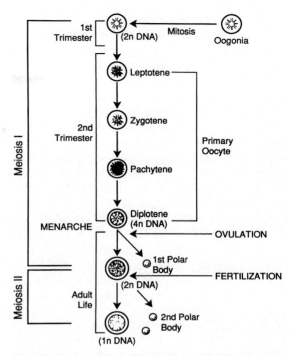

Figure 4-2 Life cycle of the oocyte. During the first trimester of fetal life, the oogonium undergoes mitosis. During the second trimester, meiosis I is initiated but arrested at the diplotene stage (4n DNA). Following menarche, at the time of ovulation, meiosis resumes in one ovum with the formation of the first polar body (2nd DNA). Meiosis II is initiated at the time of fertilization and completed with the formation of the second polar body (1n DNA). Fusing with the male pronucleus restores the nuclear content to 2n DNA. *(Reproduced, with permission, from Carr BR. Disorders of the ovary and female reproductive tract. In: Wilson JD, Foster DW, eds. William's textbook of Endocrinology, 8th ed. Philadelphia, Pa, W.B. Saunders, 1992:733–798.)*

rounding stroma. Later, meiosis is triggered to continue by meiosis-inducing substance.[10]

The conversion of oogonia into primary oocytes and the subsequent formation of primordial follicles are continued until 6 months after birth. Oocytes that are not incorporated into follicles undergo degeneration, which explains why most oocytes have disappeared by birth. The primordial follicles are first located at the inner part of the cortex near the medulla. At approximately 20 weeks of fetal life, the follicles begin to grow under the influence of gonadotropins. The need for gonadotropic influence for normal development of the ovary is suggested by the reduced follicular development seen in both the anencephalic human fetus and in monkeys following fetal hypophysectomy.[11] The primordial follicle is first surrounded by layers of granulosa cells, giving rise to the development of primary follicles. By the seventh month of gestation, follicle maturation reaches the antrum stage and is located at the outer part of the cortex.

The early human ovary, by the eighth week of gestation, has limited capacity to produce steroids when examined in vivo or in vitro. Luteinizing hormone (LH)/human chorionic gonadotropin (hCG)–binding sites are not detected in human fetal ovaries, and LH, follicle-stimulating hormone (FSH), and hCG do not stimulate steroidogenesis in vitro, suggesting that any steroidogenic enzyme expression at this stage of development is independent of gonadotropin control.[12]

The primitive form of the genital ducts, namely, the wolffian ducts (male) and the müllerian ducts (female), do not arise simultaneously. The wolffian duct develops first from the mesonephros and in the fetus destined to be a female may participate in formation of the müllerian ducts. Loss of the wolffian duct is due to the lack of locally produced androgen. While degeneration of the wolffian duct begins soon after appearance of the ovary, it is not completed until the beginning of the third trimester of pregnancy. In the female, the müllerian duct gives rise to the fallopian tubes, uterus, and upper third of the vagina. By 10 weeks, the uterus has differentiated into an upper part, the corpus, and a lower part, the cervix. Although the cervix and corpus are initially the same length, the cervix is two-thirds the total length by birth. Development of the müllerian duct is independent of gonadal hormone secretion because the ducts develop normally in fetuses without gonads.[10]

▶ CHILDHOOD AND PREMENARCHEAL OVARY

The mean ovarian weight increases from 250 mg at birth to reach a mean weight of approximately 4000 mg by menarche. The increase in size and weight of the ovaries are due to an increase in the amount of stroma, size of follicles, and number of follicles that occurs due to continuing growth of the ovary. Final maturation of the ovarian follicles occurs during puberty in response to increasing levels of gonadotropins. The two major hormones responsible for follicular development and the initiation of ovulation are FSH and LH.

There are significant variations in the levels of gonadotropin during the different stages of life in women (Fig. 4-3). Indeed, the hypothalamus, pituitary, and ovary of the fetus, newborn, and prepubertal child are functional and capable of secreting hormones. During the second trimester of fetal development, the plasma levels of gonadotropins rise to levels similar to those observed in menopause.[13] This peak in fetal gonadotropin levels is associated with maximal development of follicles. In addition, during the second trimester of pregnancy, the hypothalamic-pituitary axis (gonadostat) undergoes maturation and becomes more sensitive to the high levels of circulating steroid hormones, namely, estrogen and progesterone, that are secreted by the placenta. These steroids cause gonadotropins to fall to low levels prior to birth. Following birth, the levels of gonadotropins rise abruptly due to separation from the placenta, which results in a decrease in estrogen and progestogen levels and loss of negative feedback. The elevated levels of gonadotropins in the newborn persist for the first few months of life, declining to low levels by 1 to 3 years of life.[14] An explanation for the low gonadotropin levels during the childhood years is the increased sensitivity of the hypothalamic-pituitary axis to circulating low levels of gonadal steroids. In addition, evidence obtained from normal children suggests that the prepubertal hypothalamic axis is much

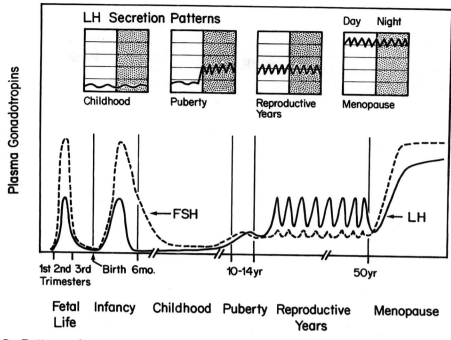

Figure 4-3 Pattern of gonadotropin secretions during different stages of life in women. Abbreviations: FSH, follicle stimulating hormone; LH, lutenizing hormone. The secretory patterns of LH during the waking hours (clear area) and night (stippled area) for each stage are indicated in the upper inserts. *(Reproduced, with permission, from Carr Br, Wilson JD. Disorders of the ovary and female reproductive tract. In: Wilson JD, Braunwald E, Isselbacher KJ, et al, eds. Harrison's Principles on Internal Medicine, 12th ed. New York, N.Y., McGraw-Hill, 1991:1776-1795.)*

more sensitive to estrogen treatment than the adult feedback mechanism.[15] There appears also to be an intrinsic role of the central nervous system (CNS) in decreasing gonadotropin levels. This is suggested by the fall in gonadotropins that occurs between ages 5 and 11 in the absence of a gonad or in children with gonadal dysgenesis.[16] The ability of gonadotropin-releasing hormone (GnRH) [also known as LH-releasing hormone (LHRH)] to stimulate the level of gonadotropins in agonadal children suggests that a central nonsteroidal substance is acting to inhibit the hypothalamic axis.[17] However, to date, no physiologic inhibitors of GnRH secretion have been identified in humans or primates.

Although basal gonadotropin secretion in prepubertal females is diminished, small pulses are detected at 2- to 3-hour intervals.[18] During puberty, the pituitary becomes more sensitive to infusions of GnRH, and the LH and FSH response to GnRH increases in an age-depended manner. The progression into puberty appears to be preceded by three major developments: (1) adrenarche (onset of adrenal androgen secretion), (2) decreased sensitivity of the hypothalamic-pituitary axis, and (3) gonadarche, the increased release of GnRH from the medial basal hypothalamus, leading to increased pituitary gonadotropin release and estrogen secretion by the ovary.

The increase in secretion of adrenal androgens occurs prior to significant quantitative and qualitative alterations in gonadotropin secretion. The levels of androstenedione, dehydroepiandrosterone, and dehydroepiandrosterone sulfate increase in children beginning at approximately 6 to 8 years of age. A decline in the expression of 3β-hydroxysteroid dehydrogenase in the reticularis zone of the human adrenal occurs after age 5, which may explain in part the rise in adrenal androgen levels.[19] This increase in secretion of androgens by the adrenal cortex is termed *adrenarche,* a process that appears independent of corticotropin (ACTH) stimulation. A number of other peptide and protein hormones have been proposed as alternative adrenal androgen–stimulating factors involved in the initiation of adrenarche, but conclusive evidence for such a hormone does not currently exist. Adrenal androgens (preandrogens) actually have little androgenic effect until they are converted to more potent androgens (true androgens) in peripheral or target tissues. True androgens (testosterone and dihydrotestosterone) can then exert biologic effects in target tissues that express androgen receptors.

Adrenal androgens and their metabolites may be responsible for the initial growth spurt and are responsible for the development of axillary and pubic hair. Because of the close association of the onset of adrenarche and gonadarche, some believe that adrenarche is an important initiating event in the increased secretion of GnRH and gonadotropin by the hypothalamic-pituitary axis. However, there is also considerable evidence that the controlling mechanisms that initiate and regulate adrenarche and gonadarche are independent. In girls with hypothalamic amenorrhea, such as Kallmann syndrome (olfactogenital dysplasia), or hypergonadotropic hypogonadism (e.g., gonadal dysgenesis), adrenarche normally occurs in the absence of gonadarche. Premature pubarche (also called *premature adrenarche*) results in the premature development of pubic and axillary hair before age 8 and is not associated with premature gonadarche. In children with absence of adrenarche due to adrenal hypofunction (Addison disease), gonadarche still occurs.[20]

Factors that regulate the onset of gonadarche and increased secretion of LH and FSH are complex but are believed to be initiated by a decreased responsiveness of the CNS-hypothalamic-pituitary axis to circulating levels of steroid hormones. Other potential initiators of puberty include loss of neuronal inhibition or increase of neuronal stimulation by neurotransmitters. One of the first signs of increased pubertal gonadotropin release is a sleep-associated surge of LH release[21] (see Fig. 4-3). Similar sleep-related LH pulses are also reported to occur in children with idiopathic precocious puberty, in agonadal subjects during the return of elevation of gonadotropins after age 11, and in women with anorexia nervosa during early stages of recovery.[22] An increased secretion of estrogen occurs, leading to a positive feedback in LH secretion and eventually to ovulation and then menarche.

Several lines of evidence suggest that the attainment of a pulsatile secretion of GnRH is critical for the initiation of puberty. In rhesus monkeys in which the hypothalamus has been destroyed, gonadotropin hormones decline. If these monkeys are treated with pulsatile GnRH given at hourly intervals, LH and FSH pulsatile secretion is reestablished.[23] In addition, infantile female rhesus monkeys treated with pulsatile injections of GnRH undergo pubertal maturation.[23] In women at puberty, an increase in pulse frequency and amplitude of LH release occurs. The infusion of pulsatile GnRH will initiate puberty in women with sexual infantilism (e.g., Kallmann syndrome).[24] Finally, the administration of GnRH analogues causes regression of pubertal changes in girls with isosexual precocious puberty.[25] The levels of FSH rise early in puberty, whereas those of LH lag behind, rising later. Prior to puberty, the ratio of FSH to LH is greater than 1, and at the end of puberty, the ratio is reversed (i.e., FSH/LH <1) until menopause, when the FSH/LH ratio is again greater than 1 (Table 4-1). The level of estradiol (more than 90 percent derived from

▶ **TABLE 4-1:** FSH/LH RATIO IN FEMALES

Fetal life	>1
Childhood	>1
Reproductive life	<1
Menopause	>1

the ovary) increases progressively throughout puberty, apparently following the increase in serum FSH levels. The level of bioactive LH is greater during early puberty than is immunologic LH. This discrepancy may be due to alterations in the amount of glycosylation of LH that alter immunoreactivity.[26] In addition to ovarian feedback on the hypothalamus and pituitary by steroid hormones, ovarian-derived peptide factors such as inhibin also appear to be involved in regulating gonadotropin levels. Serum inhibin levels increase and parallel FSH levels during puberty in girls.[27] Inhibin is secreted in two forms, A and B, each with a molecular weight of 32,000. It is postulated that FSH stimulates granulosa cells to secrete inhibin and that the levels rise until adulthood, at which time the inhibin-FSH negative-feedback relationship is established (described below).

The development of female secondary sexual characteristics occurs at puberty as the result of increased release of estradiol. The rise in estrogen levels is responsible for the initiation of accelerated growth (growth spurt) and female secondary characteristics, i.e., development of breasts, maturation of the female internal and external genitalia, and development of the female habitus. Androgens derived from the ovary (and, to a lesser degree, adrenal androgens) regulate axillary and pubic hair development. The age of initiation of puberty, as well as the rate of progression, will vary within the population. Most girls start with breast development between the ages of 10 and 11, followed by the development of pubic and axillary hair. A growth spurt ensues, and a peak growth rate is attained at a median age of 11.4 years. In part, the increase in height and growth during puberty is regulated by hormonal changes that include growth hormone, insulin-like growth factor I (IGF-I), and estrogen. Growth hormone stimulates production of IGF-I, particularly within the liver. IGF-I-levels increase progressively during puberty. The increase in IGF-I is mediated indirectly by an increase in sex steroids, which are believed to stimulate an increased secretion of growth hor-

mone. If, on the other hand, IGF-I levels do not rise, a growth spurt does not occur, as demonstrated by African pygmies.[28]

The culmination of puberty is the onset of regular, spontaneous, predictable, cyclic ovulatory menses. The age of menarche is variable and determined in part by socioeconomics as well as genetic factors, general health, nutrition, geography, and altitude.[20,29] In the United States, the mean age of menarche has decreased at a rate of 3 to 4 months per decade over the last 100 years and is now 12.7 years, a decrease believed to be due primarily to improved nutrition.[30] Frisch and colleagues analyzed growth and development of 169 girls. They observed that at a mean or "critical" body weight of 48 kg, menarche occurred.[30] However, other investigators, as well as Frisch, proposed that additional factors are also important in determining the onset of menarche and the maintenance of ovulatory menses. These include: percent of body fat, percent of body water, ratio of lean to fat, and lean body mass, as well as body "shape." Obese girls with a body weight 20 to 30 percent above ideal experience menarche earlier than do women of normal weight. In contrast, women with decreased body fat associated with participation in certain sports or ballet, malnutrition, and chronic debilitating diseases commonly experience delayed menarche. Although the theory of "critical" body weight is still speculative and controversial, the theory of a metabolic signal related to body composition appears to be an important factor in the maturation or activation of the hypothalamic GnRH pulse generator.[20] One of these metabolic signals may be leptin secreted by adipose tissue.[31]

▶ OVARY OF THE REPRODUCTIVE YEARS

Structure of the Adult Ovary

Adult human ovaries are oval with the following dimensions: length, 2 to 5 cm; width, 1.5 to 3 cm; and thickness, 0.5 to 1.5 cm. The weight of each ovary of normal women during the reproductive years is 5 to 10 g (average 7 g). The ovaries lie in approximation with the posterior and lateral pelvic walls and are attached to the posterior surface of the broad ligament by a peritoneal fold named the *mesovarium*. Blood vessels, nerves, and lymphatics traverse the mesovarium and enter the ovary at its hilum. The ovary consists of three distinct regions: an outer cortex containing the ovarian follicles, a central medulla consisting of ovarian stroma, and an inner hilum around the area of attachment of the ovary to the mesovarian.

The components and function of the adult ovary are illustrated schematically in Figure 4-4.

Follicles

The follicles are embedded in the connective tissue of the ovarian cortex and are either inactive or growing. Most follicles are inactive throughout the reproductive life of women and are termed *primordial follicles* (Fig. 4-5). In each cycle, several primordial follicles initiate growth and undergo significant changes in size,

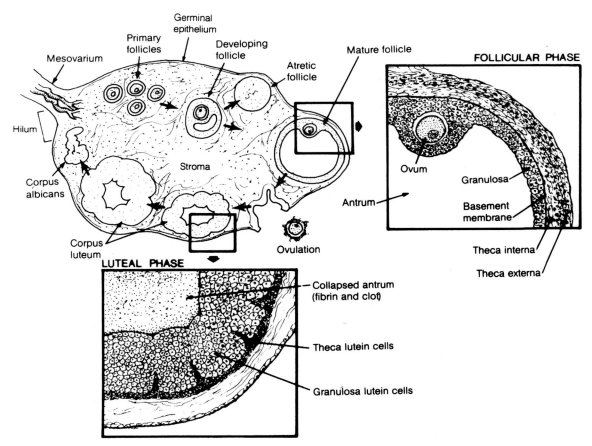

Figure 4-4 Developmental changes in the adult ovary during a complete menstrual cycle. *(Reproduced with permission, from Carr BR, Wilson JD. Disorders of the ovary and female reproductive tract. In: Wilson JD, Braunwald E, Isselbacher KJ, et al, eds. Harrison's Principles of Internal Medicine, 12th ed. New York, N.Y., McGraw-Hill, 1991:1776– 1795.)*

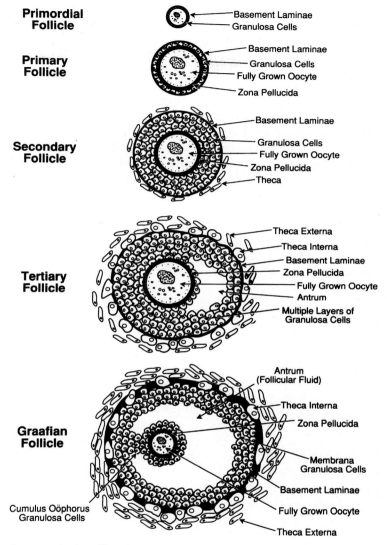

Figure 4-5 Stucture and classification of the ovarian follicle during growth and development. *(Adapted in part, with permission, from Erickson GF, Magoffin DA, Dyer CA, Hofeditz C. The ovarian androgen cells: A review of structure/functionrelationships. Endocrine rev. 6:371, 1985.)*

structure, and function. The growing follicles are divided into five stages: primary, secondary, tertiary, graafian, and atretic. The first two stages of growth can occur in the absence of gonadotropin secretion and thus appear to be under intraovarian control.[32] However, for a follicle to enter the tertiary stage, there is a dependence on gonadotropin secretion.

During each cycle, an ovum is selected from the pool of primordial follicles. Primordial follicles are composed of a single layer of granulosa cells and a single immature oocyte arrested in the diplotene stage of the first meiotic division. These follicles are separated from the surrounding stroma by a thin basal lamina (basement membrane). The oocyte is surrounded by a single layer of spindle-shaped cells with cytoplasmic processes that reach the basal lamina, providing a route for transfer of nutrients. Because of the basal lamina, the oocyte and granulosa cells do not have a blood supply and thus exist in a microenvironment without direct contact with other cells.

One of the first signs of follicular recruitment is a change in the spindle-shaped cells that surround the oocyte. These cells become cuboidal and undergo successive mitotic divisions, giving rise to a multilayered stratum granulosa or *zona granulosa*. In addition, the oocyte enlarges and secretes a mucoid substance containing glycoproteins that surrounds the oocyte. This substance is called the *zona pellucida* and can be seen to separate the granulosa cells from the oocyte. These changes represent differentiation of the primordial follicle into a *primary follicle* (see Fig. 4-5).

A *secondary follicle* results from the proliferation of granulosa cells, development of the theca, and completion of oocyte growth. The proliferation of granulosa cells is associated with differentiation of stroma cells outside the basal lamina. These cells become arranged in concentric perifollicular layers and constitute the theca (see Fig. 4-5). The *theca interna* consists of the cells immediately adjacent to the basal lamina, whereas the theca cells that merge with the surrounding stroma are named the *theca externa*. During development of the secondary follicle, the follicle acquires an independent blood supply that consists of arterioles that terminate at the basal lamina in a capillary bed. The granulosa cells and oocyte remain avascular because the blood supply does not penetrate the basement membrane. One distinct morphologic feature of the granulosa cells, the Call-Exner bodies, appears during development of the secondary follicle. Little is known about the physiologic importance of these bodies or how they form.

Formation of the *tertiary follicle* is associated with further hypertrophy of the theca and the appearance of a fluid-filled space among the granulosa cells named the *antrum* (see Fig. 4-5). The fluid consists of a plasma filtrate and the secretory products of granulosa cells, some of which are found in concentrations greater than those in peripheral blood. Gap junctions allow small molecules to pass from one cell to another, allowing for cell-to-cell communication and synchronized coordination of ovarian function.

FSH stimulates the tertiary follicle to increase rapidly in size and form the *mature or graafian follicle* (see Fig. 4-5). During this stage, the granulosa and oocyte are still contained within the basal lamina and remain devoid of direct vascularization. The antral fluid increases in volume, and the oocyte, surrounded by an accumulation of granulosa cells called the *cumulus oophorus,* occupies a polar position within the follicle. At this stage of development, the mature graafian follicle is ready to release the ova during a process called *ovulation.*

Follicles that progress beyond primordial follicles will either develop into a dominant mature graafian follicle destined to ovulate or degenerate through a process called *atresia.* As a result of atresia, the oocyte and granulosa cells within the basal lamina are replaced by fibrous tissue. The theca cells, in contrast to the cells within the basal lamina, do not die but return to the pool of cells consisting of ovarian interstitial or stromal cells. Atresia generally is thought to occur secondary to the absence of certain hormones or growth factors that were formed by the mature dominant follicle. Atresia of follicles is an apoptotic process or programmed cell death.[33]

Ovum

Oocyte growth continues, and meiosis is completed in the mature graafian follicle. In addition, there is an accumulation of nutritional, as well as genetic, information that will be required by the developing zygote following fertilization. Oocyte growth is linear until the follicle reaches the tertiary stage and then ceases to grow further.[34]

Granulosa cells play an integral role in the growth of the oocyte.[34] The oocyte is surrounded by a group of granulosa cells called the *corona radiata* that interacts with the oocyte by gap junctions. The zona pellucida (consisting of three different glycoproteins) forms between the corona radiata and the oocyte during formation of the primary follicle and exhibits a variety of biologic functions, including receptors for sperm and blockage of polyspermy, and improves the ability of the embryo to move freely in the fallopian tube on its passage to the uterus.[35]

The resumption of meiosis occurs following the preovulatory surge of LH (see Fig. 4-2). The ability of oocytes of mature follicles to undergo meiosis when placed in culture supports the hypothesis of an in vivo inhibitory influence for meiosis prior to ovulation. The resumption of meiosis in the mature oocyte is characterized by loss of the nuclear or germinal membrane, condensation of chromatin, separation of homologous chromosomes, and arrest at metaphase II. Meiosis is completed with the release of the second polar body at the time of fertilization. High concentrations of estradiol in follicular fluid are required for normal meiotic maturation.

Stroma

The ovarian stroma consists of three specific cell types: contractile cells; connective tissue cells, which function to give structural support; and interstitial cells. The interstitial cells secrete sex steroid hormones (principally androgens) and undergo morphologic changes in response to LH and hCG. Interstitial cells are derived from mesenchymal cells of the ovarian stroma.[36] The human ovary contains four major categories of interstitial cells: (1) primary interstitial, (2) secondary interstitial, (3) thecal interstitial, and (4) hilus cells.

The primary interstitial cells are the first interstitial cells to develop in the ovary and are identifiable only between 12 to 20 weeks of fetal life. These cells resemble premature Leydig cells of the fetal testis and have an ultrastructural appearance of steroid-secreting cells. Secondary interstitial cells are derived from the thecal cells of atretic follicles that undergo hypertrophy. These large epithelial cells maintain the active steroidogenic features of thecal interstitial cells from which they are derived and retain their responsiveness to LH. However, as opposed to thecal interstitial cells, secondary interstitial cells are innervated and respond to catecholamines that stimulate structural changes and hormone secretion. Cell transformation from mesenchymal cells is influenced locally by the secondary follicle and appears to be under control of gonadotropin stimulation. During development, these cells markedly increase in size and develop ultrastructural changes characteristic of steroid-secreting cells. Thecal interstitial cells give rise to secondary interstitial cells following follicular atresia, as stated earlier.[36]

The hilum of the ovary contains a specific type of interstitial cell known as the *hilus cell*. These cells contain crystalloids of Reinke and are virtually indistinguishable morphologically from Leydig cells of the testes.[37] Hyperplastic or neoplastic changes in hilus cells occasionally result in virilization associated with excessive amounts of testosterone secretion. Indeed, normal hilus cells have been shown to synthesize and secrete testosterone in response to LH.[38] The function of hilus cells is unclear but because of their close association with nerve fibers and blood vessels, they may influence ovarian function.

Corpus Luteum

The mature corpus luteum (yellow body) develops from a mature graafian follicle following ovulation (Figs. 4-4 and 4-6). A series of biochemical and morphologic changes known as *luteinization* occurs in the cells of the granulosa and theca interna at the time of the preovulatory surge of LH. These cells undergo

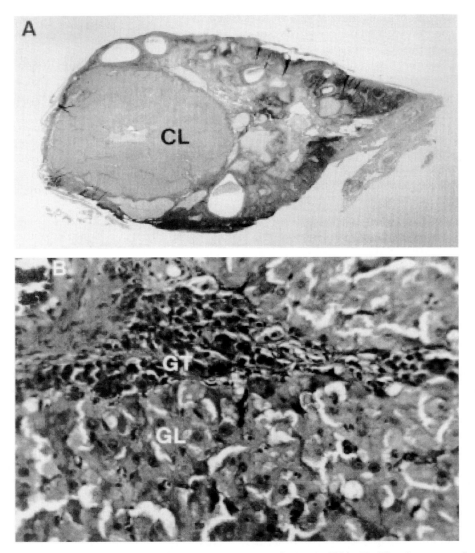

Figure 4-6 A Photomicrograph of a human corpus luteum (CL). B. The larger, pale-staining granulose-lutein cells (GL) can readily be distinguished from the smaller, dark-staining theca-lutein cells (TL). *(Reproduced, with permission, from Carr BR. Disorders of the ovary and female reproductive tract. In: Wilson JD, Foster DW, eds. William's Textbook of Endocrinology, 8th ed. Philadelphia, Pa., W.B. Saunders, 1992: 733–798.)*

hypertrophy and exhibit increased nuclear activity under the influence of LH.[39] The basement membrane separating the granulosa from the theca breaks down after ovulation has occurred. Thereafter, vascularization of the granulosa cells occurs from invading blood vessels and capillaries, leading to formation of the corpus luteum. The events leading to development of the corpus luteum have been well described.[39] First, proliferation of the granulosa cells occurs during the day after ovulation. Capillary invasion of the granulosa cells begins

▶ **TABLE 4-2:** DATES IMPORTANT IN THE LIFETIME OF THE CORPUS LUTEUM

Day 1	Proliferation of granulosa cells
Day 2	Capillary invasion
Days 7–8	Maximal capillary enlargement
Days 13–14	Luteolysis/apoptosis initiated in absence of pregnancy

on day 2 following ovulation and reaches the central cavity by day 4. Hemorrhage into the cavity can occur on any day, and fibroblasts appear in the central cavity by day 5. The center of the mature corpus luteum, the antrum, is filled with a fibrin clot. Maximal capillary enlargement or dilation is attained by days 7 to 8 at a time that corresponds to maximal progesterone secretion (up to 40 mg/d)[40] (Table 4-2). The cells that comprise the corpus luteum are derived from cells that compose the follicle, namely, the granulosa and theca. The granulosa cells enlarge and are called *granulosa-lutein cells,* whereas smaller cells called *theca-lutein cells* develop from theca cells. In addition, so-called K cells are found scattered throughout the corpus luteum and are believed to represent macrophages.

In the absence of pregnancy, the corpus luteum undergoes degeneration. This process is called *luteolysis* and is first apparent by the eighth day following ovulation. During luteolysis, the granulosa-lutein cells shrink, and the theca cells appear more prominent. Later, both cells undergo cell death, possibly involving the process of apoptosis. The remaining corpus luteum consists of dense connective tissue called the *corpus albicans.*

Ovarian Physiology

Hypothalamic-Pituitary-Ovarian Axis
The hypothalamus plays a critical role in the complex interplay that allows reproductive function in women[41] (Fig. 4-7). The hypothalamus communicates with the pituitary by a portal vascular system. The primary direction of blood flow is from the hypothalamus to the pituitary. This vascular system thus acts as a conduit for the hormones released from the hypothalamus that can control pituitary function. Interruption of this hypothalamic-pituitary connection leads to a decline in gonadotropin levels and eventually to atrophy of the ovaries and a decline in ovarian hormone secretion. Evidence also suggests that a retrograde flow occurs in the portal vessels, providing a short feedback loop of the pituitary on hypothalamic function.[42]

GnRH, a decapeptide, is the principal hypothalamic releasing factor that regulates reproductive function. It was proposed originally that separate releasing hormones existed for LH and FSH, but evidence now supports the

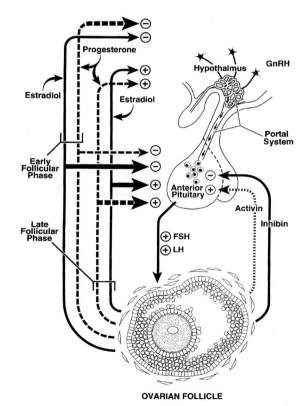

OVARIAN FOLLICLE

Figure 4-7 The regulation of feedback mechanisms of hypothalamic-pituitary-ovarian axis. (-, —progesterone.) Primary action (large arrow), secondary action (small arrow).

view that there is only one GnRH, LHRH. Moreover, GnRH analogues modulate both LH and FSH but neither selectively.[43] The variations in response of LH and FSH following GnRH infusions are believed to be due to the feedback exerted by ovarian hormones on the hypothalamic-pituitary axis. The release of GnRH by the hypothalamus is influenced by neurons from other regions of the brain whose terminals end in the arcuate nucleus.[23] Neurotransmitters such as epinephrine and norepinephrine increase GnRH release, whereas dopamine and serotonin, as well as endogenous opioid peptides, inhibit GnRH release.[44] A number of other hormones, in particular gut-related peptide hormones, also modulate GnRH release.[44]

The half-life of GnRH is 2 to 4 minutes, and metabolic clearance of GnRH averages approximately 800 L/m^2 per day.[45] Because LH and FSH are secreted in pulsatile bursts, it follows that GnRH release is also pulsatile.[23] Hypothalamic-pituitary portal venous blood collected from monkeys and sheep demonstrates that GnRH is secreted in a pulsatile fashion at frequencies of 70 to 90 minutes.[46,47] Investigators have shown that the pulsatile secretion pattern of GnRH is a prerequisite for normal secretion of pituitary gonadotropins.[23] This concept is supported by experimental evidence in the rhesus monkey by stimulating gonadotropin secretion following destruction of the arcuate nucleus. The reactivation of LH and FSH release requires that GnRH be infused at intervals of approximately 1 hour. Infusion of GnRH pulses of a lesser or greater frequency or following continuous infusion failed to stimulate the release of LH and FSH. The pulsatile release of GnRH is required but plays only a permissive role in the midcycle surge of gonadotropins, which is regulated primarily by ovarian hormone feedback at the level of the pituitary.[48] These observations have been confirmed in humans. The pulsatile administration of GnRH to women with GnRH deficiency reproduces the hormonal changes observed during the menstrual cycle, resulting in ovulation and pregnancy.[49]

GnRH acts on the gonadotropes of the pituitary to stimulate the release of LH and FSH. GnRH stimulates release of gonadotropins following high-affinity binding to the GnRH receptor via cyclic adenosine monophosphate (cAMP)–independent pathways that require calcium and activation of protein kinase C.[50] GnRH regulates (1) synthesis and storage of gonadotropins, (2) activation or movement of gonadotropins from reserve to a pool ready for secretion, and (3) immediate release of gonadotropins. LH, FSH, TSH, and hCG are glycoproteins composed of two polypeptide chains named α and β. There appears to be a single gene for the expression of the α-subunit that is similar for all glycoproteins and contains 92 amino acids.[51] The β chains for each glycoprotein hormone are unique and provide specific biologic activity for each hormone. The α- and β-subunits must combine for full expression of biologic activity. The half-life of FSH is greater than that of LH, determined in part by the higher sialic acid content of the FSH.[52]

Three types of secretory patterns can be distinguished due to the variations and frequency of gonadotropin release: *Trigintan* and *circatrigintan* are low-frequency changes during the normal menstrual cycle, occurring every 30 days. *Diurnal* are intermittent frequency changes in gonadotropin secretion that recur every 24 hours. These changes are minimal in adult women but are marked during sleep in girls at the initiation of puberty, as discussed previously. *Circhoral* are high-frequency changes in gonadotropin secretion characterized by pulses of gonadotropins at approximately every hour.[23]

Follicle growth, ovulation, and maintenance of the corpus luteum are regulated by the coordinated secretion of FSH and LH. As discussed previously, the release of FSH and LH requires continuous pulsatile release of GnRH from the hypothalamus. In addition, the release of LH and FSH is affected both positively and negatively by estrogen and progesterone, and at least two gonadal protein hormones also modulate FSH release. Whether estrogen and progesterone stimulate or inhibit gonadotropin release depends on the level of exposure and the duration of the steroid.

Ovarian steroid and peptide hormones can exert a negative feedback on both the hypothalamus and the pituitary (see Fig. 4-7). A decline in ovarian hormone secretion during menopause or following castration causes increased secretion of LH and FSH. The negative feedback exerted by estrogen on the pituitary appears to depend on the concentration of estrogen. Progesterone inhibits FSH and LH at high concentrations and primarily at the level of the hypothalamus.[53] Both inhibin and follistatin selectively inhibit FSH secretion.

Gonadal steroid and peptide hormones are also able to exert positive effects on gonadotropin secretion (see Fig. 4-7). This positive feedback is important in regulation of the LH surge required to induce ovulation and is regulated by a sharply rising level of estrogen in the late proliferative phase. There are two requirements for the positive effect of estrogen on production of LH: (1) an estradiol concentration of over 200 pg/mL and (2) a sustained level of estradiol for at least 48 to 50 hours.[54] Progesterone is also responsible for the midcycle FSH surge.[55] Progesterone at low concentrations will stimulate LH release but only after previous exposure to estrogen. In addition, granulosa cell secretion of activin stimulates FSH release.

Ovarian (Steroid) Hormones

PROGESTOGENS

The principal progestogens are 21-carbon steroids (Fig. 4-8) and include pregnenolone, progesterone, and 17α-hydroxyprogesterone. Pregnenolone has little biologic activity but is important as the precursor of all steroid hormones. Progesterone is the principal secretory steroid of the corpus luteum and is responsible for induction of secretory activity and decidual development in the endometrium of the estrogen-primed uterus. Progesterone is required for implantation of the fertilized ovum

and maintenance of pregnancy. Progesterone also inhibits uterine contractions and increases the basal body temperature. 17α-Hydroxyprogesterone is also secreted by the corpus luteum but has little biologic activity.

ESTROGENS

Estrogens are 18-carbon steroids characterized by the presence of an aromatic A ring, a phenolic hydroxyl group at C-3, and either a hydroxyl group (estradiol) or a ketone group (estrone) (see Fig. 4-8). The principal and most potent estrogen secreted by the ovary is 17β-estradiol. Although estrone is also secreted by the ovary, the principal source of estrone is the extraglandular conversion of circulating androstenedione. Estriol (16-hydroxyestradiol) is the most abundant estrogen in urine and arises from hepatic metabolism of estrone and estradiol. Obesity and hypothyroidism are associated with an increase in estriol formation.[56] Catechol estrogens are formed by hydroxylation of estrogens at the C-2 or C-4 position. The physiologic role of catechol estrogen is unclear at present, but low body weight and hypothyroidism are associated with increased formation of catechol estrogen. Estrogens, through activation of their receptor, promote development of the secondary sexual characteristics of women and promote uterine growth, thickening of the vaginal mucosa, thinning of the cervical mucus, and development of the ductal system of the breast.

ANDROGENS

The ovary (principally thecal cells) secretes a variety of C_{19} steroids, including dehydroepiandrosterone, androstenedione, testosterone, and dihydrotestosterone. The principal C_{19} steroid secreted by thecal cells is androstenedione (see Fig. 4-8). Part of the androstenedione is released into plasma, and the remainder is converted to estrone by the granulosa cells. In addition, androstenedione can be converted to estrone or testosterone in peripheral tissues. Only testosterone and dihydrotestosterone are true androgens capable of

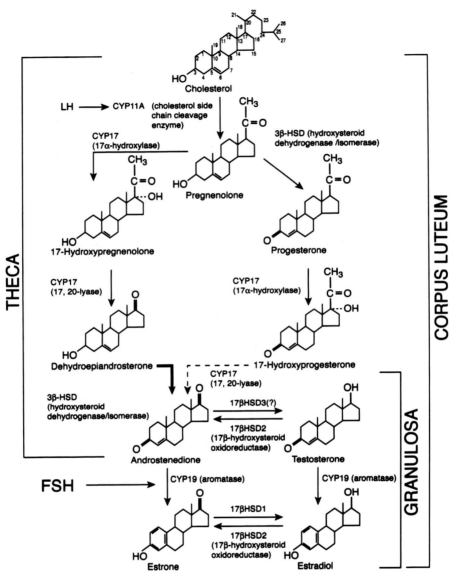

Figure 4-8 The key enzymes and pathways of steroid hormone biosynthesis in the human ovary. The principal products for the theca are noted by the bracket on the left side of the corpus luteum and granulosa cells on the right. The major sites of the action of LH and FSH are designated by horizontal arrows. The bold arrow indicates that the principal pathway in the theca is from DHEA to androstenedione because the metabolism of 17-hydroxyprogesterone is limited in the human ovary. *(Reproduced, with permission, from Carr BR. Disorders of the ovary and female reproductive tract. In: Wilson JD, Foster DW, eds.* William's Textbook of Endocrinology, *8th ed. Philadelphia, Pa., W. B. Saunders, 1992: 733–798.)*

high-affinity binding to the androgen receptor. Thus the ability to convert androstenedione to active sex steroids is critical for activation of target tissue androgen receptors. Excessive production of C_{19} steroids by the ovary or adrenal can cause sexual ambiguity in newborns and hirsutism or virilization in women.

Steroid Hormone Biosynthesis

Steroids formed by the ovary, as well as other steroid-producing organs, are derived from cholesterol. There are several sources of cholesterol that can provide the ovary with substrate for steroidogenesis. These include: (1) plasma lipoprotein cholesterol, (2) cholesterol synthesized de novo within the ovary, and (3) cholesterol from stores of cholesterol esters within lipid droplets. Considerable evidence suggests that the primary source of cholesterol used by the ovary is the uptake of lipoprotein cholesterol.[57,58] In the human ovary, low-density lipoprotein (LDL) cholesterol is the principal source of cholesterol used for steroidogenesis.[57] LH stimulates the activity of adenylate cyclase, increasing cAMP production, which serves as a second messenger to increase LDL receptor mRNA and the binding and uptake of LDL cholesterol, as well as the formation of cholesterol esters.[57,58] cAMP-activated steroidogenic acute regulatory (StAR) protein increases the intracellular transport of cholesterol to the inner mitochondria membrane.[59] The conversion of cholesterol to pregnenolone within the mitochondria is the rate-limiting step in ovarian steroidogenesis and is catalyzed by the cholesterol side-chain cleavage enzyme complex consisting of cytochrome P450 side-chain cleavage (CYP11A), adrenodoxin, and flavoprotein.

The granulosa, theca, and corpus luteum cells possess the complete enzymatic complement required for sex steroid formation. The preferred pathway of steroid synthesis in the human corpus luteum is the Δ^4 pathway, which involves the conversion of pregnenolone to progesterone (see Fig. 4-8). Recent studies suggest that in the human ovarian follicle the Δ^5 pathway is the preferred pathway for the for-

mation of androgens and estrogens because theca cells of the human ovary metabolize 17α-hydroxypregnenolone to a greater extent than 17α-hydroxyprogesterone.[60] However, the predominant steroid secreted differs among each of these cell types, so the corpus luteum forms progesterone and 17α-hydroxyprogesterone, the theca and stromal cells secrete androgen, and the granulosa cells secrete predominantly estrogen. The determination of which steroid is secreted by each cell type includes the level of gonadotropin and gonadotropin receptors; the activity, amount, and expression of steroidogenic enzymes; and the vascularity and availability of LDL cholesterol. Evidence suggests that the rate of steroid production during the menstrual cycle is related to the amount of follicular and luteal cell content of five key steroid-metabolizing enzymes: CYP11A, 3β-hydroxysteroid dehydrogenase (3β-HSD), 17α-hydroxylase/17,20 lyase cytochrome (CYP17), aromatase (CYP19), and 17β-hydroxysteroid dehydrogenase (17β-HSD type 1).[61] These enzymes are responsible for the conversion of cholesterol to pregnenolone, pregnenolone to progesterone, pregnenolone to 17-hydroxypregnenolone, 17-hydroxypregnenolone to dehydroepiandrosterone, dehydroepiandrosterone to androstenedione, androstenedione to estrone, and estrone to estradiol (Figs. 4-9 and 4-10). LH acts acutely to regulate the first step in steroid hormone biosynthesis by regulating the conversion of cholesterol to pregnenolone, and FSH acts to increase the conversion of androgens to estrogens. Chronically, these hormones act to regulate the expression of the necessary steroid-metabolizing enzymes. Recently, the immunohistochemical localization, in situ hybridization, and expression of mRNA species encoding CYP11A, 3β-HSD, CYP17, CYP19, and 17β-HSD type 1 have been determined in human follicles and corpora lutea throughout the menstrual cycle[61] (see Fig. 4-9). The expression of CYP11A mRNA is present in most stages of follicular development and located in both granulosa and theca interna cells of the follicle. There is a marked increase in

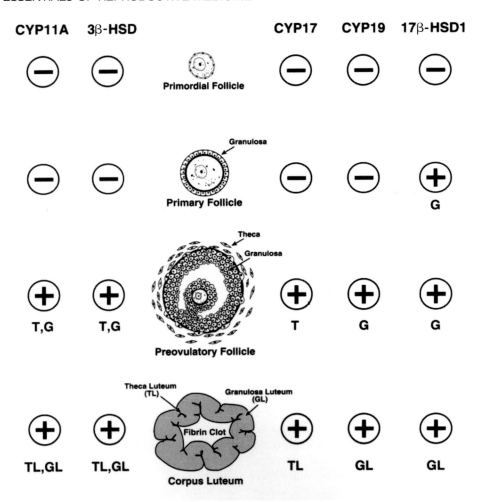

Figure 4-9 The localization and expression of the principal enzymes involved in steroidogenesis: CYP11A (cholesterol side-chain cleavage enzyme), 3β-HSD (3β-hydroxysteroid dehydrogenase), CYP17 (17α-hydroxylase), CYP19 (aromatase), 17β-HSD1 (17β-hydroxysteroid dehydrogenase type 1). (− = absent; + = present; T = theca cell; G = granulosa cell; TL = theca luteum cell; GL = granulosa luteum cell.) *(Reproduced, with permission, from Carr BR. Disorders of the Ovary and Female Reproductive Tract. In: Wilson JD, Foster DW, eds. William's Textbook of Endocrinology. Philadelphia, Pa., W. B. Saunders Co. In press.)*

the expression of CYP11A mRNA in corpora lutea in both the theca-lutein and granulosa-lutein cells as localized by immunohistochemistry. There is little expression of 3β-HSD and CYP11A in the corpus luteum, which is consistent with the enormous increase in the secretion of progesterone during the luteal phase of the cycle. The pattern of expression of CYP17 is similar in follicles and corpora lutea

(see Fig. 4-9). CYP17 can be localized only in the theca interna cells of the follicle and the theca-lutein cells of the corpus luteum but is virtually absent from granulosa and granulose-lutein cells.

The expression of CYP19 is seen only in mature follicles and is localized in granulosa cells, consistent with the marked rise in estrogen biosynthesis prior to ovulation. CYP19

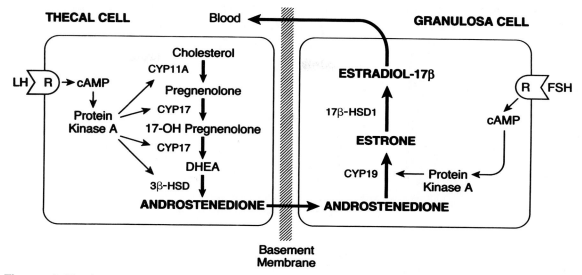

Figure 4-10   A new look at the two-cell/two-gonadotropin hypothesis in the human ovary and principal metabolic pathways (cAMP = cyclic adenosine monophosphate; CYP11A = cholesterol side-chain cleavage enzyme; CYP17 = 17α-hydroxylase; CYP19 = aromatase; DHEA = dehydroepiandrosterone; 17βHSD = 17β hydroxysteroid dehydrogenase.)   *(Reproduced, with permission, from Carr BR. Disorders of the Ovary and Female Reproductive Tract. In: Wilson JD, Foster DW, eds. William's Textbook of Endocrinology. Philadelphia, Pa: W. B. Saunders Co. In press.)*

mRNA is greatest in corpora lutea and localized in granulosa-lutein cells (see Fig. 4-9). 17β-HSD type 1 is localized in granulosa cells and converts estrone to estradiol (see Fig. 4-9). The results of studies on the expression of the mRNA encoding the various steroidogenic enzymes are consistent with previous reports of enzymatic activity in human ovaries.[61] The amount of immunoreactive CYP19 and mRNA also was shown to be stimulated by FSH in human granulosa cells.[62]

These observations help to explain the rationale for the predominance of estrogen secreted by granulosa cells and the corpus luteum, the secretion of androgens by the theca, and the secretion of progesterone by both types of corpus luteum cells of the ovary. The reports of the steroidogenic capacities of isolated granulosa and theca cells led to the two-cell/two-gonadotropin theory (see Fig. 4-10), which states that the theca cells produce C_{19} steroids in response to LH (predominantly androstenedione) and that FSH stimulates granulosa cells to aromatize the preformed an-

drostenedione to produce estrone. The final step involves 17β-HSD type 1, which converts estrone to estradiol.

The availability of LDL cholesterol also plays a regulatory role in the levels of steroid hormones secreted in the various cell types of the human ovary. The granulosa cells of the follicle are avascular and devoid of a blood supply, as discussed previously. The granulosa cells do not have ready access to plasma LDL, and because of its large molecular weight, only very low levels of LDL are found in follicular fluid bathing granulosa cells[57,63] (Fig. 4-11). Thus the granulosa cells have limited ability to form progesterone in large quantities characteristic of the luteal phase. Following ovulation, extensive vascularization of the follicle takes place, providing increased amounts of cholesterol to the luteinized granulosa cells. The increased availability of LDL to the granulosa-lutein cells now provides the ability for these cells to secrete increased quantities of progesterone during the luteal phase of the menstrual cycle. Corpus luteum tissue treated

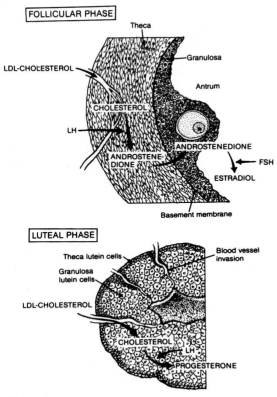

Figure 4-11 Cellular interactions in the ovary during the follicular phase (top) and luteal phase (bottom). (LDL, low-density lipoprotein; FSH, follicle-stimulating hormone; LH, lutenizing hormone.) *(Reproduced, with permission, from Carr BR, MacDonald PC, Simpson ER, The role of lipoproteins in the regulation of progesterone secretion by the human corpus luteum. Fertil Steril. 38:303, 1982.)*

with hCG stimulates progesterone secretion in vitro, as well as the number of LDL binding sites.[64] In addition, women with abetalipoproteinemia who have low levels of LDL cholesterol have extremely low levels of progesterone secretion during the luteal phase.[65]

Regulation of Ovarian Steroidogenesis by Gonadotropins

FSH and LH are required for estrogen synthesis, and the amount of estrogen produced depends on the relative exposure of each gonadotropin. FSH receptors are present exclusively on the granulosa cell. FSH also stimulates the activity of aromatase and the mRNA for CYP19 in granulosa cells that convert androgens produced by the theca cells into estrogens, as discussed previously. Enhanced secretion of estradiol causes an increase in the activation and number of estradiol receptors, which causes further proliferation of granulosa cells and follicular growth.[66] In the mature follicle, FSH in concert with estradiol causes an increase in LH receptors on granulosa cells. LH acts to augment progesterone secretion by granulosa cells, which stimulates FSH release at midcycle. The binding of gonadotropins to their respective plasma membrane receptors stimulates secretion of adenylate cyclase (see Fig. 4-10). Following ovulation, the number of LH receptors in the lutein cells increases, and the FSH receptor numbers and FSH responses decrease.[66] Taken together, these observations emphasize the important roles of autocrine and paracrine actions of steroids and the two-cell/two-gonadotropin hypothesis discussed earlier.

Extragonadal Steroidogenesis

The application of isotopic dilution methods has provided insight into the complexity of the processes involved in understanding the secretion rate (SR), production rate (PR), and the metabolic clearance rate (MCR) of steroid hormones. The concept of extragonadal hormone formulation using the following principles has clarified the regulation of plasma levels of steroid hormones in women, particularly of plasma estrogens[67] (Fig. 4-12). The amount of hormone released by an endocrine gland into the circulation per unit of time is the SR. Steroid hormones also may be derived from the extragonadal or peripheral conversion of a precursor steroid that may be secreted by the original or by another endocrine gland. The PR of a hormone is that rate at which the hormone enters the circulation and is determined by the SR plus hormone formation at extraglandular sites. If a hormone is derived exclusively via

SOURCES OF CIRCULATING ESTROGENS IN WOMEN

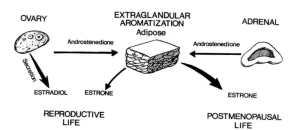

Figure 4-12   Various sources of circulating estrogens in women during reproductive and postmenopausal life.   *(Adapted, with permission, from Carr BR, MacDonald PC. Estrogen treatment of postmenopausal women. In: Stollerman GH, ed. Advances in Internal Medicine, vol 28. Chicago, Ill., Year Book Medical Publishers, 1983:491–508.)*

glandular secretion, the SR and PR are equal. However, when the hormone is formed from peripheral conversion as well as from secretion, the PR will be greater than the SR. The MCR is the volume of blood per unit of time that is irreversibly cleared of a hormone. The blood PR of a hormone equals the MCR multiplied by the concentration of the hormone in blood (PR = MCR × C).

The SR and PR of steroid hormones can be determined by a variety of techniques.[68] The most common technique involves the intravenous infusion of a radiolabeled hormone until a constant level of that hormone is attained in blood. The PR or the total entry of this hormone into the circulation can be calculated from the specific activity of the hormone in plasma. In the instance in which a steroid hormone is derived from more than one precursor steroid, infusion of each of these radiolabeled hormones makes it possible to calculate their relative contributions to the blood PR of the hormone.[67] The plasma concentrations, PR, MCR, and SR of ovarian steroid hormones in normal women are presented in Table 4-3.

The origin of plasma estrogens has been clarified using these methods, as discussed previously. In normal women of reproductive age, the vast majority of plasma estradiol is derived by direct secretion from the ovary. There is little, if any, estradiol formed from testosterone by extraglandular conversion. On the other hand, little estrone is formed by direct ovarian secretion, and most estrone circulating in plasma originates from extraglandular conversion from androstenedione and to a minor extent from estradiol[67] (see Fig. 4-12). The primary site of extraglandular aromatization of androstenedione to estrone occurs in adipose tissue and is influenced by age, liver function, and thyroid dysfunction.

The importance of the extragonadal formation and prohormone concept of estrogen formation is highlighted by a number of clinical conditions. The amount of extraglandular hormone production of estrogen can increase to a level that can interfere with the normal feedback mechanisms and produce disturbances of the ovarian cycle. The formation of estrogens by the placenta during pregnancy depends entirely on C_{19} steroids (prohormones) secreted by the fetal adrenal gland and to a lesser extent on the maternal adrenal.[67,68] In nonpregnant premenopausal women, estrone is formed by androstenedione secreted by the ovary and adrenal. In menopausal women, the ovarian contribution of prohormone (androstenedione) is negligible, but these women still have considerable estrone circulating in blood formed by extraglandular conversion of androstenedione secreted by the adrenals. An increase in estrogen formation occurs with aging and obesity that can yield enough estrogen to produce endometrial hyperplasia and bleeding. Similar findings can occur in premenopausal women with polycystic ovary disease or ovarian tumors associated with increased secretion of androstenedione.

Ovarian Steroid Hormone Transport

Most steroids secreted by the ovary and peripheral tissues are bound to plasma proteins. The bulk of steroid hormones is bound to albumin or specific globulins (>97 to 98 percent). For example, most testosterone is bound

► **TABLE 4-3:** CONCENTRATION, METABOLIC CLEARANCE RATES (MCRs), PRODUCTION RATES (PRs), AND OVARIAN SECRETION RATES (SRs) OF STEROIDS IN BLOOD

Compound	MCR of Compound in Peripheral Plasma (L/day)	Phase of Menstrual Cycle	Concentration in Plasma		PR of Circulating Compound (mg/d)	SR by Both Ovaries (mg/d)
			nmol/L	µg/dL		
Estradiol	1350	Early follicular	0.2	0.006	0.081	0.07
		Late follicular	1.2–2.6	0.033–0.019	0.445–0.945	0.4–0.8
		Midluteal	0.7	0.020	0.270	0.25
Estrone	2210	Early follicular	0.18	0.005	0.110	0.08
		Late follicular	0.5–1.1	0.015–0.045	0.331–0.662	0.25–0.38
		Midluteal	0.4	0.011	0.243	0.16
Progesterone	2200	Follicular	3.0	0.095	2.1	1.5
		Luteal	36	1.13	25.0	24.0
20α-Hydroxyprogesterone	2300	Follicular	1.5	0.05	1.1	0.8
		Luteal	7.5	0.25	5.8	3.3
17-Hydroxyprogesterone	2000	Early follicular	0.9	0.03	0.6	0–0.3
		Late follicular	6	0.20	4.0	3–4
		Midluteal	6	0.20	4.0	3–4
Androstenedione	2010		5.6	0.159	3.2	0.8–1.6
Testosterone	690		1.3	0.038	0.26	
Dehydroepiandrosterone	1640		17	0.490	8.0	0.3–3

Reproduced, with permission, from Tagatz GE, Gurpide E. Hormone secretion by the normal human ovary. In Greep RP, Astwood EB (eds), Handbook of Physiology, Section 7: Endocrinology, Vol II, Part 1. American Physiological Society. Baltimore: Williams & Wilkins, 1973:603–613.

to sex hormone–binding globulin (SHBG) and to a lesser degree to albumin. Estradiol exhibits a lower binding affinity to SHBG than does testosterone; thus most estradiol is bound to serum albumin (60 percent), whereas 38 percent is bound to SHBG and 2 to 3 percent is free.[69] It is assumed that the protein-bound hormone is inactive and that only the free hormone is active and directly available to enter target tissues, but recent evidence suggests that the transport of steroid hormones could be more complex.[70]

SHBG, a β-globulin, is formed by the liver and has a molecular weight of about 95,000. It has a high affinity (10^{-9} mol/L) and low binding capacity (one binding site per molecule).[71] Dihydrotestosterone followed by testosterone have the highest binding affinity for SHBG, whereas estradiol has one-third the affinity of dihydrotestosterone to SHBG. In contrast, dehydroepiandrosterone (DHEA) and progesterone have negligible affinity to SHBG. The MCR of sex steroids is inversely related to the affinity to SHBG, and thus alterations in the concentration of SHBG influence sex steroid metabolism and target tissue action.[71] The level of SHBG and thus the level of free hormone may be altered by a variety of clinical conditions. Levels of SHBG are increased by estrogens (pregnancy and oral contraceptive pills) and thyroid hormones (hyperthyroidism) but lowered by androgens, hypothyroidism, and obesity.[72] Also, women have double the concentration of SHBG of men, which appears to be due to the higher estrogen levels observed in women.

Mechanisms of Steroid Hormone Action

The concentration of steroid hormones in the circulation is low, and for target cells to respond, specific steroid receptors are required for steroid hormone action. Steroid hormones have low molecular weights and, because of their hydrophobic nature, enter cells by diffusion, although carrier-mediated transport may occur. The affinity, specificity, and concentration of steroid receptors in target cells allow a low concentration of steroid hormones to produce biologic responses. Estrogen can enter any cell, but only in specific target tissues, such as the uterus, is estrogen action observed due to the presence of estrogen receptors. In contrast, in most cells, estrogens are not able to manifest a response due to the lack of estrogen receptor expression.

Steroid hormones enter the target cell and localize in the nucleus and become associated with a nuclear steroid receptor. The nuclear steroid receptor consists of a number of units: a steroid hormone–binding domain (C terminus), a DNA-binding domain, a hinge region, and a transcription-activation functional domain at the N terminus. Active transformation occurs after nuclear binding and involves a conformational change in the receptor and the activated steroid-nuclear receptor complex. This complex then interacts with specific DNA sequences known as *steroid response elements* (SREs). Next, interaction of the nuclear hormone-receptor complex with DNA leads to synthesis of mRNA and finally protein synthesis in the cytoplasm, which causes specific cellular responses.

There are two estrogen receptors (ERα and ERβ). The classic receptor is ERα, localized in the vagina, uterus, and breast. ERβ is localized in the breast and granulosa cells of women. There are two progesterone receptors, A and B. In most cells, B is the positive regulator of progesterone-responsive genes, whereas binding to A inhibits B activity.

Nonsteroidal Hormones and Growth Factors of the Ovary

A number of nonsteroidal hormones and growth factors are produced by the ovary and appear to modulate local steroidogenesis via autocrine and paracrine mechanisms. In addition, some of these factors may influence hypothalamic and pituitary secretion of gonadotropin via an endocrine mechanism. A list of nonsteroidal hormones and their proposed functions is presented in Table 4-4. Recognition

► **TABLE 4-4:** NONSTEROIDAL FACTORS PRODUCED BY THE OVARY THAT MAY REGULATE ENDOCRINE-AUTOCRINE OR PARACRINE REGULATION OF OVARIAN FUNCTION

Nonsteroidal Factor	Proposed Function
Activin	Stimulates FSH release, inhibits P450c17 in theca, increases granulosa LH receptors
Angiogenic factors	Neovascularization of corpus luteum
Eicosanoids	Ovulation, corpus luteum regulation
Follicular-regulating protein (FRP)	Atresia, aromatase inhibitor, inhibition of FSH action
Follistatin	Suppresses FSH release
FSH-binding inhibitor (FSH BI)	Inhibits binding of FSH to receptor, atresia
GnRH-like peptides	Stimulatory and inhibitory actins on FSH and LH, regulation of atresia
Growth factors	
Epidermal growth factors (EFGs)	Mitogenic-granulosa, inhibits steroidogenesis, atresia
Fibroblast growth factors (FGFs)	Mitogenic, inhibits steroidogenesis, atresia
Insulin-like growth factors (IFGs)	Mitogenic, stimulate steroidogenesis, modulate corpus luteum
Growth hormone	
Growth hormone–releasing hormone	
IGF-1, IGF2	
IGF-binding proteins	
Platelet-derived growth factor (PDGF)	Unknown, enhances steroidogenesis?
Transforming growth factors (TGFs)	
TGF-α	Growth regulation, inhibits steroidogenesis
TGF-β	Stimulates FSH release, stimulates steroidogenesis-granulosa, inhibits steroidogenesis
Growth differentiating factor 9 (GDF-9)	Secreted by oocyte and stimulates follicular develpment
Bone morphogenic protein 16 (BMP-16)	Secreted by oocyte, stimulates proliferation of granulosa cells by FSH-independent mechanism, inhibits FSH receptors in granulosa cells.
Inhibin	Inhibits FSH release, increases P450cc in theca
LH-binding inhibitor (LH BI)	Inhibits binding of LH to receptor, atresia
Luteinization inhibitor	Inhibits corpus luteum development and function
Antimüllerian hormone	Inhibits oocyte maturation
Oocyte maturation inhibitor (OM1)	Inhibits meiosis
Orphan nuclear receptors	
Steroidogenic factor 1 (SF-1)	Stimulates P450 enzyme expression
Liver receptor homologue (LRH-1)	Stimulates P450 enzyme expression
Oxytocin (corpus luteum)	Modulates progesterone secretion, regulates life span of corpus luteum
Pro-opiomelanocortin (POMC)–derived peptides	Unknown
Relaxin	Remodeling of reproductive tract, modulates corpus luteum
Renin-angiotensin	Ovulation, regulation of steroidogenesis (rat), no receptors of action in human granulosa

Continued

▶ **TABLE 4-4:** NONSTEROIDAL FACTORS PRODUCED BY THE OVARY THAT MAY REGULATE ENDOCRINE-AUTOCRINE OR PARACRINE REGULATION OF OVARIAN FUNCTION *(Continued)*

Nonsteroidal Factor	Proposed Function
Substance P	Regulation of ovarian blood flow
Tissue-type plasminogen activator (tPA)	Ovulation, atresia
Vascular endothelial growth factor	Angiogenesis
Vasoactive intestinal peptide	Stimulates steroidogenesis
Vasopressin	Unknown

(Reproduced with permission, from Carr BR. Disorders of the ovary and the female reproductive tract. In: Wilson JD, Foster DW, eds. William's Textbook of Endocrinology, *8th ed. Philadelphia, Pa., W. B. Saunders, 1992: 733–798,*

that only one follicle is destined to ovulate and that the rest are destined to undergo atresia supports the view of a complex intra-ovarian regulation of follicle growth of a single follicle and inhibition of growth of the remaining follicles. Some of these nonsteroidal factors, as well as steroids produced by the dominant follicle, may play a role in local regulation of follicular growth.

▶ MENOPAUSAL OVARY

Successive cycles of ovulation and atresia eventually deplete the ovarian content of its folli-cles (Fig. 4-13). This leads to menopause, the final episode of menstrual bleeding in women. The median age of menopause is 50 to 51 years.[73] The term *menopause* commonly refers to the period of the climacteric encompassing the transition between the reproductive years up to and beyond the last episode of menstrual bleeding. The predominant event during menopause is the cessation of cyclic ovarian function, which in turn affects various endocrine, somatic, and psychological changes (see Chap. 28).

The average age of menopause has remained constant, suggesting that menopausal age is unrelated to the onset of menarche, socioeconomic

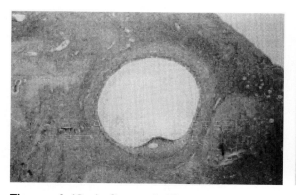
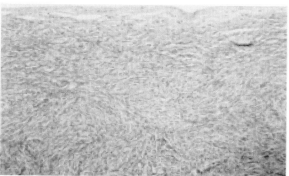

Figure 4-13 Left panel: Photomicrograph of histologic section of an ovary obtained from a woman during reproductive life. Note the large graafian follicle with single ovum in the center of the photograph and a group of primary follicles in the upper right corner (×33). Right panel: Ovary obtained from a postmenopausal woman. Note the absence of germ cells and prominent ovarian stroma (×132).   *(Reproduced, with permission, from Carr BR, MacDonald PC. The menopause and beyond. In:Andres R, Bierman EL, Hazzard WR, eds. Principles of Geriatric Medicine. New York, N.Y. McGraw-Hill, 1985: 325-336.)*

conditions, race, parity, height, or weight.[74] However, menopause may occur earlier in women who smoke. Since the life expectancy of women usually extends 30 years beyond menopause and occupies one-third of the life of women, the medical and economic impacts of these changes are significant.

During menopause, the continuous loss of ovarian follicles results in a decrease in estrogen secretion. The ovary of postmenopausal women is reduced in size, weighing less than 2.5 g, and is wrinkled or prunelike in appearance. Furthermore, the loss of ova and follicles results in a reduction of the cortical area. Rarely, a few immature follicles undergoing maturation or atresia may be seen at the corticomedullary junction for up to 5 years or more after the last menses.[75]

A reduction in the responsiveness of the ovary to gonadotropins is apparent several years prior to the cessation of menstruation. Compared with younger women, FSH and LH levels are elevated in perimenopausal women still experiencing follicular growth and ovulatory menstrual cycles. Following cessation of follicular development, a decrease in 17β-estradiol and inhibin secretion occurs, two factors responsible for negative feedback of the hypothalamus and pituitary. The absence of the negative-feedback mechanism allows gonadotropin levels to rise with FSH, rising earlier and to a greater extent than LH. Two possible explanations for the difference in gonadotropin levels exist. First, the decrease in inhibin levels may be responsible for higher FSH levels, or second, the greater sialic acid content of FSH may decrease its clearance rate.[52] Intravenous infusion of GnRH in postmenopausal women elicits an exaggerated increase in the release of both FSH and LH, similar to women with other forms of ovarian failure.[76]

In contrast to gonadotropins, the mean levels of ovarian steroid hormones decrease from premenopause to postmenopause. Prior to menopause, plasma androstenedione is derived equally from both the adrenal and ovary, but after menopause, the ovarian contribution is minimal, and plasma androstenedione levels fall by 50 percent.[77] As discussed previously, circulatory estrogens in premenopausal ovulating women are derived from two sources. Greater than 60 percent of estrogen is produced by direct ovarian secretion as estradiol; the remainder is estrone, derived from the extraglandular conversion of androstenedione. After menopause, the ovarian estrogen contribution from both sources is reduced, and the extraglandular formation of estrone from adrenal androstenedione secretion predominates (see Fig. 4-12). As expected, removal of the ovaries in postmenopausal women does not result in a significant decline in estrogen or androstenedione levels. Because adipose tissue is a major site of extraglandular estrogen production, estrogen levels in obese postmenopausal women may equal or surpass those in premenopausal women.[78] Here, the predominant form of estrogen in postmenopausal women is estrone rather than estradiol.

The decrease in estrogen formation triggers vasomotor instability (hot flashes), atrophy of the urogenital epithelium, a reduction in size of the reproductive organs and breasts, an increased risk of cardiovascular disease, and osteoporosis.[79,80] Hot flashes are characterized by periods of warmth and heat followed by profuse sweating. The frequency, duration, and intensity of vasomotor symptoms vary, but in most women they begin to subside 2 to 5 years following menopause. The pathogenesis of the hot flash or flush is complex and appears to involve catecholamines, prostaglandins, endorphins, and other neuropeptides following cessation of estrogen secretion.[81]

There is a close temporal relationship between estrogen deprivation and the development of osteoporosis. Loss of bone, both trabecular and cortical, due to osteoporosis may result in mechanical fragility and fracture. Following menopause, bone loss proceeds at a rate of 1 to 2 percent each year.[82] By age 80, women have lost 50 percent of their bone mass. It has been estimated that 25 percent of women sustain a vertebral or hip fracture between the ages of 60 and 90.[83] Such fractures are a major cause of mortality and morbidity. A number of factors influence the development of osteoporosis, including diet, activity, smoking, general health, and most important, estrogen deprivation.

The principal cause of death in postmenopausal women is cardiovascular disease.[84] Studies comparing postmenopausal women with premenopausal controls indicate that postmenopausal women are at greater risk for cardiovascular disease.[85–87] Lower high-density lipoprotein (HDL) and high LDL cholesterol levels are present in postmenopausal women. Likewise, women who undergo oophorectomy and are not treated with estrogen have an increased risk of cardiovascular disease.[88] There is currently a controversy over whether estrogen-replacement therapy reduces the risk of death from cardiovascular disease.[89]

▶ THE NORMAL MENSTRUAL CYCLE

Spontaneous, cyclic, predictable, and regular menstruations are the hallmarks of ovulatory menstrual cycles. Ovulatory menstrual cycles result from carefully regulated interactions of the hypothalamus, pituitary, ovaries, and female genital tract. The menstrual cycle can be divided into two phases: a follicular or proliferative phase and a luteal or secretory phase (Fig. 4-14).

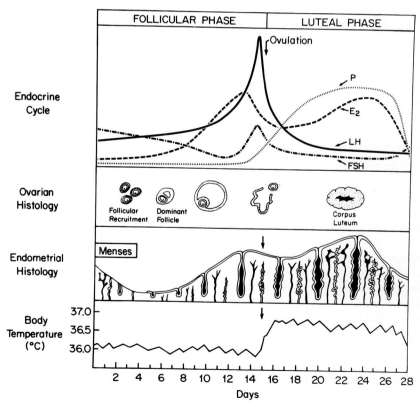

Figure 4-14 Hormonal ovarian, endometrial, and basal body temperature changes and relationship throughout the normal menstrual cycle. *(Reproduced, with permission, from Carr BR, Wilson JD. In: Wilson JD, Braunwald E. Isselbacher KJ, et al, eds. 1991: 1776.)*

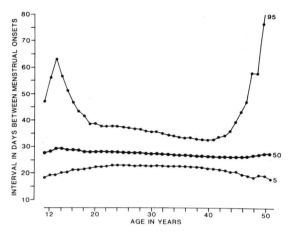

Figure 4-15 Menstrual cycle length in relation to age. The median and 5th and 95th percentiles are indicated. *(Data reproduced from Treloar AE, Boynton BE, Behn BG, et al, 1967:77 as adapted by Baird DT. Amenorrhea, anovulation and dysfunctional uterine bleeding. In: Degroot LJ, ed. Endocrinology. Philadelphia, Pa.,W.B. Saunders, 1989: 1950-1968.)*

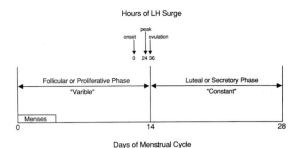

Figure 4-16 Relationship of the LH surge and menstrual cycle length. *(Modified, with permission, from Yen SSC. The human menstrual cycle. In Yen SSC, Jaffe RB, eds. Reproductive Endocrinology, 2nd ed. Philadelphia, Pa., W.B. Saunders, 1986: 203.)*

Menstrual cycle length is determined from the first day of the onset of menstrual bleeding until the onset of menstruation in the subsequent cycle. The median length of the menstrual cycle in reproductive-age women is 28 days, and the range is 25 to 35 days. The length of the menstrual cycle varies most at the extremes of reproductive life, namely, following menarche and preceding menopause (Fig. 4-15). Immediately after menarche, menstrual cycles are often prolonged and unpredictable due to poor or defective follicular development and often result in anovulatory or luteal-deficient cycles. Likewise, just prior to the onset of menopause, menstrual cycles are anovulatory and prolonged and unpredictable.[90] The least variability of menstrual cycle length is found between the ages of 20 and 30. Most studies comparing the relative length of the follicular and luteal phases have found that the length of the luteal phase is remarkably constant and lasts 13 to 14 days.[91] The length of the follicular phase may vary from 10 to 16 days, which

explains the variation in the length of normal menstrual cycles (Fig. 4-16 and Table 4-5).

▶ PHASES OF THE NORMAL MENSTRUAL CYCLE

Follicular Phase

Initiation of follicular growth, or folliculogenesis, begins during the last few days of the luteal phase of the previous menstrual cycle and ends with ovulation. During this period, plasma progesterone and estrogen levels decline because of the demise of the corpus luteum, and FSH levels rise. The rise in FSH in the late luteal phase is also associated with a dramatic fall in the level of inhibin A and inhibin B[92] (Fig. 4-17). The rise in FSH initiates the development of follicles and the next menstrual cycle. Ovulation probably occurs randomly dur-

▶ TABLE 4-5: CHARACTERISTICS OF THE NORMAL MENSTRUAL CYCLE

Mean: 28 days; range: 25–35 days
Follicular phase: 14 days, range: 10–16 days
Secretory phase: 14 days
Menstruation: 4–6 days
Blood loss: 30 mL, range: 10–80 mL

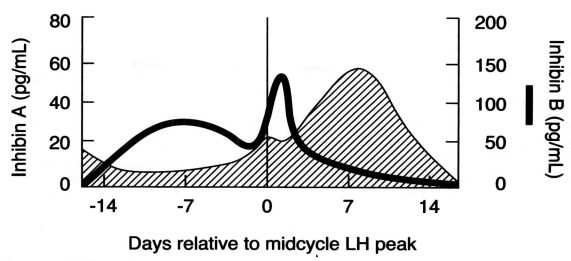

Days relative to midcycle LH peak

Figure 4-17 Comparison of inhibin A and inhibin B levels through the menstrual cycle in relation to the midcycle LH peak (0). *(Courtesy of Groom et al.[92])*

ing consecutive cycles, not preferentially to one ovary or the other.

After the onset of menses, development of the follicle continues, but FSH levels decline as a result of the negative feedback of estrogens and the rise of inhibin B secreted by the developing follicle. The decline in FSH—together with secretion by the growing follicle of additional intraovarian protein hormones, which include growth factors, cytokines, and a variety of other protein hormones (as discussed earlier)—is believed to promote steroidogenesis favoring the dominant follicle, while possibly inhibiting adjacent follicles from growing.

Three specific stages have been described in the development of a dominant follicle.[93] The first stage is recruitment. From a pool of nonproliferating follicles, a cohort of follicles is recruited during days 1 to 4 of the menstrual cycle in response to FSH. Once this stage is attained, the recruited follicles must either continue on to ovulate or undergo atresia. The following stage is selection, and it occurs when one follicle ovulates and the others undergo atresia. This stage occurs between days 5 and 7 of the menstrual cycle. In the final stage of development—dominance—the dominant folli-

cle grows and continues to suppress other ovarian follicles. This stage occurs between days 8 and 12 of the cycle and ends at the time of ovulation, ranging from days 13 to 15 (Fig. 4-18).

During the proliferative phase, estrogen levels rise parallel to the growth of the follicle and the number of granulosa cells. The granulosa cells are the exclusive source of FSH receptors. As discussed previously, the increase of FSH in the late luteal phase of the previous cycle leads to an increase in the number of FSH receptors and, subsequently, to an increase in estradiol secretion by the granulosa cells[94–97] (Table 4-6).

Small antral follicles do not form estradiol. This may be due to the presence of the enzyme 5α-reductase, which converts testosterone to the nonaromatizable androgen dihydrotestosterone, and the absence of aromatase.[98] Larger antral follicles, particularly the dominant follicle with its larger quantity of aromatase, secrete more estrogens. This change in the microenvironment and balance of androgens and estrogens of the ovary appears to be important in selection of the dominant follicle. The process of atresia in smaller follicles may be

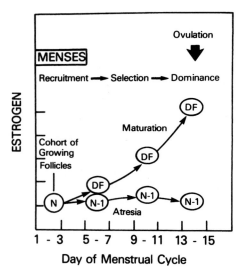

Figure 4-18   Time course for the recruitment, selection, and ovulation of the dominant ovarian follicle (DF) with onset of atresia among other follicles of the cohort (N1). *(Reproduced, with permission, from Hodgen GD, 1982:281)*

due to an excess amount of dihydrotestosterone, which appears to inhibit aromatization.

The fluid bathing the granulosa cells contains a large number of ovarian steroids and other protein hormones. In large follicles (>8 mm in diameter), the FSH, estrogen, and progesterone levels in follicular fluid are extremely high. In small follicles, the levels of androgens are higher than they are in large follicles and the follicular fluid. These observations support the hypothesis of microenvironmental control of follicular growth by hormones in the follicular fluid (Table 4-7).

Gonadotropin secretion varies during the menstrual cycle. As discussed earlier, FSH levels, which are elevated in the early part of the follicular phase, decline until just before ovulation. In contrast, LH levels are low in the first part of the follicular phase, but in the presence of increased estrogen, LH secretion begins to increase by the midfollicular phase as a result of positive feedback from estrogen. Secretion of LH in response to LH-releasing hormone increases markedly from the early to the late follicular phase. The frequency of spontaneous LH pulses varies during the menstrual cycle. During the early part of the cycle, LH pulses appear to be of constant amplitude and occur in frequencies of around 60 to 90 minutes. During the late follicular phase, just before the midcycle surge of LH, LH pulse frequency increases, and LH amplitude also may increase[97] (Fig. 4-19).

Ovulation

The onset of the LH surge resulting from increasing secretion of estrogen by preovulatory follicles is a relatively precise predictor of the time of ovulation, occurring some 34 to 36 hours before release of the ovum from the fol-

▶ **TABLE 4-6:** CHARACTERISTICS OF THE FOLLICULAR AND LUTEAL PHASES

Follicular Phase	Luteal Phase
FSH levels rise late in luteal phase and decline during follicular phase	LH and FSH levels low
LH levels rise in late follicular phase and peak at ovulation	Estrogen levels exhibit modest secondary peak
Estrogen levels rise during follicular phase and fall at the initiation of LH surge	Progesterone levels peak at mid-luteal phase
Inhibin B levels rise and fall in follicular phase; inhibin A levels are low in follicular phase	Inhibin B levels fall
Progesterone levels are low in follicular phase	Inhibin A levels peak at mid-luteal phase

► **TABLE 4-7:** SUBSTANCES FOUND
IN FOLLICULAR FLUID

Plasma proteins
Steroid-binding proteins
Enzymes
  Side-chain cleavage enzyme
  3β-Hydroxysteroid dehydrogenase
  17α-Hydroxylase
  C_{17-20} Lyase
  17β-Hydroxysteroid dehydrogenase
  20α-Hydroxysteroid dehydrogenase
  Aromatase
  Plasminogen (proteases)
Mucopolysaccharides (proteoglycans)
  Hyaluronic acid
  Chondroitin sulfate acid
  Heparin sulfate
Steroids
  Estrogens
  Androgens
  Progestins
Pituitary hormones
  Follicle-stimulating hormone
  Luteinizing hormone
  Prolactin
  Oxytocin
  Vasopressin
Nonsteroidal ovarian factors
  Inhibin
  Follicular protein (aromatase inhibitor)
  Oocyte meiosis inhibitor
  Luteinization inhibitor
  Luteinization stimulator

*Reproduced, with permission, from Yen SSC. The
human menstrual cycle. In Yen SSC, Jaffe RD (eds),
Reproductive Endocrinology. Philadelphia: Saunders,
1986:208.*

licle.[99] The peak of LH secretion occurs 10 to
12 hours before ovulation (see Fig. 4-16). The
LH surge stimulates resumption of the meiosis
process in the ovum with release of the first
polar body. Luteinization of the granulosa cells
increases progesterone secretion via another
messenger within the follicle cyclic adenosine
monophosphate (cAMP). Spontaneous luteinization occurs in the absence of LH when granulosa cells are removed from the follicle and

cultured. This finding has led to the hypothesis that oocyte maturation inhibitor or luteinization inhibitor prevents ovulation and that the
effects of these factors are overcome at the
time of ovulation.[100]

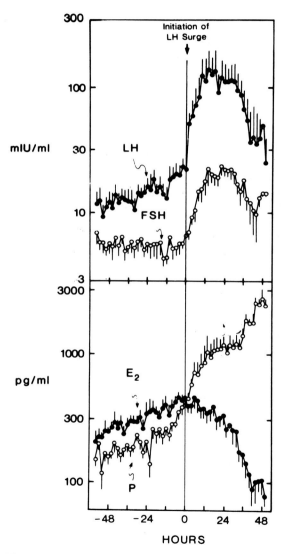

Figure 4-19 Changes in gonadtropins and
ovarian steroids at midcycle, just prior to ovu-
lation. The initiation of LH surge is at time 0.
Abbreviations: E2, estrogen; p, progesterone.
*(Reproduced, with permission, from Hoff JD,
Quigley ME, Yen SSC, 1983:792.)*

Just before ovulation, the follicle becomes vascularized. At this time there appears to be a protrusion of the follicular wall (the stigma), and this is the site of rupture with release of the oocyte-cumulus complex. The precise mechanism of follicular rupture is complex. It appears that progesterone and cAMP augment or activate proteolytic enzymes (e.g., collagenase, plasmin) that digest the collagen in the follicular wall, resulting in distensibility and thinning just before ovum release. There is no evidence that an increase in follicular pressure causes follicular rupture, but measurements have not been determined at the precise instance of rupture of the follicle.[101] Prostaglandins and other related substances reach a peak concentration in follicular fluid just before ovulation.[102] These substances are believed to be involved in rupture of the follicle, possibly by stimulating smooth muscle contraction and thereby aiding the extrusion of the oocyte-cumulus mass. It is known that women treated with prostaglandin synthetase inhibitors often retain the ovum, fail to ovulate, and develop a "luteinized unruptured follicle."[103]

Immediately before the LH peak, estradiol levels in the plasma fall rapidly. The fall in LH may be due to downregulation of its own receptors or to direct inhibition by an increase in progesterone secretion. The ovulatory peak of FSH, which is thought to be stimulated by progesterone, may have a variety of functions, including stimulating the plasminogen activator and increasing granulosa cell receptors.[104] The postovulatory fall in LH could be due to the loss of positive feedback caused by a decline in estrogen levels or by the depletion of LH content in the pituitary.

Luteal Phase

During the preovulatory surge of LH, a series of morphologic and chemical changes (a process referred to as *luteinization*) occurs in the cells of the granulosa and theca. During luteinization, these cells undergo hypertrophy and exhibit increased size and synthesis of hormones under LH stimulation. After ovulation, the basement membrane separating the granulosa from the theca breaks down, and blood vessels and capillaries invade the granulosa cells. The growth of blood vessels may be due to a variety of described angiogenic factors expressed in the developing corpus luteum. The morphologic change of the corpus luteum, or yellow body, has been well characterized and was discussed earlier.

The pattern of hormone secretion by the corpus luteum is different from that of the follicle. After ovulation, estrogen levels decrease. This decrease is followed by a secondary rise of estradiol that reaches a peak at the midluteal phase, which is followed by a secondary decrease toward the end of the menstrual cycle. The rise in estradiol parallels the pattern of progesterone secretion (see Table 4-6). Studies of the ovarian venous blood draining the corpus luteum suggest that the corpus luteum is the source of hormone secretion during the luteal phase. The role of LH as a primary luteotropic agent was first established in studies of hypophysectomized women.[105] In these women, after induction of ovulation, the length of the luteal phase and the amount of progesterone secreted were entirely dependent on repeated injections of LH. The administration of LH or hCG during the luteal phase can extend the functional life span of the corpus luteum and the secretion of progesterone for up to 2 weeks.[106]

The secretion of progesterone during the luteal phase is episodic, and the pulses of LH correspond with pulses of progesterone.[107] The frequency and amplitude of LH secretion during the luteal phase regulate the luteal phase function.[108] A reduction in FSH during the follicular phase, however, is associated with a shortened luteal phase, smaller corpora lutea, and reduced responses of dispersed corpus luteum cells in vitro.[109] In addition, the continued administration of LH-releasing hormone analogues during either the follicular phase or the luteal phase reduces the life span of the corpus luteum. A reduction in LH concentration, pulse frequency, and pulse amplitude also reduces the length of the luteal phase.[110] The corpus luteum of primates, however, can recover from a transient withdrawal of LH, depending on the age of the corpus luteum. Progesterone secretion in the luteal phase is correlated with the number of LH and hCG receptors and basal activity of adenylate cyclase.[111]

The role of other luteotropic factors in women is less clear. Prolactin does not appear to be luteotropic in women (in contrast to what happens in rats), but defective luteal function occurs when prolactin levels are either elevated or significantly suppressed by bromocriptine, although the mechanism is not understood. In addition, PGE_2 appears to be inhibitory to granulosa cells in vitro.[112] The secretion of relaxin, inhibin, and oxytocin by the human corpus luteum may modulate corpus luteum function, but it appears not to play a role in the maintenance of early pregnancy because agonadal women treated with estrogen and progesterone alone have carried pregnancy to term after donor embryo transfer.[113]

In the absence of pregnancy, the function of the corpus luteum declines rapidly 9 to 11 days after ovulation, but the mechanism of luteolysis remains unclear. Both PGF_2 and exogenous estrogens appear to be luteolytic in nonhuman primates as well as in women.[114,115] However, antiestrogens and aromatase inhibitors do not decrease the length of the luteal phase or alter corpus luteum function.[117] In addition, the fact that estrogen receptors are absent in the luteal cells of women indicates that estrogen does not play a role in luteal regression.

▶ EFFECT OF HORMONES ON THE FEMALE REPRODUCTIVE TRACT DURING THE MENSTRUAL CYCLE

The interrelationships of the hypothalamic-pituitary-ovarian axis give rise to fluctuations in estrogen and progesterone that produce striking effects on the tissues of the reproductive tract. The most characterized alterations occur in the endometrium. The changes in endometrial histology throughout the menstrual cycle are such that dating of the endometrium is possible[117] (Fig. 4-20 and Table 4-8).

The proliferative phase is less precisely dated and consists of growth of the endometrium up to 5 mm thickness. During the proliferative phase, the glands are narrow and tubular, and mitosis and pseudostratification are present. Two days after ovulation (cycle day 16), glycogen accumulates in the basal portion of the glandular epithelium. The nuclei appear to be displaced to the midportion of the cells, resulting in a pseudostratified configuration. In tissues fixed with formalin, glycogen is solubilized, leaving large vacuoles in the base of the cells. The development of subnuclear vacuolation of the glandular epithelium is evidence that a functional, progesterone-producing corpus luteum has been formed. By day 17, the glands are visibly more tortuous and dilated. On day 18, the vacuoles in the epithelium are smaller and often located along the nuclei, and glycogen is now apparent in the apex of the cells. Intraluminal secretion is present, and pseudostratification and vacuolation have nearly disappeared by day 19. On cycle days 21 and 22, the endometrial stroma becomes edematous. By day 23, stromal cells surrounding the spiral arterioles enlarge, and mitoses are visible. Day 24 is characterized by predecidual changes in the stromal cells around the spiral arterioles and increased mitoses. By day 25, predecidual changes in the stromal cells begin under the surface epithelium. By day 27, the upper half of the endometrial stroma is a solid sheet of well-developed decidualized cells. Differentiation of the decidua is accompanied by a marked increase in lymphocytic infiltration, and menstruation begins on day 28.

The breakdown of the endometrium occurs in cycles where conception fails to occur and corpus luteum function ceases with a resulting

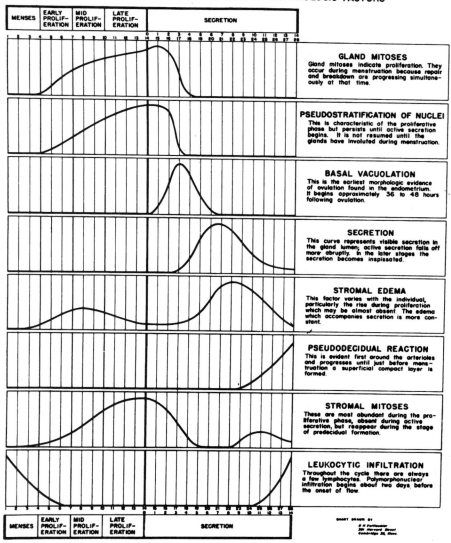

Figure 4-20 Dating of the Enodthelium. *(Reproduced, with permission, from Noyes RW, Hertig AW, Rock J, 1950:3.76)*

decrease of estrogen and progesterone levels. These hormonal changes induce three endometrial events: vascular alterations, loss of tissue, and menstruation. In association with shrinkage of the height of the endometrium, a concomitant decrease in blood flow of the spi-

ral vessels and vasodilatation ensue. The spiral vessels feeding the endometrium undergo rhythmic cycles of vasoconstriction and vasodilatation. This results in necrosis of the blood vessels and eventually leads to endometrial ischemia and cell death.[118,119] Menstrua-

▶ **TABLE 4-8:** HISTOLOGIC CHARACTERISTICS OF THE ENDOMETRIUM DURING THE MENSTRUAL CYCLE

> **Proliferative phase**
>   Gland mitosis
>   Pseudostratification of nuclei
>   Stromal mitosis
> **Secretory phase**
>   Basovacuolation (early)
>   Secretion
>   Stromal edema
>   Pseudodecidual reaction (late)
>   Leukocyte infiltration (late)

tion follows and consists of blood and desquamation of superficial endometrial tissues. Menstrual flow lasts 4 to 6 days, and the average amount of blood lost is 30 mL/cycle.[120] By the midfollicular phase, estrogen secretion by the ovarian follicles increases and induces endometrial healing. Vasoconstriction occurs, and platelets and clot formation develop over the denuded endometrial vessels.

The development of necrosis and vasospasm of the spiral vessels is thought to be due to prostaglandins. Prostaglandins are present in large quantities in secretory endometrium and menstrual blood.[121] The infusion of $PGF_{2\alpha}$ into women during the luteal phase will induce endometrial necrosis and subsequent bleeding.[122] Prostaglandin release is believed to be secondary to a disruption of the lysosomal membranes in the endometrial cell.[122] This is followed by the liberation of phospholipids and subsequent synthesis of $PGF_{2\alpha}$. Interestingly, the use of prostaglandin synthetase inhibitors decreases the amount of menstrual bleeding in normal women and women using contraceptive devices. The inability of menstrual blood to coagulate is thought to be due to the presence of fibrinolytic activity.[123]

The levels of steroid receptors for estrogen and progesterone vary markedly during the menstrual cycle. Estrogen receptor content of the endometrium is high during the prolifera-

tive phase and declines in the secretory phase due to the action of progesterone formed by the corpus luteum.[124] Because estrogen stimulates the formation not only of estrogen receptors but also of progesterone receptors, the content of progesterone receptors increases during the late proliferative phase, peaks at ovulation, and declines less rapidly than the estrogen receptors during the secretory phase.

In addition to steroid receptors, the activities of endometrial steroidogenic enzymes also vary during the menstrual cycle, particularly the activity of 17β-hydroxysteroid type II (17β-HSD type II). 17β-HSD type II stimulates the conversion of the potent estrogen 17β-estradiol to the less potent estrogen estrone. The activity of 17β-HSD type II is enhanced during the secretory phase, resulting in a decline of the endometrial content of estradiol and an increase in the content of estrone.[125] Thus by progesterone's inhibitory action on the estrogen receptor and its stimulatory action on 17β-HSD the effect of estrogen action on secretory endometrium is diminished.

The endocervical glands undergo cyclic changes that are more similar to the changes in vaginal epithelium than in the endometrium. Following the menses, the amount of mucus secreted by the endocervical gland is limited and viscous. The quantity of mucus increases up to 30-fold in response to increasing levels of estrogen secreted by the follicle during the latter half of the follicular phase. The quality of endocervical mucus also changes and becomes watery and elastic. A fine thread of mucus can be demonstrated by stretching a drop of secretion (spinnbarkeit). Also, a characteristic ferning or palm-leaf arborization can be demonstrated in mucus dried on a microscope slide. Progesterone secretion during the luteal phase reverses the effects of estrogen on the cervical mucus.

Vaginal epithelial cells are also influenced by cyclic changes in estrogen and progesterone levels. In the early follicular phase, exfoliated vaginal epithelial cells are basophilic and contain vesicular nuclei. When estrogen levels increase in the latter half of the follicular phase, vaginal epithelial cells become acidophilic with pyknotic nuclei. During the luteal phase with increasing levels of progesterone, the percentage of acidophilic cells decreases, and the number of leukocytes increases. A number of indices to characterize vaginal cytology are also available.

KEY POINTS

1. The maximal number of oocytes during a woman's life is 6 to 7 million. The time that this level is reached is at 20 weeks of fetal life.

2. Meiosis I is arrested at the diplotene stage of oocyte development during fetal life. Meiosis I resumes at ovulation, and meiosis II is initiated at the time of fertilization.

3. The FSH/LH ratio changes during the lifetime of women. During fetal life the ratio is greater than 1, during childhood greater than 1, during reproductive life less than 1, and after menopause greater than 1.

4. The documentation of ovulation is strongly supported in a woman who provides a history of spontaneous, predictable, cyclic menstrual periods.

5. Granulosa cells of the follicle do not have a direct blood supply. This is so because granulosa cells are separated from the theca cell layer by a basal lamina.

6. The lifetime of the human corpus luteum is 14 days. On day 1, proliferation of granulosa cells occurs. On day 2, capillary invasion begins, and on day 7 to 8, maximum capillary enlargement occurs. On day 13 to 14, luteolysis is initiated, and apoptosis follows.

7. The key enzymes involved in steroidogenesis are differentially expressed in granulosa and thecal cells. In the granulosa cell, CYP19 and 17β-HSD type 1 are expressed, and in the thecal cell, CYP17.

8. The postmenopausal ovary is uniquely different from the premenopausal ovary. The postmenopausal ovary contains either absent or rare follicles, absent estrogen secretion, and reduced androgen secretion.

9. The characteristics of the normal menstrual cycle include a mean of 28 days (range 25 to 35 days). The follicular phase mean is 14 days (range 10 to 16 days), and the secretory phase is fixed at 14 days. Menstruation lasts 4 to 6 days, and mean blood loss is 30 mL (range 10 to 80 mL).

10. The characteristic changes in the endometrium vary significantly throughout the menstrual cycle. The proliferative phase is characterized by glandular and stromal mitoses and pseudostratification of nuclei. The secretory phase is characterized by basovacuolization, secretion, stromal edema, and later, pseudodecidual reaction and leukocyte infiltration.

REFERENCES

1. Gillman J. The development of the gonads in man, with a consideration of the whole fetal endocrines and the histogenesis of ovarian tumors. *Contrib Embryol Carney Inst Wash* 1948; 32:67.
2. Kuwana T, Maeda-Suga H, Fujimoto T. Attraction of chick primordial germ cells by gonadal anlage in vitro. *Anat Rec* 1986;215:403.
3. Baker TG. A quantitative and cytological study of germ cells in the human ovaries. *Proc R Soc Lond [B]* 1963;158:417.
4. Lyon MF. Gene action in the X chromosome of the mouse *(Mus musculus). Nature* 1961;190: 372.
5. Singh RP, Carr DH. The anatomy and histology of XO human embryos and fetuses. *Anat Rec* 1966;155:369.
6. Peters H, Byskov AG, Grinsted J. Follicular growth in fetal and prepubertal ovaries in humans and other primates. *Clin Endocrinol Metab* 1978;3:469.
6a. Johnson J, Canning J, Kaneko T, Pru J, Tilly J. Germline Stem Cells and follicular renewal in

the postnatal mammalian ovary. *Nature* 2004; 428:145.

7. Wartenberg H. Development of the early human ovary and the role of the mesonephros in the differentiation of the cortex. *Anat Embryol* 1982;165:253.

8. Baker TG, Franchi LL. The fine structure of oogonia in oocytes in human ovaries. *J Cell Sci* 1967;2:213.

9. Tsafriri A, Dekel N, Bar-Armi S. The role of oocyte maturation inhibitor in follicular regulation of oocyte maturation. *J Reprod Fertil* 1982;64:541.

10. Byskov AG, Hoyer PE. Embryology of mammalian gonads and ducts, in Knobil E, Neill JD (eds), *The Physiology of Reproduction,* 2d ed. New York: Raven Press, 1994, p 487.

11. Guylas BJ, Hodgen GD, Tullner WW, Ross GT. Effects of fetal and maternal hypophysectomy on endocrine organs and body weight in infant monkey *(Macaca mulatta)* with particular emphasis on oogenesis. *Biol Reprod* 1977; 16:216.

12. Molsberry RL, Carr BR, Mendelson CTR, Simpson ER. Human chorionic gonadotropin binding to human fetal testes as a function of gestational age. *J Clin Endocrinol Metab* 1982;55: 791.

13. Faiman C, Winter JSD, Reyes FI. Patterns of gonadotropins and gonadal steroids throughout life. *Clin Obstet Gynecol* 1976;3:467.

14. Winter JSD, Hughes IA, Reyes FI, Faiman C. Pituitary-gonadal steroid concentrations in man from birth to two years of age. *J Clin Endocrinol Metab* 1976;42:679.

15. Yanovski JA, Cutler GB. The preproductive axis pubertal activation, in Adashi EY, Rock JA, Rosenwaks Z (eds), *Reproductive Endocrinology, Surgery, and Technology*. Philadelphia: Lippincott-Raven, 1996, p 76.

16. Conte FA, Grumbach MM, Kaplan SL. A diphasic pattern of gonadotropin secretion in patients with the syndrome of gonadal dysgenesis. *J Clin Endocrinol Metab* 1975;40:670.

17. Roth JC, Kelch RP, Kaplan SL, Grumbach MM. FSH and LH response to luteinizing hormone–releasing factor in prepubertal and pubertal children, adult males and patients with hypogonadotropic and hypergonadotropic hypogonadism. *J Clin Endocrinol Metab* 1973; 37:680.

18. Jakacki RI, Kelch RP, Sauder SE, et al. Pulsatile secretion of luteinizing hormone in children. *J Clin Endocrinol Metab* 1982;55:453.

19. Gell JS, Carr BR, Sasano H, et al. Adrenarche results from development of a 3β-hydroxysteroid dehydrogenase–deficient adrenal reticularis. *J Clin Endocrinol Metab* 1998;83:3695.

20. Miller WL, Styne DM. Female puberty and its disorders, in Yen SSC, Jaffe RB, Barbieri RL (eds), *Reproductive Endocrinology,* 4th ed. Philadelphia: Saunders, 1999, p 388.

21. Boyer RM, Rosenfeld RS, Kaplan S, et al. Simultaneous augmentation secretion of luteinizing hormone and testosterone during sleep. *J Clin Invest* 1974;54:609.

22. Kapen S, Boyer RM, Hellman L, Weitzman ED. Twenty-four-hour patterns of luteinizing hormone secretion in humans: Ontogenic and sexual considerations. *Prog Brain Res* 1975;42:103.

23. Knobil E. The neuroendocrine control of the menstrual cycle. *Recent Prog Horm Res* 1980; 36:53.

24. Crowley WF, McArthur JW. Stimulation of the normal menstrual cycle in Kallmann's syndrome by pulsatile administration of luteinizing hormone-releasing hormone (LHRH). *J Clin Endocrinol Metab* 1980;51:173.

25. Witchel SF, Barns-Barlor RG, Lee PA. Treatment of central precocious puberty: Comparison of urinary gonadotropin excretion and gonadotropin-releasing hormone (GnRH) stimulation tests in monitory GnRH analogue therapy. *J Clin Endocrinol Metab* 1996;81:1353.

26. Burstein S, Schoff-Blass E, Blass J, Rosenfield RL. Changing ratio of bioactive to immunoactive LH through puberty. *J Clin Endocrinol Metab* 1985;61:508.

27. Lockwood GM, Muttukrishna S, Ledger WL. Inhibins and activins in human ovulation, conception and pregnancy. *Hum Reprod Update* 1998;4:284.

28. Merimee TJ, Zapf J, Hewlett B, Cavalli-Sforz LL. Insulin-like growth factors in pygmies. *N Engl J Med* 1987;316:906.

29. Marshall WA, Tanner JM. Variations in pattern of pubertal changes in girls. *Arch Dis Child* 1969;44:291.

30. Frisch RE, McArthur JW. Menstrual cycles: Fatness as a determinant of minimum weight for height necessary for their maintenance at onset. *Science* 1974;185:949.

31. Castracane VD, Henson MC: Leptin and reproduction. *Semin Reprod Med* 2002;20:85.

32. Eshkol A, Lunenfeld B, Peters H. Ovarian development in infant mice: Dependence on gonadotropic hormones, in Butt WR, Crooke AC, Ryle M (eds), *Gonadotropins and Ovarian Development*. London: Livingstone, 1970, p 249.

33. Tilly JL, Kowalski KJ, Johnson A, et al. Involvement of apoptosis in ovarian follicular atresia and postovulatory regression. *Endocrinology* 1993;132:294.

34. Eppig JJ. A comparison between oocyte growth in coculture with granulosa cells and oocytes with granulosa cell–oocyte junctional contact maintained in vitro. *J Exp Zool* 1979;209:345.

35. Bleil JD, Wassermann PM. Structure and function of the zona pellucida: Identification and characterization of the proteins of the mouse oocyte's zona pellucida. *Dev Biol* 1980;76:185.

36. Erickson FG, Magoffen D, Dyer CA, Hofeditz C. The ovarian androgen producing cells: A review of structure/function relationships. *Endocr Rev* 1985;6:371.

37. Upadhyay S, Zamboni L. Ectopic germ cells: Natural model for the study of germ cell sexual differentiation. *Proc Natl Acad Sci USA* 1982;79:6584.

38. Dawson AB, McCabe M. The interstitial tissue of the ovary in infantile and juvenile rats. *J Morphol* 1951;88:543.

39. Corner GW Jr. Histological dating of human corpus luteum of menstruation. *Am J Anat* 1956;8:377.

40. Gillim SW, Christensen AK, McLennon CE. Fine structure of the human menstrual corpus luteum at its stage of maximum secretory activity. *Am J Anat* 1970;126:409.

41. Ying SY: Inhibins, activins, and follistatins: Gonadal proteins modulating the secretion of follicle-stimulating hormone. *Endocr Rev* 1988;9:267.

42. Oliver C, Mical RS, Porter JC. Hypothalamic-pituitary vasculature: Evidence for retrograde blood flow in the pituitary stalk. *Endocrinology* 1977;101:598.

43. Conn PM, Crowley WF Jr. Gonadotropin-releasing hormone and its analogues. *N Engl J Med* 1991;342:93.

44. Marshall JC. Regulation of gonadotropin secretion, in DeGroot LJ (ed), *Endocrinology*. Philadelphia: Saunders, 1989, p 1903.

45. Huseman CA, Kelch RP. Gonadotropin resonse and metabolism of synthetic gonadotropin-releasing hormone (GnRH) during constant infusion of GnRH in men and boys with delayed adolescence. *J Clin Endocrinol Metab* 1978;47:1325.

46. Carmel PW, Araki S, Ferin M. Pituitary stalk portal blood collection in rhesus monkeys: Evidence for pulsatile release of gonadotropin releasing hormone (GnRH). *Endocrinology* 1976;99:243.

47. Clarke IJ, Cummins JT. The temporal relationship between gonadotropin-releasing hormone (GnRH) and luteinizing hormone (LH) secretion in ovariectomized ewes. *Endocrinology* 1982;11:1737.

48. Knobil E, Plant TM, Wildt TL, et al. Control of the rhesus monkey menstrual cycle: Permissive role of hypothalamic gonadotropin releasing hormone. *Science* 1980;207:1371.

49. Leyendecker G, Wildt TL, Hansmen M. Pregnancies following chronic intermittent pulsatile administration of GnRH. *J Clin Endocrinol Metab* 1980;51:1214.

50. Con PM. The molecular basis of gonadotropin-releasing hormone action. *Endocr Rev* 1986;7:3.

51. Fiddes JC, Talmadge K. Structure, expression, and evolution of the genes for human glycoprotein hormones. *Recent Prog Horm Res* 1984;40:43.

52. Kholer PO, Ross GT, Odell WD. Metabolic clearance and production rates of human luteinizing hormone in pre- and post-menopausal women. *J Clin Invest* 1968;47:38.

53. Wildt TL, Hutchinson JS, Marshall G, et al. On the site of action of progesterone in the blockade of the estradiol-induced gonadotropin discharge in the rhesus monkey. *Endocrinology* 1981;109:1293.

54. Filcori M, Santoro N, Merriam GR, Crowley WF Jr. Characterization of the physiological pattern of episodic gonadotropin secretion throughout the human menstrual cycle. *J Clin Endocrinol Metab* 1986;62:1136.

55. Liu JH, Yen SSC. Induction of midcycle gonadotropin surge by ovarian steroids in women: A critical evaluation. *J Clin Endocrinol Metab* 1983;57:797.

56. Fishman J, Hellman L, Zumoff B, Gallager TF. Influence of thyroid hormone on estrogen metabolism in man. *J Clin Endocrinol Metab* 1962;22:389.

57. Carr BR, MacDonald PC, Simpson ER. The role of lipoproteins in the regulation of progesterone secretion by the human corpus luteum. *Fertil Steril* 1982;38:303.

58. Gwynne JT, Strauss JF. The role of lipoproteins in steroidogenesis and cholesterol metabolism in steroidogenic glands. *Endocr Rev* 1982;3:299.

59. Clark BJ, Soo SC, Caron KM. Hormonal and developmental regulation of the steroidogenic acute regulatory protein. *Mol Endocrinol* 1995;9:1346.

60. McAllister JM, Kerin JFP, Trant JM, et al. Regulation of cholesterol side-chain cleavage and 17α-hydroxylase/lyase activities in proliferating human theca interna cells in long-term monolayer culture. *Endocrinology* 1989;125:1959.

61. Suzuki T, Sasono H, Tamura M, et al. Temporal and spatial localization of steroidogenic enzymes in premenopausal human ovaries: In situ hybridization and immunohistochemical study. *Mol Cell Endocrinol* 1993;97:135.

62. Steinkampf MP, Mendelson CR, Simpson ER. Effects of epidermal growth factor and insulin-like growth factor I on the levels of mRNA encoding aromatase cytochrome P-450 of human ovarian granulosa cells. *Mol Cell Endocrinol* 1988;59:93.

63. Carr BR, Sadler RK, Rochelle DB, et al. Plasma lipoprotein regulation of progesterone biosynthesis by human corpus luteum tissue in organ culture. *J Clin Endocrinol Metab* 1981;52:875.

64. Ohasi M, Carr BR, Simpson ER. Lipoprotein binding sites in human corpus luteum membrane fractions. *Endocrinology* 1982;110:1477.

65. Illingworth DR, Corbin DK, Kemp ED, Keenan EJ. Hormone changes during the menstrual cycle in abetalipoproteinemia: Reduced luteal phase progesterone in a patient with homozygous hypobetalipoproteinemia. *Proc Natl Acad Sci USA* 1982;79:6685.

66. Hsueh AJW, Adashi EY, Jones PBC, Welsh TH Jr. Hormonal regulation of the differentiation of culture ovarian granulosa cells. *Endocr Rev* 1984;5:76.

67. Baird DT, Horton R, Longcope C, Tait JF. Steroid dynamics under steady state conditions. *Rec Prog Horm Res* 1969;25:611.

68. Siiteri PK, MacDonald PC. Placental estrogen biosynthesis during human pregnancy. *J Clin Endocrinol Metab* 1966;26:751.

69. Rosner W. Sex steroid transport: Binding proteins, in Adashi EY, Rock JA, Rosenwaks Z (eds), *Reproductive Endocrinology, Surgery, and Technology.* Philadelphia: Lippincott-Raven, 1996, p 605.

70. Mendel CM. The free hormone hypothesis: Distinction from the free hormone transport hypothesis. *J Androl* 1992;13:108.

71. Iqbal MJ, Johnson MW. Purification and characterization of human sex hormone-binding globulin. *J Steroid Biochem* 1979;10:535.

72. Anderson DC. Sex hormone-binding globulin. *Clin Endocrinol (Oxf)* 1974;3:69.

73. *A Statistical Portrait of Women in the US,* Publication 58, Current Population Report, Special Studies Series, Washington: US Department of Commerce, Bureau of the Census, 1976.

74. Utian WH. *Menopause in Modern Perspective.* New York: Appleton-Century-Crofts, 1980.

75. Nagamani M, Stuart CA, Doherty NG. Increased steroid production by ovarian stromal tissue of postmenopausal women with endometrial cancer. *J Clin Endocrinol Metab* 1992;74:172.

76. Scaglia H, Medina M, Pinto-Ferriera AL, et al. Pituitary LH and FSH secretion and responsiveness in women of old age. *Acta Endocrinol (Kbh)* 1976;81:673.

77. Judd JL. Hormonal dynamics associated with the menopause. *Clin Obstet Gynecol* 1976;19:775.

78. Hemsell DL, Grodin JM, Brenner PF, et al. Plasma precursors of estrogen: II. Correlation of the extent of conversion of plasma androstenedione to estrone with age. *J Clin Endocrinol Metab* 1974;38:476.

79. Brincat M, Moniz CJ, Studd JWW, et al. The long-term effects of the menopause and of administration of sex hormones on skin collagen and skin thickness. *Br J Obstet Gynecol* 1985;92:256.

80. Barrett-Connor E, Brown WV, Turner J, et al. Heart disease risk factors and hormone use in postmenopausal women. *JAMA* 1979;241:2167.

81. Meldrum DR. The pathophysiology of postmenopausal symptoms. *Semin Reprod Endocrinol* 1983;1:11.

82. Riggs BL, Wahner HW, Melton LJ III, et al. Rates of bone loss in the appendicular and axial skeletons of women. *J Clin Invest* 1986;77:1487.

83. Alderman BW, Weiss NS, Daling JR, et al. Reproductive history and postmenopausal risk of hip and forearm fracture. *Am J Epidemiol* 1986;124:262.

84. Henderson BE, Ross RK, Paganini-Hill A, Mack TM. Estrogen use and cardiovascular disease. *Am J Obstet Gynecol* 1986;154:1181.

85. Matthews KA, Meilahn E. Kuller LH, et al. Menopause and risk factors for coronary heart disease. *N Engl J Med* 1989;321:641.

86. Colditz GA, Willett WC, Stampfer MJ, et al. Menopause and the risk of coronary heart disease in women. *N Engl J Med* 1987;316:1105.

87. Matthews KA, Meilahn E. Kuller, et al. Menopause and risk factors for coronary heart disease. *N Engl J Med* 1989;321:641.

88. Colditz GA, Willett WC, Stampfer MJ, et al. Menopause and the risk of coronary heart disease in women. *N Engl J Med* 1987;316:1105.

89. Writing Group for the Women's Health Initiative Investigators. Risk benefits of estrogen plus progestin in healthy postmenopausal women: Principal results from the Women's Health Initiative Randomized Controlled Trial. *JAMA* 2002;288:321.

90. Treloar AE, Boynton BE, Behn BG, Brown RW. Variations of the human menstrual cycle throughout reproductive life. *Int J Fertil* 1967;12:77.

91. Presser HB. Temporal data relating to the human menstrual cycle, in Ferin M, Halber F, Richart RM, et al (eds), *Biorhythms and Human Reproduction*. London: Wiley, 1974, p 145.

92. Groome NP, Illingworth PJ, O'Brien M, et al. Measurement of dimeric inhibin B throughout the human menstrual cycle. *J Clin Endocrinol Metab* 1996;81:1401.

93. Hodgen GD. The dominant ovarian follicle. *Fertil Steril* 1982;38:281.

94. Dorrington JH, Armstrong DT. Effects of FSH on gonadal functions. *Recent Prog Horm Res* 1979;39:301.

95. Zeleznik AJ, Midgley AR Jr, Reichert LE Jr. Granulosa cell maturation in the rat: Increased binding of human chorionic gonadotropin following treatment with follicle-stimulating hormone in vivo. *Endocrinology* 1974;95:818.

96. Fink G. Gonadotropin secretion and its control, in Knobil E, Neill JD (eds), *The Physiology of Reproduction*. New York: Raven Press, 1988, p 1349.

97. Carr BR. Disorders of the ovaries and female reproductive tract, in Wilson JD, Foster DW, Kronenberg HM, Larsen PR (eds), *Williams' Textbook of Endocrinology,* 9th ed. Philadelphia: Saunders, 1998, p 751.

98. McNatty KP, Makris A, Reinhold VN, et al. Metabolism of androstenedione by human ovarian tissue in vitro with particular reference to reductase and aromatase activity. *Steroids* 1979;34:429.

99. Hoff JD, Quigley ME, Yen SSC. Hormonal dynamics at midcycle: A reevaluation. *J Clin Endocrinol Metab* 1983;57:792.

100. Channing CP, Schaerf FW, Anderson LD, Tsafriri A. Ovarian follicular and luteal physiology, in Greep RO (ed), *International Review of Physiology,* Vol 22. Baltimore: University Park Press, 1980, p 117.

101. Lipner H, Espey LL. Mechanism of mammalian ovulation, in Knobil E, Neill JD (eds), *The Physiology of Reproduction,* 2d ed. New York: Raven Press, 1994, p 727.

102. Yoshimura Y, Wallach EE. Studies on the mechanisms of mammalian ovulation. *Fertil Steril* 1987;47:22.

103. Murdoch WJ, Cavender JL. Effect of indomethacin on the vascular architecture of preovulatory ovine follicles: Possible implication in the luteinized unruptured follicle syndrome. *Fertil Steril* 1989;51:153.

104. Yen SS. The human menstrual cycle: neuroendocrine regulation, in Yen SS, Jaffe RB, Barbieri RL (eds), *Reproductive Endocrinology: Physiology, Pathophysiology and Clinical Management,* 4th ed. Philadelphia: Saunders, 1999, p 191.

105. Vande Wiele RL, Bogumil J, Dyrenfurth I, et al. Mechanisms regulating the menstrual cycle in women. *Recent Prog Horm Res* 1970;26:63.

106. Segaloff A, Sternberg WH, Gaskill CJ. Effects of luteotrophic doses of chorionic gonadotropin in women. *J Clin Endocrinol Metab* 1951;11:936.

107. Filicori M, Butler JP, Crowley WF Jr. Neuroendocrine regulation of the corpus luteum in the human. *J Clin Invest* 1984;73:1638.

108. McNeely MJ, Soules MR. The diagnosis of luteal phase deficiency. *Fertil Steril* 1988;50:1.

109. Stouffer RL, Hodgen GD. Induction of luteal phase defects in rhesus monkeys by follicular fluid administration at the onset of the menstrual cycle. *J Clin Endocrinol Metab* 1980;51:669.

110. Sheehan KL, Casper RF, Yen SSC. Luteal phase defects induced by an agonist of luteinizing hormone–releasing factor: A model for fertility control. *Science* 1982;215:170.

111. Rojas FJ, Moretti-Rojas I, Balmaceda JP, Asch RH. Regulation of gonadotropin-stimulable adenyl cyclase of the primate corpus luteum. *J Steroid Biochem* 1989;32:175.

112. Hahlin M, Dennefors B, Johanson C, Hamberger L. Luteotropic effects of prostaglandin E_2 on the human corpus luteum of the menstrual cycle and early pregnancy. *J Clin Endocrinol Metab* 1988;66:909.

113. Lutjen P, Trounson A, Leeton J, et al. The establishment and maintenance of pregnancy using in vitro fertilization and embryo donation in a patient with primary ovarian failure. *Nature* 1984;308:174.

114. Auletta FJ. The role of prostaglandin $F_{2\alpha}$ in human luteolysis. *Contemp Obstet Gynecol* 1987;30:119.

115. Wentz AC, Jones GS. Transient luteolytic effect of prostaglandin $F_{2\alpha}$ in the human. *Obstet Gynecol* 1973;42:172.

116. Ellinwood WE, Resko JA. Effect of inhibition of estrogen synthesis during the luteal phase on function of the corpus luteum in rhesus monkeys. *Biol Reprod* 1983;28:636.

117. Noyes RW, Hertig AW, Rock J. Dating the endometrial biopsy. *Fertil Steril* 1950;1:3.

118. Sixma JJ, Cristiens GCML, Hospels AS. The sequence of hemostatic events in the endometrium during normal menstruation, in Dicefalusy E, Fraser IS, Webb FTG (eds), *WHO Symposium on Steroid Contraception and Endometrial Bleeding*. Geneva: World Health Organization, 1980, p 86.

119. Wilborn WH, Flowers CE Jr. Cellular mechanisms for endometrial conservation during menstrual bleeding. *Semin Reprod Endocrinol* 1984;2:307.

120. Hallberg L, Hogdahl A, Nilsson L, Rybo G. Menstrual blood loss: A population study. *Acta Obstet Gynecol Scand* 1966;45:320.

121. Schwarz BE. The production and biologic effects of uterine prostaglandins. *Semin Reprod Endocrinol* 1983;1:189.

122. Turksoy RN, Safaii HS. Immediate effect of prostaglandin $F_{2\alpha}$ during the luteal phase of the menstrual cycle. *Fertil Steril* 1975;26:634.

123. Todd AS. Localization of fibrinolytic activity in tissues. *Br Med Bull* 1964;20:210.

124. Lessey BA, Killam AP, Metzger DA, et al. Immunohistochemical analysis of human uterine estrogen and progesterone receptors throughout the menstrual cycle. *J Clin Endocrinol Metab* 1988;67:334.

125. Tseng L, Masella J. Cyclic changes of estradiol metabolic enzymes in human endometrium during the menstrual cycle, in Kimball FA (ed), *The Endometrium*. New York: SP Medical and Scientific Books, 1980, p 211.

CHAPTER 5

Reproductive Genetics

Lawrence C. Layman

Genetics has expanded so rapidly in recent years that it has become even more daunting to the practicing reproductive clinician. It is assumed that the clinician has a basic understanding of genetics. The purpose of this chapter is not to cover every aspect of reproductive genetics but to discuss practical clinical genetics as will pertain to the practicing reproductive endocrinologist. Relevant topics include preconception counseling regarding the risk for rubella, neural tubal defects, and in vitro fertilization (IVF); mutations in human disease; chromosomal abnormalities; genetic basis of infertility; and preimplantation genetic diagnosis.

▶ PRECONCEPTION COUNSELING: RUBELLA, NEURAL TUBE DEFECTS, AND IN VITRO FERTILIZATION

Rubella

Rubella infection is known to cause congenital anomalies if there is exposure in mothers who are not immune. The congenital rubella syndrome (CRS) consists of mental retardation, microcephaly, congenital defects of the heart and eye, and deafness. Exposure in the first trimester may confer a malformation rate of approximately 50 percent, whereas second- and third-trimester effects are less.[1] In the United

States, Hispanic women and foreign-born women who enter the country are the individuals most at risk of giving birth to a child with CRS.[2] A rubella titer should be performed on patients who may become pregnant and who have not had one in the last year because the achievement of immunity after vaccination, although very high, is not 100 percent. If the patient is not immune, a rubella vaccine can be offered and the titer repeated subsequently to document immunity. Since the vaccine is a live attenuated virus, avoiding pregnancy for 3 months after pregnancy was recommended previously. However, since no cases of CRS have been reported following vaccination, the more recent recommendation is to wait 1 month after immunization before attempting pregnancy.[3] There is no contraindication to giving the rubella vaccine postpartum, and administration of the vaccine in pregnancy is not an indication for pregnancy termination.[3]

Neural Tube Defects and Folate Intake

Spina bifida and anencephaly are the most common neural tube defect (NTD) abnormalities, but the spectrum also may include other central nervous system (CNS) abnormalities (encephalocele, iniencephaly, craniorrhachisis). Most NTDs are multifactorial, but 20 percent may have additional anomalies, whereas up to 10 percent may be caused by teratogens or single-gene defects.[4] NTDs also may be more common in patients with recurrent abortion.

Although folate is contained within many foods, it is now recommended that all patients contemplating pregnancy should take 400 μg/day supplemental folic acid.[4] Most over-the-counter vitamins contain at least 400 μg folate per tablet, which has been shown to reduce the risk of NTDs such as spina bifida and anencephaly by about 50 percent in those without a prior family history of such defects.[4] The folic acid ideally should be started 3 months prior to conception and continued throughout at least the first trimester of pregnancy.

The ascertainment of a family history of NTD is important because the recurrence risk is increased over the general U.S. population risk of 1 to 2 per 1000. With one prior affected child, the recurrence risk is about 2 to 3 percent; with two affected children, it approaches 5 to 6 percent. If the parent has an NTD, the recurrence risk is about 1 percent. These recurrence risks are empirical risks assuming no preconception folic acid treatment. If the patient has had a prior child with an NTD, 4 mg folate per day is the recommended dose. This higher dose also should be considered in other types of patients at risk for NTDs, such as those with diabetes (particularly uncontrolled diabetes) or those who take medications (e.g., valproate) for seizures. In these patients, the risk of NTD is reduced by more than 70 percent with folate administration.[4]

Impact of In Vitro Fertilization

Couples should be aware that the background rate of birth defects is in the 2 to 4 percent range, so any discussion of genetic disease or medications taken during pregnancy should be centered on this baseline rate. In vitro fertilization (IVF) with intracytoplasmic sperm injection (ICSI) has been reported to increase the birth defect rate slightly, particularly with regard to sex chromosome abnormalities (0.4 versus 0.2 percent), structural autosomal abnormalities (0.4 versus 0.07 percent), and inherited structural aberrations, which are mostly paternal.[5] In addition, there is some preliminary evidence that IVF, with or without ICSI, may increase the prevalence of imprinting disorders such as Angelman syndrome and Beckwith-Wiedemann syndrome.[6] For some genes, there is unequal expression of maternal and paternal alleles (i.e., only one allele is active). For reasons that are not well understood, perhaps because of exposure to embryo culture medium, this process is disrupted, and genetic disease occurs. These preliminary findings await larger, prospective studies for confirmation.

▶ MUTATIONS IN HUMAN GENETIC DISEASE

Although some gene mutations in human disease may be tested for clinically by Southern blot analysis, most are now detected using the more rapid and versatile polymerase chain reaction (PCR) methodology. A Southern blot is a membrane in which restriction-enzyme-digested DNA is immobilized from a patient. To study the gene of interest, a single-stranded DNA probe must be labeled and hybridized to the blot to detect deletions or insertions. Since Southern blots require more DNA and more laboratory time and resources, usually they are used only for diseases in which deletions are common. The PCR generates a large number of copies of the DNA fragment of interest. so it can be studied without the need for a labeled DNA probe. Gel electrophoresis and DNA sequencing of the PCR product will identify the precise nucleotide change present.

Although often detectable by Southern blot analysis, deletions generally comprise only about 10 percent of all gene mutations. Some notable exceptions include steroid sulfatase deficiency (90 percent are due to whole-gene deletions), Duchenne muscular dystrophy (DMD; 60 percent have deletions of the dystrophin gene), and cystic fibrosis (CF; 60 to 70 percent have a three-base-pair deletion). The deletions of steroid sulfatase deficiency may be detected by Southern blot analysis, whereas the smaller deletions of DMD and CF may be detected using PCR techniques.

Point mutations comprise the largest percentage of gene mutations in human disease. The effect of the point mutation depends on the type of mutation. A missense mutation is present if the point mutation changes an amino acid, but it may or may not affect protein function depending on the location or the type of amino acid change. Proof that missense mutations cause the phenotype of a particular disease generally requires that the mutation be studied in an in vitro assay system to determine if it affects protein function. Nonsense mutations occur when the mutation introduces a translation termination codon so that the resulting protein is truncated and dysfunctional. Three codons (TGA, TAG, and TAA in DNA) signify the termination of translation in the ribosomes. If a wild-type TAC is mutated to a TAA, a stop codon will be produced at that particular codon, and translation will not proceed beyond that point. Frameshift mutations are deletions or insertions of bases that are not an exact multiple of three, so the genetic code is altered beyond the mutation. Amino acids downstream will be changed completely, and the probability of a premature stop codon is markedly increased. A silent mutation occurs when the point mutation does not change the amino acid. Occasionally, silent mutations can affect transcription and cause human disease. In addition, nonsense and missense mutations may have detrimental effects on expression similar to splice-site (exon-intron junction) mutations.

Point mutations may be similar in all affected individuals (as in sickle cell anemia), but this is exceedingly rare. The norm is exemplified by β-thalassemia, in which a number of point mutations, usually unique to particular families, are present. In addition, ethnic background affects the prevalence of certain mutations. For example, in Tay-Sachs disease (TSD), three mutations comprise more than 90 percent of all identified mutations in the hexosaminidase A gene in Ashkenazi Jews. However, in non-Jewish individuals, these three mutations account for only about 20 percent of mutations causing this disorder.

Another more recently recognized type of mutation is triplet-repeat expansion. Some genes normally have a certain number of repeated copies of three bases that do not result in an abnormal phenotype. However, when these repeats increase in number beyond a certain threshold, presumably by expansion in germ cells or during early postmitotic events, a disease phenotype results. An example relevant to reproductive endocrinologists is the fragile X syndrome, an X-linked dominant disease with reduced penetrance that consists of mental retardation, macroorchidism, and somewhat subtle facial features (enlarged jaw and ears). Females may have premature ovarian failure (see below). The *FMR1* gene located at a fragile site on the X chromosome (Xq27) normally contains 5 to 50 repeats of a CGG triplet-repeat sequence. Carrier females possess an increased number of triplet repeats called a *premutation* (50 to 200 repeats). These carrier females are more likely to have an expansion of the triplet repeat (>200 and often >1000 repeats), and when this occurs, fragile X syndrome results in males. Many other diseases are caused by the expansion of triplet-repeat sequences, including Huntington disease, Friedreich ataxia, myotonic dystrophy, and Kennedy disease.

Identification of triplet-repeat expansion mutations explains a feature of autosomal diseases termed *anticipation*. Anticipation refers to the observation that disease severity increases through successive generations. An example is a woman with mild myotonic dystrophy (mild facial weakness) who has a child with severe congenital myotonic dystrophy who dies of severe heart disease. In general, as the number of triplet repeats increases, the more severe the phenotype is in subsequent generations.

► ETHNIC-SPECIFIC GENETIC DISEASES

As mentioned earlier, certain ethnic groups have increased risks for specific genetic disorders: (1) African origin: sickle cell anemia and thalassemia; (2) Mediterranean origin: thalassemias; (3) French-Canadian origin: Tay-Sachs disease; (4) English/Irish, South American, and Northern China origin: NTDs; (5) Caucasian: CF; and (6) Ashkenazi Jewish origin: Tay-Sachs disease, Canavan disease, Gauche-disease, and CF. All these diseases are autosomal recessive except NTDs, which usually are multifactorial. Screening tests are available and may be offered for each of these diseases. Universal screening for CF has now become part of daily practice and is done by screening for the 25 most common mutations in the *CFTR* gene (see below).

A complete blood count (CBC) and hemoglobin screen can be used to screen for sickle cell anemia and both α- and β-thalassemia. A hemoglobin electrophoresis will detect sickle protein due to the point mutation in the β-globin gene, and it also will detect additional clinically significant variant β-globin molecules, including hemoglobin C. The normal adult hemoglobin consists of both hemoglobin A (about 98 percent) and hemoglobin A2 (2 to 3 percent). Thalassemia causes a microcytic anemia, so a mean corpuscular volume (MCV) of less than 80 cubic micrometers could indicate a carrier for α- or β-thalassemia. If the hemoglobin A2 is increased (>3.5 percent), the patient could be a carrier for β-thalassemia. If the hemoglobin electrophoresis is normal but the patient has microcytic indices that are not due to iron deficiency, the diagnosis of α-thalassemia should be considered. This is typically performed by demonstration of α-globin gene deletions by molecular genetic methods.

The diagnosis of other ethnic-specific diseases is accomplished by either biochemical or molecular methods. Tay-Sachs disease usually is screened for by using a serum test for hexosaminidase A (cultured white blood cells are needed if the patient is pregnant or taking oral contraceptives).[7] In uncertain instances, DNA testing also can be performed for Tay-Sachs disease. For Ashkenazi Jewish individuals, a "Jewish panel" consisting of Tay-Sachs disease, Canavan disease, Gauche-disease, and CF may be done, usually by molecular methods (dot-blot hybridization to allele-specific probes testing for the most common mutations).

Cystic Fibrosis Screening

CF is the most common autosomal recessive disorder in Caucasians, occurring in 1 in 2500 to 1 in 3300 liveborns. Mutations in the CF transmembrane regulator *(CFTR)* gene on 7q31 cause thick mucus secretions in the lungs, digestive system, reproductive tract, and sweat glands. Pulmonary disease is the most significant cause of death, resulting in a mean survival rarely exceeding 30 years of age. About 85 percent of CF patients also have pancreatic insufficiency, and other manifestations include chronic sinusitis, nasal polyps, pancreatitis, liver disease, and congenital bilateral absence of the vas deferens (CBAVD).[8]

The American College of Medical Genetics (ACMG) and the American College of Obstetricians and Gynecologists (ACOG) recently began recommending that a broader screening of CF be offered.[9] Previously, CF screening was offered to patients with a family history or an affected partner. However, both the ACOG and the ACMG stated that all pregnant women and all women attempting pregnancy should have screening made available to identify potential carriers.[9] Practically speaking, this amounts to discussing CF with every patient seen as part of an infertility evaluation. Screening may be sequential (test one partner and then the other if positive), or both members of the couple may be tested simultaneously (possible results are positive/positive, positive/negative, and negative/negative). If both partners are carriers, then there is a 25 percent risk of an affected child with each pregnancy.

Of special interest to the reproductive endocrinologist are patients with CBAVD who should be assumed to have CF until proven otherwise, and screening both the male with CBAVD and his partner is essential. Universal screening, as proposed by the ACOG and the ACMG, should circumvent this problem because everyone should be offered screening. However, since not all couples may elect to have screening, the reproductive endocrinologist must make certain that the couple in which a male has CBAVD gets screened or be able to counsel the patient if they decline to be tested. Even though the male with CBAVD may not have pulmonary disease, his progeny may develop CF. The genetics of CBAVD is discussed further below.

Although more than 1000 different mutations have been detected in the 230-kb, 27-exon *CFTR* gene, recommended screening for CF is by DNA analysis of 25 panethnic mutations, each with a frequency of at least 0.1 percent in the U.S. population[8,9] (Fig. 5-1). The ΔF508 is by far the most common *CFTR* mutation in Caucasians with CF, accounting for 60 to 70 percent. The mutations are included in the panel if they are known to cause CF regardless of whether the disease is mild or severe. The methods are PCR-based using allele-specific oligonucleotide methodology, which is usually automated in most laboratories. It should be noted that offering screening for additional mutations (an extended mutation panel) currently provides no increase in the detection rate of CF and is not recommended. Since the mutations included in the panel must have a prevalence of 0.1 percent in the U.S. population, any of the additional mutations will have a frequency less than this.[8,9]

Some benign variants that do not cause CF can result in false-positive results with some laboratory methods. When certain mutations are identified in the homozygous state (ΔF508

Deletions	Missense	Nonsense	Splice mutants
ΔF508	R117H	R553X	3120+1G→A
ΔI507	G85E	R1162X	621+1G→T
2184delA	R334W	G542X	3849+10kbC→T
3659delC	G551D	W1282X	2789+5G→A
1078delT	R347P		1717-1G→A
	I148T		1898+1G→A
	N1303K		711+1G→T
	A455E		
	R560T		

Figure 5-1 The recommended mutation panel of 25 *CFTR* mutations for CF is shown, based on the category of mutations (deletions, missense, nonsense, and splicing).

or ΔI507) in a potential carrier and hence should not be homozygous, then the laboratory should know to test for F508C (a true CF allele), as well as for I506V and I507V, which are benign asymptomatic variants. Likewise, if R177H is detected, the laboratory then should test for 5T/7T/9T (see CBAVD below). These are called *reflex tests*—they are done only in the presence of specific mutations and are not meant to be run as part of the initial CF screening panel.[8,9] Laboratory testing should be done by approved laboratories testing for the 25 mutations (see Fig. 5-1). The report should include the patient's ethnicity, indication, mutations tested, and the method of testing. If the test is positive, the laboratory should recommend that the partner be tested, and if negative, it should provide an estimate of the residual risk (i.e., the risk for CF that remains considering that not all *CFTR* mutations can be detected with the screening panel used in the carrier). Baseline carrier rates are 1 in 29 for European Caucasians and 1 in 65 for African Americans. CF testing is a high-complexity laboratory procedure, and quality assurance guidelines have been published by the ACMG, College of American Pathologists (CAP), and NIH-DOE Task Force on Genetic Testing.[9]

There are some specific problems that occur with CBAVD (see below), but it is important to remember that it is not the intention of CF screening to screen for CBAVD.[15,16] Any uncertainties in analyzing the report should prompt the clinician to refer the couple to a geneticist. Additionally, each of the following should be referred to a genetics center for testing and counseling: positive/negative couples wanting additional information, those with a family history of CF, otherwise healthy males with CBAVD mutations (unless the reproductive endocrinology and infertility (REI) physician is comfortable interpreting and explaining the data), and positive/positive couples regarding risks, prognosis, and options.[16]

► CHROMOSOMAL ABNORMALITIES

Mitosis/Meiosis: An Overview

A brief review of mitosis and meiosis is important to grasp an understanding of chromosomal abnormalities that may occur in reproductive endocrine patients. Mitosis is the process by which somatic cells, which contain the diploid ($2n$) number of chromosomes, replicate their DNA to the tetraploid ($4n$) complement and then divide into two identical daughter cells, each containing the diploid number of chromosomes. Prior to entering mitosis, the nuclear genome first replicates its DNA, proceeding through five stages: prophase, prometaphase, metaphase, anaphase, and telophase. Each daughter cell will represent an exact copy of the parent cell.

Germ cells contain the haploid ($1n$) number of chromosomes, and they must retain their haploid number prior to fertilization or chromosomal abnormalities will result. Meiosis is composed of two different divisions, meiosis I and meiosis II. Germ cells pass through meiosis I (the reduction division), during which the diploid number of chromosomes is reduced to the haploid number, and then into meiosis II, which occurs without intervening DNA replication. Similar to mitosis, DNA replication occurs prior to the initiation of meiosis, and the process is similar between the two types of replication. However, prophase in meiosis is much more complicated than in mitosis and has a number of additional stages (leptotene, zygotene, pachytene, diplotene, and diakinesis). In prophase I, recombination (or crossing over) occurs between homologous chromosomes, permitting genetic diversity. Meiosis II is similar to mitosis, except that the haploid number of chromosomes is present such that each daughter cell will have the haploid number of chromosomes. In contrast to mitosis, daughter cells in meiosis are not identical because recombination has occurred.

It is important to recognize that sex-specific differences in meiosis occur in male and female gametes. Primary oocytes in the fetus are arrested in a suspended state in the dictyotene stage of prophase I of meiosis I occurring at midgestation and do not resume the process of meiosis I until the dominant follicle is stimulated by gonadotropins in the mature adult. Meiosis I is completed with the luteinizing hormone (LH) surge, at which time the oocyte enters meiosis II. Meiosis is not completed until fertilization occurs. In meiosis I in the female, one primary oocyte yields a secondary oocyte and the first polar body. In meiosis II, the secondary oocyte results in an ovum and the second polar body. In contrast, in the male, spermatozoa do not form until after puberty, and each primary spermatocyte in meiosis I produces two secondary spermatocytes. In meiosis II, each secondary spermatocyte forms two spermatids, which later differentiate into mature spermatozoa.

Meiotic and Mitotic Errors

Meiotic errors result in aneuploid offspring. If nondisjunction (failure of a pair of homologous chromosomes to separate) occurs, one daughter cell will have 22 chromosomes, which, if that cell is fertilized, will cause monosomy in the embryo. The other daughter cell will have 24 chromosomes, causing trisomy. If one chromosome is not released from the spindle (anaphase lag) and is lost, monosomy also may occur with fertilization of that germ cell. The possibility of nondisjunction increases with advancing maternal age, which then increases the probability of trisomies (see below). Although it varies for each particular chromosome, in general, meiosis I errors in the female account for most of the trisomies that are seen in the clinical setting. If nondisjunction occurs in mitosis, two different cell lines (mosaicism) may arise in the individual. This may occur in patients with gonadal dysgenesis, in which nondisjunction in the 47,XXY zygote could

produce a 45,X/47,XXY cell line (all three cell lines could be present depending on how late in gonadal dysgenesis mitosis nondisjunction occurred). If anaphase lag occurs in a 46,XY individual, 45,X/46,XY mosaicism could result.

Indications for Karyotype

Advanced Maternal Age

An increased risk of chromosomally abnormal offspring is well known to be associated with advancing maternal age, notably trisomy 21, 18, and 13. Sex chromosome abnormalities 47,XXY (Klinefelter syndrome) and 47,XXX also are associated with advanced maternal age. It is also extremely important to determine if there is a family history of chromosomal abnormalities because they may increase the age-related risks. If the couple has had a prior trisomic fetus, the recurrence risk approximates 1 percent. In addition, miscarriage rates increase with advancing maternal age, with a 10 to 15 percent risk for a woman in her 20s, which increases gradually to approach 30 to 40 percent by age 40. Most of the increase in miscarriage rates with advancing maternal age is the result of an increasing incidence of chromosomal abnormalities in the fetus (see below).

In contrast to advanced maternal age, advanced paternal age does not appear to carry an increased risk of trisomy. However, the collective risk for autosomal dominant diseases such as Marfan syndrome, neurofibromatosis, achondroplasia, and Apert syndrome is increased. In addition, there is an increased risk of X-linked recessive diseases (including hemophilia A and B, Duchenne muscular dystrophy, and others) in maternal grandsons when the grandfather was at advanced age when his daughter was conceived (the so-called grandfather effect). However, the risk for any individual disease is small in the absence of a positive family history, which makes screening for advanced paternal age impractical.

Spontaneous Abortion and Recurrent Abortion

It is well known that about one-half of first trimester losses have chromosomal abnormalities, a rate that decreases with advancing pregnancy: 40 percent at 12 to 15 weeks, 20 percent at 16 to 19 weeks, 12 percent at 20 to 23 weeks, 8 percent at 24 to 28 weeks, 5 percent at more than 28 weeks, and about 0.5 percent at term. It must be emphasized that the distribution of chromosomal abnormalities in recurrent aborters cannot be assumed to be the same as that in women who have had a spontaneous abortion. It is possible that recurrent euploidy, recurrent aneuploidy, or even mixed euploidy/aneuploidy could occur, unfortunately, in patients having repeated losses. There is no large study examining successive abortions from a large group of patients with recurrent abortion. Boue and colleagues[10] karyotyped 1500 spontaneous abortions and suggested that recurrent aneuploidy is unlikely to be common in couples with recurrent abortion because repeated aneuploidy may occur by chance alone. When couples with a previous chromosomally abnormal abortion conceive, there does not appear to be an increased risk for another chromosomally abnormal abortion, suggesting that recurrent aneuploidy is uncommon.[11] Both of these large studies suffer from ascertainment bias because the samples were obtained from those submitted to a cytogenetics laboratory. Needed is a comprehensive prospective study of multiple abortuses from the same women with recurrent pregnancy losses.

Couples with recurrent abortion are at increased risk for either of two types of translocations, robertsonian and reciprocal, each of which may be balanced or unbalanced. A *balanced* translocation is one in which the individual has an apparently normal phenotype, which indicates that little or no chromosomal material was lost. An *unbalanced* translocation results in detrimental phenotypic effects, which often include mental retardation and a variety of somatic anomalies.

Robertsonian translocations involve the acrocentric chromosomes (those with very small short arms), numbers 13 to 15, 21, and 22. In a robertsonian translocation, the long arms from two different chromosomes join, and presumably the short arms are absent (Fig. 5-2). Individuals with a balanced robertsonian translocation have 45 chromosomes. Individuals with an unbalanced robertsonian translocation have 46 chromosomes, and therefore, they have trisomy for the particular translocated chromosome (i.e., trisomic for the long arm). If the partial trisomy involves chromosome 21, the Down syndrome phenotype is observed. Since 3 to 4 percent of all Down syndrome patients (95 percent have trisomy 21) may have an unbalanced translocation, performing a karyotype on the affected in-

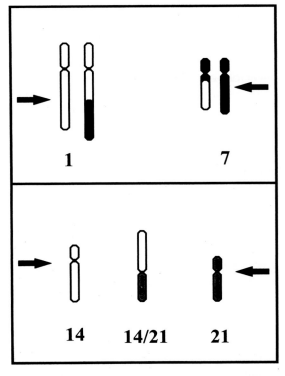

Figure 5-2 A balanced reciprocal translocation involving chromosomes 1 and 7 is shown in the top. A balanced robertsonian translocation involving chromosomes 14 and 21 is shown on the bottom.

dividual is important in counseling the couple for recurrence risks.

A reciprocal translocation results when two different chromosomes break and exchange material (see Fig. 5-2). Individuals with a balanced reciprocal translocation possess 46 chromosomes, whereas those with an unbalanced translocation have deletions/duplications. Since translocations are expected to result in a mixed history of normal children, miscarriages, and abnormal liveborns, chromosomal analysis should be considered particularly for these families.

With recurrent pregnancy loss, defined as two or more losses or one loss and a malformed fetus, approximately 4 percent of either member of the couple will carry a balanced translocation. This is approximately a 10-fold to 30-fold increase over the prevalence in couples without recurrent pregnancy loss.[12] If a balanced translocation is present, there is an increased risk of a chromosomally abnormal liveborn, which depends on the translocation but can be estimated. If the translocation is the more common reciprocal translocation (about two-thirds of those identified in recurrent aborters), the risk of an abnormal liveborn is usually similar for most translocations whether the man or the woman carries the translocation and ranges from 5 to 20 percent. However, if the translocation is robertsonian and involves chromosome 21, the risk is greater if the woman carries the translocation. If the mother carries the robertsonian translocation, the risk for having a child with Down syndrome is 10 to 15 percent, whereas if the father carries it, the risk ranges from 0 to 2 percent. For other robertsonian translocations that do not involve chromosome 21, the risks to offspring are much less. A 13;14 translocation is the most common robertsonian translocation, and the risk for trisomy 13 is low.

Several investigators have reported skewed X inactivation more commonly in women with recurrent abortion than in controls.[13,14] Normally X inactivation is random, but it appears that highly skewed X inactivation (>90 percent preferential inactivation) occurs more commonly in women with recurrent abortion (~15 percent) versus controls (~5 percent). If this occurs, it would be expected that there would be preferential inactivation of the mutant allele and lethality to males that inherit the mutant allele. These hypotheses remain controversial because not all investigators have found an increased risk of skewed X inactivation in women with recurrent abortion.

Premature Ovarian Failure

When a reproductive-age woman presents with primary amenorrhea and elevated gonadotropins, a karyotype is indicated regardless of age. More than 50 percent of these women will have chromosomal abnormalities, most notably a 46,XY (Swyer syndrome) or 45,X cell line (Turner syndrome).[15] The presence of a Y cell line in this setting confers a high risk of germ cell tumor (20 to 25 percent for women with Swyer syndrome and 15 percent for women with 45,X/46,XY karyotype). Patients with a 45,X cell line, either singly or in mosaic forms, present most commonly with short stature (<63 inches if a Y cell line and usually <60 inches without a Y cell line), and 90 to 95 percent have no secondary sex characteristics. Cardiac (50 percent of patients) and renal (30 percent) anomalies also occur in women with a 45,X cell line. Cardiac anomalies include coarctation of the aorta, biscuspid aortic valve, and aortic dilatation. Instances of ruptured aortas have been reported in women with Turner syndrome who conceived through donor-egg IVF. Patients with Swyer syndrome (46,XY gonadal dysgenesis) have normal stature, absent breast development, and streak gonads. Since the testis is nonfunctional, no antimüllerian hormone (AMH) is produced, and a normal vagina and uterus are present.

For women with secondary amenorrhea and gonadal failure, the probability of a chromosomal abnormality is markedly less.[15] However, certain clinical features indicate the possibility of a chromosomal abnormality. Patients measuring <63 inches should be considered for a karyotype because they could be one of the 5 to 10 percent of patients with Turner syndrome who have had normal puberty and menses. In addition, deletions of the X chromosome, usually of the long arm,[16] may be inherited by daughters, which may increase their risk of premature ovarian failure. Most of these women are <63 inches tall. Women with premature ovarian failure and 46,XX on karyotyping have an increased risk of being a carrier for fragile X syndrome (see "Genetics Basis of Human Infertility" below).

If all males with elevated gonadotropins are karyotyped, approximately 10 to 15 percent will have a chromosome abnormality, with 47,XXY and 46,XX being the most common defects.[15] Males with Klinefelter syndrome (47,XXY) have some pubertal development, which may be arrested rather than absent. Testosterone is typically low or low normal, gonadotropins are elevated, and small, fibrotic testes are present. Males with Klinefelter syndrome are at increased risk for diabetes, testicular tumors, and breast cancer, so increased surveillance for these disorders is indicated. 46,XX males also have hypergonadotropic hypogonadism and are phenotypic males because the sex-determining region of the Y chromosome (SRY) on Yp has translocated to the X chromosome in male meiosis I. Since Yq is absent in these males, they lack the putative spermatogenesis genes and are azoospermic.

A karyotype is usually not necessary in men or women with idiopathic hypogonadotropic hypogonadism (IHH) unless multiple congenital anomalies are present or there is suspicion for Prader-Willi syndrome (deletion 15q11-q13).[15]

Severe Oligospermia/Azoospermia

A karyotype should be considered for men with severe oligospermia or azoospermia because several percent may have chromosomal abnormalities, principally translocations.[15] Although they are unlikely to be the cause of the severe oligospermia/azoospermia, there is the potential risk for pregnancy losses if conception occurs and, of greater concern, liveborns with congenital anomalies. Y chromosome deletion analysis also could be considered for males with sperm counts <5 million/mL (see Cystic Fibrosis Testing for Congenital Bilateral Absence of the Vas Deferens under "Genetic Basis of Human Infertility"). Occasionally, a 47,XXY karyotype will be observed in severe oligospermic males with normal puberty and normal gonadotropins.

Multiple Congenital Anomalies

Patients with multiple congenital anomalies and mental deficiency often have chromosome abnormalities, and a karyotype is indicated in these patients. In addition to trisomies, partial deletions of autosomes (including 18q- or 13q-) could be present.

▶ GENETIC BASIS OF HUMAN INFERTILITY

The molecular basis for human infertility remains largely unknown. Most of the known human gene mutations cause both absent or impaired pubertal development and subsequent infertility[17] (Table 5-1). This is in contrast to the patients seen in practice, who have had normal pubertal development. Currently, it is not practical to test clinically for most of the described genetic causes of infertility. However, several mutations deserve specific mention because of their importance in daily practice.

Cystic Fibrosis Testing for Congenital Bilateral Absence of the Vas Deferens

Congenital bilateral absence of the vas deferens (CBAVD) occurs in about 1 to 2 percent of infertile men. Most investigators have demonstrated that about three-quarters of men with CBAVD have mutations or disease-associated variations in the *CFTR* gene.[18,19] The principal risk for these men and their partners is having a child with classic CF. Both members of the

►**TABLE 5-1:** GENE DEFECTS CAUSING HUMAN INFERTILITY

	Gene	Chromsome	Disease	Inheritance
I. Hypothalamus	*KAL1*	Xp22.32	Kallmann syndrome	XLR
	NROB1	Xp21.3	AHC/IHH	XLR
	LEP	7q31.3	Leptin deficiency/IHH	AR
	LEPR	1p31	Leptin resistance/IHH	AR
	KAL2 (FGFR1)	8p11.2-p11.1	Kallmann syndrome	AD
II. Pituitary	*NROB1*	Xp21.3	AHC/IHH	XLR
	GNRHR	4q21.2	GnRH resistance/IHH	AR
	FSHB	11p13	Isolated FSH deficiency	AR
	LHB	19q13.3	Isolated LH deficiency	AR
	PROP1	5q35.2	Combined pituitary defic.	AR
	HESX1	3p21.2-p21.1	Septo-optic dysplasia	AR, AD
	LHX3	9q34.3	Combined pituitary defic.	AR
III. Gonad Y chromosome	*SRY*	Yp11.3	Swyer syndrome	YL
	USP9Y	Yq11.2	Severe oligo-/azoospermia	YL
	DBY	Yq11.2	Severe oligo-/azoospermia	YL
	DAZ	Yq11	Severe oligo-/azoospermia	YL
	RBMY	Yq11	Severe oligo-/azoospermia	YL
X chromosome	45,X		Turner syndrome	Sporadic
	POF1	Xq26-28	Premature ovarian failure	Sporadic or XLD
	POF2	Xq22	See DIAPH2	?
	DIAPH2	Xq22	Disrupted in 1 case of POF	?
	FMR1	Xq27	Fragile X syndrome	XLD
Autosomal	*LHR*	2p21	LH resistance	AR
	FSHR	2p21-p16	FSH resistance	AR
	HSD17B3	9q22	17-Ketosteroid reductase deficiency	AR
	SRD5A2	2p23	5a-Reductase type II deficiency	AR
	CYP21A2	6p21.3	CAH: 21-OH deficiency	AR
	CYP17	10q24.3	CAH: 17-OH deficiency	AR
	STAR	8p11.2	Congenital lipoid hyperplasia	AR
	CYP19	15q21.1	Aromatase deficiency	AR
	CYP11A1	15q23-q24	Congenital lipoid hyperplasia	AD
	HSD3B2	1p13.1	CAH: Type II 3β-HSD deficiency	AR
	AIRE	21q22.3	APECED	AR, AD
	NR5A1	9q33	Undermasculinization	AD
	WT1	11p13	Frasier and Denys-Drash syndrome	AD
	SOX9	17q24.3-q25.1	Sex reversal; campomelic dysplasia	AD
	AMH	19p13.3	Persistent müllerian ducts	AR
	AMHR2	12q13	Persistent müllerian ducts	AR
	DNAH5	5p15-p14	Primary ciliary dyskinesia; Kartagener syndrome	AR
	DHH	12q13.1	Gonadal dysgenesis with minifascicular neuropathy	AR
IV. Outflow obstruction	CFTR	7q31-q32	CBAVD—cystic fibrosis	AR
	AR	Xq11.2-q12	Androgen insensitivity	XLR

Abbreviations: AD = autosomal dominant; AHC = adrenal hypoplasia congenita; APECED = autoimmune polyendocrinopathy-candidiasis-ectodermal dystrophy; AR = autosomal recessive; CBAVD = congenital bilateral absence of the vas deferens; DIAPH2 = Diaphenous 2; FSH = follicle stimulating hormone; GnRH = gonadotropin releasing hormone; 3β-HSD = 3β-hydroxysteroid dehydrogenase; IHH = idiopathic hypogonadotropic hypogonadism; LH = luteinizing hormone; 17-OH = 17-hydroxylase (CYP17); 21-OH = 21-hydroxylase (CYP21); XLD = X-linked dominant; XLR = X-linked recessive; YL = Y-linked.

couple should be screened for *CFTR* mutations, and appropriate counseling should be performed. If both are carriers, there is a 25 percent risk of having a child with CF depending on the mutation. Even if the male has only one CF mutation and the female is not found to be a carrier, it is better to be cautious and refer them to a geneticist for counseling. About 20 percent of men with CBAVD have renal anomalies, and in one study, no CF mutations were found in this group of patients, although the number of mutations tested was small.[20]

When universal screening for CF began in 2001, it was already recognized that population screening would reveal some alleles that may cause CBAVD.[8,9] It must be emphasized that the purpose of the population screening is to identify CF, not CBAVD. The genetics of CBAVD is extremely complicated, making counseling difficult.[8,9] In the original reports, no CBAVD patients had homozygosity for the ΔF508 mutation, the most common *CFTR* mutation, occurring in 60 to 70 percent of patients with classic CF. About 20 percent of men with CBAVD have two of the *CFTR* mutations found in CF patients, many of which are missense (genotypes of severe/mild or mild/mild alleles). There is also an intron 8 mutation in which the number of T's can either be 5, 7, or 9 on each allele (designated as 5T/7T/9T). When the 5T allele is present, exon skipping of exon 9 occurs, making the mRNA smaller, which would then truncate the protein (Fig. 5-3). The most common genotype in men with CBAVD is compound heterozygosity for a CF mutation on one allele and 5T on the other allele (~30 percent of affected patients).

The R117H mutation in the population screening panel is included because it can cause CF if present in combination with other more severe *CFTR* mutations.[8,9] If the R117H is found, a reflex test is done for the 5T/7T/9T allele (Fig. 5-4). If a 5T allele is observed, the parents should be tested to see if it is on the same allele as R117H (in cis) or on the other allele (trans). This is so because a 5T cis to R117H is a CF allele such that if the female car-

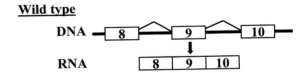

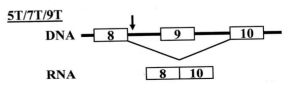

Figure 5-3 The effect of the 5T/7T/9T *CFTR* allele in intron 8 is shown. The wild type *(above)* is shown—only exons 8 to 10 are shown of the gene, which are then copied into mRNA (which also includes exons 8, 9, and 10). An arrow *(below)* marks the position of the polymorphism. If the 5T allele is present, exon 9 will be excluded from the mRNA (exon skipping).

ries a CF mutation, there will be a 25 percent risk of CF in the offspring.[8,9] The complexity of the genetics of CF is made obvious by the varying phenotypes seen with homozygosity for the 5T allele, which can cause either no symptoms, CBAVD, or rarely, a mild CF phenotype. The presence of a 5T allele decreases mRNA stability, and it is known that if the level is 1 to 3 percent, classic CF will be present.[18]

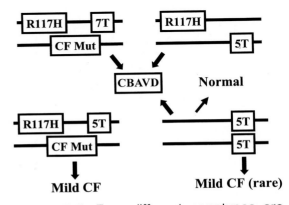

Figure 5-4 Four different genotypes are shown that may cause CBAVD. See text for discussion.

If the level of mRNA is more than 8 to 12 percent, there is no phenotype, and if the levels are intermediate, the phenotype could range from no symptoms, to CBAVD, to mild CF. It also should be noted that congenital unilateral absence of the vas deferens (CUAVD) also may be a milder form of CF. The 5T allele is present in approximately 5 percent of the general population, 25 percent in males with CAUVD, and 40 percent of males with CBAVD.[18]

The recommendations from the ACMG and the ACOG are to screen only for the 25 mutations with a frequency of at least 0.1 percent in the U.S. population and to use the 5T/7T/9T as a reflex test.[9] However, in practice, many laboratories can reduce costs by running it in the primary test and, as shown earlier, can cause tremendous complexity in interpretation.[8] It should be remembered that the primary goal of universal screening is to detect CF, not CBAVD.

Spermatogenesis Genes

Putative spermatogenesis genes on the Y chromosome (Fig. 5-5) have been mapped to the azoospermia factor (AZF) region on Yq11 (SRY is on the Yp arm). From proximal to distal are AZFa, AZFb, and AZFc. In AZFa, spermatogenesis genes include *USP9Y* (ubiquitin-specific protease 9 on the Y chromosome) and *DBY* (dead box Y). In AZFb, the *RBMY* gene complex (RNA-binding motif on the Y chromosome) are located, and in AZFc, the *DAZ* (deleted in azoospermia) genes reside.[21] *DAZ* was the first spermatogenesis gene to be characterized.[22]

Several of the spermatogenesis genes are multicopy genes, whereas others are single-copy genes. There appear to be four to six copies of the *DAZ* gene and about 20 to 50 *RBMY* genes/pseudogenes.[21] Both *DBY* and *USP9Y* are single-copy genes. There has been tremendous difficulty in dissecting out the important regions of the Y chromosome involved in spermatogenesis because of the large number of repeated sequences and the variation in

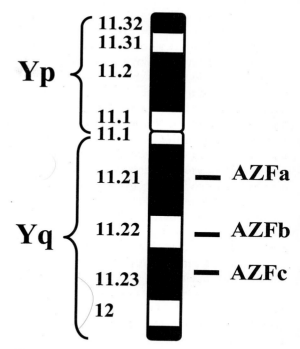

Figure 5-5 The Y chromosome is shown, along with the locations of the AZF regions (a–c). The short (p) arm and the long (q) arm are indicated, along with the chromosomal bands.

study design. For example, deletions of the AZF regions of Yq largely have been determined by studying sequence-tagged sites (STSs), which are simply markers for specific chromosomal regions. The more STSs that are studied, the higher is the likelihood of finding deletions. In general, deletions of the AZF regions tend to occur more frequently in infertile males, but they have been reported occasionally in fertile males.

Proof that the AZF region contains genes for spermatogenesis arose from demonstration of an intragenic mutation in the *USP9Y* gene, also known as *DFFRY* (*Drosophila* fat facets–related, Y-linked because of its homology to the corresponding gene in *Drosophila*).[23] A de novo four-base-pair deletion was identified in an infertile male that was absent in his fertile brother. These clinical findings and in vitro analysis suggested that the *USP9Y* mutation caused the spermatogenic failure. In a reanalysis of a previously published study, these investigators also identified another single-gene deletion of *USP9Y* associated with spermatogenic failure.

A review of the nearly 5000 infertile males screened for Y chromosome mutations in the literature indicated that approximately 8.2 percent of infertile males and 0.4 percent of fertile males have deletions of one or more AZF regions.[21] However, the specific prevalences ranged from 1 to 35 percent in individual studies. In this review, AZFc deletions were the most common (60 percent), followed by AZFb (16 percent) and AZFa (5 percent). In the remainder, deletions of more than one of the regions were present (most commonly involving AZFc). Most mutations were found in men with azoospermia (84 percent) or severe oligospermia (14 percent), defined as less than 5 million sperm per milliliter.[21] Interpretation of the AZF deletion data was extremely challenging because (1) deletions were identified in both infertile and fertile males, (2) multigene clusters of *DAZ* and *RBM* complicate the analysis, (3) different clinical phenotypes (i.e., sperm parameters) were studied, (4) there was incomplete assembly of Y chromosome contigs due to repeated sequences, and (5) there was a lack of complete data on fertile control males.

Several years ago, a double-blind molecular study was published in which full endocrine parameters and semen analyses were known for 138 consecutive men seen for IVF/ICSI, 100 fertile men, and 107 young Danish men in the military.[24] Of 21 STSs for AZFa to AZFc studied, no deletions were found in men with a normal semen analysis or in any men with a count of more than 1 million/mL. Deletions of AZFc were identified in 17 percent of men with idiopathic azoospermia/cryptoozoospermia (<1 million/mL) and in 7 percent with nonidiopathic azoospermia/cryptoozoospermia.[24] Interestingly, no deletions of AZFa or AZFb were found in any of the men studied, suggesting that the genes in the AZFc region may be the most important for spermatogenesis. A larger, more recent study had similar findings.[25]

It appears reasonable to discuss Y chromosome deletions with couples. The principal risk to offspring appears to be that male progeny could inherit the same deletion of Yq and be infertile, which has been reported.[26] It does not appear that fertilization and pregnancy rates are affected.[25]

Fragile X Syndrome in Women with Premature Ovarian Failure

In sporadic patients with premature ovarian failure, approximately 2 to 3 percent will be carriers of the fragile X permutation allele, whereas in patients with familial premature gonadal failure, approximately 12 to 15 percent will be carriers.[17] Although the fragile site on Xq28 may be detected by karyotype in which the cells are grown in medium deficient in folate, DNA testing is the standard means of diagnosis. Fragile X syndrome is one of the triplet-repeat expansion diseases in which the normal *FMR1* gene CCG repeats increase from the normal of less than 50, to 50 to 200 repeats in fragile X carriers (premutation), and to greater than 200 repeats for affected males (full mutation).[17] Fragile X syndrome is an X-linked dominant disease with reduced penetrance.

Determination of fragile X carrier status is important to establish because other family members could be carriers at risk for having males with the full mutation, i.e., manifesting mental deficiency, abnormal facies, and macroorchidism.

Hypogonadotropic Hypogonadism and Kallmann Syndrome in Males

Males with Kallmann syndrome have anosmia and hypogonadotropic hypogonadism and also may have midline facial defects, unilateral renal agenesis, and neurologic deficits such as synkinesia and oculomotor and cerebellar dysfunction. Kallmann syndrome is an X-linked recessive disorder caused by mutations in the *KAL1* gene, which probably accounts for about 10 to 15 percent of IHH in males with anosmia.[27,28] More recently, an autosomal dominant form of Kallmann syndrome was found to be caused by mutations in the fibroblast growth factor receptor 1 gene (*FGFR1,* also known as *KAL2*).[29] For IHH males without anosmia, mutations in the gonadotropin-releasing hormone receptor *(GnRHR)* gene are the most commonly recognized genetic defect. *GnRHR* mutations account for only 5 to 10 percent of all males with IHH.[30,31]

► PREIMPLANTATION GENETIC DIAGNOSIS

Preimplantation genetic diagnosis (PGD) is an alternative to prenatal diagnosis with the purpose of reducing the risk of severe genetic disease.[32] Preimplantation genetic diagnosis–aneuploid screening (PGD-AS) constitutes a specific application of PGD designed to improve IVF outcome by screening for aneuploidies. To obtain DNA for PGD, three different procedures have been used: polar body, cleavage stage, or blastocyst biopsy.[32]

Polar body diagnosis may be performed on oocytes completing meiosis I, and this is suitable for genetic diagnosis in the female only. The principal disadvantage is that confirmation of the genotype in the embryo will not be possible unless tested for by prenatal diagnosis. Misdiagnosis could result if recombination occurs. Embryo biopsy is the procedure used by most centers and permits genetic diagnosis of disorders affecting both males and females. The biopsy is usually obtained from a cleavage-stage biopsy (eight-cell embryos) removing one to two cells. Because of potential problems with attempting to establish a diagnosis with only a few cells (see below), ideally, more cells could be obtained by a blastocyst biopsy because blastocysts contain up to 300 cells. In addition, a blastocyst biopsy can be taken from the trophectoderm, which is more accessible and will give rise to the embryo proper. However, blastocyst biopsy has not been performed by as many centers because of the difficulty of culturing blastocyst cells and the concern with thawing blastocysts that have been biopsied.[32] These techniques have resulted in pregnancies, and it is likely that results will improve with more time and experience.

Two techniques have been used to analyze the biopsied cells obtained for PGD: PCR and fluorescent in situ hybridization (FISH). Laboratories that perform these procedures should have proper credentialing and report the specific methods used, as well as their interpretation. However, it is extremely important that practicing reproductive endocrinologists understand the uses and limitations of the molecular analysis of cells for PGD.

Polymerase Chain Reaction

The PCR is best suited for detecting gene mutations in single-gene disorders and has been used for sexing embryos, although this latter indication largely has been replaced by FISH.[32] To test for single-gene mutations by PCR, the exact mutation being sought must be known prior to the IVF cycle, and the PCR conditions already must be optimized. It is mandatory that appropriate positive and negative controls be included with each PCR, or the results cannot be trusted. Laboratory problems may be encountered, including (1) failed amplification, (2) sample contamination, and (3) allele dropout, and the potential for these must be appreciated by the reproductive endocrinologist. In addition, many programs perform intracytoplasmic sperm injection (ICSI) any time PGD using PCR is planned because it is possible that additional sperm embedded in the zona could result in misdiagnosis.[32]

Because of the small amount of starting DNA template available for PGD, usually several picograms, instead of the several hundred nanograms normally used for PCR studies, an increased number of PCR amplification cycles is necessary. In single-cell (or several-cell) PCR, 35 to 60 cycles are often necessary, an increase over the typically 30 cycles used for standard PCR (when the sample is not the limiting factor). An alternative is to use nested or heminested primers in two different PCRs to gain specific amplification of small amounts of template (Fig. 5-6). More recently, the sensitivity of single-cell PCR has been enhanced about 1000-fold using fluorescent-labeled primers that require shorter cycling times.[32]

Contamination is minimized by meticulous technique and the use of a negative control (i.e., a tube containing all reagents except for DNA). If the negative control reveals amplification, suggesting contamination with foreign DNA, then amplification of the other samples cannot be trusted. Since shorter cycling times may be used with fluorescent PCR, the likelihood for contamination is reduced.

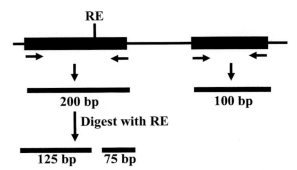

Figure 5-7 A multiplex PCR method is shown whereby one polymorphic fragment is amplified and then digested with a restriction enzyme (RE), yielding two different-sized products. Also included in the same reaction tube is a second PCR, which defines the DNA fragment of interest. See text.

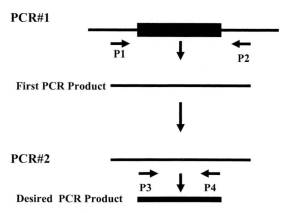

Figure 5-6 Nested PCR is shown. In the first reaction, primers P1 and P2 amplify a fragment that is then amplified in a second PCR using two primers (P3 and P4) that are internal (nested) to the original primers. The PCR product from the second PCR yields the desired fragment.

Allele dropout refers to the preferential amplification of only one allele, with little or no amplification of the other allele. Although problematic for the detection of both autosomal dominant and recessive disorders, as might be expected, this is more significant with the evaluation of autosomal dominant disorders. If an incorrect diagnosis occurs in an autosomal dominant condition, it could result in the placement of an abnormal embryo if the unamplified allele contains the mutation. To circumvent this problem, simultaneous amplification of another nearby polymorphic fragment (multiplex PCR) may be performed (Fig. 5-7). As mentioned earlier, fluorescent PCR also will increase the sensitivity of single-cell PCR.[32]

The diagnostic accuracy of PCR and FISH for PGD has been examined by bodies such as the European Society for Human Reproduction (ESHRE) PGD Consortium.[16] In data from 1999–2001, there were 5 PCR misdiagnoses of mendelian disorders from 81 (6.2 percent) patients who had post-PGD prenatal or postnatal diagnoses. Only about half of all patients having PGD had any confirmatory testing.[16] Additionally, consideration must be given for those in whom a biopsy could not be obtained and for those in whom a diagnosis was not possible (see below).

Fluorescent in Situ Hybridization (FISH)

FISH involves the fluorescent labeling of a single-stranded probe and hybridization to denatured DNA from a metaphase spread, individual cells, or tissue. FISH has a number of potential uses in PGD, which include (1) sexing embryos in X-linked disorders when no PCR test is available for gene diagnosis, (2) chromosome translocations, (3) numerical chromosome abnormalities, and (4) other chromosome abnormalities, as in PGD-AS.[32]

Procedural problems with FISH may occur with numerical counting when testing for aneuploidy.[32] When using FISH with single interphase cells, it is very difficult to be certain of the number of signals (therefore chromosomes) when only one cell is being examined. If only one signal is seen in FISH, this could be due to monosomy for that particular chromosome or, alternatively, due to signal overlap or the failure of hybridization of one of the chromosomes. Similarly, more than two signals could be due to trisomy but also could be due to technical problems of signal splitting or anomalous fluorescence. To improve diagnostic capability, the simultaneous use of at least three probes, one each for the X and Y chromosomes and an autosome such as chromosome 18, may be used. However, each laboratory must perform rigorous quality controls to maximize diagnostic accuracy because it is known that if 100 normal diploid cells are examined, there will not be 100 pairs of signals for each chromosome. Hence the diagnostic capability will be improved when more cells can be analyzed.

FISH-based methods for detecting translocations usually involve probes that flank or span the translocation. Since polar bodies just after egg retrieval have condensed metaphase chromosomes, chromosome painting probes may be used in combination with centromeric (α-satellite repeats) and locus-specific probes. Unfortunately, these probes are not useful for cleavage-stage or blastocyst-stage cells because the chromosomes may not be in metaphase and are not as condensed. Another method uses subtelomeric probes that are specific for the translocated chromosomes, along with a centromeric probe to a chromosome region proximal to the breakpoints. Subtelomeric and proximal probes permit the identification of unbalanced translocations in interphase cells but cannot distinguish between noncarriers or balanced translocations.[32,33]

In the ESHRE PGD Consortium report, the results on 8 of 145 (5.5 percent) patients undergoing PGD with FISH and who had a subsequent prenatal or antenatal diagnostic procedure were incorrect.[16] FISH misdiagnoses included two trisomies, one mosaic trisomy, one monosomy, and one balanced and one unbalanced translocation. In addition, a misdiagnosis of a trisomy 21 occurred during aneuploidy screening.[16] As with PCR, correct confirmation of the FISH diagnosis was performed in less than half those women who had undergone PGD.

Currently, the role of FISH in the detection of translocations is unclear because 50 to 70 percent of embryos formed from balanced reciprocal translocation carriers will be unbalanced.[32] Reported success rates vary, but data from three large centers indicate a clinical pregnancy rate of 29 percent per retrieval.[32] Other authors report that they were able to reduce the risk of miscarriage by using PGD[33]; however, it is unclear whether PGD results in improved liveborn rates compared with normal conception without intervention because more than half of embryos will be abnormal and may be selected against naturally. Even though PGD-AS has been performed in a large number of IVF cycles, a clear increase in the rate of liveborn pregnancies has yet to be demonstrated in any of the randomized, prospective studies published to date. Hence, since IVF with PGD is invasive and expensive, it will be important to delineate its precise role in clinical medicine.[32]

ESHRE PGD Consortium

Interpreting the results of PGD using PCR and FISH remains problematic in clinical practice. Of 1197 cycles reported by the ESHRE PGD Consortium from 1999–2001, about 6 percent of PCR diagnoses and 5.5 percent of FSH diagnoses were found to be incorrect when either prenatal or postnatal confirmatory procedures were performed.[16] It also must be remembered that less than half these patients had any confirmatory test, so the misdiagnosis rate may be underestimated. However, these data do not mean that 94 percent of all patients received the proper diagnosis. In the ESHRE PGD Consortium, the overall clinical pregnancy rate was 17 percent per egg retrieval, a biopsy was successful in 97 percent, and the diagnosis could be obtained in only 86 percent of cases.[16] Overall, this amounts to a correct diagnosis in about 85 percent of all patients who underwent PGD. Patients who wish to consider PGD should be counseled that about 15 percent of the time the correct diagnosis will not be able to be reached.

► CONCLUSIONS

An understanding of genetics is now required for every practicing reproductive endocrinologist. The health care professional should assess the family history and background risk for genetic disease in the patient or couple attempting pregnancy prior to treatment. Assessing rubella immunity, discussing folic acid supplementation and background birth defect rates, and universal screening for CF should be provided for patients. Indications for karyotype and genetic screening based on ethnic factors also should be reviewed. If PGD is being entertained, a thoughtful, thorough discussion should occur between the physician and the couple. By considering the genetic aspects of infertility, the couple will have a better understanding and more realistic expectations about their fertility treatment.

KEY POINTS

1. It is extremely important to ascertain genetic risk prior to couples/individuals seeking fertility treatment, including a discussion of folic acid supplementation and rubella immunity.

2. A karyotype should be considered in a variety of clinical situations, including gonadal failure, multiple congenital anomalies, mental retardation, recurrent abortion, and severe oligospermia/azoospermia.

3. The risk for ethnic-specific diseases should be ascertained from the history so that testing can be offered prior to pregnancy.

4. Men with azoospermia should be considered to have congenital bilateral absence of the vas deferens (CBAVD), a mild allelic form of CF, until proven otherwise.

5. CF screening should be discussed with couples/individuals undergoing an infertility evaluation. The clinician should understand the mutation panel and how to counsel patients who are carriers.

6. The clinician should understand that preimplantation genetic diagnosis by FISH or PCR has certain pitfalls that currently limit its widespread use.

REFERENCES

1. Rubella and pregnancy (ACOG Technical Bulletin Number 171, August 1992). *Int J Gynaecol Obstet* 1993;42:60–66.
2. Reef SE, Frey TK, Theall K, et al. The changing epidemiology of rubella in the 1990s: On the verge of elimination and new challenges for control and prevention. *JAMA* 2002;287:464.
3. Revised ACIP recommendation for avoiding pregnancy after receiving a rubella-containing vaccine. *MMWR Morb Mortal Wkly Rep* 2001; 50:1117.
4. Botto LD, Moore CA, Khoury MJ, et al. Neural tube defects. *N Engl J Med* 1999;341:1509–1519.
5. Van Steirteghem A, Bonduelle M, Devroey P,

et al. Follow-up of children born after ICSI. *Hum Reprod Update* 2002;8:111–116.

6. DeBaun MR, Niemitz EL, Feinberg AP. Association of in vitro fertilization with Beckwith-Wiedemann syndrome and epigenetic alterations of LIT1 and H19. *Am J Hum Genet* 2003;72:156–160.

7. Screening for Tay-Sachs disease. American College of Obstetricians and Gynecologists Committee Opinion on Genetic Screening for Hemoglobinopathies Number 162, November 1995 (replaces Number 93, March 1991), Committee on Genetics, 1995.

8. Richards CS, Bradley LA, Amos J, et al. Standards and guidelines for CFTR mutation testing. *Genet Med* 2002;4:379–391.

9. Grody WW, Cutting GR, Klinger KW, et al. Laboratory standards and guidelines for population-based cystic fibrosis carrier screening. *Genet Med* 2001;3:149–154.

10. Boue J, Bou A, Lazar P. Retrospective and prospective epidemiological studies of 1500 karyotyped spontaneous human abortions. *Teratology* 1975;12:11–26.

11. Warburton D, Kline J, Stein Z, et al. Does the karyotype of a spontaneous abortion predict the karyotype of a subsequent abortion? Evidence from 273 women with two karyotyped spontaneous abortions. *Am J Hum Genet* 1987; 41:465–483.

12. Fryns JP, Van Buggenhout G. Structural chromosome rearrangements in couples with recurrent fetal wastage. *Eur J Obstet Gynecol Reprod Biol* 1998;81:171–176.

13. Sangha KK, Stephenson MD, Brown CJ, et al. Extremely skewed X-chromosome inactivation is increased in women with recurrent spontaneous abortion. *Am J Hum Genet* 1999;65: 913–917.

14. Lanasa MC, Hogge WA, Kubik C, et al. Highly skewed X-chromosome inactivation is associated with idiopathic recurrent spontaneous abortion. *Am J Hum Genet* 1999;65:252–254.

15. Layman LC, Reindollar RH. The genetics of hypogonadism. *Infertil Reprod Med Clin North Am* 1994;5:53–68.

16. ESHRE Preimplantation Genetic Diagnosis Consortium. Data collection III (May 2001). *Hum Reprod* 2002;17:233–246.

17. Layman LC. Genetic causes of human infertility. *Endocr Metab Clin North Am* 2003;32: 549–572.

18. Chillon M, Casals T, Mercier B, et al. Mutations in the cystic fibrosis gene in patients with congenital absence of the vas deferens. *N Engl J Med* 1995;332:1475–1480.

19. Dork T, Dworniczak B, Aulehla-Scholz C, et al. Distinct spectrum of CFTR gene mutations in congenital absence of vas deferens. *Hum Genet* 1997;100:365–377.

20. Augarten A, Yahav Y, Kerem BS, et al. Congenital bilateral absence of vas deferens in the absence of cystic fibrosis. *Lancet* 1994;344: 1473–1474.

21. Foresta C, Moro E, Ferlin A. Y chromosome microdeletions and alterations of spermatogenesis. *Endocrol Rev* 2001;22:226–239.

22. Reijo R, Lee T-Y, Salo P, et al. Diverse spermatogenic defects in humans caused by Y chromosome deletions encompassing a novel RNA-binding protein gene. *Nature Genet* 1995;10: 1290–1293.

23. Sun C, Skaletsky H, Birren B, et al. An azoospermic man with a de novo point mutation in the Y-chromosomal gene USP9Y. *Nature Genet* 1999;23:429–432.

24. Krausz C, Rajpert-de Meyts EW, Frydelund-Larsen L, et al. Double-blind Y chromosome microdeletion analysis in men with known sperm parameters and reproductive hormone profiles:microdeletions are specific for spermatogenic failure. *J Clin Endocrinol Metab* 2001;86:2638–2642.

25. Peterlin B, Kunej T, Sinkovec J, et al. Screening for Y chromosome microdeletions in 226 Slovenian subfertile men. *Hum Reprod* 2002; 17:17–24.

26. Komori S, Kato H, Kobayashi S, et al. Transmission of Y chromosomal microdeletions from father to son through intracytoplasmic sperm injection. *J Hum Genet* 2002;47:465–468.

27. Franco B, Guioli S, Pragliola A, et al. A gene deleted in Kallmann's syndrome shares homology with neural cell adhesion and axonal pathfinding molecules. *Nature* 1991;353:529–536.

28. Legouis R, Hardelin J, Levilliers J, et al. The candidate gene for the X-linked Kallmann syndrome encodes a protein related to adhesion molecules. *Cell* 1991;67:423–435.

29. Dode C, Levilliers J, Dupont JM, et al. Loss-of-function mutations in FGFR1 cause autosomal dominant Kallmann syndrome. *Nature Genet* 2003;33:463–465.

30. Layman LC, Cohen DP, Jin M, et al. Mutations in the gonadotropin-releasing hormone receptor gene cause hypogonadotropic hypogonadism. *Nature Genet* 1998;18:14–15.

31. Beranova M, Oliveira LM, Bedecarrats GY, et al. Prevalence, phenotypic spectrum, and modes of inheritance of gonadotropin-releasing hormone receptor mutations in idiopathic hypogonadotropic hypogonadism. *J Clin Endocrinol Metab* 2001;86:1580–1588.

32. Braude P, Pickering S, Flinter F, et al. Preimplantation genetic diagnosis. *Nature Rev Genet* 2002;3:941–953.

33. Munne S, Sandalinas M, Escudero T, et al. Outcome of preimplantation genetic diagnosis of translocations. *Fertil Steril* 2000;73:1209–1218.

CHAPTER 6

Endocrinology of Pregnancy

C. RICHARD PARKER, JR.

The consequences of pregnancy on the maternal endocrine milieu are substantial. Most of the changes have been clearly linked to either maintenance of the uterine environment in a state that is favorable for continuance of the pregnancy or modification of maternal homeostasis to ensure proper nutritional support for the developing fetus and preparation for lactation after delivery. Most, if not all, of the endocrine changes in the pregnant woman are directly attributable to hormonal signals emanating from the fetoplacental unit. Unquestionably, estrogens and progesterone are among the most important hormones for implantation and pregnancy maintenance in humans and other species, and many endocrine changes during pregnancy are a consequence of the altered production of estrogen and progesterone.

▶ ESTROGEN/PROGESTIN PRODUCTION IN PREGNANCY

Whereas pregnancy maintenance in later pregnancy (8 weeks to term) is independent of the ovary[1] and is achieved via estrogen and progesterone production in the fetoplacental unit, early pregnancy depends on hormonal interactions between the trophoblast and ovary for maintenance of estrogen and progesterone production. Thus pregnancies with deficient or absent ovarian function should be supplemented with exogenous progesterone (and possibly for up to the first 10 to 12 weeks of gestation); 1 to 2 mg estradiol and 50 to 100 mg progesterone daily have proved successful in pregnancies achieved through assisted reproduction techniques with donor eggs.[2,3]

In contrast to the expected decline in maternal serum levels of estrogens, progesterone, and 17-hydroxyprogesterone (17-OHP) that usually occurs 10 to 12 days after ovulation in the infertile ovarian cycle (Fig. 6-1), with fertilization and implantation, production of these steroids is maintained and increased somewhat for the first 6 to 8 weeks of pregnancy (Fig. 6-2) by the corpus luteum under the influence of human chorionic gonadotropin (hCG) produced in the trophoblast (detailed elsewhere). The demise of the steroidogenic capacity of the corpus luteum of pregnancy occurs at about 8 to 10 weeks of gestation and is heralded by a reduction in maternal serum levels of hCG and of 17-OHP but no decline in serum levels of progesterone. For the duration of pregnancy, maternal serum levels of progesterone and estrogens are maintained by de novo placental progesterone formation, possibly under the influence of hCG, and by placental aromatization of estrogen precursors provided by the maternal and fetal adrenal cortices.[4] The patterns of maternal serum progesterone and estrogens

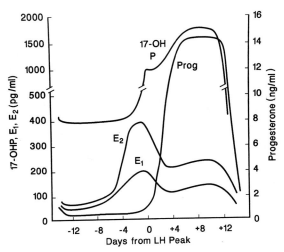

Figure 6-1 Serum levels of estrone (E₁), estradiol (E₂), 17-hydroxyprogesterone (17-OHP), and progesterone (P) in women during the ovulatory cycle. Data are presented in relation to the timing of the LH surge. *(Adapted from Carr BR, Parker CR Jr, Madden JD, et al. J Clin Endocrinol Metab 1979;49:346, and unpublished studies by the author.)*

(estrone, estradiol, and estriol) throughout the latter two-thirds of normal pregnancy are shown in Figure 6-3.

Whereas the placenta is capable of producing progesterone somewhat autonomously, the placenta is an incomplete endocrine tissue with respect to estrogen production[5] primarily as a consequence of lacking 17-hydroxylase/17,20-desmolase activities that are essential for conversion of pregnenolone or progesterone (C₂₁ steroids) into androgens (C₁₉ steroids). Consequently, placental estrogen production ultimately depends on the rate of adrenal steroidogenesis of both mother and fetus. The interactions among maternal, fetal, and placental compartments in estrogen and progesterone formation are illustrated in Figure 6-4.

Progesterone

Trophoblastic tissue usually has very low capacity for de novo cholesterol biosynthesis.[6]

Thus, as indicated earlier, progesterone normally is produced in the placenta (as it is in the corpus luteum) from cholesterol contained in low-density lipoprotein (LDL).[7,8] In steroidogenic tissues of humans and several other species, circulating LDL is assimilated via the classic LDL receptor pathway, which then provides the cholesterol in such lipoprotein particles for use by the cells for substrate in steroid formation and probably other purposes as well. Usually, maternal LDL is present in high quantities, and thus abundant substrate is available to the placenta, which also has an abundance of LDL receptors.[9] However, in circumstances of absent or negligible maternal serum LDL, placental progesterone formation may be compromised. For example, in a case of hypobetalipoproteinemia, the abnormally low, yet still substantial, quantities of progesterone produced[10] likely were achieved by a compensatory increase in de novo cholesterol synthesis in the placenta or use of fetal LDL and/or maternal high-density lipoprotein (HDL). Neither fetal well-being nor the status of estrogen production in pregnancy appears to be important to the orderly formation of progesterone in the trophoblast. Thus progesterone production is not attenuated by fetal anencephaly,[11] which gives rise to impaired fetal estrogen precursor production[12] or, at least acutely, fetal demise.[13] Indeed, progesterone production is striking in molar pregnancies and choriocarcinoma.[14]

In addition to serving to prepare the uterus for implantation, progesterone also appears to serve other functions once pregnancy is established. Progesterone appears to be important in maintaining uterine quiescence during pregnancy by actions on uterine smooth muscle.[15] Progesterone also can be inhibitory to uterine prostaglandin production,[16] which otherwise would promote uterine contractions and cervical ripening. The high local concentration of progesterone probably contributes to the immunologically privileged status of the pregnant uterus.[17] Also, progesterone plays an important role in remodeling the cellular architecture and

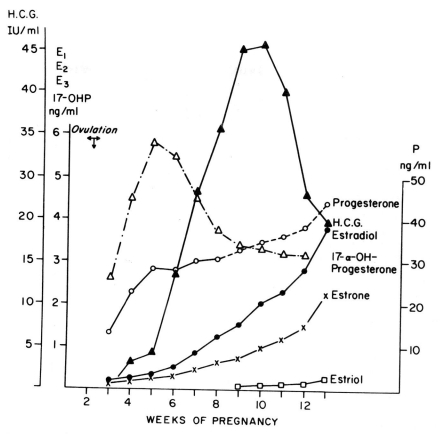

Figure 6-2   Serum levels of estrogens, pro-gestins, and hCG in women during the first trimester of pregnancy.   *(Reproduced, with permission, from Tulchinsky D, Hobel CJ. Am J Obstet Gynecol 1973;17:884.)*

secretory activity of the lining of the cervix to create a barrier to the penetration of pathogens into the uterus. Although it has been proposed that progesterone may serve as an important substrate for production of glucocorticoids in the fetal adrenal, such a role seems unlikely because the fetal adrenal has an exceptionally high rate of LDL cholesterol uptake, a high rate of de novo cholesterol biosynthesis, and the ability to produce prodigious quantities of cortisol in cell culture in the absence of added proges-terone.[18] Moreover, despite the finding that adrenal tissue of anencephalic fetuses contains, on a weight-adjusted basis, normal levels of steroidogenic enzymes and enzyme mRNA[19] and

essentially normal rates of placental progesterone formation in such circumstances, umbilical cord serum levels of glucocorticoids and mineralo-corticoids in anencephalics are subnormal.[11,20,21]

Estrogens

The high rate of estrogen production in human pregnancy is unparalleled in the mammalian kingdom. Urinary estriol excretion at term is about 1000-fold higher than in nonpregnant women.[22] In nonpregnant premenopausal women, serum levels of estrone and estradiol range from 0.05 to 0.4 ng/mL, whereas estriol

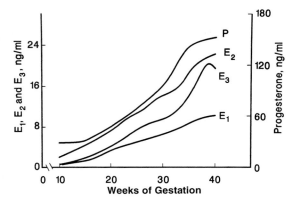

Figure 6-3 Serum levels of estrone (E₁), estradiol (E₂), estriol (E₃), and progesterone (P) in women during the second and third trimesters of normal pregnancy. *(Adapted from Parker CP Jr, Illingworth DP, Bissonnette J, Carr BP. N Engl J Med 1986;314:557, and unpublished studies by the author.)*

is virtually undetectable (<0.01 ng/mL). During pregnancy, however, serum levels of estrone and estradiol rise from 0.5 to 1 ng/mL in the first few weeks of pregnancy, when they are derived from the corpus luteum, to 10 to 30 ng/mL at term,[23] being produced primarily in the placenta from maternal and fetal adrenal precursor dehydroepiandrosterone sulfate (DS). Although maternal and fetal adrenals contribute about equally to maternal serum estrone and estradiol, the fetal adrenal, by means of 16-hydroxylation of DS in fetal liver, is the source of about 90 percent of estriol produced in pregnancy.[4]

In addition to the discordant contribution of maternal and fetal precursors to placental estrogen formation, the three major estrogens appear to be released into maternal and fetal blood differentially. Whereas estradiol is released in greater proportion into maternal blood, estrone is preferentially released into

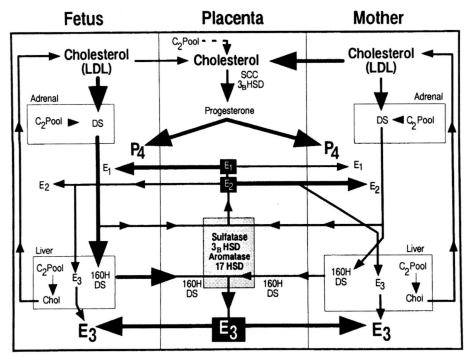

Figure 6-4 Relative contributions of the fetal, placental, and maternal compartments to estrogen and progesterone production in human pregnancy.

the umbilical vessels in humans.[24,25] The differences in fetal and maternal serum levels of estrogens and progesterone are shown in Table 6-1.

As can be seen, whereas estradiol is the predominant unconjugated estrogen in maternal serum, estriol predominates in the fetus. The estrone-estradiol ratio in maternal serum is approximately 0.5, and that in umbilical cord serum is about 2.0. Although the serum concentrations of estrone and estradiol may vary significantly from individual to individual, the ratios just noted for fetal and maternal sera are reasonably consistent in normal pregnancies at both term and midgestation. Another estrogen, estetrol, which is the 15α-hydroxylated derivative of estriol, also is present in maternal plasma; this unique estrogen appears to derive solely from fetal precursors.[26]

Since maternal estrogens, especially estriol (E₃) and estetrol, largely are derived from fetal precursors, it was once thought that monitoring of maternal serum or urinary estrogens might provide a means of assessing fetal well-being. Although such an approach was based on sound theoretical grounds and low or declining estrogen levels often correctly identified fetuses whose statuses were deteriorating, such a prognostic device has been found largely to be impractical, even in medical centers equipped to provide rapid turnaround of test results. This is due to the findings that maternal serum levels of estriol vary substantially over the course of a day[27] and that maternal serum estrogen levels can be increased artificially, despite fetal jeopardy, in women having renal disease.[28] Apart from a deteriorating intrauterine environment, there are several other circumstances in which there are low levels of estrogens in maternal serum and urine. Any developmental defect in which fetal adrenal function is compromised, e.g., anencephaly or congenital absence of adrenal, will be associated with markedly low levels of maternal estrogens, particularly estriol. Also, adrenal suppression due to glucocorticoid treatment leads to low maternal estrogen levels. Antibiotics that affect gastrointestinal flora and thus impair hydrolysis of biliary estrogen conjugates can lead to reduced urinary estrogen levels without necessarily altering estrogen levels in maternal serum. Estrogen levels are severely reduced in cases of placental sulfatase deficiency.[29] In this X-linked syndrome, which primarily affects males and has a frequency of 1 in 2000 to 6000 pregnancies, there is inability of the placenta to hydrolyze the sulfate moiety from DS or 16-OH-DS, which is required prior to conversion to estrogens. Many pregnancies affected by this disorder proceed beyond term, are resistant to labor induction, and require cesarean section.[29] A past history of postterm pregnancies, cesarean sections, and ichthyosis in relatives should be sufficient to lead the physician to perform antenatal testing. Low levels of maternal serum or urinary estrogens, increased DS and low estrogen levels in amniotic fluid, and failure of maternal estrogen levels to rise appropriately after a bolus intravenous injection of DS are predictive of the disorder.[29] Although there is merit to studies that use estrogen measurements in investigating the biochemistry and physiology of normal and abnormal pregnancy, estrogen measurements purely for assessment of fetal well-being seem to be a poor substitute for other modern monitoring techniques.

In addition to the causes mentioned of hypoestrogenism in pregnancy, another cause of estrogen deficiency in pregnancy has been

▶**TABLE 6-1:** CONCENTRATIONS OF UNCONJUGATED ESTROGENS AND PROGESTERONE IN MATERNAL VENOUS AND UMBILICAL CORD SERA AT TERM

	E₁	E₂	E₃	P
Maternal	10–13	18–24	16–20	100–140
Fetal	10–15	6–7	90–115	500–1000

Hormone values are in ng/mL and are representative of the range of mean values obtained in various published and unpublished studies of the author. Abbreviations: E₁, estrone; E₂, estradiol; E₃, estriol; P, progesterone.

described recently—placental aromatase deficiency due to mutations in the fetal aromatase gene (reviewed in ref. 30). Unlike the situations in which estrogen production is reduced due to diminished fetal adrenal DS production or to an inability to cleave the sulfate moiety of DS or 16-OH-DS, fetal aromatase deficiency is likely associated with high rates of adrenal androgen production and placental sulfatase activity as occurs normally. In such circumstances, the failure of the placenta to convert the substantial supply of maternally and fetally derived adrenal androgens into estrogens instead gives rise to accentuated conversion of such precutsors into more potent androgens. Consequently, this rare disorder has been found to be associated with maternal virilization during the latter half of pregnancy and masculinization of affected female fetuses in utero. Sexual differentiation in utero of an affected male was apparently normal.

Whereas human pregnancy is uniquely characterized by the massive levels of estrogen produced, the exact roles of estrogen in pregnancy are unclear. Based on the observations that pregnancies with marked estrogen deficiency, as in those complicated by fetal anencephaly or placental sulfatase deficiency, often proceed substantially beyond term,[29] it seems likely that estrogens are important in the timely onset of parturition. A definitive role in this process for estrogen, however, is not established in humans. The stimulatory effects of estrogen on phospholipid synthesis and turnover, prostaglandin production, and enhanced formation of lysosomes in the uterine endometrium, as well as estrogen modulation of adrenergic mechanisms in uterine myometrium, may be means whereby estrogen acts in the timing of labor onset.[31] Estrogens also stimulate uterine blood flow,[32] which is clearly important in maintaining a favorable intrauterine environment. Estrogens also are important in preparing the breast for lactation.[33] There also is evidence that estrogen plays a role in fetal development and organ maturation, such as, along with other substances, increasing the capacity for fetal lung surfactant production.[34]

▶ PLACENTAL PROTEIN/PEPTIDE HORMONES

Human Chorionic Gonadotropin

Human chorionic gonadotropin (hCG) is a glycoprotein having a molecular mass of approximately 38,000 Da. It is structurally related to the pituitary hormones luteinizing hormone (LH), follicle-stimulating hormone (FSH), and thyroid-stimulating hormone (TSH), being composed of two non-covalently-linked subunits, α and β, that are encoded by two separate mRNAs.[35,36] The α subunit of hCG contains 92 amino acids, has a mass of 16,000 Da, and is virtually identical to that of LH, FSH, and TSH. The β subunit of hCG, which confers biologic specificity to the molecule by virtue of containing the bulk of the determinants required for binding to cell surface receptors,[37] has a molecular mass of 23,000 Da and shares considerable sequence homology with LHβ, which is somewhat smaller. A family of eight genes on chromosome 19 codes for the β subunits of hCG and LH—one for LH and seven for hCG, of which only two or three are actively expressed.[36,38] The unique sequence of the extended C-terminal portion of β-hCG confers immunologic specificity to hCG, allowing it to be quantified in radioimmunoassays (RIAs) distinct from LH when antisera against the hCG β subunit are used. Because of the extensive glycosylation of hCG, this hormone has a long half-life in the circulation[39] and is thus preferable to LH when administered to stimulate the gonads in vivo.

Although it was proposed initially to derive from the cytotrophoblast, intact hCG is now recognized to be produced primarily by syncytiotrophoblastic cells.[43] hCG is produced by all types of trophoblastic tissues, including those from hydatidiform mole, chorioadenoma destruens (invasive mole), and choriocarcinoma, even those not associated with recent pregnancy.[41] Although excess free hCGβ appears to be produced in the first few weeks of gestation,[42,43] thereafter the α subunit is produced in excess of the β subunit, and the α:β-subunit ratio appears to increase with advancing gestation.[42] Thus most hCG in the circulation during most of pregnancy is either intact hCG or free hCGα, with little, if any, hCGβ present in serum.

The most widely recognized roles of hCG are: (1) stimulating the corpus luteum to produce progesterone, estrogens, and relaxin[44] and (2) maintaining corpus luteum life span beyond the normal 10 to 14 days.[45] A role for hCG in placental steroidogenesis is controversial. hCG appears to be responsible for early masculinization of male fetuses by virtue of stimulating testosterone secretion by the fetal testis[46]; a role of hCG in ovarian development is not established. Subsequent fetal gonadal stimulation probably is achieved by fetal pituitary LH and FSH, the plasma concentrations of which are not maximal until 20 to 25 weeks and then decline thereafter.[47] The studies of several investigators are suggestive that hCG also is immunosuppressive and that the high local concentrations of hCG (perhaps in concert with progesterone) in the placenta may be important in preventing the rejection of the fetal allograft by the maternal host.[48] The direct immunosuppressive actions of hCG, however, have been the subject of continuing debate since highly purified hCG was found by some investigators to be without activity in this regard.[49]

Placental production of hCG appears to be autonomous of extraplacental influences. Production of hCG in vitro has been found to be augmented by cyclic AMP,[50] epidermal growth factor,[51] and the LH-releasing factor gonadotropin-releasing hormone (GnRH).[52] It is feasible that GnRH, produced in cytotrophoblast,[52] is the trophic stimulus to hCG production in neighboring syncytiotrophoblast. Maximal placental concentrations of GnRH occur at the time of maximal hCG production and then decline after 20 weeks of gestation. It also is possible that the increasing production of placental progesterone and/or estrogens acts via a negative-feedback mechanism

to reduce placental hCG production at the end of the first trimester.[53] Such an arrangement is analogous to GnRH regulation of pituitary LH production.

Detectable amounts of hCG are produced as early as 6 days after ovulation,[43,54] and with implantation, there is a dramatic and progressive rise in maternal serum hCG levels (Fig. 6-5). During the first 4 to 5 weeks of pregnancy, serum hCG levels double each 1.3 to 2.0 days,[54,55] achieving maximal levels of 10,000 to 100,000 mIU/mL [first international reference preparation (IRP)] at 8 to 10 weeks of pregnancy, which then decline to 10,000 to 20,000 mIU/mL by 20 weeks and remain reasonably stable throughout the remainder of pregnancy.[100] The serum concentration of hCG at the time of the first expected menses after ovulation ranges from 50 to 250 mIU/mL.[54]

The clinical utility of hCG measurement is based on the finding that deviation from normal levels early in pregnancy can be diagnostic of several disorders. In cases of suspected ectopic pregnancy, hCG analysis can establish the presence or absence of pregnancy and, if values are abnormally low and fail to rise appropriately, can be diagnostic of ectopic pregnancy in a vast majority of cases.[56] Confirmation of intrauterine pregnancy is now possible at serum hCG titers of about 2000 mIU/mL by use of vaginal ultrasound. hCG measurements can be of utility in predicting the outcome of patients with threatened abortion. Women having first-trimester abortions generally had hCG levels that declined to low levels and/or failed to rise at an appropriate rate.[43,57,58] In addition to serving as a diagnostic aid in gestational trophoblastic disease (values often exceed 200,000 MIU/mL),[58,59] serum hCG levels are extremely useful in monitoring response to therapy. In general, serum hCG should be undetectable (<5 mIU/mL first IRP) within 13 to 15 weeks after evacuation of molar pregnancy.[58,59] Many patients who ultimately will be found to have persistent trophoblastic disease or choriocarcinoma, however, may be identified much earlier based on the failure of their hCG levels to

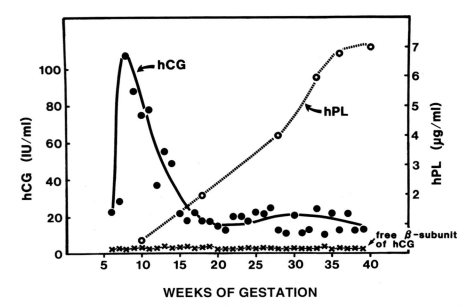

Figure 6-5 Serum levels of hCG and hPL in women during pregnancy. *(Reproduced, with permission, from Pritchard JA, MacDonald PC, Gant NF (eds). Williams' Obstetrics, 17th ed. New York: Appleton-Century-Crofts, 1985:121.)*

decline in an orderly fashion.[60] It has even been proposed that women who develop persistent disease often may be identified at the time of evacuation by virtue of having excessive levels of the free β subunit in relation to total hCG levels in serum.[61]

Recently, a fragment of the β subunit of hCG that consists of residues 6 to 40 disulfide linked to residues 56 to 92 and two N-linked sugar chains lacking sialic acid has been found in urine. High levels of this β-core fragment have been detected in urine of pregnant women and women having trophoblastic disease and certain other cancers.[62,63] Since little, if any, β-core fragment is detectable in serum, it has been assumed that the peptide in urine primarily represents a degradation product of intact hCG or of β subunit that is formed in kidney and possibly other tissues.[64] A recent study in which it has been proposed that serum β-core fragment is masked by associated macromolecules, thus preventing its detection in RIAs,[65] again raises questions about the ori-

gin and pathophysiologic significance of this interesting substance.

Human Chorionic Somatomammotropin

Human chorionic somatomammotropin (hCS), initially termed *human placental lactogen* (hPL), was isolated in the early 1960s from human placenta and found to have lactogenic activities in experimental animals.[66] This single-chain polypeptide contains 191 amino acids and two disulfide bonds and has a molecular mass of approximately 22,000 Da; the amino acid sequence of hCS shares a high degree of homology with growth hormone and somewhat less homology with prolactin.[67] The growth hormone/hCS gene family on chromosome 17 consists of five genes, two coding for hGH and three for hCS, one of which is a pseudogene.[68,69]

hCS appears to be produced exclusively by syncytiotrophoblast cells, suggesting that it is a product of fully differentiated trophoblast.[40] Since the concentration of hCS mRNA in syncytial cells remains relatively constant throughout gestation,[70] the increasing placental content of hCS and the progressive rise in maternal serum hCS levels during gestation appear to be due to increasing numbers of such cells as the trophoblast grows during gestation.[71] Thus serum hCS levels correlate well with placental mass, and due to its short half-life in contrast to that of hCG, hCS would seem to be a potentially useful marker of placental function. hCS is measurable in maternal serum early in pregnancy (although not as early as hCG), and serum levels rise continually thereafter in contrast to those of hCG (see Fig. 6-5). At term, hCS is the most abundant protein secretory product of the placenta; maternal serum levels range from 5 to 15 µg/mL,[71] and about 20 percent of the translatable mRNA in term placenta is that of hCS.[72]

The regulation of synthesis and secretion during pregnancy and the physiologic role of hCS are, for the most part, unclear. Most studies have failed to demonstrate a role of other hormones, neuropeptides, and neurotransmitters as stimulators or inhibitors of hCS production. Placental hCS production, aside from being related to placental mass and viability, may be regulated to a degree by nutritional factors. Thus maternal starvation leads to increased maternal levels of hCS.[73] Regulation of hCS production by nutritional factors seems to fit in with its postulated role in regulating maternal metabolism, particularly of lipid and carbohydrates.[74] hCS has been shown to be lipolytic in humans and other species, to augment insulin release in response to carbohydrate load in humans, and to augment glucose use in adipose tissue. Such actions could serve to ensure adequate energy stores for the mother and glucose for the fetus in states of nutritional deprivation and accentuate establishment of energy stores in the fed state. Whereas hCS has structural homology to growth hormone and prolactin, the growth-promoting and lactogenic activity of this protein appears to be very limited in humans. Since normal pregnancies and well-developed infants have occurred in circumstances of very low to absent hCS (hPL) production due to gene defects,[75] hCS may serve as an evolutionary redundancy for pituitary growth hormone and prolactin rather than a critical element for pregnancy maintenance. It is not known, however, whether the preceding pregnancies would have had good outcomes in the face of nutritional deprivation.

Soon after its initial identification and establishment of hCS as a placental secretory product, numerous studies were conducted in the 1960s and 1970s to determine whether maternal serum hCS (hPL) levels might provide insights into fetoplacental health. The findings of many such studies are summarized in Table 6-2.

A consideration of the above-mentioned findings leads one to the view that maternal serum hCS levels are related primarily to placental size and/or the integrity of the utero/

▶**TABLE 6-2:** RELATION OF MATERNAL hCS LEVELS TO PREGNANCY CONDITIONS

Pregnancy Condition	Maternal Serum hCS (hPL) Levels
Diabetes mellitus	Normal to high, even with IUFD
Rh disease	Normal to high, even with IUFD
Dysmaturity	Often reduced
Multiple gestation	High
Pregnancy-induced	Often low, severity-related hypertension
Fetal distress	Often low if due to causes other than nuchal cords
Late first/second-trimester abortion	Low in most cases after bleeding
Growth retardation	Low
Molar pregnancy	Normal to high

placental vasculature. Consequently, impending fetal demise will not necessarily be heralded by low levels of hCS. On the other hand, low or declining hCS levels often are associated with "placental insufficiency" or disruption in delivery of the peptide to the maternal bloodstream. Such phenomena are now readily recognized by other means of monitoring, suggesting that hCS measurement currently is of marginal utility in the management of obstetric complications. There is, however, much to be learned about the physiologic role of this substance in fetal development and pregnancy homeostasis.

Human Chorionic Thyrotropin

In the late 1960s, a proteinaceous substance that shared several characteristics with pituitary TSH was isolated from human placenta. Despite initial enthusiasm about the potential significance of human chorionic thyrotropin (hCT), subsequent studies have failed to confirm its existence and/or secretion by the placenta.[76] Thus it has been suggested that the mild hyperthyroid state in early pregnancy and in some cases of hydatidiform mole and choriocarcinoma is likely attributable to the weak thyroid-stimulating activity of hCG.[77]

Pro-opiomelanocortin-Related Peptides

The presence of pro-opiomelanocortin (POMC)–derived peptides in human placenta, including corticotropin (ACTH), β-lipotropin, and β-endorphin, was first suggested in the 1970s. Subsequently, the placenta has been confirmed as a site of POMC peptide synthesis and post-translational processing to such end products.[78] The responsiveness of placental POMC peptide production to the corticotropin-releasing hormone (CRH),[79] as well as the presence of locally produced CRH in the placenta,[80,81] is strongly suggestive of a CRH–POMC peptide axis in the placenta. Interestingly, glucocorticoids have been found to stimulate, rather than inhibit, placental CRH formation.[81] Whether placental CRH and POMC peptide products serve autocrine/paracrine roles or traditional hormonal functions in the maternal and/or fetal compartments is an interesting yet unresolved issue at present.[82,83]

Other Placental Proteins and Peptides

As recently reviewed by Petraglia and associates,[84] the human placenta has been found to produce insulin-like growth factors I and II. Moreover, placental protein 12, which was isolated from the placenta and found to be present in maternal and fetal sera and amniotic fluid, is now recognized to be identical to one of the insulin-like growth factor–binding proteins (IGFBPs). Placenta also has been found to contain relaxin, inhibin, and activin, each of which was assumed initially to be derived exclusively from the ovary, as well as transforming growth factors.

As mentioned earlier, placental tissue has been shown to be a site of synthesis of two peptides, GnRH and CRH, that were described initially as hypothalamic peptides that regulated pituitary function. Other biologically active peptides, traditionally thought of as neuropeptides, also are now known to be present (and likely produced) in placental tissue, including a thyrotropin-releasing hormone (TRH)–like substance, β-endorphin, oxytocin, somatostatin, dynorphin, enkephalin, neuropeptide Y, and growth hormone–releasing hormone (GH-RH). The contributions of these substances to the endocrine milieu of the maternal and fetal compartments are not known at present. However, the wide array of such potent substances that are elaborated by the placenta should continue to provide exciting research topics in the future.

Decidual Prolactin

The decidua, which is formed in uterine endometrium in the late luteal phase, even in nonfertile cycles, and comprises the maternal portion of the placenta, has been found to be the site of production of a protein identical to human pituitary prolactin.[85,86] It also now seems clear that the prodigious quantities of immunoreactive prolactin present in amniotic fluid are derived from the decidua rather than from maternal or fetal pituitary glands.[87] The gestational profile of amniotic fluid prolactin differs markedly from that in maternal (and fetal) serum, being highest at midgestation and then declining to lower levels in the latter third of gestation (Fig. 6-6). Nevertheless, amniotic fluid levels of prolactin are still higher than are those in maternal and fetal sera at term. The gestational profile of amniotic fluid prolactin parallels both decidual content in vivo and decidual capacity for synthesis of prolactin in vitro.[87,88] Unlike pituitary prolactin, production of decidual prolactin is not reduced by dopamine or its agonists and is not increased by TRH.[89] The factors that serve to regulate decidual prolactin production in vivo are unresolved. Several lines of experimental evidence are suggestive that decidual prolactin serves to regulate amniotic fluid volume and osmolarity.[90] Despite encouraging results in the rhesus monkey, there seems to be no relation between ammotic fluid prolactin levels and lung maturation in the human.[91]

▶ MATERNAL SERUM SCREENING FOR FETAL ANOMALIES

Although the theoretical basis for such an association is unclear, several investigators have found recently that women pregnant with fetuses having trisomy 21 tend to have increased serum hCG levels in early pregnancy.[92] α-Fetoprotein (AFP) is a globular protein that is produced first by the yolk sac and then in great

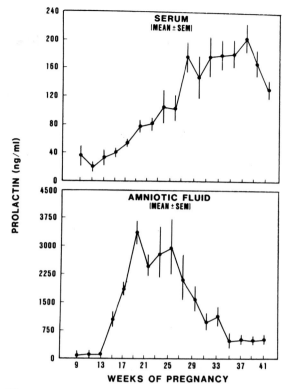

Figure 6-6 Concentration of prolactin in maternal serum and amniotic fluid during human pregnancy. *(Reproduced, with permission, from Kletsky OA, Rossman F, Bertofli SL, et al. Am J Obstet Gynecol 1985;151:878.)*

abundance by the fetal liver during gestation. Under normal circumstances, very little AFP escapes the fetal compartment into maternal serum. In instances of epithelial defects, however, such as with neural tube defects, high maternal serum levels of AFP have been noted, giving rise to the common screening procedures for such anomalies in early gestation. On the other hand, it has been found that decreased concentrations of AFP, cited as multiples of the normal median (MoM) in maternal serum, are often associated with fetal Down syndrome (trisomy 21). Further study of other analytes revealed that maternal levels of certain hormones, notably unconjugated estriol and hCG, also were frequently abnormal in instances of Down syndrome: Estriol was reduced to 0.71 MoM, whereas hCG was increased to 2.11 MoM. This triple screening protocol, usually conducted between 15 and 18 weeks of gestation, can detect approximately 60 percent of fetal Down syndrome cases at a 5 percent screen-positive rate.[92,93] This pattern of AFP, estriol, and hCG levels in Down syndrome is analogous to that expected with a younger gestational age than would be indicated from other obstetric findings. The physiologic mechanism responsible for the apparent "immaturity" of the fetus and the fetoplacental unit in trisomy 21 is unclear. The profiles of serum AFP, estriol, and/or hCG in women bearing fetuses with other abnormalities also have been noted to be altered to varying degrees.[94] In most cases, explanations for the causes of altered production and/or passage of such substances into the maternal compartment are lacking at present.

▶ MATERNAL ENDOCRINE GLANDS

Adrenal

Maternal plasma levels of several adrenal steroids are increased progressively during pregnancy (Fig. 6-7). The increase in cortisol[95,96] is largely attributable to increased levels of corticosteroid binding globulin (CBG). If cortisol production is indeed increased in pregnancy, the stimulus is unclear. Although immunoreactive ACTH levels are higher in late gestation than earlier,[96] such values are lower than or equivalent to ACTH levels in nonpregnant women.[97] The relative contributions of pituitary versus placental ACTH to maternal plasma ACTH during pregnancy are unclear. A similar reduction in ACTH and increased plasma cortisol levels also have been noted to occur in women treated with estrogen/progestin-containing oral contraceptives.[97] Despite the increased serum cortisol levels in pregnant women, clinical evidence of hypercortisolism is rare. Aldosterone production also

is increased in pregnancy in association with increased plasma renin activity and angiotensin II levels.[95] Production of another potent mineralocorticoid, 11-deoxycorticosterone (DOC), also is strikingly increased in pregnancy.[95,98] Rather than deriving from the maternal adrenal, however, the bulk of DOC produced in pregnancy appears to originate from extraadrenal 21-hydroxylation of placental progesterone,[98,99] a process that is mediated by estrogen.[11,13] Maternal serum levels of adrenal androgen, especially DS, decline progressively throughout pregnancy[100] due to markedly increased 16-hydroxylation and placental use of DS and 16-OH-DS in estrogen formation.[4]

Cushing syndrome in pregnancy, which is rare as a consequence of infertility in many affected individuals, is difficult to recognize because many clinical signs, e.g., striae, fluid retention, weight gain, glucose intolerance, and hypertension, are seen frequently in normal pregnant women.[101,102] Laboratory analysis of total and free cortisol, along with ACTH, in plasma will be of assistance in the diagnosis and also will help to identify the site of the defect: adrenal versus pituitary/extrapituitary ACTH excess. Computed tomography (CT) and magnetic resonance imaging (MRI) of the pituitary and adrenal MRI or ultrasonography also are helpful; adrenal CT, however, is not recommended due to the risk of radiation exposure to the fetus. Treatment options are the same as for nonpregnant women, and in the absence of carcinoma as the cause, every attempt should be made to delay therapeutic intervention until after delivery.

Adrenal insufficiency, Addison's disease, also is rare in pregnancy.[102] In individuals affected prior to pregnancy, replacement-therapy requirements may be reduced in pregnancy. Diagnosis of Addison's disease having its onset during pregnancy, like Cushing syndrome, can be difficult due to the similarity of symptoms of pregnancy to those of the disorder, e.g., nausea, vomiting, and lethargy. Diagnosis can be confirmed by cortisol analysis, and treatment is as for nonpregnant women. Supple-

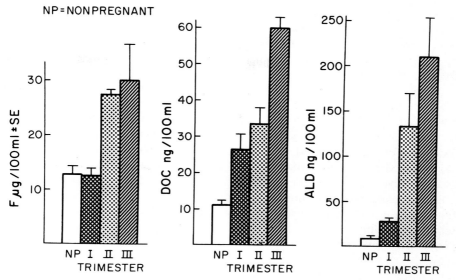

NP = NONPREGNANT

Figure 6-7 Concentration of cortisol (F), deoxycorticosterone (DOC), and aldosterone (ALD) measured sequentially in women during pregnancy and 3 months postpartum (NP). *(Reproduced, with permission, from Nolten WE, Lindheimer MD, Oparil S, Ehrlich EN. Am J Obstet Gynecol 1978;132:414.)*

mental glucocorticold therapy during labor is advisable. Since exogenous glucocorticoids (treatment for Addison's disease) or excess endogenous glucocorticoids (resulting from Cushing syndrome) can lead to suppression of the fetal adrenal, adrenal insufficiency in the neonate is a possible, albeit rare, occurrence.[103]

Thyroid

As with the adrenal, there is biochemical evidence of increased thyroid function during pregnancy; serum levels of thyroxine (T_4) and triiodothyronine (T_3) are increased due to estrogen-induced increases in thyroxine-binding globulin (TBG). On the other hand, free T_3 and T_4 and TSH are not increased in pregnancy, but there is evidence for a transient rise in serum bioactive TSH in early pregnancy that corresponds to the time of maximal serum levels of hGG. Hyperthyroidism, which occurs in about 2 of every 1000 pregnancies, can be due to acute thyroiditis, Graves' disease, toxic goi-

ter, and gestational trophoblastic disease.[104] Since pregnancy in normal individuals is characterized by an increase in metabolic state and slight enlargement of the thyroid gland, diagnosis of mild hyperthyroidism is often difficult. Laboratory analyses of total and free T_3 and T_4, T_3 uptake, and thyroid-stimulating immunoglobulins (TSIs) are usually helpful. Although normally there is little placental transfer of T_4, T_3, or TSH to the fetus,[105] transfer of TSIs to the fetus can cause thyroid disorders in the neonatal period.[106] Therapy for hyperthyroidism in pregnancy includes antithyroid drugs, which must be titrated carefully in view of the potential for affecting the fetal thyroid, and surgery.

Hypothyroidism is rarer in pregnancy than is hyperthyroidism; infertility, early spontaneous abortion, and congenital defects of the fetus are common in hypothyroid women.[107,108] Proper management of hypothyroidism with adequate replacement therapy can prevent abnormalities of pregnancy and fetal development.[107,108] Replacement doses of T_4 are equivalent to or slightly greater than those used in nonpregnant women.[108,108] In diagnosing hypothyroidism in pregnancy, one must be aware that some indices of thyroid function are normally increased in pregnancy.

Parathyroid

Fetal requirements for minerals used in bone formation are substantial, particularly in the third trimester of pregnancy. Consequently, the active transfer of calcium and phosphorus from the maternal compartment to the fetus[109] leads to a progressive lowering of total calcium in maternal plasma.[110] Maternal serum parathyroid hormone (PTH) levels rise during gestation[110,111]; variable responses of calcitonin, however, have been reported during pregnancy.[112] As might be expected, maternal serum levels of 1,26-dihydroxyvitamin D are increased about twofold in term pregnant women compared with those in nonpregnant individuals.[113]

Hypo- and hyperparathyroidism are both rare in pregnant women[114,115] and can be treated as is appropriate for nonpregnant women. Occasionally, fetal and newborn hyperparathyroidism occurs with maternal hypoparathyroidism; the long-term prognosis for most affected infants is good.[116] Maternal hyperparathyroidism is associated with significant risk for spontaneous abortion, stillbirth, and neonatal death.[117]

Pancreas

Pregnancy leads to striking changes in metabolism and maternal adaptations to ensure adequate nutritional support to the fetus. Early in pregnancy, and probably in response to increased estrogen and progestin levels, there is pancreatic β-cell hyperplasia and increased insulin secretion.[118,119] This leads to increased glycogen storage, decreased hepatic glucose production, increased glucose use, and relative hypoglycemia. Later in pregnancy, under the influence of hCS, glucocorticoids, and continued enhancement of insulin production, a relative glucose intolerance and insulin resistance occur.[120] Increased glucagon production also is noted to occur late in pregnancy.[121] These hormonal alterations appear to be essential elements in providing for normal nutrient supply to the developing fetus. Consequently, diabetes mellitus or gestational diabetes can, in the absence of proper management, have devastating effects on fetal development and neonatal outcome.[122]

Anterior Pituitary

As mentioned earlier, maternal plasma levels of TSH are similar in pregnant and nonpregnant women. On the other hand, pituitary production of gonadotropins, LH, and FSH and responsiveness to GnRH are blunted during pregnancy[123] likely as a result of the negative-feedback effect of the massive quantities of estrogens and progesterone produced in pregnancy. Also, as alluded to earlier, maternal plasma levels of ACTH are lower than or similar to those in nonpregnant women.[96,97] There is a tendency for ACTH levels to be lowest in early pregnancy and rise thereafter; substantial increases occur with labor and vaginal delivery.[97] Plasma levels of other POMC peptide–derived peptides, β-endorphin and β-lipotropin also are similar throughout pregnancy to those in nonpregnant women except at the time of labor and delivery, when they clearly are increased.[124,125] The striking increase in POMC peptides that occurs with labor is presumed to be a stress response. Interestingly, several investigators have reported that maternal plasma levels of CRH are higher than in nonpregnant women by the second trimester, rise through term, and then decline rapidly following delivery.[126,127] It is likely that the CRH in pregnancy plasma derives mostly from the placenta; the physiologic role of CRH in maternal plasma is, however, unclear because there is no evidence for major increases in pituitary POMC peptide production in pregnancy except at the time of labor and delivery.

Whereas pituitary production of growth hormone is low in pregnancy,[128] there is hypertrophy and hyperplasia of the lactotrophs in maternal pituitary and progressively increased prolactin production, with plasma levels at term being 10 to 20 times those in nonpregnant women.[129] The pregnancy-associated changes in the lactotrophs likely are due to increased estrogen production in pregnancy.[130] The antepartum increases in prolactin, as well as the maintenance of prolactin production after delivery, appear to be critical for normal lactation.[33] Since estrogen is stimulatory to the lactotroph, there has been concern that prolactinomas in pregnancy may enlarge markedly. In women having such tumors, however, complications during pregnancy have been few.[102] Conservative management with careful observation to detect tumor growth is recommended.

▶ FETAL ENDOCRINOLOGY

The development and unique characteristics of fetal endocrine tissues are intriguing topics of continuing investigation. Some facets of the endocrine milieu of the pregnant woman are determined to a large degree by the activity of fetal endocrine tissues, particularly the fetal adrenal gland. Thus a discussion of the endocrinology of pregnancy would be incomplete without a consideration of fetal endocrinology.

Hypothalamus/Pituitary

The anatomic basis for hypothalamic-pituitary interactions via the hypothalamic-hypophyseal vasculature is established in the developing hu-man by the late first/early second trimester.[131] Moreover, peptide-releasing/inhibiting factors and catecholamines are present in the hypothalamus, and a full array of traditional hormones is present in the anterior/intermediate and posterior lobes of the pituitary early in gestation.[47,132–135] The development of a functionally

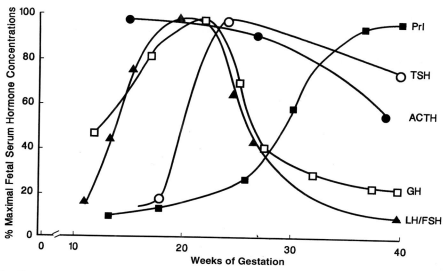

Figure 6-8 Ontogeny of pituitary hormones in human fetal serum. *(Adapted from data described in refs. 47 and 138-140.)*

intact hypothalamus/pituitary system is probably not necessary for the anterior pituitary to develop the capacity to produce its hormones because cultured pituitary tissue from very early fetuses is able to elaborate characteristic hormones,[136] and the pituitary of anencephalic infants also is capable of producing many of the usual pituitary hormones, although the levels are reduced.[137]

The developmental pattern of pituitary hormone secretion is quite varied in the fetus (Fig. 6-8). Maximal serum levels of gonadotropins, LH, and FSH occur at about 20 weeks of gestation and then decline to virtually undetectable levels at term. Whereas there is little sex-related difference in serum LH, female fetuses have higher levels of FSH than do males at midgestation.[47,138] Serum TSH levels are low until about 20 weeks, reach maximal levels at 24 to 25 weeks, and then decline slightly thereafter.[139] The pattern of growth hormone secretion is somewhat analogous to that of TSH, being highest at midgestation.[47] On the other hand, fetal serum prolactin levels are low until the late second trimester and then rise progressively through term.[47,140] There is little established about developmental patterns of POMC peptides in fetal blood. High levels of ACTH have been found at midgestation, and thereafter, plasma ACTH levels appear to decline[141]; confirmation of this paradoxical pattern is presently lacking. Developmental patterns in fetal blood of β-endorphin, β-lipotropin, or α-melanocyte-stimulating hormone (α-MSH), which appears to exist as a deacetylated form in fetal pituitary,[142] are not established.

Gonads

Steroid production in the human fetal testis, morphologically identifiable by 6 to 7 weeks of gestation, is initiated before 10 weeks of gestation, is maximal at 15 to 16 weeks, and then declines dramatically to low levels by 20 to 25 weeks.[138] Since fetal plasma gonadotropin levels are low at the time of increasing steroidogenic activity of the testis,[47,138] it seems likely that hCG, which is present in high quantities in fetal blood at this time,[263] is responsible for the differentiation and early steroid secretion by the fetal testis. The early fetal testis contains abundant hCG receptors, and hCG clearly augments steroid secretion in vitro.[143] The period of maximal testosterone production in vivo is accompanied by maximal levels of testicular hCG receptors,[143] LDL binding, and de novo cholesterol biosynthesis[144] in vitro. On the other hand, it is likely that continued gonadal activity, at least through 15 to 20 weeks, depends on the transient surge of fetal pituitary gonadotropin secretion that occurs at this time.[47,138] The importance of fetal pituitary gonadotropins in fetal testicular function is exemplified by the defects in sexual maturation that frequently occur in anencephalic fetuses: decreased numbers of Leydig cells, hypoplastic external genitalia, and undescended testes.[145] Production of testosterone and the müllerian inhibiting factor (MIF) by the testis of the early male fetus accomplishes male sexual differentiation: stimulation of embryonic wolffian duct system (testosterone) and external genitalia (5α-dihydrotestosterone), and regression of the müllerian ducts.

The fetal ovary, morphologically distinct by 7 to 8 weeks of gestation, appears to have the capacity for steroid production during the first and second trimesters.[146] On the other hand, hormone production by the fetal ovary does not appear to play a role in female sexual maturation: Wolffian ducts regress spontaneously in the absence of testosterone, and development of the müllerian duct system and the female external genitalia can occur even in the agonadal fetus.[147]

Thyroid

Since the placenta is essentially impermeable to thyroid hormones and TSH,[139] the fetal thyroid system develops and functions au-

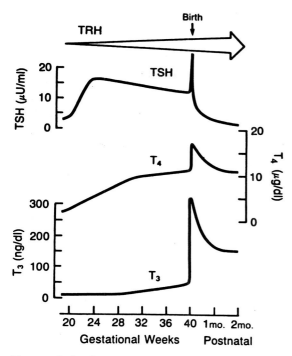

Figure 6-9 Ontogeny of TSH, thyroxine (T$_4$), and triiodothyronine (T$_3$) in fetal and neonatal serum. The increasing impact of TRH on the pituitary-thyroid axis also is depicted. *(Reproduced, with permission, from Fisher DA. Clin Perinatol 1983;10:615.)*

tonomously of the maternal compartment. By 10 to 12 weeks of gestation, the fetal thyroid is histologically distinct, concentrates radioiodine, and can synthesize iodothyronines; the fetal pituitary contains TSH, and the fetal hypothalamus contains TRH.[139] Nevertheless, pituitary secretion of TSH and thyroid hormone production are limited until about 18 to 20 weeks of gestation (Fig. 6-9). Thereafter, probably in response to increased release of hypothalamic TRH and/or increased pituitary sensitivity, a marked increase in TSH secretion occurs through about 28 to 30 weeks.[139,148] Thyroid production of T$_4$ is increased beginning at about 20 weeks and progressively through term despite the slight decline in TSH levels from 30 to 40 weeks. T$_3$ formation, however, is limited until the last few weeks of ges-

tation; the bulk of hepatic metabolism of T$_4$ proceeds through reverse T$_3$, resulting in high levels of reverse T$_3$ in fetal serum during the second and early third trimesters.[149] The decline in reverse T$_3$ and the increase in T$_3$ levels in fetal blood that occur during the last 10 weeks of gestation likely are the result of glucocorticoid actions on thyroid-metabolizing enzyme systems in fetal liver.[150] A striking surge in TSH, T$_4$, and T$_3$ levels in serum occurs shortly after birth (see Fig. 6-9).

Adrenal

Because of its involvement in estrogen production in human pregnancy and its importance in the onset of parturition, at least in the sheep,[151] the adrenal has been the most widely studied endocrine tissue of the fetus. The human fetal adrenal is disproportionately large and contains a unique zone, the fetal zone, that comprises about 80 percent of the cortical mass at term. The fetal zone then regresses soon after birth.[152] The changes in adrenal volume throughout fetal life and into young adulthood are depicted graphically in Figure 6-10. Although there are no data to demonstrate common mechanisms, there are interesting parallels between the growth and pattern of

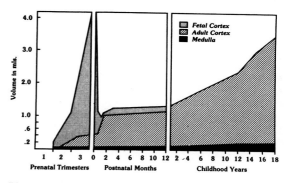

Figure 6-10 Size of the adrenal gland and its component parts during fetal life, infancy, and childhood. *(Reproduced, with permission, from Carr BR, Simpson ER. Endocr Rev 1981;2:306.)*

androgen production by the fetal adrenal and the adrenal during puberty.

The inner fetal zone is composed of eosinophilic cells having a relatively large cytoplasmic-nuclear ratio. The outer zone cells, thought to give rise to the three zones of cells of the postnatal adrenal, compose the neocortex and have a smaller cytoplasmic-nuclear ratio. In addition to the histologic differences in the two cortical zones of the fetal adrenal, the zones differ with respect to several functional characteristics (Table 6-3).

Based on the results of numerous studies using organotypic or cell culture of fetal zone tissue, it is clear that the fetal zone produces the full complement of steroids produced by the adult adrenal. Yet, as a result of the low levels of 3β-hydroxysteroid dehydrogenase (3β-HSD)/Δ4,5-isomerase,[153] which may be due in part to estrogen inhibition of this pathway, and the presence of high levels of dehydroepiandrosterone sulfotransferase,[154] the fetal zone primarily produces Δ5-sulfated steroids such as DS and pregnenolone sulfate and relatively little gluco- or mineralocorticoids. Indeed, it appears that even in the neocortex, there is little 3β-HSD/Δ4,5-isomerase until the later stages of gestation.[153] The neocortex, on the other hand, primarily produces C_{21} Δ4 steroids such as cortisol and little of the Δ5-sulfated steroids.[155] Interestingly, when exposed to ACTH in culture, fetal zone production of DS, usually high already, is enhanced only slightly, whereas production of cortisol is

increased three- to fivefold compared with initial rates of secretion. On the other hand, ACTH treatment of neocortex cells substantially increases DS production, as well as cortisol synthesis (Fig. 6-11).

It seems clear that the fetal adrenal depends on ACTH in vivo. The adrenal of anencephalic infants, who have deficient production of ACTH, is very small[156] and produces low amounts of steroids.[12,20] Fetal ACTH and adrenal steroidogenesis are suppressed by maternal glucocorticosteroid therapy,[157] whereas production of 17-OHP is increased markedly in circumstances of congenital adrenal hyperplasia due to 21-hydroxylase deficiency.[158] Yet ACTH treatment of fetal adrenal tissue in vitro leads to a pattern of production that differs from that produced at the initiation of culture (see Fig. 6-11), as well as from that seen in umbilical cord blood (high DS, low cortisol). Thus it is conceivable that factors in addition to ACTH are important regulators of the fetal adrenal in vivo.

Several hormones, including hCG, growth hormone, hPL, and prolactin, as well as ACTH-related peptides derived from POMC peptides, have been studied for their potential role as modulators of fetal adrenal growth and/or steroidogenesis. To date, there is little convincing evidence that non-POMC peptide hormones influence the human fetal adrenal. The possability that N-terminal fragments of POMC peptides and large-molecular-weight forms of POMC peptide fragments that contain the ACTH sequence, which has been shown to be active in studies of adrenal tissue from experimental animals and, therefore, might regulate fetal adrenal function, has yet to be addressed fully. Peptides, other than ACTH 1–39, that stimulate DS and cortisol production by human fetal adrenal tissue have been detected in fetal pituitary extracts; one appeared to be similar to ACTH 1–38, whereas the other appeared to be unrelated to ACTH or MSH.[159] An 18-amino-acid sequence (POMC 79–96) that is part of the joining peptide of POMC peptides has been found to be without activity in cultures of fetal[160] or adult[161] human adrenal tissues.

▶**TABLE 6-3:** FUNCTIONAL ASPECTS OF FETAL AND NEOCORTICAL ZONES OF THE HUMAN FETAL ADRENAL

	Fetal Zone	Neocortex
Major steroid	DHEA-S	Cortisol
Adenyl cyclase	1X	2X
Protein kinase	2X	1X
LDL binding	2X	1X
Cholesterol synthesis	2X	1X
3β-HSD	1X	4X
P45017α	3X	1X

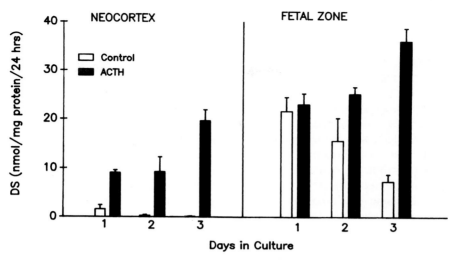

Figure 6-11 Production of DS and cortisol by fetal adrenal cell cultures in the presence and absence of ACTH. *(Reproduced, with permission, from Doody KM, Carr BR, Rainey WE, et al. Endocrinology 1990;126:2487.)*

Apart from responding to ACTH and possibly to other POMC-derived peptides, the fetal adrenal, like other steroidogenic tissues, may be regulated by cytokines and growth factors.[162] Both fibroblast growth factor and epidermal growth factor have been shown to stimulate proliferation of fetal adrenal cells, as has conditioned medium from human placental cultures, which likely contains a host of growth factors. On the other hand, ACTH generally is considered antimitotic to the fetal adrenal. Interestingly, however, ACTH has been found to interfere with the inhibitory effects of transforming growth factor β on poliferation of cultured fetal adrenal cells.[163]

Although the fetal adrenal expresses a high rate of de novo cholesterol biosynthesis in vitro and can support steroidogenesis in the absence of exogenous precursors, it also possesses extensive capacity for uptake and metabolism of LDL; both mechanisms of providing cholesterol are stimulated by ACTH.[18] Moreover, adrenal steroidogenesis in vitro is preferentially enhanced in the presence of LDL compared with that seen with high-density lipoprotein (HDL) or very low-density lipoprotein (VLDL). Indirect in vivo evidence for a role of LDL cholesterol in fetal adrenal steroidogenesis, which is substantial, is derived from several observations[12,164,165] of an inverse correlation between concentrations of adrenal steroids and LDL cholesterol (but not HDL or VLDL cholesterol) in fetal blood. Thus it appears likely that in vivo the fetal adrenal obtains cholesterol for use in steroidogenesis via the LDL receptor pathway, and the rate of adrenal LDL uptake for steroid production, in turn, regulates fetal plasma LDL concentrations.

In addition to the extensive in vitro studies of the human fetal adrenal, there have been many in vivo analyses of fetal adrenal activity during normal and abnormal pregnancy. In uncomplicated pregnancies, umbilical cord plasma levels of DS and cortisol are reasonably stable during the late second and early third trimester. During the last 6 to 10 weeks of gestation, however, there are striking increases in the concentrations of DS and cortisol in fetal blood.[166,167] Fetal plasma cortisol is derived both from fetal and maternal adrenals,[168] which makes it difficult to correlate fetal adrenal activity with fetal plasma cortisol levels in various physiologic or pathophysiologic circumstances. On the other hand, fetal plasma DS, which arises from fetal adrenal production, appears to be indicative of fetal responses to pregnancy conditions. For example, umbilical cord plasma levels of DS have been found to be reduced in pregnancies with specific medical complications such as hypertension, Rh disease, and syphilis, as well as in pregnancies in which fetal growth is retarded.[166] In such circumstances, characterized by reduced fetal DS levels, often there is subnormal estrogen production and morphologic evidence for reduced volume of the fetal zone of the fetal adrenal.[26,169] Whereas several pregnancy complications give rise to reduced fetal DS production and possible maldevelopment of the fetal zone, fetal serum or newborn urinary levels of cortisol and its metabolites seem to be normal or even increased in many such circumstances.[166] Cortisol levels in the fetus or newborn, however, may not be indicative of fetal adrenal activity.

As mentioned earlier, the mechanisms responsible for the growth and pattern of steroidogenesis by the human fetal adrenal are not established. Although short-term correlations between fetal pituitary ACTH production and fetal adrenal activity are evident, e.g., after maternal glucocorticoid treatment, there is little established concerning fetal pituitary ACTH production in relation to pregnancy complications. Somewhat paradoxically, fetal plasma immunoreactive ACTH levels appear to decline over the latter half of gestation,[141] whereas fetal adrenal growth and steroid production, particularly that of the fetal zone, are markedly enhanced. Consequently, there is much yet to learn about the control of growth and function of the fetal adrenal in normal and complicated pregnancy.

► SUMMARY

Human pregnancy is characterized by numerous physiologic adaptations in the maternal compartment. Many of these adaptations are in response to the altered hormonal milieu of pregnancy. There are changes in the rate of formation and/or clearance of most, if not all, hormones that are usually secreted in the non-pregnant state. The discovery of redundant production in the placenta of hormones that are identical or structurally similar to those found in the pituitary and hypothalamus has opened up new avenues of research. Whereas great strides have been made in defining the endocrine changes that occur during pregnancy, our understanding of the causes for such changes is less well developed. Great insights into the normal regulation of the maternal, placental, and fetal endocrine units have been made in the past based on the results of studies of pregnancies that are complicated by maternal, placental, and fetal abnormalities. Continued study of pregnancy anomalies likely will be the source of new discoveries about the endocrinology of pregnancy.

KEY POINTS

1. Whereas estrogen production in pregnancy is determined in part by the status of the fetus, placental progesterone production appears to be independent of fetal well-being.

2. Strikingly suppressed levels of estrogens, particularly of estriol, in maternal serum can arise as a consequence of placental sulfatase deficiency, aromatase deficiency, fetal anencephaly, fetal demise, and fetal exposure to glucocorticosteroids.

3. The evolution of serum hCG levels at various timepoints can be of considerable diagnostic value in conditions of ectopic pregnancy, threatened abortion, and response to therapy in the context of molar pregnancy, persistent trophoblastic disease, or choriocarcinoma.

4. The placenta produces a wide array of protein/peptides that are identical to or very similar to hormones elaborated by the pituitary gland and the hypothalamus; the

physiologic role(s) of many of these placental products are ill-defined.

5. Diagnosis of many endocrine disorders is more difficult in pregnancy since symptoms of many are similar to common complaints in pregnant women and serum levels of many hormones are normally increased in pregnancy.

6. Whereas the fetal adrenal cortex, particularly the cells of the fetal zone, is the source of the bulk of dehydroepiandrosterone and its sulfate that are used as precursors for placental estrogen formation in pregnancy, the factors that regulate the growth and steroidogenesis of the fetal adrenal have yet to be firmly established.

REFERENCES

1. Csapo Al, Pulkkinen MO, Wiest WG. Effects of luteectomy and progesterone replacement therapy in early pregnant patients. *Am J Obstet Gynecol* 1973;115:759.

2. Schmidt CL, de Ziedler D, Gagliardi CL, et al. Transfer of cryopreserved-thawed embryos: The natural cycle versus controlled preparation of the endometrium with gonadotropin-releasing hormone agonist and exogenous estradiol and progesterone (GEEP). *Fertil Steril* 1989;52:609.

3. Sauer MV, Paulson RJ, Lobo RA. A preliminary report on oocyte donation extending reproductive potential to women over 40. *N Engl J Med* 1990;323:1157.

4. Siiteri PK, MacDonald PC. Placental estrogen biosynthesis during human pregnancy. *J Clin Endocrinol Metab* 1966;26:751.

5. Simpson ER, MacDonald PC. Endocrine physiology of the placenta. *Annu Rev Physiol* 1981;43:163.

6. Zelewski L, Villee CA. The biosynthesis of squalene, lanosterol, and cholesterol by minced human placenta. *Biochemistry* 1966;5:1805.

7. Hellig H, Gattereau D, Lefebvre Y, Bolt E. Steroid production from plasma cholesterol: 1. Conversion of plasma cholesterol to placental progesterone in humans. *J Clin Endocrinol Metab* 1970;30:624.

8. Winkel CA, Snyder JM, MacDonald PC, Simpson ER. Regulation of cholesterol and progesterone synthesis in human placental cells in culture by serum lipoproteins. *Endocrinology* 1980;106:1054.

9. Malassine A, Besse C, Roche A, et al. Ultrastructural visualization of the internalization of low density lipoprotein by human placental cells. *Histochemistry* 1987;87:457.

10. Parker CR Jr, Illingworth DR, Bissonnette J, Carr BR. Endocrine changes during pregnancy in a patient with homozygous familial hypobetalipoproteinernia. *N Engl J Med* 1986;314:557.

11. Parker CR Jr, Carr BR, Casey ML et al. Extraadrenal deoxycorticosterone production in hypoestrogenic pregnancies: Serum concentrations of progesterone and deoxycorticosterone in anencephalic fetuses and in women pregnant with an anencephalic fetus. *Am J Obstet Gynecol* 1983;147:415.

12. Parker CR Jr, Carr BR, Winkel CA, et al. Hypercholesterolemia due to elevated low density lipoprotein cholesterol in newborns with anencephaly and adrenal atrophy. *J Clin Endocrinol Metab* 1983;57:37.

13. MacDonald PC, Cutter S, MacDonald C, et al. Regulation of extra-adrenal steroid 21-hydroxylase activity: Increased conversion of plasma progesterone to deoxycorticosterone during estrogen treatment of women pregnant with a dead fetus. *J Clin Invest* 1982;69:469.

14. Teoh ES, Das NP Dawood MY, Ratsum SS. Serum progesterone and serum chorionic gonadotropin in hydatidiform mole and choriocarcinoma. *Acta Endocrinol* 1972;70:791.

15. Roberts JM, Lewis VL, Riemer RK. Hormonal control of uterine adrenergic response, in Bottari J, Thomas P, Vokser A, Vokser R (eds), *Uterine Contractility*. New York: Masson, 1984:161–173.

16. Cane EM, Villee CA. The synthesis of prostaglandin F by human endometrium in organ culture. *Prostaglandins* 1975;9:281.

17. Siiteri PK, Febres F, Clemens LE, et al. Progesterone and maintenance of pregnancy: Is progesterone nature's immunosuppressant? *Ann NY Acad Sci* 1977;286:384.

18. Carr BR, Simpson ER. Lipoprotein utilization and cholesterol synthesis by the human fetal adrenal gland. *Endocr Rev* 1981;2:306.

19. Simpson ER, Carr BR, John ME, et al. Cholesterol metabolism in the adrenals of normal and anencephalic fetuses, in Albrecht E, Pepe GJ (eds), *Perinatal Endocrinology*. Ithaca, NY: Perinatology Press, 1985, p 161.

20. Montserrat de MF, Osathanondh R, Tulchinsky D. Plasma cortisol and cortisone in pregnancies with normal and anencephalic fetuses. *J Clin Endocrinol Metab* 1976;43:80.

21. Parker CR Jr, Carr BR, Winkel CA, et al. Umbilical cord plasma concentrations of deoxycorticosterone sulfate in anencephalic fetuses. *Am J Obstet Gynecol* 1984;150:754.

22. Brown JB. Urinary excretion of estrogen during pregnancy, lactation and the re-establishment of menstruation. *Lancet* 1956;1:704.

23. Loriaux H, Ruder J, Knab DR et al. Estrone sulfate, estrone, estradiol and estriol plasma levels in human pregnancy. *J Clin Endocrinol Metab* 1972;35:887.

24. Tulchinsky D. Placental secretion of unconjugated estrone, estradiol and estriol into the maternal and the fetal circulation. *J Clin Endocrinol Metab* 1973;36:1079.

25. Gurpide E, Marks C, de Ziegler, D, et al. Asymmetric release of estrone and estradiol derived from labeled precursors in perfused human placentas. *Am J Obstet Gynecol* 1982;144:551.

26. Tulchinsky D, Frigoletto FD Jr, Ryan KJ, Fishman J. Plasma estetrol as an index of fetal well-being. *J Clin Endocrinol Metab* 1975;40:560.

27. Patrick J, Challis J, Campbell K, et al. Circadian rhythms in maternal plasma cortisol and estriol concentrations at 30 to 31, 34 to 35, and 38 to 39 weeks of gestational age. *Am J Obstet Gynecol* 1980;136:325.

28. Carrington ER, Oesterling MJ, Adams FM. Renal clearance of estriol in complicated pregnancies. *Am J Obstet Gynecol* 1970;106:1131.

29. Bradshaw KD, Carr BR. Placental sulfatase deficiency: Maternal and fetal expression of steroid sulfatase deficiency and X-linked ichthyosis. *Obstet Gynecol Surv* 1986;41:401.

30. Bulun SE. Aromatase deficiency in women and men: Would you have predicted the phenotypes? *J Clin Endocrinol Metab* 1996;81:867.

31. Casey ML, Winkel CA, Porter JC, et al. Endocrine regulation of the initiation and maintenance of parturition. *Clin Perinatol* 1983;10:709.

32. Resnik R, Killam AP, Battaglia FC, et al. The stimulation of uterine blood flow by various estrogens. *Endocrinology* 1974;94:1192.

33. Martin RH, Oakey RE. The role of antenatal estrogen in postpartum human lactogenesis: Evidence from estrogen deficient pregnancies. *Clin Endocrinol* 1982;17:403.

34. Parker CR Jr, Hankins GD, Guzick DS, et al. Ontogeny of unconjugated estriol in fetal blood and the relation of estriol levels at birth to the development of respiratory distress syndrome. *Pediatr Res* 1987;21:386.

35. Bahl OP, Carlsen RB, Bellisario R, et al. Human chorionic gonadotropin: amino acid sequence of the α and β subunits. *Biochem Biophys Res Commun* 1972;48:416.

36. Naylor SL, Chin WW, Goodman HM, et al. Chromosome assignment of genes encoding the α and β subunits of glycoprotein hormones in man and mouse. *Somat Cell Mol Genet* 1983;9:757.

37. Strickland TW, Puett D. Contribution of subunits to the function of luteinizing hormone/human chorionic gonadotropin recombinants. *Endocrinology* 1981;109:1933.

38. Talmadge K, Boorstein WR, Vamvakopoulos NC, et al. Only three of the seven human chorionic gonadotropin beta subunit genes can be expressed in the placenta. *Nucl Acids Res* 1984;12:8415.

39. Yen SSC, Llerena O, Little B, et al. Disappearance rates of endogenous luteinizing hormone and chorionic gonadotropin in man. *J Clin Endocrinol Metab* 1968;28:1763.

40. Hoshina M, Boothby M, Hussa R, et al. Linkage of human chorionic gonadotropin and placental lactogen biosynthesis to trophoblast differentiation and tumorigenesis. *Placenta* 1985;6:163.

41. Morrow CP. Postmolar trophoblastic disease: Diagnosis, management, and prognosis. *Clin Obstet Gynecol* 1984;27:211.

42. Cole LA, Kroll TG, Ruddon RW, et al. Differential occurrence of free beta and free alpha subunits of human chorionic gonadotropin (hCG) in pregnancy sera. *J Clin Endocrinol Metab* 1984;58:1200.

43. Hay DL. Discordant and variable production of human chorionic gonadotropin and its free α- and β-subunits in early pregnancy. *J Clin Endocrinol Metab* 1985;61:1195.

44. Bryant-Greenwood GD. Relaxin as a new hormone. *Endocr Rev* 1982;3:62.

45. Hanson FW, Powell JE, Stevens VC. Effects of HCG and human pituitary LH on steroid secretion and functional life of the human corpus luteum. *J Clin Endocrinol Metab* 1971; 32:211.

46. Huhtaniemi IT, Korenbrot CC, Jaffe RB. HCG binding and stimulation of testosterone biosynthesis in the human fetal testis. *J Clin Endocrinol Metab* 1977;44:963.

47. Kaplan SL, Grumbach MM, Aubert ML. The ontogenesis of pituitary hormones and hypothalamic factors in the human fetus: Maturation of central nervous system regulation of anterior pituitary function. *Recent Prog Horm Res* 1976;32:161.

48. Billingham RE. Transplantation immunity and the maternal-fetal relation. *N Engl J Med* 1964; 270:667.

49. Gundert D, Metz WE, Hilgenfeldt U, et al. Inability of highly purified preparations of human chorionic gonadotropin to inhibit the phytohemagglutinin induced stimulation of lymphocytes. *FEBS Lett* 1975;53:309.

50. Hussa RO, Story MT, Pattillo RA. Cyclic adenosine monophosphate stimulates secretion of human chorionic gonadotropin and estrogens by human trophoblast in vitro. *J Clin Endocrinol Metab* 1974;38:338.

51. Benveniste R, Speeg KV, Carpenter G, et al. Epidermal growth factor stimulates secretion of human chorionic gonadotropin by cultured human choriocarcinoma cells. *J Clin Endocrinol Metab* 1978;46:169.

52. Siler-Khodr TM, Kang IA, Khodr GS. Current topic: Symposium on placental endocrinology: 1. Effects of chorionic GnRH on intrauterine tissues and pregnancy. *Placenta* 1991;12:91.

53. Iwashita M, Watanabe M, Adachi T, et al. Effect of gonadal steroids on gonadotropin-releasing hormone stimulated human chorionic gonadotropin release by trophoblast cells. *Placenta* 1989;10:103.

54. Lenton EA, Neal LM, Sulaiman R. Plasma concentrations of human chorionic gonadotropin from the time of implantation until the second week of pregnancy. *Fertil Steril* 1982;37:773.

55. Pittaway DE, Reisch RL, Wentz AC. Doubling times of human chorionic gonadotropin increase in early viable intrauterine pregnancies. *Am J Obstet Gynecol* 1985;152:299.

56. Romero R, Kadar N, Copel JA, et al. The value of serial human chorionic gonadotropin testing as a diagnostic tool in ectopic pregnancy. *Am J Obstet Gynecol* 1986;155:392.

57. Nygren KG, Johansson EDB, Wide L. Evaluation of the prognosis of threatened abortion from the peripheral plasma levels of progesterone, estradiol and human chorionic gonadotropin. *Am J Obstet Gynecol* 1973;116:916.

58. Jovanovic L, Dawood MY, Landesman R, et al. Hormonal profile as a prognostic index of early threatened abortion. *Am J Obstet Gynecol* 1978;130:274.

59. Ho Yuen B, Cannon W. Molar pregnancy in British Columbia: Estimated incidence and postevacuation regression patterns of the beta subunit of human chorionic gonadotropin. *Am J Obstet Gynecol* 1981;139:316.

60. Schlaerth JB, Morrow CP, Kletzky OA, et al. Prognostic characteristics of the serum radioimmunoassay beta subunit human chorionic gonadotropin titer regression curve following molar pregnancy. *Obstet Gynecol* 1981;58:478.

61. Khazaeli MB, Hedavat MM, Hatch KD, et al. Radioimmunoassay of free β-subunit of human chorionic gonadotropin as a prognostic test for persistent trophoblastic disease in molar pregnancy. *Am J Obstet Gynecol* 1986;155:320.

62. Birken S, Armstrong EG, Kolks MA, et al. Structure of the human chorionic gonadotropin β-subunit fragment from pregnancy urine. *Endocrinology* 1988;123:572.

63. Cole LA, Wang YX, Elliott M, et al. Urinary hCG free β-subunit and β-core fragment: A new marker of gynecological cancers. *Cancer Res* 1988;48:1356.

64. Wehmann RE, Blithe DL, Akar AH, et al. Disparity between β-core levels in pregnancy urine and serum: Implications for the origin of urinary β-core. *J Clin Endocrinol Metab* 1990; 70:371.

65. Kardana A, Cole LA. Serum HCG β-core fragment is masked by associated macromolecules. *J Clin Endocrinol Metab* 1990;71:1393.

66. Ito Y, Higashi K. Studies on the prolactin-like substance in human placenta, part II. *Endocrinol Jpn* 1961;8:279.

67. Bewley TA, Dixon JS, Li CH. Sequence comparison of human pituitary growth hormone,

human chorionic somatomammotropin, and ovine pituitary growth and lactogenic hormones. *Int J Pept Protein Res* 1972;4:281.

68. Owerbach D, Rutter WJ, Martial JA, et al. Genes for growth hormone chorionic somatomammotropin and growth hormone–like gene on chromosome 17 in humans. *Science* 1980;209: 289.

69. Barrera-Saldana HA, Seeburg PH, Saunders GE. Two structurally different genes produce the same secreted human placental lactogen hormone. *J Biol Chem* 1983;258:3787.

70. Hoshina M, Boothby M, Boime I. Cytological localization of chorionic gonadotropin α and placental lactogen mRNAs during development of the human placenta. *J Cell Biol* 1982;93:190.

71. Friesen HG, Suwa S, Pare P. Synthesis and secretion of placental lactogen and other proteins by the placenta. *Recent Prog Horm Res* 1969;25:161.

72. McWilliams D, Callahan RC, Boime L. Human placental lactogen mRNA and its structural genes during pregnancy: Quantitation with a complementary DNA. *Proc Natl Acad Sci USA* 1977;74:1024.

73. Tyson JE, Austin KL, Farinholt JW. Prolonged nutritional deprivation in pregnancy: Changes in human chorionic somatomammotropin and growth hormone secretion. *Am J Obstet Gynecol* 1971;109:1080.

74. Grumbach MM, Kaplan SL, Sciarra JJ, et al. Chorionic growth hormone–prolactin (CGP): Secretion, disposition, biological activity in man, and postulated function as the "growth hormone" of the second half of pregnancy. *Ann NY Acad Sci* 1968;148:501.

75. Nielsen PV Pedersen H, Kampmann EM. Absence of human placental lactogen in an otherwise uneventful pregnancy. *Am J Obstet Gynecol* 1979;135:322.

76. Harada A, Hershman JM. Extraction of human chorionic thyrotropin (hCT) from term placentas: Failure to recover thyrotropic activity. *J Clin Endocrinol Metab* 1978;47:681.

77. Kenimer JG, Hershman JM, Higgins HP. The thyrotropin in hydatidiform moles is human chorionic gonadotropin. *J Clin Endocrinol Metab* 1975;40:482.

78. Odagiri ED, Sherrell Bj, Mount CD, et al. Human placental immunoreactive corticotropin, lipotropin and β-endorphin: Evidence for a common precursor. *Proc Natl Acad Sci USA* 1979;76:2027.

79. Petraglia F, Sawchenko P, Rivier J, et al. Evidence for local stimulation of ACTH secretion by corticotropin-releasing factor in human placenta. *Nature* 1987;328:717.

80. Grino M, Chrousos GP, Margioris AN. The corticotropin releasing hormone gene is expressed in human placenta. *Biochem Biophys Res Commun* 1987;148:1208.

81. Robinson BG, Emanuel RL, Frim DM, et al. Glucocorticoid stimulates expression of corticotropin-releasing hormone gene in human placenta. *Proc Natl Acad Sci USA* 1988; 85:5244.

82. Challis JRG, Matthews SG, Van Meir C, et al. Current topic: The placental corticotropin-releasing hormone–adrenocorticotropin axis. *Placenta* 1995;61:147.

83. Maclean M, Brisits A, Davies J, et al. A placental clock controlling the length of human pregnancy. *Nature Med* 1995;1:4460.

84. Petraglia E Calza L, Garuti GC, et al. New aspects of placental endocrinology. *J Endocrinol Invest* 1990;13:353.

85. Maslar IA, Riddick DH. Prolactin production by human endometrium during the normal menstrual cycle. *Am J Obstet Gynecol* 1979;135:751.

86. Golander A, Hurley T, Barrett J, et al. Synthesis of prolactin by human decidua in vitro. *J Endocrinol* 1979;82:263.

87. Kletzky OA, Rossman E Bertolli SI, et al. Dynamics of human chorionic gonadotropin, prolactin, and growth hormone in serum and amniotic fluid throughout normal human pregnancy. *Am J Obstet Gynecol* 1985;151: 878.

88. Luciano AA, Varner MW. Decidual, amniotic fluid, maternal and fetal prolactin in normal and abnormal pregnancies. *Obstet Gynecol* 1984;63:384.

89. Golander A, Barrett J, Hurley T, et al. Failure of bromocriptine, dopamine, and thyrotropin-releasing hormone to affect prolactin secretion by human decidual tissue in vitro. *J Clin Endocrinol Metab* 1979;49:787.

90. Ogren L, Talamantes E. Prolactins of pregnancy and their cellular source. *Int Rev Cytol* 1988;112:1.

91. Hatjis CG, Wu CH, Gabbe SG. Amniotic fluid prolactin levels and lecithin/sphingomyelin ra-

tios during the third trimester of human gestation. *Am J Obstet Gynecol* 1981;139:435.

92. Heyl PS, Miller W, Canick JA. Maternal serum screening for aneuploid pregnancy by alpha-fetoprotein, hCG, and unconjugated estriol. *Obstet Gynecol* 1990;76:1025.

93. Sailer DN, Canick JA. Maternal serum screening for fetal Down syndrome: Clinical aspects. *Clin Obstet Gynecol* 1996;39:783.

94. Sailer DN, Canick JA. Maternal serum screening for fetal Down syndrome: The detection of other pathologies. *Clin Obstet Gynecol* 1996;39:793.

95. Nolten WE, Lindheimer MD, Oparil S, et al. Deoxycorticosterone in normal pregnancy: 1. Sequential studies of the secretory patterns of deoxycorticosterone, aldosterone, and cortisol. *Am J Obstet Gynecol* 1978;132:414.

96. Carr BR, Parker CR Jr, Madden JD, et al. Maternal plasma adrenocorticotropin and cortisol relationships throughout human pregnancy. *Am J Obstet Gynecol* 1981;139:416.

97. Carr BR, Parker CR Jr, Madden JD, et al. Plasma levels of adrenocorticotropin and cortisol in women receiving oral contraceptive steroid treatment. *J Clin Endocrinol Metab* 1979;49:346.

98. Parker CR Jr, Everett RB, Quirk JG, et al. Hormone production in pregnancy in the primigravida: II. Plasma concentrations of deoxycorticosterone throughout pregnancy in normal women and in women who developed pregnancy induced hypertension. *Am J Obstet Gynecol* 1980;138:626.

99. Winkel CA, Milewich L, Parker CR Jr, et al. Conversion of plasma progesterone by deoxycorticosterone in men, nonpregnant and pregnant women and adrenalectomized subjects: Evidence for steroid 21-hydroxylase in non-adrenal tissues. *J Clin Invest* 1980;66:803.

100. Milewich L, Gomez-Sanchez C, Madden JD, et al. Dehydroisoandrosterone sulfate in peripheral blood of premenopausal, pregnant and postmenopausal women and men. *J Steroid Biochem* 1978;9:1159.

101. Grimes EM, Fayez JA, Miller GL. Cushing's syndrome and pregnancy. *Obstet Gynecol* 1973;42:550.

102. van der Spuy ZM, Jacobs HS. Management of endocrine disorders in pregnancy: II. Pituitary, ovarian and adrenal disease. *Postgrad Med J* 1984;60:312.

103. Kreines K, Devaux WD. Neonatal adrenal insufficiency associated with maternal Cushing's syndrome. *Pediatrics* 1971;47:516.

104. Burrow GN. Hyperthyroidism during pregnancy. *N Engl J Med* 1978;298:150.

105. Fisher DA, Lehman H, Lackey C. Placental transport of thyroxine. *J Clin Endocrinol Metab* 1964;24:393.

106. Zakarija M, McKenzie JM. Pregnancy associated changes in the thyroid stimulating antibody of Graves' disease and the relationship to neonatal hyperthyroidism. *J Clin Endocrinol Metab* 1983;57:1036.

107. Pekonen F, Teramo K, Ikonen E, et al. Women on thyroid hormone therapy: Pregnancy course, fetal outcome, and amniotic fluid thyroid hormone level. *Obstet Gynecol* 1984;63:635.

108. Van der Spuy ZM, Jacobs HS. Management of endocrine disorders in pregnancy: I. Thyroid and parathyroid disease. *Postgrad Med J* 1984;60:245.

109. Shauberger CW, Pitkin RM. Maternal-perinatal calcium relationships. *Obstet Gynecol* 1979;53:74.

110. Pitkin RM, Reynolds WA, Williams GA, et al. Calcium metabolism in pregnancy: A longitudinal study. *Am J Obstet Gynecol* 1979;133:781.

111. Drake TS, Kaplan RA, Lewis TA. The physiologic hyperparathyroidism of pregnancy: Is it primary or secondary? *Obstet Gynecol* 1979;53:746.

112. Pitkin RM. Endocrine regulation of calcium homeostasis during pregnancy. *Clin Perinatol* 1983;10:575.

113. Kumar R, Cohen WR, Silva P, et al. Elevated 1,26-dihydroxyvitamin D plasma levels in normal human pregnancy and lactation. *J Clin Invest* 1979;63:342.

114. Lowe DK, Orwoll ES, McClung MR, et al. Hyperparathyroidism and pregnancy. *Am J Surg* 1983;145:611.

115. Juan D. Hypocalcemia: Differential diagnosis and mechanisms. *Arch Intern Med* 1979;139:1166.

116. Landing BH, Kamoshita S. Congenital hyperparathyroidism secondary to maternal hypoparathyroidism. *J Pediatr* 1970;77:842.

117. Johnstone RE II, Kreindler T, Johnstone RE. Hyperparathyroidism during pregnancy. *Obstet Gynecol* 1972;40:580.

118. Costrini NV, Kalkhoff RK. Relative effects of pregnancy, estradiol and progesterone on

plasma insulin and pancreatic islet insulin secretion. *J Clin Invest* 1971;50:992.

119. Kalkhoff RK. Metabolic effects of progesterone. *Am J Obstet Gynecol* 1982;142:735.

120. Phelps RL, Metzger BE, Freinkel N. Carbohydrate metabolism in pregnancy: XVII. Diurnal profiles of plasma glucose, insulin, free fatty acids, triglycerides, cholesterol and individual amino acids in late normal pregnancy. *Am J Obstet Gynecol* 1981;140:730.

121. Hollingsworth DR. Alterations of maternal metabolism in normal and diabetic pregnancies: Differences in insulin-dependent, non-insulin-dependent, and gestational diabetes. *Am J Obstet Gynecol* 1983;146:417.

122. Soler NG, Soler SM, Malins JM. Neonatal morbidity among infants of diabetic mothers. *Diabetes Care* 1978;1:340.

123. Reyes FI, Winter JS, Faiman C. Pituitary gonadotropin function during human pregnancy: Serum FSH and LH levels before and after LHRH administration. *J Clin Endocrinol Metab* 1976;42:590.

124. Genazzani AR, Facchinetti F, Parrini D. β-Lipotropin and β-endorphin plasma levels during pregnancy. *Clin Endocrinol* 1981;14:409.

125. Goland RS, Wardlaw SL, Stark RI, et al. Human plasma β-endorphin during pregnancy, labor and delivery. *J Clin Endocrinol Metab* 1981;52:74.

126. Campbell EA, Linton EA, Wolfe CDA, et al. Plasma corticotropin-releasing hormone concentrations during pregnancy and parturition. *J Clin Endocrinol Metab* 1987;64:1054.

127. Goland RS, Wardlaw SL, Blum M, et al. Biologically active corticotropin-releasing hormone in maternal and fetal plasma during pregnancy. *Am J Obstet Gynecol* 1988;159:884.

128. Spellacy WN, Buhi WC, Birk SA. Human growth hormone and placental lactogen levels in mid-pregnancy and late postpartum. *Obstet Gynecol* 1970;36:238.

129. Tyson JE, Hwang P Guyda H, Friesen HG. Studies of prolactin secretion in human pregnancy. *Am J Obstet Gynecol* 1972;113:14.

130. Franks S. Regulation of prolactin secretion by estrogens: Physiological and pathological significance. *Clin Sci* 1983;65:457.

131. Thliveris JA, Currie RW. Observations on the hypothalamohypophyseal portal vasculature in the developing human fetus. *Am J Anat* 1980;157:441.

132. Nobin A, Bjorklund A. Topography of the monoamine neuron systems in the human brain as revealed in fetuses. *Acta Physiol Scand* 1973;388(suppl):1.

133. Fisher DA. Maternal-fetal neurohypophyseal system. *Clin Perinatol* 1983;10:695.

134. Bugnon C, Fellman D, Gouger A, et al. Corticoliberin neurons: Cytophysiology, phylogeny and ontogeny. *J Steroid Biochem* 1984;20:183.

135. Ackland J, Ratter S, Bourne G, et al. Proopiomelanocortin peptides in the human fetal pituitary. *Regul Pept* 1983;6:51.

136. Siler-Khodr TM, Morgenstern LL, Greenwood FC. Hormone synthesis and release from human fetal adenohypophyses in vitro. *J Clin Endocrinol Metab* 1974;39:891.

137. Allen JP, Greer MA, McGilvra R, et al. Endocrine function in an anencephalic infant. *J Clin Endocrinol Metab* 1974;38:94.

138. Reyes FI, Boroditsky RS, Winter JSO, et al. Studies on human sexual development: II. Fetal and maternal serum gonadotropin and sex steroid concentrations. *J Clin Endocrinol Metab* 1974;38:612.

139. Fisher DA, Dussault JH, Sack J, et al. Ontogenesis of hypothalamic-pituitary-thyroid function and metabolism in man, sheep and rat. *Recent Prog Horm Res* 1977;33:59.

140. Winters AJ, Colston C, MacDonald PC, et al. Fetal plasma prolactin levels. *J Clin Endocrinol Metab* 1975;41:626.

141. Winters AJ, Oliver C, Colston C, et al. Plasma ACTH levels in the human fetus and neonate as related to age and parturition. *J Clin Endocrinol Metab* 1974;39:269.

142. Tilders FJH, Parker CR Jr, Barnea A, et al. The major immunoreactive α-melanocyte-stimulating hormone (α-MSH)–like substance found in human fetal pituitary tissue is not α-MSH but may be desacetyl α-MSH (adrenocorticotropin 1–13 NH$_2$). *J Clin Endocrinol Metab* 1981;52:319.

143. Huhtaniemi IT, Korenbrot CC, Jaffe RB. HCG binding and stimulation of testosterone biosynthesis in the human fetal testis. *J Clin Endocrinol Metab* 1977;44:963.

144. Carr BR, Parker CR Jr, Ohashi M, et al. Regulation of human fetal testicular secretion of testosterone: Low density lipoprotein–

cholesterol and cholesterol synthesized de novo as steroid precursor. *Am J Obstet Gynecol* 1983; 146:241.

145. Bearn JG. Anencephaly and the development of the male genital tract. *Acta Paediatr Acad Sci Hung* 1968;9:159.

146. Payne AH, Jaffe RB. Androgen formation from pregnenolone sulfate by the human fetal ovary. *J Clin Endocrinol Metab* 1974;39:300.

147. Jost A. Problems of fetal endocrinology: The gonadal and hypophyseal hormones. *Recent Prog Horm Res* 1953;8:379.

148. Klein AH, Oddie TH, Parslow M, et al. Developmental changes in pituitary thyroid function in the human fetus and newborn. *Early Hum Dev* 1982;6:321.

149. Isaac RM, Hayek A, Standefef JC, et al. Reverse triiodothyronine to triiodothyronine ratio and gestational age. *J Pediatr* 1979;94:477.

150. Osathanondh R, Chopra IJ, Tulchinsky D. Effects of dexamethasone on fetal and maternal thyroxine, triiodothyronine, reverse triiodothyronine and thyrotropin levels. *J Clin Endocrinol Metab* 1978;47:1236.

151. Challis JRG, Brooks AN. Maturation and activation of hypothalamic-pituitary-adrenal function in fetal sheep. *Endocr Rev* 1989;10:182.

152. Johannison E. The fetal adrenal cortex in the human. *Acta Endocrinol* 1968;58(suppl 130):7.

153. Parker CR Jr, Faye-Petersen O, Stankovic AK, et al. Immunohistochernical evaluation of the cellular localization and ontogeny of 30-hydroxysteroid dehydrogenase/Δ6,4-isomerase in the human fetal adrenal gland. *Endocr Res* 1995;21:69.

154. Parker CR Jr, Stankovic AK, Falany CN, et al. Immunocytochemical analyses of dehydroepiandrosterone sulfotransferase in cultured human fetal adrenal cells. *J Clin Endocrinol Metab* 1995;80:1027.

155. Pepe GJ, Albrecht ED. Regulation of the primate fetal adrenal cortex. *Endocr Rev* 1990;11:151.

156. Benirschke K. Adrenals in anencephaly and hydroencephaly. *Obstet Gynecol* 1956;8:412.

157. Parker CR Jr, Atkinson MW, Owen J, et al. Dynamics of the fetal adrenal, cholesterol, and apolipoprotein B responses to antenatal betamethasone therapy. *Am J Obstet Gynecol* 1996;174:562.

158. Pang S, Levine LS, Decerquist LL, et al. Amniotic fluid concentrations of Δ4- and Δ5-steroids in fetuses with congenital adrenal hyperplasia due to 21-hydroxylase deficiency and in anencephalic fetuses. *J Clin Endocrinol Metab* 1980;51:223.

159. Brubaker PL, Baird AL, Bennett HPJ, et al. Corticotropic peptides in the human fetal pituitary. *Endocrinology* 1982;111:1150.

160. Mellon SH, Shively JE, Miller WL. Human proopiomelanocortin (79–96), a proposed androgen stunulatory hormone, does not affect steroidogenesis in cultured human fetal adrenal cells. *J Clin Endocrinol Metab* 1991;72:19.

161. Penhoat A, Sanchez P, Jaillard C, et al. Human pro-opiomelanocortin (79–96), a proposed cortical androgen stimulating hormone, does not affect steroidogenesis in cultured human adult adrenal cells. *J Clin Endocrinol Metab* 1991;72:23.

162. Mesiano S, Jaffe RB. Developmental and functional biology of the primate fetal adrenal cortex. *Endocr Rev* 1997;18:378.

163. Stankovic AK, Grizzle WE, Stockard CR, et al. Interactions between transforming growth factor β and adrenocorticotropin in growth regulation of human fetal zone cells: Possible involvement of adenylate cyclase. *Am J Physiol* 1994;266:E495.

164. Parker CR Jr, Simpson ER, Bilheimer DW, et al: Inverse relation between low-density lipoprotein-cholesterol and dehydroisoandrosterone sulfate in human fetal plasma. *Science* 1980;208:512.

165. Parker CR Jr, Carr BR, Simpson ER, et al. Decline in the concentration of low-density lipoprotein cholesterol in human fetal plasma near term. *Metabolism* 1983;32:919.

166. Parker CR Jr. Dehydroepiandrosterone and dehydroepiandrosterone sulfate production in the human adrenal during development and aging. *Steroids* 1999;64:640.

167. Murphy BEP. Human fetal serum cortisol levels related to gestational age: Evidence of a midgestational fall and steep late gestational rise, independent of sex or mode of delivery. *Am J Obstet Gynecol* 1982;144:276.

168. Beitins IZ, Bayard F, Ances IG, et al. The metabolic clearance rate, blood production, interconversion, and transplacental passage of cortisol and cortisone in pregnancy near term. *Pediatr Res* 1973;7:509.

169. Bech K. Morphology of the fetal adrenal cortex, and maternal urinary oestriol excretion in pregnancy. *Acta Obstet Gynecol Scand* 1971; 50:215.

CHAPTER 7

Embryology and Morphogenesis of Reproduction

Hugh S. Taylor

► **REPRODUCTIVE TRACT EMBRYOLOGY**

Sex Determination

Reproductive medicine, as we know it, arises from human sexual dimorphism. The early embryo is phenotypically identical in both sexes; sexual dimorphism arises only after several weeks of gestation. Sexual development is a specialization of particular organ systems in response to a chromosomal complement determined at the time of fertilization in humans. In other species, the sex of an adult is determined not by a distinct chromosomal complement but by the number of chromosomes or by environmental factors such as temperature. It is therefore not surprising that the reproductive tract is relatively plastic and that disorders of reproductive tract development occur with some frequency. A knowledge of reproductive tract development is an essential foundation for understanding reproductive tract anomalies.

The genetic sex of all mammals is normally determined by the X or Y chromosome present in the sperm. While this fact is well known, it was not until the early twentieth century that it was established that the chromosomal complement resulted in sexual identity. The presence of a Y chromosome results in a male phenotype, whereas the absence results in a female phenotype. This suggests the existence of a Y chromosome—specific gene product resulting in male development. Specifically, the presence of the Y chromosome results in differentiation of the embryonic somatic cells of the gonad into testes rather than into ovaries.

The Klinefelter and Turner syndromes provide evidence of a Y chromosome contribution to male sex determination. Klinefelter syndrome results from the chromosomal complement 47,XXY; these individuals have two X chromosomes but are still male. Turner syndrome results from a 46,X karyotype, but these individuals are still female. These syndromes and their associated abnormalities will be discussed in Chapter 8. There are also reports of XY females and XX males that result from loss or gain of the specific region of the Y chromosome responsible for sex determination. This gain is thought to occur during meiosis due to crossing over, whereas loss can be due to mutation.[1]

The sex-determining region of the Y chromosome, *SRY*, was identified by mapping the chromosomal region responsible for sex reversal and cloning the gene of interest.[2,3] This gene is found in normal XY males and in rare XX phenotypic males. XY females have been shown to have mutations in this gene.[4,5] The *SRY* gene has been demonstrated to be sufficient to determine the male phenotype in mice. When the murine equivalent of the *SRY* gene, termed *Sry*, is transferred into XX mice, these XX embryos (transgenic for the *Sry* gene) developed as males; this is despite lacking all other genes of the Y chromosome. The *SRY* gene encodes a transcription factor that regulates genes responsible for testicular development. These transgenic mice, although phenotypically male, are infertile. Additional Y chromosome genes are necessary for spermatogenesis.

Gonadal Development

The human gonad first develops through an indifferent phase, possessing neither distinctly male nor female characteristics. This is unique in human embryology; once an organ primordia is defined, it typically is restricted to one developmental pathway. The indifferent gonad can differentiate into either an ovary or a testis. The fate of the gonad is specified by the *SRY* gene product. In all other reproductive organs (discussed below), sexually dimorphic development depends not directly on chromosomal complement but on the presence of either the male or female gonad. The indifferent gonad develops in close association with the mesonephros, an embryonic kidney that contributes to both the male and female reproductive tract (Fig. 7-1). Germ cells induce cells of the mesonephros to form the genital ridge. This gonadal rudiment appears in the intermediate mesoderm during week 4 and remains indifferent until week 7. The genital ridge is the site of epithelial proliferation into the loose connective tissue underlying it. These epithelial cells will form the sex cords that eventu-

ally surround the migrating germ cells during week 6. If germ cells do not develop and reach the mesonephros, the gonad does not form. Gonad development is a distinct process from development of the external and internal genitalia, and disorders of each are not necessarily associated.

Sexual dimorphism is first apparent in the behavior of the sex cords. Male sex cords continue to proliferate while the indifferent sex cords of the female gonad degenerate. In the male, the sex cords proliferate into connective tissue through week 8. The male cords fuse to form a network of medullary sex cords and end in the rete testis. In the testis these epithelial cords separate from surface epithelium from which they originated and are enveloped by extracellular matrix termed the *tunica albuginea*. During fetal life and after birth until puberty, the cords are solid. Afterward, the germ cells are enveloped by the cords. At puberty, the cords cannulate to form the seminiferous tubules. Sperm produced in the testis are transferred via the seminiferous tubules to the rete testis and the efferent ducts; these remnants of the mesonephric kidney link the testis to the wolffian duct—the former collecting tubule of the mesonephric kidney. In males, the wolffian duct persists as the vas deferens. The mesenchymal cells of the testis differentiate into Leydig cells, whereas the cords form Sertoli cells.

In the female, the initial sex cords degenerate and are replaced by new epithelial proliferation, resulting in a new set of sex cords. These cortical sex cells superficially penetrate the mesenchyme, remaining near the outer cortex of the ovary—the location of the female germ cells. Rather than forming an interconnected network, these cords form distinct clusters surrounding germ cells. This is the initial origin of the ovarian follicles. The epithelial sex cords differentiate into granulosa cells, whereas the mesenchymal cells form the thecal cells.

Germ cells develop initially at some distance from the gonads and later migrate to the

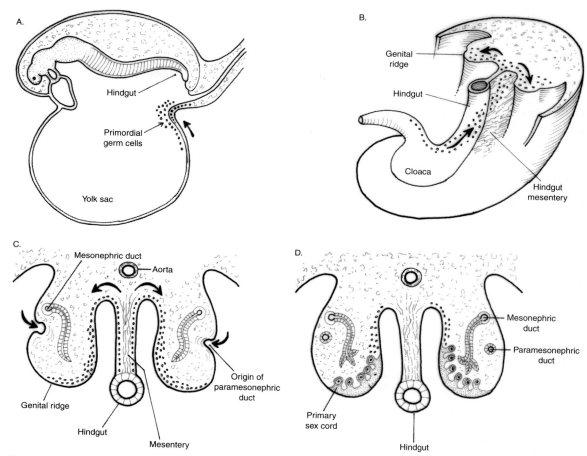

Figure 7-1 Migration of the primordial germ cells from the yolk sac to the hindgut. Arrow indicates direction of migration. From the hindgut, the primordial germ cells traverse the hindgut mesentery and migrate to the genital ridge. The primordial germ cells accumulate in the mesenchyme of the gonadal ridge. The paramesonephric duct begins to invaginate lateral to the mesonephros. During the sixth week the primordial germ cells become incorporated in the primary sex cords. The paramesonephric duct has fully formed next to the mesonephric duct.

site of gonadal formation, where the germ cells ultimately will differentiate into eggs or sperm. This separation may serve to exclude the germ cells from developmental signals of early embryogenesis and maintain their uniquely undifferentiated state. While the gonad develops from the mesoderm lining the abdominal cavity at the genital ridge, the primordial germ cells appear during the fourth week of development in the endoderm of the yolk sac. They migrate from the yolk sac, along the dorsal mesentery of the hindgut, and arrive at the genital ridge by the sixth week (see Fig. 7-1). There they invade the medial genital ridge and become invested in the primitive gonad. The mechanisms controlling migration and proliferation of the germ cells are not fully known. In mice, the steel protein and its receptor, Kit, have been demonstrated to play a role. Kit is expressed in migrating germ cells, whereas the Kit ligand, steel, is expressed along the path of germ cell migration. Mutation of either of the genes for these proteins can cause a decrease in germ cell numbers reaching the genital ridge, demonstrating the requirement for signals guiding the germ cells to their eventual destination.

Development of the Internal Genitalia

Without gonads, all internal genitalia develop as female, regardless of chromosomal sexual identity. Associated with the mesonephros are the paired wolffian ducts that open to the cloaca.[6] Parallel to each wolffian duct is a müllerian duct also ending in the cloaca. The wolffian duct arises from the mesonephric ducts of the mesonephric kidney, which does not exist in the adult. The müllerian ducts are also known as the *paramesonephric ducts*. The müllerian ducts arise from an invagination of the epithelium on the surface of the mesonephric duct in the urogenital ridge; they develop in a location parallel to the mesonephric ducts (Fig. 7-2). Müllerian duct development begins with prolif-

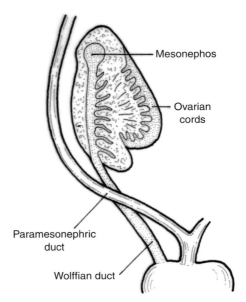

Figure 7-3 The mesonephros, mesonephric duct, and paramesonephric duct coexist at 8 weeks along with an indifferent gonad.

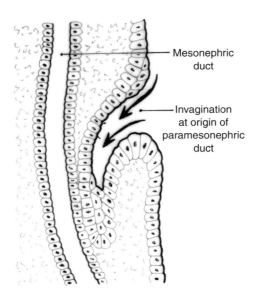

Figure 7-2 The mesonephric duct induces the development of the paramesonephric duct. The paramesonephric duct forms from an invagination and subsequent fusion of the coelomic epithelium.

eration of the coelomic epithelium at the cranial end of the urogenital ridge and lateral to the regressing wolffian duct. The wolffian duct directs müllerian duct development. Both pairs of ducts exist simultaneously in early human development, from 5 to 8 weeks, prior to gonadal differentiation (Fig. 7-3).

Formation of the male internal genitalia requires Leydig cell production of testosterone to prevent wolffian duct regression. In the absence of testosterone, the wolffian ducts degenerate. Also required is antimüllerian hormone (AMH, also known as *müllerian inhibiting substance* or *MIS*), which is produced by the Sertoli cells and results in regression of the müllerian duct. In the absence of AMH, the müllerian duct persists. It is therefore the active production of these two factors by the testis that results in male internal genitalia and the absence of these two hormones in the female that results in female internal genitalia. In the absence of any gonadal stimulation, all embryos develop female internal genitalia, i.e., regression of the wolffian ducts and persistence of the müllerian duct.

In the presence of testosterone, the wolffian duct differentiates into the epididymis, vas deferens, and seminal vesicles. The wolffian duct therefore depends on active testosterone secretion from the testis. The androgen receptor is essential to mediate the effects of testosterone. This is evident in patients with androgen insensitivity. These individuals have an XY karyotype, make SRY, and therefore form testis that produces testosterone. However, they lack a functional androgen receptor; therefore, the wolffian duct cannot respond to the testosterone produced and regresses. Failure of compete regression of the wolffian duct in a normal XX female can result in cystic structures along its course. These most commonly appear as Gärtner's duct cysts along the lateral wall of the vagina.

In contrast to the wolffian duct, the müllerian duct persists in the absence of external signals and must be directed to degenerate in males. The testis secretes AMH that specifically causes degeneration and resorption of the müllerian duct in males. AMH is a 560-amino-acid glycoprotein made in Sertoli cells.[7,8] It belongs to the transforming growth factor β (TGF-β) family of proteins and acts as a local signal targeting the müllerian duct. AMH blocks the function of the epidermal growth factor (EGF) receptor, causing regression of EGF receptor–regulated development; the müllerian duct depends on EGF signaling for development.

In the absence of gonads (i.e., in the absence of testosterone and AMH production), female internal genitalia will develop. In patients with androgen insensitivity, the testis is present, makes AMH, and causes müllerian regression. Androgen insensitivity therefore results in failure to support the wolffian duct and simultaneous active regression of the müllerian duct due to secretion of AMH. These individuals therefore have neither male nor female internal genitalia.

In the absence of AMH, the müllerian ducts develop into fallopian tubes, uterus, cervix, and upper vagina. While estrogen is necessary to attain a fully developed uterus, the differentiation into unique (however smaller) morphologic structures does not require estrogen or the estrogen receptor. Mice with a targeted disruption of estrogen receptor α (ERα) have rudimentary genitalia with a distinct oviduct, uterus, cervix, and vagina.[9] The genetic basis of this differential pattern of müllerian duct segmentation has been described recently.

Developmental patterning genes have been highly conserved throughout evolution. All multicellular animals share the same genes that ultimately determine the body plan along undifferentiated developmental axes. The HOX genes establish cellular identities along undifferentiated axes of all higher multicellular animals.[10] The müllerian duct and wolffian duct are two such seemingly uniform undifferentiated tissue axes. HOX genes give differential identity to the various segments of these developmental axes, leading to distinct external and internal genital structures such as fallopian tubes, uterus, cervix, and vagina.

The phenomenon that led to discovery of the HOX genes was observed over a century ago when Bateson described the transformation of one body structure into another in the fruit fly. Less than two decades ago, the genetic basis for these transformations was identified in the "selector" or HOX genes. Mutations in these genes often resulted in transformation of one body structure into another; this led to the concept that HOX genes are master regulators of tissue identity along all body axes. These genes have been shown to give rise to tissue identity along several body axes, including the central nervous system, vertebrae, limbs, and the reproductive tract. Humans have 39 HOX genes arranged in four parallel clusters, termed HOXA, HOXB, HOXC, and HOXD. Each cluster exhibits a spatial colinearity; the genes are arranged on the chromosome in the same order (3'–5') as they are expressed (cranial to caudal) along the body axes.

HOX genes are transcription factors. They regulate gene expression, resulting in appropriate determination of body segment identity. The order and differential expression of HOX genes along previously differentiated axes leads to proper development of appropriate region-specific body structures. HOX genes of groups

9 to 13 are expressed in restricted domains along the axes of the developing wolffian and müllerian ducts.[11,12] *HOXA9* is expressed in areas destined to become the fallopian tube, *HOXA10* in the developing uterus, *HOXA11* in the primordia of the lower uterine segment and cervix, and *HOXA13* in the future upper vagina. The expression of these *HOX* genes in their designated location along the müllerian ducts leads to the development of appropriate adult structures, as demonstrated in Figure 7-4. Genes of the *HOXC* and *HOXD* cluster are also expressed in the developing müllerian duct and likely contribute further to the specification of tissue identity during development. Similar *HOX* expression leads to segmental identity of the wolffian duct.[13]

The importance of *HOX* genes in development of the human reproductive tract is demonstrated by alterations in the reproductive tract seen in women with mutations in the *HOXA13* gene.[14] Some of these women have hand-foot-genital syndrome. This is typified by müllerian fusion defects such as didelphic or bicornuate uterus (to be discussed later).

The nonsteroidal estrogen diethylstilbestrol (DES) alters reproductive tract development. DES has been shown to alter the expression pattern of *HOXA* genes in the müllerian duct.[15] In utero, DES exposure shifts *HOXA9* expression from the oviducts to the uterus and decreases both *HOXA10* and *HOXA11* expression in the uterus. The uterus thus could be imparted with a developmental identity more similar to those structures in which *HOXA9* is normally expressed, e.g., the fallopian tube. The T-shaped uterus seen in women exposed to DES could represent a narrow and more branched structure, similar to the structure of the fallopian tube. Uterine development therefore is directed toward an identity similar to that structure where *HOXA9* is normally expressed and looses the typical uterine structure normally driven by *HOXA10* and *HOXA11* expression. Alteration of normal patterns of *HOX* gene expression and other developmental

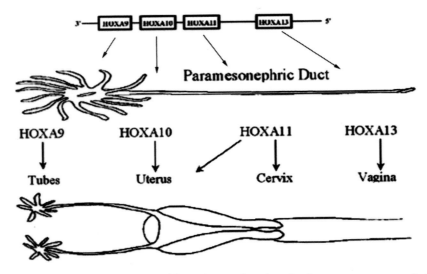

HOX Code of the Developing Müllerian System

Figure 7-4 *HOX* genes give segmental identity to the developing paramesonephric (müllerian) duct. Expression of a particular *HOX* gene in a segment of this duct leads to appropriate development of adult structures.

genes likely accounts for the developmental anomalies induced by DES.

At approximately 9 weeks of gestation, after müllerian duct fusion and formation of the uterine horns, the caudal end of the müllerian duct contacts the urogenital sinus. This induces proliferation of the endoderm called the *sinovaginal bulb* (Fig. 7-5). This proliferation continues between the müllerian duct and the urogenital sinus, forming the vaginal plate. By 18 weeks, the sinovaginal bulb forms a lumen between the urogenital sinus and the lower müllerian tract. The vaginal fornices and upper third of the vagina are thought to be of müllerian origin, whereas the lower two-thirds of the vagina is derived from the sinovaginal bulbs. The hymen consists of remnants of tissue separating the urogenital sinus from the lumen of the vagina. It consists of cells originating in both the vaginal and urogenital sinus.

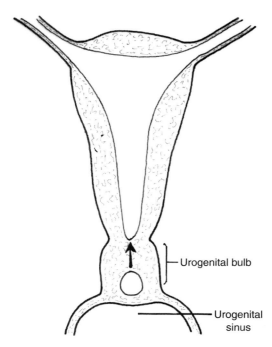

Figure 7-5 After contact of the fused müllerian ducts with the urogenital sinus, the urogenital bulb will proliferate, forming the lower vagina.

— Urogenital bulb

— Urogenital sinus

Development of the External Genitalia

The external genitalia begin to form during the fourth week. Mesenchymal cells migrate around the cloaca to form the labioscrotal swellings. Fusion of these swellings eventually forms the genital tubercle. The genital tubercle will form the clitoris or glans penis. By the sixth week of gestation, the urethral folds are distinct from the more posterior anal folds, whereas laterally the labial scrotal folds form. At the end of the sixth week, the anus develops from the dorsal cloaca, and the ventral portion becomes the urogenital fold. Without androgen stimulation, the urogenital folds do not fuse and become the labia minora, whereas the labial scrotal folds remain as distinct labia majora. In the male, testosterone is converted to 5α-dihydrotestosterone (DHT) via the action of 5α-reductase in the urogenital swellings but not in the wolffian duct. DHT is required for male external genitalia development. In the absence of androgen signal, as in androgen insensitivity (discussed earlier), the external genitalia remain female.

In males with 5α-reductase deficiency, newborns have produced AMH and testosterone. The internal genitalia therefore are male; the müllerian ducts have regressed, and wolffian duct–derived structures are present. However, due to the lack of DHT, the external genitalia have remained female in appearance. There is, however, only a blind vaginal opening and an enlarged clitoris. Affected children are assigned a female gender and typically are raised as such. Interestingly, at puberty, the genitalia become responsive to higher levels of testosterone, causing obvious masculinization and often leading to a change of gender identity.

▶ DEVELOPMENTAL ANOMALIES OF THE FEMALE REPRODUCTIVE TRACT

Developmental reproductive disorders due to altered chromosomal complement, absence of the gonads, or enzyme deficiencies will be discussed primarily in Chapter 8. This chapter will focus on clinically observed anomalies of the internal and external genitalia. Most anomalies of the reproductive tract result from disordered development of the müllerian or vaginal primordium near the eighth week of gestation. These typically involve a defect in the migration or fusion of the müllerian structures or their complete absence. Müllerian anomalies are present in approximately 2 to 3 percent of births.[16–22]

Anomalies of the Lower Female Reproductive Tract

Anomalies of the External Genitalia

Minor congenital malformations of the external genitalia are uncommon and may not be detected at birth. Major vulvar anomalies may result in sexual ambiguity at birth and will be discussed subsequently with androgen disorders. Some may be a sign of life-threatening enzyme deficiencies that must be recognized promptly and treated. Major congenital malformations of the external genitalia should prompt the search for additional anomalies, especially in the rest of the urogenital tract.

Clitoral hypertrophy generally is caused by androgen exposure. In utero, androgen exposure resulting in clitoral enlargement may be due to fetal adrenal enzyme disorders, maternal enzyme disorders, androgen-producing tumors, or exogenous androgen exposure. Clitoral hypertrophy should prompt an evaluation of androgen excess and localization and identification of the etiology for excess androgen exposure. Deficiencies of the 21-hydroxylase enzyme (discussed later) accounts for approximately 90 percent of these cases; deficiencies of 3β-hydroxysteroid dehydrogenase or 11-hydroxylase are far less common. Androgen-secreting maternal tumors can masculinize the external genitalia and are typically ovarian in origin but also can be adrenal in origin. However, despite markedly elevated maternal an-

drogen levels in the affected pregnancy, the majority of female offspring are not masculinized. In contrast to patients with congenital adrenal hyperplasia, further postnatal virilization does not occur in those affected by a maternal source of androgen. The most common cause of excessive ovarian production of androgens in pregnancy is a luteoma. This is a hyperplastic response of the luteinized thecal cells to human chorionic gonadotropin (hCG) stimulation, typically regressing spontaneously after pregnancy. Ingestion of testosterone, progestins derived from testosterone, or other androgens also can result in clitoral hypertrophy; the synthetic steroids are aromatized less effectively by the placenta and therefore are more likely to cause clitoromegaly.

The labia majora are derived from the labioscrotal folds. Labial size depends primarily on fat content. Fusion of the labioscrotal folds, as normally occurs in males, also may occur as a result of androgen exposure. Acquired labial adhesions primarily involve the labia minora and are often a consequence of vulvitis in prepubertal girls. Labial fusion is characterized by a thick perineum that includes the labia majora, whereas labial adhesions are characterized typically by adherence of the labia minora along a thin vertical translucent line. Labial adhesions respond to topical estrogen, whereas labial fusion requires surgical correction.

Asymmetric development of the labia occurs to some degree in 12 percent of women. Labial hypertrophy is subjective and common. Correction is not needed except in the extreme, when there is interference with daily activity or clothing. Imperforate hymen results from failure of the sinus tubercle to regress. This anomaly may present as a mucocele prepubertally or as a hematocolpos after menarche. These are easily corrected surgically.

Anomalies of the Nonmüllerian Portion of the Vagina

Congenital anomalies of the vagina often present at puberty with lack of menstruation or with obstruction to attempted intercourse. A common anomaly of the vagina is due to failure of complete regression of the wolffian duct. A remnant or sinus of the wolffian duct is typically cystic and parallels the müllerian duct. Vaginal wolffian remnants are seen in the lateral vaginal wall and are referred to as *Gärtner's duct cysts*. Other wolffian duct remnants such as peritubal cysts, epoophoron, or paroophoron may be seen at the time of surgery. Typically, Gärtner's duct cysts are clinically insignificant; however, in the extreme, they can cause obstruction of menstrual flow.

In the absence of virilization and in the presence of otherwise normal female secondary sexual characteristics, a blind vaginal opening suggests either congenital absence of the vagina or androgen-insensitivity syndrome. Androgen insensitivity, as discussed previously, occurs in 46,XY individuals with defective androgen receptors, normal or low-normal male serum testosterone levels, and lack of external genitalia masculinization. Müllerian regression, however, is seen in these individuals. In XX individuals, congenital absence of the vagina can occur either in isolation or with the absence of all müllerian structures (müllerian agenesis, also known as *Mayer-Rokitansky-Küster-Hauser syndrome*).

Failure of the fused müllerian ducts to fuse subsequently with the urogenital sinus results in a transverse vaginal septum. Indicative of the embryologic point of fusion of these two structures, the vaginal septum typically occurs between the middle and upper third of the vagina.[23] However, the septum can occur anywhere along the vagina, perhaps indicating that several distinct developmental defects can alter the point of fusion or lead to proliferation of the vaginal mesoderm to the point of occlusion. Transverse vaginal septa vary widely in size and may affect most of the vagina.[24] Differentiation from imperforate hymen or vaginal agenesis typically is assessed on examination; however, ultrasound and magnetic resonance imaging (MRI) are helpful in confirming the diagnosis.[25,26] It is imperative to distinguish a transverse vaginal septum from an imperforate hymen. The imperforate hymen often is accompanied by a mucocele or a hematocolpos and typically will bulge during a Valsalva maneuver. While surgical correction of the imperforate hymen is accomplished fairly easily, resection of a transverse vaginal septum requires more extensive training. Müllerian anomalies commonly are accompanied by other anatomic abnormalities of the urinary and gastrointestinal tract. Depending on the length of the septum, the surgeon must be prepared for possible skin grafting or complete vaginal reconstruction. Evaluation includes MRI to delineate the extent of the lesion, including the length of the septum.

Reconstruction of vaginal anomalies should take into account the anatomy of surrounding structures (including gastrointestinal and genitourinary), the extent of the lesion, accompanying müllerian anomalies, and any functional defect caused by the lesion. Vaginal agenesis may be corrected without surgery using vaginal dilators. The Frank procedure involves the patient applying daily pressure at the introitus using progressively larger dilators.[27] This technique has been successful within several months.[28] An alternative technique described by Ingram uses a dilator fixed to a bicycle seat with the patient allowing her body weight to assist in the application of pressure.[29] These techniques require patient motivation and must be continued or replaced by frequent coitus to maintain vaginal patency.

Surgical correction is used for patients with absent vagina who decline or have failed conservative therapy. The McIndoe procedure involves sharp dissection of the peritoneal body followed by blunt dissection superiorly to the level of the inferior parietal peritoneum. An artificial vaginal mold is inserted with an inverted split-thickness skin graft that is sutured to the mold. The graft is typically left in place for 10 days while the patient remains at bed rest with bladder catheterization. The Williams vulvovaginoplasty similarly creates a neovagina but uses the patient's own vulvar skin to line the canal. It is particularly effective for patients with considerable scar formation or poor tissue integrity.

Müllerian Anomalies

Classification of Müllerian Anomalies

The most widely used classification system of müllerian anomalies is that established by the American Society for Reproductive Medicine (ASRM),[30] as demonstrated in Figure 7-6. It can be divided into anomalies involving (1) agenesis or hypoplasia of the müllerian tract, (2) failure of müllerian duct fusion, and (3) failure to resorb the intervening tissue between the fused müllerian ducts. Class I defects involve hypoplasia or agenesis of segments of the müllerian tract. These anomalies, which specifically result in segmental developmental defects, may arise from aberrant control of developmental identity of individual müllerian tract components; this identity is regulated by *HOX* genes. Class II defects are characterized by unilateral hypoplasia or agenesis of structures derived from a single müllerian duct. Class III defects arise from failed fusion of the müllerian ducts, resulting in the didelphic uterus. The didelphic uterus consists of two completely separate hemiuteri. The class IV defect is the bicornuate uterus resulting from incomplete fusion of the müllerian ducts; the bicornuate uterus has a single cavity and an unfused fundus. Class V anomalies consist of a persistent septum as a result of failed resorption of the median tissue between the fused müllerian ducts. Class VI is the arcuate uterus resulting from resorption of most, but not all, of the septum. Finally, class VII consists of diethylstilbestrol (DES)–induced anomalies. One review combining several studies estimated a mean distribution of specific anomalies as follows: bicornuate uterus, 37 percent; arcuate uterus, 15 percent; incomplete septum, 13 percent; uterine didelphys, 11 percent; complete septum, 9 percent; and unicornuate uterus, 4.4 percent.[31]

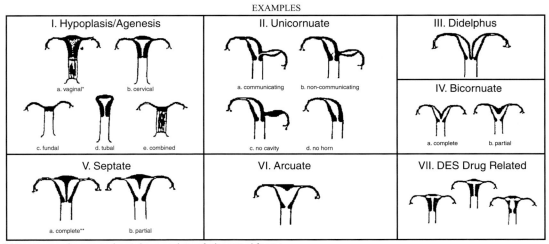

THE AMERICAN FERTILITY SOCIETY CLASSIFICATION OF MÜLLERIAN ANOMALIES

* Uterus may be normal or take a variety of abnormal forms.
** May have two distinct cervices

Figure 7-6 The spectrum of clinically observed müllerian anomalies as classified by the American Society for Reproductive Medicine. (Adapted from *Fertil Steril* 1989;51:199–201.)

Anomalies of the Müllerian Portion of the Vagina

A longitudinal vaginal septum results from failure of the tissue between the fused müllerian ducts to regress. Failure of fusion may result in the appearance of two vaginal canals. Presence of two vaginal canals should prompt evaluation of the upper müllerian tract for a uterine septum or uterus didelphys (discussed below). Most communicating longitudinal septa are asymptomatic, whereas a noncommunicating septum may result in symptoms secondary to menstrual outflow obstruction. The vaginal septum is often missed on examination because rapid placement of the speculum obscures the entrance to the second canal that may appear similar to vaginal rugae when compressed. Patients presenting at menarche with pelvic pain, dysmenorrhea, or a purulent vaginal discharge should be evaluated for a vaginal septum. These patients often are misdiagnosed because of unilateral menstrual flow. The retrograde flow may result in accumulation of tubal and peritoneal menstrual blood and endometriosis. The finding of a müllerian fusion defect should prompt evaluation of the urinary tract for associated anomalies.

Uterine Anomalies

Uterine developmental anomalies are fairly common. They have been estimated to occur in 2 to 3 percent of women.[16,17,19,20,22,32,33] The precise incidence is unknown because many go undiagnosed. Uterine anomalies are reported to have significant effects on reproductive success. However, detection depends on the method used for diagnosis, as well as patient selection. Exploration of the uterus after delivery determined the rate of uterine anomalies to be 3 percent,[34] whereas testing of women with recurrent pregnancy losses with imaging techniques such as hysterosalpingogram (HSG), ultrasound, or MRI revealed that approximately one-quarter had an anomaly.[35] The overall incidence of uterine defects appears to be similar in both fertile and infertile women at 2 to 5 percent.[31] However, uter-

ine anomalies are more common in women with first-trimester losses (5 to 10 percent) and very common in women with later adverse reproductive outcomes, such as recurrent loss, preterm delivery, and malpresentation. In these women, the incidence is estimated to be approaching 27 percent.

Since these uterine anomalies are common and may have significant effects on reproductive outcome, each will be discussed individually.

Hypoplasia or agenesis of the müllerian ducts may involve the vagina, cervix, fundus, fallopian tubes, or a combination of these. Cervical and tubal ageneses are both rare. Patients with tubal agenesis present with infertility and can be treated with in vitro fertilization and embryo transfer (IVF/ET). Patients with cervical agenesis present with recurrent cyclic pain. Attempts to treat cervical agenesis by creation of an outflow tract largely have been unsuccessful. Patients with congenital absence or hypoplasia of the uterus also typically lack the vagina as well. Normal ovaries and external genitalia are typical of the Mayer-Rokitansky-Küster-Hauser syndrome. As described earlier, differential diagnosis includes androgen insensitivity, transverse vaginal septum, and imperforate hymen. These can be distinguished by karyotype and testosterone levels or by the presence of hematocolpos on rectal examination or ultrasound. Major urinary tract anomalies such as absence of a kidney or pelvic kidney occur in 15 percent of patients, whereas two to three times as many have minor defects.[36] Individuals with an absent or hypoplastic uterus may be treated with IVF (because they have ovarian function) and a surrogate gestational carrier.

The unicornuate uterus results from asymmetric development of the müllerian ducts. One side develops normally, while the contralateral side fails to develop. Rudimentary uterine horns result from incomplete development of the contralateral müllerian duct. A rudimentary horn may communicate with the unicornuate uterus or may be obstructed or solid. Approximately 75 percent of rudimentary horns do not communicate with the contralateral functional hemiuterus and can result in hematometra, retrograde menstruation, and endometriosis. Renal anomalies are present in the majority of patients with unicornuate uterus and invariably occur ipsilateral to the absent hemiuterus.[37] An obstructed hemiuterus is often diagnosed at menarche; patients present with increasing dysmenorrhea and pelvic mass. In the absence of a rudimentary horn or lack of functional endometrial tissue in the rudimentary horn, these patients are typically asymptomatic and fertile.[38] Recurrent pregnancy loss, preterm labor, and malpresentation are common in women with unicornuate uterus.[38-40] Pregnancies can occur in a rudimentary horn and have a survival rate of only 1 to 2 percent. The uterine horn ruptures prior to 20 weeks of gestation in 90 percent of pregnancies, typically resulting in life-threatening hemorrhage.[41]

Failure of the müllerian ducts to fuse results in a double uterus or uterus didelphys. Each separate uterine horn is accompanied by its own cervix and fallopian tube. Typically the didelphic uterus is accompanied by vaginal septum. Renal anomalies are less common than in patients with unicornuate uterus. Occasionally, obstruction of one hemivagina may result in hematocolpos presentating soon after menarche, but most are asymptomatic. Patients may have difficulty with tampon use or experience dyspareunia depending on the extent of the vaginal septum. As with all nonobstructive müllerian anomalies, infertility is not typical of the didelphic uterus; rather, this anomaly is associated with pregnancy loss, malpresentation, and preterm labor.

Incomplete fusion of the müllerian ducts results in a bicornuate uterus. In these individuals, müllerian duct fusion occurs caudally but not to the fundus, resulting in a single cervix and lower uterine segment with two separate fundi. A vaginal septum is rarely seen, and urinary tract anomalies occur in less than 10 percent of patients.[42] These patients also typically are asymptomatic prior to pregnancy and are fertile. Pregnancy loss and obstetric complications are not uncommon, but live birth rates of greater than 52 to 85 percent have been reported.[43-45]

Failure of resorption of the intervening midline tissue after müllerian duct fusion results in a septate uterus.[46] This common congenital uterine anomaly is highly variable, with the extent of the septum ranging from partial to complete. A partial septum projecting caudally from the fundus is most common. A complete septum can divide the entire uterine cavity and is seen in less than 10 percent of patients with this anomaly.[47] The septum can divide the cervix and continue into the vagina. Urinary tract anomalies occur in approximately 20 percent of patients with a septate uterus. Again, pregnancy loss and obstetric complications are associated with this anomaly. Most patients are asymptomatic, and most septa are not detectable on physical examination; therefore, the true incidence of septate uterus is difficult to ascertain. The septum itself is fibrous with a poor blood supply.

The arcuate uterus represents a minimal failure of müllerian duct fusion in the fundus. The arcuate uterus is often diagnosed incidentally and can be considered a normal variant, unlikely to be a cause of impaired reproduction.

Unlike most uterine anomalies that result from failure of the müllerian duct to either form, fuse internally, or subsequently resorb, exposure to DES results in craniocaudal defects. DES affects developmental gene expression along the müllerian duct, causing inappropriate segmentation. DES was used in women with recurrent or threatened abortion or otherwise poor obstetric history until the early 1970s. Females exposed in utero often had müllerian anomalies. Typical findings are a T-shaped uterine cavity or a constricted cavity along with cervical and vaginal defects.[48-51] Affected women have an increased incidence of adverse obstetric outcomes.[52] Vaginal adenosis and a propensity to develop vaginal clear cell carcinoma result from a caudal displacement of the squamocolumnar junction.[51-53] Cervical hoods, hypoplasia, collars, and ridges result from failure of the vaginal plate to develop the vaginal fornices.[54] The T-shaped uterus has been hypothesized to result from misexpression of developmental control genes (e.g., *HOX* genes, *Wnt* genes). *HOXA9,* typically expressed in the fallopian tube, is instead expressed in the developing uterus, resulting in an incomplete caudal displacement of the uterotubal junction.[15]

▶ DIAGNOSIS AND TREATMENT OF UTERINE ANOMALIES

Women with uterine anomalies have an increased incidence of spontaneous abortion, preterm labor, and malpresentation.[42,55] In the absence of endometriosis from an obstructed outflow tract, these anomalies are not a significant cause of infertility.[6] Anomalies with an obstructive component often are diagnosed after menarche; however, most uterine anomalies are diagnosed incidentally or during evaluation of recurrent pregnancy loss or obstetric complications. A careful physical examination, hysterosalpingogram, ultrasound, MRI, and laparoscopy may be helpful in the diagnosis of uterine anomalies and subsequent classification.[56–63] Additionally, because of the high incidence of accompanying urinary tract anomalies, an intravenous pyelogram (IVP) should be performed on all patients diagnosed with a uterine anomaly. While an MRI may characterize the kidney, it is insufficient to characterize

the course of the ureter or to identify a duplication of the ureter.

A high index of suspicion is necessary to diagnose a uterine anomaly in most instances. An anomaly should be considered in the differential diagnosis in patients with early-onset, severe dysmenorrhea, a nonovarian pelvic mass presenting soon after menarche, repeated pregnancy loss, repeated unexplained preterm labor, malpresentation, or fetal growth retardation. Complete evaluation is more informative in the nongravid state.

The unicornuate uterus is difficult to identify on physical examination. The diagnosis typically is suggested by an HSG that demonstrates a solitary, laterally displaced cavity and a single fallopian tube. When a unicornuate uterus is suspected after HSG, careful evaluation looking for a second vaginal canal or obstructed canal is warranted. Differential diagnosis includes complete septum or didelphys. Additionally, the possibility of a rudimentary horn should be evaluated. Sonography often incorrectly diagnoses a unicornuate uterus, and a rudimentary horn may be mistaken for a myoma.[57,64] MRI has excellent sensitivity and specificity and is the best noninvasive means of diagnosing unicornuate uterus[65] (Fig. 7-7A). Laparoscopy may be necessary if the diagnosis

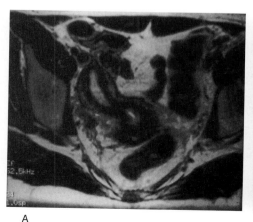 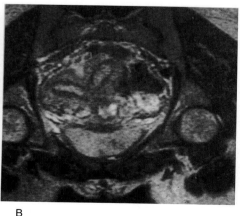

A   B

Figure 7-7 MRI demonstrates unicornuate and bicornuate uterus. *A.* Unicornuate uterus as seen as a single hemiuterus displaced to the right. *B.* The bicornuate uteri demonstrate a single caudal uterine cavity and unfused fundus.

is uncertain with imaging studies. Surgery is indicated only for the removal of a functional rudimentary horn, thereby avoiding the risk of pregnancy therein and reducing potential reflux resulting in endometriosis.[39,41,63,66,67]

The diagnosis of didelphic uterus often is made after identification of a double vagina or cervix or an irregularly contoured duplication of the uterus. Differential diagnosis includes a complete septum extending through the cervix, appearing as a double cervix and perhaps vagina. While there is no proven treatment for didelphic uterus, a septate uterus is easily repaired hysteroscopically, and therefore, definitive diagnosis is imperative. The HSG is not helpful in differentiating a didelphic uterus from a complete septum (Fig. 7-8). The two cervixes can be separately infused with contrast material, which will identify two separate uterine cavities with a single tube originating from each. While the didelphic uterus generally has an acute angle between the cavities, this distinction is not sufficient to distinguish the two entities. Ultrasound is helpful but also insufficient for diagnosis.[57,68,69] MRI can be used accurately to diagnose a didelphic uterus and to distinguish it from a septate uterus. However, MRI often cannot distinguish clearly the vaginal anatomy. As mentioned earlier, if the diagnosis remains uncertain after imaging studies, laparoscopy can be performed to confirm the diagnosis. While metroplasty has been advocated for didelphic uterus, data show no efficacy of this procedure in improving pregnancy outcome, and surgical correction generally should not be attempted.

A bicornuate uterus typically is found incidentally at laparoscopy or HSG (see Fig. 7-7B).

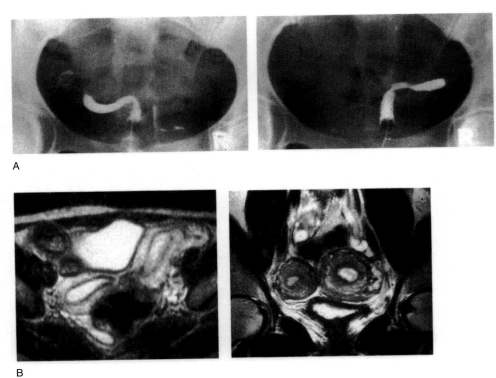

Figure 7-8 Diagnosis of the didelphic uterus. *A.* Each hemiuterus demonstrated on HSG. *B.* MRI defines two distinct cavities in two separate hemiuteri.

Differential diagnosis includes a didelphic uterus and an incomplete septum.[70] A bicornuate uterus may be suspected by palpation of two uterine horns on physical examination but can readily be distinguished from didelphic uterus. Septate and bicornuate uterus cannot be distinguished on HSG because both will demonstrate the appearance of two uterine horns. Differentiating these conditions is essential because the septum is amenable to surgical correction, whereas the bicornuate uterus is not. Ultrasonography, while often suggestive, is not sufficient to outline the fundal contour. As with other anomalies, MRI is extremely accurate in elucidating the nature of the uterine anatomy. A normal fundus distinguishes septum from the biphid fundus of the bicornuate uterus. While it was believed previously that the low-intensity signal in the septum, indicating the lack of myometrium, would distinguish the two, it has been demonstrated recently that the septum can contain myometrium.[60,71] Diagnosis also can be made accurately with simultaneous laparoscopy and hysteroscopy. While the Strassman procedure was advocated for unification of a bicornuate uterus, it is not without complications, and data on efficacy are lacking.[31]

Septate uterus is a common anomaly for which treatment is readily available.[72] The septum may vary from minimal to complete. A partial uterine septum that divides the cranial portion of the cavity to various degrees is most common. On HSG, a partial septate uterus cannot be distinguished with complete certainty from a bicornuate uterus, as discussed earlier[73] (Fig. 7-9). A complete septum, present in 8 percent of patients with a septate uterus, completely divides the cavity and may divide the cervix and vagina as well.[47] The complete septum with a divided cervix must be distinguished from a didelphic uterus. Associated urinary tract anomalies occur in approximately 20 percent of patients with a septate uterus.

Septate uteri are associated with poor reproductive outcomes, similar to that found in

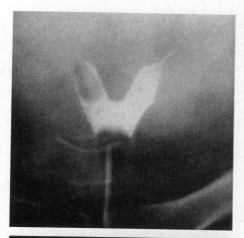

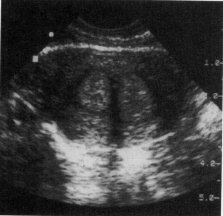

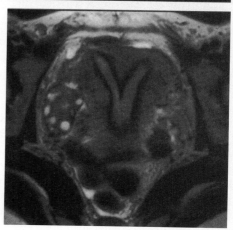

Figure 7-9 The septate uterus as imaged by HSG (top), Ultrasound (center), or MRI (bottom).

women with other uterine anomalies.[74] The etiology of the compromised reproductive outcome was thought to arise from implantation on a fibrous septum. Biopsies of the septum, however, have revealed muscular tissue in the septum. Repeated pregnancy losses may be due to the abnormal vascularization of the septum and surrounding myometrium.[75]

The Jones metroplasty involves removing a wedge that includes the septum, whereas the Tompkins metroplasty involves bivalving the uterus.[76,77] These techniques have been replaced almost completely by hysteroscopic resection of the septum.[74] The hysteroscopic approach not only is less invasive but also does not require subsequent caesarean section for obstetric delivery.[78,79]

Hysteroscopy is accompanied typically by a laparoscopy. Laparoscopy confirms the diagnosis of septate uterus and can be used to monitor the hysteroscopic procedure. With the use of a dimmed light source, the proximity of the hysteroscope to the fundus can be ascertained, thereby reducing the risk of uterine perforation. Similarly, laparoscopic assistance can limit complications in the event of perforation. The experienced surgeon may forego laparoscopy if the diagnosis is ensured by prior laparoscopy or MRI. The procedure is best scheduled in the early proliferative phase or after suppression of endometrial proliferation with a gonadotropin-releasing hormone (GnRH) agonist, GnRH antagonist, or a progestin. The septum and tubal ostia are identified prior to resection. A midline incision is made with scissors or a modified straight resectoscope (Fig. 7-10). The septum retracts as it is divided, and typically there is little need for resection. Minimal bleeding typically is encountered due to the relative avascularity of the septum; bleeding is usually indicative of having gone past the septum into the myometrium. The resection is complete when a normal-appearing fundus is created.[80,81]

Surgical correction of the complete septum is a more challenging procedure. Dye placed into one uterine cavity may be helpful at iden-

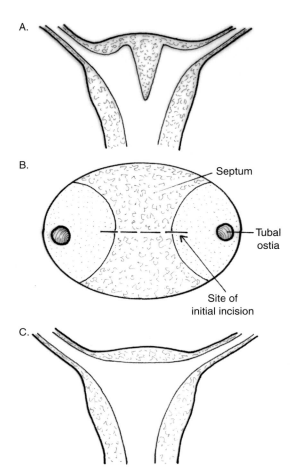

Figure 7-10 *A.* The partial septate uterus. Hysteroscopic view of the uterine septum. An incision is made in the midline connecting the tubal ostia. *B.* The uterine cavity after correction of the septum.

tifying entry into the second cavity (Fig. 7-11). The portion of the septum that extends through a double cervix should be left intact to avoid future cervical incompetence. Following resection of the uterine septum, adequate estrogen stimulation is used to enhance endometrial proliferation and to prevent intrauterine synechia. Conjugated equine estrogens (2.5 mg bid) or the equivalent is suggested, particularly in those patients who received GnRH agonist or antagonist preoperatively.[82] An intrauterine device,

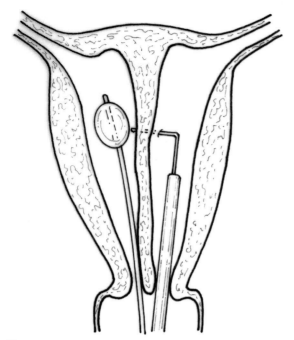

Figure 7-11 One hysteroscopic approach to the repair of a complete uterine septum.

pediatric Foley catheter (trimmed of its protruding end), or a specific uterine-shaped balloon can be used to maintain cavity integrity after more extensive resections. A postoperative HSG can evaluate the technical success of the procedure. Successful pregnancies have been reported in up to 86 percent of patients after hysteroscopic resection (similar to normal pregnancy rates).[83]

▶ SUMMARY

The human urogenital tract develops from a well-orchestrated developmental program. Components include sex chromosome complement, developmental genes, cell segmental identity genes, and alteration by epigenic factors. Knowledge of the origin of the reproductive tract, including the müllerian system, allows better understanding of the diverse array of anomalies encountered clinically.

KEY POINTS

1. The fate of the gonad is specified by the presence or absence of the *SRY* gene on the Y chromosome.

2. Development of the male internal genitalia depends on local testosterone production by the gonad. Regression of the müllerian duct depends on the production of AMH by the testicle. In the absence of testosterone and AMH, the müllerian duct persists, and the female reproductive tract develops.

3. Development of the external genitalia is mediated by the absence or presence of dihydrotestosterone (DHT).

4. Differential segmental identity of the reproductive tract is determined by the expression of *HOX* and other developmental genes.

5. Developmental anomalies of the female reproductive tract are common. They typically result from failure of genesis or fusion or resorption of segments of the embryonic reproductive tract. Common anomalies include vaginal septa or the unicornuate, bicornuate, septate, or didelphic uterus. Additionally, the T-shaped uterus is associated with in utero DES exposure.

6. Nonobstructive uterine anomalies typically result in an increased incidence of spontaneous abortion, preterm labor, and malpresentation. Obstructive lesions of the female reproductive tract may present with a pelvic mass and severe dysmenorrhea. A high index of suspicion is necessary to diagnose uterine anomalies promptly in most instances.

7. While HSG and ultrasound have a role in diagnosing uterine anomalies, the gold standard is laparoscopy and hysteroscopy. However, MRI has excellent sensitivity and may be substituted for surgery, reserving laparoscopy for instances in which the diagnosis is uncertain.

> 8. Surgical repair is indicated for the vaginal and the uterine septum. It also may be indicated for removal of the rudimentary horn coincident with a unicornuate uterus.

► ACKNOWLEDGEMENTS

Imaging (HSG, ultrasound, and MRI) courtesy of Professor Shirley McCarthy, Yale University School of Medicine.

REFERENCES

1. Schafer AJ, Goodfellow PN. Sex determination in humans. *Bioessays* 1996;18:955–963.
2. Page DC, De La Chapelle A, Weissenbach J. Chromosome Y–specific DNA in related human XX males. *Nature* 1985;315:224–226.
3. Sinclair AH, Berta P, Palmer MS, et al. A gene from the human sex-determining region encodes a protein with homology to a conserved dna-binding motif. *Nature* 1990;346:240–244.
4. Berta P, Hawkins JR, Sinclair AH, et al. Genetic evidence equating *SRY* and the testis-determining factor. *Nature* 1990;348:448–450.
5. Jager RJ, Anvret M, Hall K, Scherer G. A human XY female with a frame shift mutation in the candidate testis-determining gene *SRY*. *Nature* 1990;348:452–454.
6. Larsen WJ. *Development of the Urogenital System: Human Embryology*. New York: Churchill Livingstone, 1993.
7. Cate RL, Mattaliano RJ, Hession C, et al. Isolation of the bovine and human genes for müllerian inhibiting substance and expression of the human gene in animal cells. *Cell* 1986;45:685–698.
8. Tran D, Muesy-Dessole N, Josso N. Antimullerian hormone is a functional marker of fetal sertoli cells. *Nature* 1977;269:411–412.
9. Mueller SO, Korach KS. Immortalized testis cell lines from estrogen receptor (ER) α knockout and wild-type mice expressing functional ERα or ERβ. *J Androl* 2001;22:652–664.
10. McGinnis W, Krumlauf R. Homeobox genes and axial patterning. *Cell* 1992;68:283–302.
11. Taylor HS. The role of *HOX* genes in the development and function of the female reproductive tract. *Semin Reprod Med* 2000;18:81–89.
12. Taylor HS, Vandenheuvel GB, Igarashi P. A conserved *HOX* axis in the mouse and human female reproductive system: Late establishment and persistent adult expression of the *HOXA* cluster genes. *Biol Reprod* 1997;57:1338–1345.
13. Warot X, Fromental-Ramain C, Fraulob V, et al. Gene dosage–dependent effects of the *HOXA-13* and *HOXD-13* mutations on morphogenesis of the terminal parts of the digestive and urogenital tracts. *Development* 1997;124:4781–4791.
14. Mortlock DP, Innis JW. Mutation of *HOXA13* in hand-foot-genital syndrome. *Nature Genet* 1997;15:179–180.
15. Block K, Kardana A, Igarashi P, Taylor HS. In utero diethylstilbestrol (DES) exposure alters *HOX* gene expression in the developing müllerian system. *FASEB J* 2000;14:1101–1108.
16. Ashton D, Amin HK, Richart RM, Neuwirth RS. The incidence of asymptomatic uterine anomalies in women undergoing transcervical tubal sterilization. *Obstet Gynecol* 1988;72:28–30.
17. Byrne J, Nussbaum-Blask A, Taylor WS, et al. Prevalence of müllerian duct anomalies detected at ultrasound. *Am J Med Genet* 2000;94:9–12.
18. Heinonen PK, Saarikoski S, Pystynen P. Reproductive performance of women with uterine anomalies: An evaluation of 182 cases. *Acta Obstet Gynacol Scand* 1982;61:157–162.
19. Maneschi F, Zupi E, Marconi D, et al. Hysteroscopically detected asymptomatic müllerian anomalies: Prevalence and reproductive implications. *J Reprod Med* 1995;40:684–688.
20. Simon C, Martinez L, Pardo F, et al. Müllerian defects in women with normal reproductive outcome. *Fertil Steril* 1991;56:1192–1193.
21. Rock JA, Schlaff WD. The obstetric consequences of uterovaginal anomalies. *Fertil Steril* 1985;43:681–692.
22. Green LK, Harris RE. Uterine anomalies: Frequency of diagnosis and associated obstetric complications. *Obstet Gynecol* 1976;47:427–429.
23. Spence JE. Vaginal and uterine anomalies in the pediatric and adolescent patient. *J Pediatr Adolesc Gynecol* 1998;11:3–11.
24. Rock JA. Anomalous development of the vagina. *Semin Reprod Endocrinol* 1986;4:13–31.
25. Moore KL, Persaud TV. *The Developing Human: Clinically Oriented Embryology*. Philadelphia: Saunders, 2003.

26. Vainright JR Jr, Fulp CJ Jr, Schiebler ML. MR imaging of vaginal agenesis with hematocolpos. *J Comput Assist Tomogr* 1988;12:891–893.

27. Frank RT. Formation of artificial vaginal without operation. *Am J Obstet Gynecol* 1938;35:1053–1055.

28. Costa EMF, Mendonca BB, Inacio M, et al. Management of ambiguous genitalia in pseudohermaphrodites: New perspectives on vaginal dilation. *Fertil Steril* 1981;67:229–232.

29. Ingram JM. The bicycle seat stool in the treatment of vaginal agenesis and stenosis: A preliminary report. *Am J Obstet Gynecol* 1981;140:867–873.

30. Golan A, Langer R, Bukovsky I, Caspi E. Congenital anomalies of the müllerian system. *Fertil Steril* 1989;51:747–755.

31. Acien P. Incidence of müllerian defects in fertile and infertile women. *Hum Reprod* 1997;12:1372–1376.

32. Sanfilippo JS, Wakim NG, Schikler KN, Yussman MA. Endometriosis in association with uterine anomaly. *Am J Obstet Gynecol* 1986;154:39–43.

33. Rock JA, Schlaff WD. The obstetric consequences of uterovaginal anomalies. *Fertil Steril* 1985;43:681–692.

34. Greiss FC, Mauzy CH. Genital anomalies in women. *Am J Obstet Gynecol* 1961;82:330–339.

35. Harger JH, Archer DF, Marchese SG, et al. Etiology of recurrent pregnancy losses and outcome of subsequent pregnancies. *Obstet Gynecol* 1983;62:574–581.

36. Jones HW Jr, Rock JA. *Reparative and Constructive Surgery of the Female Generative Tract.* Baltimore: Williams & Williams, 1983.

37. Woolf RB, Allen WM. Concomitant malformations. *Obstet Gynecol* 1953;1953:236–265.

38. Semmens JP. Congenital anomalies of female genital tract: Functional classification based on review of 56 personal cases and 500 reported cases. *Obstet Gynecol* 1962;19:328–350.

39. Andrews MC, Jones HW J. Impaired reproductive performance of the unicornuate uterus: Intrauterine growth retardation, infertility, and recurrent abortion in five cases. *Am J Obstet Gynecol* 1982;144:173–176.

40. Beernink FJ, Beernink JR, Chinn A. Uterus unicorns with uterus solidaris. *Obstet Gynecol* 1976;47:651–653.

41. O'Leary JL, O'Leary JA. Rudimentary horn pregnancy. *Obstet Gynecol* 1963;22:371–375.

42. Rock JA, Jones H W Jr. The clinical management of the double uterus. *Fertil Steril* 1977;28:798–806.

43. Thompson JP, Smith RA, Welch JS. Reproductive ability after metroplasty. *Obstet Gynecol* 1966;28:363–368.

44. Ludmir J, Samuels P, Brooks S, Mennuti MT. Pregnancy outcome of patients with uncorrected uterine anomalies managed in a high-risk obstetric setting. *Obstet Gynecol* 1990;75:906–910.

45. Buttram VC Jr. Müllerian anomalies and their management. *Fertil Steril* 1983;40:159–163.

46. Homer HA, Li TC, Cooke ID. The septate uterus: A review of management and reproductive outcome. *Fertil Steril* 2000;73:1–14.

47. Hassiakos DK, Zourlas PA. Transcervical division of uterine septa. *Obstet Gynecol Surv* 1990;45:165–173.

48. Rennell CL. T-Shaped uterus in diethylstilbestrol (DES) exposure. *AJR* 1979;132:979–980.

49. Decherney AH, Cholst I, Naftolin F. Structure and function of the fallopian tubes following exposure to diethylstilbestrol (DES) during gestation. *Fertil Steril* 1981;36:741–745.

50. Kipersztok S, Javitt M, Hill MC, Stillman RJ. Comparison of magnetic resonance imaging and transvaginal ultrasonography with hysterosalpingography in the evaluation of women exposed to diethylstilbestrol. *J Reprod Med* 1996;41:347–351.

51. Goldberg JM, Falcone T. Effect of diethylstilbestrol on reproductive function. *Fertil Steril* 1999;72:1–7.

52. Herbst AL, Ulfelder H, Poskanzer DC. Adenocarcinoma of the vagina: Association of maternal stilboestrol therapy with tumor appearance in young women. *N Engl J Med* 1971;284:878–881.

53. Kaufman RH, Adam E, Hatch EE, et al. Continued follow-up of pregnancy outcomes in diethylstilbestrol-exposed offspring. *Obstet Gynecol* 2000;96:483–489.

54. Lin PC, Bhatnagar KP, Nettleton GS, Nakajima ST. Female genital anomalies affecting reproduction. *Fertil Steril* 2002;78:899–915.

55. Raga F, Bauset C, Remohi J, et al. Reproductive impact of congenital müllerian anomalies. *Hum Reprod* 1997;12:2277–2281.

56. Troiano RN, Mccarthy SM. State of the art:. Muellerain duct anomalies: Imaging and clinical issues. *Radiology* (in press).

57. Nicolini U, Bellotti M, Bonazzi B, et al. Can ultrasound be used to screen uterine malformations? *Fertil Steril* 1987;47:89–93.

58. Pellerito JS, Mccarthy SM, Doyle MB, et al. Diagnosis of uterine anomalies: Relative accuracy of MR imaging, endovaginal sonography, and hysterosalpingography. *Radiology* 1992;183: 795–800.

59. Goldberg JM, Falcone T, Attaran M. Sonohysterographic evaluation of uterine anomalies noted on hysterosalpingography. *Hum Reprod* 1998;12:2151–2152.

60. Kupesic S, Kurjak A. Ultrasound and Doppler assessment of uterine anomalies, in *Ultrasound and Infertility*. Pearl River, NY: Parthenon, 2000.

61. Raga F, Bonilla-Musoles F, Blanes J, Osborne NG. Congenital müllerian anomalies: Diagnostic accuracy of three-dimensional ultrasound. *Fertil Steril* 1996;65:523–528.

62. Wu MH, Hsu CC, Huang KE. Detection of congenital müllerian duct anomalies using three-dimensional ultrasound. *J Clin Ultrasound* 1997;25:487–492.

63. Fedele L, Zamberletti D, Vercellini P, et al. Reproductive performance of women with unicornuate uterus. *Fertil Steril* 1987;47:416–419.

64. Valdes C, Malini S, Malinak LR. Ultrasound evaluation of female genital tract anomalies: A review of 64 cases. *Am J Obstet Gynecol* 1984; 149:285–292.

65. Brody JM, Koelliker SL, Frishman GN. Unicornuate uterus: Imaging appearance, associated anomalies, and clinical implications. *AJR* 1998;171:1341–1347.

66. Heinonen PK. Unicornuate uterus and rudimentary horn. *Fertil Steril* 1997;68:224–230.

67. Rolen AC, Choquette AJ, Semmens JP. Rudimentary uterine horn: Obstetric and gynecologic implications. *Obstet Gynecol* 1966;27: 806–813.

68. Fedele L, Ferrazzi E, Dorta M, et al. Ultrasonography in the differential diagnosis of "double" uteri. *Fertil Steril* 1988;50:361–364.

69. Fedele L, Dorta M, Brioschi D, et al. Magnetic resonance evaluation of double uteri. *Obstet Gynecol* 1989;74:844–847.

70. Tulandi T, Arronet GH, Mcinnes RA. Arcuate and bicornuate uterine anomalies and infertility. *Fertil Steril* 1980;34:362–364.

71. Zreik TG, Troiano RN, Ghoussoub RA et al. Myometrial tissue in uterine septa. *J Am Assoc Gynecol Laparosc* 1998;5:155–160.

72. Fedele L, Bianchi S. Hysteroscopic metroplasty for septate uterus. *Obstet Gynecol Clin North Am* 1995;22:473–489.

73. Reuter KL, Daly DC, Cohen SM. Septate versus bicornuate uteri: Errors in imaging diagnosis. *Radiology* 1989;172:749–752.

74. Daly DC, Walters CA, Soto-Albors CE, Riddick DH. Hysteroscopic metroplasty: Surgical technique and obstetric outcome. *Fertil Steril* 1983; 39:623–628.

75. Raziel A, Arieli S, Bukovsky I, et al. Investigation of the uterine cavity in recurrent aborters. *Fertil Steril* 1994;62:1080–1082.

76. Jones HW Jr, Ges J. Double uterus as an etiologic factor in repeated abortion. *Am J Obstet Gynecol* 1953;65:325–339.

77. Tompkins P. Comments on the bicornuate uterus and twinning. *Surg Clin North Am* 1962; 42:1049–1062.

78. Gray SE, Roberts DK, Franklin RR. Fertility after metroplasty of the septate uterus. *J Reprod Med* 1984;29:185–188.

79. Decherney AH, Russell JB, Graebe RA, Polan ML. Resectoscopic management of müllerian fusion defects. *Fertil Steril* 1986;45:726–728.

80. Musich JR, Behrman SJ. Obstetric outcome before and after metroplasty in women with uterine anomalies. *Obstet Gynecol* 1978;52: 63–66.

81. Fedele L, Bianchi S, Marchini M, et al. Residual uterine septum of less than 1 cm after hysteroscopic metroplasty does not impair reproductive outcome. *Hum Reprod* 1996;11: 727–729.

82. Perino A, Mencaglia L, Hamou J, Cittadini E. Hysteroscopy for metroplasty of uterine septa: report of 24 cases. *Fertil Steril* 1987;48:321–323.

83. Valle RF, Sciarra JJ. Hysteroscopic treatment of the septate uterus. *Obstet Gynecol* 1986;67: 253–257.

Disorders of the Endocrine System

CHAPTER 8

Disorders of Sexual Development

Lorna Timmreck, David A. Ryley, and Richard H. Reindollar

At conception, every embryo has the potential to develop into either a male or a female. An orderly sequence of embryonic events must proceed for normal sexual differentiation of the gonads, internal ductal system, and external genitalia to occur. This developmental sequence proceeds along a predictable timetable for both male and female sexual differentiation, as shown in Figures 8-1 and 8-2.[1] This process is remarkably conserved from generation to generation because disorders in sexual development are noted only rarely at birth. As we continue to learn more about genes that regulate developmental processes, we can further our understanding of how and when abnormalities may occur.

Many intersex disorders have been identified and described[2] (Table 8-1). Such disorders result when the sequence of sexual development is disrupted in some way. Predictable defects are then present in the gonads, internal ductal system, and external genitalia. Because the defects occur in such a predictable fashion, the physician can quickly make a differential diagnosis with minimal ancillary testing when presented with an individual who has a disorder of sexual development. With continued advances in molecular medicine, not only do we have a better understanding of the genes involved in the pathogenesis of some of these disorders, but we also have the ability to provide rapid diagnosis, often within the first day of a newborn's life.

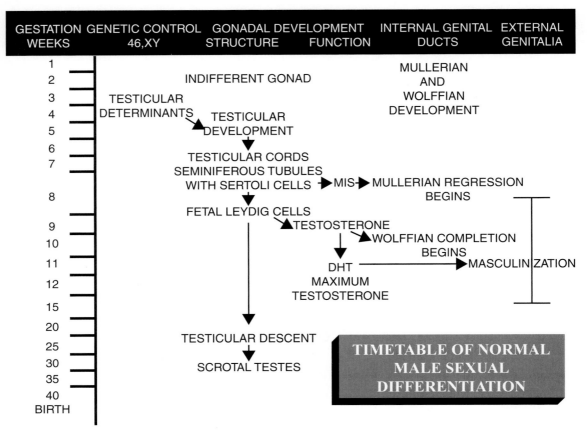

Figure 8-1 Timetable of normal male sexual differentiation. Understanding the timing of abnormalities in this developmental pathway allows prediction of the phenotype of the gonadal, internal ductal, and external genitalia. *(Modified, with permission, from Reindollar RH, et al.[1])*

When presented with an individual with an intersex disorder, one must consider both the medical and psychosocial consequences inherent in the diagnosis. It should be considered a medical emergency when a child is born with ambiguous genitalia. Prompt evaluation, diagnosis, and treatment must be initiated to addresses the individual's medical needs as well as the emotional needs of both patient and family. Such a plan is crucial in the assignment of sex of rearing and the initiation of counseling that will facilitate a healthy transition from infant to adolescent to adult.[3]

▶ NORMAL SEXUAL DIFFERENTIATION

Figures 8-1 and 8-2 display the ordered sequence of male and female sexual differentiation. An abnormality of development can occur at any of these steps. When an abnormality does occur, the resulting phenotype follows a predictable pattern depending on the developmental stage in which the error took place. By understanding this disordered sequence, one can predict the manner in which the gonads, internal ductal system, and external genitalia thus would be affected.

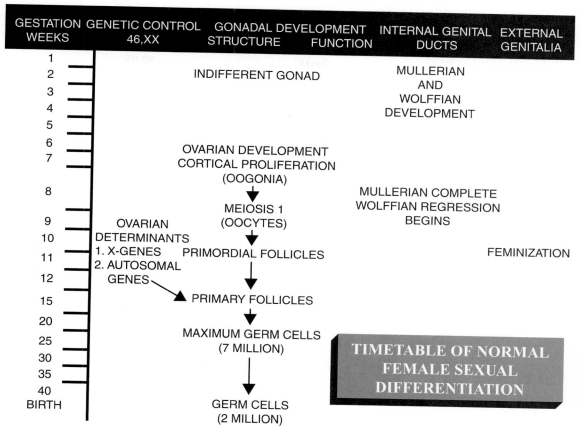

Figure 8-2 Timetable of normal female sexual differentiation. Understanding the timing of abnormalities in this developmental pathway allows prediction of the phenotype of the gonadal, internal ductal, and external genitalia. *(Modified, with permission, from Reindollar RH, et al.[1])*

Every embryo at conception has bisexual potential. The undifferentiated gonads may develop in the embryonic medullary region to form testes or in the cortical region to form ovaries. Both wolffian and müllerian internal ductal primordia are present, and the external genitalia of the emerging fetus can undergo either masculinization or feminization.

In both 46,XX and 46,XY embryos, the primordial germ cell is first identified as a large polyhedral cell in the yolk sac. These cells move by ameboid motion to the dorsal mesentery and then onto the undifferentiated genital ridge. From this point onward the two different characteristics between the development of

a male fetus and a female fetus are the presence or absence of (1) gonadal determinant genes required to initiate gonadal development and (2) function of the respective gonads during intrauterine life. For testicular development to begin, testicular determinant genes must be activated very early in the timetable of sexual differentiation. Ovarian determinant genes, although likely playing an active role in gonadal morphogenesis, are required only at later stages of development. If testicular determinant genes do not function, ovarian development will begin irrespective of the embryo's genetic sex. The developing testes produce and secrete the steroid hormone testosterone and the

▶ **TABLE 8-1:** ABNORMALITIES OF SEXUAL DIFFERENTIATION

Historical Classification	Abnormalities by Karyotype
Male pseudohermaphroditism	I. Deletion syndromes without Y cell lines (45,X)
	II. Deletion syndromes with Y cell lines (45,X/46,XY)
	III. 46,XY
	a. Gonadal dysgenesis (Swyer syndrome)
	b. MIS deficiency
	c. Empty pelvis/agonadia
	d. LHβ/LH receptor mutations
	e. Steroid enzyme gene mutations
	1. Cholesterol side-chain cleavage enzyme
	2. 3β-Hydroxysteroid dehydrogenase
	3. 17α-Hydroxylase
	4. 17,20-Lyase
	5. 5α-Reductase
	f. Androgen insensitivity
	1. Complete
	2. Incomplete
	g. Nonendocrine/non-sex chromosomal abnormalities*
	h. 46,XY True hermaphrodite†
True hermaphrodite	IV. 46,XX/46,XY True hermaphrodite†
	V. 46,XX
	a. 46,XX True hermaphrodite†
Female pseudohermaphroditism	b. 46,XX sex-reversed male
	c. Congenital adrenal hyperplasia
	1. 21-Hydroxylase deficiency
	2. 11β-Hydroxylase deficiency
	d. Fetal/placental aromatase deficiency
	e. Exposure to maternal androgens*
	1. Drug
	2. Tumor of pregnancy
	f. Nonendocrine/non-sex-chromosomal abnormalities*

Disorders are presented by historical classification and by karyotype. The latter is in order of occurrence during embryogenesis (refer to Figs. 8-1 and 8-2).

* Occurs at variable times during development.

† Exact timing of event is likely to be early in embryogenesis.

Modified, with permission, from Reindollar RH[2].

non-steroid müllerian-inhibiting substance (MIS). These hormones directly and indirectly guide the development of the internal ductal systems and external genitalia. To the best of our knowledge, however, the developing ovaries are not endocrinologically active during intrauterine life. In fact, the internal ductal system and external genitalia of a female fetus develop in the absence of ovarian hormone production. See Chap. 7 for a complete discussion of müllerian development.

Male Sexual Differentiation

The sexual differentiation of a male fetus has been studied extensively and is known to proceed according to a well-described sequence of events (see Fig. 8-1). This pathway allows for development of the testes, wolffian system, and external genitalia, as well as regression of the müllerian system. The genetic events that make this pathway possible appear to be triggered by *SRY* (sex-determining region of chromosome Y) gene products,[4,5] although it is possible that genes upstream in expression to *SRY* also exist and are required in this process. The *SRY* gene is located in the sex-determining region of the Y chromosome. Once *SRY* initiates activity, several downstream genes are activated and likely work collaboratively for continued male testicular development.[6] It is believed that the protein product of *SRY* serves as a transcription factor that initiates activity in these downstream genes.[7]

Pertinent genes activated by *SRY* may include *MIS*,[8] dosage-sensitive sex-reversal gene *(DSS)*,[9,10] *SOX9*,[11–13] and the Wilms' tumor *(WT-1)* gene.[14–17] The SRY protein is known to bind to the *MIS* promoter region. Patients with campomelic dysplasia (46,XY karyotype, female phenotype, and a broad spectrum of bony abnormalities) have mutations in the *SOX9* gene located in the autosomal sex-reversal locus *(SRA1)* on the long arm of chromosome 17.[11–13] This gene appears to be involved in both testicular formation and bony development.

The endocrinologically active developing testes guide development of the internal ductal system and the external genitalia. The Sertoli cells produce the first hormone of the testes, MIS. One of the many functions of this protein[18] is to arrest and disrupt development of the müllerian system by apoptosis. Subsequently, the Leydig cells develop and begin to produce androgens. Testosterone production by the Leydig cells is triggered initially by placental human chorionic gonadotropin (hCG) production and then later by fetal luteinizing hormone (LH). 5α-Reductase acts peripherally to convert testosterone into dihydrotestosterone (DHT). Both testosterone and DHT require the presence of a functional androgen receptor to exert their effects. During early fetal development, 5α-reductase is not produced within the developing wolffian system[19]; it is testosterone alone that stimulates completion of the developing internal wolffian ducts. In contrast, 5α-reductase is present within the external genitalia, and DHT is responsible for masculinization of the external genitalia.[20]

Classic experiments by Jost and colleagues[21] illustrate that the effect of MIS and testosterone on the developing wolffian and müllerian systems are local and unilateral. These studies demonstrated that unilateral removal of a testis from a developing male rabbit resulted in the development of a müllerian system on that side and a wolffian system on the side of the remaining testis. When a fetal testis was removed from a male rabbit and transplanted into a fetal female rabbit adjacent to a developing ovary, the associated müllerian system regressed, whereas the wolffian system continued to develop on that side. The same principles exist for humans, as demonstrated by individuals with various intersex disorders.

Development of male external genitalia depends on the production of DHT and the presence of androgen receptors on the target tissues. This development likely begins around 9 weeks of gestation and is completed early during the second trimester. The labioscrotal folds fuse, and the urethral groove is enveloped into the genital tubercle, which subsequently elongates to form a penis. The testes descend in the third trimester of pregnancy, usually beginning around 32 weeks of gestation. Stimuli required for testicular descent include locally produced testosterone, gubernaculum development with the associated "pulling" of the testes toward the scrotum, and possibly, MIS.

Female Sexual Differentiation

Figure 8-2 represents the pathway for normal female sexual differentiation. In contrast to male sexual development, specific genes that direct female sexual development have yet to be identified. While these genes certainly exist, it is suspected that they are broad-spectrum developmental genes, in contrast to the step-specific genes involved in male sexual differentiation.

The ovary begins its development in the absence of either testicular or ovarian determinant genes. Additionally, the ovary does not appear to produce substantial amounts of hormones in utero that are essential to further guide the development of the internal or external genitalia. The müllerian system develops into the fallopian tubes, uterus, and upper portion of the vagina unless exposed to MIS. In the absence of androgens, female external genitalia develop.

Germ cell division and maturation differ between the ovary and the testis. A maximum complement of approximately 6 million germ cells is attained in the female fetus by 20 weeks of gestation through an aggressive mitotic effort. Germ cell replenishment in the female appears to be limited to intrauterine life, in contrast to spermatogenesis, which occurs throughout adult life. Preservation of the germ cells likely depends on ovarian determinant genes located on both arms of the X chromosomes, as well as the autosomes. These genes direct the development of a primitive granulosa cell layer that surrounds the primordial germ cell and likely provides a mechanical barrier to premature oocyte loss. In addition, these genes probably direct and maintain meiotic arrest in the diplotene stage of prophase I.

The importance of both having X chromosomes in female sexual differentiation is illustrated by comparing the germ cells in fetuses with 45,X Turner syndrome with those of 46,XX fetuses. By midgestation, the number of germ cells in 45,X and 46,XX fetuses are comparable. However, the usual single granulosa cell layer incompletely surrounds the germ cells present in the 45,X fetus, and the germ cells may herniate through the defective granulosa layer.[22] This is likely one mechanism for the more rapid germ cell loss that is seen in 45,X fetuses compared with those with a 46,XX karyotype. Another hypothesis is that the ovarian determinant genes produce meiotic inhibitors

and that absence or nonfunction of these genes is associated with early oocyte attrition. Candidates include the recently described premature ovarian failure-1 (POF1) and POF2 genes.[23–25] Previously, reports of 46,XX nontwin sisters who were concordant for gonadal dysgenesis promoted the concept that other autosomal ovarian determinant genes exist.[3] No doubt some of these sisters may have premutations for fragile X syndrome, an X-linked locus recently recognized as one of the more common causes of premature ovarian failure.

In summary, female sexual differentiation seemingly occurs in a somewhat independent fashion when compared with male sexual development, a dependent step-specific process (see Figs. 8-1 and 8-2). While female differentiation is certainly not a passive event, as we have long been taught, the specific genes that initiate and guide female sexual differentiation have yet to be identified.

► ABNORMALITIES OF SEXUAL DIFFERENTIATION

Patient Classification

Patients with abnormalities of sexual differentiation historically have been classified as either pseudohermaphrodites or true hermaphrodites (see Table 8-1). A *pseudohermaphrodite* has external genitalia that contradict the karyotypic sex. Thus a male pseudohermaphrodite has a 46,XY karyotype and undermasculinized external genitalia. A female pseudohermaphrodite has a 46,XX karyotype and masculinized external genitalia. A *true hermaphrodite* is an individual who has internal gonadal tissue comprised of both ovarian and testicular elements. Histologically, gonadal tissue from a true hermaphrodite must display both ovarian follicles and seminiferous tubules. Because overlap exists between these syndromes, the term *pseudohermaphrodite* should be considered an anachronism. Rather, it is easier to consider these disorders based solely on the patient's karyotype and the timing of the defect during development, as reflected in Table 8-1. The following discussion of the various abnormalities of sexual differentiation will be directed by the karyotype of the individual and the time during development at which the insult occurs.

X Chromosome Deletion Syndromes (Turner Syndrome)

Deletion syndromes refer to conditions in which an X chromosome is partially or completely missing and can occur in the presence or absence of a Y cell line. The classic karyotype of Turner syndrome is 45,X, but most patients with Turner syndrome actually have mosaicism: A 45,X cell line is associated with either an X or a Y chromosome that can be structurally normal or abnormal. 45,X/46,XY is the most common form of mosaicism; other variants include 45,X/46,XX and 45,X/46,X,i(Xq).[3]

Abnormal gonadal development is present in patients with Turner syndrome to varying degrees. The ovarian remnants usually are represented by streaks that are often devoid of all follicles. Fifteen percent of these patients have enough follicles to mount a pubertal response, whereas 5 percent have enough follicles to allow ovulation and the maintenance of regular menses for a variable period of time. One percent of these patients can achieve a spontaneous pregnancy. Initially, these individuals have a normal complement of oocytes in utero. Loss of a portion or all of the ovarian determinant regions on the X chromosome is associated with incomplete generation of an intact germ cell–granulosa cell membrane.[22] Unarrested meiotic activity occurs. These oocytes appear to be unprotected by the poorly developed granulosa cell membrane. Streak ovaries usually are formed by this rapid and early attrition.

Müllerian system and external genitalia development proceeds normally in these patients with bilateral streak gonads. Additional common stigmata of these patients include cardio-vascular and renal anomalies, short stature (<63 inches), high-arched palate, short fourth metacarpals, cubitus valgus, shield chest, and multiple pigmented nevi. The most common cardiovascular abnormalities include coarctation of the aorta, bicuspid aortic valves, and predisposition to develop dilatation and dissection of the aorta. Recently, the X-linked *SHOX* gene has been implicated in the etiology of short stature in Turner syndrome.[26,27] In the presence of a 45,X/46,XY karyotype, gonadal development may range from bilateral streaks to a unilateral streak with contralateral immature testis to bilateral immature testes.[3,28,29] If present, the testes may be found either in the labioscrotum or intraabdominally. The presence of a unilateral streak gonad and contralateral testis is described as *mixed gonadal dysgenesis*.[3,28,29] The phenotype of the internal and external genitalia depends on the adjacent gonadal tissue and follows the rules of development outlined by the rabbit experiments of Jost. A streak gonad is accompanied by a müllerian system, whereas an immature testis is accompanied by variable development of a wolffian system. The external genitalia undergo masculinization to varying degrees both in utero and at puberty. For patients with an intraabdominal testis, minimal masculinization (clitoromegaly) usually occurs. This is understandable because the testes do not produce sufficient amounts of testosterone to promote their descent. The presence of a unilateral descended testis in other patients signifies a more functional gonad, producing higher levels of testosterone. For them, genital ambiguity is usually present. If bilateral descended testes are present, a normal male phenotype is often found.

If an intraabdominal dysgenetic gonad is left in place, 15 to 25 percent of patients will experience neoplastic gonadal tumor formation.[30,31] The most common such tumor is a gonadoblastoma, although malignant germ cell tumors such as dysgerminoma, yolk sac tumor, and choriocarcinoma also can occur.[3,32] Because of the significant risk of malignant transformation at any age, all these patients require gonadectomy at the time of diagnosis. Alternatively, a male with 45,X/46,XY gonadal dysgenesis and bilaterally descended testes appears to have a very low risk for malignant transformation. These patients are followed more easily because of the ready ability to examine and palpate the testes.

Individuals with 45,X/46,XY gonadal dysgenesis and bilaterally descended testes usually are given a male sex of rearing because they are usually phenotypically normal males. For individuals with genital ambiguity at birth, however, consideration should be given to assignment to a female sex of rearing. In such patients, penile reconstructive surgery only rarely may be satisfactory, the risk of gonadal neoplasm is significant; and they are typically infertile as adults. Issues surrounding sex-of-rearing assignment will be addressed later in this chapter.

▶ 46,XY ABNORMALITIES OF SEXUAL DIFFERENTIATION

46,XY Gonadal Dysgenesis (Swyer Syndrome)

When one of the earliest steps in male sexual differentiation (see Fig. 8-1 and Table 8-1) is disrupted, 46,XY gonadal dysgenesis, or Swyer syndrome, results.[33,34] Two theories exist regarding how this disorder occurs. Normally, germ cells must first migrate to the genital ridge before they can further direct gonadal differentiation. In some patients with Swyer syndrome, it is thought that the germ cells fail to migrate to the genital ridge. Subsequent testicular development cannot occur, and streak gonads form. Other patients with Swyer syndrome have a mutation in one of the genes that directs testicular differentiation.[35,36] As a result, the germ cells organize in the ovarian cortex rather than the medullary region of the undifferentiated gonad and undergo rapid loss. There is a complete loss of germ cells in pa-

tients with a Y cell line. Mutations have been identified in the SRY gene in 15 percent of patients with Swyer syndrome.[35–38] Given that most patients with Swyer syndrome do not have mutations in SRY, mutations in other genes involved in testicular morphogenesis likely exist. An X-linked form has been reported, and it is felt that genes downstream in expression to SRY are critical in gonadal development.[3,34,39,40] These patients have a normal müllerian system and are phenotypically female.

Women with 46,XY gonadal dysgenesis typically present with delayed pubertal development as opposed to genital ambiguity.[3] They tend to be taller than their peers for two reasons. The absence of sex steroid production, if undiagnosed and untreated, allows the bony epiphyses to remain open longer, allowing additional growth. Also, Y chromosome–related statural genes likely contribute to an increased adult height. On laboratory evaluation, gonadotropin levels are significantly elevated, and karyotype reveals a 46,XY chromosomal complement. Of all patients with a Y cell line and dysgenetic testes, these patients are at the highest risk (25 to 35 percent) of malignant transformation of their gonadal streaks. Gonadectomy therefore is required at the time of diagnosis. Rarely, some of these patients display varying degrees of masculinization or feminization around the time of puberty due to the production of testosterone or estrogen by a germ cell tumor.[41,42]

Persistent Müllerian Duct Syndrome

In normal male sexual differentiation, once the SRY gene is expressed and downstream genes are activated, germ cell migration and testicular differentiation occur. Subsequently, MIS is produced, and a local tissue effect causes arrested development of the müllerian system. Individuals with persistent müllerian duct syndrome (also known as *uteri inguinale*) have either absent MIS production or absent tissue effect caused by mutations in the genes encoding MIS or the MIS receptor.[18,43–45] When this occurs as an isolated defect, testicular development and testicular androgen production are otherwise normal. The end result is the persistence of the müllerian system in a phenotypically normal male.

These patients generally present with either unilateral or bilateral cryptorchidism or an inguinal hernia[43] resulting from anatomic interference of the persistent müllerian structures with normal descent of the testes. The functionally normal testes are adjacent to fallopian tubes, uterus, and upper portion of a vagina. Removal of the müllerian structures may cause sterility as a result of damage occurring to the adjacent wolffian system during the attempted surgical repair. Additionally, abnormal development of the vas deferens may be the consequence of persistent mullerian development.

Agonadia (Testicular Regression Syndrome)

In this syndrome, the testes begin to develop normally and produce MIS, resulting in müllerian regression. Following the initiation of MIS production but prior to androgen biosynthesis, the testes disappear or regress (see Fig. 8-1). It has been hypothesized that this regression is caused by an undetermined vascular or environmental insult. Given the fact that this is a bilateral event and always complete, it is more likely the result of a pertubation of development at the molecular level. In addition to the normal regression and absence of the müllerian system, the wolffian system also fails to develop due to nonexistent androgen production. Both the testes and internal genitalia are therefore absent. Similarly, the external genitalia do not masculinize. This has been described as "empty pelvis syndrome."

These individuals are phenotypically female and usually present in adolescence because they do not undergo normal pubertal changes. Laboratory testing reveals significantly elevated gonadotropins along with a 46,XY karyotype. Exploration of the pelvis demonstrates absence of both the gonads and an internal ductal system. Variations of this disorder exist, the phenotype being dependent on the time during sexual development that testicular regression occurs.[46,47]

▶ ABNORMALITIES ASSOCIATED WITH DEFECTS IN ANDROGEN PRODUCTION OR FUNCTION IN 46,XY INDIVIDUALS

46,XY individuals with abnormalities in androgen function usually have normal testicular differentiation and development along with normal MIS production. In addition to normal testicular development, appropriate regression of müllerian structures occurs. Such defects include inadequate stimulation of androgen biosynthesis, abnormalities of androgen biosynthesis, and androgen receptor malfunction (see Fig. 8-1).

Abnormal Androgen Stimulation: Luteinizing Hormone Receptor Gene Mutation

Luteinizing hormone (LH) receptors are present on the Leydig cells and are required for testicular androgen production. The elevated maternal levels of hCG during pregnancy initially stimulate the LH receptor on Leydig cells before fetal production of LH has begun. Mutations of the gonadotropin-releasing hormone (GnRH) receptor gene and the LHβ gene have been identified in 46,XY individuals. Because the hCG of pregnancy is sufficient to initiate androgen biosynthesis in the fetal testes at the LH receptor, these individuals are normally masculinized in fetal life. They are not identified by genital ambiguity at birth but by delayed puberty years later. Alternatively, a mutation that inactivates the LH receptor gene in a 46,XY individual is usually associated with a complete lack of masculinization. In these patients, the hCG of pregnancy cannot stimulate fetal androgen biosynthesis via the LH receptor, and these individuals have a phenotype similar to that seen in androgen-insensitivity syndrome.[48] The absence of androgens in utero leads to the undermasculinization of the external genitalia, generally resulting in a normal female phenotype at birth.

Androgen Biosynthetic Defects

When an enzyme involved in androgen biosynthesis[2] (Fig. 8-3) is absent or deficient, decreased androgen production results and is associated with varying degrees of undermasculinization. The responsible enzyme defects can occur at any point along this pathway, and

the deficiency can be partial or complete. The resulting undermasculinization of external genitalia can range from slight to absolute genital ambiguity. It may consist of abnormal testicular descent (unilaterally or, more often, bilaterally), a significantly underdeveloped phallus, and/or a blind vaginal pouch that represents the remnant of the understimulated prostatic utricle. These enzyme deficiencies usually result from autosomal recessive mutations.

Cholesterol Side-Chain Cleavage Enzyme (P450scc) Deficiency

With this high block in steroidogenesis, negligible androgens are produced, and thus no external genital masculinization is present.[49–54] If an affected newborn having this enzyme deficiency is not detected promptly, adrenal failure also will occur. Recently, a patient with con-

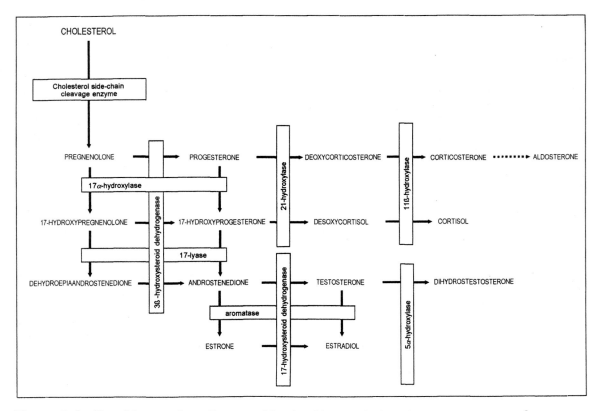

Figure 8-3   Steroidogenesis pathway.   *(Used, with permission, from Reindollar RH.[2])*

genital adrenal insufficiency was found to harbor two different mutations of the cholesterol side-chain cleavage enzyme gene (CYP11A).[55] This is the first identification of any mutation within this gene, the affected individual being a compound heterozygote.

3β-Hydroxysteroid Dehydrogenase (3β-HSD) Deficiency

Deficiency of this enzyme is associated with increased production of weak androgens such as dehydroepiandrostenedione (DHEAS) and a decrease in the more potent androgens androstenedione and, eventually, testosterone. These individuals have a significant degree of undermasculinization and external genital ambiguity,[56–64] and they are usually raised as females. Of note, adrenal failure may occur if a newborn goes unrecognized and untreated. The 3β-HSD enzymatic activity is mediated by two genes: *3β-HSD type I (HSD3B1) and type II (HSD3B2)*. Mutations in the *3β-HSD-II* gene have been identified in patients with this deficiency.[54]

17α-Hydroxylase Deficiency and 17,20-Lyase Deficiency

A single enzyme (P450c17α) has been identified that has both 17α-hydroxylase and 17,20-lyase enzyme activity, determined by the *CYP17* gene.[65] Different mutations within this gene are responsible for each enzyme deficiency.[51,66–69] These enzyme deficiencies also represent a high block in steroidogenesis in which negligible androgens are produced, and external genital masculinization is not present.[54,70–81] Individuals with 17α-hydroxylase deficiency also may develop hypokalemic hypotension secondary to the excessive accumulation of mineralocorticoid precursors (e.g., deoxycorticosterone).

17-Hydroxysteroid Dehydrogenase (17-HSD) Deficiency

A deficiency in 17-HSD (also called *17-ketoreductase*) results in an increase in the production of the weaker androgens DHEA and androstenedione and a reduction in the production of testosterone and, eventually, DHT. These individuals have significant undermasculinization of the external genitalia to the degree of genital ambiguity.[82–87] They are usually assigned a female sex of rearing. If left untreated, these individuals may experience gynecomastia secondary to the conversion of excess androstenedione to estrone. Several mutations in the 17-HSD gene have been identified in these patients.[82,88]

5α-Reductase Deficiency

Once the testes have developed normally, testosterone is produced by the Leydig cells, and 5α-reductase acts peripherally to convert testosterone to a more potent androgen, DHT. Both testosterone and DHT stimulate the same androgen receptor, but the lower dissociation constant of DHT allows it to occupy the receptor longer than testosterone, thereby increasing its potency. If 5α-reductase is deficient, testosterone levels may be normal or increased. Both internal and external genitalia development is affected in a predictable fashion.[89–101] The presence of testosterone allows for normal internal wolffian system development and variable but reduced masculinization of the external genitalia. This phenotype is predictable given the fact that 5α-reductase activity is not involved in the development of the internal wolffian system. These individuals are usually given a female sex of rearing.

At puberty, it is not uncommon for patients with 5α-reductase deficiency to undergo a significant degree of masculinization if their testes have not been removed. While the enzyme deficiency persists, at this point there is a significant increase in the amount of testosterone produced by the testes, which is concordant with normal puberty. The increased amount of testosterone is sufficient to stimulate a local tissue effect and compensate for the deficient DHT production, resulting in further masculinization of the external genitalia, possibly including the development of a functional penis. This phenomenon was identified previously in a large kindred in the Dominican Republic, with affected individuals known as *guevedoces,* meaning "testis at twelve."[99,100] Even though many of these individuals had been given a female sex of rearing at birth, sufficient masculinization occurred at puberty and allowed conversion to male gender identity and a change in the sex of rearing.

Two genes have been identified that encode 5α-reductase: *5α-reductase 1* and *5α-reductase 2*.[102–105] The *5α-reductase 2* gene is responsible for the genital production of DHT, and mutations in this gene are likely associated with the above-described syndrome. The *5α-reductase 1* gene is functional in the liver, whether or not its activity in peripheral tissues contributes significantly to testosterone metabolism has not been fully elucidated.

Androgen Receptor Defects (Androgen-Insensitivity Syndrome)

Individuals with androgen-insensitivity syndrome (AIS) have a defect in the final step in the pathway of male sexual development. These individuals have normal testicular development, normal MIS production with associated müllerian duct regression, normal androgen production by the testes, and peripheral conversion to DHT[106,107] (see Fig. 8-1). Despite the presence of androgens, the androgen receptor is either defective or absent, and thus varying degrees of undermasculinization occur. A wide spectrum of phenotypic findings is associated with this disorder, varying from complete to partial androgen insensitivity.

The androgen-receptor gene is located on the X chromosome, and both complete and incomplete androgen-insensitivity syndromes are inherited in an X-linked recessive fashion. Studies evaluating the androgen receptor in these individuals have revealed variable levels of androgen-receptor binding ranging from absent to normal.[106–108]

Much is known about the nature of the androgen receptor and the mutations within

it that lead to this disorder. The androgen-receptor gene is comprised of eight exons, and mutations have been detected throughout the entire gene, most of which are point mutations.[109] While a few, unrelated families share the same mutation within the androgen-receptor gene, most families with AIS have unique mutations.[106,107,110,111] Since there are no common mutations that exist in AIS, it is not possible to make the diagnosis by screening for a single-gene defect. However, knowledge of the different types of mutations has helped provide better understanding regarding differences in receptor function. Most of the mutations identified are located in the steroid-binding domain of the gene, resulting in nucleotide alterations that encode for the portion of the receptor responsible for androgen binding. The remainder of the mutations are found in the DNA-binding domain. For these latter patients, prior androgen-receptor binding assays have demonstrated normal androgen-receptor function. However, the androgen-receptor complex cannot bind to the DNA and have its effect. This is a malfunction commonly referred to as a *postreceptor defect*.

Complete Androgen-Insensitivity Syndrome (CAIS)

In utero, 46,XY individuals with CAIS have total absence of masculinization. A blind-ending vaginal pouch is present. While normal testes are present either abdominally, inguinally, or in the labioscrotal folds, spermatogenesis is either incomplete or absent. The testes have a 2 to 22 percent chance of malignant transformation if left in place after the completion of puberty. Seminomas are the most common tumors and are likely related to the cryptorchid location of the otherwise normal testes.[112,113] Malignant transformations rarely develop prior to puberty, and it is recommended that intraabdominal testes remain in place until after puberty because they play an important role in the development of female secondary sexual characteristics. The spontaneous nature of these pubertal changes enhances normal psychosocial development. Androgens produced by the testes are converted to estrogens, which stimulate the growth of breast tissue. Additionally, breast development may be stimulated more than usual due to the absence of normal androgen inhibition. Consequently, these individuals often develop abundant breast tissue, which is composed of a large amount of adipose rather than glandular tissue. They also have sparse pubic hair and are relatively tall[106,107] compared with 46,XX females, likely due to the presence of Y chromosome-related statural genes.

Incomplete Androgen Insensitivity Syndrome (IAIS)

IAIS presents as a very broad spectrum of phenotypic findings. It is much less common than CAIS. These individuals may have some degree of clitoromegaly, partial fusion of the labioscrotal folds, and a vaginal pouch.[106,107] Usually they have been given a female sex of rearing and differ from individuals with CAIS when they reach puberty. At puberty, pubic hair increases, and clitoral enlargement occurs. Breast development also occurs, although not to the same degree as seen in individuals with CAIS. In IAIS, breast development at puberty is somewhat inhibited by the presence of androgens.

In addition to phenotypic females, 46,XY individuals with IAIS also can present as phenotypic males. A spectrum exists for the phenotypic males. Some may present with degrees of undermasculinization with or without hypospadias, and others may present with a normal male appearance with isolated gynecomastia or infertility.[106,112,114,115] While axillary and pubic hair may be normal, chest and facial hair is sparse. The spectrum of phenotypic findings for the undermasculinized males has been referred to collectively as *Reifenstein syndrome.*

Nonendocrine Genital Ambiguity

Even in the presence of a normal pathway for male sexual differentiation (see Fig. 8-1), ab-normalities of sexual development can still occur. These defects typically are isolated and may include absence of the gonads or penis; disorganized growth, such as duplicate phallus, epispadias, or cloacal formation; or abnormal placement of the scrotum relative to the phallus. Potential etiologies include environmental insults, amniotic band syndrome, congenital rubella, major chromosomal defects (e.g., deletion of the long arm of chromosome 13), and developmental gene abnormalities.

▶ TRUE HERMAPHRODITISM

A true hermaphrodite has the presence of both ovarian and testicular gonadal tissue. The most common karyotype associated with true hermaphroditism is 46,XX, followed by 46,XX/46,XY. A 46,XY karyotype is found only rarely in these patients.[116,117]

The phenotype of a 46,XX true hermaphrodite includes a unilateral ovotestis with a contralateral ovary or testis or bilateral ovotestes.[117] Very few of these patients carry any detectable Y chromosomal DNA.[118,119] The presence of testicular tissue in the absence of the Y chromosome *SRY* gene is evidence that other genes involved in testicular development must exist.

46,XX/46,XY and 46,XY true hermaphrodites usually have a unilateral ovary and a contralateral testis.[117] The phenotypes of 46,XX/46,XY and 46,XY true hermaphrodites are so similar that it is suspected that the 46,XY individuals may, in fact, have undetected 46,XX cell lines. 46,XX/46,XY individuals are most likely chimeras, i.e., comprised of two or more cell lines that originated from different embryos. A chimera is likely formed by one of two mechanisms: (1) separate 46,XX and 46,XY fetuses that have undergone whole-body fusion in utero and (2) concurrent fertilization of the secondary oocytes or ovum along with the first or second polar body.[120] A case report exists of a 46,XX/46,XY true hermaphrodite resulting after transfer of two embryos at in vitro fertilization (IVF).[121]

In the gonads of true hermaphrodites, the ovarian component typically is better developed anatomically and more functional than the testicular component.[117] The gonadal location varies from abdominal to inguinal to scrotal. The nature of the internal ductal system (müllerian or wolffian) depends on the ipsilateral gonad and its degree of differentiation. The testicular products, MIS and testosterone, determine to what degree the internal ductal systems are masculinized or feminized. In the presence of an ovary or ovotestis, a müllerian system usually develops that likely will function at puberty unless surgically altered. When a wolffian system develops ipsilaterally with the mullerian system, abnormalities such as a hemiobstructed uterine horn or cervical aplasia may occur. External genitalia are ambiguous and usually are undermasculinized due to an inadequate amount of testosterone.

The consensus on sex of rearing has changed throughout the years. Previously, these individuals were raised as males due to the somewhat masculinized ambiguous genitalia. However, even in the presence of exogenous testosterone supplementation along with increasing endogenous androgen production at puberty, masculinization usually was incomplete, leading to later issues of gender identity. Puberty in these individuals commonly presents with breast development and cyclic menstruation. Ovarian follicles can reach maturity, and ovulation can occur spontaneously. Case reports indicate that at least six true hermaphrodites raised as females have achieved pregnancy. It is now recommended that a true hermaphrodite diagnosed at birth usually be given a female sex of rearing, and preservation of ovarian tissue and müllerian structures should be attempted.

▶ 46,XX ABNORMALITIES OF SEXUAL DIFFERENTIATION

A phenotype in 46,XX individuals ranging from genital ambiguity to that of a completely normal male can result from in utero exposure to endogenous or exogenous androgens. Less commonly, this results from the anomalous expression of testicular determining genes.

46,XX Sex-Reversed Male

In this disorder, male sexual differentiation occurs in the presence of a 46,XX karyotype, resulting in a sex-reversed male. Usually, varying lengths of DNA from the Y chromosome are interchanged with the X chromosome during meiotic pairing. The *SRY* gene is abnormally translocated from the short arm of the Y chromosome to the X chromosome in 60 percent of 46,XX sex-reversed males. For those 46,XX males who lack *SRY,* it is likely that downstream Y, X, or autosomal testicular determining factor genes are present and/or activated.[122,123] The presence of *SRY* guides the undifferentiated gonad to develop along testicular lines, and testicular hormone function approximates normal.[124–126] Because of the near-normal testicular function, MIS is produced, the müllerian system regresses, and androgen production directs the development of the internal wolffian system, as well as masculinization of the external genitalia. Spermatogenesis, however, is absent due to the fact that the encoding genes are located on the long arm of the Y chromosome and are not also translocated to the X chromosome. These individuals have a normal male phenotype and usually remain undiagnosed until puberty or at the time of a later infertility evaluation. The adult testes are usually small and may be cryptorchid. Pubic hair is present but may be more female than male in its distribution. The penis may be small, and hypospadias is present in less than 10 percent of these individuals. Semen analysis reveals azospermia due to absent spermatogenesis.

Classic Congenital Adrenal Hyperplasia

Classic congenital adrenal hyperplasia (CAH) results from an enzymatic defect in the steroidogenesis pathway and represents one of the most common and potentially most serious abnormalities of sexual differentiation in the 46,XX individual.[54,127] A defect in the gene CYP21, encoding the enzyme P450C21 which determines 21-hydroxylase (21-OH) activity, occurs most commonly with an incidence of 1 in 5000 to 15,000 births in the United States and Europe.[127] Deficiencies of 11β-OH (CYP11B1) and 3β-HSD (HSD3B2) are diagnosed less frequently. When any of these enzyme deficiencies are present, cortisol production is either significantly decreased or absent. As a result, negative feedback to the pituitary is reduced, and the pituitary responds by increasing its production and secretion of adrenocorticotropic hormone (ACTH). Constant adrenal stimulation by ACTH leads to hyperplasia of the gland and an excess production of cortisol precursors and androgens (see Fig. 8-3).

Adrenal development in utero occurs by the third month of gestation at a time when the ovaries are functioning normally, the wolffian system has already regressed, and the müllerian system is completing its development. The presence of high adrenal androgens in utero adversely affects development of the external genitalia in a 46,XX fetus, resulting in varying degrees of genital ambiguity. In a 46,XY fetus with a similar enzymatic defect, the external genitalia are not adversely affected because their normal development depends on the presence of androgens, although they may be enlarged. The degree to which the external genitalia are masculinized in a 46,XX individual depends on the timing and level of androgen exposure in utero. The phenotypic spectrum ranges from minimal clitoromegaly and labioscrotal fusion to varying degrees of hypospadias and marked clitoral hypertrophy.[127–130] In severe cases, the urethral orifice is displaced, and the enlarged clitoris looks like a normal penis.

Evaluation of the gonads in a newborn with genital ambiguity can facilitate an expeditious diagnosis. While normal ovaries may herniate, they do not descend into the labioscrotum.

Testes, on the other hand, normally descend into the labioscrotum. If a newborn has unilateral or bilateral inguinal or scrotal masses suggesting gonadal descent into the labioscrotum in the presence of ambiguous genitalia, then this individual is not a 46,XX individual with CAH. If a newborn is identified with bilateral undescended gonads and has either genital ambiguity or normal male external genitalia, this infant should be considered to have CAH until proven otherwise. Remember that a 46,XY newborn can have CAH but will not present with genital ambiguity.

If left untreated, both 46,XX and 46,XY individuals with CAH will continue to masculinize after birth. Excess androgens also will be converted to estrogens, causing accelerated linear growth during childhood before premature epiphyseal fusion. These individuals are tall as children and short as adults. When treated, 46,XX patients with CAH may be fertile as adults.

21-Hydroxylase-Deficient CAH

Classic 21-OH deficiency exists as either a "salt wasting" or a "simple virilizing" form.[127–130] Seventy-five percent of individuals with CAH due to 21-OH deficiency have the salt-wasting variety. At birth, these infants may develop hyponatremia, hyperkalemia, elevated urinary sodium concentration, low serum and urinary aldosterone concentrations, and a resulting elevated plasma rennin activity. If undiagnosed, a catastrophic salt-wasting crisis may occur as early as 2 weeks of life. This will manifest as poor feeding, diarrhea, and lethargy before developing into hypotension, hypoglycemia, and cardiovascular collapse, resulting in death if undiagnosed. Because 46,XY males with CAH do not present with genital ambiguity, historically they are diagnosed less commonly with 21-OH deficiency at birth and are more likely to present in full-blown crisis. The 46,XX females with CAH usually are identified at birth because of the presence of genital ambiguity and generally are treated before a full salt-wasting crisis develops.

Simple virilizing 21-OH deficiency presents with varying degrees of genital ambiguity in a 46,XX individual at birth; further masculinization can occur throughout childhood if the patient is left untreated. Today, newborn screening for CAH in most states obviates these risks of delayed diagnosis.

Genes involved in 21-OH deficiency include *CYP21,* the active gene, and *CYP21P,* the pseudogene. These genes are located on the short arm of chromosome 6 adjacent to the genes encoding components of complement (*C4A* and *C4B*), HLA-B, and HLA-DR. The pseudogene is an inactive 21-OH gene containing nearly a dozen different point mutations. Each of these mutations separately alters 21-OH activity to varying degrees. Because of the close proximity of *CYP21* to *CYP21P,* mismatching and recombination during meiosis can result in either a complete deletion of *CYP21* or a reshuffling of any or all of the *CYP21P* mutations into *CYP21*. The latter defects are called *conversion mutations* because the active *CYP21* gene is, in essence, converted to a form of the pseudogene by this recombination error. Thus deletion and conversion mutations have been found in the *CYP21* gene that render it inactive or less active and cause various forms of 21-OH deficiency.[129] Diagnosis of these gene mutations in the past relied on the genetic linkage to the HLA region.[129,131,132] These linkage studies have the potential for misdiagnosis (i.e., 1 percent risk) because of recombination during meiosis and have been replaced by methodologies that identify specific causative mutations.[133]

Most affected CAH patients are compound heterozygotes and harbor different mutations on each of their two *CYP21* alleles. These patients phenotypically tend to manifest the least deleterious of their gene mutations.[134] For example, in the presence of a classic salt-wasting mutation on one chromosome and a classic simple virilizing mutation on the other chromosome, the patient usually will display the simple virilizing phenotype, the less severe mutation in this case. If a patient had a classic salt-wasting mutation on one chromosome and a nonclassic mutation on the other chromosome, that individual will express the nonclassic mutation (see below).

The molecular findings for 21-OH deficiency are relevant to prenatal and preconceptional counseling. A 46,XX woman with nonclassic 21-OH deficiency may, in fact, harbor a classic mutation at one of her *CYP21* alleles.[134,135] The classic mutation may be passed to her offspring with the potential for development of genital ambiguity or salt wasting should the father similarly contribute a classic mutation. Reproductive-age women with nonclassic adrenal hyperplasia therefore should be counseled accordingly. Nonclassic adrenal hyperplasia is discussed further in Chap. 13.

11β-Hydroxylase Deficiency

11β-OH deficiency is relatively infrequent and accounts for approximately 16 percent of classic CAH.[130] As deoxycorticosterone accumulates, salt retention increases, and hypertension occurs. Hypertension is the distinguishing feature of this form of CAH.

Two genes have been identified that encode 11β-OH: *CYP11B1* and *CYP11B2*. Mutations causing 11β-OH deficiency have been found primarily in *CYP11B1,* with a few mutations identified in *CYP11B2*.[136]

3β-Hydroxysteroid Dehydrogenase Deficiency

First described by Bongiovanni and Kellenbenz in 1962,[137] the inherited deficiency of 3β-hydroxysteroid dehydrogenase/Δ^5-Δ^4-isomerase (3β-HSD) accounts for about 1–10% of cases of all cases of CAH.[138] This autosomal recessive disorder 3β-HSD deficient CAH results from mutations in the HSD3B2 gene affecting the 3β-HSD Type 2 enzyme, and generally presents with salt wastage. In contrast to 21-OH and 11β-OH deficiencies, in which the defect is restricted to affecting adrenal function, the severe form of 3β-HSD deficiency impairs steroidogenesis in both the adrenals and the gonads. In females, mild virilization of external genitalia may be present in some by the effect of androgen metabolite of excess DHEA secreted from the affected fetal adrenals, although generally no obvious masculinization is apparent. Alternatively, in males 3β-HSD deficiency results in incomplete masculinization of the external genitalia. About two-thirds of the reported patients are 46,XY. During childhood, mild signs of androgen excess (such as premature pubarche) develop in both sexes, primarily due to the conversion of 3β-HSD Type 2 precursors being converted to active androgens by the normal 3β-HSD type I isoenzyme.

The nonclassic form of this disorder is extremely rare, and is usually diagnosable in children with premature pubarche with 17-hydroxypregnenolone levels at or >~290 nmol/liter (or ~54 SD above Tanner II pubic hair stage matched control levels).[139] To date no adult women with androgen excess and normal genitalia have been diagnosed with the non-classic form of 3β-HSD deficiency, although the frequent finding of supranormal 17-hydroxypregnenolone levels appears to be related primarily to insulin-resistant polycystic ovary syndrome.[140]

Androgen Excess Syndromes

Exposure to excessive amounts of androgens can masculinize the external genitalia of a 46,XX fetus that otherwise has normal sexual differentiation. The placenta has a remarkable ability to aromatize androgens, except DHT, to estrogens. Thus, even in the presence of significantly elevated levels of maternal androgens, placental aromatase activity prevents unintended masculinization of the fetus. Specific situations do exist, however, in which mother or fetus may be subject to masculinization by circulating androgens.

Endogenous Androgens

A maternal androgen-producing tumor may cause masculinization of a female fetus if there is 5α-reductase activity in the tumor leading to excessive DHT production. Aromatization of

this androgen is not able to occur because of the hydrogen saturation of the number 5 carbon atom in the molecule, and large amounts of DHT therefore can accumulate. It has been postulated but never proven that masculinization of a female fetus also can occur when the production rate of testosterone surpasses the placenta's ability to aromatize it to estrogen. The luteoma of pregnancy is the most common tumor known to masculinize a female fetus due to its 5α-reductase activity with excessive production of DHT. Prior cases of genital ambiguity in a 46,XX infant labeled as idiopathic likely were caused by an undiagnosed luteoma of pregnancy. Rarely, other maternal ovarian or adrenal testosterone-producing tumors such as arrhenoblastomas, Leydig cell tumors, and metastatic epithelial tumors have been associated with masculinization of a female fetus.

Exogenous Androgens

Synthetic testosterone derivatives (ethisterone, norethindrone, and danocrine) were used previously to treat conditions such as endometriosis. If taken during pregnancy, these nonaromatizable androgens can masculinize a female fetus.

Aromatase Deficiency

Placental aromatase deficiency results from recessive mutations in the gene that encodes this enzyme *(CYP19)*.[141–143] High fetal levels of adrenal androgens or their metabolites (e.g., DHEAS) normally are present in both male and female fetuses because of the physiologic deficiency in fetal adrenal 3β-HSD activity. Fetal DHEAS is shunted to the placenta, where it undergoes conversion to androstenedione and testosterone with subsequent aromatization to estrogens. In the absence of placental aromatase activity, these placental androgens are not aromatized. Consequently, both the mother and female fetus may undergo variable degrees of androgenization. A 46,XY male fetus with placental aromatase deficiency has a normal phenotype, and the mother may present with androgenization.

Idiopathic Genital Ambiguity

There are some 46,XX individuals who display varying degrees of genital ambiguity at birth but are otherwise normal. While commonly they have been diagnosed as having idiopathic genital ambiguity, their masculinized external genitalia likely resulted from a luteoma of pregnancy, as noted earlier. It is also possible that somatic cell mutations, de novo mutations, or environmental teratogens may cause genital ambiguity in an otherwise normal 46,XX individual.

► IDENTIFICATION AND EVALUATION OF INTERSEX DISORDERS

Delivery of a newborn with a disorder of sexual development should be considered a medical emergency. As with any birth defect, parents understandably may feel guilt, fear, or sadness. Specific dilemmas that may confront these parents include decisions regarding sex of rearing, development of a healthy gender identity (defined as the individual's perception of his or her gender), and determination of the future fertility of the newborn. For the clinician, recognition of the metabolic consequences of untreated salt-wasting CAH, if present, is crucial.

Delivery Room Identification and Reaction

When a child is delivered with abnormal genitalia, the obstetrician must act promptly to identify and address the situation. A disorder of sexual development may present with a range of genital findings, such as minimal clitoromegaly, isolated cryptorchidism, hypospadias, or overt ambiguity. Prompt diagnosis, treatment, and long-term follow-up are essential in ensuring that gender identity is concordant with sex of rearing. The delivery of a newborn with ambiguous genitalia requires an appropriate response from the clinician. Unfortunately, the unexpected nature of this rare clinical presentation makes this difficult. If the genetic sex of an infant is not obvious, it is best to postpone assignment of a sex of rearing until further information is obtained, optimally within 24 h. This prompt diagnosis is possible with current cytogenetic and molecular techniques (see Chap. 5).

The initial discussion with the parents should include an explanation of in utero genital development, specifically that male and female genitalia appear nearly identical until midgestation. It further should be explained that they have given birth to a boy or a girl but that the genitalia have not completed the developmental process. For this reason, male and female genitalia may appear similar. In either case, surgery will be corrective.

As tempting as it may be to provide an educated guess for the parents about the sex of the baby, the obstetrician is encouraged to resist such an urge. These initial judgments can result in incorrect sex-of-rearing assignments, necessitating reassignment to the opposite sex later and predisposing to long-term psychosocial conflict. Changing the sex of rearing should be avoided at all costs so as to prevent the family from casting doubt on the accuracy of the sex-of-rearing assignment. This approach will enhance the subsequent development of gender identity and long-term emotional well-being of both the patient and the family.

There are two exceptions for which it is usually safe to assign the sex of rearing in the delivery room. The infant that has minimal clitoral hypertrophy with a normal-appearing urethral and vaginal orifices usually can be assigned a female sex of rearing. In addition, the infant with a normal-size penis, hypospadias, and unilateral cryptorchidism usually is safely assigned a male sex of rearing. For all other forms of genital ambiguity, it is unwise to quickly assign a sex of rearing in the delivery room. Although tempting, it would be incorrect to give a male sex of rearing to an infant with a normal-appearing penis, scrotum, and *bilateral* cryptorchidism. Although this child may be an otherwise normal male, this phenotype is also consistent with a normal fertile female who has intraabdominal ovaries and CAH.

Delivery Room Evaluation

Maternal History

A review of the maternal history should include questions regarding maternal ingestion of androgenic compounds and the perinatal development of hyperandrogenism, i.e., acne or hirsutism. Review of a family history may reveal instances of similarly affected relatives or infants (e.g., CAH or AIS). CAH may be suspected if there is a family history of unexplained neonatal death.

Neonatal Evaluation

The expeditious diagnostic evaluation of the newborn should be designed to answer the following questions: (1) Is the ambiguity part of a syndrome? (2) Does the infant have CAH? (3) Is a testis or testes present? and (4) Can an exact diagnosis be made?

Syndromes associated with a chromosomal abnormality or viral infection, such as congenital rubella, usually are associated with a spectrum of somatic malformations beyond the reproductive tract. They commonly involve the limbs (especially hands and feet), facial features (especially the eyes and lips/palate), and heart. Identification of at least one testis in an ambiguous infant rules out CAH and the potential for a salt-wasting crisis. Ambiguity associated with CAH occurs only in 46,XX individuals who have intraabdominal ovaries. An infant with an identifiable testis or testes is more likely to have one of the 46,XY syndromes (see Table 8-1) or to be a true hermaphrodite, none of which results in neonatal death. Finally, having an exact diagnosis will allow the clinical team the opportunity to provide complete counseling about the disorder,

focusing on associated somatic, metabolic, or neoplastic abnormalities. Also, a detailed discussion pertaining to pubertal progression, fertility, and risk of recurrence, in addition to issues related to psychosexual development, can be initiated.

Neonatal Physical Examination

Beginning with an assessment of the entire body, identification of findings such as the stigmata of Turner syndrome may provide initial clues to the diagnosis. The clinician should carefully examine the left side of the body compared with the right side looking for differences that may exist in chimerism, such as skin mottling or different eye colors. Chimerism results from whole-body fusion of two different fetuses and may be seen, albeit rarely, in patients with true hermaphroditism. A classic "blueberry muffin" appearance to the skin would suggest congenital rubella syndrome, although routine prenatal screening has nearly eliminated the occurrence of this disorder.

Evaluation of the external genitalia must first identify the degree of ambiguity. Isolated anatomic abnormalities such as an abnormally located scrotum or bifid genital tubercle suggest a nonhormonal and non-sex chromosomal insult. Evaluation of the genital tubercle by stretching it to measure its maximum length and width will help differentiate between an undermasculinized penis and an overmasculinized clitoris. A normal newborn penis is 3 to 4 cm in length on average and usually has a midline frenulum. A normal newborn clitoris usually has two lateral folds and is $<1 \times 1$ cm in size. Determining the location of the urethral orifice (e.g., penile, hypospadic, or perineal) provides further information regarding the degree of masculinization.

To determine whether or not a testis or testes are present, the examiner should carefully examine the inguinal canal and labioscrotal areas. It is important to remember that only gonads with testicular elements will descend beyond the external inguinal ring. Normal testicular descent does not occur until approximately 32 to 34 weeks of gestation, and newborn males delivered prematurely may need to be reexamined in the first few weeks of life to identify the presence or absence of testicular descent. Elements of the internal genitalia (e.g., portions of the müllerian system associated with MIS deficiency) may herniate into the inguinal canal. One should attempt to distinguish herniated gonadal versus nongonadal structures.

The examiner also should attempt to determine whether müllerian system structures are present or absent. If a normal vagina, cervix, and uterus can be identified, then one can conclude that, at least on one side, a testis does not exist. The presence of müllerian structures can be identified in the delivery room by two methods. A rectal examination can help to identify a uterus, and the perineal orifice can be probed to distinguish the urinary system from the internal genitalia. By passing a pediatric catheter into the urethra, one can identify its location. With this catheter still in place, a second catheter such as a pediatric feeding tube can be passed through the same opening and directed posteriorly in an attempt to identify the vagina. The presence of clear mucus in the second canal confirms the presence of a vagina because only the columnar epithelium of the müllerian system will produce mucus. Usually it is abundant because of placental steroids and will be drawn spontaneously into the feeding tube. Outside of the delivery room, pelvic ultrasonography, cystoscopy/vaginoscopy, and magnetic resonance imaging (MRI) can provide more definitive information about the gonads and internal genitalia.

Laboratory Assessment

Initial laboratory testing is directed toward determining the presence or absence of CAH. Elevated serum 17α-hydroxyprogesterone levels will establish this diagnosis, and this test can be performed expeditiously in most centers. Electrolytes in the serum and urine should be followed in order to identify the classic salt-wasting findings of hyponatremia and hyper-

kalemia that should develop in 7 to 10 days. Chromosomal analysis is crucial to facilitate diagnosis and assign sex of rearing. Rapid fluorescent in situ hybridization (FISH) can be used to identify the presence or absence of a Y chromosome.

To help identify the presence of functioning testicular tissue, serum testosterone levels can be measured. A normal or elevated testosterone concentration in the presence of a normal 17α-hydroxyprogesterone concentration confirms the presence of testicular tissue.[64,144] MIS levels also can be used to detect the presence of testes.[145,146] The newborn male has the highest levels, 30 to 70 ng/mL, and these drop at puberty to 2 to 5 ng/mL. In the newborn female, MIS levels are undetectable but will rise at puberty to the same level as seen in pubertal males. A normal or high testosterone concentration in the presence of MIS confirms that testicular elements are present. A karyotype will further direct the diagnosis to 45,X/46,XY gonadal dysgenesis, true hermaphroditism (if 46,XY or 46,XX), and androgen insensitivity or 5α-reductase deficiency (if 46,XY). Low testosterone levels in the presence of MIS and a 46,XY karyotype suggest a deficiency in one of the enzymes of steroidogenesis, 45,X/46,XY gonadal dysgenesis, or true hermaphroditism.

Additional studies on the newborn may include measuring androgens (androstenedione, testosterone, and DHT) before and after hCG stimulations, 500 IU administered intramuscularly for 5 days. Short-term application of testosterone cream to the genital tubercle will help to assess the competency of the androgen receptor. In addition to a karyotype, a sample of blood should be collected for DNA extraction and analyzed or storage for later analysis. Nearly all the 46,XY disorders of sexual differentiation and the various forms of CAH are associated with mutations within their respective genes.

Maternal serum levels of DHEAS, testosterone, and DHT are used to diagnose an androgen-producing tumor or an androgenizing luteoma of pregnancy. Serum estrogen concentrations, when decreased, are consistent with placental aromatase deficiency. These laboratory studies should be obtained from the mother immediately following delivery, in addition to cord blood sampling.

▶ TREATMENT AND COUNSELING

A team approach will best meet the medical needs of the newborn and the emotional needs of the family. This team should be composed of a pediatrician, a reproductive endocrinologist, a urologist, and a psychologist and should be coordinated by the most knowledgeable individual present. During the early days of the baby's life, it is essential that the team work together to gain the trust of the parents while pursuing the definitive diagnosis. This relationship is critical not only in the newborn period but also in future years as close follow-up is maintained.

Except for initiation of steroid replacement in the newborn with CAH, the two most important considerations for subsequent long-term management in all newborns with genital ambiguity are: (1) determination of the sex of rearing and (2) the counseling needs of the patient's family.

Sex-of-Rearing Assignment

Guidelines to assist in the assignment of sex of rearing were developed originally by Money and Hampson in 1955[147] and have been refined since. Changing the sex of rearing after the neonatal period is suspected to have adverse psychological consequences in the long term. Among individuals with disorders of sexual development, gender identity appears to develop independently of gonadal morphology, sex chromosome status, and external genital configuration. Money and Hampson suggested previously that gender identity develops concordant with sex of rearing when this is as-

signed prior to the age of 18 months. However, a gathering body of case reports of intersex patients, some of whom have discordant gender identity and others homosexuality, suggests that androgenization and masculinization of the brain may occur in utero in an androgenic hormonal environment.[148] Implications of this concept are that gender-identity problems more likely arise should the child be raised ambiguously once this programming has been established.

Expert opinion suggests that the recommendations put forth by Money and Hampson in 1955 are obsolete and that new approaches need to be considered.[149,150] At the very least, an expedient sex-of-rearing assignment should be made when the available information provides the clinician with reassurance that a change in this assignment is unlikely to be necessary. A sex-of-rearing assignment should be made with the intent that it will never be changed. The following two factors have been used previously for sex-assignment decisions: (1) the individual should be able to perform sexually concordant with the assigned sex, and (2) if raised as a male, the patient should be able to stand to urinate. Of course, other important issues may be involved in these decisions based on the specific etiology of the genital ambiguity.

One should be made aware of the emerging controversy over the appropriateness of physicians and parents making these surgical decisions for the patient versus allowing the patient to make his or her own decision as their sense of gender identity evolves from childhood through adolescence. Long-term follow-up studies of the emotional health of intersex individuals are lacking, and case reports of intersex individuals unhappy with the sex of rearing assigned at birth are mounting. The latter emerging concept would imply that any surgical repair should be delayed until that time. However, it is difficult to understand how such delays could possibly help to prevent gender-identity problems. Dealing with the persistence of ambiguous genitalia through childhood and adolescence would no doubt be very difficult.

Most of the proponents of surgical delay appear to be patients who have had gender-identity problems. One wonders whether this seemingly vocal minority of intersex patients may have had unique situations predisposing them to these unfortunate gender-identity issues. Encouragingly, most patients with intersex disorders seemingly do well.

Counseling

The family should be counseled regarding the possible etiology of the sexual ambiguity, the implications of sex of rearing, and the potential need for corrective surgery. Future sexual development, sexual performance, and the fertility potential of the child also should be discussed in detail. These conversations must be tailored to the family's education level. While genetic and karyotypic information may be helpful in some situations, it may be harmful in others. There is never a situation that would benefit from descriptors such as *true hermaphrodite* or *male pseudohermaphrodite*. Once the sex of rearing has been established, the child always should be referred to only as a boy or a girl.

The following discussion is suggested for approaching the conversation with family members: "Most females have 46 chromosomes, both of which are X chromosomes, and most males have 46 chromosomes, one an X chromosome and the other a Y chromosome. Occasionally, men are identified who have two X chromosomes and no Y chromosomes, usually during an infertility evaluation. Occasionally, women are identified who have an X chromosome and a Y chromosome, and depending on the nature of the disorder, they may be able to gestate a pregnancy via donor egg with assisted reproductive technology (e.g., 46,XY gonadal dysgenesis) or spontaneously progress through puberty (e.g., androgen insensitivity)." Stressing female qualities, such as potential fertility and spontaneous breast development, is helpful in these discussions. The appropriate question to ask a family once sex of rearing has been determined and counseling has been initiated is, "What are you going to name your child?" If the parents select a gender-ambiguous name such as Kimberly, Courtney, Tommie, or Toni, it is likely that they are still not confident in the sex assignment. This should be addressed immediately in further counseling, and consideration should be given to selecting a more gender-specific name.

Genetic counseling is also very important in these families. For some disorders, recurrence is unlikely, whereas other disorders are more likely to recur. Most enzyme deficiencies are the result of homozygous autosomal recessive mutations and thus carry a 25 percent risk for recurrence in subsequent pregnancies. In a subsequent pregnancy, 21-OH deficiency can be detected in utero by measuring amniotic fluid levels of 17α-hydroxyprogesterone.[151] However, since genital formation is completed by the early second trimester, data from an amniocentesis may be useful for selecting pregnancies that would benefit from antenatal glucocorticoid suppression. Hence the decision for antenatal treatment is based primarily on the result of the genetic analysis of the parents and prior pregnancy outcome. If CAH is suspected, high-dose maternal glucocorticoids can be initiated early in the first trimester to suppress fetal adrenal androgen production and prevent masculinization of a 46,XX fetus.[152] If the fetus is found by chorionic villus sampling (CVS) or early amniocentesis to be an unaffected female or a male, maternal glucocorticoid suppressive therapy may be stopped. Preimplantation genetic diagnosis (PGD) is also now being used to identify affected embryos with a few of these disorders (e.g., 21-OH deficiency), allowing only the transfer of embryos that are found to be unaffected.

Surgical Correction

It has been considered ideal for the newborn to be brought home from the hospital with the external genitalia concordant with sex of rearing and that corrective surgery be performed immediately following delivery during the same hospitalization. Recent experience suggests that families are less likely to choose a gender-ambiguous name after corrective surgery has been performed. Surgery may involve reduction clitoroplasty or removal of the gonads from the labioscrotal folds. If gonad(s) are present intraabdominally, they may be left in place temporarily but not indefinitely. Usually, creation of a neovagina should be deferred until adolescence due to the possibility of postoperative closure and scarring unless continued vaginal dilation is performed postoperatively. Only surgeons who are well trained in these techniques should perform these procedures. The aggressive, early surgical approach of many pediatric surgeons has been questioned recently. However, until long-term studies are available, decisions regarding early timing of surgery still should be considered seriously and should be based on a multidisciplinary team approach that includes the family.

Long-Term Management

Ideally, the same team of clinicians that initiated treatment in infancy should provide long-term follow-up. Specific issues requiring attention include consistent psychological support, expedient management of problems related to gender identity, monitoring for the potential development of malignancy, facilitation of normal pubertal development, and preservation of fertility, if possible.

Vigilant monitoring for the occurrence of a neoplasm is required because patients with a Y cell line may undergo malignant transformation of their gonads. Screening tests may include serum measurements of α-fetoprotein, hCG, and lactate dehydrogenase (LDH). Imaging studies such as pelvic ultrasound or computed tomographic (CT) scanning also may be helpful.

Pubertal onset should occur in these patients at a time that is age appropriate with their peers. If spontaneous puberty does not begin by 10 years of age (i.e., if the gonads have been removed previously), exogenous steroid replacement should be initiated.

Fertility and future reproduction are possible in many of these patients. Females with CAH will have preserved fertility if recognized and treated early. Occasionally, true hermaphrodites may have enough ovarian follicles to initiate puberty, ovulate, menstruate, and even achieve pregnancy. In other agonadal patients who have a preserved uterus, the use of donor egg and assisted reproductive technologies is a means to gestate a pregnancy. Recent evidence is accumulating, however, that patients with Turner syndrome may have a maternal mortality of 20 percent or greater in this setting because of the increased risk of aortic dissection, rupture, and death.[153]

▶ THE ROLE OF PRENATAL ULTRASOUND IN THE DIAGNOSIS OF AMBIGUOUS GENITALIA

The diagnosis of ambiguous genitalia in utero has become increasingly common with the routine use of second-trimester ultrasonography. However, it may be difficult to confirm the diagnosis of ambiguous genitalia in utero because there is great variability in the proficiency of ultrasonographers. Vigilant adherence to the use of follow-up ultrasound scanning is, however, one tool that can identify a fetus at risk.[154] Most fetuses suspected of having ambiguous genitalia in utero are born as normal-appearing females. If ambiguous genitalia are detected antenatally, then the most likely cause is CAH, which can be diagnosed by measuring the intraamniotic levels of 17α-hydroxyprogesterone via amniocentesis.[155,156] Antenatal treatment may then allow for an amelioration of the genital abnormality. Chromosomal studies may be performed on amniotic fluid and also can provide helpful information. A 46,XX fetus with ambiguous genitalia could have CAH, exposure to excess androgens, or true hermaphroditism, all of which are likely best assigned a female sex of rearing. A 46,XY fetus, however, makes the decision of sex of rearing much more difficult because this largely depends on both the size of the genitals and the placement of the urethra. The suspicion of ambiguous genitalia in utero can provide expectant parents with the privacy to initiate discussions on sex of rearing and generate expectations for the delivery room that otherwise were unavailable before the advent of routine prenatal ultrasound.

KEY POINTS

1. At conception, every embryo has bisexual potential to develop into either a male or a female.

2. An orderly sequence of embryonic events must proceed for normal sexual differentiation of the gonads, internal ductal system, and external genitalia to occur.

3. Predictable phenotypes result from gene mutations or environmental insults occurring at specific points in the pathway of sexual differentiation.

4. For testicular development to begin, testicular determinant genes must be activated very early in the timetable of sexual differentiation. If testicular determinant genes do not function, ovarian development will begin irrespective of the embryo's genetic sex.

5. The sexual differentiation of a male fetus proceeds according to a well-described sequence of events requiring the presence of: (a) *SRY* and related testicular genes and their expression, (b) bilateral MIS production, (c) bilateral testicular testosterone for wolffian development, (d) peripheral 5α-reductase activity converting testosterone to DHT for development of the external genitalia; and (e) functional androgen receptors at the target tissue to translate the hormone signals into the end-organ event of masculinization.

6. Ovarian determinant genes, likely playing an active role in gonadal morphogenesis, have yet to be characterized.

7. The developing ovaries are not endocrinologically active, as are the testes, during intrauterine life. The internal and external genitalia of a female fetus develop in the absence of ovarian hormone production.

8. Germ cell division and maturation differ between the ovary and the testis. Germ cell replenishment in the female is limited to intrauterine life. Spermatogenesis occurs throughout adult life. In the female, preservation of the germ cells likely depends on ovarian determinant genes located on both arms of the X chromosomes, as well as the autosomes. The genes encoding spermatogenesis are located on the long arm of the Y chromosome.

9. Delivery of a newborn with a disorder of sexual development should be considered a medical and psychosocial emergency. Accurate diagnosis, prompt treatment, and close long-term follow-up are essential in ensuring that gender identity is concordant with sex of rearing. Changing the sex of rearing should be avoided at all costs during the newborn and childhood years.

10. The expedient recognition and treatment of CAH are crucial because of the risk of a salt-wasting crisis and death.

11. The infant with an identifiable testis or testes does not have CAH. Ambiguity associated with CAH only occurs in 46,XX individuals who have intraabdominal ovaries. Elevated serum 17α-hydroxyprogesterone levels will establish this diagnosis. The infant with an identified gonad in the inguinal canal or within the labioscrotom is likely to have one of the 46,XY syndromes or be a true hermaphrodite, none of which result in neonatal death.

12. One should not make a hurried decision in the delivery room about a newborn's sex (i.e., sex of rearing) for babies identified with genital ambiguity. In addition, one should be careful in labeling an infant with a normal-appearing penis yet bilateral undescended testes as a normal male. The latter infant may be a 46,XX female with CAH and intraabdominal ovaries.

13. Corrective surgery by experienced clinicians historically has been performed during the delivery hospitalization. Recent controversy surrounds this long-held tenet, some advocate waiting until adolescence when the individual can verbalize gender identity. In the absence of long-term studies to support the latter, and with a majority of prior satisfactory outcomes, there appears no compelling reason to change this step of management in all but the most difficult of situations. That controversy exists is even further evidence for the need of a team approach from the time of birth until gender identity is well established to allow decision making that seems appropriate for each specific situation.

14. Long-term follow-up requires reinforcement of sex of rearing and management of problems related to gender identity, monitoring for the development of malignancy, facilitation of normal pubertal development, and preservation of fertility, if possible.

REFERENCES

1. Reindollar RH, Tho SP, McDonough PG. Abnormalities of sexual differentiation: Evaluation and management. *Clin Obstet Gynecol* 1987; 30:697–713.

2. Reindollar RH. Normal and abnormal sexual differentiation, in Lobo RA, et al (eds), *Mishell's Textbook of Infertility, Contraception, and Reproductive Endocrinology*. Malden, MA: Blackwell Science, 1997:255–277.

3. Reindollar RH, Byrd JR, McDonough PG. Delayed sexual development: A study of 252 patients. *Am J Obstet Gynecol* 1981;140:371–380.

4. Sinclair AH, et al. A gene from the human sex-determining region encodes a protein with homology to a conserved DNA-binding motif. *Nature* 1990;346:240–244.

5. Ferguson-Smith MA. Abnormalities of human sex determination. *J Inherit Metab Dis* 1992; 15:518–525.

6. Salas-Cortes L, et al. SRY protein is expressed in ovotestis and streak gonads from human sex-reversal. *Cytogenet Cell Genet* 2000;91:212–216.

7. Dubin RA, Ostrer H. *SRY* is a transcriptional activator. *Mol Endocrinol* 1994;8:1182–1192.

8. Haqq CM, et al. Molecular basis of mammalian sexual determination: Activation of müllerian inhibiting substance gene expression by *SRY*. *Science* 1994;266:1494–1500.

9. Bardoni B, et al. A dosage sensitive locus at chromosome Xp21 is involved in male-to-female sex reversal. *Nature Genet* 1994;7: 497–501.

10. Ramkissoon Y, Goodfellow P. Early steps in mammalian sex determination. *Curr Opin Genet Dev* 1996;6:316–321.

11. Wagner T, et al. Autosomal sex reversal and campomelic dysplasia are caused by mutations in and around the *SRY*-related gene *SOX9*. *Cell* 1994;79:1111–1120.

12. Foster JW, et al. Campomelic dysplasia and autosomal sex reversal caused by mutations in an *SRY*-related gene. *Nature* 1994;372:525–530.

13. Tommerup N, et al. Assignment of an autosomal sex reversal locus *(SRA1)* and campomelic dysplasia *(CMPD1)* to 17q24.3-q25.1. *Nature Genet* 1993;4:170–174.

14. Melo KF, et al. An unusual phenotype of Frasier syndrome due to IVS9 + 4C>T mutation in the *WT1* gene: Predominantly male ambiguous genitalia and absence of gonadal dysgenesis. *J Clin Endocrinol Metab* 2002;87:2500–2505.

15. Klamt B, et al. Frasier syndrome is caused by defective alternative splicing of *WT1* leading to an altered ratio of *WT1±KTS* splice isoforms. *Hum Mol Genet* 1998;7:709–714.

16. Barbaux S, et al. Donor splice-site mutations in *WT1* are responsible for Frasier syndrome. *Nature Genet* 1997;17:467–470.

17. Parker KL, Schimmer BP, Schedl A. Genes essential for early events in gonadal development. *EXS* 2001;91:11–24.

18. Lee MM, Donahoe PK. Müllerian inhibiting substance: A gonadal hormone with multiple functions. *Endocr Rev* 1993;14:152–164.

19. Siiteri PK, Wilson JD. Testosterone formation and metabolism during male sexual differentiation in the human embryo. *J Clin Endocrinol Metab* 1974;38:113–125.

20. Wilson JD, et al. The role of gonadal steroids in sexual differentiation. *Recent Prog Horm Res* 1981;37:1–39.

21. Jost A, et al. Studies on sex differentiation in mammals. *Recent Prog Horm Res* 1973;29:1–41.

22. Jirasek JE. Principles of reproductive embryology, in Simpson JL (ed), *Disorders of Sexual Differentiation: Etiology and Clinical Delineation*. New York: Academic Press, 1976: 466.

23. Davison RM, Fox M, Conway GS. Mapping of the *POF1* locus and identification of putative genes for premature ovarian failure. *Mol Hum Reprod* 2000;6:314–318.

24. Sala C, et al. Eleven X chromosome breakpoints associated with premature ovarian failure *(POF)* map to a 15-Mb YAC contig spanning Xq21. *Genomics* 1997;40:123–131.

25. Bione S, et al. A human homologue of the *Drosophila melanogaster diaphanous* gene is disrupted in a patient with premature ovarian failure: Evidence for conserved function in oogenesis and implications for human sterility. *Am J Hum Genet* 1998;62:533–541.

26. Ogata T, Matsuo N, Nishimura G. *SHOX* haploinsufficiency and overdosage: Impact of gonadal function status. *J Med Genet* 2001;38: 1–6.

27. Binder G, et al. Tall stature, gonadal dysgenesis, and stigmata of Turner's syndrome caused by a structurally altered X chromosome. *J Pediatr* 2001;138:285–287.

28. Gantt PA, et al. A clinical and cytogenetic study of fifteen patients with 45,X/46XY gonadal dysgenesis. *Fertil Steril* 1980;34:216–221.

29. Kofman S, et al. Clinical and endocrine spectrum in patients with the 45,X/46,XY karyotype. *Hum Genet* 1981;58:373–376.

30. Simpson JL, Photopulos G. The relationship of neoplasia to disorders of abnormal sexual differentiation. *Birth Defects* 1976;12:15–50.

31. Schellhas HF. Malignant potential of the dysgenetic gonad, part 1. *Obstet Gynecol* 1974; 44:289–309.

32. Troche V, Hernandez E. Neoplasia arising in dysgenetic gonads. *Obstet Gynecol Surv* 1986; 41:74–79.

33. Swyer GI. Male pseudohermaphroditism: A hitherto undescribed form. *BMJ* 1955;4941: 709–712.

34. Espiner EA, et al. Familial syndrome of streak gonads and normal male karyotype in five phenotypic females. *N Engl J Med* 1970;283:6–11.

35. Jager RJ, et al. A human XY female with a frame shift mutation in the candidate testis-determining gene *SRY*. *Nature* 1990;348:452–454.

36. Muller J, Schwartz M, Skakkebaek NE. Analysis of the sex-determining region of the Y chromosome *(SRY)* in sex-reversed patients: Point mutation in *SRY* causing sex reversal in a 46,XY female. *J Clin Endocrinol Metab* 1992;75: 331–333.

37. Beer-Romero P, Fusaris RRK, Gray MR, Page DC. Mutations identified by rapid screening of the *SRY* locus in 46,XY gonadal dysgenesis and true hermaphrodite patients with denaturing gradient gel electrophoresis (DGGE). Society for Gynecologic Investigation, 39th Annual Meeting San Antonio, TX, 1992; abstract 146.

38. Schaffler A, et al. Identification of a new missense mutation (Gly95Glu) in a highly conserved codon within the high-mobility group box of the sex-determining region of the Y gene: Report on a 46,XY female with gonadal dysgenesis and yolk-sac tumor. *J Clin Endocrinol Metab* 2000;85:2287–2292.

39. Somkuti SG, et al. 46,XY monozygotic twins with discordant sex phenotype. *Fertil Steril* 2000;74:1254–1256.

40. Ogata T, Matsuo N. Testis determining gene(s) on the X chromosome short arm: Chromosomal localisation and possible role in testis determination. *J Med Genet* 1994;31:349.

41. Davidoff F, Federman DD. Mixed gonadal dysgenesis. *Pediatrics* 1973;52:725–742.

42. Reindollar RH, Davis AJ, Otkin LB, Smith DM, Bayer SR. Steroid secretion from neoplastic gonads of two unrelated patients with 46,XY gonadal dysgenesis and spontaneous pubertal development. Society for Gynecologic Investigation, 38th Annual Meeting, San Antonio, TX. 1991; abstract 257.

43. Josso N, et al. Persistence of müllerian ducts in male pseudohermaphroditism and its relation-

ship to cryptorchidism. *Clin Endocrinol (Oxf)* 1983;19:247–258.

44. Guerrier D, et al. The persistent müllerian duct syndrome: a molecular approach. *J Clin Endocrinol Metab* 1989;68:46–52.

45. Knebelmann B, et al. Antimüllerian hormone bruxelles: A nonsense mutation associated with the persistent müllerian duct syndrome. *Proc Natl Acad Sci USA* 1991;88:3767–3771.

46. Parks GA, et al. "True agonadism": A misnomer? *J Pediatr* 1974;84:375–380.

47. Cleary RE, et al. Endocrine and metabolic studies in a patient with male pseudohermaphroditism and true agonadism. *Am J Obstet Gynecol* 1977;128:862–867.

48. Laue L, et al. A nonsense mutation of the human luteinizing hormone receptor gene in Leydig cell hypoplasia. *Hum Mol Genet* 1995;4: 1429–1433.

49. Camacho AM, et al. Congenital adrenal hyperplasia due to a deficiency of one of the enzymes involved in the biosynthesis of pregnenolone. *J Clin Endocrinol Metab* 1968;28: 153–161.

50. Degenhart HJ, et al. Evidence for deficient 20-cholesterol-hydroxylase activity in adrenal tissue of a patient with lipoid adrenal hyperplasia. *Acta Endocrinol (Copenh)* 1972;71:512–518.

51. Kirkland RT, et al. Congenital lipoid adrenal hyperplasia in an eight-year-old phenotypic female. *J Clin Endocrinol Metab* 1973;36:488–496.

52. Koizumi S, et al. Cholesterol side-chain cleavage enzyme activity and cytochrome P-450 content in adrenal mitochondria of a patient with congenital lipoid adrenal hyperplasia (Prader disease). *Clin Chim Acta* 1977;77:301–306.

53. Hauffa BP, et al. Congenital adrenal hyperplasia due to deficient cholesterol side-chain cleavage activity (20,22-desmolase) in a patient treated for 18 years. *Clin Endocrinol (Oxf)* 1985; 23:481–493.

54. Chantilis SJ, Bradshaw KD. Clinical and molecular aspects of steroidogenic enzyme deficiencies. *Infertil Reprod Med Clin North Am* 1994;81–104.

55. Katsumata N, et al. Compound heterozygous mutations in the cholesterol side-chain cleavage enzyme gene *(CYP11A)* cause congenital adrenal insufficiency in humans. *J Clin Endocrinol Metab* 2002;87:3808–3813.

56. Zachmann M, et al. Unusual type of congenital adrenal hyperplasia probably due to deficiency of 3β-hydroxysteroid dehydrogenase: Case report of a surviving girl and steroid studies. *J Clin Endocrinol Metab* 1970;30: 719–726.

57. Janne O, Perheentupa J, Vihko R. Plasma and urinary steroids in an eight-year-old boy with 3β-hydxysteroid dehydrogenase deficiency. *J Clin Endocrinol Metab* 1970;31:162–165.

58. Rosenfield RL, et al. The response to human chorionic gonadotropin (hCG) administration in boys with and without Δ5-3β-hydroxysteroid dehydrogenase deficiency. *J Clin Endocrinol Metab* 1974;39:370–374.

59. Janne O, et al. Testicular endocrine function in a pubertal boy with 3β-hydroxysteroid dehydrogenase deficiency. *J Clin Endocrinol Metab* 1974;39:206–209.

60. Schneider G, et al. Persistent testicular Δ5-isomerase-3β-hydroxysteroid dehydrogenase (5-3β-HSD) deficiency in the Δ5-3β-HSD form of congenital adrenal hyperplasia. *J Clin Invest* 1975;55:681–690.

61. Rosenfield RL, et al. Pubertal presentation of congenital Δ5-3β-hydroxysteroid dehydrogenase deficiency. *J Clin Endocrinol Metab* 1980;51:345–353.

62. Lobo RA, Goebelsmann U. Evidence for reduced 3β-ol-hydroxysteroid dehydrogenase activity in some hirsute women thought to have polycystic ovary syndrome. *J Clin Endocrinol Metab* 1981;53:394–400.

63. Bongiovanni AM. Acquired adrenal hyperplasia: With special reference to 3β-hydroxysteroid dehydrogenase. *Fertil Steril* 1981;35:599–608.

64. Pang S, et al. Non-salt-losing congenital adrenal hyperplasia due to 3β-hydroxysteroid dehydrogenase deficiency with normal glomerulosa function. *J Clin Endocrinol Metab* 1983;56: 808–818.

65. Bradshaw KD, et al. Characterization of complementary deoxyribonucleic acid for human adrenocortical 17α-hydroxylase: A probe for analysis of 17α-hydroxylase deficiency. *Mol Endocrinol* 1987;1:348–354.

66. Yanase T, et al. Combined 17α-hydroxylase/17,20-lyase deficiency due to a stop codon in the N-terminal region of 17α-hydroxylase cytochrome P-450. *Mol Cell Endocrinol* 1988; 59:249–253.

67. Yanase T, et al. Combined 17α-hydroxylase/17,20-lyase deficiency due to a 7-base-pair duplication in the N-terminal region of the cytochrome P450$_{17\alpha}$ (CYP17) gene. *J Clin Endocrinol Metab* 1990;70:1325–1329.

68. Biason A, et al. Deletion within the *CYP17* gene together with insertion of foreign DNA is the cause of combined complete 17α-hydroxylase/17,20-lyase deficiency in an Italian patient. *Mol Endocrinol* 1991;5:2037–2045.

69. Ahlgren R, et al. Compound heterozygous mutations (Arg 239----stop, Pro 342----Thr) in the *CYP17* (P450$_{17\alpha}$) gene lead to ambiguous external genitalia in a male patient with partial combined 17α-hydroxylase17,20-lyase deficiency. *J Clin Endocrinol Metab* 1992;74:667–672.

70. Goldsmith O, Solomon DH, Horton R. Hypogonadism and mineralocorticoid excess: The 17-hydroxylase deficiency syndrome. *N Engl J Med* 1967;277:673–677.

71. New MI. Male pseudohermaphroditism due to 17α-hydroxylase deficiency. *J Clin Invest* 1970; 49:1930–1941.

72. Kershnar AK, et al. Studies in a phenotypic female with 17α-hydroxylase deficiency. *J Pediatr* 1976;89:395–400.

73. Jones HW Jr, et al. A genetic male patient with 17α-hydroxylase deficiency. *Obstet Gynecol* 1982;59:254–259.

74. Morimoto I, et al. An autopsy case of 17α-hydroxylase deficiency with malignant hypertension. *J Clin Endocrinol Metab* 1983;56:915–919.

75. Dean HJ, Shackleton CH, Winter JS. Diagnosis and natural history of 17α-hydroxylase deficiency in a newborn male. *J Clin Endocrinol Metab* 1984;59:513–520.

76. Zachmann M, et al. Steroid 17,20-desmolase deficiency: A new cause of male pseudohermaphroditism. *Clin Endocrinol (Oxf)* 1972;1: 369–385.

77. Goebelsmann U, et al. Male pseudohermaphroditism consistent with 17,20-desmolase deficiency. *Gynecol Invest* 1976;7:138–156.

78. Forest MG, Lecornu M, de Peretti E. Familial male pseudohermaphroditism due to 17-20-desmolase deficiency: I. In vivo endocrine studies. *J Clin Endocrinol Metab* 1980;50: 826–833.

79. Zachmann M, Werder EA, Prader A. Two types of male pseudohermaphroditism due to 17,20-desmolase deficiency. *J Clin Endocrinol Metab* 1982;55:487–490.

80. Larrea F, et al. Hypergonadotrophic hypogonadism in an XX female subject due to 17,20-steroid desmolase deficiency. *Acta Endocrinol (Copenh)* 1983;103:400–405.

81. Kaufman FR, et al. Male pseudohermaphroditism due to 17,20-desmolase deficiency. *J Clin Endocrinol Metab* 1983;57:32–36.

82. Saez JM, et al. Familial male pseudohermaphroditism with gynecomastia due to a testicular 17-ketosteroid reductase defect: I. Studies in vivo. *J Clin Endocrinol Metab* 1971;32:604–610.

83. Virdis R, et al. Endocrine studies in a pubertal male pseudohermaphrodite with 17-ketosteroid reductase deficiency. *Acta Endocrinol (Copenh)* 1978;87:212–224.

84. Imperato-McGinley J, et al. Male pseudohermaphroditism secondary to 17β-hydroxysteroid dehydrogenase deficiency: Gender role change with puberty. *J Clin Endocrinol Metab* 1979; 49:391–395.

85. Rosler A, Kohn G. Male pseudohermaphroditism due to 17β-hydroxysteroid dehydrogenase deficiency: Studies on the natural history of the defect and effect of androgens on gender role. *J Steroid Biochem* 1983;19:663–674.

86. Leinonen P, et al. Male pseudohermaphroditism due to deficiency of testicular 17-ketosteroid reductase. *Acta Paediatr Scand* 1983;72:211–214.

87. Ulloa-Aguirre A, et al. Endocrine and biochemical studies in a 46,XY phenotypically male infant with 17-ketosteroid reductase deficiency. *J Clin Endocrinol Metab* 1985;60: 639–643.

88. Andersson S, et al. Molecular genetics and pathophysiology of 17β-hydroxysteroid dehydrogenase 3 deficiency. *J Clin Endocrinol Metab* 1996;81:130–136.

89. Opitz JM, et al. Pseudovaginal perineoscrotal hypospadias. *Clin Genet* 1972;3:1–26.

90. Imperato-McGinley J, et al. Steroid 5α-reductase deficiency in man: An inherited form of male pseudohermaphroditism. *Science* 1974; 186:1213–1215.

91. Moore RJ, Griffin JE, Wilson JD. Diminished 5α-reductase activity in extracts of fibroblasts cultured from patients with familial incomplete male pseudohermaphroditism, type 2. *J Biol Chem* 1975;250:7168–7172.

92. Imperato-McGinley J, Peterson RE. Male pseudohermaphroditism: The complexities of male phenotypic development. *Am J Med* 1976; 61:251–272.

93. Imperato-McGinley J, et al. Male pseudohermaphroditism secondary to 5α-reductase deficiency: A model for the role of androgens in both the development of the male phenotype and the evolution of a male gender identity. *J Steroid Biochem* 1979;11:637–645.

94. Peterson RE, et al. Male pseudohermaphroditism due to steroid 5α-reductase deficiency. *Am J Med* 1977;62:170–191.

95. Leshin M, Griffin JE, Wilson JD. Hereditary male pseudohermaphroditism associated with an unstable form of 5α-reductase. *J Clin Invest* 1978;62:685–691.

96. Imperato-McGinley J, et al. Androgens and the evolution of male-gender identity among male pseudohermaphrodites with 5α-reductase deficiency. *N Engl J Med* 1979;300:1233–1237.

97. Pang S, et al. Dihydrotestosterone and its relationship to testosterone in infancy and childhood. *J Clin Endocrinol Metab* 1979;48: 821–826.

98. Savage MO, et al. Familial male pseudohermaphroditism due to deficiency of 5α-reductase. *Clin Endocrinol (Oxf)* 1980;12:397–406.

99. Imperato-McGinley J, et al. Steroid 5α-reductase deficiency in a 65-year-old male pseudohermaphrodite: The natural history, ultrastructure of the testes, and evidence for inherited enzyme heterogeneity. *J Clin Endocrinol Metab* 1980;50:15–22.

100. Imperato-McGinley J, et al. Hormonal evaluation of a large kindred with complete androgen insensitivity: Evidence for secondary 5α-reductase deficiency. *J Clin Endocrinol Metab* 1982;54:931–941.

101. Price P, et al. High-dose androgen therapy in male pseudohermaphroditism due to 5α-reductase deficiency and disorders of the androgen receptor. *J Clin Invest* 1984;74:1496–1508.

102. Andersson S, Bishop RW, Russell DW. Expression cloning and regulation of steroid 5α-reductase, an enzyme essential for male sexual differentiation. *J Biol Chem* 1989;264:16249–16255.

103. Jenkins EP, et al. Genetic and pharmacological evidence for more than one human steroid 5α-reductase. *J Clin Invest* 1992;89:293–300.

104. Jenkins EP, et al. Characterization and chromosomal mapping of a human steroid 5α-reductase gene and pseudogene and mapping of the mouse homologue. *Genomics* 1991;11:1102–1112.

105. Andersson S, et al. Deletion of steroid 5α-reductase 2 gene in male pseudohermaphroditism. *Nature* 1991;354:159–161.

106. Griffin JE. Androgen resistance: The clinical and molecular spectrum. *New Engl J Med* 1992; 326:611–618.

107. Wilson JD. Syndromes of androgen resistance. *Biol Reprod* 1992;46:168–173.

108. Rosa S, et al. Complete androgen insensitivity syndrome caused by a novel mutation in the ligand-binding domain of the androgen receptor: Functional characterization. *J Clin Endocrinol Metab* 2002;87:4378–4382.

109. Gottlieb B, et al. Update of the androgen receptor gene mutations database. *Hum Mutat* 1999;14:103–114.

110. McPhaul MJ, et al. Genetic basis of endocrine disease: 4. The spectrum of mutations in the androgen receptor gene that causes androgen resistance. *J Clin Endocrinol Metab* 1993;76:17–23.

111. Gottlieb B, Beitel LK, Trifiro MA. Variable expressivity and mutation databases: The androgen receptor gene mutations database. *Hum Mutat* 2001;17:382–388.

112. Muller J. Morphometry and histology of gonads from twelve children and adolescents with the androgen insensitivity (testicular feminization) syndrome. *J Clin Endocrinol Metab* 1984; 59:785–789.

113. Morris JM, Mahesh VB. Further observations on the syndrome, "testicular feminization." *Am J Obstet Gynecol* 1963;87:731–748.

114. Akin JW, et al. Evidence for a partial deletion in the androgen receptor gene in a phenotypic male with azoospermia. *Am J Obstet Gynecol* 1991;165:1891–1894.

115. Grino PB, et al. A mutation of the androgen receptor associated with partial androgen resistance, familial gynecomastia, and fertility. *J Clin Endocrinol Metab* 1988;66:754–761.

116. Johnson JG, Byrd JR, McDonough PG. True hermaphroditism with peripheral blood and gonadal karyotyping. *Obstet Gynecol* 1979;54: 549–553.

117. van Niekerk WA, Retief AE. The gonads of human true hermaphrodites. *Hum Genet* 1981; 58:117–122.

118. Tho SP, et al. Absence of the testicular determining factor gene *SRY* in XX true hermaphrodites and presence of this locus in most subjects with gonadal dysgenesis caused by Y aneuploidy. *Am J Obstet Gynecol* 1992;167: 1794–1802.

119. Berkovitz GD, et al. The role of the sex-determining region of the Y chromosome *(SRY)* in the etiology of 46,XX true hermaphroditism. *Hum Genet* 1992;88:411–416.

120. Verp MS, et al. Chimerism as the etiology of a 46,XX/46,XY fertile true hermaphrodite. *Fertil Steril* 1992;57:346–349.

121. Strain L, et al. A true hermaphrodite chimera resulting from embryo amalgamation after in vitro fertilization. *N Engl J Med* 1998;338:166–169.

122. Kolon TF, Ferrer FA, McKenna PH. Clinical and molecular analysis of XX sex-reversed patients. *J Urol* 1998;160:1169–1172; discussion 1178.

123. Slaney SF, et al. An autosomal or X-linked mutation results in true hermaphrodites and 46,XX males in the same family. *J Med Genet* 1998; 35:17–22.

124. de la Chapelle A. Analytic review: Nature and origin of males with XX sex chromosomes. *Am J Hum Genet* 1972;24:71–105.

125. de la Chapelle A. The etiology of maleness in XX men. *Hum Genet* 1981;58:105–116.

126. Schweikert HU, et al. Clinical, endocrinological, and cytological characterization of two 46,XX males. *J Clin Endocrinol Metab* 1982; 54:745–752.

127. White PC, New MI, Dupont B. Adrenal 21-hydroxylase cytochrome P-450 genes within the MHC class III region. *Immunol Rev* 1985; 87:123–150.

128. New MI, et al. The adrenal cortex, in Kaplan SA (ed), Clinical Pediatric Endocrinology. Philadelphia: Saunders, 1990; pp 181–234.

129. Reindollar RH, Gray MR. The molecular basis of 21-hydroxylase deficiency. *Semin Reprod Endocrinol* 1991;9:34–45.

130. New MI. Female pseudohermaphroditism. *Semin Perinatol* 1992;16:289–297.

131. Reindollar RH, et al. Prenatal diagnosis of 21-hydroxylase deficiency by the complementary deoxyribonucleic acid probe for cytochrome P-450C-21OH. *Am J Obstet Gynecol* 1988;158: 545–547.

132. Mornet E, et al. First trimester prenatal diagnosis of 21-hydroxylase deficiency by linkage analysis to HLA-DNA probes and by 17-hydroxyprogesterone determination. *Hum Genet* 1986;73:358–364.

133. Reindollar RH, et al. Rapid identification of deoxyribonucleic acid sequence differences in cytochrome P-450 21-hydroxylase *(CYP21)* genes with denaturing gradient gel blots. *Am J Obstet Gynecol* 1992;166:184–191.

134. Speiser PW, New MI. Genotype and hormonal phenotype in nonclassical 21-hydroxylase deficiency. *J Clin Endocrinol Metab* 1987;64:86–91.

135. White PC, New MI, Dupont B. HLA-linked congenital adrenal hyperplasia results from a defective gene encoding a cytochrome P450–specific for steroid 21-hydroxylation. *Proc Natl Acad Sci USA* 1984;81:7505–7509.

136. White PC, Curnow KM, Pascoe L. Disorders of steroid 11β-hydroxylase isozymes. *Endocr Rev* 1994;15:421–438.

137. Bongiovanni A, Kellenbenz G. The adrenogenital syndrome with deficiency of 3 beta-hydroxysteroid dehydrogenase. *J Clin Invest* 1962;41:2086–2092.

138. Pang S. Congenital adrenal hyperplasia owing to 3 beta-hydroxysteroid dehydrogenase deficiency. *Endocrinol Metab Clin North Am* 2001; 30:81–99.

139. Lutfallah C, Wang W, Mason JL, et al. Newly proposed hormonal criteria via genotypic proof for type II 3 beta-hydroxysteroid dehydrogenase deficiency. *J Clin Endocrinol Metab* 2002; 87:2611–22.

140. Carbunaru G, Prasad P, Scoccia B, et al. The hormonal phenotype of nonclassic 3 beta-hydroxysteroid dehydrogenase (HSD3β) deficiency in hyperandrogenic females is associated with insulin-resistant polycystic ovary syndrome and is not a variant of inherited HSD3β2 deficiency. *J Clin Endocrinol Metab* 2004;89:783–94.

141. Shozu M, et al. A new cause of female pseudohermaphroditism: placental aromatase deficiency. *J Clin Endocrinol Metab* 1991;72:560–566.

142. Harada N, et al. Biochemical and molecular genetic analyses on placental aromatase (P-450$_{AROM}$) deficiency. *J Biol Chem* 1992;267: 4781–4785.

143. Conte FA, et al. A syndrome of female pseudohermaphrodism, hypergonadotropic hypogo-

nadism, and multicystic ovaries associated with missense mutations in the gene encoding aromatase (P450$_{arom}$). *J Clin Endocrinol Metab* 1994;78:1287–1292.

144. Meyers-Seifer CH, Charest NJ. Diagnosis and management of patients with ambiguous genitalia. *Semin Perinatol* 1992;16:332–339.

145. Hudson PL, et al. An immunoassay to detect human müllerian inhibiting substance in males and females during normal development. *J Clin Endocrinol Metab* 1990;70:16–22.

146. Josso N, et al. An enzyme linked immunoassay for antimüllerian hormone: A new tool for the evaluation of testicular function in infants and children. *J Clin Endocrinol Metab* 1990;70:23–27.

147. Money J, Hampson J, Hampson J. Hermaphroditisim: Recommendations concerning assignment of sex, change of sex and psychologic management. *Bull John Hopkins Hosp* 1955;97:284–291.

148. Nordenstrom A, et al. Sex-typed toy play behavior correlates with the degree of prenatal androgen exposure assessed by *CYP21* genotype in girls with congenital adrenal hyperplasia. *J Clin Endocrinol Metab* 2002;87:5119–5124.

149. Creighton S. Consensus statement on 21-hydroxylase deficiency from the Lawson Wilkins Pediatric Endocrine Society and the European Society for Paediatric Endocrinology. *Horm Res* 2002;58:188–195; *Horm Res* 2003;59:262.

150. Creighton S, et al. Regarding the consensus statement on 21-hydroxylase deficiency from the Lawson Wilkins Pediatric Endocrine Society and the European Society for Paediatric Endocrinology. *J Clin Endocrinol Metab* 2003; 88:3455; reply 3456.

151. Nagamani M, et al. Maternal and amniotic fluid 17α-hydroxyprogesterone levels during pregnancy: Diagnosis of congenital adrenal hyperplasia in utero. *Am J Obstet Gynecol* 1978; 130:791–794.

152. Hughes IA. Congenital adrenal hyperplasia: 21-Hydroxylase deficiency in the newborn and during infancy. *Semin Reprod Med* 2002; 20:229–242.

153. Karnis MF, et al. Risk of death in pregnancy achieved through oocyte donation in patients with Turner syndrome: A national survey. *Fertil Steril* 2003;80:498–501.

154. Pinhas-Hamiel O, et al. Prenatal diagnosis of sex differentiation disorders: The role of fetal ultrasound. *J Clin Endocrinol Metab* 2002; 87:4547–4553.

155. Forest MG, Betuel H, David M. Prenatal treatment in congenital adrenal hyperplasia due to 21-hydroxylase deficiency: Update 88 of the French Multicentric Study. *Endocr Res* 1989; 15:277–301.

156. New MI, et al. Prenatal diagnosis for congenital adrenal hyperplasia in 532 pregnancies. *J Clin Endocrinol Metab* 2001;86:5651–5657.

CHAPTER 9

Disorders of Puberty and Amenorrhea

KAREN BRADSHAW AND BRUCE R. CARR

► PHYSIOLOGY OF PUBERTY

Puberty is a period during which many dramatic hormonal changes occur. Of these, it is clear that changes controlling the secretion of growth hormone and gonadal steroids play central roles. Growth hormone (GH) is produced by the somatotropes of the anterior pituitary gland. GH synthesis and release are underregulated by growth hormone–releasing hormone (GHRH), which is released by the nerve endings of the hypothalamic GHRH neurons into the hypophyseal portal circulation. In response to pulses of GHRH, the pituitary releases pulses of GH into the systemic circulation. GH exerts its effects by binding to high-affinity receptors on the surfaces of responsive cells. Although GH certainly modulates some biologic processes directly, in many tissues the actions of GH are modulated indirectly through the action of growth factors that are produced in response to the action of GH, specifically insulin-like growth factor I (IGF-I) and its complex series of binding proteins. Serum levels of IGF-I rise in concert with age-related increases in mean GH levels.[1]

At the onset of puberty, increased activity of the gonadotropin-releasing hormone (GnRH) pulse generator causes a progressive rise in the mean concentration of gonadotropins, resulting from an increase in the frequency and amplitude of GnRH pulses (see below). This increase is first detected as nocturnal gonadotropin pulses, but as puberty progresses, gonadotropin pulses also increase during daytime until adult mean gonadotropin levels and pulsatility are achieved. Figure 9-1 depicts pulsatile luteinizing hormone (LH) release throughout the pubertal stages.

Although a number of lines of evidence indicate that there are complex hormonal interactions that mediate the somatic changes of puberty, the interplay between the sex steroid and GH axes can be seen most clearly in studies of the patterns of growth of individuals with genetic defects that alter the function of the GnRH and/or GHRH axes. Boys with absent gonadal function at the time of puberty and a normal GH axis (e.g., patients with an isolated deficiency of gonadotropins) manifest normal growth rates when treated with testosterone alone.[2] Administration of androgens alone to patients with combined defects of the gonadal and GH axes (e.g., patients with panhypopituitarism) does not reestablish a normal rate of growth. Normal growth rates are observed only when such patients are treated with both GH and gonadal steroids.[2]

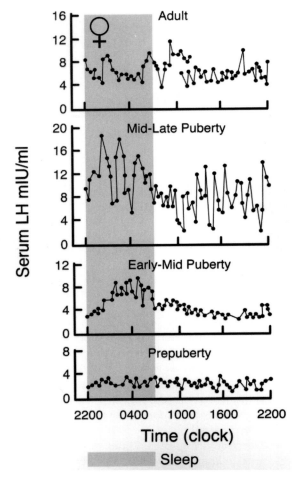

Figure 9-1 Serum LH levels throughout the pubertal stages. Note nocturnal release initially in early puberty. *Adapted from E.O. Reiter Slide Atlas of Endocrinology, Grower Medical Publishing, London, p. 12.20, 1988.*

Other hormone levels change with onset and progression of puberty. As a result of increased estrogen concentrations, sex hormone–binding globulin is higher during puberty than in childhood. The gonadal peptide inhibin, structurally related to transforming growth factor β (TGF-β), lowers the levels of follicle-stimulating hormone (FSH). This product of Sertoli and granulosa cells increases with advancing puberty in both sexes.[1] Concentra-

tions of the glycoprotein antimüllerian hormone (AMH) show marked sexual dimorphism. AMH is produced in Sertoli cells, and levels are relatively high in newborn boys but undetectable in girls. In contrast, the hormone becomes very low in boys during puberty, at which time AMH concentrations increase in girls.[3]

The role of estrogens in the process of skeletal maturation in both boys and girls had been postulated for some time. As an example, effective suppression of the rapid skeletal maturation seen in boys with gonadotropin-independent forms of precocious puberty requires inhibition of aromatase activity to reduce serum estradiol concentrations, in addition to the need for antiandrogens to interfere with androgen action.[4] Furthermore, a female patient with the genetic deficiency of aromatase activity did not exhibit a pubertal growth spurt and exhibited delayed skeletal maturation, indicating that estrogen, not androgens, is normally required for these events.[3]

Inferences drawn from such cases regarding the importance of estrogen in promoting skeletal maturation in both sexes are reinforced by contrasting the patterns of pubertal development in the syndromes of androgen and estrogen resistance. Patients with complete androgen insensitivity syndrome have a normal pubertal growth spurt with the onset of pubertal gonadal function.[5] In contrast, in males with estrogen resistance due to an inactivating mutation of the estrogen receptor, the epiphyseal growth plates do not fuse, and bone mineralization is markedly decreased. Thus the effects of gonadal steroids in male pubertal development are not mediated via the androgen receptor but by estrogen formed by aromatization of androgens.[6]

These considerations emphasize the complex hormonal interactions that characterize the process of puberty. It is clear that the normal functioning of each of these components is necessary for normal pubertal development to occur. As described below, a variety of conditions can disrupt normal pubertal growth, development, and maturation.

Maturation of the Hypothalamic-Pituitary-Gonadal Axis

Maturation of the reproductive system occurs in a phasic manner in humans, and in higher primates it occurs in several distinct stages. The first stage, which begins during fetal life and lasts until late infancy, is characterized by development of the neuroendocrine systems responsible for regulation of the reproductive system. GnRH neurons develop in the rostral forebrain associated with the olfactory placode. These neurons migrate to an area in the arcuate nucleus of the hypothalamus destined to become the GnRH pulse generator. These neural cells develop intrinsic and unregulated pulsatile activity by about 11 weeks of gestation. During this stage, the reproductive system appears to be fully active, with gonadotropin and sex steroid hormone concentrations being measurable in fetal plasma. Concentrations of LH and FSH peak at about 4 to 5 months of gestational age. Later in gestation, negative feedback from gonadal steroids begins to regulate the pulse generator, and by term, gonadotropin levels (and, by inference, the activity of the GnRH pulse generator) are low.[7]

At the time of delivery, the infant is separated from the dominant source of estrogenic sex steroids, the placenta, and owing to withdrawal of this negative feedback, the levels of gonadotropins rise. This increase is responsible for a transient secondary gonadal stimulation occurring in the first months following birth. Although occurring in both boys and girls, this is observed most readily in female infants, in whom there may be prolonged neonatal breast budding.

By 6 months of postnatal age, gonadotropin and sex steroid concentrations in plasma have again declined to low levels, and the third stage of maturation is initiated. This stage lasts throughout childhood and is characterized by low plasma concentrations of LH, FSH, and sex steroids. From a physiologic perspective, the prepubertal stage of development presents apparent contradictions. Measurements of go-nadotropins and sex steroids during fetal development suggest that the hypothalamic-gonadal axis has developed completely in utero and that it is regulated by steroid hormones during the latter stages of pregnancy. Despite this, during the prepubertal period, gonadotropins remain low, even when sex steroid concentrations are extremely low, such as in patients with Turner syndrome or in castrated children.[3] That serum gonadotropin concentrations remain low under such conditions suggests that additional inhibitory mechanisms in the central nervous system (CNS)/hypothalamus have developed. Early studies to explain these different regulatory behaviors focused on examining the sensitivity of the hypothalamus and pituitary to feedback inhibition by gonadal steroids. These investigations demonstrated that the levels of estrogen and androgen required to inhibit LH and FSH secretion in young prepubertal animals and in humans are consistently lower than those required to suppress gonadotropin levels to an equivalent extent in adult castrated animals.[1] Differences in the sensitivity of regulation of gonadotropin secretion in young prepubertal and adult animals have been described in a number of different species. Although these studies appear to explain the prepubertal quiescence of gonadotropin secretion, other observations suggest that additional mechanisms also may be operative. Although mean serum concentrations of gonadotropins are low during the prepubertal period, the reproductive system is not completely inhibited because spontaneous LH pulses occur at a low frequency in normal children.

The fourth stage, puberty itself, results from reactivation of the reproductive axis. There is a reemergence of GnRH secretion that activates maturation of the pituitary-gonadal axis.[8] Although a great deal of effort has been expended to identify the signals that control the onset of puberty, it appears that the mechanisms responsible for the initiation of pubertal events are extremely complex. There is growing evidence that attainment of a certain body mass or composition likely is linked with leptin levels. The effect of increased leptin levels on the initiation of puberty appears to be secondary to the suppression of the neuropeptide Y by leptin, thus releasing its inhibition of the pituitary gonadotropin axis. Neural signals derived from centers within the CNS that serve as a biologic clock may be involved.

The onset of puberty is heralded by striking increases in nocturnal LH secretion, manifested by an increase in the amplitude and frequency of LH pulses. These increases in LH precede rises in sex steroid concentrations and the development of secondary sex characteristics. As pubertal maturation progresses, the amplitude and frequency of gonadotropin pulses also increase during the day in a pattern similar to that seen at night until the final stage of sexual maturation, adulthood, is reached. The mechanism underlying the relative suppression and subsequent pubertal activation of hypothalamic GnRH is unknown. In females, this results in the regular cyclic variations of gonadotropins, estrogen, and progesterone characteristic of the menstrual cycle. Pulsatile GnRH stimulates pituitary FSH and LH secretion, ultimately stimulating gonadal steroid production and gametogenesis in males and females (Fig. 9-2) In the ovary, FSH stimu-

Hormonal Changes In Puberty

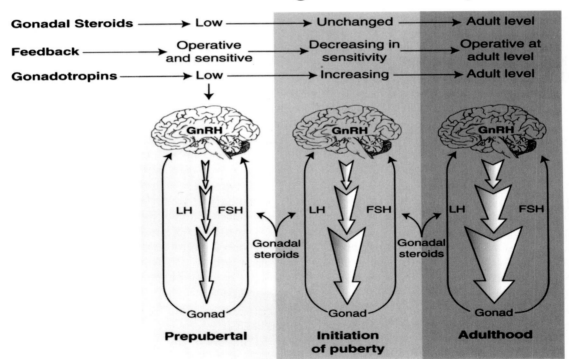

Figure 9-2 The changes in sensitivity of the hypothalamic gonodostat. In the prepubertal state, the concentration of sex steroids and gonadotropins is low; the hypothalamic gonadostat is functional but highly sensitive to low levels of sex steroids. With the onset of puberty, there is decreased sensitivity of the hypothalamus to negative feedback by sex steroids, increased release of luteinizing hormone-releasing factor (LRF), and enhanced secretion of gonadotropins. In adults, the negative-feedback mechanism in the hypothalamus is less sensitive to feedback by sex steroids (adult set point), and adult levels of gonadotropins and sex steroids are present. *(Copyright by the University of Texas Southwestern Medical Center at Dallas and Karen Bradshaw, M.D., 2000. Reprinted with permission.)*

lates follicular maturation and estrogen production through aromatization of androgens, whereas LH stimulates production by theca cells, triggers ovulation, and maintains progesterone production by the corpus luteum. In males, the same regular pulses of GnRH establish a pattern characterized by relatively constant levels of testosterone and gonadotropins, with minimal diurnal variation. In the testis, FSH acts on Sertoli-Leydig cells to initiate spermatogenesis, and LH acts on the Leydig cells to stimulate testosterone production.[9]

The hypothalamic-pituitary-adrenal (HPA) axis also has some minor input into the physiologic process of puberty through secretion of adrenal androgens (adrenarche). However, the major involvement of the HPA axis in puberty is its potential pathologic influence, primarily in accelerating its onset and/or progress.[9]

▶ CLINICAL ASPECTS OF NORMAL PUBERTY

Characteristics of Normal Pubertal Development

The age at which the somatic change of puberty begins is variable. In the United States and most industrialized countries, pubertal changes usually begin between 8 and 13 years of age in girls and between 9 and 14 years of age in boys.[10] This variability in the time of onset is due to a variety of genetic and environmental influences. Approximately 5 percent of a given population will have the onset of puberty at an age outside this range and will be considered to have either precocious or delayed puberty.[11]

In girls, the first somatic change that usually occurs is the beginning of breast development (thelarche), although in a minority of instances pubic hair growth (pubarche) is the initial event. Figure 9-3 outlines the mean age of pubertal milestones in girls. Thelarche and pubarche occur at mean ages of 10.9 and 11.2 years, respectively. Although the process of pubertal development is in fact a continuum, for descriptive purposes it is usually recorded

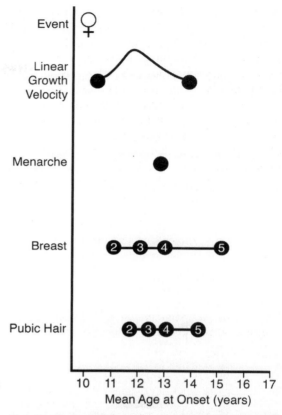

Figure 9-3 Mean age of onset of pubertal milestones in girls. (Numbers 2, 3, 4, etc. denote Tanner stage.) *Adapted from E.O. Reiter Slide Atlas of Endocrinology, Grower Medical Publishing, London, p. 12.6, 1988.*

in terms of a series of distinct stages, the five stages of breast and pubic hair development outlined by Marshall and Tanner being the most commonly employed scheme[11] (Table 9-1 and Fig. 9-4). In parallel with the somatic changes of puberty, the resulting increase in FSH, LH, and GnRH causes ovarian stimulation. This, along with endogenous estrogen, allows fat accumulation to thicken the mons pubis and labia majora; the clitoris enlarges, the hymen thickens, and the vaginal orifice enlarges. The perineal tissue is smoother and more elastic, and the vaginal tissue becomes thicker, keratinized (evidenced clinically by lightening of the color of the mucosa from a deep red to a pale pink), and more rugated.

▶ **TABLE 9-1:** STAGES OF DEVELOPMENT OF SECONDARY SEXUAL CHARACTERISTICS

Boys: Genital (penis) development
Stage 1. Prepubertal: Testes, scrotum, and penis of about same size and proportion as in early childhood.
Stage 2. Enlargement of scrotum and testes; skin of scrotum reddens and changes in texture.
Stage 3. Enlargement of penis, at first mainly in length; further growth of testes and scrotum.
Stage 4. Increased size of penis with growth in breadth and development of glans; testes and scrotum larger; scrotal skin darkened.
Stage 5. Genitalia adult in size and shape.

Girls: Breast development
Stage 1. Prepubertal: Elevation of papilla only.
Stage 2. Breast bud stage: Elevation of breast and papilla as small mound. Enlargement of areola diameter.
Stage 3. Further enlargement and elevation of breast and areola, with no separation of their contours.
Stage 4. Projection of areola and papilla to form a secondary mound above level of breast.
Stage 5. Mature stage: Projection of papilla only, related to recession of areola to general contour of breast.

Both sexes: Pubic hair
Stage 1. Prepubertal: Vellus over pubes is not further developed than over abdominal wall.
Stage 2. Sparse grown of long, slightly pigmented, downy hair, straight or slightly curled, chiefly at base of penis or along labia.
Stage 3. Considerably darker, coarser, and more curled hair; hair spreads sparsely over junction of pubes.
Stage 4. Hair now adult in type, but area covered is still considerably smaller than in adult; no spread to medial surface of thighs.
Stage 5. Adult in quantity and type with distribution of horizontal (or classically "feminine") pattern.
Stage 6. Spread up linea alba (male-type pattern).

The volume of the ovaries and the size of the uterus enlarge as well. Adrenal production of dehydroepiandrostenedione (DHEAS) occurs and is involved in pubic hair growth. After a variable period, averaging about 2 years from the onset of breast development, most of the processes of pubertal maturation are complete, and menarche (the first menstrual period) occurs. Average age of menarche in the United States is 12.8 years, but since the timing of these events are variable, it may occur as late as 14.5 years in normal girls.[10] Further, it is during this period that the most rapid increases in bone mineralization occur.

As in girls, puberty in boys is often described as a series of five distinct stages based on testicular size, penile development, and dis-tribution and character of pubic hair. In boys, the first physical evidence of puberty is an increase in testicular size. Measurement of the testes (length and width) or estimation of testicular volume using a Prader orchidometer allows for early detection of pubertal onset. Testicular volume of 4.0 mL (or length of 2.5 cm), representing the onset of puberty, is noted at an average age of about 11.5 years. Testicular enlargement is followed by scrotal thinning, development of pubic hair, and penile enlargement. Adult testicular volumes and penile dimensions generally are achieved by about 16 years of age; however, there is quite marked individual variation, young men completing their sexual maturation anywhere between the ages of 14 and 18 years.

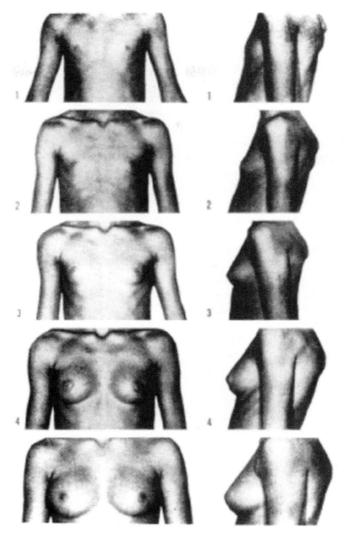

Figure 9-4 Sequence of breast development in girls during this process of puberty. The Tanner stage of breast development is indicated by the number. *(Reprinted with permission, from Mashall WA, Tanner JM. Arch Dis Child. 1969;44:291.)*

In addition to the appearance and development of secondary sexual characteristics in both boys and girls, puberty represents a period during which marked changes in body size and composition occur. Prior to the onset of puberty, the bodies of boys and girls are comprised of similar proportions of adipose tissue and muscle. By the end of puberty, boys have a higher percentage of muscle and a lower percentage of fat relative to girls.

Variations of Normal Puberty

The transition to puberty begins across a wide range of ages, and sexual maturation can be varied among young adults. The factors that regulate the hypothalamic-pituitary-gonadal axis and modulate the timing of puberty remain elusive, but it is evident that some regulation is under genetic control. Studies have shown that the transition from childhood quiescence to the adolescent pattern of GnRH secretion is a gradual process.[12] Notably, the incontrovertible sign of puberty, age at menarche, has remained unchanged.[13]

Fairly common forms of partial premature pubertal development are the isolated development of pubic hair (premature pubarche) and the isolated development of breasts (premature thelarche) (Table 9-2). Although these are benign conditions, such patients must be followed closely in order to monitor for progression to constitutional precocious puberty (CPP). Precocious pubarche is most often a benign condition secondary to early adrenarche. Balducci and colleagues[14] studied 171 subjects with isolated precocious pubarche. Mild errors of steroidogenesis (21-hydroxylase or 3β-hydroxysteroid dehydrogenase) were present in 12 percent of patients, as diagnosed by adrenocorticotropic hormone (ACTH) stimulation tests. In the majority of these, basal 17-OH progesterone levels were higher than in pubertal norms and were felt to be a good screening test to determine which patients should undergo ACTH stimulation testing. In some patients, premature pubarche may predict the future development of chronic anovulation and androgen excess associated with polycystic ovarian syndrome.

Premature thelarche typically is associated with some degree of FSH secretion, antral follicular development, and ovarian function that is greater than that measured in age-matched prepubertal controls. The prevalence of ovar-

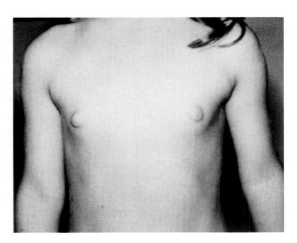

Figure 9-5 Precocious thelarche in a 5-year-old girl. All hormonal studies were normal. Her pubertal development began at 10 years of age.

ian microcysts detected by ultrasonography is increased in these girls; however, plasma estradiol is commonly unmeasurable despite genitourinary cytology that shows evidence of estrogenization.[15] Premature thelarche usually occurs in the first 2 years of life and regresses before puberty. Children who present with breast development later are more likely to have some degree of continued breast development, representing an early stage of precocious puberty (Fig. 9-5). Once breast development is stimulated much beyond the breast bud stage and reaches early adolescent proportions, breast contour generally does not regress. Approximately 10 to 15 percent of these girls develop CPP, but in the majority of patients the breast bud is a transient event that warrants only close follow-up for the appearance of other pubertal signs.[11]

▶ **TABLE 9-2:** ISOLATED FORMS OF PRECOCIOUS PUBERTY IN GIRLS

Premature thelarche
Premature adrenarche
Premature pubarche

▶ PRECOCIOUS PUBERTAL DEVELOPMENT

The development of progressive isosexual secondary sexual characteristics before the age of 8 years in girls and before the age of 9 years in boys is termed *precocious puberty.*[16] Precocious puberty is characterized by early and progressive sexual development accompanied by advancement of skeletal maturation as measured by a bone age. The rapid linear growth that characterizes precocious puberty is associated with premature and rapid skeletal maturation and fusion of the epiphyses. In many cases this results in short adult stature compared with genetic height potential. Signs of early physical maturation should not be dismissed. Young girls may experience psychological and social difficulty when physical maturation exceeds that of their peers. It is important that young girls are educated and adequately prepared for their menses, which typically will follow breast development by approximately 2 years.[13]

There are two major classes of isosexual precocity: disorders that result from early reactivation of the hypothalamic-pituitary-gonadal axis (referred to as *gonadotropin-dependent* or *central precocious puberty;* Table 9-3) and those which do not (referred to as *gonadotropin-*

▶ **TABLE 9-3:** CAUSES OF GONADOTROPIN-DEPENDENT (CENTRAL) PRECOCIOUS PUBERTY

Idiopathic precocious puberty
CNS tumors
Craniopharyngioma
Hypothalamic hamartoma
Optic glioma, astrocytoma, and others
Other CNS disorders
Static encephalopathy (secondary to infection, hypoxia, trauma etc)
Low-dose cranial radiation
Hydrocephalus
Arachnoid cyst
Septooptic dysplasia
Secondary central precocious puberty
After late treatment of congenital adrenal hyperplasia
Hypothyroidism

An overview of the causes of gonadotropin-dependent precocious puberty.

▶ **TABLE 9-4:** GONADOTROPIN-INDEPENDENT PRECOCIOUS PUBERTY

Boys
Testicular disorders
Familial male precocious puberty (testotoxicosis)
McCune-Albright syndrome
Leydig cell adenomas
Human chorionic gonadotropin–secreting tumors
Androgen-secreting teratomas
Girls
Ovarian disorders
McCune-Albright syndrome
Adrenal tumors
Ovarian tumors (granulosa cell)
Simple follicular cyst
Hypothyroidism
Silver-Russell syndrome
Estrogen-containing medications

An overview of the causes of gonadotropin-independent precocious puberty. This term is used interchangeably with the term *peripheral precocious puberty.*

independent precocious puberty; Table 9-4). Most girls who present with precocious puberty have central gonadotropin-dependent precocious puberty that results from secretion of GnRH from the hypothalamus. Although CPP is much more common among females than males, boys with this form of precocious puberty are more likely to be found to have an underlying CNS abnormality.[16] By contrast, most girls (90 percent) have no discernible structural CNS lesion and are thus said to have an "idiopathic" form of the disorder. The overall incidence of gonadotropin-dependent precocious puberty has increased in both sexes due to the survival of children who have received CNS irradiation for brain tumors or leukemia.[17,18]

Typically, children with central precocious puberty experience development of secondary sexual characteristics along with acceleration in linear growth and progressive bone age advancement. Diagnostic confirmation is based on demonstration of pubertal levels of

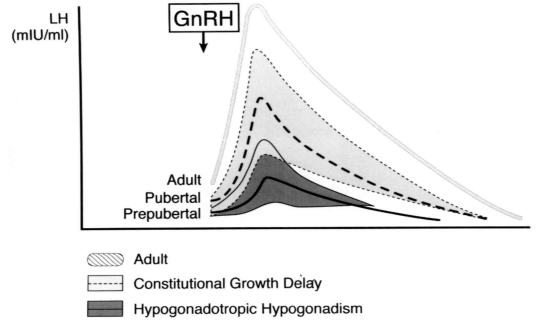

Figure 9-6 Graph of serum LH levels following GnRH stimulation. Adult, constitutional, and hypogonadal curves are shown. Pubertal response is depicted as LH >10 mIU/mL after stimulation. *Adapted from E.O. Reiter Slide Atlas of Endocrinology, Grower Medical Publishing, London, p. 12.50, 1988.*

gonadotropin and sex steroid secretion. Diagnosis of central precocious puberty classically is made when magnetic resonance imaging (MRI) is negative and a significant LH response occurs following GnRH stimulation that is two to three times higher than the prepubertal response. Typically, stimulated LH levels rise to 10 mIU/mL in CPP (Fig. 9-6).

Evaluation of patients with early pubertal development should begin with a detailed history focused on the occurrence of prior CNS trauma, radiation, seizure activity, exposure to exogenous sex steroids in cosmetics or food, or a positive family history. In girls, physical examination should focus on determining whether the development reflects androgen action, estrogen action, or both. Diagnostic evaluation should begin with an x-ray to assess bone age as a marker for sex steroid hormone action. In general, when skeletal age is concordant with chronologic age, continued close observation may be elected (Fig. 9-7).

When secondary sexual characteristics are associated with an advanced bone age, measurements of estradiol, testosterone, and thy-

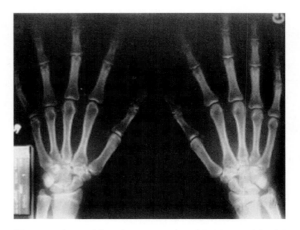

Figure 9-7 Hand x-ray of a 15-year-old girl with isolated gonadotropin deficiency. She is 65 in tall. The epiphyses have not closed, and an adult height of 66 in is forecast.

roid hormone should be obtained, and a GnRH stimulation test may be indicated to differentiate between central (gonadotropin-dependent) and peripheral (gonadotropin-independent) causes of precocious puberty.[12] In most cases, the diagnosis of gonadotropin-dependent precocious puberty, particularly in younger children, warrants obtaining an MRI or computed tomographic (CT) scan of the head.

Gonadotropin-Dependent Precocious Puberty

Idiopathic Precocious Puberty (Central)

In girls, most cases of precocious puberty are central (gonadotropin dependent) in origin and are believed to be due to premature idiopathic maturation of the hypothalamic-pituitary-ovarian axis. In perhaps two-thirds of cases, no recognizable cause of the disorder can be found. In these cases, the pattern of development and progression parallels that of normal pubertal development, although the onset is at an early age (Fig. 9-8).

CENTRAL NERVOUS SYSTEM DISORDERS

Lesions of the CNS are well recognized as causing CPP. Common causes include static encephalopathy due to infection, hypoxia, trauma, or irradiation during infancy or early childhood[17] (see Table 9-3). A less common but important cause of CPP is a CNS tumor. Hypothalamic hamartomas are benign tumors that have been shown to contain measurable GnRH. As such, they may be considered to be acting as ectopic GnRH pulse generators that have escaped from the normal inhibitory influences exerted in the prepubertal period on the centers that normally secrete GnRH. These small tumors are diagnosed more frequently in boys than in girls and are visualized most easily using MRI because some may only be 2 or 3 mm in size. These tumors tend to grow slowly, if at all, and uncommonly cause neurologic symptoms. Symptomatic hamartomas are associated with gelastic or laughing seizures. Precocious

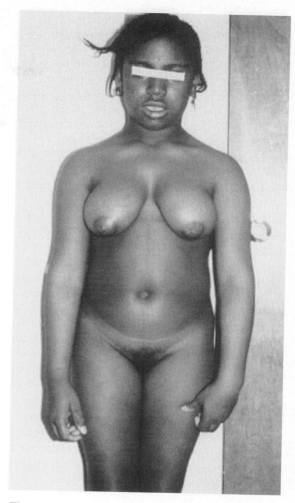

Figure 9-8 A 6-year-old girl with idiopathic precocious puberty. Her menarche occurred at 7 years of age.

sexual development is adequately controlled with GnRH agonists in patients with hamartomas. Optic and hypothalamic gliomas, astrocytomas, ependymomas, and craniopharyngiomas also may cause CPP possibly by impinging on the neural pathways that inhibit the GnRH pulse generator in childhood. Treatment for these tumors is surgical.

The chance of finding CNS pathology in either sex is inversely proportional to the age of the child, with the greatest yield in children younger than 4 years of age. Kappy et al.[15]

found that in girls whose pubertal development began after 6 years of age, any CNS pathology was already known or clinically evident, suggesting that routine MRI in these children will less likely have positive findings. In contrast, Pescovitz and coworkers[16] reported that in a series of 4000 children referred to the National Institutes of Health (NIH), about 33 percent of the girls and over 90 percent of the boys had an identifiable lesion of the CNS visible on CT scan or MRI. This high prevalence of CNS lesions likely reflects the referral population.

Cranial irradiation has dose-dependent effects on many hypothalamic-pituitary functions. While doses of cranial irradiation exceeding 50 Gy to the hypothalamic-pituitary axis may render a child gonadotropin-deficient, lesser doses of irradiation have been associated with early puberty in both sexes. Low-dose cranial irradiation (18 to 24 Gy) employed in the CNS prophylactic treatment of acute lymphoblastic leukemia is associated with a downward shift in the distribution of ages at pubertal onset and menarche in girls.[17,18] CPP is rare in boys treated in this manner.

The pathophysiology of CPP in nonhamartomatous lesions of the CNS is not yet established. It is possible that neural defects located near the hypothalamus cause precocious puberty by interfering with tonic CNS inhibition of the hypothalamic-pituitary gonadal axis. It is also possible that focal derangements of the cellular environment in the vicinity of GnRH neurons may be causally related to the premature activation of GnRH secretion. Junier et al.[19] have speculated that neurotrophic or mitogenic activities produced locally in response to brain injury may be involved in the process. They suggest that the response of GnRH neurons to hypothalamic injury consists of three phases. In the initial stage, some of the neurons lose mature morphologic characteristics, reverting to a presumably more immature condition. An intermediate phase occurs in which morphologic differentiation is reestablished, and an increased synthesis of TGF-β by reactive astrocytes enhances GnRH release without affecting GnRH gene expression through a process that may involve glial release of prostaglandins. The final phase is described as associated with a rise in sex steroid caused by the GnRH-dependent increase in basal LH release that activates GnRH neurons to secrete gonadotropins in an episodic manner. A rare cause of isosexual precocity is virilizing hyperplasia resulting from 21-hydroxylase deficiency in girls in whom treatment is delayed until ages 4 to 8. After initiation of glucocorticoid replacement, such patients may undergo true isosexual precocious puberty.

Treatment of Gonadotropin-Dependent Precocious Puberty

Long-term complications of true idiopathic precocious puberty include compromised adult height and psychosocial and behavioral issues. Studies have proven that adult height is improved with treatment if treatment is instituted prior to epiphyseal closure[20] (Table 9-5).

Historically, medroxyprogesterone and cyproterone acetate were used in an attempt to suppress activation of the hypothalamic-pituitary-gonadal axis. Neither of these agents was satisfactory because they were not fully effective in inhibiting pubertal or skeletal maturation or improving adult height.

Recognition that the continuous, nonpulsatile presentation of GnRH to the pituitary gonadotropes induced a state of secondary hypogonadism led to the development and use of potent GnRH agonists in the therapy of precocious puberty. These gonadotropin-releasing hormone analogues (GnRHas) represent the first truly effective treatment for CPP.[21] Significant reductions in basal and peak (GnRH-stimulated) serum FSH and LH concentrations occur within the first month of GnRHa therapy. In parallel with these changes, a reduction in plasma concentrations of estradiol (in girls) and testosterone (in boys) occurs after the first month and persists while the drug is administered. Importantly, the effects of these drugs are reversible. Following withdrawal of GnRHa

► **TABLE 9-5:** DIAGNOSTIC TESTS AND TREATMENT OF SEXUAL PRECOCITY

Diagnostic tests
  History and physical examination
  Bone age
  CNS imaging
  Sonography of ovaries
  CT scan of adrenal (if virilized)
  Thyroid function tests
  Estradiol
  FSH, LH, hCG
  Testosterone, DHEAS, 17-hydroxyprogesterone (if virilized)

Treatment
  Isosexual precocity
    True precocious puberty
      Constitutional: LHRH analogues/progestagens
      Organic brain disease: Surgery, radiation, LHRH analogues/progestogens
      Congenital adrenal hyperplasia (delayed treatment): LHRH analogues/progestogens
    Precocious pseudopuberty
      Ovarian tumors: Surgery
      Adrenal tumors: Surgery
      McCune-Albright syndrome: Testolactone, ketoconazole
      Silver-Russell syndrome: LHRH analogues/progestogens
      Estrogen-containing medications: Discontinue use
    Isolated forms of pubertal development: Observation
  Heterosexual precocity
    Ovarian tumors: Surgery
    Adrenal tumors: Surgery
    Congenital adrenal hyperplasia: Glucocorticoids

Abbreviations: CNS, central nervous system; CT, computed tomography; DHEAS, dehydroepiandrosterone sulfate; FSH, follicle-stimulating hormone; hCG, human chorionic gonadotropin; LH, luteinizing hormone; LHRH, luteinizing hormone-releasing hormone

therapy, gonadotropin and gonadal steroid concentrations return to their pretreatment levels.

Institution of GnRHa therapy results in a decrease in growth velocity, usually to within a range that is appropriate for the child's skeletal maturation. The slowing of linear growth is accompanied in most cases by slowing of skeletal maturation, one of the primary aims of such treatment. Preservation of or an increase in adult height can be achieved in some children with gonadotropin-dependent precocious puberty treated with GnRHas.[22] Most investigators, using the tables of Bayley and Pinneau, reported increases in the predicted final height of patients during the course of GnRHa ther-

apy, with a mean increase of 5 cm. Most studies suggest that the greatest improvement in predicted adult height is obtained in children whose bone ages are relatively young at the onset of treatment, indicating the need for early diagnosis and intervention. Therapy with GnRHa does not substantially affect adult height in girls who enter puberty between the ages of 6 and 8 years.[13] The length of time that such therapy is continued depends on bone age and estimates of final height in individual patients. Although concern has been raised regarding the possible effect of pubertal suppression on skeletal mineralization, an important feature of normal puberty, evidence available to date indicates no significant problem. Bone mineral density was evaluated (BMD) in female patients treated with GnRHas for gonadotropin-dependent precocious puberty who had completed therapy and subsequently had attained a bone age of greater than 14 years. They found that BMDs were not different from those of a control population of girls with the same bone ages.[23,24]

The physical effects of pubertal suppression with GnRHas are not limited to the effects on bone development. The majority of girls experience no increase in breast development, and a third show regression to an earlier Tanner stage, correlating with a reduction in ovarian and uterine size. Some girls experience transient vaginal bleeding approximately 2 to 4 weeks after initiation of GnRHa therapy due to estrogen withdrawal. Effects on pubic hair are less predictable, although most children show either no progression or a minor degree of regression. Some children show an increase in pubic hair that correlates with the timing of normal adrenarche.[25]

Most recent studies indicate that not all patients need to be treated. It is obvious that any girl with physical signs of precocious puberty, such as rapidly advancing bone age, decreased predicted height, and a pubertal response to gonadotropin testing, should be treated with GnRHas to suppress pubertal progression and improve adult height. Treatment is not well defined in girls with an equivocal evaluation. There is a need for close follow-up but not always a need for treatment.[20]

Furthermore, in those who need treatment, during GnRHa therapy for CPP, growth is sometimes suppressed to a subnormal velocity. It is speculated that this a result of the estrogen concentration being decreased (suppressed by the analogue) to below normal prepubertal levels. A recent pilot study suggests that this hypothesis is true. A look at 13 girls over 2 years evaluated growth and bone maturation among those with CPP and compared treatment with GnRHa with and without estrogen. The study shows that supplementation with minidose estrogen replacement is safe and effective (for at least 2 years) in maintaining normal prepubertal growth without acceleration of bone maturation or pubertal development.[26]

Gonadotropin-Independent Precocious Puberty

Gonadotropin-independent forms of precocious puberty are about one-fifth as common as gonadotropin-dependent forms of precocious puberty. Gonadotropin-independent precocious puberty is characterized by increased production of gonadal steroids, causing the typical physical changes of puberty, in the absence of reactivation of the hypothalamic-pituitary axis.[10] This form of precocious puberty includes conditions that mimic the effect of pituitary gonadotropins on gonadal function, such as those in which there is secretion of gonadotropins from nonpituitary sources. Table 9-4 lists conditions associated with gonadotropin-independent precocious puberty. Isosexual precocious pseudopuberty, or incomplete isosexual precocity, occurs when girls feminize as a consequence of endogenous estrogen production or exogenous estrogen exposure but do not ovulate or have cyclic menses. Ovarian cysts or tumors that secrete estrogen (granulosa or thecal cell tumors) are the most frequent cause. The Peutz-Jeghers syndrome of intestinal polyps and mucocutaneous pigmentation is associated with ovarian tumors that secrete estrogen (or androgen that is converted to estrogen at extraglandular sites) and cause precocious pseudopuberty. Most ovarian tumors can be diagnosed by rectoabdominal examination, but ultrasonography, CT scan, or laparoscopy also may be of help.

Most tumors are unilateral and benign and can be cured by oophorectomy. Gonadotropin levels are suppressed, and the LH response to GnRH is blunted. The presence of ovarian cysts can cause problems in diagnosis. Ultrasonography may be helpful to differentiate a benign cyst from a cystic solid ovarian tumor, but exploratory laparotomy ultimately is necessary in most cases, with the recognition that unnecessary removal of a benign cyst may lead to adhesions and infertility later in life. Follicular growth of up to 3 cm may occur in patients with true precocious puberty as a consequence of increased gonadotropin secretion and is not an indication for exploration. Ovarian teratomas, choriocarcinomas or germinomas, and hepatoblastomas that secrete pure hCG do not appear to cause precocious puberty in girls unless estrogen is secreted concomitantly by the tumor (i.e., hCG or LH in the absence of FSH does not stimulate ovarian estrogen secretion). Rarely, feminizing tumors of the adrenal can cause isosexual precocious puberty either by formation of estrogen directly or by secretion of androgens that are aromatized to estrogens in extraglandular sites.

The second type of incomplete isosexual precocity that may be associated with increased gonadotropin secretion is hypothyroidism. Hypothyroidism usually is associated with delayed pubertal development and amenorrhea, but occasionally patients present with precocious puberty, galactorrhea, and ovarian cysts. In addition to increased levels of thyrotropin, gonadotropin and prolactin levels are also increased; the cause for the enhanced gonadotropin secretion is unknown. In most cases bone age is retarded, and pituitary hypersecretion and retardation of bone development respond to thyroid hormone replacement.

Molecular mechanisms underlying two forms of gonadotropin-independent precocious puberty, familial Leydig cell hyperplasia in boys and McCune-Albright syndrome, have been described recently.

McCune-Albright Syndrome

McCune-Albright syndrome (MAS) is characterized classically by the clinical triad of cutaneous hyperpigmentation (café-au-lait spots), polyostotic fibrous dysplasia, and isosexual precocious puberty.[27] Although it is stated that at least two of the features of the triad must be present to make the diagnosis, this guideline

should be interpreted with caution because the features may develop over time. The condition occurs distinctly less frequently in boys than in girls, who comprise 90 percent of affected patients. In contrast to those with CPP, these girls not uncommonly present with vaginal bleeding as the first sign of their sexual development. A pattern of variable involvement of hormone-secreting cells occurs in patients with MAS. The endocrine abnormalities are characterized by excessive function of the hormone secreted. The most common endocrine manifestation of MAS is precocious puberty, often associated with ovarian cysts. A waxing and waning course of the precocious puberty is not uncommon. Depending on the specific cell types affected, a number of other endocrine disturbances may occur. These include hyperthyroidism (due to nodular or follicular thyroid hyperplasia) in 20 to 40 percent of patients, hypercortisolism (due to nodular adrenal hyperplasia), and GH- or prolactin-secreting pituitary adenomas.[28]

The peculiar bone lesion of MAS (polyostotic fibrous dysplasia) may occur in any bone, including long bones, the skull, and the pelvis, and result in pathologic fracture or severe disfigurement. Malignant degeneration occurs in up to 4 percent of lesions. The usually large, pigmented cutaneous lesions (café-au-lait patches) have irregular, "serrated" outlines. Their distribution, like the variable involvement of endocrine tissues, reflects an underlying genetic mosaicism that results from a postzygotic somatic cell mutation occurring after a number of cell divisions have taken place. Common sites of occurrence of the café-au-lait patches include the forehead, the neck and upper back, the shoulder and upper arm, the lumbosacral region, and the buttocks. The patches often follow a distribution that is not dermatomal but in fact relates to the lines of Blaschko, which are thought to represent the patterns of dorsal and ventral outgrowth of two different cell populations during early embryogenesis. The hyperpigmentation is present in the basal epidermis; the number and size of melanocytes are normal, but the melanosomes are enlarged. The skeletal and cutaneous involvement in MAS is commonly asymmetric, and the skin lesions often stop abruptly at the midline.

The diverse clinical abnormalities of MAS have in common the involvement of cells that respond to extracellular signals through activation of the hormone-sensitive adenylate cyclase system, the membrane-bound enzyme that catalyzes formation of the intracellular second messenger cyclic AMP.[27] However, these endocrine disturbances are not accompanied by increased plasma concentrations of the relevant trophic or stimulatory hormones. Thus girls with precocious puberty caused by MAS have ovarian enlargement and follicular hyperplasia but have low serum levels of LH and FSH and a prepubertal response of LH to the administration of GnRH.[28]

The basis of the gonadotropin-independent nature of the precocious sexual development in MAS was elucidated by identification of mutations that activate the intracellular second-messenger pathways by which the trophic hormones such as gonadotropins and thyrotropin signal. The activity of the hormone-sensitive adenylate cyclase system is regulated primarily by two guanine nucleotide–binding proteins (G proteins), one inhibitory and the other stimulatory. Schwindinger and colleagues[29] identified a mutation in the gene encoding the α subunit of the stimulatory G protein that regulates adenylate cyclase activity. A heterozygous guanine-to-adenine transition was found in exon 8 of the gene encoding the α subunit of G_s, predicting the replacement of arginine by histidine at position 201 of the mature protein.[30] This amino acid is located within a critical region of the $G_{s\alpha}$ protein, and the substitution causes a marked decrease in the intrinsic GTPase activity of $G_s\alpha$, prolonging survival of the active conformation of the enzyme and resulting in constitutive activation of adenylate cyclase activity. The consequent increased production of cyclic AMP explains the increases in endocrine organ function typical of this disease because this system mediates the stimulatory effects of many hormones (e.g., gonadotropins, thyrotropin, adrenocorticotropin, and GHRH). Mutations also have been detected in the hyperpigmented skin lesions, which commonly colocalize with the bone lesions, but their role in the pathogenesis remains unclear. Inactivating mutations of $G_s\alpha$ are associated with pseudohypoparathyroidism.

These findings are consistent with the hypothesis that a spontaneous mutation early in gestation produced an abnormal monoclonal cell population. Therefore, the variable clinical presentation of MAS is due to the varying degrees of somatic mosaicism of this genetic alteration that otherwise would represent an autosomal dominant lethal defect. Because of this mosaicism, MAS is not inherited.

Familial Male Precocious Puberty

Although the endocrine disturbances are confined to the testes, a similar mechanism characterizes another GnRH-independent form of precocious puberty, familial male precocious puberty (FMPP) or familial testotoxicosis.[31] This disorder is inherited as an autosomal dominant, male-limited pattern and is characterized by the onset of puberty (testicular enlargement) before 4 years of age. Testosterone production and Leydig cell hyperplasia occur autonomously in the context of low, prepubertal levels of LH. The clinical hallmark of this disorder is the relatively modest enlargement of the testes for the degree of virilization. Affected adult men are often short, due to early epiphyseal fusion; however, they are otherwise healthy and have normal fertility. Although LH concentrations are low in childhood, they are normal in adulthood, indicating that normal maturation of the hypothalamic-pituitary-gonadal axis occurs. The disorder is not expressed in heterozygous females because estrogen production by ovarian follicles requires coordinated stimulation by both LH and FSH; thus activation of the LH pathway alone has no significant effect.

The pathogenesis of this gonadotropin-independent form of precocious puberty has been traced to heterozygous mutations within specific segments of the gene encoding the receptor for LH and hCG (the LH/hCG receptor).[32] The LH/hCG receptor is a member of the seven-transmembrane family of G protein–coupled receptors. Unlike the inactivating mutations of the LH receptor, which can occur in many parts of the molecule, most of the activating mutations of the LH receptor have resulted in amino acid substitutions within the fifth and sixth transmembrane helices and the cytoplasmic loop that connects them. Shenker[33] found a mutation that resulted in replacement of the native aspartate with glycine at position 578 in the sixth transmembrane helix of the protein. In vitro studies of the mutant receptor containing the Asp578-to-Gly substitution demonstrated marked increase in cyclic AMP production in the absence of li-gand. It is presumed that the structural changes induced in the LH receptor by these amino acid substitutions shift these portions of the receptor to a conformation that mimics the conformation of the normal LH receptor activated by LH.[34] This conformation of the mutant LH receptor leads to the agonist-independent production of cyclic AMP and thereby to autonomous testosterone production by the Leydig cells of affected boys. Other mutations in the receptor also have been described.[35–37]

Ectopic Hormone Production

hCG-secreting germ cell tumors have been thought to cause precocious puberty exclusively in boys. Due to the extensive structural homology of the β subunits of hCG and LH, the excess hCG acting through the LH receptor stimulates Leydig cell production of testosterone.

Non-CNS tumors causing gonadotropin-independent precocious puberty in females also have been described. In such instances, the pubertal development is traced most often to the presence of a granulosa cell ovarian tumor or an adrenal tumor that produces excess estrogen. There is one report of a Sertoli-Leydig cell tumor in a 4 month-old who represented after resection prior to age 1 with symptoms of CPP. Molecular characterization reveals the presence of genes specific for granulosa and Leydig cells. The relative expression of these genes, in addition to the histology, suggests that this tumor may result from a dysdifferentiation of a primordial follicle.[38]

As discussed earlier, congenital adrenal hyperplasia (CAH), most commonly due to deficiency of 21-hydroxylase, is another cause of early virilization. It is distinguished by absence of testicular enlargement in boys (hence the designation *pseudopuberty*) and virilization without feminization in girls. Virilization is due to maturation of the HPA axis from increased androgen levels present before adequate cortisol replacement.[38]

Treatment of Gonadotropin-Independent Forms of Precocious Puberty

Because patients with these forms of precocious puberty demonstrate pubertal development that is independent of pituitary gonadotropin secretion, GnRHa therapy is ineffective, at least as part of initial management (see Table 9-5). As such, even though the molecular lesions are different, treatments for FMPP and MAS are instead focused on directly inhibiting the synthesis or action of sex steroids.

In boys with FMPP, this has been approached through administration of inhibitors of steroidogenesis, such as the antifungal agent ketoconazole. This compound inhibits the enzyme that catalyzes the cleavage of the 20–22 bond of the cholesterol molecule and thus inhibits the synthesis of both androgens and estrogens. An alternative approach has been to employ drugs that block the actions of androgen at the level of the androgen receptor itself. Although more potent drugs are now available, published reports have used spironolactone (a drug that has demonstrated modest activity as a competitive inhibitor of androgen receptor function).[28] Results using this drug have been somewhat disappointing but have been more encouraging when it is coupled with testolactone.

Testolactone is an aromatase inhibitor that blocks the enzyme (P450 aromatase) that catalyzes aromatization of testosterone—the rate-limiting step in estrogen biosynthesis. This process reduces the high estrogen concentrations responsible for the accelerated skeletal maturation typical of this condition.[39] Of note, the early maturation of the hypothalamus induced by exposure to high levels of sex steroids may result in activation of the endogenous GnRH pulse generator, leading to the development of gonadotropin-dependent CPP secondary to the preexisting gonadotropin-independent precocious puberty. In such instances, the addition of GnRHa therapy is required to prevent progression of pubertal development and skeletal maturation.

Treatment of girls with precocious puberty due to MAS employs drugs that inhibit the synthesis of estrogen (aromatase inhibitors). The longest-term studies of this type have used testolactone. The availability of more potent aromatase inhibitors (e.g., Arimidex) may improve the effectiveness of such approaches in the future. The approach to inhibition of testosterone synthesis in boys with precocious puberty caused by MAS is similar to that employed in the treatment of patients with FMPP. Addition of a GnRH analogue is required for patients with MAS who develop secondary CPP.

Contrasexual Development

Contrasexual (or *heterosexual*) *development* refers to feminization in males and virilization in females and can occur at any age, either prepubertally or postpubertally. Evaluation consists of a careful history and physical examination followed by measurement of gonadal and adrenal steroids and, in more subtle cases, ACTH stimulation testing to identify cryptic or atypical forms of CAH.[21] Depending on the pattern of steroid hormone excess detected, imaging of the adrenals, gonads, or liver may be required. Gynecomastia is the most common manifestation of feminization and in pubertal boys is usually a benign self-limited condition; however, gynecomastia in a prepubertal boy is clearly pathologic. When associated with hypogonadism, Klinefelter syndrome should be considered and a karyotype obtained. In most cases, estrogen concentrations are not increased. However, in patients in whom there is a measurably high estrogen concentration, the source of excess estrogen may be a neoplasm (e.g., adrenal, hepatic, or testicular), an abnormality of steroid metabolism, or increased extraglandular conversion of C_{19} steroids to C_{18} estrogens such as occurs in the presence of significant obesity (gynecomastia is more common in obese boys). Exposure to exogenous estrogens is another uncommon cause of feminization in males.

Females with virilization may have adrenal or gonadal sources of androgen excess causing development of sexual hair, clitoromegaly, acne, and hirsutism. The most common cause of virilization in prepubertal girls is CAH due to deficiency of 21-hydroxylase activity. Most will suffer from the nonclassic form (i.e., late-onset or attenuated CAH), although some girls actually may have simple virilizing classic CAH missed at birth. Other virilizing forms of CAH include 3β-hydroxysteroid dehydrogenase and 11β-hydroxylase deficiencies. Severely advanced skeletal maturation is a common accompaniment of the virilization in affected girls, and these conditions can be further complicated by the development of secondary CPP. Virilizing adrenal adenoma or ovarian neoplasms are associated with elevated levels of dehydroepiandrosterone sulfate, androstenedione, or testosterone. β-hCG and α-fetoprotein also may be increased and should be measured as markers for ovarian, testicular, and hepatic tumors in virilized girls and feminized boys.

▶ DELAYED PUBERTY

Delayed puberty is defined as a failure to begin sexual maturation at an age that is 2 standard deviations above the mean age of the onset of puberty within a specific population. In the United States, the ages of 13 years for girls and 14 years for boys serve as practical guidelines to determine the need for evaluation.[3] The search for a diagnosis should differentiate between constitutional delay, hypogonadotropic hypogonadism, and hypergonadotropic hypogonadism. Obtaining a careful history and physical examination and determining serum gonadotropin levels are the first steps toward finding the correct diagnosis among the diverse causes of delayed puberty (Table 9-6).

Evaluation of Delayed Puberty

A careful history and physical examination should be performed whenever a patient or his or her parents express concern about physical development. In the United States, a girl who does not demonstrate pubertal development by age 13 satisfies the definition of delayed puberty and should be medically examined. Adolescent boys mature sexually at a slightly slower rate than girls; consequently, the time to examine boys for delayed puberty begins at 14 years of age.[8] The initial evaluation of delayed puberty

should include questions about functional disorders such as anorexia or bulimia, excessive exercise, or chronic disease. Functional disorders are common causes of delayed puberty, but this diagnosis should remain a diagnosis of exclusion.[40] An assessment of psychosocial health also should be included. Other pertinent information to obtain about the patient's past medical history may include the following:

1. *Family history:* Any other relatives with delayed puberty; heights of family members; age of menarche and fertility status of female relatives; any family members with genetic abnormalities such as CAH, androgen receptor insensitivity, or gonadal dysgenesis; any relatives with thyroiditis or Addison disease
2. *Neonatal history:* Birth weight and any birth trauma, congenital anomalies, lymphedema, or hypopituitarism
3. Previous surgery, radiation, or chemotherapy
4. *Review of systems:* Any neurologic symptoms, ability to smell, weight gain or loss, chronic disease, eating disorders, or substance abuse

▶ **TABLE 9-6:** CAUSES OF DELAYED PUBERTY

Constitutional delay

Hypogonadotropic hypogonadism (low gonadotropin levels, low sex steroid levels)
    Isolated gonadotropin deficiency
    Kallmann syndrome and variants
    Functional gonadotropin deficiency
        Chronic systemic disease and malnutrition
        Anorexia nervosa
        Exercise-induced amenorrhea
    CNS disorders
        Tumors
        Radiation therapy
        Anatomic defects (e.g., septooptic dysplasia)

Hypergonadotropic hypogonadism (low gonadotropin levels, low sex steroid levels)
    Gonadal dysgenesis and variants
    Primary ovarian failure (females)
    Primary testicular failure (males)
    Klinefelter syndrome (males)

5. Amount, type, and intensity of exercise, emotional, or psychological stress
6. Age of initiation and rate of growth spurt, pubic hair growth, and breast development (if any)
7. Prior growth charts, if available[41]

In contrast to complete pubertal delay, some girls will present with normal or incomplete pubertal maturation and the absence of menstruation. This condition is classified as primary or secondary amenorrhea. Amenorrhea will be discussed in detail later in this chapter. The evaluation of amenorrhea is somewhat different than that for delayed puberty, but many overlapping causes exist[42] (Tables 9-7 and 9-8).

The physical examination should begin with vital signs and height and weight. Growth data plotted on appropriate charts can help make the initial diagnosis and measure treatment success. A general sense of the health and well-being of the patient should be assessed. The patient should be evaluated for congenital disorders such as midline facial defects, scoliosis, or somatic stigmata of Turner syndrome. The thyroid should be palpated for masses or tenderness. Tanner staging of breast development and examination of the nipples for galactorrhea should be recorded. A neurologic examination of optic fundi, cranial nerves, visual fields, and sense of smell also may be incorporated.

The gynecologic examination should begin with Tanner staging of pubic hair growth. The physician should inspect the clitoris for enlargement and the hymeneal ring for patency.

▶ **TABLE 9-7:** CLASSIFICATION OF AMENORRHEA

1. Anatomic defects
2. Ovarian failure (hypergonadotropic hypogonadism)

3. Chronic anovulation
   With estrogen present
   With estrogen absent (hypogonadotropic hypogonadism)

The color of the vagina, degree of vaginal rugation, and presence or absence of mucus can indicate the degree of estrogen effect. If congenital obstruction or absence of the outflow tract is suspected, visualization of the vagina and cervix may be attempted. Vaginal examination or rectovaginal examination may be used to palpate the uterus and ovaries.

Laboratory tests are ordered based on the suspected differential diagnoses. First, determination of FSH and LH levels, used in assessing gonadal function, helps to differentiate between hypogonadotropic versus hypergonadotropic hypogonadism. A hypogonadal patient with elevated gonadotropin levels is described as hypergonadotropic, reflecting gonadal failure. Second, karyotyping can determine genetic abnormalities associated with hypergonadotropic hypogonadism.[1] In patients with amenorrhea, it is always important to exclude pregnancy. Determination of gonadotropin levels and clinical assessment of estrogen status allow for initial categorization and diagnosis in patients with amenorrhea (see Tables 9-7 and 9-8).

Variations of Normal Puberty: Constitutional Delay

Constitutional delay of puberty, a benign variant of normal puberty, occurs more commonly in boys than in girls. The pattern of pubertal development in affected children is normal, although its onset is delayed with respect to the population as a whole. In conjunction with delayed pubertal development, these children are short stature (approximately 2 to 3 standard deviations below the mean height for age), which reflects delayed skeletal maturation (2 to 4 years behind chronologic age).[42] These children generally demonstrate sexual maturation that is more commensurate with their bone ages than with their chronologic ages. Adult height and sexual maturation are achieved significantly later; many individuals with constitutional delay report continued linear growth into their late teens or early twenties. Family history

▶ **TABLE 9-8:** CLASSIFICATION OF AMENORRHEA (NOT INCLUDING DISORDERS OF CONGENITAL SEXUAL AMBIGUITY)

I. Anatomic defects (outflow tract)
   A. Labial agglutination/fusion
   B. Imperforate hymen
   C. Transverse vaginal septum
   D. Cervical agenesis, isolated
   E. Cervical stenosis, iatrogenic
   F. Vaginal agenesis, isolated
   G. Müllerian agenesis (Mayer-Rokitansky-Küster Hauser syndrome)
   H. Complete androgen resistance (testicular feminization)
   I. Endometrial hyperplasia or aplasia, congenital
   J. Asherman syndrome (intrauterine synechiae)
II. Ovarian failure (hypergonadotropic hypogonadism)
   A. Gonadal agenesis
   B. Gonadal dysgenesis
      1. Abnormal karyotype
         a. Turner syndrome 45,X
         b. Mosaicism
      2. Normal karyotype
         a. Pure gonadal dysgenesis
            i. 46,XX
            ii. 46,XY (Swyer syndrome)
   C. Ovarian enzymatic deficiency
      1. 17α-Hydroxylase deficiency
      2. 17,20-Lyase deficiency
      3. Aromatase deficiency
   D. Premature ovarian failure
      1. Idiopathic-premature aging
      2. Injury
         a. Mumps oophoritis
         b. Radiation
         c. Chemotherapy
      3. Resistant ovary
         a. Idiopathic
         b. Mutations of FSH receptor
         c. Mutations of LH receptor
      4. Autoimmune disease
      5. Galactosemia
III. Chronic anovulation with estrogen present
   A. Polycystic ovarian syndrome (PCOS)
   B. Adrenal disease
      1. Cushing syndrome
      2. Adult-onset adrenal hyperplasia
   C. Thyroid disease
      1. Hypothyroidism

2. Hyperthyroidism
   D. Ovarian tumors
      1. Granulosa-theca cell tumors
      2. Brenner tumors
      3. Cystic teratomas
      4. Mucinous/serous cystadenomas
      5. Krukenberg tumors
IV. Chronic anovulation with estrogen absent (hypogonadotropic hypogonadism)
   A. Hypothalamic
      1. Tumors
         a. Craniopharyngioma
         b. Germinoma
         c. Hamartoma
         d. Hand-Schüller-Christian disease
         e. Teratoma
         f. Endodermal sinus tumors
         g. Metastatic carcinoma
      2. Infection and other disorders
         a. Tuberculosis
         b. Syphilis
         c. Encephalitis/meningitis
         d. Sarcoidosis
         e. Isolated gonadotropin deficiency
            i. Kallmann syndrome
            ii. Idiopathic hypogonadotropic hypogonadism
         f. Chronic debilitating disease
      3. Functional
         a. Stress
         b. Weight loss/diet
         c. Malnutrition
         d. Psychologic eating disorders (anorexia nervosa, bulimia)
         e. Exercise
         f. Pseudocyesis

Continued

▶ **TABLE 9-8:** CLASSIFICATION OF AMENORRHEA (NOT INCLUDING DISORDERS OF CONGENITAL SEXUAL AMBIGUITY) *(Continued)*

B. Pituitary	b. Arterial aneurysm
1. Tumors	3. Necrosis
a. Prolactinomas	a. Sheehan syndrome
b. Other hormone-secreting pituitary tumors	b. Panhypopituitarism
(ACTH, thyrotropin-stimulating hormone,	4. Inflammatory/infiltrative
growth hormone, gonadotropin)	a. Sarcoidosis
c. Nonfunctional tumors (craniopharyngioma)	b. Hemochromatosis
d. Metastatic carcinoma	c. Lymphocyte hypophysitis
2. Space-occupying lesions	5. Gonadotropin mutations
a. Empty sella	(FSH)

Adapted from Carr BR. Disorders of the ovary and female reproductive tract. In Wilson and Foster (eds), Williams Textbook of Endocrinology. Philadelphia: Saunders, 1992, pp. 733–798.

often reveals other affected relatives, most often males.[43]

Hypogonadotropic Hypogonadism

Hypogonadotropic hypogonadism, a defect in the pulsatile release of gonadotropins, may result from a variety of hypothalamic or pituitary pathologies. For example, defective or absent GnRH–secreting neurons within the hypothalamus can fail to secrete GnRH, an essential hormone for stimulation of pituitary gonadotropin secretion. In contrast, pituitary disorders such as tumors or hypophysitis can cause direct failure of pituitary gonadotropin secretion.

During embryogenesis, the olfactory nerves and terminal nerve develop from the olfactory placodes in the rostral forebrain. The olfactory nerves associate with the terminal nerve and vomeronasal nerve to create a bridge between the olfactory epithelium and the forebrain. The cells that will become GnRH-synthesizing neurons arise from the olfactory placodes, move from the nasal epithelium through the cribriform plate of the nose, and then migrate along the olfactory tract–forebrain bridge to reach the preoptic and hypothalamic areas; here they differentiate to become the GnRH-secreting neurons. These GnRH-secreting neurons, dispersed throughout the medial basal hypothalamus,

transduce neural signals into hormonal signals, the pulsatile secretion of GnRH. Given the developmental connection between olfactory and GnRH neurons, it is interesting to note the relationship between olfactory acuity and reproduction in animals, evidenced by the importance of pheromones in sexual attraction. Defects in development or migration of GnRH neurons may lead to Kallmann syndrome and its variants.[40]

Kallmann Syndrome and Variants

Isolated gonadotropin deficiency may occur sporadically or in a familial pattern. Kallmann syndrome is the association of hypogonadotropic hypogonadism with anosmia or hyposomia. In this genetic disorder, fetal GnRH-secreting neurons fail to migrate from the olfactory placode to the medial basal hypothalamus, resulting in agenesis or hypoplasia of the olfactory bulbs and tracts. First described in 1856, Kallmann syndrome is uncommon, occurring in only 1 in 10,000 males and 1 in 50,000 females. Three modes of transmission have been identified: X-linked, autosomal recessive, and autosomal dominant.[44–46]

Typical clinical features of Kallmann syndrome include delayed puberty, eunuchoid habitus, gynecomastia in males, and a reduced sense of smell (often unrecognized by the patient). In males, cryptorchism and a small penis are present in infancy. Females may display complete or partial defects. They may present with sexual infantilism and anosmia or a reduced sense of smell, delayed menarche, or irregular menses. Other clinical features of Kallmann syndrome include unilateral renal agenesis in up to 40 percent of affected individuals; midline facial anomalies such as cleft lip, high-arched or cleft palate, or other forms of imperfect facial fusion; short metacarpals; pes cavus; cerebellar ataxia; sensorineural deafness; epilepsy; and synkinesis (mirror movements of the hands).[47] MRI may demonstrate hypoplasia of the olfac-

tory gyri and absent olfactory bulbs and tracts (Fig. 9-9). When analyzed histologically, the olfactory epithelium of these patients is thinner than normal and contains fewer neurons. Neurons that were present lacked cilia, were immature, or showed signs of degeneration.

The X-linked form of Kallmann syndrome found in males has been studied most extensively. Positional cloning studies by Legouis and colleagues[46] led to isolation and characterization of the defective gene in this form. The Kallmann gene (*KAL1* or *KALIG1*) is located at Xp22.3 and encodes a 680-amino-acid

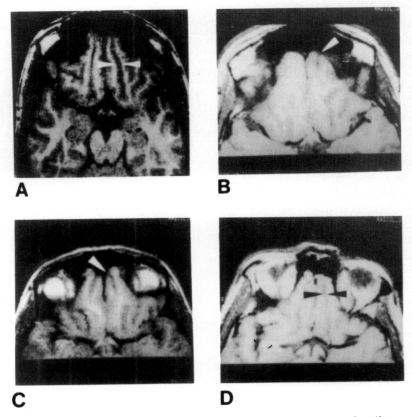

Figure 9-9 Transverse MRI images through the rhinencephalon comparing the normal anatomy of olfactory sulci *(A)* with the findings in three patients with Kallmann syndrome *(B–D)*. Rudimentary sulci *(B, C)* and hypoplastic sulci *(D)* are denoted by arrowheads. *(Adapted from Klingmuller D, Dewes W, Krahe T, et al. Magnetic resonance imaging of the brain in patient with anosmia and hypothalamic hypogonadism (Kallmann's syndrome).* J Clin Endocinol Metab *1987;65:581–584. Copyright © 1987, by The Endocrine Society.)*

protein that is apparently extracellular in location. This gene is thought to escape, at least partially, X inactivation. An inactive homologous pseudogene *(KALP)* is located on the Y chromosome at Yq11. Studies of patients with the X-linked form of Kallmann syndrome show genetic heterogeneity, and all but one of the mutations reported to date predict the absence or marked truncation of the encoded protein. In a study of 21 men with the X-linked form of the disorder, Hardelin and coworkers detected a range of abnormalities within the *KAL1* gene, including large deletions in two families and nine different point mutations in other affected individuals, resulting in the introduction of premature termination codons into the DNA sequence.[48] To date, the genetic causes of the other forms of Kallmann syndrome (i.e., non-X-linked) have not been defined. Studies of individuals with Kallmann syndrome associated with cytogenetic abnormalities, however, have suggested possible loci for genes responsible for the autosomal dominant form of Kallmann syndrome.[44] It is likely that the genetic defects will be traced to other genes that participate in pathways affecting GnRH-secreting neuron migration.

Girls with Kallman syndrome or other forms of hypogonadotropic hypogonadism are given oral estradiol in doses that mimic normal puberty to initiate breast development and sexual maturation. After 6 to 9 months, progesterone taken in a cyclic pattern will effect endometrial shedding. Estradiol doses are increased approximately every 6 months until breast development is optimized, and then oral contraceptives may be used for hormone replacement. When fertility is desired, treatment with either pulsatile GnRH delivered by a pump or injectable gonadotropins may be given. Treatment with supplemental testosterone, given orally to boys with Kallmann syndrome, will induce virilization, whereas intranasal GnRH or intramuscular chorionic gonadotropin treatment can stimulate actual endogenous sex steroid production and even reproductive capability.[40]

Isolated Gonadotropin Deficiency

A number of families have been identified in which affected members have isolated gonadotropin deficiency without the features of Kallmann syndrome. The inheritance pattern is autosomal recessive.[49] Although not yet reported in humans, this defect likely results, as has been observed in the hypogonadal *(Hpg)* mouse, from a GnRH deficiency caused by mutations in the gene that encodes GnRH.[45]

Isolated FSH Deficiency

A small number of patients have been reported to have isolated deficiencies of FSH. A woman with an isolated deficiency of FSH who presented with primary amenorrhea and infertility was found to have a mutation in the gene encoding the β subunit of FSH. The 2-base-pair deletion caused a frame shift in the coding sequence, resulting in formation of a truncated FSH β-subunit protein that lacks regions required for coupling with the α subunit of FSH and for binding to the FSH receptor.[50]

Functional Gonadotropin Deficiency

Severe systemic disease, chronic disorders, and malnutrition are associated with delayed onset of puberty or failure to progress through the stages of puberty. When body weight measures less than 80 percent of ideal weight for height, a functional gonadotropin deficiency may occur. Examples include the functional gonadotropin deficiencies associated with an-orexia nervosa and exercise-induced amenorrhea. In such instances, normal hypothalamic-pituitary-gonadal function returns after restoration of normal body mass and normal psych-ological functioning.[3,42]

CNS Disorders

Mass lesions, such as sellar or suprasellar tumors (e.g., craniopharyngiomas), commonly disturb pubertal development, causing either precocious puberty or delayed puberty. These tumors cause delayed puberty by impairing hypothalamic or pituitary function. In addition to abnormalities of pubertal development, children with craniopharyngiomas may have growth failure, polydipsia, polyuria, and visual disturbances.[3]

Hypergonadotropic Hypogonadism

Primary gonadal failure is associated with elevated gonadotropins due to the absence of negative-feedback effects of the gonadal sex steroids.[51] The most common causes of hypergonadotropic hypogonadism are associated with genetic or somatic abnormalities, although isolated idiopathic gonadal failure may present with delayed puberty but without other abnormal physical findings.[1]

Mutations of the LH and FSH Receptors

The receptors for the gonadotropins LH/hCG and FSH are both members of the seven-transmembrane domain family of G protein–coupled receptors. Specific defects in the gonadal response to gonadotropins have been traced in several pedigrees to mutations of the genes that encode the FSH and LH/hCG receptors. In males, rather than being associated with delayed puberty, mutations in the gene encoding the LH/hCG receptor are associated with a form of male pseudohermaphroditism termed *Leydig cell hypoplasia* (LCH). This disorder is characterized by a female phenotype in the presence of a 46,XY karyotype, decreased serum testosterone and increased serum LH levels, and a lack of testosterone secretion in response to hCG administration. LH/hCG gene mutations that result in premature termination or amino acid replacement can create errors in the transmembrane regions of the receptor protein and can produce this phenotype.[52–56]

The discovery of inactivating mutations in the LH receptor in patients with LCH and defective fetal masculinization is to be expected. Several interesting aspects of LH receptor mutations deserve comment. First, two patients with LCH had a 46,XX sibling who was a phenotypically normal adult female with amenorrhea and cystic ovaries. This presentation suggests an LH receptor defect that allowed normal pubertal development but impaired cyclic ovarian function.[53] Second, finding a missense mutation of the LH receptor in a phenotypic male infant who was evaluated for a small but normally formed penis implies that the range of altered phenotypes associated with LH receptor abnormalities may be broader than those initially identified.[53,54,56]

An uncommon form of hypergonadotropic hypogonadism is 46,XX gonadal dysgenesis. Affected girls, who typically present with pubertal failure, are of normal stature and have no phenotypic features of Turner syndrome. The condition appears to be genetically heterogeneous, and both sporadic and familial cases have been reported. One familial variant, Perrault syndrome, has sensorineural hearing loss associated with the hypogonadism. A candidate recessive gene on chromosome 2, the ovarian dysgenesis 1 gene *(ODG1)* was identified by analysis of a large cohort of affected Finnish patients. The disorder is common in this population (1 in 8300 females) and is inherited in an autosomal recessive manner. Aittomaki and colleagues[50] recently discovered a missense mutation in the gene encoding the FSH receptor in affected families. The FSH receptor gene is located at 2p21, coinciding with the *ODG1* locus. A limited number of families with such defects have been described to date.[57] The mutation in the FSH receptor gene in this group is an arginine-to-valine substitution at amino acid 189, located in the extracellular ligand-binding domain of the receptor. The mutation segregated with the affected phenotype and had a dramatic effect on the binding of ligand and the stimulation of cyclic AMP production. Of interest, the affected males in the pedigrees were phenotypically normal and half were fertile, suggesting that variable defects in spermatogenesis may be the only discernible effect in males with this disorder.[50]

Klinefelter Syndrome

The most common form of delayed puberty and primary testicular failure in males is Klinefelter syndrome (47,XXY karyotype), which occurs with an incidence of 1 in 1000 men.[40] Male sexual differentiation is normal; testicular function remains relatively normal until approximately the age of puberty and declines thereafter. Patients with Klinefelter syndrome do not usually present with delayed puberty, although affected patients may demonstrate a slowing or arrest of pubertal development as testicular function declines. Supplemental testosterone is then required.[47]

Turner Syndrome/Gonadal Dysgenesis

Turner syndrome, 45,X gonadal dysgenesis, is associated with short stature, female phenotype, and delayed or absent pubertal development (Fig. 9-10). Patients have streak gonads consisting of fibrous tissue without germ cells (germ cells may be present in infancy). Other classic but variable phenotypic features include ptosis; low-set ears; micrognathia; a short, "webbed" neck; a broad, shieldlike chest; hypoplastic areolae; short fourth and/or fifth metacarpals; cubitus valgus; structural anomalies of the kidney; many pigmented nevi; hypoplastic, hyperconvex fingernails and toe- nails; and left-sided cardiovascular anomalies, coarctation of the aorta being the most common. Pubic hair may appear late and usually is somewhat sparse.[41]

These phenotypic features reflect this syndrome's central theme of disordered growth that begins in utero and worsens progressively from early childhood onward. Patients have no pubertal growth spurt and attain a mean final height that is approximately 20 cm shorter than that of the reference population. Short stature, although a classic feature of Turner syndrome, is not a feature of hypergonadotropic hypogonadism forms that occur without karyotypic abnormalities. Because GH usually is normal in Turner syndrome, the short stature is likely caused by a subtle form of skeletal dysplasia. This dysplasia may result from imbalances in gene expression caused by the absent X chromosome segments. GH treatment increases growth rates and the final adult height of many affected patients.[3]

In Turner syndrome, serum gonadotropin concentrations increase between birth and 4 years of age, decrease toward the normal range in prepubertal patients, and then rise to castrate levels after 9 or 10 years of age.[3]

Variant forms of gonadal dysgenesis are associated with a number of mosaic phenotypes, usually including a 45,X line, in addition to more complex X chromosomal rearrangements. Girls and women with these karyotypes may have phenotypic features typical of the classic syndrome of 45,X gonadal dysgenesis or may have fewer manifestations. Swyer syndrome (46,XY complete gonadal dysgenesis) patients have streak gonads and delayed puberty similar to patients with Turner syndrome.[3] They do not, however, have the short stature or in most cases the other phenotypic features typical of Turner syndrome. Gonadal tumors are rare in 45,X patients, but gonadal malignancies have been reported in women with chromosomal mosaicism involving the Y chromosome. Chromosomal analysis should be obtained in all cases of amenorrhea associated with ovarian failure. If a Y chromosome is found, the streak gonad should be removed completely because of the increased incidence of gonadal tumors (gonadoblastoma, embryonal cell carcinoma or seminoma) in these patients.[3] Approximately 90 percent of individuals with gonadal dysgenesis, associated with deletion of genetic material in the X chromosome, never have menstrual bleeding. The remaining 10 percent have sufficient residual follicles to experience menses and, rarely, fertility. The menstrual and reproductive lives of these individuals invariably are brief.[40]

Other causes of primary ovarian failure include radiation therapy, chemotherapy, and premature menopause. Patients with Addison disease, in addition to their adrenal failure, may have autoimmune oophoritis and other features of autoimmune disease. Primary amenorrhea is a common presenting feature of women with androgen-insensitivity syndrome (phenotypic females with 46,XY genotype and androgen resistance). A defect of cytochrome

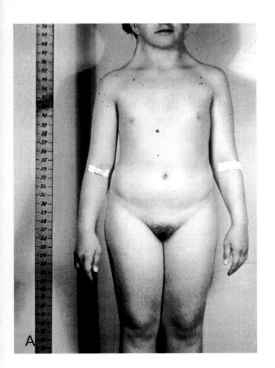

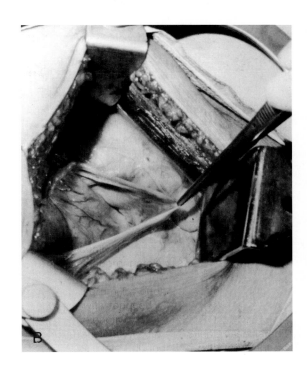

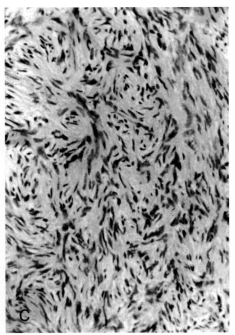

Figure 9-10 Turner syndrome. *A.* Patient with stigmata of gonadal dysgenesis, including short stature, sexual infantilism, webbed neck, and broadly spaced nipple. *B.* Streak ovary (held by forceps). *C.* Microscopic section of a streak ovary demonstrating fibrous replacement of ovarian structures and absence of germ cells and follicles. *(From Carr BR. Disorders of the ovaries and female reproductive tract, in Wilson JD, Foster DW, Kronenberg HM, Larsen PR (eds), Williams' Textbook of Endocrinology, 9th ed. Philadelphia: Saunders, 1998: pp 751–817, with permission.)*

P450 for 17α-hydroxylase *(CYP17)* will be manifest by delayed puberty and primary amenorrhea in a phenotypic female (regardless of genotype), hypokalemia, and hypertension. The hypertension and hypokalemia are caused by increased production of deoxycorticosterone (DOC). Defects in only the 17,20-lyase activity of *CYP17* are characterized by delayed puberty and primary amenorrhea alone.[58]

Breast development in female patients with delayed puberty may be induced by estrogen-replacement therapy using either a conjugated equine estrogen (such as Premarin), a synthetic estrogen (such as ethinyl estradiol), or micronized estradiol at slowly increasing doses until feminization is achieved. The initial dose should be quite low (i.e., 0.3 mg conjugated equine estrogen CEE). Thereafter, a progestin is required to induce endometrial cycling. After adequate breast development is attained, a low-dose combined oral contraceptive pill may be used. Estrogen-replacement therapy in Turner syndrome is more complex, requiring coordination with GH administration to optimize adult height attainment.

▶ AMENORRHEA

Although a complaint commonly seen with disorders of delayed puberty, amenorrhea also may be a symptom of other disorders. *Amenorrhea* is defined as the absence of menarche in girls 16 years of age, irrespective of the presence or absence of secondary sexual characteristic development, or the absence of menstruation for 6 months in a woman with previous periodic menses. Amenorrhea may not always be an abnormal symptom. During the lifetime of a woman, amenorrhea normally occurs prior to puberty, during pregnancy and lactation, and following menopause. The average age of menarche in the United States is 12.8 years.[59] By 16 years of age, approximately 98 percent of American girls have begun menstruating. Women who do not fulfill these criteria also should be evaluated if (1) the girl

and/or her family are greatly concerned, (2) no breast development has occurred by 15 years of age, or (3) any sexual ambiguity or virilization is present. Amenorrhea is usually categorized as either primary (in a girl who has never menstruated) or secondary (in a girl or woman who menstruates for a variable length of time and then ceases). Some disorders present as both primary and/or secondary amenorrhea. Thus, categorizing the symptom of amenorrhea into primary and secondary types is less helpful than classifying disorders based on the following physiologic derangements: (1) anatomic defects, (2) ovarian failure, and (3) chronic anovulation with or without estrogen present (see Table 9-7 and 9-8).

Evaluation of Amenorrhea

A general scheme for the evaluation of women with amenorrhea is given in Figure 9-11. If the patient also has congenital ambiguous genitalia as well as amenorrhea, she should be evaluated as described in Chapter 8. In the initial examination, special attention should be given to three features: (1) degree of maturation of the breasts, the pubic and axillary hair, and the external genitalia, (2) the current estrogen status, and (3) the presence or absence of a uterus. Women with amenorrhea should be evaluated for the possibility of pregnancy. Even when history and physical examination are not suggestive, it is prudent to exclude pregnancy by measuring urinary or serum hCG concentration. Adolescents who fear reprisal from parents and authority figures may falsely deny prior sexual activity.[60] Once pregnancy is excluded, the cause of amenorrhea frequently can be diagnosed on the basis of the history and physical examination. For example, in women with clear-cut primary amenorrhea and sexual infantilism, the essential differential diagnoses are gonadal dysgenesis and hypopituitarism. In addition, the diagnosis of gonadal dysgenesis (Turner syndrome) or anatomic defects of the outflow tract (müllerian agenesis,

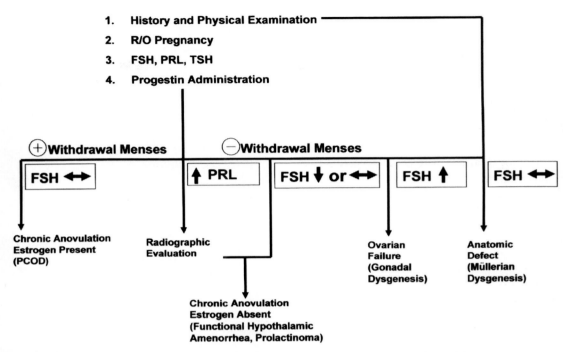

1. **History and Physical Examination**
2. **R/O Pregnancy**
3. **FSH, PRL, TSH**
4. **Progestin Administration**

⊕**Withdrawal Menses**   ⊖**Withdrawal Menses**

FSH ⟷   ↑ PRL   FSH ↓ or ⟷   FSH ↑   FSH ⟷

Chronic Anovulation Estrogen Present (PCOD)

Radiographic Evaluation

Chronic Anovulation Estrogen Absent (Functional Hypothalamic Amenorrhea, Prolactinoma)

Ovarian Failure (Gonadal Dysgenesis)

Anatomic Defect (Müllerian Dysgenesis)

Figure 9-11   Flow diagram for the evaluation of women with amenorrhea. The most common diagnosis for each category is shown in parentheses.

testicular feminization, and cervical stenosis) is frequently suggested on the basis of physical findings. When a specific cause is suspected, it is appropriate to proceed directly to confirm the diagnosis (such as obtaining a chromosomal karyotype or measurement of plasma gonadotropins). It is also useful to measure serum prolactin levels during the initial evaluation.

Estrogen status is evaluated by determining the level of estrogenization of the vagina and cervix. Adequate estrogenization is evident if the vaginal mucosa is moist and rugated and the cervical mucus is abundant. Microscopic examination of the vaginal cells will show a pattern of mature squamous cells. A hypoestrogenic environment will be associated with a pale pink, atrophic vagina, scant mucus within the cervix, and immature squama on microscopic examination. If these criteria are indeterminate, a progestational challenge is indicated, most often administration of 10 mg of

medroxyprogesterone acetate by mouth once or twice daily for 5 days or 200 mg of progesterone in oil intramuscularly. (It should be emphasized that progestin should never be administered until pregnancy is excluded.) If estrogen levels are adequate (and the outflow tract is intact), menstrual bleeding should occur within 1 week of ending the progestin treatment. If withdrawal bleeding occurs, the diagnosis is chronic anovulation with estrogen present, usually polycystic ovary syndrome.

If no withdrawal bleeding occurs, the nature of the subsequent workup depends on the results of the initial prolactin assay. If plasma prolactin level is elevated or if galactorrhea is present, CT scan or MRI of the pituitary sella should be undertaken.

When the plasma prolactin level is normal in a woman who does not develop withdrawal bleeding after progestin administration, measurement of plasma gonadotropins is required.

If the gonadotropin levels are elevated in these women, the diagnosis is ovarian failure. If the gonadotropins are in the low or normal range, the diagnosis is either hypothalamic-pituitary dysfunction or anatomic defect. As indicated previously, the diagnosis of anatomic defects of the outflow tract is usually suspected or established on the basis of the history and physical findings. However, when the physical findings are not clear-cut, it is useful to administer cyclic estrogen plus progestin (1.25 mg oral conjugated estrogens per day for 3 weeks followed by 10 days of progestin). If no bleeding occurs, the diagnosis of Asherman syndrome or other anatomic defect of the outflow tract is strongly suggested. If withdrawal bleeding occurs following the estrogen-progestin regimen, the diagnosis of chronic anovulation with estrogen absent (functional hypothalamic amenorrhea) is suggested. Radiologic evaluations of the pituitary-hypothalamic areas should be performed, irrespective of the prolactin level, because of the danger of overlooking a pituitary-hypothalamic tumor and because the diagnosis of functional hypothalamic amenorrhea is one of exclusion[3] (Fig. 9-11; see also Table 9-6).

Anatomic Defects

Anatomic or obstructive defects of the female genital outflow tract can preclude menstrual bleeding. Congenital obstructive defects of the vagina, imperforate hymen, and transverse vaginal septa also can cause amenorrhea (Figs. 9-12 and 9-13). These women frequently have accumulation of menstrual blood behind the obstruction and may have cyclic or monthly worsening of abdominal pain.

More extensive anomalies of the female genital tract involve absence of the uterus and vagina (also called *müllerian agenesis* or *dysgenesis* or *Mayer-Rokitansky-Küster-Hauser syndrome*) that occurs second in frequency only to gonadal dysgenesis as a cause of primary amenorrhea.[42] Women with müllerian agenesis have a 46,XX karyotype and normal female secondary sex characteristics, including

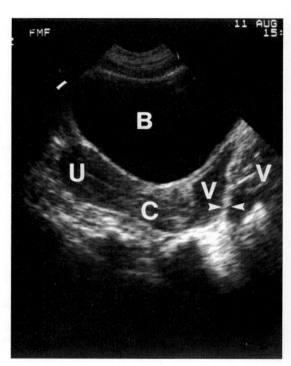

Figure 9-12 Transabdominal ultrasonographic study demonstrating a transverse vaginal septum. Arrowheads denote the location and width of the transverse septum. (B = bladder; U = uterus; C = cervix; V = vagina.) Menstrual blood is located between the septum and the cervix. *(From Doody KM, Carr BR. Amenorrhea. Obstet Gynecol Clin North Am 1990;17: pp 361–387, with permission.)*

breast development and pubic hair. They have normal ovarian function, including cyclical ovulation, but lack a vagina and have severe hypoplasia of the uterus. Disorders of the outflow tract are discussed more fully in Chapter 19. One diagnostic problem is to distinguish müllerian agenesis from testicular feminization, also known as complete *androgen resistance*. In androgen resistance, affected 46,XY individuals have intraabdominal testes, a blind-ending vaginal pouch, an absent uterus and feminized breasts (gynecomastia), but scant pubic and axillary hair. In this disorder, a defective androgen receptor cannot bind testosterone, resulting in profound resistance to the action of circulatory androgens. Androgen resistance can

Anatomical Defects

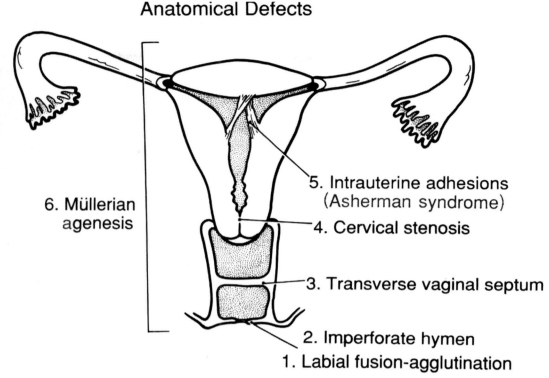

6. Müllerian agenesis

5. Intrauterine adhesions (Asherman syndrome)

4. Cervical stenosis

3. Transverse vaginal septum

2. Imperforate hymen

1. Labial fusion-agglutination

Figure 9-13 Diagrammatic representation of causes of amenorrhea resulting from disorders of the female reproductive (outflow) tract. (*From Carr BR. Disorders of the ovaries and female reproductive tract, in Wilson JD, Foster DW, Kronenberg HM, Larsen PR (eds), Williams' Textbook of Endocrinology, 9th ed. Philadelphia: Saunders, 1998: pp 751–817, with permission.*)

be diagnosed by demonstrating a male level of serum testosterone or a 46,XY karyotype.[43]

Other abnormalities of the uterus that cause amenorrhea include obstruction caused by scarring and stenosis of the cervix, often resulting from surgery, electrocautery, or cryosurgery. Destruction of the endometrium (Asherman syndrome) may follow a therapeutic abortion complicated by infection or a vigorous curettage, commonly performed to stop postpartum hemorrhage. Tuberculous endometritis and uterine surgery are rare causes of Asherman syndrome. The diagnosis is confirmed by finding filling defects and intrauterine synechiae either using hysterosalpingography or direct visualization with hysteroscopy.[41]

Treatment of outflow tract disorders is surgical. Repair of vaginal agenesis or vaginal septa results in normal menstruation and potential fertility only if an intact uterus is present. With müllerian agenesis, a functional vagina may be created by vaginal dilation or by vaginal creation using a split-thickness skin graft (McIndoe procedure).[58]

Ovarian Failure (Hypergonadotropic Hypergonadism)

Primary ovarian failure is characterized by pubertal delay, primary amenorrhea, and elevated plasma gonadotropins (hypergonadotropic hypogonadism). Causes of ovarian failure have been described earlier in this chapter and include gonadal dysgenesis, 17α-hydroxylase deficiency, 17,20-desmolase deficiency, premature ovarian failure, and the resistant ovary syndrome. Treatment of ovarian failure is directed at estrogen-progesterone replacement to augment or maintain secondary sexual characteristics, prevent osteoporosis, and lower the risk of cardiovascular disease.[41]

Chronic Anovulation

The most common cause of secondary amenorrhea is chronic anovulation, a disorder in which ovaries fail to secrete estrogen in a normal cyclic pattern. Women can be separated clinically into those who produce sufficient estrogen to bleed following progesterone withdrawal therapy and those who fail to produce enough estrogen to bleed after taking progesterone and who often have hypothalamic-pituitary dysfunction.

Chronic Anovulation with Estrogen Present (Hypogonadotropic Hypogonadism)

Women with chronic anovulation who experience withdrawal bleeding after taking progesterone are said to be in a state of chronic anovulation with estrogen present due to the acyclic production of estrogen, largely estrone, by extraglandular aromatization of circulating androstenedione. This disorder, called *polycystic ovarian syndrome* (PCOS), is characterized by pubertal-onset androgen excess, obesity, and amenorrhea or oligomenorrhea.[61] The uterine bleeding that occurs in subjects with PCOS is unpredictable with respect to onset, duration, and amount. This dysfunctional uterine bleeding associated with PCOS is usually due to estrogen breakthrough.[43] PCOS is described in greater detail in Chapter 13.

Chronic Anovulation with Estrogen Absent

Women with chronic anovulation who have low or absent estrogen production and do not bleed after progesterone withdrawal usually have hypogonadotropic hypogonadism due to either pituitary disease or any of several organic or functional disorders of the CNS. They may present with pubertal delay and primary amenorrhea or with secondary amenorrhea depending on the timing of the insult to the CNS.[3]

Hypogonadotropic hypogonadism associated with defects of olfaction is Kallmann syndrome, which was described earlier in this chapter. A number of rare hypothalamic lesions, including craniopharyngioma, germinoma (pinealoma), glioma, Hand-Schüller-Christian disease, teratomas, endodermal sinus tumors, tuberculosis, sarcoidosis, and metastatic tumors, can suppress or destroy the hypothalamus, leading to the development of hypogonadotropic hypogonadism. CNS trauma and radiation also can cause hypothalamic amenorrhea and deficiencies in secretion of GH, thyroid hormone, and ACTH.[41]

More commonly, gonadotropin deficiency leading to chronic anovulation is believed to come from functional disorders of the hypothalamus or higher centers. Stress, in the form of rigorous exercise such as jogging or ballet, extreme dieting, or emotional events can lead to low or low-normal gonadotropin and estrogen levels. Anorexia nervosa, an extreme form of weight loss, is characterized in young women by the development of chronic anovulation and amenorrhea; distorted attitudes toward eating, weight gain, and body image; self-induced vomiting; and emaciation. Amenorrhea in anorexia nervosa can precede, follow, or appear coincidentally with the loss of body weight. During a patient's successful recovery, gonadotropin increases mimic those of normal puberty. In addition, chronic debilitating diseases such as end-stage kidney disease, malignancy, and malabsorption syndromes can lead to hypogonadotropic hypogonadism and amenorrhea by a hypothalamic mechanism.[42]

Treatment of chronic anovulation due to hypothalamic disorders includes reversal of the stressful situation or correction of weight loss if possible. Estrogen-replacement therapy to induce and maintain normal secondary sexual characteristics is recommended for women with the Kallmann syndrome who do not desire pregnancy. When pregnancy is desired, physicians can give exogenous gonadotropins. In other instances, the primary disease of the hypothalamus directs therapy.

Disorders of the pituitary can lead to secondary amenorrhea and the estrogen-deficient form of chronic anovulation by two mechanisms: direct interference with gonadotropin secretion by lesions that either obliterate or interfere with the gonadotrope cells (chromophobe adenomas, Sheehan syndrome) or inhibition of gonadotropin secretion due to excess prolactin (prolactinoma). A tenth or more of amenorrheic women have increased levels of serum prolactin, and more than one-half of women with both galactorrhea and amenorrhea have elevated prolactin levels. When tumors of any size are associated with symptoms of amenorrhea or galactorrhea, however, therapy should be considered, and when visual field defects or severe headaches are present, neurosurgical evaluation is mandatory. Most prolactinomas are treated successfully with medical therapy. Bromocriptine and other dopamine agonists are used routinely to suppress prolactin production from pituitary adenomas. Therapy is usually associated with return to menstruation and potential for fertility.[43]

KEY POINTS

1. The first sign of increased gonadotropin secretion is during sleep.

2. Evidence supporting the role of estrogen in regulating skeletal maturation includes estrogen receptor- and aromatase-deficient males who developed delayed skeletal maturation and early-onset osteoporosis.

3. GnRH neurons develop in the forebrain and migrate to the hypothalamus. Defects in this process may lead to hypogonadotropin hypogonadism and loss of smell. This disorder is known as Kallmann syndrome.

4. After birth, gonadotropin levels rise due to withdrawal of placental sex steroids and remain elevated for 6 months to a year and then remain low until puberty.

5. One genetic defect associated with Kallmann syndrome is in the *KAL1* gene.

6. LH receptor defects in 45,XY males are associated with a female phenotype, low levels of testosterone, high levels of LH, and unresponsiveness to hCG administration.

7. Females with a 46,XX karyotype and LH receptor defects present with normal female development but exhibit amenorrhea and cystic ovaries.

8. Characteristics of Turner syndrome include failure of secondary sexual characteristics, short stature, webbed neck, shield chest, fourth short metacarpal, pigmented nevi, and cardiac anomalies.

9. Patients with 46,XY Swyer syndrome or pure gonadal dysgenesis have a female phenotype, failure of development of secondary sexual characteristics, and absence of a uterus but exhibit streak gonads that must be removed (Y karyotype) due to risk of malignancy.

10. Evaluation of amenorrhea requires clinical assessment; determination of gonadotropin, βhCG, TSH, and prolactin levels; and progestin withdrawal testing.

11. Müllerian agenesis or dysgenesis is associated with normal female secondary characteristics, 46,XX karyotype, normal pubic hair, and absence of vagina and uterus. Androgen resistance (testicular feminization) is associated with female secondary characteristics, 46,XY karyotype, and absence of pubic hair, vagina, and uterus.

12. The first sign of puberty in females is breast development and in males is testicular growth.

13. The most common cause of isosexual precocity in girls is constitutional.

14. Gonadotropin-independent precocious puberty suggests a risk of ovarian tumor as the source.

15. McCune-Albright syndrome is characterized by a triad of: café-au-lait spots, polyostotic fibrous dysplasia, and precocious puberty due to a defect in the $G_s\alpha$ protein.

16. Familial testotoxicosis is associated with isosexual male precocity and is due to activation of the LH receptor.

17. The primary treatment of constitutional sexual precocity is GnRH agonists.

REFERENCES

1. Plant TM. Puberty in primates, in Knobil E, Neill JD (eds), *The Physiology of Reproduction,* 2d ed. New York: Raven Press, 1994; pp 453–485.
2. Kappy MS, Ganong CS. Advances in the treatment of precocious puberty. *Adv Pediatr* 1994;41:223–261.
3. Bradshaw KD, Quigley CA. Disorders of pubertal development, in Jameson JL (ed), *Principles of Molecular Medicine.* Totowa, NJ: Humana Press, 1998; pp 569–580.
4. Laue L, Jones J, Barnes KM, et al. Treatment of familial male precocious puberty with spironolactone, testolactone, and deslorelin. *J Clin Endocrinol Metab* 1993;76:151–155.
5. Zachman M, Prader A, Sobel EH, et al. Pubertal growth in patients with complete androgen insensitivity: Indirect evidence for the importance of estrogen in girls. *J Pediatr* 1986; 108:694–697.
6. Smith EP, Boyd J, Frank GR, et al. Estrogen resistance caused by a mutation in the estrogen-receptor gene in a man. *N Eng J Med* 1994; 331:1056–1061.
7. Winter JSD, Hughes IA, Reyes FI, Faiman C. Pituitary-gonadal relations in infancy: 2. Patterns of serum gonadal concentrations in man from birth to two years of age. *J Clin Endocrinol Metab* 1976;42:679–686.
8. Palmert MR, Boepple PA. Variations in the timing of puberty: Clinical spectrum and genetic investigation. *J Clin Endocrinol Metab* 2001;86:2364–2368.
9. Kalantaridou SN, Chrousos GP. Monogenic disorders of puberty. *J Clin Endocrinol Metab* 2002;87:2481–2494.
10. Plant TM. Puberty in primates, in Knobil E, Neill JD (eds), *The Physiology of Reproduction,* 2d ed. New York: Raven Press, 1994; pp 453–485.
11. Bates GW. Normal and abnormal puberty, in Carr BR, Blackwell RE (eds), *Textbook of Reproductive Medicine,* 2d ed. Stamford, CT: Appleton and Lange, 1998; pp 93–112.
12. Palmert MR, Boepple PA. Variations in the timing of puberty: Clinical spectrum and genetic investigation. *J Clin Endocrinol Metab* 2001; 86:2364–2368.
13. Hillard PJA. Menstruation in young girls: A clinical perspective. *Obstet Gynecol* 2002;99: 655–662.
14. Balducci R, Boscherini B, Mangiantini A, et al. Isolated precocious pubarche: An approach. *J Clin Endocrinol Metab* 1994;79:582–589.
15. Kappy MS, Ganong CS. Advances in the treatment of precocious puberty. *Adv Pediatr* 1994;41:223–261.
16. Pescovitz OH, Comite F, Hench K, et al. The NIH experience with precocious puberty: Diagnostic subgroups and response to short-term luteinizing hormone releasing hormone analogue therapy. *J Pediatr* 1986;108:47–54.
17. Burstein S. Growth disorders after cranial radiation in childhood (editorial). *J Clin Endocrinol Metab* 1994;78:1280–1281.
18. Ogilvy-Stuart AL, Clayton PE, Shalet SM. Cranial irradiation and early puberty. *J Clin Endocrinol Metab* 1994;78:1282–1286.
19. Junier MP, Hill DF, Costa ME, et al. Hypothalamic lesions that induce female precocious puberty activate glial expression of the epidermal growth factor receptor gene: Differential regulation of alternatively spliced transcripts. *J Neurosci* 1993;13:703–713.
20. Klein KO. Precocious puberty: Who has it? Who should be treated? *J Clin Endocrinol Metab* 1999;84:411–414.

21. Lee PA. Advances in the management of precocious puberty. *Clin Pediatr* 1994;33:54–61.

22. Paul D, Conte FA, Grumbach MM, Kaplan SL. Long-term effect of gonadotropin-releasing hormone agonists therapy on final and near-final height in 26 children with true precocious puberty treated at a median age of less than 5 years. *J Clin Endocrinol Metab* 1995;80:546–551.

23. Van der Sluis IM, Boot AM, Krenning EP, et al. Longitudinal follow-up of bone density and body composition in children with precocious or early puberty before, during, and after cessation of GnRH agonist therapy. *J Clin Endocrinol Metab* 2002;87:506–512.

24. Neely EK, Bachrach LK, Hintz RL, et al. Bone mineral density during treatment of central precocious puberty. *J Pediatr* 1995;127:819–822.

25. Shankar RR, Pescovitz OH. Precocious puberty. *Adv Endocrinol Metab* 1995;6:55–89.

26. Lampit M, Golander A, Guttmann H, Hochberg Z. Estrogen minidose replacement during GnRH agonist therapy in central precocious puberty: A pilot study. *J Clin Endocrinol Metab* 2002;87:687–690.

27. Feuillan PP, Foster CM, Pescovitz OH, et al. Treatment of precocious puberty in the McCune-Albright syndrome with the aromatase inhibitor testolactone. *N Engl J Med* 1986;315:1115–1119.

28. Holland FJ, Fishman L, Bailey JD, Fazekas AT. Ketoconazole in the management of precocious puberty not responsive to LHRH analogue therapy. *N Engl J Med* 1985;312:1023–1027.

29. Schwindinger WF, Francomano CA, Levine MA. Identification of a mutation in gene encoding the α subunit of the stimulatory G protein of adenylyl cyclase in McCune-Albright syndrome. *Proc Natl Acad Sci USA* 1992;89:5152–5156.

30. Kalantaridou SN, Chrousos GP. Monogenic disorders of puberty. *J Clin Endocrinol Metab* 2002;87:2481–2494.

31. Furui K, Suganuma N, Tsukahara S-I, et al. Identification of two point mutations in the gene coding luteinizing hormone (LH) β-subunit, associated with immunologically anomalous LH variants. *J Clin Endocrinol Metab* 1994;78:107–113.

32. Kawate N, Kletter GB, Wilson BE, et al. Identification of constitutively activating mutation of the luteinising hormone receptor in a fam-

ily with male limited gonadotrophin independent precocious puberty (testotoxicosis). *J Med Genet* 1995;32:553–554.

33. Shenker A. G protein–coupled receptor structure and function: the impact of disease-causing mutations. *Baillieres Clin Endocrinol Metab* 1995;9:427–451.

34. Shenker A, Laue L, Kosui S, et al. A constitutively activating mutation of the luteinizing hormone receptor in familial male precocious puberty. *Nature* 1993;365:652–654

35. Kosugi S, Van Dop C, Geffner ME, et al. Characterization of heterogeneous mutations causing constitutive activation of the luteinizing hormone receptor in familial male precocious puberty. *Hum Mol Genet* 1995;4:183–188.

36. Latronico AC, Anasti J, Arnhold IJ, et al. A novel mutation of the luteinizing hormone receptor gene causing male gonadotropin-independent precocious puberty. *J Clin Endocrinol Metab* 1995;80:2490–2494.

37. Laue L, Chan WY, Hsueh AJ, et al. Genetic heterogeneity of constitutively activating mutations of the human luteinizing hormone receptor in familial male-limited precocious puberty. *Proc Natl Acad Sci USA* 1995;92:1906–1910.

38. Choong CS, Fuller PJ, Chu S, et al. Sertoli-Leydig cell tumor of the ovary, a rare cause of precocious puberty in a 12-month-old infant. *J Clin Endocrinol Metab* 2002;87:49–56.

39. Laue L, Jones J, Barnes KM, et al. Treatment of familial male precocious puberty with spironolactone, testolactone, and deslorelin. *J Clin Endocrinol Metab* 1993;76:151–155.

40. Grumbach MM, Styne DM. Puberty: ontongeny, neuroendocrinology, physiology, in Willson JD, Foster DW (eds), *Williams' Textbook of Endocrinology,* 8th ed. Philadelphia: Saunders, 1992; p 1139.

41. Emans SJH, Goldstein DP. *Pediatric and Adolescent Gynecology.* Boston: Little, Brown, 1990.

42. Carr BR, Bradshaw KD. Disorders of the ovary and female reproductive tract, in Braunwald E, Fauci AS, Kasper DI (eds), *Harrison's Principles of Internal Medicine,* 15th ed. New York: McGraw-Hill, 2001; p 2154.

43. Speroff L, Glass RH, Kase NG. *Clinical Gynecologic Endocrinology and Infertility,* 6th ed. Philadelphia: Lippincott Williams & Wilkins, 1999.

44. Duke VM, Winyard PJ, Thorogood P, et al. *KAL,* a gene mutated in Kallmann's syndrome, is

expressed in the first trimester of human development. *Mol Cell Endocrinol* 1995;110:73–79.

45. Hardelin JP, Petit C. A molecular approach to the pathophysiology of the X-linked Kallmann's syndrome. *Baillieres Clin Endocrinol Metab* 1995;9:489–507.

46. Legouis R, Cohen-Salmon M, Del Castillo I, Petit C. Isolation and characterization of the gene responsible for the X chromosome–linked Kallmann syndrome. *Biomed Pharmacother* 1994;48:241–246.

47. Winters SJ. Expanding the differential diagnosis of male hypogonadism. *N Engl J Med* 1992; 326:193–195.

48. Hardelin JP, Levilliers J, Blanchard S, et al. Heterogeneity in the mutations responsible for X chromosome linked Kallmann syndrome. *Hum Mol Genet* 1993;2:373–377.

49. Kalantaridou SN, Chrousos GP. Monogenic disorders of puberty. *J Clin Endocrinol Metab* 2002;87:2481–2494.

50. Aittomäki K, Lucena JLD, Pakarinen P, et al. Mutation in the follicle-stimulating hormone receptor gene causes hereditary hypergonadotropic ovarian failure. *Cell* 1995;82:959–968.

51. Burstein S. Growth disorders after cranial radiation in childhood (editorial). *J Clin Endocrinol Metab* 1994;78:1280–1281.

52. Clayton RN. Molecular genetics, hypogonadism and luteinizing hormone. *Clin Endocrinol* 1992;34:201–202.

53. Furui K, Suganuma N, Tsukahara S-I, et al. Identification of two point mutations in the gene coding luteinizing hormone (LH) β-subunit, associated with immunologically anomalous LH variants. *J Clin Endocrinol Metab* 1994;78:107–113.

54. Latronico AC, Anasti J, Arnhold IJP, et al. Testicular and ovarian resistance to luteinizing hormone caused by inactivating mutations of the luteinizing hormone. *N Eng J Med* 1996;334: 507–512.

55. Laue L, Wu SM, Kudo M, et al. A nonsense mutation of the human luteinizing hormone receptor gene in Leydig cell hypoplasia. *Hum Mol Genet* 1995;4:1429–1433.

56. Weiss J, Axelrod L, Whitcomb RW, et al. Hypogonadism caused by a single amino acid substitution in the β subunit of luteinizing hormone. *N Engl J Med* 1992;326:179–183.

57. Matthews CH, Borgato S, Beck-Peccoz P, et al. Primary amenorrhoea and infertility due to a mutation in the β-subunit of follicle-stimulating hormone. *Nature Genet* 1993;5:83–86.

58. Bradshaw KD, Waterman MR, Couch RT, et al. Characterization of complementary deoxyribonucleic acid for human adrenocortical 17α-hydroxylase: A probe for analysis of 17α-hydroxylase deficiency. *Mol Endocrinol* 1987; 1:348–354.

59. Carr BR. The normal menstrual cycle: The coordinated events of the hypothalamic-pituitary-axis and the female reproductive tract, in Carr BR, Blackwell RE (eds), *Textbook of Reproductive Medicine,* 2d ed. Stamford, CT: Appleton and Lange, 1998; p 233.

60. Hillard PJA. Menstruation in young girls: A clinical perspective. *Obstet Gynecol* 2002;99:655–662.

61. Yen SSC. Polycystic ovary syndrome: (hyperandrogenic chronic anovulation), in Yen SSC, Jaffe RB, Barbieri RL (eds), *Reproductive Endocrinology: Physiology, Pathophysiology, and Clinical Management,* 4th ed. Philadelphia: Saunders, 1999; p 413.

CHAPTER 10

Disorders of the Hypothalamic System

Richard E. Blackwell

A number of metabolic and anatomic conditions can lead to dysfunction of the hypothalamic-pituitary axis. The most common causes are chronic hypothalamic anovulation disturbing the pulse rhythm of the arcuate nucleus and prolactinomas that cause dysfunction of anatomy and biochemistry.

The classic studies from Knobil's laboratory demonstrated that the arcuate nucleus fires in a circhoral (once per hour) rhythm. This delivers gonadotropin-releasing hormone (GnRH) through the hypothalamic portal system to the gonadotropes, which results in the hourly pulsatile release of luteinizing hormone (LH) and follicle-stimulating hormone (FSH). This can be duplicated in the monkey model by the delivery of pulsatile GnRH. Alteration of the GnRH pulse frequency results in a decline in gonadotropin secretion and in functional disorders of the hypothalamus. GnRH pulse frequency drops from one surge per hour to one surge every 3 hours.[1,2]

▶ CHRONIC HYPOTHALAMIC ANOVULATION

Yen has called the most common cause of anovulation *chronic hypothalamic anovulation.*[3]

This involves an alteration in GnRH pulse frequency to the point that ovulation fails to occur. The features of this particular syndrome involve normal gonadotropins with an appropriate LH/FSH ratio and the ability of the endometrium to respond appropriately to a progesterone challenge with bleeding. This type of disorder is treated frequently with clomiphene citrate if pregnancy is desired or a cyclic progesterone or progestogens or an oral contraceptive agent.

Hypothalamic Anovulation

Hypothalamic anovulation is a different disorder from chronic hypothalamic anovulation. Individuals with this type of disorder have low gonadotropin levels with an inverted LH/FSH ratio such that FSH is greater than LH. Normally, one finds this type of ratio only in certain stages of puberty and menopause. The features of this disorder are amenorrhea, failure of ovulation, and failure of the endometrium to respond to a progestogen challenge with bleeding. Individuals who wish to conceive are best treated with gonadotropins, and those who do not desire pregnancy may be treated with cyclic estrogen/progestogens

▶ **TABLE 10-1:** TYPES OF CNS-MEDIATED
OVULATION DYSFUNCTION

- Chronic hypothalamic anovulation (CHA)
- Hypothalamic anovulation
  Stress-related
  Exercise-related
  Eating disorders (low body weight)
  Combination of above
- Pseudocyesis

or birth control pills with adequate estrogen
expression.[4]

There are three conditions that deserve discussion that could produce either chronic hypothalamic anovulation or hypothalamic amenorrhea depending on severity. These are stress-related amenorrhea, exercise-associated amenorrhea, and eating disorders such as anorexia nervosa (Table 10-1).

Stress-Related Amenorrhea

Various forms of stress have been shown to result in alterations of the positive and negative input that is received by the arcuate nucleus.[5] GnRH pulse frequency decreases from one pulse per hour to one pulse per 3 hours. This is a gradual process that can present clinically with altered menstrual cycle length, delayed ovulation, dysfolliculogenesis, oligoovulation, anovulation, and ultimately, amenorrhea. Classically, 60 percent of infertility was thought to be associated with stress; however, it is probably closer to 2 percent. Nevertheless, trim women with inappropriate body fat-lean mass ratios who are avid exercisers frequently have a stress-induced ovulatory dysfunction as part of their overall infertility problem. The appropriate treatment of these disorders ranges from ovulation induction with clomiphene citrate to induction of withdrawal bleeding with progesterone to total replacement therapy with cyclic estrogen/progesterone.

Exercise Amenorrhea

Exercise has been shown to have a profound effect on menstrual cycle length, onset, and ovulation. For instance, prepubertal ballerinas have a delay in the onset of menarche approximately 30 percent of the time. Certain activities associated with low body weight such as long-distance running, ballet, and gymnastics result in more menstrual dysfunction than swimming or cycling. For instance, runners who reach a level of 70 miles per week have a 50 percent rate of amenorrhea, whereas cyclists might have a comparable 10 to 12 percent. If untrained individuals are subjected to strenuous exercise and calorie restriction simultaneously, menstrual dysfunction can be induced rapidly. Therefore, in individuals who wish to conceive, it is advisable to have them limit their physical activity, although at times this is very difficult to achieve. If the individuals are unable to comply with this form of therapy, gonadotropins will override the ovulatory defect. On the other hand, these individuals are at increased risk for stress fractures, and at times, severe bone loss can occur with extremes of exercise. It is advisable that these individuals be treated with cyclic estrogen/progesterone if pregnancy is not desired.[6]

Eating Disorders

Observations of Frisch et al. demonstrated that there is a critical threshold in body mass composition required for normal menstrual function.[7,8] It is hypothesized that 48-kg body weight is required for the institution of puberty. A woman who loses 15 percent of her ideal body weight will often become amenorrheic. For example, a woman who is 5 ft, 4 in tall should have a minimum body weight of 114 lb. The addition of stress or exercise will amplify the effect of low body weight.

Anorexia nervosa is perhaps the most extreme form of eating disorder.[9] It is a psychosomatic condition characterized by extreme weight loss usually greater than 25 percent, a body image disturbance, and an intense fear of obesity. These individuals may or may not simultaneously experience bulimia; therefore, the condition can present with either severe dietary restriction or binge eating followed by vomiting. Although 95 percent of individuals who are anorectic are female, the condition has been described in male athletes, usually long-distance runners or individuals who participate in sports such as crewing, where weight is critical. Individuals with these disorders are almost always Caucasian, from the middle and upper classes; the incidence of anorexia increased from 0.64 percent per 100.000 to about 1 to 1.2 percent per 100,000. It has been estimated that 18 percent of high school and college students have experienced periods of bulimia, and the *Diagnostic and Statistical Manual,* Vol. 4 (DSM-4), suggests that 1 to 2 percent of the female population has a problem with anorexia.[10,11] Anorexia traditionally occurs under the age of 16, with a bimodal distribution of 13 to 14 years and 17 to 18 years. Bulimia usually begins later at 17 to 25 years.[12]

These conditions pose significant health risks. These individuals have hypothermia, bradycardia, cardiac arrhythmias, hypotension, hypokalemia, dry skin, increased β-carotene levels, hyperactivity, obsessive-compulsive behavior, osteopenia and osteoporosis, elevated hepatic enzymes, anemia, and leukopenia. Further, vomiting induced in the bulimic phase can result in tears of the gastroesophageal system (Mallory-Weiss syndrome), and in the most profound forms, 9 percent of patients with this disorder die secondary to cardiac arrhythmias and hypotension. Further, suicide has been reported in 2 to 5 percent of patients with the chronic form of anorexia nervosa. Osteoporosis may be profound and develop rapidly in these individuals. I have seen individuals who have had a reduction in height of up to 5 in within a 5-year period. The therapy for these individuals is replacement of their estrogen/progesterone, psychological counseling, and antipsychotic medication, where needed. At times these individuals must be hospitalized for invasive feeding techniques.[13]

Pseudocyesis

Pseudocyesis is a peculiar disorder that disrupts menstrual cycle function. It was described by John Goode and derives from the Greek *pseudes,* meaning "false," and *kyesis,* meaning "pregnancy."[14] It has been described as imaginary or phantom pregnancy, with individuals demonstrating amenorrhea or oligomenorrhea, morning sickness, abdominal bloating, enlargement of the breasts, galactorrhea, and often softening of the cervix with congestion. These patients have been demonstrated to have abnormal hormone secretion, including hyperprolactinemia and decreased levels of LH and FSH. The symptoms resolve when the patients are demonstrated not to be pregnant.

Central Nervous System Tumors and Other Disorders

A number of conditions can result in disruption of normal menstrual function. These include any tumor of the central nervous system (CNS) from astrocytomas to gliomas to pinealomas. One also can get disruption of menstrual cycle function with temporal arteritis, cavernous sinus thrombosis, infiltrative disorders such as histiocytosis X (Hand-Schüller-Christian syndrome), and tubercle-forming disorders such as tuberculosis or von Recklinghausen's disease. These may affect input into the arcuate nucleus, the arcuate nucleus itself, or the hypothalamic-pituitary portal track. These conditions are treated medically or surgically dependent on their nature[15] (Table 10-2).

▶ **TABLE 10-2:** DISEASES THAT ALTER CNS ANATOMY AND PRODUCE OVULATORY DYSFUNCTION

- All tumors
- Temporal arteritis
- Cavernous sinus thrombosis
- Histiocytosis X
- Tuberculosis
- Syphilis
- Von Recklinghausen's disease

▶ PITUITARY DISORDERS

A number of functional disorders affect the activity of the pituitary, including isolated gonadotropin deficiency, postpartum pituitary necrosis (Sheehan's syndrome), pituitary apoplexy, and head trauma (Table 10-3).

Isolated Gonadotropin Deficiency

Isolated gonadotropin deficiency (Kallmann syndrome) is characterized by an absence of the secretion of GnRH, which leads to hypo-

▶ **TABLE 10-3:** PITUITARY DISEASE

- Isolated gonadotropin deficiency
- Sheehan syndrome
- Pituitary apoplexy
- Trauma
- Craniopharyngioma
- Empty sella syndrome
- Pituitary tumors
  Nonfunctioning
    Null cell
    Subtype III
  Functioning
    Prolactinomas
    Growth hormone–secreting
    ACTH-secreting
    TSH-secreting
    Gonadotropin-secreting
    Mixed
- Sarcoidosis

gonadotropic hypogonadism with unicoid features. In some cases the individuals have anosmia, and the disorder can be inherited through an autosomal dominant pattern.[16] The defect appears to be due to a failure of GnRH neurons to form completely in the medial olfactory placode of the developing nose or failure to migrate from the olfactory bulb to the mediobasal hypothalamus during embryogenesis. Gonadotropins in these patients may be in the low or normal range, and levels of other pituitary hormones will be normal. However, these individuals will present with failure to undergo gonadarche. The diagnosis is made by administering a GnRH bolus and measuring the release of gonadotropins. In general, these individuals are treated with cyclic estrogen and progesterone to allow them to complete puberty. When pregnancy is desired, either pulsatile GnRH delivered via a pump or gonadotropins will result in folliculogenesis and ovulation.

Postpartum Pituitary Necrosis (Sheehan Syndrome)

Postpartum pituitary necrosis can be a life-threatening endocrine emergency.[17] Autopsy studies of obstetric patients who died between 12 hours and 34 days following delivery revealed that approximately 25 percent were found to have necrosis of the anterior pituitary. This syndrome was described by both Simmonds and Sheehan. In almost all cases, pituitary necrosis is preceded by a massive obstetric hemorrhage characterized by circulatory collapse, hypotension, and shock. It seems to occur more frequently in diabetics. The pituitary gland, which is enlarged during pregnancy, seems to be susceptible to severe hypotensive episodes. The pathogenesis of the disorder remains unclear. Clinically, patients with pituitary necrosis have partial or total deficiency of one or more pituitary hormones or may demonstrate panhypopituitarism. These individuals may demonstrate hypoadrenalism with symptoms of hypotension, nausea, vomiting, lethargy, or hypothyroidism. Pituitary reserve can be evaluated with provocative testing using thyrotropin-releasing hormone (TRH), GnRH, growth hormone releasing hormone (GRH), and corticotropin releasing hormone (CRH). In general, once the deficiency has been identified, replacement hormones such as cortisone acetate or Synthroid can be administered.

Pituitary Apoplexy

Pituitary apoplexy is characterized by acute hemorrhagic infarction of the pituitary gland.[18] Patients complain of a sudden onset of severe retroorbital headache, visual and pupillary disturbances, and depressed sensorium. The symptoms can mimic other neurologic disorders, such as basal artery occlusion, hypertensive encephalopathy, or cavernous sinus thrombosis. Magnetic resonance imaging (MRI) or computed tomographic (CT) scanning reveals hemorrhage in the pituitary area. Surgical decompression may be required, but many of these patients will have prolactinomas, and intervention with a dopamine agonist such as bromocriptine, pergolide mesylate, or cabergoline will arrest the process.

Posttraumatic Hypopituitarism

Severe head trauma such as that experienced in a automobile accident may result in damage to the hypothalamic portal system. These individuals may present with hyperprolactinemia as well as diabetes insipidus. The most common initial symptoms are hypogonadism, amenorrhea, loss of pubic and axillary hair, anorexia, weight loss, and galactorrhea.

Anatomic Lesions

A number of tumors may affect the pituitary gland or areas adjacent to the sella turcica. The craniophrayngioma is generally manifested in children, although one-third of patients are adults.[19] These lesions arise from remnants of Rathke's pouch and are composed of stratified squamous epithelium. These lesions may reach 8 to 10 cm in diameter; they demonstrate an aggressive growth pattern affecting the optic chiasm, hypothalamus, and third ventricle. Many of these lesions are supersellar in nature, and 50 percent of them are calcified, which facilitates the diagnosis. Craniopharyngiomas are not endocrine active, and individuals affected with them usually present with complaints of vomiting, headache, visual loss, and diabetes insipidus. The lesions are diagnosed with either CT scan or MRI. Surgery is the primary therapy for these lesions, although it is difficult to achieve complete resection. When total excision can occur, occurrence rates are described as low. Postoperative radiation usually is used in individuals in whom tumor resection is incomplete.

Empty Sella Syndrome

Empty sella syndrome generally is associated with hyperprolactinemia, ovulatory dysfunction, and galactorrhea.[20] On radiographic studies, an area of low attenuation is seen in the pituitary fossa, and it has been suggested that there are two potential etiologies for the syndrome: (1) a herniation of the membranes through the diaphragm sella and (2) an infarction of a pituitary tumor. There is no specific treatment for this disorder other than suppression of the hyperprolactinemia with a dopamine agonist and/or replacement-hormone therapy with estrogen/progesterone.

Pituitary Tumors

Between 10 and 23 percent of the general population are thought to have pituitary tumors. Ten percent of all intracranial neoplasms involve the pituitary. However, Costello has suggested from autopsy studies that approximately 25 percent of individuals have pituitary tumors; the incidence is greater in men than in women.[21] Further, it has been suggested that if radiographic imaging is carried out randomly on the population, approximately 27 percent of individuals will be found to have a lesion that has been described in the internal medicine literature as an "incidentaloma."

Nonfunctioning Tumors

There are a number of nonfunctioning tumors of the pituitary gland that deserve mention. The most common is the null cell tumor. These tend to be large lesions that grow slowly, they can be associated with low-grade hyperprolactinemia, and often individuals are treated with bromocriptine for extended periods of time before these lesions grow large enough to warrant surgical intervention. A second tumor is the subtype III lesion, which is an aggressive tumor that grows rapidly. There is a tumor described as the "invasive adenoma" that closely resembles a meningoma and grows along dural planes. It has been suggested that these lesions can metastasize, but it is unclear whether some of these reports in fact may have been describing meningomas.[22,23]

Functional Pituitary Tumors

The prolactinoma is the most common functional pituitary tumor found in humans. These lesions result from expansion of lactotropes, which generally are found in the lateral aspects of the pituitary gland. These lesions may grow outward through bone structure and penetrate the cavernous sinus or extend superiorly to affect the optic chiasm. Lesions less than 10 mm in size are classified as *microadenomas* (Fig. 10-1); lesions larger than 10 mm are classified as *macroadenomas* (Fig. 10-2). The behavior of these two lesions varies greatly, the microadenoma having a much more benign course than that demonstrated by the macroadenoma.

Patients with pituitary tumors generally present with ovulatory dysfunction approximately 5 years before they develop galactorrhea. If

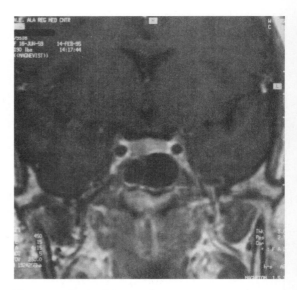

Figure 10-1 Magnetic resonance image demonstrating a pituitary microadenoma.

these lesions are seen early in life, disruption of the pubertal process can occur, and it is not uncommon to find large pituitary tumors in patients who have just gone through puberty yet fail to menstruate or have one or two menstrual cycles prior to the onset of amenorrhea. Alternatively, the patient with a prolactinoma may present with a polyendocrinopathy because lesions have been described that can produce both growth hormone and prolactin, and it should be remembered that there are adrenocorticotropic hormone (ACTH)–, thyroid-stimulating hormone (TSH)–, and gonadotropin-secreting adenomas as well. The workup of the patient with a prolactinoma consists of measurement of serum prolactin levels on multiple occasions; measurement of TSH to rule out compensated hypothyroidism, which can present with thyrotrope hypertrophy; and evaluation of the central nervous system with either CT scan or an MRI. Radiologists generally prefer the MRI (Fig. 10-3); however, most CT scans and MRI images cut at approximately 2 mm, which is adequate to differentiate whether one is dealing with a microadenoma or a macroadenoma. Obviously, in the era of managed care,

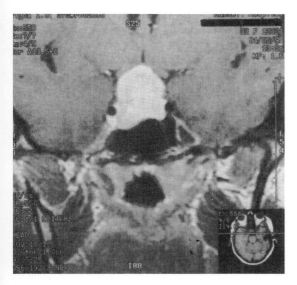

Figure 10-2 Magnetic resonance image demonstrating a pituitary microadenoma with involvement of the carotid artery.

the CT scan may be the method of choice. Visual field examinations using Goldman-Bowl perimetry (Fig. 10-4) should be restricted to individuals with demonstrated macroadenomas. Individuals with these types of lesions will present with superior bitemporal hemianopsia approximately 68 percent of the time. A lesion that does not extend outside the sella cannot possibly affect the optic chiasm; therefore, it is pointless to obtain such a study in these patients.

The etiology of prolactinomas is unclear. It has been suggested that these lesions acquire blood supply that is outside the normal hypothalamic portal pathway, thus decreasing the delivery of dopamine to the lactotropes.[24] Other studies have suggested alterations in various oncogenes. It has been suggested that there are receptor abnormalities in these lesions, and in fact, tumors have been described that do not have D_2 receptors on their surfaces.[25] Errors in signal transduction have been described; therefore, it is possible that these lesions represent the end result of multiple dysfunctions.

Treatment of Prolactinomas

The treatment of prolactinomas depends on the size of the lesion and the goals of the patient. Traditionally, neurosurgical resection was carried out, which resulted in greater than 90 percent cure rate in patients with microadenomas and approximately a 30 to 40 percent failure rate in patients with macroadenomas.[26] Unfortunately, many of the patients who were cured of their tumor still had hyperprolactinemia; therefore, medical therapy was required.

For individuals who desire medical therapy, dopamine agonists were introduced in the mid-1970s. The prototype drug bromocriptine (Parlodel Novartis) binds to both D_1 and D_2 receptors and inhibits the synthesis and secretion of prolactin.[27] Because of the D_1 activities, individuals frequently have hypotension, nausea, and nasal stuffiness. Dysphoria is also a common complaint when using this drug. The dose range generally is 2.5 to 10 mg, although when treating Parkinson's disease doses of 140 to 180 mg per day have been used. Bromocriptine should be administered at night to block the nocturnal surge of prolactin and should be started at dose levels of 1.25 mg and increased slowly over several weeks. The vaginal delivery of this drug has been advocated to attenuate side effects; however, I have not found this to be successful.

Pergolide mesylate (Permax, Eli Lilly Co.) is approved for the treatment of Parkinson's disease; however, it is used worldwide for the treatment of hyperprolactinemia.[28] This is active in a dose range of 50 to 100 μg once a day, and it is a nonergoline dopamine agonist. It has similar side effects to Parlodel, but individuals respond slightly differently to these drugs, and it is an alternative therapy. Cabergoline (Dostinex, Pharmacia) was developed in Europe; it is a pure D_2 receptor agonist and therefore has minimal side effects.[29] Its dose range is 0.25 to 0.5 mg twice a week. The side effects of this drug are minimal, but the drug is quite expensive (Table 10-4).

▶ **TABLE 10-4:** DOPAMINE AGONISTS

Bromocriptine (Parlodel)	D_1, D_2	1.25–20 mg bid–qid
Pergolide (Permax)	D_1, D_2	50–100 μg qd
Cabergoline (Dostinex)	D_2	0.125–0.5 mg 2×/wk

Patients who go on dopamine agonist therapy generally require long-term treatment. Weaning a patient from this drug is a trial-and-error process, and in general, when one stops the dopamine agonist, prolactin levels rise. I have followed over 1000 patients with pituitary tumors and have never seen an individual who was suppressed initially with a dopamine agonist escape suppression. Therefore, the long-term follow-up of these individuals is customized based on clinical response. In general, the patient with a microadenoma who receives no treatment will have a 10 percent growth of the tumor, a 30 percent resolution of the tumor, and 60 percent of the time there will be no change.[30] These individuals can be followed through pregnancy as any other obstetric patient because numerous studies have demonstrated that these lesions do not cause a problem during gestation.[31] The macroadenoma, on the other hand, can grow aggressively during pregnancy, and there are two schools of thought regarding their management. In general, on the west coast patients are kept on dopamine agonist therapy throughout pregnancy. On the east coast there is a tendency to follow these patients expectantly with visual field examinations every 2 months. The measurement of prolactin during pregnancy is of no value in following these patients because

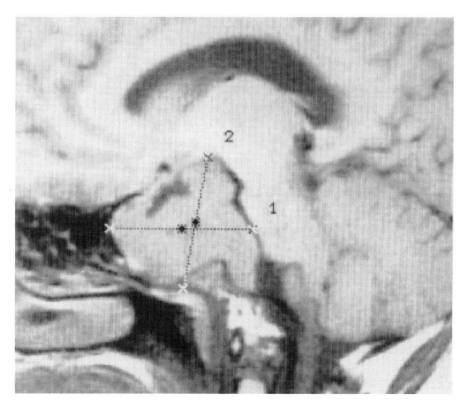

Figure 10-3 Demonstration of a large pituitary macroadenoma by MRI.

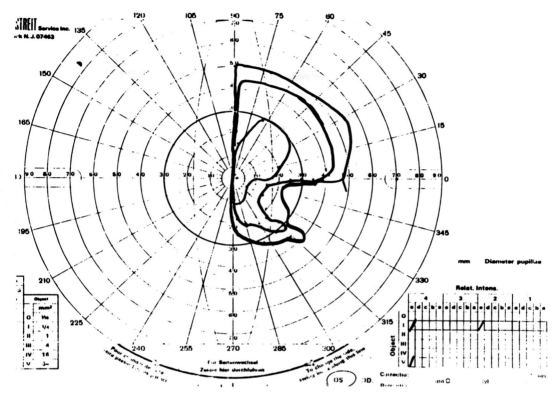

Figure 10-4 Visual field deficit in one eye of a patient with a large prolactinoma. Note the extremely limited field of vision encircled by the indicated border. In the opposite eye (visual field not shown), the patient had lost total vision.   *(Reproduced, with permission, from Blackwell, RE Diagnosis and Management of Prolactinomas Fert Steril 43:5, 1985.)*

prolactin levels generally rise to between 250 and 400 ng/mL during normal gestation.

The use of radiographic imaging also deserves mention. Since microadenomas grow slowly, there is no point in reimaging these individuals any sooner than every 10 years unless they have a change in symptoms. One can argue that when they are on dopamine agonist therapy, there is no point in reimaging them at all. The patient with a macroadenoma should be reimaged after about 6 months of therapy if the pituitary tumor is no longer visible or is now of a microadenoma size, and if individuals stay on therapy, one could argue that they do not need reimaging unless they have increased symptoms. The use of multiple nonindicated images is to be discouraged.

Growth Hormone-Secreting Tumors

Tumors that secrete growth hormone often present with insidious clinical alterations usually involving the face, hands, and feet. Bone growth is stimulated, with soft tissue proliferation usually resulting in enlargement of the nose, jaw, and superorbital ridges. Carpal tunnel syndrome sometimes develops with paresthesias of the hands, and the voice may deepen due to thickening of the vocal cords. Hypertension is encountered in one-fourth of patients, obesity in one-half, and enlargement is seen in the cardiac, hepatic, and renal systems. Patients are diagnosed by an elevated growth hormone level or abnormal response to a glucose load. The treatment of these lesions involves destruction of the tumor with either surgery, radiation, or suppression of tumor growth with somatostatin.[32,33]

ACTH-Secreting Tumors

ACTH-secreting tumors are somewhat rare with small lesions less than 1 cm. Ovulatory dysfunction usually occurs due to the presence of hypercorticalism, and urinary free cortisol levels can be expected to be greater than 150 μg/d. These lesions generally are treated by transsphenoidal pituitary resection.[34] Treatment of patients with pituitary irradiation in the face of persistent or recurrent Cushing's disease after unsuccessful transsphenoidal surgery can be expected to produce a remission rate of about 82 percent with long-term follow-up.

TSH-Secreting Tumors

The TSH-secreting pituitary adenoma is a rare cause of hyperthyroidism. The introduction of ultrasensitive TSH immunoassays have simplified their diagnosis. The availability of such tools aids in the early recognition of these tumors and prevents misdiagnosis and treatment. However, no single diagnostic test is pathopneumonic of the disease, and an elevation in the α-subunit level, elevation in serum sex hormone-binding globulin, absence or impaired TSH response to TRH, and triiodothyronine (T_3) suppression test are all used for markers in making the diagnosis of a TSH-secreting tumor. Most of these tumors are quite small (in the range of 3 mm) and therefore difficult to detect by either CT scanning or MRI. These tumors are generally treated surgically with irradiation therapy used for failure.[35]

Gonadotropin-Secreting Tumors

In the past it was considered that gonadotropin-secreting pituitary tumors were exceedingly rare, occurring primarily in men. Recently it has been demonstrated that these lesions are not uncommon and may comprise the majority of nonfunctioning tumors in women. Daneshdoost and colleagues described a series of patients with gonadotropin-secreting microadenomas that were all menopausal. TRH administration significantly increases FSH, LH, LHα, and LHβ subunit in some but not all cases. The most consistent response was the elevation of LHβ, which occurs 68 percent of the time.[36]

▶ CONCLUSION

Disorders of the hypothalamic-pituitary axis encompass a wide range of anatomic lesions and functional disorders. Physical findings, liberal use of the endocrine laboratory, and radiographic imaging allow differentiation of these disorders, which can be managed by medical therapy or surgery, with irradiation treatment being reserved for refractory cases.

KEY POINTS

1. Chronic hypothalamic anovulation is the most common ovulatory disorder and is characterized by normal gonadotropin levels and withdrawal bleeding in response to progesterone challenge.

2. Psychogenic amenorrhea generally is related to altered body weight, stress, and extremes in exercise. The condition is characterized by low gonadotropin levels with an FSH level greater than LH and a failure to withdraw to progesterone challenge.

3. Arcuate nucleus pulse frequency is generally maintained at one pulse per hour. However, slowing the rate to one pulse every 3 hours will result in ovulatory dysfunction.

4. The acquisition of a body weight of 48 kg is necessary for the institution of puberty. Individuals who lose 15 percent of their body weight often will become amenorrheic.

5. Anorexia nervosa is associated with weight loss greater than 25 percent of ideal, disturbed body image, and an intense fear of obesity.

6. Any space-occupying lesion of the hypothalamic portal system can cause disruption in ovulation.

7. The craniopharyngioma usually presents in children. The lesions are frequently large, and 50 percent of them are calcified.

8. Between 10 and 23 percent of the general population have pituitary tumors.

9. The most common nonfunctioning tumors are the null cell lesion, which tends to be large and grows slowly, and the subtype III lesion, which can be aggressive and grows rapidly.

10. The prolactinoma is the most common functional pituitary tumor found in humans.

11. The workup of the prolactinoma consists of the measurement of two serum prolactin levels, a TSH level, and the imaging of the sella turcica with either CT scanning or MRI.

12. Treatment of prolactinomas is directed at stimulation of the D_2 receptor. Activation of this receptor decreases both the synthesis and secretion of prolactin.

13. The microadenoma is a lesion less than 1 cm, the macroadenoma is a lesion greater than 1 cm. The microadenoma is a nonaggressive lesion, and the macroadenoma should be treated aggressively.

REFERENCES

1. Belchetz PE, et al. Hypophyseal responses to continuous and intermittent delivery of hypothalamic gonadotropin-releasing hormone. *Science* 1978;202:631.

2. Plant TM, Krey LC, Moossy J, et al. The accurate nucleus and the control of the gonadotropin and prolactin secretion in the female rhesus monkey *(Macaca mulatta)*. *Endocrinology* 1998;102:52.

3. Lachelin GCL, Yen SSC. Hypothalamic chronic anovulation. *Am J Obstet Gynecol* 1978;130:825.

4. Berga S, Mortola J, Gierton L, et al. Neuroendocrine aberrations in women with functional hypothalamic amenorrhea. *J Clin Endocrinol Metab* 1989;68:301.

5. Reame NE, Sauder SE, Case GD, et al. Pulsatile gonadotropin secretion in women with hypothalamic amenorrhea: Evidence that reduced frequency of gonadotropin secretion is the mechanism of persistent anovulation. *J Clin Endocrinol Metab* 1985;61:851.

6. Sanborn CF, Martin BJ, Wagner WW. Is athletic amenorrhea specific to runners? *Am J Obstet Gynecol* 1982;143:859.

7. Frisch RE, Wyshak G, Vincent L. Delayed menarche and amenorrhea in ballet dancers. *N Engl J Med* 1980;303:17.

8. Frisch RE. Body fat, menarche, and reproductive ability. *Semin Reprod Endocrinol* 1985; 3:45.

9. Vigersky RA, Loriaux D, Anderson AE, Lipsett MR. Anorexia nervosa: Behavioral and hypothalamic aspects. *Clin Endocrinol Metab* 1976; 5:517.

10. Crisp AH, Palmer RL, Kaluey RS. How common is anorexia nervosa? A prevalence study. *Br J Psychiatry* 1976;128:549.

11. Willis J, Grossman S. Epidemiology of anorexia nervosa in a defined region of Switzerland. *Am J Psychiatry* 1983;140:564.

12. Fairburn C. A cognitive behavioral approach to the treatment of bulimia. *Psychol Med* 1981; 11:707.

13. Patton G. Mortality in eating disorders. *Psychol Med* 1988;18:947.

14. Barglow P. Pseudocyesis: A paradigm of psychophysiological interactions. *Arch Gen Psychiatry* 1964;24:221.

15. Braunstein GD, Kohler PO. Pituitary function in Hand-Schüller-Christian disease; evidence for deficient growth hormone release in patients with short stature. *N Engl J Med* 1972; 286:1225.

16. Kallman F, Schonfeld WA, Barrera SW. Genetic aspects of primary eunuchoidism. *Am J Ment Defic* 1944;48:203.

17. Sheehan HL, Davis JC. Pituitary necrosis. *Br Med Bull* 1968;24:59.

18. Reid RL, Quigley ME, Yen SSC. Pituitary apoplexy: A review. *Arch Neurol* 1985;42:712.

19. Banna M. Craniopharyngioma: Based on 160 cases. *Br J Radiol* 1976;49:206.

20. Hsu TH, Shapiro JR, Tyson JE, et al. Hyperprolactinemia associated with empty sella syndrome. *JAMA* 1976;235:2002.

21. Costello RT. Subclinical adenoma of the pituitary gland. *Am J Pathol* 1936;12:205.

22. Sheng HZ, Zhadanov AB, Mosinger B Jr, et al. Specifications of pituitary cell lineages by the LIM homeobox gene *Lhx3*. *Science* 1996;272:1004.

23. Kovacs K, Scheithauer BW, Horvath E, Lloyd RV. The World Health Organization classification of adenohypophyseal neoplasms. *Cancer* 1996;78:502.

24. Schechter J, Goldsmith P, Wilson C, et al. Morphological evidence for the presence of arteries to human prolactinomas. *J Clin Endocrinol Metab* 1988;67:713.

25. Spada A, Basser M, Reza-Elahi F, et al. Differential transduction of dopamine signal in different subtypes of human growth hormone–secreting adenomas. *J Clin Endocrinol Metab* 1994;78:411.

26. Serri O, Basio E, Beauregard H, et al. Recurrence of hyperprolactinemia after selective transsphenoidal adenomectomy in women with prolactinomas. *N Engl J Med* 1983;309:280.

27. Molitch ME, Elton RL, Blackwell RE, et al. Bromocriptine as primary therapy for prolactin-secreting macroadenomas: Results of a prospective multicenter study. *J Clin Endocrinol Metab* 1985;60:698.

28. Blackwell RE, Bradley EL, Kline LB, et al. Comparison of dopamine agonists in the treatment of hyperprolactinemic syndrome: A multicenter study. *Fertil Steril* 1981;39:744.

29. Molitch ME. Medical management of prolactin-secreting pituitary adenomas. *Pituitary* 2002;5:56–65.

30. Weiss MH, Teal J, Gott P, et al. Natural history of microprolactinomas: Six-year follow-up. *Neurosurgery* 1983;12:180.

31. Bronstein MD, Salgado LR, de Castro Musolino NR. Medical management of pituitary adenomas: The special case of management of the pregnant woman. *Pituitary* 2002;5:99.

32. Shimon I, Nass D, Gross DJ. Pituitary macroadenoma secreting thyrotropin and growth hormone: Remission of bihormonal hypersecretion in response to lanreotide therapy. *Pituitary* 2001;4:265.

33. Mahamoud-Ahmed AS, Suh JH, Mayberg MR. Gamma knife radiosurgery in the management of patients with acromegaly: A review. *Pituitary* 2001;4:223.

34. Estrada J, Boronat M, Melgo M, et al. The long-term outcome of pituitary irradiation after unsuccessful transsphenoidal surgery in Cushing's disease. *N Engl J Med* 1997;336:172.

35. Beck-Peccoz P, Brucker-Davis F, Persani L, et al. Thyrotropin-secreting pituitary tumors. *Endocr Rev* 1996:17:610.

36. Shomali ME, Katznelson L. Medical therapy of gonadotropin-producing and nonfunctioning pituitary adenomas. *Pituitary* 2002;5:89.

CHAPTER 11

Disorders of the Adrenal

LYNNETTE K. NIEMAN

The adrenal gland is a major source of steroid and catecholamine hormones, and over- or underproduction of these hormones results in clinical disorders. These disorders can be classified by the type of hormone abnormality and by the area of the adrenal gland that functions abnormally.

Steroid hormones are synthesized in the adrenal cortex, which has three functional zones distinguished by the presence of specific steroidogenic enzymes that restrict hormone production (Fig. 11-1). In adults, the outermost layer, the glomerulosa, produces aldosterone and other mineralocorticoids, which regulate sodium resorption in the kidney and thus affect salt and water metabolism. The expression of CYP11B2, aldosterone synthase, is restricted to this functional zone. The regulation of aldosterone synthesis is primarily under the control of the renin-angiotensin system, via increased expression of CYP11B2 (Fig. 11-2). Renin is secreted by the renal juxtaglomerular cells in response to hypotension and low oncotic fluid pressure and is suppressed by hypertension and high salt intake. Renin cleaves angiotensin I from angiotensinogen, and angiotensin-converting enzyme converts angiotensin I into the biologically active form, angiotensin II. Angiotensin II increases peripheral vascular resistance and stimulates aldosterone secretion, which leads to sodium retention and increased plasma volume.

The middle functional layer of the adrenal cortex, the fasciculata, secretes cortisol, a glucocorticoid that regulates energy balance and many intracellular processes. Cortisol synthesis is regulated by adrenocorticotropin (ACTH), which increases cholesterol delivery to the mitochondrial steroidogenic enzymes and increases the synthesis of the CYP enzymes, including CYP11B1, which encodes for 11β-hydroxylase, which converts 11-deoxycortisol to cortisol. ACTH secretion by pituitary corticotropes, in turn, is increased by the hypothalamic secretion of corticotropin-releasing hormone (CRH). Both ACTH secretion and CRH secretion are inhibited by hypercortisolism and increased by hypocortisolism, thus maintaining homeostasis (Fig. 11-3).

The innermost cortical layer, the reticularis, synthesizes androgens such as androstenedione and dehydroepiandrosterone (DHEA) and represents about 50 percent of androgen production in premenopausal women. ACTH stimulates synthesis of these hormones.

The catecholamines epinephrine and norepinephrine, the major products of the adrenal medulla, regulate blood pressure, cardiac output, and vascular tone. Disorders of the adrenal medulla generally do not involve the cortex. The opposite is true in general, although recent data suggest that normal cortical function is essential for normal medullary development because examination of the adrenal glands from

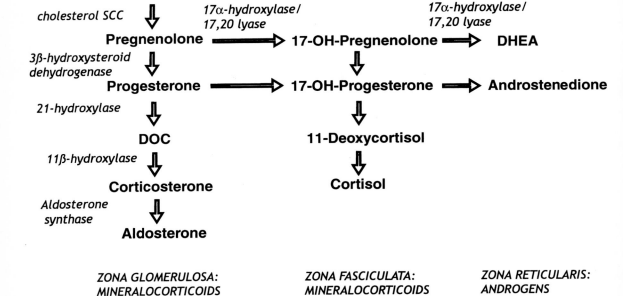

Figure 11-1 Steps in steroidogenesis in the three functional layers of the adrenal cortex: the glomerulosa, fasciculata, and reticularis.

a patient with poorly controlled congenital adrenal hyperplasia showed disordered morphology in the medulla.[1]

▶ FUNCTIONAL DISORDERS OF THE ADRENAL CORTEX: ADRENAL INSUFFICIENCY

Etiology of Adrenal Insufficiency

Adrenal insufficiency is a clinical syndrome caused by insufficient production of mineralocorticoid and/or glucocorticoid.[2] It may be caused by physical disruption of the adrenal glands, termed *primary adrenal insufficiency,* or by inadequate ACTH stimulation, termed *secondary adrenal insufficiency.* Disorders that affect the structure of the adrenal cortex tend to affect all three functional layers, resulting in decreased production of glucocorticoids, min-

eralocorticoids, and androgens. By contrast, disorders that affect CRH and/or ACTH production result only in decreased glucocorticoids (and androgens) because mineralocorticoid secretion does not depend on ACTH stimulation.

A number of disorders may destroy the adrenal cortex and cause primary adrenal insufficiency, including autoimmune attack, infections, and space-occupying lesions such as metastases or hemorrhage[3,4] (Table 11-1). One important genetic diagnosis to consider in young men is adrenoleukodystrophy, a rare X-linked condition characterized by deficiency of peroxisomal membrane adrenoleukodystrophy protein. A deficiency of this protein results in accumulation of very long-chain fatty acids (VLCFAs) in the central nervous system (CNS) and the adrenal glands, as well as increased circulating levels that can be detected as an increase in plasma C26:0 fatty acids. The clinical

▶ **TABLE 11-1:** CAUSES OF ADRENAL INSUFFICIENCY AND ANCILLARY TESTS

Specific Cause	Suggestive Clinical Features	Useful Ancillary Tests
Primary adrenal insufficiency	Hyperpigmentation, orthostatic hypotension	Hypokalemia, elevated ACTH
Idiopathic autoimmune destruction	The most common cause (80%) in developed countries, with or without other endocrinopathy as below	Antibodies to 21-hydroxylase are present; radiographically, these adrenal glands are small
Polyglandular failure type I[10]	Hypoparathyroidism, mucocutaneous candidiasis, vitiligo; age <20 years	
Polyglandular failure type II[9]	Insulin-dependent diabetes, autoimmune thyroid disease, alopecia areata, vitiligo; age >40 years	Radiographically, these adrenal glands are small
Infections: tuberculosis, systemic fungal diseases, and AIDS-associated opportunistic infections such as CMV[8]	15% of patients in U.S. series	These adrenal glands tend to be large on CT scan and may be calcified
Space-occupying adrenal lesions	Metastases from carcinoma of lung, breast, kidney, gut, lymphoma,[3] or possible hemorrhage (heparin use)[4]	Abnormal shape of adrenal glands on CT; evidence of hemorrhage
Bilateral adrenalectomy or treatment with steroidogenesis inhibitors	Ketoconazole, mitotane, aminoglutethimide, trilostane, and metyrapone all reduce cortisol levels[39]	
Adrenoleukodystrophy	X-linked—screen males; in child-hood, cognitive and gait disturbances, in adults, spastic paraparesis[5,6]	Deficiency of peroxisomal very long-chain acyl-CoA synthetase leads to elevated plasma C26:0 fatty acid levels
Genetic disorders in children	These are discussed in a recent review[7]	
Secondary adrenal insufficiency		
Suppression of the adrenal axis by exogenous or endogenous glucocorticoids	Medication history, history of Cushing's syndrome	Adrenal glands are small on CT
Structural lesions of the hypothalamus or pituitary gland (tumors, destruction by infiltrating disorders, x-irradiation, and lymphocytic hypophysitis)	Other pituitary deficiencies	Adrenal glands are normal or small on CT; MRI/CT may show pituitary or hypothalamic lesion
Isolated ACTH deficiency[55]		

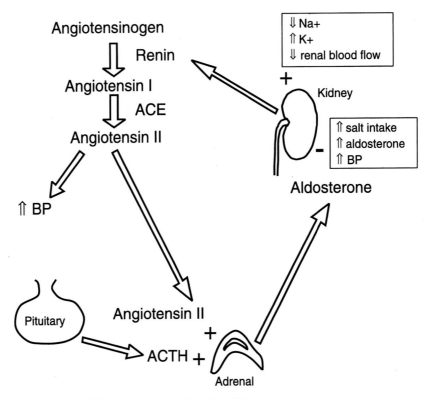

Figure 11-2 Regulation of the renin-angiotensin-aldosterone system.

phenotype varies, so the childhood form is characterized by cognitive and gait disturbances, and the adult form is characterized by spinal cord and peripheral nerve demyelination. In both, accumulation of VLCFAs in the adrenal cortex inhibits signal transduction by ACTH.[5,6] A number of rare congenital adrenal disorders that usually are diagnosed in childhood are the topic of a recent review.[7] Apart from congenital adrenal hyperplasia, reviewed below, these genetic disorders will not be considered further.

In underdeveloped countries where tuberculosis is common, it is the most common cause of adrenal insufficiency. However, other granulomatous diseases such as histoplasmosis, coccidioidomycosis, and blastomycosis, as well as acquired immune deficiency syndrome (AIDS)– associated infections such as

cytomegalovirus, also may destroy the gland.[8] One clue to an infectious etiology is enlarged glands on computed tomographic (CT) scans.

In developed countries where tuberculosis is uncommon, autoimmune etiologies, including isolated adrenal insufficiency and autoimmune syndromes, represent more than 80 percent of the cases of adrenal insufficiency[9,10] (see Table 11-1).

Secondary adrenal insufficiency is caused most often by exogenous or endogenous glucocorticoids, which suppress the hypothalamic-pituitary-adrenal axis. Long-standing exposure to hypercortisolism reduces CRH and ACTH, resulting in adrenal atrophy. When glucocorticoids are withdrawn, the glands, although intrinsically normal, cannot make enough glucocorticoid until the axis recovers.[11] Struc-

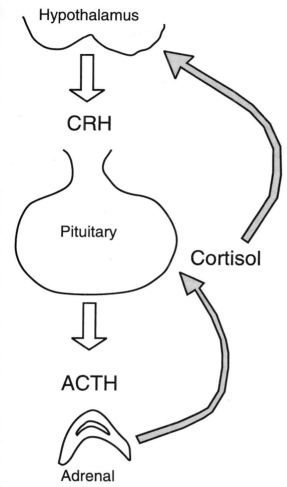

Hypothalamus

CRH

Pituitary

Cortisol

ACTH

Adrenal

Figure 11-3 Regulation of the hypothalamic-pituitary-adrenal axis.

tural lesions of the hypothalamus or pituitary gland also may interfere with CRH and/or ACTH secretion (see Table 11-1).

Clinical Features of Adrenal Insufficiency

Acute primary adrenal insufficiency presents with orthostatic hypotension, fever, hyperkalemia, hypernatremia, and hypoglycemia. It may be mistaken for septic shock. Patients with this presentation often have an acute disorder such as metastatic growth, hemorrhage, or infection. By contrast, patients with a chronic form of primary adrenal insufficiency complain of chronic malaise, fatigue, anorexia, weight loss, salt craving, and joint and back pain. Darkening of the skin in sun-exposed areas, as well as the creases of the hands, extensor surfaces, recent scars, buccal and vaginal mucosa, and nipples, is a hallmark feature caused by increased proopiomelanocortin production. The biochemical features are similar to those of the acute presentation. Clinical features of secondary adrenal insufficiency are similar to those listed earlier, but without skin darkening or features of mineralocorticoid deficiency.

Testing for Adrenal Insufficiency

A screening serum cortisol value is helpful but does not correctly categorize all patients, so additional testing is often necessary.[12] Patients with acute adrenal insufficiency may have a normal or subnormal plasma cortisol concentration, which is inappropriate in the setting of acute stress. If this diagnosis is suspected in a hypotensive patient, a cortisol value should be obtained when an intravenous line is inserted for fluid administration. Values of less than 18 μg/dL (500 nmol/L) suggest adrenal insufficiency.

There is no consensus on a single "best" diagnostic test for chronic adrenal insufficiency. If a screening cortisol value is less than 3 μg/dL (83 nmol/L) or more than 19 μg/dL (524 nmol/L), the diagnosis is virtually established or excluded, respectively.[12] However, many patients have intermediate values and require additional tests.

The best studied tests for evaluation of adrenal sufficiency use synthetic ACTH or insulin as a provocative stimulus. ACTH directly tests the ability of the adrenal glands to respond. Thus, in the setting of mild or recent secondary adrenal insufficiency, in which the adrenal glands are not atrophic, there may be a normal or near-normal response to the conventional 250-μg supraphysiologic dose of ACTH.[13] Because of this, a lower-dose test using 1 μg has been advocated.[12] With this lower dose, glands with only partial atrophy may have a subnormal response. The disadvantage of this test is that there is no commercial preparation of the lower dose of ACTH, so the drug must be diluted on site, raising issues of accurate dose delivery.[14] Others advocate use of the insulin tolerance test (ITT), based on its ability to test the entire axis.[15] Hypoglycemia tests the entire adrenal axis by stimulating CRH and hence ACTH release, which, in turn, stimulates cortisol. However, the ITT has the disadvantage that it may precipitate angina or seizures in vulnerable individuals and therefore may not be a good choice in older patients. Because of the potential need to treat hypoglycemia, the test requires additional medical personnel and is more costly than the ACTH tests. One problem with all these tests is that there is no agreement about the cutoff point for a normal response[12,14,16,17] (Table 11-2).

Having made the diagnosis of adrenal insufficiency, its etiology—primary or secondary—may be determined by measurement of plasma ACTH. These levels will be low (<10 pg/mL) in secondary disease and above the normal range in primary disorders. Additionally, hypokalemia and elevated plasma renin activity distinguish patients with primary forms of the disorder. All patients should then be considered for further testing to determine a specific etiology (see Table 11-1). An autoimmune cause of primary adrenal insufficiency may be diagnosed if antibodies to 21-hydroxylase (CYP21A2) are present.[18] In males, a VLCFA measurement will detect adrenoleukodystrophy.[6] Patients with secondary adrenal insufficiency should be evaluated for pituitary and hypothalamic structural lesions and for additional hormone deficiencies.

Treatment of Adrenal Insufficiency

Treatment of adrenal insufficiency involves physiologic replacement of the deficient steroids. Patients with acute adrenal insufficiency should receive fluid resuscitation and medical care as appropriate in addition to "stress" doses of hydrocortisone given intravenously (100 mg every 8 hours). This dose provides supraphysiologic glucocorticoid and mineralocorticoid activity.

For patients who are not acutely ill, hydrocortisone (12 to 15 mg/m² daily) provides glucocorticoid replacement in a way that can be easily titrated and given as divided doses during the day. Many patients do best by taking the medication as soon as possible in the morning; for those with afternoon fatigue, a split dose (two-thirds in the morning and one-third in the afternoon) may alleviate this complaint. Other glucocorticoids, especially prednisone (5 to 7.5 mg/d), have a longer half-life and may be superior to hydrocortisone in relieving fatigue (Table 11-3). However, the few avail-

▶ **TABLE 11-2:** TESTS FOR ADRENAL INSUFFICIENCY

Agent	Dose	Route	Time of Day	Time of Sampling	Cutoff Point for Normal
ACTH	250 μg	IV or IM	Any	30 min	>18–25.4 μg/dL (497–700 nmol/L)
ACTH	1 μg	IV	Not clear	To 60 min (earlier may be best)	>18–21.7 μg/dL (500–600 nmol/L)
Insulin	1–1.5 U/kg	IV	Any	0, 30, 60 min	>18 μg/dL (500 nmol/L); 18.8 μg/dL (520 nmol/L)

▶ **TABLE 11-3:** COMPARISON OF COMMONLY USED GLUCOCORTICOIDS

Agent	Biologic Half-Life (h)	Equivalent Glucocorticoid Dose (mg)	Relative Mineralcorticoid Activity
Cortisone	8–12	25	0.8
Cortisol (hydrocortisone)	8–12	20	1
Prednisone	12–36	5	0.8
Dexamethasone	36–72	0.3	0
Fludrocortisone	18–36	~2.1	250

able dosage formulations make it difficult to adjust the dose.

Patients with mineralocorticoid deficiency should receive fludrocortisone (0.05 to 0.3 mg/d). The optimal dose will vary depending on whether the glucocorticoid administered also has mineralocorticoid activity (hydrocortisone does, dexamethasone does not), as well as the salt intake of the patient.

Patients with primary adrenal insufficiency also are DHEA-deficient, and replacement of this hormone at a daily dose of 50 mg improved well-being and scores of fatigue, depression, and anxiety in one study. Women, but not men, evidenced improvement in sexual interest and the level of satisfaction with sex.[19]

Patients requiring glucocorticoid replacement therapy should receive education about the need for compliance and should wear a medical information bracelet or necklace that identifies this requirement (Medic Alert Foundation, 2323 Colorado Ave, Turlock, CA 95382; 1-800-432-5378). Patients and their families also need education about glucocorticoid adjustment during physiologic stress conditions, including emergency administration of intramuscular glucocorticoid using a kit containing prefilled syringes with injectable steroid.

Although there are few data to support the practice, glucocorticoid doses are increased during physically stressful situations. If the patient is vomiting, has severe diarrhea, or has collapsed, intramuscular glucocorticoids should be given before transport to a medical facility.

Otherwise, the daily oral dose is doubled when fever or nausea is present, although the dose need not be increased for minimal stress such as tooth extraction. For more moderately stressful situations, such as cholecystectomy, the dose is increased to 75 to 100 mg on the day of surgery, given parenterally, and tapered by 50 percent on each successive day. During maximally stressful conditions, such as major surgery, trauma, or labor and delivery, the daily hydrocortisone dose will be 100 to 300 mg with a less rapid taper.[20]

Unfortunately, there is no simple way to assess whether the replacement dose of glucocorticoids is correct. Clinical evaluation seeks to identify signs and symptoms of over- or underreplacement. In primary adrenal insufficiency, plasma ACTH levels decrease but generally remain elevated at 100 to 200 pg/mL. Plasma cortisol is cleared rapidly after hydrocortisone administration and cannot be used to judge adequacy of the dose. Similarly, urine free cortisol does not correlate well with adequate hydrocortisone dosage, although very elevated values suggest that the dose should be decreased. Development of cushingoid features or osteopenia suggest overtreatment. The mineralocorticoid dose is adjusted according to the plasma renin activity, which should be in the normal range. In patients with continued salt craving or hypotension, evaluation of renin, adjustment of fludrocortisone dosage, and addition of salt should be considered before the glucocorticoid dose is changed so as to avoid excess glucocorticoid treatment. New hirsutism, acne, or other signs of androgen excess may suggest overreplacement with DHEA.

► FUNCTIONAL DISORDERS OF THE ADRENAL CORTEX: CONGENITAL ADRENAL HYPERPLASIA (CAH)

Physiology of CAH

The congenital adrenal hyperplasias (CAHs) are a disparate group of diseases caused by a genetic deficiency of one of the enzymes needed for adrenal steroidogenesis (see Fig. 11-1). Patients with nearly complete deficiency of an enzyme (termed *classic* CAH) required for cortisol synthesis present in childhood with adrenal insufficiency. This is most problematic in patients with mutations of the 21-hydroxylase (*CYP21*) or 11β-hydroxylase (*CYP11B1* and *B2*) gene, which account for nearly all CAH cases.[21] Because of relative glucocorticoid insufficiency, ACTH levels increase and stimulate the androgen synthetic pathway. As a result, there is an increase in circulating androgens, as well as precursors just proximal to the enzymatic block, 17-hydroxyprogesterone and 11-deoxycortisol, respectively, in 21-hydroxylase and 11β-hydroxylase deficiency. As a result, severely affected girls may be virilized in utero. Most patients with the classic form of CYP21 deficiency also have salt wasting. Girls and women with nonclassic CAH have greater enzyme activity, so cortisol production is adequate, but increased adrenocorticol function causes hyperandrogenism after puberty.[22] This disorder is considered elsewhere in Chapter 13.

Testing for CYP21 Deficiency

The diagnosis of 21-hydroxylase deficiency should be considered in an infant with salt wasting, ambiguous genitalia, or hypotension and is confirmed by measurement of 17-hydroxyprogesterone before and 60 minutes after administration of 250 μg ACTH. Patients with classic and nonclassic CAH have values greater than 11 μg/L (35 nmol/L), normal individuals have values less than 3 to 9 μg/L (10 to 30 nmol/L), and heterozygote carriers have intermediate values.[21]

Prenatal diagnosis of CAH generally is considered after a couple has had an affected child and wishes to undertake prenatal treatment in a subsequent pregnancy. To do this, parental DNA samples are needed to segregate the alleles and identify the mutations. Fetal DNA obtained by chorionic villous sampling is screened for the maternal and paternal mutations and is examined for presence of the Y chromosome. This should be done in a laboratory with extensive experience.[23,24]

Treatment of Congenital Adrenal Hyperplasia

Children with classic CAH should receive replacement glucocorticoid and mineralocorticoid if they have the salt-losing form or increased plasma renin activity. Many different regimens are advocated; most use hydrocortisone 10 to 20 mg/m^2 per day and fludrocortisone 0.05 to 0.2 mg/day, aiming for mildly elevated morning 17-hydroxyprogesterone levels and normal plasma renin activity. Physical features and clinical symptoms should be monitored for evidence of excessive (e.g., decreased linear growth) or insufficient (e.g., hypotension) treatment. It is often quite difficult to reduce excess androgen without giving excess glucocorticoids. After growth is complete, children are often changed to a longer-acting glucocorticoid such as prednisone, which is continued as lifelong therapy.[21]

While patients with nonclassic CAH generally do not require treatment for adrenal insufficiency, reducing ACTH stimulus to the adrenal gland by exogenous glucocorticoid administration may reduce excess androgens that cause bone age advancement, severe acne, hirsutism, menstrual irregularity, and infertility.

Prenatal treatment seeks to minimize ambiguous genitalia in a female fetus and is accomplished by administering dexamethasone to the mother. The dexamethasone crosses the placenta and suppresses fetal ACTH and hence androgens. Because genital development occurs in the first trimester, treatment is initiated as soon as pregnancy is confirmed and is stopped if prenatal diagnostic tests reveal an unaffected female or a male fetus. Statistically, treatment will continue in only one of eight pregnancies. While this strategy works well to reduce genital ambiguity, its long-term side effects on the children are not well known, and it carries some increased morbidity for the mother. Thus many consider this a research endeavor, and all would advocate that only multidisciplinary teams with great experience institute this treatment.[24,25]

Because of genital ambiguity, many female infants require corrective surgery. This is usually done in infancy and perhaps again as needed in late adolescence or adulthood. Again, management by an experienced team is critical.

▶ DISORDERS OF THE ADRENAL CORTEX: HYPERCORTISOLISM

Cushing's syndrome is a symptom complex that reflects excessive tissue exposure to cortisol. The diagnosis cannot be made without both clinical features and biochemical abnormalities. Thus clinical features consistent with the syndrome prompt biochemical screening.[26–28]

Clinical features of Cushing's syndrome (Table 11-4) reflect the amount and duration of exposure to excess cortisol.[29] Patients may present with different combinations of these signs and symptoms (Fig. 11-4). The number and severity of the symptoms usually correlate with the duration and severity of cortisol excess. Many of these signs and symptoms are common in the general population and may lead to a misdiagnosis of psychiatric disorders, the metabolic syndrome, anovulation, simple obesity, fibromyalgia, or acute illness. For example, one study of 250 women with hirsutism found only one with Cushing's syndrome.[30]

▶ **TABLE 11-4:** FREQUENCY OF CLINICAL SIGNS AND SYMPTOMS AMONG 70 PATIENTS WITH CUSHING'S SYNDROME

Sign/Symptom	Percent
Decreased libido	100
Obesity or weight gain	97
Plethora	94
Round face	88
Menstrual changes	84
Hirsutism	81
Hypertension	74
Eccymoses	62
Lethargy, depression	62
Striae	56
Weakness	56
ECG changes or atherosclerosis	55
Dorsal fat pad	54
Edema	50
Abnormal glucose tolerance	50
Osteopenia or fracture	50
Headache	47
Backache	43
Recurrent infections	25
Abdominal pain	21
Acne	21
Female balding	13

Modified, with permission, from Plotz CM, et al.[29]

Biochemical Testing for Cushing's Syndrome

Screening tests are needed to establish the diagnosis of Cushing's syndrome.[26–28] However, the commonly used screening tests have poor diagnostic accuracy. When judged using a criterion that maximizes sensitivity (diagnosis of the disorder in patients who are affected), a number of patients without the disorder will be falsely diagnosed. One option is to follow patients over time and to screen them only as they acquire new features of the syndrome. Since Cushing's syndrome tends to progress

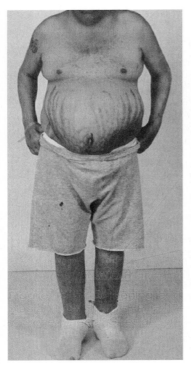
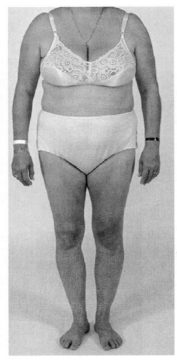
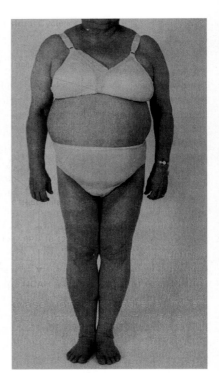

Figure 11-4 Patients with Cushing's syndrome illustrating the phenotype of centripetal obesity. Not all patients have gross centripetal obesity; some appear merely overweight.

over time, the absence of progression mitigates against the diagnosis.[29]

Signs that best predict possible Cushing's syndrome include redistribution of fat to the supraclavicular and temporal areas, proximal muscle weakness, wide (>1 cm) purple striae (Fig. 11-5), new psychiatric symptoms, decreased cognition, and decreased short-term memory. Testing also is indicated for a patient who has acquired additional cushingoid features over time.

Screening tests for Cushing's syndrome include tests of excessive cortisol production and impaired sensitivity to glucocorticoid negative feedback. Urine free cortisol (UFC) excretion over 24 hours is an integrated measure of hypercortisolism. It is increased in Cushing's syndrome, as well as in depression, anxiety, obsessive-compulsive disorder, chronic pain, severe exercise, alcoholism, uncontrolled dia-

betes, and morbid obesity.[31] In these so-called pseudo-Cushing states it is thought that central brain mechanisms stimulate CRH release with subsequent activation of the entire hypothalamic-pituitary-adrenal axis. Cortisol negative-feedback inhibition of CRH and ACTH release restrains the resulting hypercortisoluria to less than fourfold normal. Thus normal UFC excretion excludes Cushing's syndrome (apart from patients with intermittent hypercortisolism), but elevated UFC identifies patients with pseudo-Cushing states as well as Cushing's syndrome. Since UFC in pseudo-Cushing states tends not to exceed four times the upper limit of normal, higher values establish the diagnosis of Cushing's syndrome (or the more rare disorder of glucocorticoid resistance).

The methodology for measurement of UFC is moving away from immunoassays to more structurally based detection systems. Antibodies used

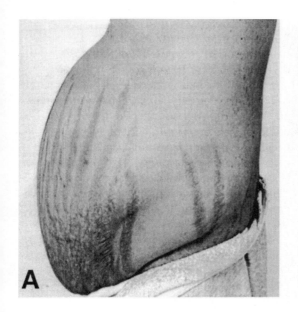
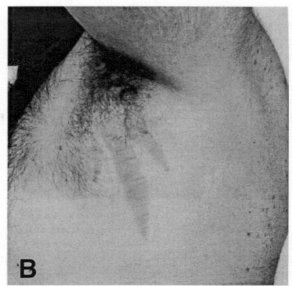
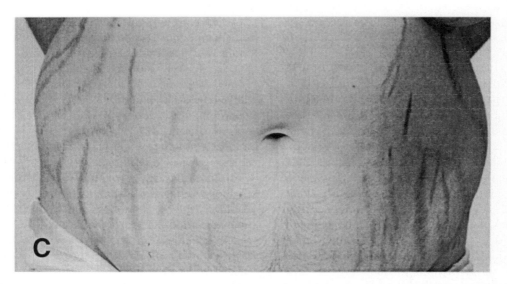

Figure 11-5 Typical striae in Cushing's syndrome. Wide (>1 cm) purple striae *(A, B)* are most specific to Cushing's syndrome, but striae may be pink and less wide *(C)*. Striae occur most often on the abdomen, but may be seen in the axilla or on the breasts, buttocks and thighs.

in immunoassays interact with cortisol and its metabolites, as well as structurally similar steroids. By contrast, liquid chromatography– mass spectroscopy (LC-MS) distinguishes cortisol from these other compounds, so the normal range is lower and more specific.[32] Because of these assay differences, it is important to interpret the results using the assay-specific normative range.

Measurement of plasma cortisol at midnight is a useful way to distinguish between pseudo-Cushing states and Cushing's syndrome with 95 percent diagnostic accuracy using a cutoff point of more than 7.5 μg/dL for the diagnosis of Cushing's syndrome.[33] Measurement of salivary cortisol at bedtime or midnight works as well as the plasma cortisol and is more convenient. However, the cutoff points used in the various studies are different, so salivary cortisol assays must be validated before they are used for this purpose.[34,35]

Measurement of plasma cortisol after administration of dexamethasone provides an index of sensitivity to glucocorticoid administration. The classic test involves oral administration of dexamethasone (1 mg) between 11 P.M. and midnight and measurement of plasma cortisol between 8 and 9 A.M. the next day. Because some patients with Cushing's disease are as sensitive to dexamethasone as normal individuals, the best criterion for interpretation is debated. Recent proposals to characterize a normal response as less than 1.8 μg/dL (50 nmol/L) will result in increased sensitivity but will greatly increase the number of false-positive results.[36] There is up to a 30 percent false-positive rate in chronic illness, obesity, psychiatric disorders, and normal individuals using a higher cutoff point (5 μg/dL).[37]

The 2-day, 2-mg dexamethasone suppression test (DST) works well to discriminate normal individuals and those with a pseudo-Cushing state from patients with Cushing's syndrome if plasma cortisol end points of 1.4 or 2.2 μg/dL are used. The test involves taking dexamethasone (500 μg) orally every 6 hours for eight doses and measuring plasma cortisol 2 or 8 hours after the last dose. The test has excellent sensitivity (90 to 100 percent) and specificity (97 to 100 percent) for discriminating Cushing's syndrome but has the disadvantage of high cost and the requirement for excellent patient compliance.[28,31] The immediate subsequent administration of CRH (1 μg/kg of body weight IV) and measurement of cortisol 15 minutes later increased the sensitivity and specificity to 100 percent in a small study of 58 patients who used values greater than 1.4 μg/dL

(38 nmol/L) to indicate Cushing's syndrome.[31] While this combined dexamethasone-CRH test has a very high diagnostic accuracy, it has the disadvantages of the 2-day DST and the added cost of CRH testing. Because of these drawbacks, in the United States these tests usually are reserved for patients with ambiguous or confusing results on UFC or the 1-mg DST. CRH is available commercially (ACTHREL, Ferring Corp.) with Food and Drug Administration (FDA)–approved labeling for the differential diagnosis of Cushing's syndrome. Use of the agent in the dexamethasone-CRH test represents an off-label use.

Any dexamethasone test may give false-positive results in patients with abnormal metabolic clearance of the drug. Alcohol, rifampin, phenytoin, and phenobarbital induce the P450 enzymes that metabolize the agent and increase its clearance, whereas renal or hepatic failure retard dexamethasone clearance. Measurement of a dexamethasone level can determine if its clearance has been altered when these medications cannot be discontinued.

Tests for the Differential Diagnosis of Cushing's Syndrome

Endogenous Cushing's syndrome is caused by primary adrenal hyperfunction (15 percent) or by excessive ACTH secretion from a tumor (85 percent)[38] (Table 11-5). Since hypercortisolism suppresses ACTH secretion from normal corticotropes, plasma ACTH values are low (<10 pg/mL) in primary adrenal disorders (adenoma, cancer, and rare bilateral hyperplasia). For this reason, measurement of plasma ACTH is the first test in the differential diagnosis of Cushing's syndrome. If values are low (<10 pg/mL), an adrenal CT scan will identify the site(s) of adrenal abnormality.

Plasma ACTH values >10 pg/mL are found in corticotropic tumors (termed *Cushing's disease*) and ectopic ACTH-secreting tumors. These patients must undergo a complex set of biochemical and radiographic tests to discrim-

▶ **TABLE 11-5:** ETIOLOGY OF CUSHING'S SYNDROME

Exogenous	Endogenous
Most common cause of Cushing's syndrome	ACTH-independent, autonomous adrenal activation (20%)
Due to prescribed glucocorticoids (oral, intramuscular or inhaled) or ACTH	Adrenal carcinoma (40–50%)
	Adrenal adenoma (40–50%)
May be factitious or iatrogenic	Rare causes: Primary pigmented nodular adrenal disease, McCune-Albright syndrome, massive macronodular adrenal disease
	ACTH-dependent, adrenal activation by excessive ACTH (80%)
	Ectopic ACTH secretion (20%)
	Corticotrope adenoma (80%)
	Ectopic CRH secretion (rare)

inate between these etiologies, ideally under the direction of an experienced endocrinology team. While inferior petrosal sinus sampling is the best test, the 8-mg DST, the CRH stimulation test, and magnetic resonance imaging (MRI) of the pituitary also may be useful. Identification of an ectopic ACTH-secreting tumor relies on imaging studies. By contrast, pituitary MRI often is normal in Cushing's disease and is not required to establish the diagnosis.[27,28,38]

Treatment of Cushing's Syndrome

The optimal treatment of Cushing's syndrome is surgical resection of the lesion that is producing excessive ACTH or cortisol. This is generally successful in primary adrenal disorders, either via unilateral or bilateral adrenalectomy, except in patients with adrenal cancer, which is often metastatic at the time of presentation. In Cushing's disease, transsphenoidal resection of a corticotropic tumor is the treatment of choice.[39] When surgery is unsuccessful or cannot be done, or when the tumor cannot be found, bilateral adrenalectomy is an option. Pituitary irradiation may be used to treat Cushing's disease, generally followed by medical steroidogenesis inhibition until the radiation takes effect. Medical therapy or adrenalectomy

also may be used for patients with metastatic cortisol- or ACTH-producing tumors or when an ectopic ACTH-secreting tumor is occult.[40]

▶ DISORDERS OF THE ADRENAL CORTEX: PRIMARY ALDOSTERONISM

Primary adrenal hyperaldosteronism presents as spontaneous hypokalemia with hypertension.[41] The diagnosis also should be considered in patients with hard-to-control hypertension and in those with an adrenal incidentaloma and hypertension, regardless of the potassium level.

Testing for Aldosteronism

As shown in Figure 11-2, aldosterone levels will increase passively if renin increases, e.g., in patients with renal artery stenosis. Because of this, increased aldosterone levels alone do not identify an aldosterone-producing adrenal tumor or hyperplasia. However, when aldosterone levels increase from a primary adrenal disorder, renin levels will decrease. Thus the diagnosis of these primary adrenal disorders requires an increased ratio of aldosterone to plasma renin activity (>20) in the setting of an elevated aldosterone value greater than 15 pg/mL. β-Adrenergic antagonists and spironolactone decrease plasma renin activity and should be discontinued for 2 to 4 weeks (6 to 8 weeks for spironolactone) if possible, but potassium should be given to maintain normal potassium levels.[42,43] Ideally, specimens are obtained after 2 hours of standing to give the best diagnostic accuracy. The diagnosis is confirmed by measurement of urinary or plasma aldosterone after oral sodium loading. A 24-hour urinary aldosterone excretion rate >10 to 14 μg/d (28 to 39 nmol/d) is considered diagnostic of primary hyperaldosteronism if the urinary sodium concentration is >250 mmol/d. Alternatively, isotonic saline (500 ml/L for 4 to 6 hours) will suppress plasma aldosterone levels to <10 ng/dL (280 pmol/L) in normal individuals but not those with hyperaldosteronism. Recognition that some patients have a more normal response has led to a more stringent al-

dosterone criterion of <5 to 8 ng/dL to exclude the disorder[44] (Table 11-6).

Tests for the Differential Diagnosis of Hyperaldosteronism

Once the diagnosis has been made, its etiology should be established so as to provide appropriate treatment. The most common causes of primary aldosteronism are adrenal hyperplasia and aldosterone-producing adenoma. Patients with an aldosterone-producing tumor are not responsive to renin-angiotensin regulation and do not respond to manipulations of this system, whereas patients with adrenal hyperplasia tend to retain normal physiologic responses. As a result, patients with an adenoma do not show an increase in aldosterone in response to upright posture, whereas patients with hyperplasia do. Additionally, plasma levels of 18-

► **TABLE 11-6:** TESTING FOR HYPERALDOSTERONISM

Test	How to Do It	Interpretation
Screening Test		
Aldosterone to plasma plasma renin activity	Specimens are obtained after 2 hours of standing	Ratio >20 suggests hyper-aldosteronism if concomitant aldosterone value >15 pg/mL
Confirmatory Tests		
Oral sodium loading	Ensure that diet has high sodium content (>200 meq/d); if unsure, give NaCl tablets, 2 g tid for 3 days; collect a 24-hour urine on the third day	A 24-hour urinary aldosterone excretion rate greater than 10–14 μg/d (28–39 nmol/d); the urinary sodium should be >250 mmol/d.
Isotonic saline infusion	Give 0.9% NaCl, 500 mL/h for 4–6 hours intravenously; measure plasma aldosterone at the end of the infusion	Plasma aldosterone levels >10 ng/dL (280 pmol/L) = hyperaldosteronism some use <5–8 ng/dL to exclude the disorder)
Tests for the Differential Diagnosis		
Adrenal vein sampling	Performed under fluoroscopy; both veins and IVC are cannulated; ACTH 250 μg given intravenously; cortisol and aldosterone measured at time 1 and 15 minutes	Aldosterone:cortisol >5 on the side of an adenoma; hyperplasia has similar values bilaterally

hydroxycorticosterone are usually more than 100 ng/dL in patients with adenoma. Unfortunately, the presence or absence of an adrenal mass does not unequivocally confirm or exclude an adenoma.[45,46] Patients with biochemical findings consistent with adenoma and imaging findings that do not show a mass should undergo bilateral adrenal vein sampling in an experienced center. This technically challenging procedure should be done with ACTH stimulation and simultaneous sampling of each adrenal vein and a peripheral vein for measurement of aldosterone and cortisol. Patients with an adenoma show a unilateral increase in the aldosterone-cortisol ratio (usually greater than fivefold), whereas those with hyperplasia tend to have similar values on each side.[47]

Glucocorticoid-remediable aldosteronism (GRA) is an important rare genetic cause of hyperaldosteronism. This disorder manifests as difficult-to-control hypertension in young individuals, often without hypokalemia, and is associated with early hemorrhagic strokes. It is caused by unequal crossing over between the 11β-hydroxylase *(CYP11B1)* and aldosterone synthase *(CYP11B2)* genes. As a result, the ACTH-responsive promoter for CYP11B1 regulates the expression of CYP11B2. It can be diagnosed via detection of the hybrid steroids 18-oxocortisol and 18-OH-cortisol in the urine. Patients suspected of having the disorder may have genetic analysis performed by calling the International GRA Registry (1-617-732-5011). Dexamethasone suppresses aldosterone levels in these patients, and this response may suggest the diagnosis.[48]

Treatment of Hyperaldosteronism

In general, patients with single aldosterone-producing tumors undergo unilateral adrenalectomy, with normalization of blood pressure in about half.[49] Patients with bilateral hyperplasia do not respond well to bilateral adrenalectomy and are treated medically with the mineralocorticoid antagonist spironolactone

(100 to 500 mg/d) or the sodium channel blocker amiloride (5 to 15 mg twice daily). Patients with GRA respond well to glucocorticoid suppression of ACTH.

▶ DISORDERS OF THE ADRENAL CORTEX: HYPERANDROGENISM

Women with excess circulating androgens or increased sensitivity to androgens present with complaints of hirsutism, acne, and/or anovulation/infertility.[50] When testosterone is secreted in great excess, women may virilize and show deepened voice, clitoromegaly, a masculinized body habitus, and alopecia. As part of the hyperandrogenic anovulation syndrome, women may develop features of the metabolic syndrome, with hyperlipidemia, hypertension, and visceral obesity.[51] While hyperandrogenism often is caused by ovarian androgen production, it is important to consider the possibility of an adrenal source. The adrenal causes of hyperandrogenism—CAH, Cushing's disease, adrenal cancer, and androgen-producing adrenal adenoma—are uncommon and may be suggested when DHEA, DHEA sulfate (DHEAS), and androstenedione are increased. Since DHEA and DHEAS levels decline throughout adult life, these values must be interpreted with age-specific normal ranges. Although a tumor is more likely if the DHEAS concentration is >500 μg/dL or the testosterone concentration is >200 ng/ml, it is not excluded at lower levels.[52] Other causes of hyperandrogenism are presented in Chapter 13.

▶ DISORDERS OF THE ADRENAL MEDULLA: PHEOCHROMOCYTOMA

Clinical Features of Pheochromocytoma

The excess catecholamine production by a pheochromocytoma classically presents as a

▶ **TABLE 11-7:** SIGNS AND SYMPTOMS THAT SUGGEST PHEOCHROMOCYTOMA

Sign or Symptom	Comments
Classic triad	Episodic headache, sweating, and tachycardia
Hypertension	Especially if difficult to control or paroxysmal
Associated signs	Papilledema, pallor, dilated cardiomyopathy, orthostatic hypotension, or anxiety attacks
Severe hyper- or hypotension during surgery or pregnancy	
In the context of familial syndromes	von Hippel–Lindau disease, neurofibromatosis, or MEN-2

triad of episodic headache, sweating, and tachycardia.[41] Nearly all patients are hypertensive, but paroxysmal hypertension occurs in only about 50 percent. Patients may have other symptoms, including papilledema, pallor, dilated cardiomyopathy, orthostatic hypotension, and anxiety attacks (Table 11-7). Depending on the spectrum of signs and symptoms, the differential diagnosis includes panic disorder, hyperthyroidism, and other causes of hypertension, headache, or heart disease. Sympathomimetic drugs (amphetamines, epinephrine, phenylpropanolamine, and monoamine oxidase inhibitors) taken with tyramine-containing foods may precipitate hypertension that mimics the symptoms of pheochromocytoma.

The diagnosis of pheochromocytoma also may be suspected on the basis of severe hyper- or hypotension during surgery or pregnancy and in the context of familial syndromes that include the condition, such as von Hippel–Lindau disease, neurofibromatosis, or multiple endocrine neoplasia type 2 (MEN-2).

Testing for Pheochromocytoma

The diagnosis of pheochromocytoma is made by measurement of plasma or urine catecholamines or metabolites such as metanephrine in a patient not taking medications that elevate these values.[41,53] An increase in plasma catecholamines in response to glucagon is highly specific (few normal individuals demonstrate

this), and lack of suppression of plasma catecholamines after clonidine is a very sensitive test. A normal response to each virtually excludes pheochromocytoma. However, there is a risk to giving an agent such as glucagon, so this testing usually is reserved for patients with equivocal results.

Having made the diagnosis, a CT scan and/or MRI is obtained to locate the tumor(s), which are usually in the adrenal medulla or the abdomen (95 percent) but may occur anywhere in the sympathetic ganglia. Occasionally, ^{123}I-meta-iodobenzylguanidine (MIBG), which is taken up by these cells, may be needed to localize the tumor. Bilateral pheochromocytomas are more likely in the associated familial disorders, von Hippel–Lindau syndrome, and MEN-2. However, a large fraction of patients with nonsyndromic pheochromocytoma have a germ-line mutation, so screening the patient and family may be reasonable.[54]

Treatment of Pheochromocytoma

These tumors should be resected because there is a chance of malignancy. Because manipulation of the tumor may release large quantities of catecholamines, an experienced surgical and anesthesiology team is necessary to reduce morbidity. Preoperative administration of α- and β-adrenergic antagonists, with or without metyrosine, which inhibits catecholamine synthesis, is used to prevent intraoperative hypertension.

KEY POINTS

1. When acute, primary adrenal insufficiency presents with hypotension, but when chronic, nonspecific features of malaise, fatigue, nausea, weight loss, and joint pain predominate. Secondary adrenal insufficiency does not include the hyperkalemia typical of primary adrenal insufficiency.

2. The diagnosis of adrenal insufficiency is likely when the morning cortisol concentration is <3 μg/dL (83 nmol/L), but most patients have values between 3 and 19 μg/dL and require testing with synthetic ACTH or insulin. The optimal dose of ACTH and the cutoff points (18 to 25 μg/dL) for the cortisol response to these stimuli are controversial.

3. Treatment of adrenal insufficiency and classic CYP21 congenital adrenal hyperplasia involves replacement of deficient steroids. Glucocorticoids are best replaced using hydrocortisone, whereas fludrocortisone provides mineralocorticoid replacement. Doses are adjusted according to clinical parameters and to normalize the plasma renin activity. Increased doses are given during extreme physical stress such as surgery or trauma.

4. Cushing's syndrome is suggested by a variety of clinical features and requires confirmation by biochemical demonstration of excess cortisol production and/or impaired sensitivity to glucocorticoid negative feedback. Apart from purple striae and proximal muscle weakness, clinical features are common in the general population. Additionally, other conditions (psychiatric disorders, exercise, pain, morbid obesity) are associated with mild hypercortisolism. Because of this, watchful waiting and observation for progression may be needed before the diagnosis can be established.

5. The differential diagnosis and treatment of Cushing's syndrome and the prenatal treatment of CAH are best carried out by an experienced multidisciplinary endocrinology team.

6. Primary aldosteronism should be suspected in patients with hypokalemia and/or hard-to-control hypertension. The diagnosis is suggested if the ratio of aldosterone to plasma renin activity is greater than 20 in the setting of a plasma aldosterone concentration of >15 pg/mL. The diagnosis is confirmed by failure of a sodium load to suppress aldosterone. Adrenal venous sampling may be needed to distinguish between the etiologies of adrenal adenoma and hyperplasia.

7. Pheochromocytoma should be suspected in patients with the classic triad of episodic headache, tachycardia, and sweating in the setting of hypertension. However, other associated signs (pallor, orthostatic hypotension, and anxiety attacks) may obscure the diagnosis, which is established by documentation of increased urinary or plasma catecholamine or metabolite concentrations.

REFERENCES

1. Merke DP, Chrousos GP, Eisenhofer G, et al. Adrenomedullary dysplasia and hypofunction in patients with classic 21-hydroxylase deficiency. *N Engl J Med* 2000;343:1362.
2. Nieman LK, Rother KI. Glucocorticoids for postnatal treatment of adrenal insufficiency and for the prenatal treatment of congenital adrenal hyperplasia, in Meikle AW (ed). *Endocrine Replacement Therapy in Clinical Practice*. Totowa, NJ: Humana Press, 1999; p 285.
3. Ihde JK, Turnbull AD, Bajourunas DR. Adrenal insufficiency in the cancer patient: Implications for the surgeon. *Br J Surg* 1990;77:1335.
4. Rao RH, Vagnucci AH, Amico JA. Bilateral massive adrenal hemorrhage: Early recognition and treatment. *Ann Intern Med* 1989;110:227.
5. Rizzo WB. X-linked adrenoleukodystrophy: A cause of primary adrenal insufficeincy in males. *Endocrinologist* 1992;2:177.

6. Moser AB, Kreiter N, Bezman L, et al. Plasma very long chain fatty acids in 3000 peroxisome disease patients and 29,000 controls. *Ann Neurol* 1999;45:100.

7. Ten S, New M, Maclaren N. Clinical review 130: Addison's disease 2001. *J Clin Endocrinol Metab* 2001;86:2909.

8. Piedrola G, Casado JL, Lopez E, et al. Clinical features of adrenal insufficiency in patients with acquired immunodeficiency syndrome. *Clin Endocrinol (Oxf)* 1996;45:97.

9. Betterle C, Volpato M, Greggio AN, et al. Type 2 polyglandular autoimmune disease (Schmidt's syndrome). *J Pediatr Endocrinol Metab* 1996;9(suppl 1):113.

10. Ahonen P, Myllarnieini S, Sipila I, et al. Clinical variation of autoimmune polyendocrinopathy-candidiasis-ectodermal dystrophy (APECED) in a series of 68 patients. *N Engl J Med* 1990; 322:1829.

11. Graber AL, Ney RL, Nicholson WE, et al. Natural history of pituitary-adrenal recovery following long-term suppression with corticosteroid. *J Clin Endocrinol Metab* 1965;25:11.

12. Grinspoon SK, Biller BM. Clinical review 62: Laboratory assessment of adrenal insufficiency. *J Clin Endocrinol Metab* 1994;79:923.

13. Cunningham SK, Moore A, McKenna TJ. Normal cortisol response to corticotropin in patients with secondary adrenal failure. *Arch Intern Med* 1983;143:2276.

14. Tordjman K, Jaffe A, Trostanetsky Y, et al. Low-dose (1 μg) adrenocorticotropin (ACTH) stimulation as a screening test for impaired hypothalamo-pituitary-adrenal axis function: Sensitivity, specificity and accuracy in comparison with the high-dose (250 μg) test. *Clin Endocrinol (Oxf)* 2000;52:633.

15. Borst GC, Michenfelder HJ, O'Brian JT. Discordant cortisol responses to exogeneous ACTH and insulin-induced hypoglycemia in patients with pituitary diseases. *N Engl J Med* 1982;302:1462.

16. Oelkers H, Diederich S, Bahr V. Diagnosis and therapy surveillance in Addison's disease: Rapid adrenocorticotropin (ACTH) test and measurement of plasma ACTH, renin activity, and aldosterone. *J Clin Endocrinol Metab* 1992; 75:259.

17. Dickstein G, Schechner C. Low-dose ACTH test: A word of caution to the word of caution: When and how to use it. *J Clin Endocrinol Metab* 1997;82:322.

18. Laureti S, Aubourg P, Calcinaro F, et al. Etiological diagnosis of primary adrenal insufficiency using an original flowchart of immune and biochemical markers. *J Clin Endocrinol Metab* 1998;83:3163.

19. Hunt PJ, Gurnell EM, Huppert FA, et al. Improvement in mood and fatigue after dehydroepiandrosterone replacement in Addison's disease in a randomized, double-blind trial. *J Clin Endocrinol Metab* 2000;85:465.

20. Coursin DB, Wood KE. Corticosteroid supplementation for adrenal insufficiency. *JAMA* 2002;287:236.

21. White PC, Speiser P. Congenital adrenal hyperplasia due to 21-hydroxylase deficiency. *Endocr Rev* 2000;21:245.

22. Merke DP, Camacho CA. Novel basic and clinical aspects of congenital adrenal hyperplasia. *Rev Endocr Metab Disord* 2001;2:289.

23. New MI, Carlson A, Obeid J, et al. Prenatal diagnosis for congenital adrenal hyperplasia in 532 pregnancies. *J Clin Endocrinol Metab* 2001;86:5651.

24. Section on Endocrinology and Committee on Genetics. American Academy of Pediatrics: Technical report: Congenital adrenal hyperplasia. *Pediatrics* 2000;106:1511.

25. Seckl JR, Miller WL. Commentary: How safe is long-term prenatal glucocorticoid treatment? *JAMA* 1997;277:1077.

26. Nieman LK. Diagnostic Tests for Cushing's syndrome. *Ann NY Acad Sci* 2002;970:112.

27. Nieman LK. Cushing syndrome, in Degroot L (ed). *DeGroot's Textbook of Endocrinology.* Philadelphia: Saunders, 2000; p 1677.

28. Newell-Price J, Trainer P, Besser M, et al. The diagnosis and differential diagnosis of Cushing's syndrome and pseudo-Cushing's states. *Endocr Rev* 1998;19:647.

29. Plotz CM, Knowlton AI, Ragan C. The natural history of Cushing's syndrome. *Am J Med* 1952;13:597.

30. Moran C, Tapia MC, Hernandez E, et al. Etiological review of hirsutism in 250 patients. *Arch Med Res* 1994;25:31.

31. Yanovski JA, Cutler GBJ, Chrousos GP, et al. Corticotropin-releasing hormone stimulation following low-dose dexamethasone administration: A new test to distinguish Cushing's syn-

drome from pseudo-Cushing's states. *JAMA* 1993;269:2232.

32. Taylor RL, Machacek D, Singh RJ. Validation of a high-throughput liquid chromatography–tandem mass spectrometry method for urinary cortisol and cortisone. *Clin Chem* 2002;48:1511.

33. Papanicolaou DA, Yanovski JA, Cutler GB Jr, et al. A single midnight serum cortisol measurement distinguishes Cushing's syndrome from pseudo-Cushing states. *J Clin Endocrinol Metab* 1998;83:1163.

34. Papanicolaou DA, Mullen N, Kyrou I, et al. Nighttime salivary cortisol: a useful test for the diagnosis of Cushing's syndrome. *J Clin Endocrinol Metab* 2002;87:4515.

35. Raff H, Raff JL, Findling JW. Late-night salivary cortisol as a screening test for Cushing's syndrome. *J Clin Endocrinol Metab* 1998;83:2681.

36. Wood PJ, Barth JH, Freedman DB, et al. Evidence for the low-dose dexamethasone suppression test to screen for Cushing's syndrome: Recommendations for a protocol for biochemistry laboratories. *Ann Clin Biochem* 1997;34:222.

37. Crapo L. Cushing's syndrome: A review of diagnostic tests. *Metabolism* 1979;28:955.

38. Nieman LK. The Evaluation of ACTH-dependent Cushing's syndrome. *Endocrinologist* 1999;9:93.

39. Melby JC. Therapy of Cushing disease: A consensus for pituitary microsurgery. *Ann Intern Med* 1998;109:445.

40. Nieman LK. Cushing's syndrome treatment, in Bardin CW (ed). *Current Therapy of Endocrinology and Metabolism.* Philadelphia: Saunders, 1996; p 609.

41. Young WF Jr. Pheochromocytoma and primary aldosteronism: Diagnostic approaches. *Endocrinol Metab Clin North Am* 1997;26:801.

42. Mulatero P, Rabbia F, Milan A, et al. Drug effects on aldosterone/plasma renin activity ratio in primary aldosteronism. *Hypertension* 2002;40:897.

43. Seifarth C, Trenkel S, Schobel H, et al. Influence of antihypertensive medication on aldosterone and renin concentration in the differential diagnosis of essential hypertension and primary aldosteronism. *Clin Endocrinol (Oxf)* 2002;57:457.

44. Holland OB, Brown H, Kuhnert L, et al. Further evaluation of saline infusion for the diagnosis of primary aldosteronism. *Hypertension* 1984;6:717.

45. Brickner RC, Knechtges TE, Kehoe ME, et al. Comparison of adrenal vein sampling and computed tomography in the differentiation of primary aldosteronism. *J Clin Endocrinol Metab* 2002;86:1066.

46. Magill SB, Raff H, Shaker JL, et al. Comparison of adrenal vein sampling and computed tomography in the differentiation of primary aldosteronism. *J Clin Endocrinol Metab* 2001;86:1066.

47. Phillips JL, Walther MM, Pezzullo JC, et al. Predictive value of preoperative tests in discriminating bilateral adrenal hyperplasia from an aldosterone-producing adrenal adenoma. *J Clin Endocrinol Metab* 2000;85:4526.

48. Litchfield WR, New MI, Coolidge C, et al. Evaluation of the dexamethasone suppression test for the diagnosis of glucocorticoid-remediable aldosteronism. *J Clin Endocrinol Metab* 1997;82:3570.

49. Meria P, Kempf BF, Hermieu JF, et al. Laparoscopic management of primary hyperaldosteronism: Clinical experience with 212 cases. *J Urol* 2003;169:32.

50. Azziz R, Carmina E, Sawaya ME. Idiopathic hirsutism. *Endocr Rev* 2000;21:347.

51. Legro RS. Polycystic ovary syndrome: Long-term sequelae and management. *Minerva Gynecol* 2002;54:97.

52. Derksen J, Nagesser SK, Meinders AE, et al. Identification of virilizing adrenal tumors in hirsute women. *N Engl J Med* 1994;331:968.

53. Lenders JW, Pacak K, Walther MM, et al. Biochemical diagnosis of pheochromocytoma: Which test is best? *JAMA* 2002;287:1427.

54. Neumann HP, Bausch B, McWhinney SR, et al. Germ-line mutations in nonsyndromic pheochromocytoma. *N Engl J Med* 2002; 346:1459.

55. Yamamoto T, Fukuyama J, Haasegawa K, et al. Isolated corticotropin deficiency in adults: Report of 10 cases and review of the literature. *Arch Intern Med* 1999;152:170.

CHAPTER 12

Disorders of the Thyroid

ROBERT HEYMANN AND GREGORY A. BRENT

► THYROID GLAND DEVELOPMENT, THYROID HORMONE SYNTHESIS, AND IODINE NUTRITION

Thyroid Gland Development

The thyroid gland develops in the midline of the anterior pharyngeal floor at 8 to 10 weeks of gestational age in close proximity to differentiating myocardium and is pulled into its final position at the base of the neck as the developing heart descends.[1] There is a lateral contribution to the developing thyroid from the fourth and fifth pharyngeal pouches, the ultimobranchial bodies, which include the precursors of the parafollicular calcitonin-producing cells (C cells). Thyroid gland development requires the action of at least three transcription factors: thyroid transcription factors 1 and 2 (TTF-1 and TTF-2) and Pax-8. Defects in the genes that produce these transcription factors have been associated with congenital absence of the thyroid, as well as other congenital defects. Cardiac anomalies are the defects associated most commonly with congenital hypothyroidism. Remnants of thyroid tissue can be found at the base of the tongue (lingual thyroid) and along the midline thyroglossal duct. However, ectopic thyroid tissue usually does not function as well as thyroid tissue located in the usual neck position.

Thyroid Hormone Physiology

The thyroid gland produces and secretes thyroid hormone in the form of thyroxine (T_4) and triiodothyronine (T_3)[2] (Fig. 12-1). The thyroidal secretion contains about 80 percent T_4 and 20 percent T_3, although this can vary as a consequence of thyroid disease or nutritional deficiencies (iodine or selenium). T_3 combines with the nuclear T_3 receptors (coded for by two thyroid hormone receptor genes, α and β) and is responsible for most of the actions of thyroid hormone.[3] T_4 may mediate some nongenomic effects that have been identified primarily in the developing brain.[4] About 60 to 70 percent of circulating T_3 is produced in peripheral tissue from the conversion of T_4, primarily by the liver.[2] Thyroid hormone contains 60 percent elemental iodine, and the ability to concentrate environmental iodine is a key adaptation of the thyroid gland and is the first step in thyroid hormone synthesis[5] (Fig. 12-2). The sodium-iodide transporter or symporter (NIS) is located at the basolateral surface of the cell and concentrates iodide 40- to 60-fold relative to the levels of this element in serum. NIS gene expression in the thyroid is regulated primarily by thyrotropin [also known as *thyroid-stimulating hormone* (TSH)], secreted by the pituitary. Iodide is transported from the follicular cells to the apical side of the cell and into the colloid, where it is incorporated into

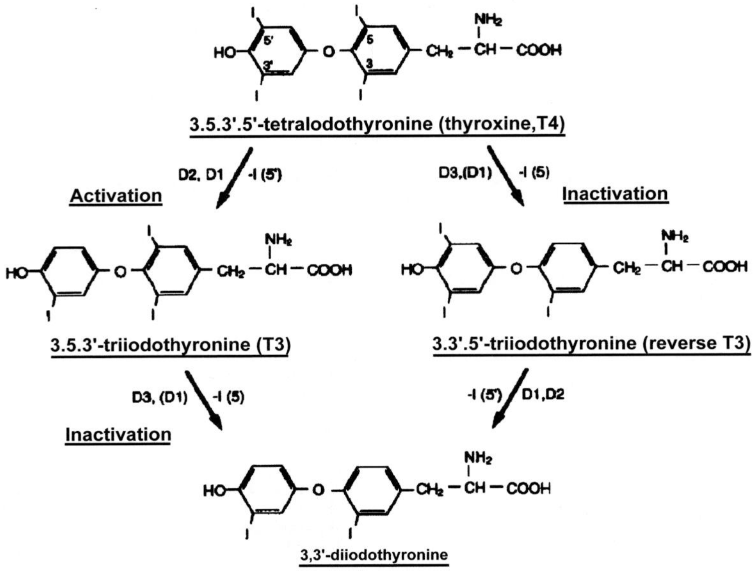

Figure 12-1 Metabolic pathways of thyroid hormone activation and disposal. The enzymes shown include types 1 (D1) and 2 (D2) 5'-deiodinase and type 3 5-deiodinase (D3). *(Reproduced, with permission, from Bianco AC et al. Endocr Rev 2002;23–38.)*

thyroglobulin (Tg) by the enzyme thyroperoxidase (TPO). Tg is a large glycoprotein with abundant tyrosine residues. Pendrin is an apical iodine transporter (AIT), and mutations in this gene are found in patients with Pendrin syndrome, an inherited condition with goiter and congenital deafness.[6]

In the thyroid colloid, iodine is added to tyrosine residues, forming 3-monoiodotyrosine (MIT) or 3,5-diiodotyrosine (DIT) (see Fig. 12-2). TPO then catalyzes the organification of iodine and the coupling of MIT and DIT. Coupling of two molecules of DIT forms T_4, and coupling of a molecule of MIT and one of DIT forms T_3. T_4 and small amounts of T_3 are then cleaved from Tg and released from the basolateral cell surface into the bloodstream, a process stimulated primarily by TSH.[1]

The thyroid contains both type 1 (D1) and type 2 (D2) 5'-deiodinase enzymes, which convert T_4 to the active form of the hormone, T_3 (see Fig. 12-1).[2] Some of the secreted T_3, therefore, comes directly from intrathyroidal T_4 to

T_3 conversion, although the majority arises from peripheral conversion of T_4 (see above). The rate of intrathyroidal conversion is increased in certain thyroid conditions, such as Graves' disease and toxic adenomas.

Thyroid function is regulated by hypothalamic-pituitary activity. The hypothalamus produces thyrotropin-releasing hormone (TRH),[7] which acts on the anterior pituitary thyrotroph cells to stimulate secretion of TSH. TSH then binds to a cellular membrane receptor in the thyroid gland, stimulating thyroid follicles to produce thyroid hormone (see Fig. 12-2) and, at sustained levels, stimulating thyroid growth. Serum levels of thyroid hormone (T_4 and T_3) provide feedback to the pituitary and hypothalamus to regulate the production and secretion of TRH and, consequently, TSH. The majority of T_3 in the pituitary, however, comes from local conversion of T_4 to T_3 by D2.[2] Serum T_4, therefore, has the most direct influence on hypothalamic-pituitary feedback, although T_3 alone at sufficiently high serum concentrations also will directly suppress TSH.

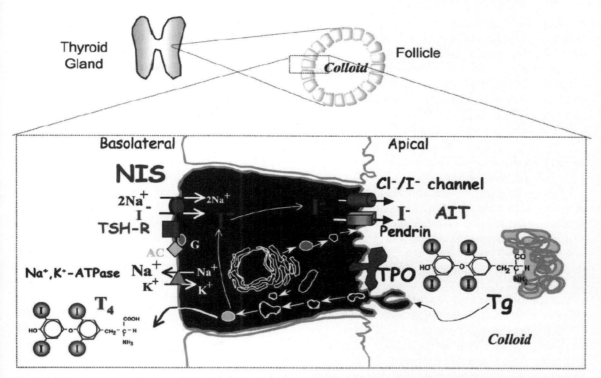

Figure 12-2   Model of thyroid follicle and biosynthetic pathways of thyroid hormone. (Abbreviations: Tg = thyroglobulin; TPO = thyroperoxidase; AIT = apical iodide transporter; TSH-R = thyrotropin receptor.) *(Reproduced, with permission, from Dohan O et al. Endocr Rev 2003; 24:48.)*

Iodine Dietary Intake

Iodine has an essential role in thyroid hormone synthesis. Diet is the primary source of elemental iodine, and adequate dietary intake depends on geographic location and food intake.[8] Mountainous areas tend to have low soil and water iodine content, whereas coastal areas generally have adequate supplies. Approximately 30 percent of the world population is at risk for iodine-deficiency disorders. The clinical manifestations of iodine deficiency include hypothyroidism and endemic goiter. This can have profound effects on pregnancy and fetal development. Iodine deficiency is the leading cause of intellectual deficiency in the world. The United States is iodine-sufficient, although a recent survey showed a reduction in dietary iodine.[9]

The World Health Organization (WHO) recommends a daily iodine intake of 150 μg but a higher level, 200 μg daily, for pregnant and lactating women. This increased requirement is due to increased renal iodine clearance and thyroid hormone degradation by the placenta and uterus during pregnancy.[10] In a recent survey, only about 60 percent of standard prenatal vitamins included these amounts of iodine.[11] Iodine deficiency prior to and during pregnancy is associated with increased rates of neonatal death and severe neurologic deficits.[12] However, the developing brain is most vulnerable to iodine deficiency in the first trimester. A spectrum of neurologic disease can occur ranging from mild intellectual impairment to cretinism with severe mental retardation, mutism, and impaired growth. Review of a number of studies concluded that the mean reduction in the intelligence quotient (IQ) of children in iodine-deficient areas averaged 13.5 points.[12]

▶ THYROID FUNCTION TESTS

A number of thyroid function tests are available to assess thyroid status. Laboratory testing is more reliable than clinical signs and symptoms of thyroid abnormalities, which are often nonspecific.[13] The clinical diagnosis and decision for treatment, however, should be based on both the thyroid function tests and the overall clinical presentation. Routine thyroid testing is influenced by the ready availability of free T_4 measurements and sensitive TSH assays by automated systems in most clinical laboratories. The core test used in thyroid evaluation includes the measurement of free T_4, total and free T_3, TSH, and TPO antibody. Provocative testing with TRH is not indicated for routine clinical thyroid evaluation and does not add any significant clinical information to that obtained from a sensitive TSH measurement.

Thyroid-Stimulating Hormone (TSH)

TSH is a highly sensitive indicator of thyroid hormone status in most situations, although in some patients TSH may not correctly reflect thyroid status.[14] These include patients with hypothalamic-pituitary disease, those receiving treatment for hyperthyroidism, patients on certain medications such as dopamine and glucocorticoids, those with acute psychiatric decompensation, and hospitalized patients.[15]

The normal range for serum TSH is usually 0.5 to 4.0 mU/L. In general, an abnormally low TSH reflects hyperthyroidism, and an elevated TSH reflects hypothyroidism. The second- and third-generation TSH assays can measure ab-

normally suppressed levels and are distinguished by their lower limit of sensitivity, around 0.1 mU/L for the second-generation and 0.01 mU/L for the third-generation assays. This lower limit of detection allows normal patients to be distinguished from those who are truly hyperthyroid. The additional sensitivity of the third-generation assay is especially useful for monitoring TSH suppression in thyroid cancer patients, in whom the goal is to achieve a subnormal TSH, and for diagnosing thyroid disease in hospitalized patients.[14]

The upper limit of normal for TSH is currently being reexamined. Since there is a log-linear relationship between serum TSH and serum T_4 concentrations, TSH levels are not "normally distributed" across a linear range in the population but "skewed" toward the lower limit. Thus the normal range for TSH is more likely to be between 0.5 and 3.0 mU/L.[16] TSH values between 0.1 and 0.5 mU/L and 4 and 10 mU/L usually reflect early or subclinical thyroid disease, although only a subset of these patients will require immediate treatment.

Thyroxine and Triiodothyronine

T_4 and T_3 circulate predominantly bound to proteins, with only 0.02 and 0.03 percent, respectively, circulating free. The free thyroid hormone is the active form and is able to exert its effects at the cellular level by binding to nuclear thyroid hormone receptors.[3] Total T_4 or T_3 is measured by radioimmunoassay or immunofluorescence assay. The normal values for total T_4 range from 5 to 11 μ/dL and from 75 to 195 ng/dL for T_3. Total T_4 and T_3 levels are influenced by high or low serum levels of thyroid hormone–binding proteins. In the circulation, T_4 and T_3 are bound primarily (in descending order of affinity) to thyroxine-binding globulin (TBG), transthyretin, and albumin. There are genetic disorders of deficient or excess TBG, as well as diseases and medications that influence TBG levels. Unbound or free thyroid hormone levels in these situations, however, generally are normal. The free T_4 or T_3 index is the product of the total T_4 or T_3 levels and the resin uptake ratio, expressed as a fraction of normal, but this index is used rarely today. The total T_4 level has been replaced largely by the free T_4 measurement. The total T_3 level continues to be useful, however, primarily in diagnosing and monitoring treatment in hyperthyroidism.

Serum free T_4 is most commonly measured by radioimmunoassay (or analog) methods using automated systems. It is generally accurate, although the measurement can be influenced by the presence of exceedingly high or low thyroid-reduced binding proteins.[18] When the direct free T_4 method does not correlate with the TSH concentration or the clinical status, a free T_4 measurement by dialysis is recommended. This is the gold standard method of assessing free T_4 and is not influenced by abnormalities in binding-protein levels or activity.

Antithyroid Antibodies

Thyroid autoantibodies are used commonly in clinical practice. These include anti-TPO antibodies, anti-Tg antibodies, and a variety of antibody measurements affecting the TSH-receptor including TSH-receptor antibodies (TSH-R Abs), thyrotropin-stimulating immunoglobulins (TSIs), and thyrotropin-binding inhibitory immunoglobulins (TBIIs).[19,20]

Anti-TPO antibodies bind to TPO, the enzyme that catalyzes the organification of iodine and iodination of the tyrosine residues of thyroglobulin. Since TPO is the antigenic component of the microsome, measurement of the anti-TPO antibody level replaces the previous antimicrosomal antibody test. In general, values above 0.5 IU/mL are considered positive, although there is some variation among assays. In the U.S. population, anti-TPO antibodies are more common in women than in men, 17 versus 8.7 percent.[16] The prevalence of anti-TPO antibody positivity also increases with age.

Anti-Tg antibodies bind to Tg, the precursor to thyroid hormone that is stored as colloid in the thyroid follicle. Positive values are above 1.0 IU/mL and are found in 15.2 percent of the female population and 11.5 percent of the male population. Anti-Tg antibodies are not predictive for the development of hypothyroidism[21] however, and are used primarily in conjunction with serum Tg measurements in thyroid cancer patients to ensure the accuracy of the Tg measurement.

Several different antibody tests are available to evaluate patients with suspected Graves' disease or to monitor response to treatment. TSI determines the magnitude of TSH receptor-stimulating activity in a sample of serum, as reflected by cyclic AMP (cAMP) production in thyroid follicular cells in an in vitro assay. TSH-R Ab and TBII assays directly assess the amount of TSH-R-binding antibody present. Most patients with Graves' disease can be diagnosed on clinical grounds and thyroid hormone and TSH levels, and the routine determination of TSH-R Abs is not recommended.[22] TSI measurement, however, can be useful in evaluating euthyroid Graves' ophthalmopathy, predicting risk for neonatal Graves' disease during pregnancy (usually measured in the second trimester) and assessing the likelihood of remission of Graves' disease while on therapy.

Conditions Influencing Thyroid Function Tests

Medications
A number of medications can influence thyroid function tests and T_4 absorption and metabolism through a variety of mechanisms.[23] Increased serum estrogen, as is seen in pregnancy or during the use of estrogen-containing medications, results in increased serum levels of TBG. This leads to an increase in total T_4 and T_3 concentration, although the free T_4 and free T_3 remain within the normal range. Hypothyroid patients may require an increased dose of T_4 if beginning estrogen-replacement

therapy or oral contraception.[24] Androgens are associated with a modest reduction in TBG levels, which can result in a small decrease in total T_4 and T_3 levels. Hypothyroid women on T_4 who were treated with androgens for breast cancer were found to require lower doses of medication.[26]

Other medications may affect the hypothalamic-pituitary-thyroid axis. Acute administration of glucocorticoids inhibits the pulsatile secretion of TSH.[27] Dopamine infusion decreases serum TSH levels.[28] Rexinoids (which bind the RXR receptor) are used for treatment of a variety of tumors and are known to suppress TSH. Chronic treatment can be associated with symptomatic central hypothyroidism requiring thyroid hormone replacement.[29] Carbamazepine, phenytoin, and phenobarbital induce cytochrome CYP3A4 and consequently increase hepatic disposal of thyroid hormone. Free T_4 levels may be slightly decreased by a direct assay, but TSH is within the normal range, and patients generally are euthyroid.[30] Selective serotonin reuptake inhibitors (SSRIs) may accelerate T_4 metabolism and increase T_4 requirements in patients on T_4 replacement, although limited data are available.[31]

Thyroid Function Tests in Nonthyroidal Illness

Patients with acute illness, surgery, or psychiatric episodes frequently have transient abnormalities in thyroid function tests.[32] In mild illness or if fasting, patients will have only low T_3 levels, in the face of normal TSH and T_4 levels, known as the *low T_3 syndrome*. This is due to decreased peripheral conversion of T_4 to T_3 by D1. With more severe illness, serum T_4 concentrations also fall, and this is referred to as the low T_4/T_3 *syndrome*. In this situation, serum thyroid hormone–binding proteins also usually are reduced, although serum free T_4 concentrations generally are normal to low, depending on the assay used.

Total serum T_4 concentrations rarely are elevated and are seen most commonly in psy-chiatric illness. Diagnosing primary thyroid disease can be difficult in inpatients, and the predictive value of thyroid function tests is reduced tenfold relative to the evaluation of outpatients.[33]

▶ HYPOTHYROIDISM

Primary hypothyroidism indicates reduced thyroid hormone production due to a defect of the thyroid gland. Alternatively, central or secondary hypothyroidism is due to defects in the pituitary or hypothalamus leading to reduced TSH stimulation of the thyroid gland. *Overt hypothyroidism* is defined as a high serum TSH concentration with a low serum free T_4 concentration.[19] *Subclinical hypothyroidism,* or *early thyroid failure,* is defined as a high serum TSH concentration with a normal-range serum free T_4 concentration.[34] The prevalence of overt and subclinical hypothyroidism in the United States is approximately 1 to 2 percent and 5 to 10 percent, respectively.

Etiologies of Hypothyroidism (Table 12-1)

Chronic Autoimmune Thyroiditis
Chronic autoimmune thyroiditis, also known as *Hashimoto thyroiditis,* is the most common cause of primary hypothyroidism.[19] The prevalence in women is five to seven times greater than in men. Prevalence increases with age, and in one study, 33 percent of women over age 70 had positive antithyroid antibodies. Patients may have an enlarged (goitrous form) or normal-sized (atrophic form) thyroid gland. The goitrous thyroid (goiter) is firm, diffusely enlarged, and often has a firm and slightly irregular surface. A lymphocytic infiltrate is present in fine-needle aspirates. High serum concentrations of anti-TPO antibodies are present in up to 80 percent of Hashimoto thyroiditis patients.[21] Reidel struma or thyroiditis is a rare variant of this disease with fibrosis of the thyroid gland and surrounding tissue. The gland

▶ **TABLE 12-1:** CONDITIONS ASSOCIATED WITH REDUCED SERUM T_4/T_3 CONCENTRATIONS

Diagnosis	Etiology	Thyroid Gland	TSH	Antibodies
Hashimoto thyroiditis	Immune-mediated destruction	Initially firm and symmetrically enlarged, ultimately becomes atrophic	Elevated	TPO
Postablation	Secondary to radioiodine, surgery, or external surgery	Absent or atrophic	Elevated	May have persistent Graves' associated antibodies
Central hypo-thyroidism	Pituitary or hypothalamic dysfunction, suppressive drugs	Normal or reduced size	Usually inappropriately "normal" for low serum T_4, often with reduced bioactivity	None
Subacute thyroiditis	Postviral (painful), immune-mediated (silent)	Slightly enlarged	Transiently elevated during hypothyroid phase	Silent, associated with transient positive TPO antibodies.

feels like a firm mass and should be distinguished from thyroid cancer, usually by fine-needle aspiration.

Progression of hypothyroid disease from subclinical to overt in women with antithyroid antibodies has been reported to be 4.3 percent per year over a 20-year study.[35] Higher initial titers of antithyroid antibodies predicted higher rates of progression from subclinical to overt disease. It is important to be aware of the association of autoimmune hypothyroidism with other autoimmune endocrine conditions, including type I diabetes (TPO antibodies are present in 30 percent of type I diabetic women), adrenal insufficiency, pernicious anemia, premature ovarian failure, and vitiligo.

Central Hypothyroidism

Central hypothyroidism is a result of disorders of TSH or TRH synthesis or release. Reduced pituitary function can be due to medications, adenoma, postpartum pituitary necrosis (Sheehan syndrome), radiation, metastatic tumors, head trauma, and pituitary surgery. Symptoms of central hypothyroidism are similar to those of primary hypothyroidism except that patients additionally may have signs of hypopituitarism, including adrenal insufficiency, hypogonadism, and amenorrhea.[7] If the cause is a pituitary adenoma, there may be signs of mass effect, including headache and visual field defects. If the pituitary adenoma is functional, there may be signs of excess hormones, e.g., prolactin, growth hormone, or cortisol. Primary hypothyroidism can be associated with significant elevations in prolactin levels and even pituitary enlargement that reverses with treatment of the hypothyroidism and normalization of the serum TSH concentration.

Diagnosis of central hypothyroidism is based on a low serum free T_4 concentration and a TSH concentration that is "inappropriately" normal or reduced. Central hypothyroidism also should be suspected when other hormonal deficiencies are identified or there is known hypothalamic or pituitary disease. Free T_4 concentration, rather than the serum TSH concentration, should be used to monitor T_4

replacment in these patients, targeting a free T_4 concentration in the upper normal range. Patients diagnosed with central hypothyroidism should have magnetic resonance imaging (MRI) of the pituitary and hypothalamus or a computed tomographic (CT) with coronal views of the pituitary.[7]

Unusual Causes of Hypothyroidism

TSH receptor–blocking antibodies are a rare cause of hypothyroidism. These antibodies can be transferred from mother to fetus and cause transient congenital hypothyroidism. About 5 percent of mothers with chronic autoimmune thyroiditis have infants with transient neonatal hypothyroidism, likely due to TSH receptor–blocking antibodies.[19]

Primary hypothyroidism occurs after thyroidectomy and after radiation. After total thyroidectomy, hypothyroidism occurs within weeks, and in partial thyroidectomy, the course is variable and depends on the amount of thyroid tissue that remains. Radioiodine therapy for Graves' disease generally is targeted to achieve hypothyroidism, although the time course for development of hypothyroidism depends on the dose of radioiodine and the size of the thyroid.[22] External radiation for treatment of Hodgkin's disease and head and neck cancers often produces hypothyroidism. Rarely, infiltrating diseases such as hemochromatosis, scleroderma, sarcoidosis, and amyloidosis can cause hypothyroidism.

Drug-Induced Hypothyroidism

Certain drugs have the potential to induce hypothyroidism.[23] Iodine or drugs containing iodine given in large quantities can lead to excessive intrathyroidal gland iodine levels that inhibit organification of iodine, a reaction known as the *Wolff-Chaikoff effect*. Normal patients are able to "escape" from this iodine load over several days, but those with thyroid disease, such as chronic autoimmune thyroiditis, may not recover and may become hypothyroid. Amiodarone, radiographic contrast materials, saturated solution of potassium iodide

(SSKI), and kelp tablets all contain large amounts of iodine and can produce these effects. Systemic absorption of betadine applied to the skin or mucosa also can induce transient hypothyroidism. Other drugs that potentially can induce hypothyroidism by impairing release or synthesis of thyroid hormone include lithium, perchlorate, propylthiouracil, methimazole, interferon-α, and interleukin 2.[23]

Clinical and Laboratory Manifestations of Hypothyroidism

The clinical presentation of a hypothyroid patient is variable and depends on the duration and severity of thyroid hormone deficiency.[13] Due to widespread serum TSH testing, hypothyroidism often is diagnosed before many of the classic symptoms and signs appear. There are many possible symptoms affecting every organ system.[36]

- *Neurologic.* Patients may complain of memory problems, mental slowing, and depression. Deep tendon reflexes show a delayed relaxation phase. Accumulation of substances in soft tissues may lead to paresthesias from nerve compression, including carpal tunnel syndrome.
- *Cardiac.* Bradycardia may be present along with mild hypertension. Electrocardiographic (ECG) changes include flattened T waves and a prolonged PR interval. If a pericardial effusion is present, the QRS-complex and P-wave amplitudes may be diminished, and cardiomegaly can be seen on radiography. The QT interval may be prolonged, leading to ventricular ectopy.[37] Myocardial contractility can be reduced. Overt heart failure is rare because cardiac output usually is sufficient to meet the reduced demand for peripheral oxygen delivery.[37]
- *Musculoskeletal/Connective Tissue.* Glycosaminoglycans can become deposited in subcutaneous tissues, resulting in facial puffi-

ness and lower extremity edema. Skin is usually dry, hair is coarse and brittle, and thinning of lateral eyebrows is sometimes seen. Patients also frequently complain of muscle aches and arthralgias.

- *Reproductive.* Menstrual irregularities occur, and menorrhagia from anovulatory cycles may be seen.[38,39] Galactorrhea can occur in severe hypothyroidism due to increases in prolactin from TRH stimulation of lactotrophs.
- *Gastrointestinal.* Peristaltic activity is decreased, leading to constipation. Patients may have modest weight gain, but this should not be greater than 5 percent of usual body weight.
- *Laboratory Test Abnormalities.* Normocytic anemia, hyponatremia, increased creatine kinase, and increased low-density lipoprotein (LDL) cholesterol can occur.

Subclinical Hypothyroidism

Subclinical hypothyroidism is defined as an elevated TSH concentration in the setting of a normal free T_4 concentration. It usually occurs with positive anti-TPO antibodies. It is most common in women over age 60, approaching 20 percent of this population.[34] Patients may have clinical features of mild hypothyroidism, but many have no noticeable symptoms. Patients who should be considered for testing include those with a family history of thyroid disease or other autoimmune diseases (especially type I diabetes) and those with the presence of goiter, infertility, menstrual irregularity, depression, and hyperlipidemia. Some potential benefits of treatment include prevention of progression to overt hypothyroidism, reduction of LDL cholesterol, improvement of some symptoms, reduction in goiter, improvement in ovulatory dysfunction, and reduction in cardiac risk. The progression to overt hypothyroidism is about 5 to 10 percent per year, with the greatest risk in those with positive anti-TPO antibodies and higher TSH levels (>12 mU/mL).[21] It is generally recommended that

treatment be initiated if the TSH concentration is >10 mU/mL or if any symptoms or associated conditions are present if the TSH concentration is from 5 to 10 mU/mL.

Treatment of Hypothyroidism

The most common form of replacement therapy is levothyroxine. Levothyroxine is well absorbed, about 80 percent of an oral dose, primarily in the small intestine. The serum half-life of levothyroxine is 7 to 10 days, so daily dosing results in relatively constant serum levels.[40] After T_4 is absorbed, it must be converted to its active form, T_3, in peripheral tissues. Formulations are color-coded and come in strengths from 25 to 300 μg. Tablets with increments of 12.5 μg are available in the most common dose range of 50 to 150 μg. With these increments, it should be possible to normalize the serum TSH concentration in essentially all patients with a single daily dose rather than alternating doses. Smaller increments between higher doses (>150 μg) can be achieved by combining dose strengths in the 50- to 150-μg range.

Less commonly used forms of replacement are liothyronine (Cytomel), containing T_3, and desiccated animal thyroid extract (thyroid USP), which contains both T_3 and T_4. There are disadvantages to using these preparations. A 60-mg tablet of thyroid USP is roughly equivalent to 80 μg of T_4 but can vary in thyroid hormone content and bioavailability. T_3 has a short half-life, and its levels can fluctuate widely. As a result, it also must be given more frequently than T_4. One study of patients with hypothyroidism on regular T_4 replacement showed some improvement in cognition and mood when changed to a combination of T_4 and T_3.[41] Relatively high doses of T_3, however, were used in this study.

The treatment goal of primary hypothyroidism is to reduce the TSH concentration to within the normal range, and most physicians recommend targeting the lower part of the normal range.[40] To achieve a normal-range serum TSH concentration, the serum free T_4 concentrations are usually within the upper normal range or slightly above normal. A full replacement dose is 1.6 µg/kg/d, approximately 75 to 125 µg/d in women and 125 to 200 µg/d in men. Young patients without heart disease may be started on the full dose of thyroid hormone. Older patients (>60 years old) can be started on a lower dose of 50 µg/d, and patients with coronary disease may be started on 25 µg/d. Most patients with hypothyroidism and coronary artery disease have no change or improve-ment in angina when taking T_4.[42] However, thyroid hormone does increase myocardial oxygen consumption and can worsen angina in some patients. It takes about 6 to 8 weeks from dosage change until steady state is achieved, so adjustments can be made based on thyroid function tests obtained during that time interval. Increases should be done in 12.5- to 25-µg increments. One should remember that in central hypothyroidism, the TSH concentration is not useful to follow, so the therapeutic goal is to bring the free T_4 concentration to within the upper normal range.

Hypothyroidism and Pregnancy

Women in the first trimester of pregnancy with positive TPO antibodies have a significantly increased rate of miscarriage, up to twice the norm.[20] This increased risk is thought to represent a greater tendency to autoimmunity rather than a direct effect of antithyroid antibodies, although studies are underway to determine if there is any direct influence of thyroid status on miscarriage rate. Women with TPO antibodies early in pregnancy are also more likely to develop postpartum thyroiditis, 30 to 50 percent, compared with 3 percent in women without positive antibodies.[20] Some investigators recommend screening with anti-TPO antibodies in the first trimester in high-risk patients to identify those at risk for subsequent postpartum thyroiditis.[4]

In women known to be hypothyroid, the T_4 dose should be titrated to a low-normal TSH concentration prior to conception. Normal maternal thyroid status is likely important in early gestation, prior to fetal thyroid gland functioning at 10 to 12 weeks. Several studies have shown that approximately 50 to 70 percent of hypothyroid women require an increase in T_4 dose, an average of 50 µg, during pregnancy.[43,44] The T_4 dose in athyrotic women (as a result of treatment for goiter or hyperthyroidism with radioiodine or surgery) is likely to require the greatest increase compared with women with early Hashimoto disease or goiter, who may need only a small increase in dose. Some hypothyroid women on T_4 may take calcium or iron supplements for the first time during pregnancy, both of which interfere with T_4 absorption.[45]

The increased T_4 dose requirement in pregnancy is likely due to a number of factors, including the increased TBG pool, increased iodine clearance by the kidney, and increased inactivation of thyroid hormone by placental and uterine type III 5-deiodinase (D3). Some women may stop T_4 replacement due to concerns of harming their developing fetus and need to be counseled about the importance of continuing T_4. Thyroid function tests should be evaluated in the first trimester, with follow-up monitoring every 4 to 6 weeks, and dose adjustments should be made as necessary to maintain the serum TSH concentration within the normal range. Testing should be more frequent if the serum TSH concentration is elevated significantly. Although there is not sufficient time to reach a steady state, it is important to document that the tests are improving with treatment. Immediately after delivery, the previously established T_4 dose can be restarted.

The primary complications of pregnancy associated with hypothyroidism are pregnancy-induced hypertension and preterm delivery (Table 12-2). A study of 150 pregnancies complicated by overt or subclincal hypothyroidism demonstrated that the incidences of miscarriage and preterm delivery were much greater in women with elevated serum TSH concen-

▶ **TABLE 12-2:** MATERNAL AND FETAL CONSEQUENCES OF MATERNAL HYPOTHYROIDISM

Maternal Complications	Fetal Complications
Ovulatory dysfunction	Low birth weight
Miscarriage (with hypothyroidism and positive TPO antibodies)	Perinatal mortality (some studies)
Pregnancy-induced hypertension	Increase in congenital anomalies (some studies)
Placental abruption	Impaired intellectual development
Preterm delivery	

trations (both overt and subclinical) compared with those on adequate T_4 replacement.[39] Term deliveries were seen in almost 95 percent of women on adequate T_4 replacement at delivery but in only 20 percent of women with inadequate T_4 replacement.

Infants with congenital hypothyroidism, when identified and started on T_4 replacement shortly after birth, generally have normal intellectual and neurologic development. The intellectual development of 7- to 9-year-old children whose mothers had an elevated TSH concentration during pregnancy was modestly but significantly reduced compared with children from euthyroid mothers.[46] These findings support the importance of maternal thyroid status.

▶ HYPERTHYROIDISM

Signs and symptoms of hyperthyroidism can vary from mild subclinical disease to overt hyperthyroidism. Hyperthyroidism is less common than hypothyroidism, with an incidence of around 0.3 percent of overt disease and 1 to 2 percent of subclinical disease. The various etiologies of hyperthyroidism are depicted in Table 12-3.

Etiologies of Hyperthyroidism

Graves' Disease

Graves' disease is the most common cause of hyperthyroidism and is 5 to 10 times more common in women than in men.[22] In Graves' disease, autoantibodies are produced that bind to and stimulate the TSH receptor. In addition to thyroid gland enlargement and overproduction of thyroid hormone, other immune manifestations include ophthalmopathy and, rarely, dermopathy. Thyroid enlargement is diffuse, and there may be an audible bruit on examination. The disease has a moderate genetic association. Although the autoimmunity trigger is not known, the disease can occur postpartum, after infections, or following stressful life events.

Ophthalmopathy (or orbitopathy) is present in 50 percent of Graves' patients by imaging studies, whereas clinical manifestations are seen in fewer. Stare and eyelid retraction are general symptoms of hyperthyroidism due to increased sympathetic sensitivity. Exophthalmos (proptosis) and periorbital edema are unique to Graves' disease. This is the result of an increase in orbital connective tissue and fat mass and can lead to diplopia. A lymphocytic infiltrate is present in the connective tissue and extraocular muscles. TSH receptors have been identified in orbital tissue, suggesting a possible direct effect of TSH on these tissues. Significant eye involvement requires an evaluation by an ophthalmologist.

The associated dermopathy is characterized by edema and raised pigmented papules. It is found most frequently over the anterolateral leg. It occurs in only 1 to 2 percent of patients with Graves' disease and usually is accompanied by severe ophthalmopathy.[22] On histopathologic examination, lymphocytic infiltration of the dermis can be seen with increased accumulation of glycosaminoglycans. Treatment in early disease with topical steroids can be effective.

▶ **TABLE 12-3:** CONDITIONS ASSOCIATED WITH ELEVATED SERUM T_4/T_3 CONCENTRATIONS

Diagnosis	Etiology	Thyroid Gland	TSH	Antibodies	Iodine Uptake
Graves' disease	Circulating antibodies that stimulate the TSH receptor	Usually symmetrically enlarged	Suppressed	TSH-receptor antibodies (Abs) thyrotropin-stimulating Ig immuno-globulins (TSIs), thyrotropin-binding inhibitory Ig immuno-globulins (TBIIs)	Increased with diffuse pattern of uptake
Toxic nodule	Most associated with acquired activating TSH-R mutation	Focal nodule/enlargement	Suppresse.0d	None	Focal increase with suppres-sion of sur-rounding tissue
Toxic goiter	Autonomous activity throughout gland	Diffuse, irregular enlargement	Suppressed	None	Increased in dif-fuse patchy pattern
Subacute thyroiditis	Postviral inflammation or immune	Slightly enlarged	Suppressed during hyperthyroid phase	Some with positive thyroperoxi-dase (TPO)	Reduced
TSH-secreting pituitary adenoma	Excess TSH despite ele-vated serum T_4/T_3	Diffusely enlarged	Inappropriately "normal" or elevated	None	Increased with diffuse pattern of uptake
Hydatidiform mole/hyper-emesis	"Spillover" stim-ulation by hu-man chori-onic gonado-tropin (hCG)	Normal to diffusely enlarged	Suppressed	None	Should be increased, but is not recom-mended
Exogenous thyroxine	Thyroid-containing products	Normal to reduced	Suppressed	None	Low
Resistance to thyroid hormone	Thyroid recep-tor β mutations	Usually enlarged	Inappropriately "normal" or elevated	Negative	Normal

Toxic Multinodular Goiter and Toxic Adenoma

Toxic multinodular goiter is more common in areas of iodine deficiency.[47] A toxic adenoma is a single hyperfunctioning nodule. It generally develops slowly and gradually leads to an increase in thyroid hormone secretion. The amount of thyroid hormone produced is proportional to the size of the tumor, and clinical hyperthyroidism generally is associated with nodules >2 cm in diameter. An acquired activating mutation of the TSH receptor gene has been identified in the majority of toxic adenomas.[48] Identifying a hyperfunctioning nodule essentially rules out the presence of a cancer in that location.

Iodine-Induced Hyperthyroidism

Iodine-induced hyperthyroidism generally occurs in patients with a preexisting nodular goiter and follows administration of or challenge with a large amount of iodine. It tends to occur in areas with iodine deficiency but also may occur in iodine-sufficient areas. The iodine load leads to excess synthesis of thyroid hormone, thus causing the hyperthyroid state, a consequence referred to as the *Jod-Basedow effect*. Sources of iodine include radiographic contrast material and amiodarone but also may include excessive intake of nutritional iodine supplements.[23]

TSH-Induced Hyperthyroidism

TSH-producing pituitary adenomas are a rare cause of hyperthyroidism. Patients will have signs of hyperthyroidism, including a goiter. TSH levels often are not markedly elevated but rather "inappropriately" normal for the level of serum T_4/T_3 elevation.[49]

Clinical and Laboratory Manifestations of Hyperthyroidism

- *Neurologic*. Symptoms include emotional lability, poor concentration, and insomnia. Fine tremor is another common finding and is due to increased adrenergic sensitivity. Deep tendon reflexes are hyperactive.

- *Cardiac*. Findings include resting tachycardia and an increase in cardiac output. Patients frequently complain of palpitations. Atrial fibrillation occurs in 10 percent of these patients,[40] and the American College of Cardiology/American Heart Association guideline is to anticoagulate these individuals to prevent stroke. Others, however, reserve anticoagulation for patients who are older or have intrinsic heart disease.

- *Musculoskeletal*. Muscle weakness can occur due to muscle catabolism. Patients may experience problems climbing stairs or rising from a sitting position, reflecting weakness of proximal muscles. Hypokalemic periodic paralysis rarely may be associated with hyperthyroidism and is more common in Asian individuals. Chronic thyrotoxicosis leads to increased bone resorption/turnover and accelerated bone loss.

- *Ocular*. Eye involvement is apparent as retraction of the upper lid due to increased sympathetic tone. Lid lag is the appearance of the sclera above the iris as the eye is brought from superior to inferior gaze. Findings of Graves' orbitopathy were discussed earlier.

- *Gastrointestinal*. Increased motility causes frequent bowel movements known as *hyperdefecation*. Weight loss can occur despite an increased appetite, although in younger patients (twenties to forties) weight gain also can be seen.

- *Skin*. Skin may be warm and moist. The skin posterior to elbows is unusually smooth and soft. In Graves' disease, infiltrative dermopathy appears as hyperpigmented papules on the lower extremities. Hair loss and hair thinning can occur. Retraction of the nail from its bed, onycholysis, is a rare feature.

- *Reproductive*. In women, oligomenorrhea and amenorrhea may occur. Thyrotoxicosis causes an increase in sex hormone–binding globulin that results in an increase in total estradiol and low-normal free estradiol concentrations. The diminished midcycle luteinizing hormone (LH) surge may be the cause of menstrual irregularities.[40] In men, the elevation in sex hormone–binding globulin and reduction in free testosterone have been associated with erectile dysfunction in a small subset of patients.

- *Presentation in the Elderly.* Hyperthyroidism in the elderly may present with fewer symptoms of adrenergic activity and is known as *apathetic hyperthyroidism.* The primary findings are unexplained weight loss and atrial tachyarrhythmias.

The diagnosis of hyperthyroidism is made clinically and confirmed by laboratory findings. Symptoms from Graves' disease generally are present for several months, and those of hyperthyroidism due to thyroiditis are of a much shorter duration. The tests usually obtained include serum TSH, free T_4, and total or free T_3. In overt hyperthyroidism, the TSH concentration is below normal, and the free T_4 and total T_3 concentrations are elevated. The magnitude of elevation of T_3 and T_4 varies among the different thyroid conditions. In Graves' disease and toxic adenomas, T_3 usually is elevated more than T_4 due to a stimulation of intrathyroidal T_4 to T_3 conversion.[43] Elevation of only serum T_3 concentration and not serum T_4 concentration is known as *T_3 toxicosis* and usually is due to an underlying toxic adenoma or toxic multinodular goiter.

A thyroid iodine uptake scan is helpful in distinguishing types of hyperthyroidism. In Graves' disease, the gland is active, and the uptake will be increased diffusely. Thyroiditis (discussed below), on the other hand, is characterized by a low uptake scan. A toxic nodule usually will be apparent on physical examination, but a scan will show a focus of increased uptake with suppression of surrounding tissue.

Subclinical Hyperthyroidism

Subclinical hyperthyroidism is defined as a subnormal serum TSH concentration (<0.1 mU/L)

and normal free T_4 and total T_3 concentrations.[50] Symptoms of hyperthyroidism are subtle or absent. The primary reasons to consider treating subclinical hyperthyroidism include prevention of development to overt disease, prevention or improved control of atrial tachyarrhythmias, reduction in symptoms, reversal of weight loss, and reduction in bone loss. There is evidence that patients with subclinical hyperthyroidism have an increased risk of atrial fibrillation. In the Framingham Study population, the relative risk of developing atrial fibrillation was 3.1 times higher in patients with a suppressed serum TSH concentration.[51]

Postmenopausal women with a suppressed TSH concentration and not receiving hormone-replacement therapy are at increased risk of bone loss and fractures.[50] Treatment should be considered in patients with artial tachyarrhythmias, osteopenia or osteoporosis, unexplained weight loss, or other symptoms. Antithyroid medication can be used initially with the goal of normalizing serum TSH concentration. If there is a good response of symptoms, definitive treatment with radioiodine can be considered. Patients with mild Graves' disease should be treated for 6 to 12 months with antithyroid drugs if there are no contraindications. The overall chance of remission is around 30 percent, but there is likely a higher rate in patients with milder disease.

Treatment of Hyperthyroidism

Graves' Disease

Antithyroid medications, radioactive iodine, and surgery are useful tools in the treatment of Graves' disease. In patients younger than age 50 without cardiovascular disease, antithyroid medications are used often as initial treatment.[52,53] Methimazole and propylthiouracil (PTU) inhibit thyroid hormone synthesis by blocking thyroid peroxidase and preventing the organification of iodide and coupling of iodothyronines. PTU has the added benefit, at high serum T_4 concentration, of blocking the peripheral deiodination of T_4 to T_3, which makes it the preferred drug in severe hyperthyroidism. Thionamides also may have an immunosuppressive effect by decreasing thyroid antigen expression. Patients may have a remission from disease if their thyroid-stimulating immunoglobulin titers decline. About one-third of patients will have long-term remission after being treated for 6 to 12 months with thionamides. Treating beyond 18 months does not increase remission rates, and the patient and physician may decide to continue oral therapy or switch to another form of therapy at that time. The most significant side effect of thionamide therapy, occuring in 3 of 1000 patients, is agranulocytosis. It is more common in patients older than the age of 40 and possibly with higher doses of medication. Patients should be instructed to stop the medication and seek medical care if sore throat, fever, or oral ulcers develop. Other rare reactions include a rash, cholestasis, and hepatitis.

In older patients or those without clinical remission from antithyroid drug therapy, radioactive iodine is a viable option. Radioactive iodine is concentrated in the thyroid gland and selectively ablates the surrounding tissue. Radioactive iodine should not be used in pregnant or lactating females because of the risk of causing hypothyroidism in the offspring. In women of reproductive age, conception should be delayed until 6 months after the therapeutic dose of radioiodine has been administered. Radioactive iodine is a safe and effective therapy in nonpregnant adults. As a consequence of effective radioiodine treatment, most patients will become hypothyroid and require lifelong T_4 replacement therapy. Radioiodine may worsen Graves' ophthalmopathy, but treatment with prednisone has been shown to reduce the incidence of worsening ophthalmopathy.[54] Approximately 10 percent of patients with Graves' disease may require a second treatment with radioactive iodine. Patients with severe hyperthyroidism should be treated with antithyroid drugs for 4 to 8 weeks prior to radioactive iodine to prevent the slight risk of a radioiodine-induced thyrotoxic crisis. Antithyroid drugs should be stopped for 3 to 5 days prior to radioiodine therapy to ensure maximal uptake of radioactive iodine in the thyroid gland. In more active disease, antithyroid therapy may be restarted 3 to 5 days after radioiodine, but these patients should be followed every 2 to 3 weeks to monitor response to treatment.

Near-total thyroidectomy may be done in patients who refuse other forms of therapy, those with large goiters, pregnant women requiring high-dose antithyroid drug, or those with a coexisting suspicious nodule. Patients should be pretreated with an antithyroid agent and iodine until euthyroid, when possible, to minimize surgical morbidity.[55]

Short-term β-blocker therapy is useful to decrease the adrenergic effects of thyrotoxicosis. It can reduce the symptoms of tremor, anxiety, and palpitations more rapidly than antithyroid medications. It should be used in combination with antithyroid medications and not as a single treatment.

Inorganic iodine can be used to inhibit the release of thyroid hormone. Its onset of action is more rapid than antithyroid drugs, but it is effective for only a few days. It can be used during thyroid crises, prior to surgery to prevent thyroid crisis, and after radioactive iodine therapy to rapidly decrease serum thyroid hormone levels.

Toxic Adenoma/Goiter

Toxic goiters may be treated with antithyroid medications, radioactive iodine, or surgery.[56] Antithyroid medications are effective in controlling the thyrotoxic state caused by these adenomas or goiters and may be used long term. However, unlike Graves' disease, remission is rare with antithyroid medications alone. Radioiodine is usually the definitive therapy for toxic goiters or adenomas. The dose of radioiodine generally is higher than that used for Graves' disease. Surgery is indicated for those with a very large multinodular goiter, those with coexisting nonfunctioning nodules, or those who need rapid correction of thyrotoxicosis.

Hyperthyroidism in Pregnancy

Hyperthyroidism occurs in 0.2 percent of pregnancies, and Graves' disease accounts for 95 percent of these cases.[57] Pregnancy complicated by poorly controlled hyperthyroidism poses a health risk (Table 12-4) and is associated with preterm delivery, spontaneous abortion, low birth weight, preeclampsia, and maternal congestive heart failure. Thyroid-stimulating immunoglobulins causing maternal Graves' disease are able to cross the placenta and induce neonatal Graves' disease in about 1 percent of patients. Persistent elevations of TSI in the second trimester are associated with increased risk of neonatal Graves' disease.

Human chorionic gonadotropin (hCG) shares a common α subunit with TSH and considerable homology with the β subunit,[58] consequently having a spectrum of effects on the thyroid (Table 12-5). The CG/LH receptor is also similar to the TSH receptor. Many patients with hydatidiform mole, associated with high levels of hCG, were found to be thyrotoxic. It was later shown that at high concentrations of hCG there is "spillover," with direct stimulation of the TSH receptor. In normal pregnancy, this produces slightly increased free T_4 levels with a resulting decrease in TSH levels in the first trimester (Fig. 12-3). The clinical significance of this increase in free T_4 is not certain, but it may be important for placental and fetal development prior to the presence of the fetal thyroid gland. In conditions where the hCG concentration is higher than in a normal pregnancy, such as multiple gestations or hyperemesis gravidarum, thyroid function tests are more significantly altered with a suppressed serum TSH concentration and an elevated serum T_4 concentration. Antithyroid drug treatment, however, does not influence the course of hyperemesis gravidarum. Choriocarcinomas and hydatidiform mole, with very high hCG levels, are associated with thyrotoxicosis.[59]

Determining the etiology of hyperthyroidism in pregnancy is more difficult than in the nonpregnant patient. hCG has thyroid-stimulating properties (see Table 12-5). Consequently, TSH levels will decrease as hCG levels rise in early pregnancy (see Fig. 12-3). However, even then an elevated free T_4 or free T_3 concentration with a low TSH concentration would indicate hyperthyroidism. In nonpregnant patients, the distinction between Graves' disease and thyroiditis usually is made with a radioiodine uptake scan. This test, however, is contraindicated during pregnancy because of the potential for the fetal thyroid to concentrate the radioiodine. A TSI titer is helpful in this instance because a positive value will be suggestive of Graves' disease. Although less common than Graves' disease, one also should consider thyroiditis, toxic nodule/goiter, a state of excess hCG (e.g., multiple-gestation or hydatidiform molar pregnancy), and exogenous thyroid hormone ingestion (see Table 12-3).

Treatment of Graves' disease during pregnancy can be challenging. Radioiodine is contraindicated, and surgery may induce premature labor. If surgery must be done, it should

▶ **TABLE 12-4:** MATERNAL AND FETAL COMPLICATIONS OF HYPERTHYROIDISM

Maternal Complications	Fetal Complications
Eclampsia	Low birth weight
Preterm delivery	Increased perinatal mortality
Congestive heart failure	Increase in congenital anomalies (some studies)
	Neonatal hypothyroidism (maternal antithyroid drug)
	Neonatal hyperthyroidism (transplacental stimulating immunoglobulin)

▶ **TABLE 12-5:** RANGE OF INFLUENCE OF hCG ON THYROID FUNCTION

Nature of hCG Elevation	Clinical Consequences and Changes in Thyroid Function Test
Physiologic elevation in the first trimester	Mild elevation of free T_4, mild reduction of TSH
Exaggerated first-trimester elevation (e.g., multiple gestations)	Greater increase in free T_4 and greater reduction in TSH, hyperemesis gravidarum
Pathologic elevation from hydatidiform mole or choriocarcinoma	Marked increase in free T_4/T_3, suppressed TSH, clinical thyrotoxicosis
TSH mutation with increased sensitivity to hCG	Gestational thyrotoxicosis

be scheduled during the second trimester, if possible. Otherwise, the therapy of choice is antithyroid medication. Propylthiouracil is used more commonly because methimazole has been associated with the development of a rare anomaly, aplasia cutis. PTU readily crosses the placenta, and in excess it can induce neonatal goiter and hypothyroidism. For this reason, the dose of PTU used in pregnancy should be as low as possible and should be adjusted to maintain the maternal free T_4 concentration in the upper normal range. Beta blockers have been used safely in pregnancy, but there are reports of intrauterine growth retardation, neonatal hypoglycemia, and respiratory depression with these drugs.

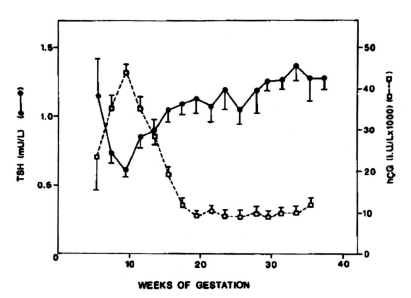

Figure 12-3 Pattern of serum concentrations of TSH and hCG in 606 healthy Belgium women throughout pregnancy. *(Reproduced, with permission, from Glinoer et al. J Clin Endocrinol Metab 1990;71:276–287.)*

▶ THYROIDITIS

Transient thyroid inflammation can be due to a number of etiologies and can be associated with thyroid hormone elevation, reduction, or elevation followed by reduction. Because thyroiditis involves the release of preformed hormone, antithyroid medications that block the synthesis of new thyroid hormone have no role in the treatment. Beta blockade may be useful in severe cases to reduce adrenergic side effects. In patients with painful subacute thyroiditis, glucocorticoid therapy can help to relieve thyroid pain. Patients with thyroiditis may develop transient hypothyroidism after 1 to 4 months that requires thyroid hormone replacement.[47]

Painful Subacute Thyroiditis

Subacute granulomatous thyroiditis (de Quervain's thyroiditis) is a transient hyperthyroid disorder in which inflammation of the thyroid gland leads to release of preformed thyroid hormone. It occurs after a viral upper respiratory illness, and symptoms include a painful goiter, hoarseness, dysphagia, and symptoms of hyperthyroidism.

Painless "Silent" Subacute Thyroiditis

This is an autoimmune-mediated transient hyperthyroidism usually not associated with thyroid pain. The hyperthyroidism lasts 1 to 2 months and is followed by euthyroidism in 50 percent of affected patients. The other 50 percent of individuals will develop hypothyroidism lasting 2 to 9 months. Although most eventually will become euthyroid, some may become hypothyroid in the future.[40] Postpartum thyroiditis is a variant of silent thyroiditis that can present 3 to 6 months after delivery.

Other Causes of Thyroiditis

Other causes of thyroiditis include radiation and neck surgery. Drugs that may cause thyroiditis include amiodarone, interferon, and lithium. Hyperthyroidism associated with thyroiditis usually is transient and requires only observation.

Postpartum Thyroiditis

Postpartum thyroiditis is a silent subacute thyroiditis. Pregnant women with positive anti-TPO antibodies are more likely to develop postpartum thyroiditis because approximately 50 percent of antibody-positive women will develop thyroiditis.[60] This disorder occurs 2 to 6 months after delivery and has at least three different patterns. The most common pattern is hypothyroidism only, affecting about 40 percent of patients. About 35 percent of patients have hypothyroidism, and 25 percent have hyperthyroidism followed by hypothyroidism occurring over a period of 4 to 8 months. These patterns are then followed by normalization in most patients. In general, the iodine uptake during hyperthyroidism is low. The only other conditions that can be associated with elevated T_4 levels and low uptake are exogenous thyroid hormone ingestion and iodine load. The hypothyroidism usually resolves spontaneously over 6 to 12 months, but about 25 percent of affected women will develop overt hypothyroidism within 4 years. These patients generally can be identified by persistent TPO positivity.

▶ GOITER

Approach to the Patient with Goiter

Goiter refers to a diffuse enlargement of the thyroid gland and can be a manifestation of a number of different underlying thyroid conditions. The conditions to consider include Graves' disease, chronic autoimmune thyroiditis, subacute thyroiditis, euthyroid multinodular goiter, and iodine deficiency. Most of these conditions can be diagnosed with history, examination, and routine thyroid function tests, including TPO antibodies. A nodular thyroid gland can be diffusely nodular or contain single or multiple localized nodules. Patients should be evaluated for underlying thyroid function, assessed for any impingement of swallowing or breathing, and evaluated for cancer risk. Discrete, solitary nodules >1.5 cm in diameter should undergo fine-needle aspiration. If diffuse or irregular thyroid enlargment is present, imaging generally includes a radioiodine uptake scan to identify any discrete "cold" areas that are suspicious for cancer, although only 10 to 20 percent of cold nodules are cancerous. A thyroid ultrasound often can complement the information from a scan and provide baseline thyroid gland dimensions to be used for follow-up. If there are any signs or symptoms of impingement of the trachea or esophagus, a neck CT or MRI should be obtained. Many older patients with multinodular goiters can develop autonomous thyroid function, usually identified by a suppressed TSH concentration.[50]

Treatment of Goiter

There are a number of treatments for goiter. Many patients with nontoxic goiter are treated initially with levothyroxine to reduce the serum TSH concentration. The reduction in size generally is modest, and treatment must be continued chronically. If the initial TSH level is elevated, however, reduction in size in response to levothyroxine can be quite significant. Radioactive iodine can be effective at reducing the size of goiters from 40 to 60 percent in volume, although large doses of radioiodine usually are required because the uptake is mod-

est. Recombinant TSH can be given, however, to increase uptake and improve the effectiveness of radioiodine therapy.[56] Larger goiters with compression of the trachea or esophagus usually are best treated with surgical removal.

▶ THYROID DISEASE AND FERTILITY

There are many reports of women with severe hypothyroidism and hyperthyroidism becoming pregnant, so thyroid disease does not necessarily interfere with fertility. Several studies, however, have found a higher incidence of thyroid dysfunction among women being evaluated for infertility. Ovulatory dysfunction is associated with hypothyroidism and in some women appears most responsive to treatment with T_4 alone. In one study of 704 women who were unable to conceive for 1 year, 2.3 percent had an elevated serum TSH concentration.[63] These women were treated with T_4 to normalize the serum TSH level. Among these women who received T_4 treatment, 70 percent were classified as having ovulatory dysfunction, and 64 percent of them became pregnant. Among the 30 percent without ovulatory dysfunction, only 30 percent became pregnant. Overall, the rate of conception is thought to be reduced in the presence of hypothyroidism.

A recent study compared over 400 women with infertility and 100 controls.[64] Although the mean TSH level was slightly higher and TPO positivity also was higher in the women with infertility, there was no overall difference in the incidence of thyroid dysfunction in the study and control groups. TPO positivity and TSH elevation were, however, significantly more common in women from couples with female-origin infertility. Women with endometriosis had the highest prevalence of TPO positivity (29 percent).

Antithyroid antibodies during pregnancy are associated with an increased rate of miscarriage. Women with antithyroid antibodies in the first trimester of pregnancy have a rate of spontaneous abortion that is twice the normal rate.[14] This is thought most likely to be an index of autoimmunity rather than a direct effect of antithyroid antibodies. Among almost 500 women who became pregnant by assisted reproductive techniques, the miscarriage rate in antibody-positive patients (anti-Tg or anti-TPO) was 32 percent compared with 16 percent in antibody-negative patients.[61] There was no significant difference in the incidence of ectopic pregnancy or the ability to achieve pregnancy between the groups. The presence of antithyroid antibodies in women with multiple previous abortions was associated with an increased risk of subsequent miscarriages.[61]

Although there is little evidence that thyroid dysfunction plays a central role in most women with infertility, there are a number of compelling reasons for evaluation of thyroid status and treatment if abnormalities are demonstrated. Some women with infertility and thyroid dysfunction, especially those with ovulatory dysfunction and possibly endometriosis, may respond to thyroid treatment. Even if T_4 treatment does not induce ovulation and conception directly, there are a number of reasons to believe that euthyroxinemia is especially important in the first trimester for normal development of the fetus. It is reasonable, therefore, to evaluate women with a serum TSH and, possibly, an anti-TPO antibody measurement. Thyroxine treatment can be initiated if abnormalities are detected, targeting a low-normal TSH.

▶ RESISTANCE TO THYROID HORMONE

The characteristic laboratory findings of resistance to thyroid hormone (RTH) are high serum concentrations of T_4 and T_3 with an inappropriately normal or slightly elevated TSH value.[65] Individuals with RTH are clinically euthyroid but usually retain cardiac sensitivity to the elevated thyroid hormone levels and often have tachycardia. There is also an association of RTH with attention deficit–hyperactivity disorder and impaired growth. The genetic defect in RTH is a point mutation in the thyroid hormone receptor β gene creating a dominant negative protein. Affected patients are heterozygous for the mutation. Selective pituitary resistance has been reported in a few patients who have elevated thyroid hormone levels, "inappropriately" normal or slightly high TSH levels, and some clinical manifestations of hyperthyroidism. The diagnosis can be based on family history, dynamic testing demonstrating a resistance to graded doses of T_3, or direct sequencing of the thyroid hormone receptor beta gene. Treatment is usually not necessary, although some physicians use T_3 supplements in selected patients.

KEY POINTS

1. Measurement of serum TSH is generally sufficient to evaluate thyroid status, but additional studies sometimes are required, including thyroid peroxidase antibodies, T_4, and T_3.

2. Subclinical hypothyroidism, an elevated serum TSH level, and a normal-range serum T_4 concentration can be associated with symptoms of fatigue, elevated cholesterol, goiter, and ovulatory dysfunction.

3. Thyroid peroxidase antibody positivity is associated with an increased risk of miscarriage.

4. T_4 therapy in infertile women with hypothyroidism is associated with conception in women with ovulatory dysfunction.

5. Women likely to have postpartum thyroiditis, the most common thyroid disorder associated with pregnancy, can be identified by measurement of thyroid peroxidase antibodies in the first trimester.

6. Many hypothyroid women who become pregnant require an increase in T_4 replacement dose that persists throughout pregnancy.

7. Incompletely treated maternal hypothyroidism during pregnancy is associated with preterm delivery and moderate intellectual deficit in offspring.

8. Hyperthyroidism in pregnancy can be treated with antithyroid drugs, usually propylthiouracil, but the maternal free T_4 concentration should be kept in the upper normal range to prevent inducing fetal hypothyroidism.

REFERENCES

1. LaFranchi S. Congenital hypothyroidism: Etiologies, diagnosis, and management. *Thyroid* 1999;9:735.

2. Bianco AC, Salvatore D, Gereben B, et al. Biochemistry, cellular and molecular biology, and physiological roles of the iodothyronine selenodeiodinases. *Endocr Rev* 2002;23:38.

3. Motomura K, Brent GA. Mechanism of thyroid hormone action: Implications for the clinical manifestations of thyrotoxicosis. *Endocrinol Metab Clin North Am* 1998;27:1.

4. Davis PJ, Davis FB. Nongenomic actions of thyroid hormone. *Thyroid* 1996;6:497.

5. Dohan O, DeLaVieja A, Paroder V, et al. The sodium/iodide symporter (NIS): Characterization, regulation, and medical significance. *Endocr Rev* 2003;24:48.

6. Kopp P. Pendred's syndrome and genetic defects in thyroid hormone synthesis. *Rev Endocr Metab Disord* 2000;1:109.

7. Gudmundsdottir A, Schlechte JA. Central hypothyroidism. *Endocrinologist* 2002;12:218.

8. Dunn JT, Dunn AD. Update on intrathyroidal iodine metabolism. *Thyroid* 2001;11:407.

9. Hollowell JG, Staehling NW, Hannon WH, et al. Iodine nutrition in the United States, trends and public health implications: Iodine excretion data from National Health and Nutrition Examination Surveys I and III (1971–1974 and 1988–1994). *J Clin Endocrinol Metab* 1998;83:3401.

10. Glinoer D. The regulation of thyroid function in pregnancy: Pathways of endocrine adaptation from physiology to pathology. *Endocr Rev* 1997;18:404.

11. Smallridge RC, Ladenson PW. Commentary: hypothyroidism in pregnancy: Consequences to neonatal health. *J Clin Endocrinol Metab* 2001; 86:2349.

12. Dunn JT, Delange F. Damaged reproduction: The most important consequence of iodine deficiency. *J Clin Endocrinol Metab* 2001;86:2360.

13. Zulewski H, Muller B, Exer P, et al. Estimation of tissue hypothyroidism by a new clinical score: Evaluation of patients with various grades of hypothyroidism and controls. *J Clin Endocrinol Metab* 1997;82:771.

14. Nicoloff JT, Spencer CA. The use and misuse of the sensitive thyrotropin assays. *J Clin Endocrinol Metab* 1990;71:553.

15. Langton JE, Brent GA. Nonthyroidal illness syndrome: Evaluation of thyroid function in sick patients. *Endocrinol Metab Clin North Am* 2002; 31:159.

16. Hollowell JG, Staehling NW, Flanders WD, et al. Serum TSH and thyroid antibodies in the United States population (1988 to 1994): National Health and Nutrition Examination Survey (NHANES III). *J Clin Endocrinol Metab* 2002; 87:489.

17. Brent GA. Maternal thyroid function: Interpretation of thyroid function tests in pregnancy. *Clin Obstet Gynecol* 1997;40:3.

18. Wang R, Nelson JC, Weiss RM, et al. Accuracy of free thyroxine measurements across natural ranges of thyroxine binding to serum proteins. *Thyroid* 2000;10:31.

19. Dayan CM, Daniels GH. Medical progress: Chronic autoimmune thyroiditis. *N Engl J Med* 1996;335:99.

20. Smallridge RC. Postpartum thyroid disease: A model of immunologic dysfunction. *Clin Appl Immunol Rev* 2000;1:89

21. Huber G, Staub J-J, Meier C, et al. Prospective study of the spontaneous course of subclinical hypothyroidism: Prognostic value of thyrotropin, thyroid reserve, and thyroid antibodies. *J Clin Endocrinol Metab* 2002;87:3221.

22. Weetman, AP. Medical progress: Graves' disease. *N Engl J Med* 2000;343:1236.

23. Surks MI, Sievert R. Drugs and thyroid function. *N Engl J Med* 1995;333:1688.

24. Arafah BM. Increased need for thyroxine in women with hypothyroidism during estrogen therapy. *N Engl J Med* 2001;344:1743.

25. Arafah BM. Decreased levothyroxine requirement in women with hypothyroidism during

androgen therapy for breast cancer. *Ann Intern Med* 1994;121:247.

26. Brabant G, Brabant A, Ranft K. Circadian and pulsatile thyrotropin secretion in euthyroid man under the influence of thyroid hormone and glucocorticoid administration. *J Clin Endocrinol Metab* 1987;65:83.

27. LoPresti JS, Eigen A, Kaptein E, et al. Alterations in 3,3'5'-trioiodothyronine metabolism in response to propylthiouracil, dexamethasone, and thyroxine administration in man. *J Clin Invest* 1989;84:1650.

28. Kaptein E, Spencer CA, Kamiel MB, et al. Prolonged dopamine administration and thyroid hormone economy in normal and critically ill subjects. *J Clin Endocrinol Metab* 1980;51:387.

29. Sherman SI, Gopal J, Haugen BR, et al. Central hypothyroidism associated with retinoid X receptor–selective ligands. *N Engl J Med* 1999; 340:1075.

30. Bongu D, Sachdev J, Kabadi UM. Effects of carbamazepine on the hypothalamic-pituitary-thyroid axis. *Endocr Pract* 1999;5:239.

31. McCowen KC, Garber JR, Spark R. Elevated serum thyrotropin in thyroxine-treated patients with hypothyroidism given sertraline. *N Engl J Med* 1997;337:1010.

32. Bryer-Ash M. Evaluation of the patient with a suspected thyroid disorder. *Obstet Gynecol Clin* 2001;28:421.

33. Attia J, Margetts P, Guyatt G. Diagnosis of thyroid disease in hospitalized patients: A systematic review. *Arch Intern Med.* 1999;159:658.

34. Cooper DS. Subclinical hypothyroidism. *N Engl J Med* 2001;345:260.

35. Vanderpump MP, Tunbridge WM, French JM, et al. The incidence of thyroid disorders in the community: A twenty-year follow-up of the Whickham Survey. *Clin Endocrinol (Oxf)* 1995; 43:55–68.

36. Hershman JM. Hyperthyroidism and hypothyroidism, in Norman Lavin (ed) *Manual of Endocrinology and Metabolism,* 3d ed. Philadelphia: Lippincott Williams & Wilkins, 2002; pp 396–409.

37. Klein I, Ojamaa K. Mechanisms of disease: Thyroid hormone and the cardiovascular system. *N Engl J Med* 2001;344:501.

38. Leung AS, Millar LK, Koonings PP, et al. Perinatal outcome in hypothyroid pregnancies. *Obstet Gynecol* 1993;81:349.

39. Abalovich M, Gutierrez S, Alcaraz G, et al. Overt and subclinical hypothyroidism complicating pregnancy. *Thyroid* 2002;12:63.

40. Mandel SJ, Brent GA, Larsen PR. Levothyroxine therapy in patients with thyroid disease. *Ann Intern Med* 1993;119:492.

41. Bunevicius R, Kazanavicius G, Zalinkevicius R, et al. Effects of thyroxine as compared with thyroxine plus triiodothyronine in patients with hypothyroidism. *N Engl J Med* 1999;340: 424.

42. Keating FR, Parkin TW, Selby JB, et al. Treatment of heart disease associated with myxedema. *Prog Cardiovasc Dis* 1961;3:364.

43. Mandel SJ, Larsen PR, Seely EW, Brent GA. Increased need for thyroxine during pregnancy in women with primary hypothyroidism. *N Engl J Med* 1990;323:91.

44. Kaplan MM. Monitoring thyroxine treatment during pregnancy. *Thyroid* 1992;2:147.

45. Singh N, Singh PN, Hershman JM. Effect of calcium carbonate on the absorption of levothyroxine. *JAMA* 2000;283:2822.

46. Haddow JE, Palomaki GE, Allan WC, et al. Maternal thyroid deficiency during pregnancy and subsequent neuropsychological development of the child. *N Engl J Med* 1999;341:549.

47. Laurberg P, Pedersen KM, Vestergaard H, et al. High incidence of multinodular toxic goiter in the elderly population in a low iodine area vs high incidence Graves' disease in the young in a high iodine intake area: Comparative surveys of thyrotoxicosis epidemiology in East Jutland Denmark and Iceland. *J Intern Med* 1991;229: 415.

48. Paschke R, Ludgate M. The thyrotropin receptor in thyroid diseases. *N Engl J Med* 1997; 337:1675.

49. Beck-Peccoz P, Brucker-Davis F, Persani L, et al. Thyrotropin-secreting pituitary tumors. *Endocr Rev* 1996;17:610–638.

50. Toft AD. Subclinical hyperthyroidism. *N Engl J Med* 2001;345:512.

51. Sawin CT, Gellar A, Wolf PA, et al. Low serum thyrotropin concentrations as a risk factor for atrial fibrillation in older patients. *N Engl J Med* 1994;331:249.

52. Franklyn JA. The management of hyperthyroidism. *N Engl J Med* 1994;330:1731.

53. Cooper DS. Antithyroid drugs. *N Engl J Med* 1984;311:1353.

54. Bartalena L, Marcocci C, Bogazzi F, et al. Relation between therapy for hyperthyroidism and the course of Graves' opthalmopathy. *N Engl J Med* 1998;338:73.

55. Chou F-F, Wang P-W, Huang SC. Results of subtotal thyroidectomy for Graves' disease. *Thyroid* 1999;9 253.

56. Nieuwlaat W-A, Hermus AR, Huysmans DA. Nontoxic, nodular goiter: New management paradigms. *Endocrinologist* 2003;13:31.

57. Kilpatrick S. Thyroid disease in pregnancy. *ACOG Pract Bull* 2001;98:879.

58. Yoshimura M, Hershman JM. Thyrotropic action of human chorionic gonadotropin. *Thyroid* 1995;5:425.

59. Goodwin TM, Montoro M, Hershman JM, et al. The role of chorionic gonadotropin in transient hyperthyroidism of hyperemesis gravidarum. *J Clin Endocrinol Metab* 1992;75:1333.

60. Stagnaro-Green A. Postpartum thyroiditis. *J Clin Endocrinol Metab* 2002;87:4042.

61. Singh A, Dantas ZN, Stone S, et al. Presence of thyroid antibodies in early reproductive failure: Biochemical versus clinical pregnancies. *Fertil Steril* 1995;63:277.

62. Pratt D, Novotny M, Kaberlein G, et al. Antithyroid antibodies and the association with non-organ-specific antibodies in recurrent pregnancy loss. *Am J Obstet Gynecol* 1993;168:837.

63. Lincoln SR, Ke RW, Kutteh WH. Screening for hypothyroidism in infertile women. *J Reprod Med* 1999;44:455.

64. Poppe K, Glinoer D, Van Steirteghem A, et al. Thyroid dysfunction and autoimmunity in infertile women. *Thyroid* 2002;12:997.

65. Weiss RE, Refetoff S. Resistance to thyroid hormone. *Rev Endocr Metab Disord* 2000;1:97.

CHAPTER 13

Androgen Excess, Hirsutism, and the Polycystic Ovary Syndrome

Ricardo Azziz

Androgen excess disorders include the polycystic ovary syndrome (PCOS), nonclassic adrenal hyperplasia (NCAH), the hyperandrogenic insulin-resistant acanthosis nigricans (HAIRAN) syndrome, and androgen-secreting neoplasms (Table 13-1). Androgen excess may result in the development of androgenic clinical features in the women affected, with the development of hirsutism, androgenic alopecia, acne, ovulatory dysfunction, and if extreme and prolonged, even virilization and masculinization. Although the most recognizable clinical feature of androgen excess is hirsutism, it should be noted that not all patients with hirsutism have evidence of androgen excess, as in the patient with idiopathic hirsutism (IH). Likewise, not all patients with an androgen excess disorder have clinically evident hirsutism, as in the Asian patient with PCOS.

► ANDROGEN BIOSYNTHESIS IN WOMEN

Androgens are C_{19} steroids secreted by the zona reticularis of the adrenal cortex and the theca and stroma of the ovaries, and they also are produced through de novo synthesis from cholesterol[1] (Fig. 13-1). In addition, circulating steroid precursors can be metabolized further in these organs or in peripheral tissues, including the liver, adipose tissue stroma, and the pilosebaceous unit (PSU) in skin, to more potent androgens [e.g., the conversion of testosterone to dihydrotestosterone (DHT)] and to estrogens via the action of aromatase, or they can be inactivated and readied for excretion via glucuronidization or sulfation. The origins of the principal circulating plasma androgens in premenopausal women are summarized in Table 13-2.

Androgens, either directly or through metabolites, can act systemically in a classic endocrine fashion or locally in a paracrine and intracrine fashion (e.g., in the PSU). Androgens exert their genomic effects through interaction with the androgen receptor, a member of the nuclear receptor superfamily. The unbound androgen receptor is a cytoplasmic protein, and on ligand binding, it translocates into the nucleus. In the nucleus it influences the transcription of target genes through a complex

▶ **TABLE 13-1:** DIFFERENTIAL DIAGNOSIS OF THE PATIENT WITH ANDROGEN EXCESS AND/OR HIRSUTISM

Disorder	Prevalence*
Polycystic ovary syndrome (PCOS)	80–90%
21-Hydroxylase-deficient nonclassic adrenal hyperplasia (NCAH)	1–10%
Hyperandrogenic–insulin resistant–acanthosis nigricans (HAIRAN) syndrome	2–4%
Drug-induced	~1%
Ovarian androgen-secreting neoplasms	1/300–1/1000
Andrenal androgen-secreting neoplasms	<1/1000
Idiopathic hirsutism	5–15%†

*Prevalence based on all patients with androgen excess.
†Prevalence based on all patients with hirsutism.

process that includes interactions with other transcription factors and coactivators. As noted, androgens also can exert their effects indirectly, though metabolites such as the estrogens.

Androgens circulate in the body bound by a variety of proteins, most important of which is sex hormone–binding globulin (SHBG). Because of its greater concentration and total amount, albumin has a much higher overall binding capacity for androgens than SHBG. However, since the affinity of androgens for SHBG is much higher, this protein binds the

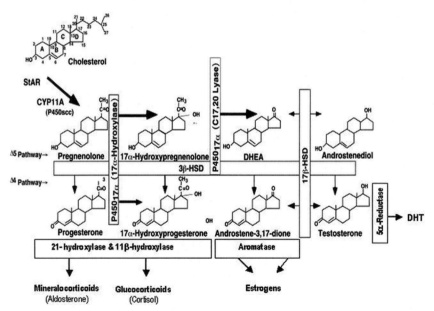

Figure 13-1 Pathways of androgen synthesis. The ovary, the testis, and the adrenal gland produce six common core steroids. The core Δ^5 steroids are pregnenolone, 17α-hydroxy-pregnenolone, and dehydroepiandrosterone. The core Δ^4 steroids are progesterone, 17α-hydroxy-progesterone, and androstenedione (androstene-3,17-dione). These core steroids are important precursors for the production of sex steroids, glucocorticoids, and mineralocorticoids.

▶ **TABLE 13-2:** PERCENT ORIGIN OF ANDROGENS IN PREMENOPAUSAL WOMEN IN THE FOLLICULAR PHASE OF THE MENSTRUAL CYCLE

Androgen*	Ovarian Theca/Stroma	Adrenal Reticularis	Pheripheral Conversion†
DHT	0	0	80 (A4), 20 (T)
T	25	20	55 (A4), 5 (DHEA)
A_4	30–50	50–70	15 (DHEA)
DHEA	25	50	25 (DHEAS)
DHEAS	0	70	30 (DHEA)

*Abbreviations: A_4 = androstenedione; DHEA = dehydroepiandrosterone; DHEAS = dehydroepiandrosterone sulfate; T = testosterone; DHT = dihydrotestosterone.

†Peripheral conversion primarily occurs in the liver, adipose tissue stroma, and pilosebaceous unit. Within parentheses are the denoted the precursors for peripheral conversion.

Modified from Vermeulen A. Androgen secretion by adrenals and gonads, in Mahesh VB, Greenblatt RB (eds), Hirsutism and Virilism. Boston: John Wright/PSG, Inc., 1983, p 17.

largest portion of circulating testosterone. Androgens bound to SHBG are essentially not bioavailable, although those complexed with albumin are more readily available for tissue interaction. The liver produces SHBG, and production is stimulated by estrogen, particularly oral forms; and inhibited by androgens and, most important, insulin. These factors lead to lower levels of SHBG and higher bioavailable androgens in males and patients with androgen excess disorders compared with healthy women. The clearance of androgens is accomplished by hepatic extraction and peripheral metabolism, which are highly dependent on the unbound portion of circulating steroid.

Androgens are affected by aging and obesity. Adrenal androgen production, particularly that of dehydroepiandrosterone (DHEA), its metabolite DHEA sulfate (DHEAS) and androstenedione, clearly decreases with age in premenopausal and postmenopausal women.[2] Testosterone levels are less affected by age and menopause, and it is clear that the ovary continues to produce a significant amount of testosterone in postmenopause.[3] Most of the decrease in circulating testosterone with age and menopause is explainable by the lower androstenedione levels. In obesity, the production rate and metabolic clearance rate of ovarian and adrenal-secreted androgens are increased, whereas circulating levels are maintained normal.[4]

▶ CLINICAL FEATURES OF ANDROGEN EXCESS

Androgen excess results in various clinical signs and symptoms, including abnormalities of the PSU (i.e., hirsutism, acne, and androgenic alopecia) and of the hypothalamic-pituitary-ovarian axis (i.e., ovulatory and menstrual dysfunction). If the androgen excess is very severe, virilization and/or masculinization also can be apparent (Table 13-3).

Androgen Excess and the PSU

The effects of androgens are most visible on the PSU. Androgens stimulate the transformation of fine, unpigmented vellus hairs to coarse, pigmented, thickened terminal hairs, a process termed *terminalization,* in skin areas sensitive to the effects of androgens. The peripheral effects of androgens are determined primarily by the intracellular actions of the enzymes 17β-ketosteroid reductase (converting androstenedione to testosterone) and 5α-reductase (converting testosterone to the more potent androgen DHT) and the androgen receptor content. Before puberty, body hair is composed primarily of fine, short, unpigmented vellus hairs. The increase in androgen production observed with pubertal development

▶ **TABLE 13-3:** CLINICAL FEATURES OF ANGROGEN EXCESS

▶ **TABLE 13-3:** CLINICAL FEATURES OF ANGROGEN EXCESS

Pilosebaceous Unit
- Hirsutism
- Acne
- Androgenic alopecia

Hypothalamic-Pituitary-Ovarian Axis
- Ovulatory dysfunction
- Oligomenorrhea
- Dysfunctional uterine bleeding
- Anovulatory infertility

Hypothalamic-Pituitary-Adrenal Axis
- Increased adrenal androgen production

Adipose Tissue
- Obesity (?)
- Android fat deposition (?)

Anabolic
- Clitoromegaly
- Virilization*
- Masculinization*

*Virilization is indicated by the presence of male-pattern balding, severe hirsutism, voice change, amenorrhea, and/or clitoromegaly. Masculinization is present when the androgen excess has resulted in a masculinized pattern of muscle and fat distribution, including reduction in breast size.

transforms some of these, mainly in androgen-sensitive areas of skin, such as the axilla and the genital triangle, into coarser, longer, pigmented terminal hairs. It should be noted that not all skin areas are androgen-sensitive. For example, the development of terminal hairs in body areas such as the eyebrows, eyelashes, and temporal and occipital scalp is relatively androgen-independent.

Hirsutism

Hirsutism is the presence of terminal (coarse) hairs in females in a malelike pattern. Excessive growth of coarse hairs of the lower forearms and lower legs alone does not constitute hirsutism, although women suffering from hirsutism may note an increase in the pigmentation and growth rate of hairs on these body areas. There are ethnic and genetic differences

that can modify the effects of androgens on skin, as demonstrated by the lesser degree of hirsutism present in Asian women with PCOS[5] (Fig. 13-2).

Hirsutism should be viewed much as polycystic ovaries are—*as a sign rather than a diagnosis.* Most commonly, hirsutism is associated with androgen excess. Some patients may have *idiopathic hirsutism,* identified as the presence of hirsutism without identifiable cause or associated abnormality. Because of its frequent association with PCOS, clinically evident androgen excess (e.g., hirsutism) is also a useful predictor of metabolic abnormalities in these women, including insulin resistance, glucose intolerance, or type 2 diabetes mellitus (DM).

Acne

The pilosebaceous unit, in addition to the hair follicle, also contains a sebaceous gland that produces an oily protective secretion called *sebum.* Androgens also cause increased sebum production and abnormal keratinization of the PSU, contributing to the development of seborrhea, folliculitis, and acne evident at puberty and in women with androgen excess. Elevations in serum androgen levels[6,7] and in the conversion rate of androgens to DHT via 5α-reductase[8] have been reported in patients with acne. Consequently, acne frequently improves following treatment with antiandrogens, oral contraceptives, or glucocorticoids.[9–11]

Androgenic Alopecia

While androgen excess can stimulate facial and body hair growth, paradoxically, androgens also can exert opposite effects on the hair follicles of the scalp, causing conversion of terminal follicles to vellus-like follicles, a process termed *miniaturization.* This effect may lead to the development of alopecia in women (and men). Scalp hair loss as a consequence of androgen excess can take two forms. In severe cases, where massive androgen excess and virilization/masculinization is present, patients can demonstrate the typical pattern of balding found in men (i.e., premature male-pattern

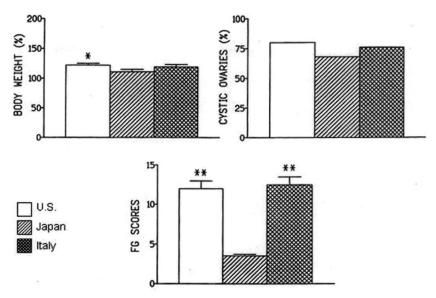

Figure 13-2   Features in PCOS women 25 each from the United States, Italy, and Japan. Note the much lower prevalence of hirsutism among Japanese women.   *(Modified from Carmina E, Koyama T, Chang L, et al. Does ethnicity influence the prevalence of adrenal hyperandrogenism and insulin resistance in polycystic ovary syndrome? Am J Obstet Gynecol 1992;167:1807–1812.)*

balding). More common, however, is the so-called androgenic (also known as androgenetic) alopecia of women, or female-pattern balding. In female androgenic alopecia, a diffuse thinning of hair throughout the sagittal scalp is noted primarily,[12] and approximately 40 percent of women with androgenic alopecia have some form of hyperandrogenemia.[13] However, if only nonhirsute women with androgenic alopecia are considered, then only 20 percent of these patients are found to be hyperandrogenemic.

Androgen Excess and Ovarian Function

A common feature of androgen excess disorders is ovulatory dysfunction, which may arise from a disruption in gonadotropin secretion or from direct ovarian effects. Androgens, indirectly through conversion to estrogens[14] and directly,[15] alter the secretion of gonadotropins

in women. However, the effect of androgens on the hypothalamic-pituitary-ovarian axis appears to depend primarily on the their aromatization to estrogens.[16] Excessive androgen levels also may inhibit follicular development directly[17,18] at the ovarian level, which may result in the accumulation of multiple small cysts within the ovarian cortex, the so-called polycystic ovary.

Androgens and the Adrenal

Adrenal androgen excess (e.g., elevated levels of DHEA and its metabolite DHEAS) is observed in 25 to 50 percent of women with androgen excess.[5,19,20] However, it is also possible that extraadrenal androgens (e.g., ovarian) may be responsible, at least in part, for the altered adrenocortical steroidogenesis and adrenal androgen excess. For example, we and others have observed a 20 to 25 percent decrease in mean DHEAS levels following long-acting gonadotropin-releasing hormone agonist (GnRH-a) suppression in PCOS women with elevated levels of this adrenal metabolite,[21,22] although elevated adrenal androgen levels in these women rarely normalize with GnRH-a suppression.[22] In a prospective study of seven healthy oophorectomized women receiving 3 weeks of parenteral exogenous testosterone, an increase in the metabolism of DHEA to DHEAS was observed, although the adrenal response to adrenocorticotropic hormone (ACTH) stimulation did not change.[23] Thus it appears that the secretion of adrenal androgens, particularly the metabolite DHEAS, can be increased by extraadrenal hyperandrogenemia, a mechanism that would serve to further maintain the androgen excess.

Obesity

Obesity has been closely associated with androgen excess, particularly PCOS. It is unclear whether obesity follows or precedes the development of androgen excess. Patients with PCOS will have more androgens available for peripheral aromatization, which can result in higher estradiol levels. In vitro, 17β-estradiol has been observed to promote human lipocyte replication.[24] In a prospective study, 10 young nonobese female-to-male transsexuals undergoing sex reassignment were studied by magnetic resonance imaging (MRI) before, 1 year after, and 3 years after of testosterone administration.[25] Therapy with testosterone in these patients was associated with only minimal changes in body weight over the course of the study, although there were important alterations in body fat distribution. After 1 year of treatment, subcutaneous fat at all levels studied (at the level of the abdomen, hip, and thigh) showed significant reductions compared with baseline, but these differences were no longer significant at 3 years. Alternatively, the mean visceral fat area did not change significantly in the first year of treatment, although subjects who gained weight in the first year of

treatment demonstrated an increase in visceral fat. By the third year of testosterone administration, the mean visceral fat depot had increased by 47 percent from baseline, and as before, the increase in visceral fat was most pronounced in the subjects who had gained weight.

Overall, these data suggest that androgen excess, either directly or via conversion to estrogens, is associated with an increase in visceral fat deposition, which may worsen the degree of insulin resistance and hyperandrogenemia in androgen excess patients. Alternatively, it is not known whether androgens themselves promote the development of obesity, although the observation that men are more obese than women of similar socioeconomic class is suggestive of this effect.[26]

Androgen Excess and Anabolic Features: Virilization and Masculinization

When androgen excess is extreme and prolonged, changes in fat and muscle distribution and masculinization of the genitalia, breasts, and facies may occur. Virilization includes the development of sagittal and frontal balding, clitoromegaly, and severe hirsutism. Furthermore, if androgen levels remain extremely elevated for a substantial period of time, particularly if begun before puberty, virilization may be accompanied by masculinization of the body habitus, with atrophy of the breasts, an increase in muscle mass, a redistribution of body fat, and a deepening of the voice. Premenopausal patients with virilization or masculinization are almost always amenorrheic. In general, virilization and/or masculinization suggests an androgen-secreting neoplasm or untreated classic (but not nonclassic; see below) adrenal hyperplasia. Occasionally, girls suffering from severe insulin resistance (i.e., HAIRAN syndrome; see below) may exhibit a moderate degree of virilization.

► POLYCYSTIC OVARY SYNDROME

By far the most common cause of androgen excess is PCOS, accounting for the vast majority of patients seen[27] (see Table 13-1). While there is continuing debate regarding the definition of PCOS, useful diagnostic criteria arose from a 1990 National Institutes of Health (NIH) conference on the subject.[28] These criteria note that PCOS should include: (1) clinical and/or biochemical evidence of hyperandrogenism, (2) ovulatory dysfunction, and (3) exclusion of other causes of androgen excess or ovulatory dysfunction, including adrenal hyperplasia, hyperprolactinemia, thyroid dysfunction, and androgen-secreting neoplasms (Table 13-4). The presence of polycystic ovaries on ultrasound was considered to be controversial and was not included as part of the definition. However, more recent proposals for the definition of this disorder have included polycystic ovaries on ultrasonography as one of the signs of the disorder.[29] Thus PCOS represents unexplained functional hyperandrogenic chronic anovulation and is primarily a diagnosis of exclusion.

► **TABLE 13-4:** CRITERIA FOR DEFINING PCOS ARISING FROM A 1990 NATIONAL INSTITUTES OF HEALTH CONFERENCE

1. Clinical and/or biochemical evidence of hyperandrogenism
2. Ovulatory dysfunction
3. Exclusion of other causes of androgen excess or ovulatory dysfunction*
4. The presence of polycystic ovaries on ultrasound was considered to be "controversial"

*Nonclassic adrenal hyperplasia, hyperprolactinemia, thyroid dysfunction, or androgen-secreting neoplasms.

From Zawadzki JK, Dunaif A. Diagnostic criteria for polycystic ovary syndrome: Towards a rational approach, in Dunaif A, Givens JR, Haseltine F, Merriam GR (eds), Polycystic Ovary Syndrome. Boston: Blackwell Scientific Publications, 1990:377–384.

PCOS appears to affect 4 to 6 percent of reproductive-age women.[30–32] A number of patient features are associated with a higher prevalence of PCOS, including a higher body mass,[33] insulin resistance,[33] type 1 or type 2 DM,[32,34,35] hirsutism,[30–32,36] oligoovulatory infertility,[37–39] and polycystic ovaries on sonography.[40,41] The risk of PCOS also may increase in women with a history of premature adrenarche,[42] gestational diabetes,[43,44] or PCOS in a first-degree relative.[45] Below are reviewed the clinical, biochemical, and metabolic features of PCOS (Table 13-5), as well as the long-term sequelae.

Clinical, Morphologic, Biochemical, and Metabolic Features of PCOS

Clinically evident PCOS tends to develop shortly after menarche and persists through most of reproductive life. Nonetheless, some patients may present initially in prepuberty with premature adrenarche, with affected girls displaying hyperinsulinemia, elevated DHEAS levels, and postmenarcheal oligomenorrhea.[42]

Ovulatory Dysfunction in PCOS

If the criteria arising from the 1990 NIH conference[28] are used, by definition, 100 percent of patients with PCOS have evidence of ovulatory dysfunction, although many may not be amenorrheic or even oligomenorrheic.[46] However, it has been suggested that PCOS (or ovarian hyperandrogenism) may be present even if ovulatory function is retained,[47] although further studies are needed. Ovulatory dysfunction in PCOS frequently results in oligoovulatory infertility. As a general rule, PCOS women represent one of the most difficult groups in which to induce ovulation both successfully and safely. Many PCOS women are unresponsive or resistant to ovulation induction with clomiphene citrate and may have an inappropriate or exaggerated response to the administration of human menopausal gonadotropins (menotropins). In part, the abnormal response

▶ **TABLE 13-5:** FEATURES OF PCOS

Clinical	
• Hirsutism	~30–80% depending on ethnicity
• Acne	~15–20%
• Androgenic alopecia	~5–10%
• Obesity	~20–60%
• Anovulation	~90–100% depending on definition
• Oligo/amenorrhea	~50–70%
Ovarian	
• Polycystic ovaries	~70–80%
Biochemical	
• Elevated LH/FSH ratio	~35–95%
• Elevated Free T	~60–80%
• Elevated Total T	~30–50%
• Elevated DHEAS	~25–70%
Metabolic	
• Hyperinsulinism	~25–60%

to ovulatory agents of PCOS patients may relate to their degree of hyperinsulinemia and obesity, as well as abnormalities of the intra-ovarian hormonal milieu and the increased number of preantral follicles.

PCOS women are at especially increased risk for developing the ovarian hyperstimulation syndrome, a syndrome including massive enlargement of the ovaries, development of rapid and symptomatic ascites, intravascular contraction, hypercoagulability, and systemic organ dysfunction. Patients with PCOS are also at greater risk for multiple gestations. These complications occur generally following treatment with menotropins, although ovarian hyperstimulation has even been reported in women with PCOS conceiving a singleton pregnancy spontaneously, or after clomiphene or pulsatile GnRH use.

Abnormalities of the PSU in PCOS

Due to the androgen excess of PCOS, these patients frequently develop hirsutism, acne, or androgenic alopecia depending on ethnicity.[5] While insulin is essential for hair follicle growth in vitro, it is unclear whether the hyperinsulinemia of PCOS directly stimulates the termi-nalization of body hairs and the development of hirsutism.

Ovarian Morphology in PCOS

In approximately 70 percent of patients with PCOS, the ovaries contain intermediate and atretic follicles measuring 2 to 5 mm in diameter, resulting in a "polycystic appearance" at sonography[5] (Fig. 13-3). Diagnostic criteria for PCOS using ovarian morphologic features have been suggested.[48] However, it should be noted that polycystic ovaries on sonography or at pathology simply may be a sign of follicular development dysfunction (Table 13-6). For example, this ovarian morphology is seen frequently in patients with other androgen excess disorders, including nonclassic[49] and classic adrenal hyperplasia.[50] It is also frequently observed in patients with hyperprolactinemia,[51] type 2 DM,[42] and bulimia nervosa,[52] independent of the presence of hyperandrogenism. Up to 25 percent of unselected women have polycystic ovaries on ultrasound, many of which are normoandrogenic and cycling regularly.[39] Hence the presence of polycystic ovaries should be considered to be only one of the possible signs of androgen excess or PCOS.

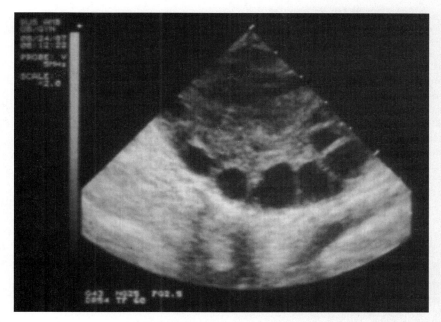

Figure 13-3   Transvaginal ultrasound visualization of a polycystic ovary. Note the string of sub-capsular follicles measuring 3–6 mm in diameter, with increased central stroma mass.   *(Courtesy of Dr. Michael Steinkampf).*

Obesity in PCOS

Overall, 20 to 60 percent of patients with PCOS will be defined as obese, the incidence varying depending on the criteria used to define overweightness. However, it should be understood that the frequency of obesity among PCOS patients may not be much higher than its prevalence in the general population of the United States when obesity is defined as 20 percent above ideal body weight. Clearly, obesity in PCOS worsens the degree of insulin resistance and hyperandrogenemia, and weight loss can improve the endocrine milieu and ovulatory function (see "Treatment of the Patient with Androgen Excess" below). The presence of android obesity is associated with an even further worsening of the insulin resistance and hyperinsulinemia in androgen excess patients.[53] However, PCOS and obesity-related oligoovulation are not identical. For example, the ovarian changes observed in women with morbid obesity are not similar to those

found in PCOS patients.[54] Overall, obesity appears to favor the development of PCOS and worsens the clinical and particularly the metabolic presentation. As such, the higher prevalence of obesity in PCOS patients may be secondary to selection bias in that women who are obese also may have a greater risk for developing PCOS. Alternatively, it is unclear that PCOS itself predisposes to the development of obesity, although data in female-to-male transsexuals suggests that androgens themselves may predispose to the development of an android type of fat distribution (see below).[25]

Biochemical Features of PCOS

Approximately 70 to 80 percent of women with PCOS demonstrate frank elevations in circulating androgens, particularly free testosterone,[55,56] and approximately 25 to 65 percent will have elevated levels of the adrenal androgen metabolite DHEAS.[5,20] Prolactin levels usually are normal, although they may be slightly

▶ **TABLE 13-6:** SYNDROMES OR DISEASE ENTITIES THAT HAVE BEEN ASSOCIATED WITH POLYCYSTIC OVARIES

Hyperandrogenism without Insulin Resistance
- Steroidogenic enzyme deficiencies
  - Congenital adrenal hyperplasia
  - Aromatase deficiency
- Androgen-secreting tumors
  - Ovarian
  - Adrenal
- Exogenous androgens
  - Anabolic steroids
  - Transsexual hormone replacement
- Other
  - Acne
  - Idiopathic hirsutism

Hyperandrogenism and Insulin Resistance
- Congenital
  - Type A syndrome
  - Type B syndrome
  - Leprechaunism
  - Lipoatrophic diabetes
  - Rabson-Mendenall syndrome
  - Polycystic ovary syndrome
- Acquired
  - Cushing's syndrome

Insulin Resistance
- Glycogen storage diseases
- Type 2 diabetes

Other
- Central nervous system
  - Trauma/Lesions
  - Hyperprolactinemia
- Nonhormonal medications
  - Valproate
  - Heriditary angioedema
  - Bulimia
  - Idiopathic (includes normoandrogenic women with cyclic menses)

elevated (generally <40 ng/mL) in a small fraction of patients.[57] The luteinizing hormone/follicle-stimulating hormone (LH/FSH) ratio is elevated in 35 to 95 percent of these patients,[58,59] depending on how it is defined. Re-

cent ovulation appears to be associated with a transient normalization in the ratio.[60] Treatment of PCOS patients with insulin sensitizers may result in lower circulating levels of LH,[61] suggesting that insulin resistance (see below) or, more likely, hyperinsulinemia is in part responsible for the gonadotropic abnormalities observed in many women with PCOS, although not all agree.[62]

Metabolic Features of PCOS

While not part of the diagnostic criteria, many PCOS women appear to be uniquely insulin-resistant.[63] Approximately 50 to 70 percent of PCOS patients demonstrate insulin resistance[64,65] and secondary hyperinsulinemia,[66] independent of body weight. In PCOS, insulin resistance usually refers to the impaired action of insulin in stimulating glucose transport[67] and in inhibiting lipolysis[68] in adipocytes, although studies of the action of insulin in myocytes and other tissues in this disorder are forthcoming. Insulin resistance in PCOS appears to be due to an intracellular defect of insulin signaling.[67,69,70] Many PCOS patients are obese, which compounds their underlying insulin resistance.

The compensatory hyperinsulinemia resulting from the underlying insulin resistance augments the stimulatory action of LH on the growth and androgen secretion of ovarian thecal cells[71] while inhibiting the hepatic production of SHBG.[72] Since insulin is also a mitogenic hormone, the elevated insulin levels may lead to hyperplasia of the basal layers of the epidermis, resulting in the development of acanthosis nigricans (a velvety, hyperpigmented change of the crease areas of the skin; Fig. 13-4) and achrocordons. Overall, insulin resistance and secondary hyperinsulinemia affect a large fraction of PCOS patients and may cause or augment the androgen excess of these patients.

Long-Term Sequelae of PCOS

Due to its associated ovulatory dysfunction, PCOS results in oligoovulatory infertility, men-

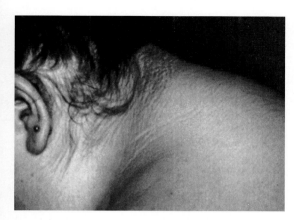

Figure 13-4 Acanthosis nigricans on the nape of the neck, a sign of hyperinsulinemia.

strual irregularity, and dysfunctional uterine bleeding. However, both menstrual irregularity[73] and hyperandrogenemia[74] appear to normalize as PCOS women approach the perimenopause. Although the endocrine and reproductive features of the disorder may improve with age, the associated metabolic abnormalities, particularly glucose intolerance, actually may worsen with age. Below are discussed common sequelae of PCOS, including type 2 and gestational DM, cardiovascular disease, and certain gynecologic cancers.

Type 2 and Gestational DM

The inherent insulin resistance present in many women with PCOS, aggravated by the high prevalence of obesity in these individuals, places these patients at increased risk for beta-cell dysfunction and impaired glucose tolerance (IGT) or type 2 DM.[75] About 30 to 40 percent of obese reproductive-age PCOS women have been found to have IGT, and about 10 percent have frank type 2 DM based on a 2-h glucose level greater than 200 mg/dL.[76] Of note is that only a small fraction of the PCOS women with either IGT or type 2 DM detected by an oral glucose tolerance test (oGTT) have fasting hyperglycemia consistent with the diagnosis of diabetes using the 1997 American Diabetes Association criteria (i.e., fasting glucose concen-

tration $\geq$ 126 mg/dL).[77] Overall, in PCOS patients it is preferable to use an oGTT to detect IGT or DM. The conversion rate to glucose intolerance over time is unknown, which makes recommendations for the frequency of screening for glucose intolerance difficult.

An increased risk of gestational DM also has been reported among women with PCOS,[78–80] although not all investigators agree.[81–83] However, with few exceptions the studies have been retrospective and included less than 50 subjects. In the largest study to date, 99 patients with PCOS were assessed retrospectively and compared with a group of controls.[78] Logistic regression analysis indicated that a body mass index (BMI) of greater than 25 kg/m^2 seemed to be the greatest predictor for gestational DM [adjusted odds ratio (OR) 5.1; confidence interval (CI) 3.2–8.3], and although PCOS remained as another independent predictor (adjusted OR 1.9; CI 1.0–3.5), it was considerably less important.

Cardiovascular Disease

Women with PCOS have a higher prevalence of risk factors for cardiovascular disease than expected, including insulin resistance (see above); impaired fibrinolysis[84]; elevations in tissue plasminogen activator antigen,[85] endothelin-1,[86] and plasma homocysteine levels[87,88]; increased vascular stiffness and a functional defect in the vascular action of insulin[89]; and diastolic dysfunction.[87] Many PCOS women also have significant dyslipidemia, with lower high-density lipoprotein (HDL) and higher triglyceride and low-density lipoprotein (LDL) levels than age-, sex-, and weight-matched controls.[90] PCOS women, at least in later life, also appear to have a higher risk of developing hypertension.[91,92] Recent studies have documented other interim risk factors, such as increased carotid artery intimal thickness,[93] to suggest that these women have evidence of atherosclerotic disease at an earlier and more advanced stage than control women. However, an increase in actual cardiovascular events in PCOS women, such as myocardial infarction, has not been observed,[94] although a higher number of nonfatal cerebrovascular disease events has.[92] It remains to be demonstrated that the increased prevalence of cardiovascular disease risk factors in PCOS translates into a higher risk for symptomatic cardiovascular disease.[95]

Endometrial Cancer

Many gynecologic cancers have been reported to be more common in women with PCOS, including ovarian, breast, and endometrial carcinomas. However, the clearest association is between PCOS and endometrial cancer because many of the risk factors for this cancer, including obesity, chronic anovulation, and hyperinsulinemia, are present in the PCOS patient. A number of early reports have noted the increased risk of PCOS patients for endometrial carcinoma,[96] although more recent analyses of published data suggest that the risk is still unclear.[97,98] Consistent with the etiologic role that PCOS potentially plays in the development of this neoplasia, in an analysis of 176 patients with endometrial cancer hirsutism, increased BMI, and hypertension were significantly more common among affected patients, and nulliparity and infertility were more frequent in younger women with endometrial cancer compared with controls.[99]

▶ HAIRAN SYNDROME

The hyperandrogenism, insulin resistance, and acanthosis nigricans (HAIRAN) syndrome is an inherited disorder of severe insulin resistance, distinct from PCOS, that actually includes many different genetic syndromes.[100] Although single point mutations of the insulin receptor are rare among these patients, some patients with this syndrome actually may suffer from a form of the familial lipodystrophy syndrome.[101] Approximately 3 to 4 percent of hyperandrogenic women suffer from these disorders.[27] These patients are diagnosed by having extremely high circulating levels of basal (>80 μU/mL)

▶ **TABLE 13-7:** FEATURES OF THE HYPERANDROGENIC–INSULIN RESISTANT– ACANTHOSIS NIGRICANS SYNDROME

- Androgen excess, which may be severe
- Extreme insulin resistance and hyperinsulinism levels*
- Acanthosis nigricans

*Basal insulin >80 μU/mL and/or glucose-stimulated insulin levels >300 to 500 μU/mL.

or glucose-stimulated (>300 to 500 μU/mL) insulin levels, although exact diagnostic criteria are lacking in part due to the heterogeneity of the syndrome (Table 13-7). Patients can be severely hyperandrogenemic, with testosterone levels reminiscent of patients with androgen-secreting neoplasms, resulting in the development of severe hirsutism and even virilization. In addition to significant hirsutism, patients also develop the characteristic dermatologic finding of acanthosis nigricans (see Fig. 13-4) due to hyperplasia of the basal cells of the epidermis. Acanthosis nigricans is principally noted in most crural areas of the body, including the back of the neck, the axilla, underneath the breasts, and even on the vulva.

Because of their high androgen levels, gonadotropins in these patients may be somewhat suppressed, resulting in persistent endometrial atrophy and amenorrhea despite the administration of a cyclic progestogen or an oral contraceptive. Because of the mitogenic effect of insulin on ovarian theca cells, the ovaries of many patients with the HAIRAN syndrome will become enlarged and hyperthecotic.[102] On ultrasound and histology the ovaries morphologically have a paucity of cortical cysts and demonstrate a thickened and enlarged theca/stroma compartment. These patients are at significant risk for developing dyslipidemia, type 2 DM, hypertension, and cardiovascular disease and are difficult to treat, although the selected use of long-acting GnRH analogues has been promising.[103] Some patients may even need surgery, either ovarian wedge resection or oophorectomy.

▶ NONCLASSIC ADRENAL HYPERPLASIA (NCAH)

While it is possible theoretically that NCAH may be due to mutations in other genes determining steroidogenic enzymes, such as *CYP11B1* (encoding for P450c11A and 11β-hydroxylase) and *HSD3B* (encoding for 3β-hydroxysteroid dehydrogenase), mutations in the genes coding for these enzymes are rarely noted in adult women presenting with androgen excess.[104,105] Principally, NCAH (also known as *late-onset congenital adrenal hyperplasia*) is a homozygous recessive disorder due to mutations in the *CYP21* gene. These mutations results in an abnormal (or absent) cytochrome P450c21 with relatively deficient of 21-hydroxylase (21-OH) activity.[49]

Overall, between 1 and 8 percent of women with androgen excess have 21-OH-deficient NCAH, depending on ethnicity.[49] Due to the lack of 21-hydroxylation, the progestogenic precursors to cortisol, 17α-hydroxyprogesterone (17-HP) and progesterone, accumulate in excess. These steroids are then metabolized to C_{19} products, principally androstenedione and testosterone (see Fig. 13-1).

Clinically and biochemically, these patients are difficult to distinguish from other hyperandrogenic patients, particularly patients with mild forms of PCOS. Circulating testosterone levels in women with NCAH usually are no different from those of PCOS patients.[106,107] Serum levels of androstenedione usually are higher in NCAH, but overlap between the two populations does not permit one to distinguish NCAH from PCOS patients.[106] DHEAS levels often are normal in 21-OH–deficient NCAH,[106] and it should not be used as a marker for this disorder. Patients with NCAH usually have LH/FSH ratios that are intermediate between those of normal women and PCOS patients.[107,108] Clinically, women with NCAH may present only

with persistent acne or may have moderate degrees of hirsutism and oligoamenorrhea, but frank virilization or even severe hirsutism is relatively rare.[107,108]

Currently, 21-OH-deficient NCAH can be screened for by using a basal 17-HP level obtained in the follicular or preovulatory phase of the menstrual cycle (Fig. 13-5). Levels below 2.0 ng/mL (6.0 nmol/L) effectively exclude the disorder,[109] whereas 90 percent of NCAH patients have basal levels higher than 2.0 ng/mL (6.0 nmol/L).[110] Among 284 consecutively seen hyperandrogenic women, the positive predictive values (PPVs) of the first and second 17-HP levels were 7.3 and 19 percent for a cutoff level of greater than 2 ng/mL.

Although the population frequency is relatively low, all patients with unexplained androgen excess should be screened for NCAH due to *CYP21* mutations because this diagnosis has a different prognosis and treatment regimen than PCOS, and requires preconception genetic counseling regarding the risks of congenital transmission. The risk of inheriting CAH or NCAH for the children of patients with NCAH depends on the genotype of the mother (homozygous versus compound heterozygote) and the probability that the father is a carrier for CYP21 mutations. Patients should be counseled that in the absence of additional data regarding the genetic status of the parents, the overall risk of a women with NCAH conceiving a child with CAH is between 1.7 and 2.3 per 1000.[49] This risk is higher in individuals, among others, who are of Ashkenazi Jewish descent or are already known to carry a defect of *CYP21*.

The treatment of androgen excess disorders is reviewed below. In brief, the therapy of NCAH should include decreasing cutaneous features of hyperandrogenism if present, such as hirsutism, acne, and alopecia; improving ovulatory function and fertility; preventing the development of anovulatory complications, such as dysfunctional bleeding and endometrial cancer; and providing genetic or preconception counseling. Although not studied systematically, younger patients with NCAH

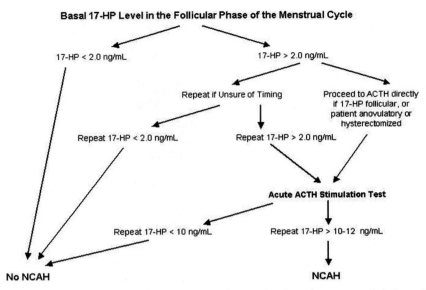

Figure 13-5 Screening and diagnostic scheme for 21-hydroxylase nonclassic adrenal hyperplasia (NCAH) (17-HP = 17-hydroxy-progesterone). *(Adapted from Azziz R, Hincapie LA, Knochenhauer ES, et al.*[110]*)*

generally respond favorably to corticosteroid replacement alone, such as with dexamethasone 0.25 mg every other day. However, many older NCAH patients also demonstrate ovarian hyperandrogenism and a PCOS-like pattern,[111] particularly those diagnosed in adulthood, and may require additional ovarian suppression. Glucocorticoid suppression is effective in improving acne and may improve the final height of affected children.[112] However, glucocorticoids alone have limited impact on establish hirsutism, and therapy should include an antiandrogen.[113] If fertility is a concern and ovulatory function is not regulated by glucocorticoid alone, clomiphene citrate or human meno-pausal gonadotropin therapy is indicated. Nonetheless, while women with NCAH may be considered subfertile, it should be stressed that many of these patients become pregnant without the need for treatment.[114]

During therapy, the levels of androstenedione represent an adequate hormonal marker, although this remains to be demonstrated in prospective studies. The levels of this steroid should be maintained at the upper limit of normal or slightly above normal to avoid the noxious effects of glucocorticoid excess. The levels of 17-HP may remain elevated despite adequate androgen suppression,[115] and consequently, 17-HP is not a good marker for monitoring therapy in NCAH patients. Alternatively, circulating DHEAS levels rapidly suppress with glucocorticoid treatment, even in the face of minimal or inadequate suppression of other androgens, such that it is also a poor marker of the adequacy of therapy.

▶ ANDROGEN-SECRETING NEOPLASMS

Androgen-secreting neoplasms (ASNs) usually originate in the ovary, although rarely they may arise in the adrenal cortex. Ovarian ASNs affect between 1 in 300 and 1 in 1000 hirsute patients.[55,56,116] The most common androgen-producing tumor in a premenopausal woman is a Sertoli-Leydig cell tumor, with thecomas and hilus cell tumors being less frequent. Hilus cell tumors are often small and can be less than 1 cm in diameter, theoretically below the range of most imaging techniques in the pelvis. In addition, 10 percent of granulosa cell tumors secrete primarily androgens instead of estrogens. Any large tumor within the body of the ovary (e.g., benign cystic teratomas, dysgerminomas, or epithelial tumors) can stimulate the production of androgens from the surrounding normal stroma. Fortunately, the vast majority of ovarian ASNs are benign.

Alternatively, adrenal ASNs generally are malignant and are associated with a high mortality rate because the majority are adrenocortical carcinomas. Nonetheless, isolated androgen-secreting adrenal adenomas also have been reported.[117] Fortunately, adrenal ASNs are rare, with an estimated incidence of 2 per 1 million persons per year, peaking in the fifth decade of life. Virilizing adrenocortical carcinomas generally produce excess glucocorticoids and mineralocorticoids, in addition to androgens, and result in the development of cushingoid features and hypertension. Alternatively, isolated virilizing adenomas tend to produce only androgens.

The presence of an ASN should be suspected when the onset of symptoms is rapid and sudden, when androgen excess presents in late life, when there is virilization and masculinization, or when there are associated cushingoid features. Nonetheless, it should be remembered that some of the younger patients with virilization who may be suspected of having an ASN actually suffer from the HAIRAN syndrome (see above). Suppression and stimulation tests can be misleading and are not encouraged for the diagnosis of these neoplasias. Overall, the single *best* predictor of an androgen-producing tumor is clinical presentation, not biochemical markers (Fig. 13-6). For example, in a recent study, we noted that the PPV of a repeat total testosterone determination above 250 ng/dL for an ASN was only 9 percent

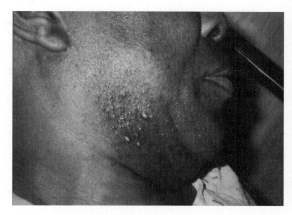

Figure 13-6 Patient with an ovarian androgen secreting neoplasm. *(Courtesy of Dr. John Porter).*

because most women with total testosterone levels above this cutoff had other abnormalities, such as the HAIRAN syndrome or PCOS.[116]

▶ IDIOPATHIC HIRSUTISM (IH)

Although IH is by definition not an androgen excess disorder, it should be considered in the differential diagnosis of these disorders. Overall, approximately 5 to 15 percent of hirsute women will be diagnosed as having IH.[46,118] The diagnosis of IH is one of exclusion, such that patients with IH are obviously hirsute but have normal circulating androgens and ovulatory function and no associated disorders.[119] While some clinicians use regular menses as a predictor of normal ovulatory function, it should be noted that approximately 40 percent of eumenorrheic hirsute women are actually anovulatory and hence do not suffer from IH.[46] Although biochemically these patients do not have an obvious elevation in circulating androgen levels, it also likely that many of these patients simply demonstrate degrees of hyperandrogenemia that may not be detectable with routine clinical androgen assays (see below). In some women with IH, the 5α-reductase activity in the skin and hair follicle is overactive, leading to the development of hirsutism in the face of normal circulating androgen levels.[119]

▶ VERY RARE CAUSES OF ANDROGEN EXCESS

Clinical signs of androgen excess also may result from the presence an ACTH-secreting tumor due to either a pituitary adenoma (i.e., Cushing's disease) or an extrapituitary (ectopic) source.[120] However, since Cushing's syndrome has an extremely low prevalence in the population (1 in 1 million) and screening tests do not have 100 percent sensitivity and specificity,[31] routine screening of all women with androgen excess for Cushing's syndrome is not indicated. Symptomatic hyperandrogenism also rarely may be the result of excess androgen intake, such as in a body builder or postmenopausal woman on androgen replacement. Severe hirsutism, and even virilization, that begins during pregnancy may be due to benign ovarian sources such as hyperreactio luteinalis (i.e., gestational ovarian theca-lutein cysts) or luteomas or to the extremely rare aromatase deficiency producing androgen excess as a result of placental inability to convert precursor androgens into estrogens. Finally, gonadal dysgenesis associated with an abnormal Y chromosome can present initially as peripubertal androgenization and amenorrhea.[121]

▶ EVALUATION OF ANDROGEN EXCESS

A history and physical examination are essential to making a diagnosis of the underlying cause of androgen excess, whereas the laboratory assessment serves primarily to confirm or exclude the various diagnoses arising from the clinical evaluation (Table 13-8).

History Taking

A thorough history should be obtained, including a discussion of drug or medication use; exposure to skin irritants; menstrual and reproductive history; onset and progression of hirsutism; change in extremity or head size, facial contour, or weight; the presence of balding, hair loss, and acne; and a family history of similar disorders, including diabetes. A family history of diabetes is an important predictor of beta cell dysfunction in the patient.[122] Lifestyle factors such as smoking, ethanol consumption, and diet and exercise histories should be recorded.

Physical Examination

The physical examination should carefully assess the patient for cushingoid features, acanthosis nigricans, balding, acne, and the degree and type of body hair distribution. One scale used commonly to score the degree of excess hair growth is based on a modification of the scale originally reported in 1961 by Ferriman and Gallwey (Fig. 13-7). Signs of virilization and masculinization should be sought, although their recognition usually is obvious. Clitoromegaly usually is defined as a clitoral index greater than 35 mm^2, where the clitoral index is the product of the sagittal and transverse diameters of the glans of the clitoris in millimeters. In normal women these diameters are in the range of 5 mm. Signs of insulin resistance on physical examination, such as obesity, particularly with an android distribution, and the presence of acanthosis nigricans and acrochordons should be sought. In women, a central or abdominal distribution of adiposity fat (the so-called apple-shaped or android obesity) has been associated with abnormal lipid profiles, increased insulin resistance compared with the gynecoid pattern, an increased risk for cardiovascular disease, and an increased index of death from all causes. Fat distribution is as-

► **TABLE 13-8:** EVALUATION OF THE PATIENT SUSPECTED OF HAVING ANDROGEN EXCESS

History
- Drug or medication use
- Exposure to topical/skin irritants
- Menstrual and reproductive history
- Onset and progression of hirsutism, acne, and/or alopecia
- Change in extremity or head size, facial contour, or weight
- Lifestyle factors, e.g., smoking, ethanol consumption, diet, and exercise
- Family history, e.g., of diabetes, CVD, hirsutism, PCOS, irregular periods

Physical
- Hirsutism score, e.g., modified F-G score
- Acne
- Alopecia/male-pattern balding
- Acanthosis and acrochordons
- Cushingoid features
- Obesity and body habitus, e.g., android versus gynecoid obesity (WHR)
- Clitoromegaly
- Signs of virilization/masculinization

Laboratory
- TSH (third generation)
- 17-HP in follicular phase of cycle
- Prolactin
- Total and free T, DHEAS, primarily if minimal or ambiguous androgenic features
- Fasting plasma glucose and/or postprandial glucose (at oGTT)
- Fasting insulin and/or postprandial insulin (at oGTT)

Abbreviations: CVD = cardiovascular disease; PCOS = polycystic ovary syndrome; TSH = thyroid-stimulating hormone; 17-HP = 17-hydroxyprogesterone; T = testosterone; DHEAS = dehydroepiandrosterone sulfate; oGTT = 75-g oral glucose tolerance test.

sessed most easily using the waist-to-hip ratio (WHR), obtained by measuring the circumferences at the narrowest point of the abdomen (i.e., the abdominal measure), generally immediately above the umbilicus, and at the widest part of the hips (i.e., the hip measures). Values greater than 0.72 (primarily android fat distribution) are considered abnormal, but increased morbidity and mortality become more noticeable at values greater than 1.0.[123]

Laboratory Evaluation of Androgen Excess

The laboratory evaluation should have the objective of excluding related and specific disorders and, if necessary, providing confirmation of androgen excess. Second, the presence of metabolic abnormalities, particularly in patients with PCOS or the HAIRAN syndrome, should be sought out. Specific related disorders that should be excluded during evaluation of the patient with suspected androgen excess are thyroid dysfunction, hyperprolactinemia, NCAH, the HAIRAN syndrome, and ASNs. Thyroid dysfunction and NCAH are excluded by measurement of a third-generation TSH level and a basal 17-HP level, respectively, the latter measured in the follicular phase of the menstrual cycle. If the 17-HP level is over 2 ng/mL, the patient should undergo an acute adrenal stimulation test to exclude 21-OH-deficient NCAH.[110] If the 17-HP level 60 minutes following ACTH administration

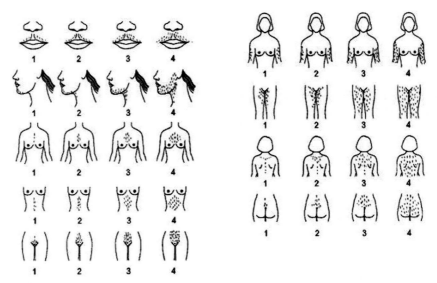

Figure 13-7 Modified Ferriman-Gallwey scale for assessing hirsutism. *(Modified from Hatch R, Rosenfield RL, Kim MH, Tredway D. Hirsutism: Implications, etiology, and management. Am J Obstet Gynecol 1981;140:815– 830.)*

is greater than 10 to 12 ng/mL, the diagnosis of 21-OH-deficient NCAH is established.

As noted previously, hirsute women claiming to have regular menstrual cycles should be evaluated for the presence of ovulatory dysfunction, most simply by obtaining a basal body temperature chart and serum progesterone concentration in the luteal phase (days 20 to 24) of the cycle. If the patient has ovulatory dysfunction, as evidenced by either a luteal progesterone level of less than 3 to 5 ng/mL in an otherwise eumenorrheic patient, or overt menstrual abnormalities, the diagnosis of PCOS should be entertained. In a woman with ovulatory dysfunction, serum prolactin and fasting insulin and glucose determinations also should be done to exclude hyperprolactinemia and the HAIRAN syndrome, respectively. ASN generally are excluded by the history and physical examination.[116,124] Rarely, will a 24-hour urine free cortisol determination be required in a patient with features suggestive of Cushing's syndrome.

The measurement of circulating androgen levels, including total and free testosterone and DHEAS, is useful primarily in the minimally or nonhirsute oligoovulatory patient to exclude the presence of androgen excess as the cause of the ovulatory dysfunction. However, these measurements have limited diagnostic utility in a patient who is frankly hirsute, and have a low PPV for adrenal or ovarian ASNs.[117]

Inappropriate gonadotropin secretion has been one of the characteristics signs of PCOS, and many clinicians have used an elevated LH/FSH ratio of 2:1 or 3:1 as a diagnostic criterion for PCOS. Nonetheless, because the measurement of gonadotropin levels at a single time point is relatively insensitive, with up to 40 percent of PCOS patients having a normal ratio, measurement of gonadotropins is not recommended for the routine evaluation of patients with suspected PCOS.

Laboratory Assessment for Metabolic Abnormalities

Metabolic abnormalities are common among women with PCOS and occur in all patients with the HAIRAN syndrome. In patients with the HAIRAN syndrome, the presence of insulin resistance is obvious, although this may not be case in women with PCOS. Unfortunately, there are no accurate, inexpensive, or reproducible tests for assessing insulin sensitivity clinically. The investigational standards are dynamic tests such as the euglycemic clamp and the frequently sampled intravenous glucose tolerance test, although these have limited applicability in the routine diagnostic evaluation of androgenic patients.

It appears that the use of a single fasting plasma glucose level, as recommended by the American Diabetes Association (ADA) in 1997,[77] is not very sensitive for detecting IGT or type 2 DM in PCOS compared with using criteria based on the liberal use of the oGTT.[125] For example, Legro and colleagues prospectively studied a population of 254 consecutive non-Hispanic white PCOS patients recruited in the United States.[76] Using the 1985 WHO criteria, 10 percent of subjects ages 25 to 35 years and 21 percent of PCOS women ages 35 to 40 years were affected with type 2 DM. Another 32 percent of all subjects were found to have IGT. Since IGT heralds the development of beta cell dysfunction with a relatively inadequate insulin secretion for the degree of reduced peripheral insulin sensitivity, the finding of IGT is a clear risk factor for type 2 DM. Importantly, 3.2 percent of the PCOS women studied would have been classified as having type 2 DM using the 1997 ADA criteria, whereas 7.5 percent could be classified as affected using the 1985 WHO diagnostic criteria.[76] Other investigators have confirmed this finding.[126,127]

Given the high prevalence of abnormalities in glucose tolerance, PCOS and HAIRAN syndrome patients should be routinely screened for IGT or frank diabetes with an oGTT using a 75-g glucose load. Considering the WHO criteria,[77] IGT is diagnosed by a normal fasting glucose level ($\leq$110 mg/dL) and a 2-hour glucose concentration of between 140 and 199 mg/dL, whereas frank diabetes is diagnosed by a fasting glucose level of 140 mg/dL or greater

or a 2-hour glucose concentration during the oGTT of 200 mg/dL or greater. Abnormal oGTT results need to be repeated for confirmation.

Although no firm guidelines exist, a plasma lipid profile should be considered in patients with PCOS, particularly those with significant insulin resistance or older than 35 years, those with the HAIRAN syndrome, and those with a strong family history of diabetes or cardiovascular disease.

Radiologic Imaging in the Evaluation of Patients with Androgen Excess

Routine ultrasound of the pelvis in patients with androgen excess generally is not indicated. As discussed earlier, polycystic ovaries can be observed with many of the androgen excess disorders and remains nonspecific. However, in hyperandrogenic patients seeking fertility treatment, an ultrasound demonstrating polycystic ovaries may be useful as a predictor for the development of ovarian hyperstimulation syndrome during ovulation induction.[128] Furthermore, a transvaginal sonogram in obese individuals to properly examine the ovaries for pathologic masses also may be appropriate.

In patients in whom an androgen-secreting tumor is suspected, a computed tomographic (CT) scan or MRI of the adrenals should be considered to exclude adrenal masses as small as 5 mm in diameter and to detect bilateral adrenal hyperplasia in the event of an ACTH-secreting tumor. However, since 2 percent of the population harbors a clinically insignificant adrenal adenoma (i.e., incidentaloma), the finding of an adrenal mass is not necessarily diagnostic for an androgen-secreting adrenal tumor and may lead to additional invasive but unnecessary procedures. Hence the radiologic examination of the adrenal should be undertaken only in patients whose symptoms are clearly suggestive of an adrenal process. Functional radiologic techniques such as selective venous catheterization or scintigraphy with

[131I]iodomethyl-norcholesterol may used, albeit rarely, for the localization of an ASN.

▶ TREATMENT OF THE PATIENT WITH ANDROGEN EXCESS

Treatment of androgen excess tends to be symptom-based. In general, we can consider four different reasons for treatment, including (1) regulation of uterine bleeding, (2) improvement of dermatologic abnormalities, (3) amelioration and prevention of associated metabolic abnormalities, and (4) treatment of anovulatory infertility (Table 13-9). Therapies used to achieve these treatment goals may include suppression of androgen production, blockade of peripheral androgen action, improvement of any associated insulin resistance and dyslipidemia, and topical, mechanical, or cosmetic measures for improving the dermatologic manifestations of these disorders. Combi-

▶ **TABLE 13-9:** THERAPEUTIC GOALS IN THE TREATMENT OF THE PATIENT WITH ANDROGEN EXCESS

Regulation of Uterine Bleeding
- OCPs
- Cyclic/continuous progestins
- Glucocorticoids
- Insulin sensitizers
- Lifestyle modification (diet and exercise)
- Ovarian surgery (ovarian drilling)

Improvement of Dermatologic Abnormalities (Hirsutism, Acne, Alopecia)
- Androgen suppression
  - OCPs
  - Long-acting GnRH analogues
- Androgen receptor antagonists
  - Spironolactone
  - Flutamide
  - Cyproterone acetate
- 5α-Reductase inhibitors
  - Finasteride
- Topical hair growth suppression
  - Ornithine decarboxylase inhibitors
- Mechanical and cosmetic means of hair reduction/destruction
  - Electrolysis
  - Laser reduction
  - Cosmetic technniques (shaving, depilating, bleaching)

Amelioration and Prevention of Associated Metabolic Abnormalities
- Insulin sensitizers
- Lifestyle modification (diet and exercise)

Treatment of Anovulatory Infertility
- Clomiphene citrate
- Gonadotropins
- GnRH pump
- Ovarian surgery (ovarian drilling)
- Lifestyle modification (diet and exercise)

nation therapy is required in the majority of patients with androgen excess. Methods of regulating uterine bleeding and improving associated dermatologic abnormalities, primarily hirsutism are reviewed below. For a full discussion of the treatment of oligoovulatory infertility see Chap. 17.

Regulation of Uterine Bleeding

The regulation of uterine bleeding reduces the risk of endometrial hyperplasia and cancer, dysfunctional uterine bleeding, and secondary anemia. In general, regulation of uterine bleeding can be achieved with oral contraceptives (OCs), cyclic or continuous progestogens in some patients with PCOS, insulin-sensitizing agents and, rarely, ovarian surgery.

Oral Contraceptives

OCs generally act by suppressing circulating gonadotropins, leading to decreased ovarian androgen production.[129] In addition, the estrogen in the birth control pill increases SHBG production, resulting in a decrease in unbound (free) testosterone levels. Furthermore, the progestin in the OC can have a beneficial antagonist effect on 5α-reductase activity and androgen receptor binding.[129] Finally, these medications also may decrease adrenal androgen production by a mechanism not yet clear. Treatment with OCs is very effective at regulating uterine bleeding and decreasing the associated risk of endometrial hyperplasia or carcinoma in patients with androgen excess, regardless of etiology. It is preferable, although not critical, to select an OC containing a progestin with low androgenic activity (e.g., norethindrone acetate, ethynodiol diacetate, desogesterol, gestodene, or norgestimate). While not specifically studied, OCs that contain 30 to 35 μg ethinyl estradiol generally minimize the occurrence of breakthrough bleeding and maximize compliance. There is some evidence that OCs can worsen insulin resistance and glucose tolerance in PCOS women,[130,131] although there

is no evidence that these effects of OCs on glucose metabolism result in an increased risk for developing type 2 DM in the general population.[132] In general, OCs remain part of the first line of therapy in the patient with androgen excess, including PCOS.

Cyclic or Continuous Progestogens

Cyclic progestogen administration is also useful to regulate uterine bleeding in androgen excess patients, particularly in amenorrheic women. However, it is not known how many progestin-induced withdrawal bleeds per year are necessary to adequately prevent the development of endometrial cancer in PCOS women. Extrapolating from the postmenopausal hormone-replacement literature, monthly treatment for a minimum of 12 days or longer may be optimal. Because progestogen administration occasionally can stimulate an ovulatory event, and because not all these patients are completely anovulatory, it may be preferable to treat sexually active women with oral micronized progesterone (100 to 200 mg twice daily) rather than a synthetic progestin.

Glucocorticoids

Glucocorticoid therapy may be beneficial in regulating menstrual bleeding in patients with NCAH, particularly if diagnosed as adolescents (see above). The lowest effective dose of glucocorticoids should be used, e.g., dexamethasone 0.25 mg daily or every other day. However, in a prospective study, a beneficial effect of glucocorticoids on ovulatory function in PCOS, regardless of basal DHEAS level.[133] Furthermore, glucocorticoids have the potential of producing weight gain and cushingoid features and worsening existing insulin resistance. Hence, the role of glucocorticoids in PCOS, at least as monotherapy, is limited.

Insulin-Sensitizing Agents

Drugs developed initially to treat type 2 DM have now also been used to treat PCOS. These include metformin[134,135] and the thiazolidinediones.[62] Other drugs such as acarbose also have been studied in PCOS with beneficial effects.

METFORMIN

Metformin was approved for the treatment of type 2 DM by the Food and Drug Administration (FDA) in 1994 but was used clinically for close to 20 years before that in other parts of the world. Metformin is a biguanide that works primarily by suppressing hepatic gluconeogenesis, but it also improves insulin sensitivity peripherally. Gastrointestinal symptoms (diarrhea, nausea, vomiting, abdominal bloating, flatulence, and anorexia) are the most common reactions to metformin, occurring in about 30 percent of treated women. There is a small risk of lactic acidosis among women taking this medication, which may be triggered by exposure to intravenous iodinated radiocontrast agents in susceptible individuals, although this adverse effect occurs primarily in patients with poorly controlled diabetes and impaired renal function. Metformin therapy has been found to improve uterine bleeding and menstrual function in 40 to approximately 100 percent of PCOS patients treated.[134–137]

Effective doses of metformin in PCOS tend to range from 1500 to 2000 mg/d, although between 15 and 30 percent of patients may suffer from gastrointestinal side effects sufficient to consider discontinuation of therapy. Beginning the medication at a lower dose and increasing it to the full dose over 2 to 4 weeks, and the use of the extended-release preparation, may result in fewer side effects.

THIAZOLIDINEDIONES

Thiazolidinediones are peroxisome proliferator–activating receptor gamma (PPAR-γ) agonists and are thought to improve insulin sensitivity through a postreceptor mechanism. In a large multicenter trial, troglitazone has been shown to have a dose-response effect in improving ovulation and menstrual dysfunction in women with PCOS.[62] This appeared to be mediated through decreases in hyperinsulinemia and free testosterone levels. Troglitazone subsequently has been removed from the worldwide market due to the potential for inducing hepatotoxicity. Newer thiazolidinediones such as rosiglitazone and pioglitazone appear to be safer in terms of hepatotoxicity but also have been associated with embryotoxicity in animal studies (both are pregnancy category C). Furthermore, there are limited studies on their effectiveness in PCOS.[138] When using these drugs, liver function tests should be monitored on a regular basis. Combination treatment with other insulin sensitizers, primarily metformin, has been shown to further improve insulin sensitivity and glycemic control in type 2 DM, although the effect of such combination therapy in women with PCOS is not clearly delineated.

Weight Loss

All patients with PCOS who are obese should be strongly advised to attempt weight lose, which will improve the response to hormonal or ovulatory therapies, improve their endocrine milieu, and most important, reduce their risk of metabolic abnormalities. Multiple studies in hyperandrogenic or PCOS women have shown that exercise[139] and/or weight loss[140,141] can lower circulating androgen levels and cause spontaneous resumption of menses,[139,140] not withstanding the other beneficial effects. These changes have been reported with a weight loss as small as 5 percent of the initial weight.[141] In patients with massive obesity, consideration may be given to surgical means of inducing weight loss, such as laparoscopic gastric bypass.

Preliminary data suggest that the type of diet (e.g., 15 to 25 percent versus 45 percent carbohydrate content) used for weight loss is significantly less important than the total amount of calories consumed.[142,143] However, a low-carbohydrate diet (25 percent) has been reported to be associated with a greater improvement in fasting blood insulin levels, the glucose-insulin ratio, and triglyceride levels,[143] suggesting that this type of diet may be more favorable in patients with insulin resistance. Firm recommendations, however, await prospective studies in women with PCOS.

Surgery

In patients with intractable uterine bleeding who have completed their childbearing, consideration may be given to a hysterectomy and bilateral salpingo-oophorectomy. In addition, ovulatory function also may improve following ovarian wedge or laparoscopic ovarian drilling procedures, although the long-term effect of these therapies on menstrual function is unclear.[144] Gjonnaess reported that of 31 anovulatory women with PCOS followed for 10 to 20 years after laparoscopic ovarian drilling, 74 percent continued to ovulate.[145] Alternatively, the same investigator indicated that laparoscopic ovarian drilling did not seem to have any major advantages over the use of OCs for the treatment of PCOS patients not seeking fertility.[146] In general, laparoscopic ovarian drilling should not be considered a first-line therapy for the treatment of menstrual dysfunction in PCOS.

Treatment of Hirsutism

The treatment of hirsutism can be complex. Optimal therapy usually requires a combination of approaches, including suppression of circulating androgens (with OCs, insulin sensitizers, or even long-acting GnRH analogues or glucocorticoids), peripheral androgen blockade (with spironolactone, flutamide, cyproterone acetate, or finasteride), and use of a topical hair growth inhibitor (eflornithine hydrochloride) or mechanical methods of hair reduction or destruction (electrology or lasers) and appropriate cosmetic measures (bleaching or chemical depilation). Acne in androgen excess patients usually can be treated with OCs alone or accompanied by topical or antibiotic therapies. The treatment of androgenic alopecia may require the use of androgen suppression in combination with androgen blockade and topical means of stimulating hair regrowth (e.g., minoxidil).

In general, combination therapies appear to produce better results than single-agent approaches.[147] The response of hirsutism to medical suppression often takes 3 to 6 months to be noticeable, and adjunctive mechanical removal methods are often necessary. However, the majority of women appear to experience improvement in their hirsutism,[27] although often less dramatically than some patients would desire. Unfortunately, there are no universally accepted techniques for assessing the response of hirsutism to treatment, although in patients who shave, depilate, or have electrolysis, assessing the interval between treatment sessions may be useful. Some of the depilatory treatments used by patients are so effective that it is difficult to ever determine baseline hirsutism and response to treatment such that the patient's subjective assessment guides therapy.

Androgen Suppression

Women with documented hyperandrogenemia theoretically would benefit most from hormonal suppression. Androgen suppression is accomplished most commonly with OCs but also may be achieved using long-acting GnRH agonists, glucocorticoids, or insulin sensitizers.

ORAL CONTRACEPTIVES

Treatment with OCs alone improves hirsutism, although the response is generally modest.[129]

LONG-ACTING GnRH AGONISTS

Treatment with a long-acting GnRH agonist may result in a greater lowering of circulating androgens than with OCs and hence theoretically may produce a greater degree of hair growth suppression. Nonetheless, comparative trials against other agents and combined-agent trials have yielded mixed results.[148,149] It should be noted that a long-acting GnRH agonist given alone, particularly if administered for greater than 6 months, results in unacceptable bone loss.[149]

GLUCORTICOIDS

Glucocorticoid suppression alone produces only modest improvements in hair growth in hirsute women[150,151] and has no real additive effect to treatment with antiandrogens.[152,153] Nonetheless, in one follow-up study of 54 patients with hirsutism and hyperandrogenism, the addition of dexamethasone to spironolactone prolonged the duration of remission of the hirsutism after discontinuation of therapy.[154] The potential benefit of glucocorticoids in prolonging the effect of antiandrogen therapy for hirsutism remains to be prospectively confirmed. Furthermore, the glucocorticoid-associated deterioration in glucose tolerance may be problematic for PCOS women, and long-term effects such as glucocorticoid-induced osteoporosis are of significant concern. In general, androgen suppression with either long-acting GnRH analogues or glucocorticoids is not recommended solely as a treatment for hirsutism.

Insulin-Sensitizing Agents

As noted above, treatment with insulin sensitizers results in significant decreases in circulating androgens in many women with PCOS. Moghetti and colleagues treated 32 PCOS patients with metformin (1500 mg/d) for an average of 11.0 ± 1.3 months (range 4 to 26 months) in a study with an open-label design.[137] These investigators noted that in women with excessive hair growth, the modified Ferriman-Gallwey (F-G) hirsutism scores were not improved with treatment, independent of any change in menstrual cycle. In another study, 10 women with PCOS and hirsutism were enrolled into a 14-month (two 6-month phases of metformin or placebo with a 2-month washout) double-blind, placebo-controlled cross-over study.[155] There was a significant improvement in hirsutism (both in F-G scores and growth velocity) at the end of the metformin phase compared with placebo.

A dose-related decrease in the mean F-G score was also observed in about 150 hirsute PCOS patients included in a randomized, placebo-controlled trial of troglitazone for the treatment of PCOS.[62] A 17 percent decrease in the modified F-G score was observed in patients treated with troglitazone (600 mg/d) for at least 24 weeks compared with a 1 percent increase for those treated with placebo (Fig. 13-8). Overall, it appears that PCOS-associated hirsutism

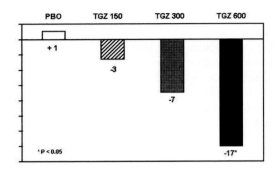

Figure 13-8 The percent decrease in hirsutism, measured by a modified Ferriman-Gallwey (F-G) score, in patients treated with placebo (PBO), troglitazone 150 mg/d (TGZ 150), troglitazone 300 mg/d (TGZ 300), and troglitazone 600 mg/d (TGZ 600). Note that the decrease in hirsutism score was significantly different from placebo with the use of troglitazone 600 mg/d. *(Reprinted with permission from Azziz R, Ehrmann D, Legro RS, et al.[62])*

may improve modestly with use of insulin-sensitizing drugs.

Androgen Receptor Antagonists

These compounds antagonize the binding of testosterone and other androgens to the androgen receptor. As a class, therefore, they are teratogenic and carry the teratogenic risk of feminization of the external genitalia in a male fetus should the patient conceive.

Spironolactone

The most commonly used antiandrogen used in the United States is spironolactone, a nonsteroidal antiandrogen that is also a diuretic and aldosterone antagonist. Spironolactone binds to the androgen receptor with 67 percent of the affinity of dihydrotestosterone.[156] It has other mechanisms of action, including inhibition of ovarian and adrenal steroidogenesis, competition for androgen receptors in hair follicles, and direct inhibition of 5α-reductase activity. Hirsutism[157,158] and even acne[9] have been successfully treated with spironolactone. The usual dose for the treatment of hirsutism is 25 to 100 mg twice a day, and the dose should be titrated to minimize the potential for side effects. About 20 percent of the women will experience increased menstrual frequency, a reason for combining this therapy with an OC.[159] Other side effects include polyuria, orthostatic hypotension, nausea, dyspepsia, and fatigue. Because it can cause and exacerbate hyperkalemia, it should be used cautiously in patients with renal impairment and should not be combined with other potassium-sparing diuretics. The medication also has potential teratogenicity as an antiandrogen, although exposure rarely has resulting in ambiguous genitalia in male infants.[160]

FLUTAMIDE

Flutamide is a nonsteroidal androgen receptor blocker approved by the FDA as adjuvant treatment for prostate cancer. Flutamide has been shown to be effective against hirsutism.[158,161] Side effects include the appearance of greenish urine, excessive dryness of skin or scalp hair, liver enzyme abnormalities, and rarely, fatal hepatotoxicity.[162] A dose of 250 mg twice daily generally is used, although a single dose of 250 mg/day may be effective in some patients.[163]

CYPROTERONE ACETATE

Cyproterone acetate (CPA) is a strong progestin that decreases testosterone and androstenedione levels through a decrease in circulating LH levels and antagonizes the effect of androgens at the peripheral level. It is an effective agent for the treatment of hirsutism.[164] Cyproterone acetate in doses of 50 to 100 mg/d, combined with 30 to 35 μg ethinyl estradiol, is as effective as the combination of spironolactone 100 mg/day and an OC in the treatment of hirsutism.[161,165] However, lower doses of CPA, as in an OC containing CPA 2 mg/day in combination with ethinyl estradiol 35 μg/day (marketed as Diane-35 in Europe and Canada

and Dianette in the United Kingdom by Schering AG, Berlin, and Berlex, Canada), seems less effective than 100 mg/day of spironolactone.[166] Side effects may include adrenal insufficiency and loss of libido. This drug is currently not available in the United States, and it unlikely that it will be approved by the FDA because it is now not under patent protection.

5α-Reductase Inhibitors

There are two forms of the enzyme 5α-reductase, type 1 predominantly found in the skin, and type 2, predominantly found in the prostate and reproductive tissues. Both forms are found in the PSU and may contribute to the development of hirsutism, acne, and alopecia. Finasteride inhibits both forms of 5α-reductase and is available as a 5-mg tablet for the treatment of prostate cancer and as a 1-mg tablet for the treatment of male alopecia. It has been found to be effective for the treatment of hirsutism in women.[158,161] Finasteride is better tolerated than other antiandrogens but has the highest and clearest risk for teratogenicity in a male fetus, so adequate contraception must be used. Overall, randomized trials have found that spironolactone, flutamide, and finasteride have similar efficacy in improving hirsutism[158,161] (Fig. 13-9).

Topical Hair Growth Suppression: Ornithine Decarboxylase Inhibitors

Ornithine decarboxylase is necessary for the production of polyamines and is also a sensitive and specific marker of androgen action in the prostate. Inhibition of this enzyme limits cell division and function, including that of the PSU. Recently, a potent inhibitor of this enzyme, eflornithine, has been found to be effective for the treatment of unwanted facial hair. Available as a 13.9% cream of eflornithine hydrochloride, it is applied to affected areas twice daily. In clinical trials, 32 percent of patients had marked improvement after 24 weeks compared with 8 percent of placebo-treated women, and the benefit was first noted at 8 weeks.[167] It appears to be well tolerated, with

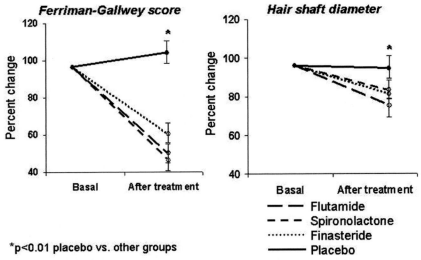

Figure 13-9 Spironolactone (100 mg/d), flutamide (250 mg/d), and finasteride (5 mg/d) were compared for the treatment of hirsutism in a randomized, double-blind, placebo-controlled trial including 40 affected women. *(Modified from Moghetti P, Tosi E, Tosti A, Negri C, Misciali C, Perrone F, Caputo M, Muggeo M, Castello R. Comparison of spironolactone, flutamide, and finasteride efficacy in the treatment of hirsutism: A randomized, double-blind, placebo-controlled trial. J Clin Endocrinol Metab 2000;85:89–94.)*

only about 2 percent of patients developing skin irritation or other adverse reactions.

Mechanical and Cosmetic Means of Hair Reduction and Destruction

Mechanical hair removal (shaving, plucking, waxing, depilatory creams, electrolysis, and laser vaporization) can assist in controlling hirsutism and often are the front line of treatment used by women. Shaving, bleaching, and chemical depilation may be useful temporary treatments for unwanted hairs. Although shaving can lead to a blunt hair end that may feel "stubble-like," it does not lead to a worsening of hirsutism.[168] Depilating agents, while useful, can result in chronic skin irritation and worsening of hirsutism if used excessively or indiscriminately. The use of plucking and/or waxing in androgenized skin areas should be discouraged because these techniques not only do not kill the hair follicles but also can induce folliculitis and trauma to the hair shaft with subsequent development of ingrown hairs and further skin damage.

ELECTROLYSIS

Electrolysis (i.e., electroepilation) has been in use for over a century and results in long-term hair destruction, albeit slowly.[169,170] The FDA recognizes electrology as providing permanent hair removal. The reported efficacy with repeated treatments is permanent destruction (alopecia or hair loss) in 15 to 50 percent of the hairs treated.[169,170] The number of treatments necessary varies with each patient.

There are three modalities of electrology. *Electrolysis* refers to the application of direct or galvanic current (DC, e.g., from a battery) using one or more sterile needles/probes to achieve chemical destruction of the hair follicle. *Thermolysis* uses alternating current (AC, e.g., as in regular electricity) whose frequency is increased and delivered through a single sterile needle/probe, creating heat that destroys the hair follicle. Thermolysis also has been called *short-wave* or *high-frequency current.* Finally, the *blend,* or *dual modality, technique* uses both types of current applied simultaneously or sequentially, generally through a single sterile needle/probe, to achieve dual-action destruction of the hair follicle. Side effects may include temporary skin irritation and, rarely, burning and scarring of the skin.

LASER HAIR REDUCTION

Hair reduction via lasers also can be useful for selected patients.[171] The main objective of laser therapy for hair removal is to selectively cause thermal damage of the hair follicle without destroying adjacent tissues, a process termed *selective photothermolysis*. Selective photothermolysis relies on the selective absorption of a brief radiation pulse to generate and confine heat at specific pigmented targets. Lasers useful in hair removal may be grouped into three categories based on the type of laser or light source each employs: (1) red light systems (694-nm ruby), (2) infrared light systems [755-nm alexandrite, 800-nm semiconductor diode, or 1064-nm neodymium:yttrium-aluminum-garnet (Nd:YAG)], and (3) intense pulsed light (IPL) sources (590 to 1200 nm). In general, laser hair removal is most successful in patients with Fitzpatrick skin colors I to IV who have dark-colored hairs.[172] However, repeated therapies are necessary, and complete alopecia is rarely achieved.[171]

In general, treatment with the ruby, alexandrite, and diode lasers or the IPL results in similar success rates, although the success rate appears to be somewhat lower for the Nd:YAG laser.[171] After laser-assisted hair removal, most patients experience erythema and edema lasting no more than 48 hours.[173] Blistering or crusting may occur in 10 to 15 percent of patients (Fig. 13-10). Temporary hyperpigmentation occurs in 14 to 25 percent of patients, and hypopigmentation occurs in 10 to 17 percent of patients. Dyspigmentation is less common with the use of longer wavelengths, as in the alexandrite and diode lasers, and longer pulse durations. Overall, laser hair removal is a promising technique for the treatment of hirsute patients. Nonetheless, it should be noted that most studies have been uncontrolled and have included fewer than 50 patients, none

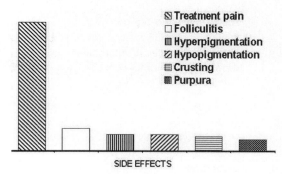

Figure 13-10 Frequency of side effects during and after Q-switched Nd:YAG, long-pulsed ruby, or alexandrite laser-assisted hair removal in a reprospective study of 900 patients. *(Modified, with permission, from Nanni CA, Alster TS. Laser-assisted hair removal: side effects of Q-switched Nd:YAG, long-pulsed ruby, and alexandrite lasers.* J Am Acad Dermatol *1999;41:165–171.)*

have been blinded, and all have studied a variety of treatment protocols, equipment, skin types, and hair colors.

KEY POINTS

1. Androgen excess (i.e., hyperandrogenism) is one of the most frequent, albeit heterogeneous, endocrine disorders of women; the most common etiology of androgen excess, PCOS, affects 4 to 6 percent of unselected reproductive-age women.

2. Androgen excess results in various clinical signs and symptoms, including abnormalities of the PSU (e.g., hirsutism, acne, and androgenic alopecia), of the hypothalamic-pituitary-ovarian axis (e.g., ovulatory and menstrual dysfunction), and of the hypothalamic-pituitary-adrenal axis (e.g., adrenal androgen excess). If the androgen excess is very severe, virilization and/or masculinization also can be apparent.

3. A common sign of androgen excess is hirsutism, although in up to 15 percent of

such patients no obvious ovulatory or endocrine abnormality may be observed (i.e., idiopathic hirsutism). Alternatively, not all women with androgen excess will have hirsutism.

4. The vast majority of androgen excess is due to PCOS, with 21-OH-deficient NCAH, the HAIRAN syndrome, androgen-secreting tumors, and drug-induced hyperandrogenism generally accounting for less than 10 percent of such patients.

5. PCOS is a diagnosis by exclusion basically defined as the presence of androgen excess (hyperandrogenemia and/or clinical evidence of androgen excess) in combined with chronic oligoanovulation after the exclusion of related disorders (e.g., 21-OH-deficient NCAH, thyroid dysfunction, and hyperprolactinemia). Polycystic-appearing ovaries alone are insufficient for the diagnosis of PCOS, nor are their absence exclusionary.

6. Approximately 50 to 70 percent of patients with PCOS suffer from insulin resistance and hyperinsulinism and are at higher risk for the development of endometrial cancer, glucose intolerance and type 2 DM, and an adverse cardiovascular risk profile.

7. The history and physical examination are essential to making a diagnosis of the underlying cause of androgen excess. The laboratory evaluation should have the objective of excluding related and specific disorders and, if necessary, providing confirmation of androgen excess. Second, the presence of metabolic abnormalities, particularly in patients with PCOS or the HAIRAN syndrome, should be sought out.

8. Treatment of androgen excess tends to be symptom-based, with reasons for treatment including (a) regulation of uterine bleeding and reduction of the risk of endometrial hyperplasia and cancer, dysfunctional uterine bleeding (DUB), and secondary anemia, (b) improvement of dermatologic abnormalities such as hirsutism, acne, and alopecia, (c) amelioration and prevention of associated metabolic abnormalities, particularly insulin resistance and hyperinsulinemia, and (d) treatment of anovulatory infertility.

9. Overall, avenues of treatment include suppression of androgen production, blockade of peripheral androgen action, improvement in any associated insulin resistance and dyslipidemia, and topical, mechanical, or cosmetic measures for improving the dermatologic manifestations of these disorders. The vast majority of patients with androgen excess will require and benefit the most from combination therapy.

REFERENCES

1. Vermeulen A. Androgen secretion by adrenals and gonads, in Mahesh VB, Greenblatt RB (eds), *Hirsutism and Virilism*. Boston: John Wright/PSG, Inc, 1983; pp 17–34.
2. Azziz R, Koulianos G. Adrenal adrogens and reproductive aging in females. *Semin Reprod Endocrinol* 1991;9:249.
3. Judd HL. Hormonal dynamics associated with the menopause. *Clin Obstet Gynecol* 1976;19:775.
4. Azziz R. Reproductive endocrinologic alterations in female asymptomatic obesity. *Fertil Steril* 1989;52:703.
5. Carmina E, Koyama T, Chang L, et al. Does ethnicity influence the prevalence of adrenal hyperandrogenism and insulin resistance in polycystic ovary syndrome? *Am J Obstet Gynecol* 1992;167:1807.
6. Lucky AW, McGuire J, Rosenfield RL, et al. Plasma androgens in women with acne vulgaris. *J Invest Dermatol* 1983;81:70.
7. Slayden SM, Moran C, Sams WMJ, et al. Hyperandrogenemia in patients presenting with acne. *Fertil Steril* 2001;75:889.
8. Lookingbill DP, Horton R, Demers LM, et al. Tissue production of androgens in women with acne. *J Am Acad Dermatol* 1985;12:481.

9. Muhlemann MF, Carter GD, Cream JJ, et al. Oral spironolactone: An effective treatment for acne vulgaris in women. *Br J Dermatol* 1986; 115:227.

10. Nader S, Rodriguez-Rigau LJ, Smith KD, et al. Acne and hyperandrogenism: Impact of lowering androgen levels with glucocorticoid treatment. *J Am A Dermatol* 1984;11:256.

11. Redmond GP, Olson WH, Lippman JS, et al. Norgestimate and ethinyl estradiol in the treatment of acne vulgaris: A randomized, placebo-controlled trial. *Obstet Gynecol* 1997;89:615.

12. Ludwig E. Classification of the types of androgenetic alopecia (common baldness) occurring in the female sex. *Br J Dermatol* 1977;97:247.

13. Futterweit W, Dunaif A, Yeh HC, et al. The prevalence of hyperandrogenism in 109 consecutive female patients with diffuse alopecia. *J Am Acad Dermatol* 1988;19:831.

14. Dunaif A, Longcope C, Canick J, et al. The effects of the aromatase inhibitor delta 1-testolactone on gonadotropin release and steroid metabolism in polycystic ovarian disease. *J Clin Endocrinol Metab* 1985;60:773.

15. Dunaif A, Scully RE, Andersen RN, et al. The effects of continuous androgen secretion on the hypothalamic-pituitary axis in woman: Evidence from a luteinized thecoma of the ovary. *J Clin Endocrinol Metab* 1984;59:389.

16. Dunaif A. Do androgens directly regulate gonadotropin secretion in the polycystic ovary syndrome? *J Clin Endocrinol Metab* 1986;63:215.

17. Spinder T, Spijkstra JJ, van den Tweel JG, et al. The effects of long term testosterone administration on pulsatile luteinizing hormone secretion and on ovarian histology in eugonadal female to male transsexual subjects. *J Clin Endocrinol Metab* 1989;69:151.

18. Amirikia H, Savoy-Moore RT, Sundareson AS, et al. The effects of long-term androgen treatment on the ovary. *Fertil Steril* 1986;45:202.

19. Wild RA, Umstot ES, Andersen RN, et al. Androgen parameters and their correlation with body weight in one hundred thirty-eight women thought to have hyperandrogenism. *Am J Obstet Gynecol* 1983;146:602.

20. Moran C, Knochenhauer ES, Boots LR, et al. Adrenal androgen excess in hyperandrogenism: Relation to age and body mass. *Fertil Steril* 1999;71:671.

21. Azziz R, Rittmaster RS, Fox LM, et al. Role of the ovary in the adrenal androgen excess of hyperandrogenic women. *Fertil Steril* 1998;69: 851.

22. Gonzalez F, Hatala DA, Speroff L. Adrenal and ovarian steroid hormone responses to gonadotropin-releasing hormone agonist treatment in polycystic ovary syndrome. *Am J Obstet Gynecol* 1991;165:535.

23. Azziz R, Gay FL, Potter SR, et al. The effects of prolonged hypertestosteronemia on adrenocortical biosynthesis in oophorectomized women. *J Clin Endocrinol Metab* 1991;72:1025.

24. Roncari DA, Van RL. Promotion of human adipocyte precursor replication by 17β-estradiol in culture. *J Clin Invest* 1978;62:503.

25. Elbers JM, Asscheman H, Seidell JC, et al. Long-term testosterone administration increases visceral fat in female-to-male transsexuals. *J Clin Endocrinol Metab* 1997;82:2044.

26. Marques-Vidal P, Ruidavets JB, Cambou JP, et al. Trends in overweight and obesity in middle-aged subjects from southwestern France, 1985–1997. *Int J Obes Relat Metab Dis* 2002;26:732.

27. Azziz R, Sanchez LA, Knochenhauer ES, et al. Androgen excess in women: Experience with over 1000 consecutive patients. *J Clin Endocrinol Metab* 2004;89:453–462.

28. Zawadzki JK, Dunaif A. Diagnostic criteria for polycystic ovary syndrome: Towards a rational approach, in Dunaif A, Givens JR, Haseltine F, Merriam GR (eds), *Polycystic Ovary Syndrome.* Boston: Blackwell Scientific, 1990; p 377

29. The Rotterdam ESHRE/ASRM Sponsored PCOS Consensus Workshop Group. Revised 2003 consensus on diagnostic criteria and long-term health risks related to polycystic ovary syndrome (PCOS). *Fertil Steril* 2004;81:19.

30. Knochenhauer ES, Key TJ, Kahsar-Miller M, et al. Prevalence of the polycystic ovary syndrome in unselected black and white women of the southeastern United States: A prospective study. *J Clin Endocrinol Metab* 1998;83:3078.

31. Diamanti-Kandarakis E, Kouli CR, Bergiele AT, et al. A survey of the polycystic ovary syndrome in the Greek island of Lesbos: Hormonal and metabolic profile. *J Clin Endocrinol Metab* 1999;84:4006.

32. Asuncion M, Calvo RM, San Millan JL, et al. A prospective study of the prevalence of the polycystic ovary syndrome in unselected Caucasian women from Spain. *J Clin Endocrinol Metab* 2000;85:2434.

33. Korhonen S, Hippelainen M, Niskanen L, et al. Relationship of the metabolic syndrome and obesity to polycystic ovary syndrome: A controlled, population-based study. *Am J Obstet Gynecol* 2001;184:289.

34. Peppard HR, Marfori J, Iuorno MJ, et al. Prevalence of polycystic ovary syndrome among premenopausal women with type 2 diabetes. *Diabetes Care* 2001;24:1050.

35. Conn JJ, Jacobs HS, Conway GS. The prevalence of polycystic ovaries in women with type 2 diabetes mellitus. *Clin Endocrinol* 2000;52:81.

36. Farah L, Lazenby AJ, Boots LR, et al. Prevalence of polycystic ovary syndrome in women seeking treatment from community electrologists. Alabama Professional Electrology Association Study Group. *J Reprod Med* 1999;44:870.

37. Hull MG. Epidemiology of infertility and polycystic ovarian disease: Endocrinological and demographic studies. *Gynecol Endocrinol* 1987;1:235.

38. Allen SE, Potter HD, Azziz R. Prevalence of hyperandrogenemia among nonhirsute oligoovulatory women. *Fertil Steril* 1997;67:569.

39. Kousta E, White DM, Cela E, et al. The prevalence of polycystic ovaries in women with infertility. *Hum Reprod* 1999;14:2720.

40. Swanson M, Sauerbrei EE, Cooperberg PL. Medical implications of ultrasonically detected polycystic ovaries. *J Clin Ultrasound* 1981;9:219.

41. Farquhar CM, Birdsall M, Manning P, et al. The prevalence of polycystic ovaries on ultrasound scanning in a population of randomly selected women. *Aust NZ J Obstet Gynaecol* 1994;34:67.

42. Ibanez L, Dimartino-Nardi J, Potau N, et al. Premature adrenarche: Normal variant or forerunner of adult disease?. *Endocr Rev* 2000;21:671.

43. Holte J, Gennarelli G, Wide L, et al. High prevalence of polycystic ovaries and associated clinical, endocrine, and metabolic features in women with previous gestational diabetes mellitus. *J Clin Endocrinol Metab* 1998;83:1143.

44. Anttila L, Karjala K, Penttila RA, et al. Polycystic ovaries in women with gestational diabetes. *Obstet Gynecol* 1998;92:13.

45. Kahsar-Miller MD, Nixon C, Boots LR, et al. Prevalence of polycystic ovary syndrome (PCOS) in first-degree relatives of patients with PCOS. *Fertil Steril* 2001;75:53.

46. Azziz R, Waggoner WT, Ochoa T, et al. Idiopathic hirsutism: An uncommon cause of hirsutism in Alabama. *Fertil Steril* 1998;70:274.

47. Chang PL, Lindheim SR, Lowre C, et al. Normal ovulatory women with polycystic ovaries have hyperandrogenic pituitary-ovarian responses to gonadotropin-releasing hormone-agonist testing. *J Clin Endocrinol Metab* 2000;85:995.

48. Polson DW, Adams J, Wadsworth J, et al. Polycystic ovaries: A common finding in normal women. *Lancet* 1988;1:870.

49. Azziz R, Dewailly D, Owerbach D. Clinical review 56: Nonclassic adrenal hyperplasia: Current concepts. *J Clin Endocrinol Metab* 1994;78:810.

50. Hague WM, Adams J, Rodda C, et al. The prevalence of polycystic ovaries in patients with congenital adrenal hyperplasia and their close relatives. *Clin Endocrinol* 1990;33:501.

51. Isik AZ, Gulekli B, Zorlu CG, et al. Endocrinological and clinical analysis of hyperprolactinemic patients with and without ultrasonically diagnosed polycystic ovarian changes. *Gynecol Obstet Invest* 1997;43:183.

52. Raphael FJ, Rodin DA, Peattie A, et al. Ovarian morphology and insulin sensitivity in women with bulimia nervosa. *Clin Endocrinol* 1995;43:451.

53. Gambineri A, Pelusi C, Vicennati V, et al. Obesity and the polycystic ovary syndrome. *Int J Obesit Relat Metab Dis* 2002;26:883.

54. Fisher ER, Gregorio R, Stephan T, et al. Ovarian changes in women with morbid obesity. *Obstet Gynecol* 1974;44:839.

55. O'Driscoll JB, Mamtora H, Higginson J, et al. A prospective study of the prevalence of clear-cut endocrine disorders and polycystic ovaries in 350 patients presenting with hirsutism or androgenic alopecia. *Clin Endocrinol* 1994;41:231.

56. Moran C, Tapia MC, Hernandez E, et al. Etiological review of hirsutism in 250 patients. *Arch Med Res* 1994;25:311.

57. Zacur HA. Prolactin abnormalities in PCOS, in Azziz R, Nestler JE, Dewailly D (eds), *Androgen Excess Disorders*. Philadelphia: Lippincott-Raven, 1997; p 287.

58. Rebar R, Judd HL, Yen SS, et al. Characterization of the inappropriate gonadotropin secretion in polycystic ovary syndrome. *J Clin Invest* 1976;57:1320.

59. Conway GS, Honour JW, Jacobs HS. Heterogeneity of the polycystic ovary syndrome: Clinical, endocrine and ultrasound features in 556 patients. *Clin Endocrinol* 1989;30:459.

60. Taylor AE, McCourt B, Martin KA, et al. Determinants of abnormal gonadotropin secretion in clinically defined women with polycystic ovary syndrome. *J Clin Endocrinol Metab* 1997;82:2248.

61. Nestler JE, Jakubowicz DJ. Decreases in ovarian cytochrome P450C17α activity and serum free testosterone after reduction of insulin secretion in polycystic ovary syndrome. *N Engl J Med* 1996;335:617.

62. Azziz R, Ehrmann D, Legro RS, et al. Troglitazone improves ovulation and hirsutism in the polycystic ovary syndrome: A multicenter, double blind, placebo-controlled trial. *J Clin Endocrinol Metab* 2001;86:1626.

63. Dunaif A. Insulin resistance and the polycystic ovary syndrome: Mechanism and implications for pathogenesis. *Endocr Rev* 1997;18:774.

64. Dunaif A, Segal KR, Futterweit W, et al. Profound peripheral insulin resistance, independent of obesity, in polycystic ovary syndrome. *Diabetes* 1989;38 :1165.

65. Legro RS, Finegood D, Dunaif A. A fasting glucose to insulin ratio is a useful measure of insulin sensitivity in women with polycystic ovary syndrome. *J Clin Endocrinol Metab* 1998;83:2694.

66. Falsetti L, Eleftheriou G. Hyperinsulinemia in the polycystic ovary syndrome: A clinical, endocrine and echographic study in 240 patients. *Gynecol Endocrinol* 1996;10:319.

67. Ciaraldi TP, el-Roeiy A, Madar Z, et al. Cellular mechanisms of insulin resistance in polycystic ovarian syndrome. *J Clin Endocrinol Metab* 1992;75:577.

68. Ek I, Arner P, Bergqvist A, et al. Impaired adipocyte lipolysis in nonobese women with the polycystic ovary syndrome: A possible link to insulin resistance? *J Clin Endocrinol Metab* 1997;82:1147.

69. Dunaif A, Segal KR, Shelley DR, et al. Evidence for distinctive and intrinsic defects in insulin action in polycystic ovary syndrome. *Diabetes* 1992;41:1257.

70. Dunaif A, Xia J, Book CB, et al. Excessive insulin receptor serine phosphorylation in cultured fibroblasts and in skeletal muscle: A potential mechanism for insulin resistance in the polycystic ovary syndrome. *J Clin Invest* 1995; 96:801.

71. Nestler JE, Jakubowicz DJ, de Vargas AF, et al. Insulin stimulates testosterone biosynthesis by human thecal cells from women with polycystic ovary syndrome by activating its own receptor and using inositolglycan mediators as the signal transduction system. *J Clin Endocrinol Metab* 1998;83:2001.

72. Nestler JE, Powers LP, Matt DW, et al. A direct effect of hyperinsulinemia on serum sex hormone–binding globulin levels in obese women with the polycystic ovary syndrome. *J Clin Endocrinol Metab* 1991;72:83.

73. Elting MW, Korsen TJ, Rekers-Mombarg LT, et al. Women with polycystic ovary syndrome gain regular menstrual cycles when ageing. *Hum Reprod* 2000;15:24.

74. Winters SJ, Talbott E, Guzick DS, et al. Serum testosterone levels decrease in middle age in women with the polycystic ovary syndrome. *Fertil Steril* 2000;73:724.

75. Ovalle F, Azziz R. Insulin resistance, polycystic ovary syndrome, and type 2 diabetes mellitus. *Fertil Steril* 2002;77:1095.

76. Legro RS, Kunselman AR, Dodson WC, et al. Prevalence and predictors of risk for type 2 diabetes mellitus and impaired glucose tolerance in polycystic ovary syndrome: A prospective, controlled study in 254 affected women. *J Clin Endocrinol Metab* 1999;84:165.

77. Anonymous. American Diabetes Association: Clinical practice recommendations 1997. *Diabetes Care* 1997;20(suppl 1):S1.

78. Mikola M, Hiilesmaa V, Halttunen M, et al. Obstetric outcome in women with polycystic ovarian syndrome. *Hum Reprod* 2001;16:226.

79. Urman B, Sarac E, Dogan L, et al. Pregnancy in infertile PCOD patients: Complications and outcome. *J Reprod Med* 1997;42:501.

80. Radon PA, McMahon MJ, Meyer WR. Impaired glucose tolerance in pregnant women with polycystic ovary syndrome. *Obstet Gynecol* 1999; 94:194.

81. Vollenhoven B, Clark S, Kovacs G, et al. Prevalence of gestational diabetes mellitus in polycystic ovarian syndrome (PCOS) patients pregnant after ovulation induction with gonadotrophins. *Aust NZ J Obstet Gynaecol* 2000;40:54.

82. Lesser KB, Garcia FA. Association between polycystic ovary syndrome and glucose intolerance during pregnancy. *J Maternal-Fetal Med* 1997;6:303.

83. Wortsman J, de Angeles S, Futterweit W, et al. Gestational diabetes and neonatal macrosomia in the polycystic ovary syndrome. *J Reprod Med* 1991;36:659.

84. Yildiz BO, Haznedaroglu IC, Kirazli S, et al. Global fibrinolytic capacity is decreased in polycystic ovary syndrome, suggesting a prothrombotic state. *J Clin Endocrinol Metab* 2002;87:3871.

85. Kelly CJ, Lyall H, Petrie JR, et al. A specific elevation in tissue plasminogen activator antigen in women with polycystic ovarian syndrome. *J Clin Endocrinol Metab* 2002;87:3287.

86. Diamanti-Kandarakis E, Spina G, Kouli C, et al. Increased endothelin-1 levels in women with polycystic ovary syndrome and the beneficial effect of metformin therapy. *J Clin Endocrinol Metab* 2001;86:4666.

87. Yarali H, Yildirir A, Aybar F, et al. Diastolic dysfunction and increased serum homocysteine concentrations may contribute to increased cardiovascular risk in patients with polycystic ovary syndrome. *Fertil Steril* 2001;76:511.

88. Loverro G, Lorusso F, Mei L, et al. The plasma homocysteine levels are increased in polycystic ovary syndrome. *Gynecol Obstet Invest* 1902;53:157.

89. Kelly CJ, Speirs A, Gould GW, et al. Altered vascular function in young women with polycystic ovary syndrome. *J Clin Endocrinol Metab* 2002;87:742.

90. Talbott E, Clerici A, Berga SL, et al. Adverse lipid and coronary heart disease risk profiles in young women with polycystic ovary syndrome: Results of a case-control study. *J Clin Epidemiol* 1998;51:415.

91. Dahlgren E, Johansson S, Lindstedt G, et al. Women with polycystic ovary syndrome wedge resected in 1956 to 1965: A long-term follow-up focusing on natural history and circulating hormones. *Fertil Steril* 1992;57:505.

92. Wild SH, Pierpoint T, Jacobs HS. Long-term consequences of polycystic ovary syndrome: Results of a 31-year follow-up study. *Hum Fertil* 2000;3:101.

93. Talbott EO, Guzick DS, Sutton-Tyrrell K, et al. Evidence for association between polycystic ovary syndrome and premature carotid atherosclerosis in middle-aged women. *Arterioscler Thromb Vasc Biol* 2000;20:2414.

94. Pierpoint T, McKeigue PM, Isaacs AJ, et al. Mortality of women with polycystic ovary syndrome at long-term follow-up. *J Clin Epidemiol* 1998;51:581.

95. Legro RS. Polycystic ovary syndrome and cardiovascular disease: a premature association? *Endocr Rev* 2003;24:302.

96. Jackson RL, Dockerty MB. The Stein-Leventhal syndrome: Analysis of 43 cases with special reference to association with endometrial carcinoma. *Am J Obstet Gynecol* 1957;73:161.

97. Hardiman P, Pillay OS, Atiomo W. Polycystic ovary syndrome and endometrial carcinoma (review). *Lancet* 2003;361:1810.

98. Farhi DC, Nosanchuk J, Silverberg SG. Endometrial adenocarcinoma in women under 25 years of age. *Obstet Gynecol* 1986;68:741.

99. Dahlgren E, Friberg LG, Johansson S, et al. Endometrial carcinoma; ovarian dysfunction: A risk factor in young women. *Eur J Obstet Gynecol Reprod Biol* 1991;41:143.

100. Barbieri RL, Ryan KJ. Hyperandrogenism, insulin resistance, and acanthosis nigricans syndrome: A common endocrinopathy with distinct pathophysiologic features. *Am J Obstet Gynecol* 1983;147:90.

101. Moller DE, Cohen O, Yamaguchi Y, et al. Prevalence of mutations in the insulin receptor gene in subjects with features of the type A syndrome of insulin resistance. *Diabetes* 1994;43:247.

102. Nagamani M, Van Dinh T, Kelver ME. Hyperinsulinemia in hyperthecosis of the ovaries. *Am J Obstet Gynecol* 1986;154:384.

103. Azziz R. The hyperandrogenic-insulin-resistant acanthosis nigricans syndrome: therapeutic response. *Fertil Steril* 1994;61:570.

104. Joehrer K, Geley S, Strasser-Wozak EM, et al. *CYP11B1* mutations causing nonclassic adrenal hyperplasia due to 11β-hydroxylase deficiency. *Hum Mol Genet* 1997;6:1829.

105. Sakkal-Alkaddour H, Zhang L, Yang X, et al. Studies of 3β-hydroxysteroid dehydrogenase genes in infants and children manifesting premature pubarche and increased adrenocorticotropin-stimulated delta 5-steroid levels. *J Clin Endocrinol Metab* 1996;81:3961.

106. Kuttenn F, Couillin P, Girard F, et al. Late-onset adrenal hyperplasia in hirsutism. *N Engl J Med* 1985;313:224.

107. Dewailly D, Vantyghem-Haudiquet MC, Sainsard C, et al. Clinical and biological phenotypes in late-onset 21-hydroxylase deficiency. *J Clin Endocrinol Metab* 1986;63:418.

108. Moran C, Azziz R, Carmina E, et al. 21-Hydroxylase-deficient nonclassic adrenal hyperplasia is a progressive disorder: A multicenter study. *Am J Obstet Gynecol* 2000;183:1468.

109. Azziz R, Zacur HA. 21-Hydroxylase deficiency in female hyperandrogenism: screening and diagnosis. *J Clin Endocrinol Metab* 1989;69:577.

110. Azziz R, Hincapie LA, Knochenhauer ES, et al. Screening for 21-hydroxylase-deficient nonclassic adrenal hyperplasia among hyperandrogenic women: A prospective study. *Fertil Steril* 1999;72:915.

111. Carmina E, Lobo RA. Ovarian suppression reduces clinical and endocrine expression of late-onset congenital adrenal hyperplasia due to 21-hydroxylase deficiency. *Fertil Steril* 1994;62:738.

112. New MI, Gertner JM, Speiser PW, et al. Growth and final height in classical and nonclassical 21-hydroxylase deficiency. *J Endocrinol Invest* 1989;12:91.

113. Spritzer P, Billaud L, Thalabard JC, et al. Cyproterone acetate versus hydrocortisone treatment in late-onset adrenal hyperplasia. *J Clin Endocrinol Metab* 1990;70:642.

114. Feldman S, Billaud L, Thalabard JC, et al. Fertility in women with late-onset adrenal hyperplasia due to 21-hydroxylase deficiency. *J Clin Endocrinol Metab* 1992;74:635.

115. Sanchez LA, Moran C, Reyna R, et al. Adrenal progestogen and androgen production in 21-hydroxylase-deficient nonclassic adrenal hyperplasia is partially independent of adrenocorticotropic hormone stimulation. *Fertil Steril* 2002;77:750.

116. Waggoner W, Boots LR, Azziz R. Total testosterone and DHEAS levels as predictors of androgen-secreting neoplasms: A populational study. *Gynecol Endocrinol* 1999;13:394.

117. Derksen J, Nagesser SK, Meinders AE, et al. Identification of virilizing adrenal tumors in hirsute women. *N Engl J Med* 1994;331:968.

118. Carmina E. Prevalence of idiopathic hirsutism. *Eur J Endocrinol* 1998;139:421.

119. Azziz R, Carmina E, Sawaya ME. Idiopathic hirsutism. *Endocr Rev* 2000;21:347.

120. Kreisberg R. Clinical problem-solving: Half a loaf. *N Engl J Med* 1994;330:1295.

121. Yukizane S, Yamakawa R, Murakami T, et al. A 15-year-old girl with pubertal masculinization due to bilateral gonadoblastoma and 45,X/46,X,+mar karyotype. *Kurume Med J* 1994;41:155.

122. Ehrmann DA, Sturis J, Byrne MM, et al. Insulin secretory defects in polycystic ovary syndrome: Relationship to insulin sensitivity and family history of non-insulin-dependent diabetes mellitus. *J Clin Invest* 1995;96:520.

123. Folsom AR, Kaye SA, Sellers TA, et al. Body fat distribution and 5-year risk of death in older women. *JAMA* 1993;269:483.

124. Surrey ES, de Ziegler D, Gambone JC, et al. Preoperative localization of androgen-secreting tumors: Clinical, endocrinologic, and radiologic evaluation of 10 patients. *Am J Obstet Gynecol* 1988;158:1313.

125. World Health Organization Report of a WHO Consultation, Part 1: *Diagnosis and Classification of Diabetes Mellitus: Definition, Diagnosis and Classification of Diabetes Mellitus and its Complications.* WHO, Geneva, 1999.

126. Ehrmann DA, Barnes RB, Rosenfield RL, et al. Prevalence of impaired glucose tolerance and diabetes in women with polycystic ovary syndrome. *Diabetes Care* 1999;22:141.

127. Weerakiet S, Srisombut C, Bunnag P, et al. Prevalence of type 2 diabetes mellitus and impaired glucose tolerance in Asian women with polycystic ovary syndrome. *Int J Gynaecol Obstet* 2001;75:177.

128. MacDougall MJ, Tan SL, Balen A, et al. A controlled study comparing patients with and without polycystic ovaries undergoing in vitro fertilization. *Hum Reprod* 1993;8:233.

129. Azziz R, Gay F. The treatment of hyperandrogenism with oral contraceptives. *Semin Reprod Endocrinol* 1989;7:246.

130. Korytkowski MT, Mokan M, Horwitz MJ, et al. Metabolic effects of oral contraceptives in women with polycystic ovary syndrome. *J Clin Endocrinol Metab* 1995;80:3327.

131. Nader S, Riad-Gabriel MG, Saad MF. The effect of a desogestrel-containing oral contraceptive on glucose tolerance and leptin concentrations in hyperandrogenic women. *J Clin Endocrinol Metab* 1997;82:3074.

132. Chasan-Taber L, Willett WC, Stampfer MJ, et al. A prospective study of oral contraceptives and NIDDM among U.S. women. *Diabetes Care* 1997;20:330.

133. Azziz R, Black VY, Knochenhauer ES, et al. Ovulation after glucocorticoid suppression of adrenal androgens in the polycystic ovary syndrome is not predicted by the basal dehydroepiandrosterone sulfate level. *J Clin Endocrinol Metab* 1999;84:946.

134. Velazquez EM, Mendoza S, Hamer T, et al. Metformin therapy in polycystic ovary syndrome reduces hyperinsulinemia, insulin resistance, hyperandrogenemia, and systolic blood pressure, while facilitating normal menses and pregnancy. *Metab Clin Exp* 1994;43:647.

135. Nestler JE, Jakubowicz DJ, Evans WS, et al. Effects of metformin on spontaneous and clomiphene-induced ovulation in the polycystic ovary syndrome. *N Engl J Med* 1998;338:1876.

136. Moghetti P, Castello R, Negri C, et al. Metformin effects on clinical features, endocrine and metabolic profiles, and insulin sensitivity in polycystic ovary syndrome: A randomized, double-blind, placebo-controlled 6-month trial, followed by open, long-term clinical evaluation. *J Clin Endocrinol Metab* 2000;85:139.

137. Morin-Papunen LC, Vauhkonen I, Koivunen RM, et al. Endocrine and metabolic effects of metformin versus ethinyl estradiol-cyproterone acetate in obese women with polycystic ovary syndrome: A randomized study. *J Clin Endocrinol Metab* 2000;85:3161.

138. Cataldo NA, Abbasi F, McLaughlin TL, et al. Improvement in insulin sensitivity followed by ovulation and pregnancy in a woman with polycystic ovary syndrome who was treated with rosiglitazone. *Fertil Steril* 2001;76:1057.

139. Jaatinen TA, Anttila L, Erkkola R, et al. Hormonal responses to physical exercise in patients with polycystic ovarian syndrome. *Fertil Steril* 1993;60:262.

140. Clark AM, Ledger W, Galletly C, et al. Weight loss results in significant improvement in pregnancy and ovulation rates in anovulatory obese women. *Hum Reprod* 1995;10:2705.

141. Kiddy DS, Hamilton-Fairley D, Bush A, et al. Improvement in endocrine and ovarian function during dietary treatment of obese women with polycystic ovary syndrome. *Clin Endocrinol* 1992;36:105.

142. Golay A, Allaz AF, Morel Y, et al. Similar weight loss with low- or high-carbohydrate diets. *Am J Clin Nutr* 1996;63:174.

143. Golay A, Eigenheer C, Morel Y, et al. Weight-loss with low or high carbohydrate diet? *Int J Obes Relat Metab Disord* 1996;20:1067.

144. Donesky BW, Adashi EY. Surgically induced ovulation in the polycystic ovary syndrome: Wedge resection revisited in the age of laparoscopy. *Fertil Steril* 1995;63:439.

145. Gjonnaess H. Late endocrine effects of ovarian electrocautery in women with polycystic ovary syndrome. *Fertil Steril* 1998; 69:697.

146. Gjonnaess H. Comparison of ovarian electrocautery and oral contraceptives in the treatment of hyperandrogenism in women with polycystic ovary syndrome. *Acta Obstet Gynaecol Scand* 1999;78:530.

147. Pittaway DE, Maxson WS, Wentz AC. Spironolactone in combination drug therapy for unresponsive hirsutism. *Fertil Steril* 1985;43:878.

148. Azziz R, Ochoa TM, Bradley ELJ, et al. Leuprolide and estrogen versus oral contraceptive pills for the treatment of hirsutism: A prospective randomized study. *J Clin Endocrinol Metab* 1995;80:3406.

149. Carr BR, Breslau NA, Givens C, et al. Oral contraceptive pills, gonadotropin-releasing hormone agonists, or use in combination for treatment of hirsutism: A clinical research center study. *J Clin Endocrinol Metab* 1995;80: 1169.

150. Emans SJ, Grace E, Woods ER, et al. Treatment with dexamethasone of androgen excess in adolescent patients. *J Pediatr* 1988;112:821.

151. Carmina E, Lobo RA. Peripheral androgen blockade versus glandular androgen suppression in the treatment of hirsutism. *Obstet Gynecol* 1991;78:845.

152. Prezelj J, Kocijancic A, Andolsek L. Dexamethasone and spironolactone in the treatment of non-tumorous hyperandrogenism . *Gynecol Endocrinol* 1989;3:281.

153. Devoto E, Aravena L, Rios R. [Treatment of hirsutism with spironolactone and with spironolactone plus dexamethasone]. [Spanish]. *Rev Med Chile* 2000;128:868.

154. Carmina E, Lobo RA. The addition of dexamethasone to antiandrogen therapy for hirsutism prolongs the duration of remission. *Fertil Steril* 1998;69:1075.

155. Kelly CJ, Gordon D. The effect of metformin on hirsutism in polycystic ovary syndrome. *Eur J Endocrinol* 2002;147:217.

156. Eil C, Edelson SK. The use of human skin fibroblasts to obtain potency estimates of drug binding to androgen receptors. *J Clin Endocrinol Metab* 1984;59 :51

157. Cumming DC, Yang JC, Rebar RW, et al. Treatment of hirsutism with spironolactone. *JAMA* 1982;247:1295.

158. Moghetti P, Tosi F, Tosti A, et al. Comparison of spironolactone, flutamide, and finasteride efficacy in the treatment of hirsutism: A randomized, double-blind, placebo-controlled trial. *J Clin Endocrinol Metab* 2000;85:89.

159. Helfer EL, Miller JL, Rose LI. Side effects of spironolactone therapy in the hirsute woman. *J Clin Endocrinol Metab* 1988;66:208.

160. Groves TD, Corenblum B. Spironolactone therapy during human pregnancy. *Am J Obstet Gynecol* 1995;172:1655.

161. Venturoli S, Marescalchi O, Colombo FM, et al. A prospective, randomized trial comparing low dose flutamide, finasteride, ketoconazole, and cyproterone acetate-estrogen regimens in the treatment of hirsutism. *J Clin Endocrinol Metab* 1999;84:1304.

162. Wysowski DK, Freiman JP, Tourtelot JB, et al. Fatal and nonfatal hepatotoxicity associated with flutamide. *Ann Intern Med* 1993;118:860.

163. Müderris II, Bayram F, Sahin Y, et al. The efficacy of 250 mg/day flutamide in the treatment of patients with hirsutism. *Fertil Steril* 1996;66:220.

164. Belisle S, Love EJ. Clinical efficacy and safety of cyproterone acetate in severe hirsutism: Results of a multicentered Canadian study. *Fertil Steril* 1986;46:1015.

165. O'Brien RC, Cooper ME, Murray RM, et al. Comparison of sequential cyproterone acetate/estrogen versus spironolactone/oral contraceptive in the treatment of hirsutism. *J Clin Endocrinol Metab* 1991;72:1008.

166. Lunde O, Djoseland O. A comparative study of Aldactone and Diane in the treatment of hirsutism. *J Steroid Biochem* 1987;28:161.

167. Schrode K, Huber F, and Staszak J. Randomized, double-blind, vehicle-controlled safety and efficacy evaluation of eflornithine 15 percent cream in the treatment of women with excessive facial hair. 58th Annual Meeting American Academy of Dermatology, San Francisco, CA, March 10–15, 2000 (abstract P291).

168. Peereboom-Wynia JD. Effect of various methods of depilation on density of hair growth in women with idiopathic hirsutism. *Arch Dermatol Forsch* 1972;243:164.

169. Peereboom-Wynia JD, Stolz E, van Joost T, et al. A comparative study of the effects of electrical epilation of beard hairs in women with hirsutism by diathermy and by the blend method. *Arch Dermatol Res* 1985;278:84.

170. Richards RN, Meharg GE. Electrolysis: Observations from 13 years and 140,000 hours of experience. *J Am Acad Dermatol* 1995;33:662.

171. Sanchez LA, Perez M, Azziz R. Laser hair reduction in the hirsute patient: a critical assessment. *Hum Reprod Update* 2002;8:169.

172. Williams R, Havoonjian H, Isagholian K, et al. A clinical study of hair removal using the long-pulsed ruby laser. *Dermatol Surg* 1998;24:837.

173. Nanni CA, Alster TS. Laser-assisted hair removal: side effects of Q-switched Nd:YAG, long-pulsed ruby, and alexandrite lasers. *J Am Acad Dermatol* 1999;41:165.

CHAPTER 14

Endocrine Aspects of Female Obesity

Barbara A. Gower

Obesity is the most prevalent nutritional disorder of affluent nations, with a broad and significant impact on many endocrinologic parameters. Although obesity is rarely the result of endocrinologic disorders, the presence of obesity is associated with a number of disturbances in androgen, estrogen, binding globulin, insulin/glucose, gonadotropin, prolactin, and growth hormone/growth factor metabolism. Additionally, the hormone leptin, produced in and secreted by adipose tissue, affects the neuroendocrine-reproductive axis both centrally and peripherally. It is possible that some or all of these physiologic alterations play a role in the genesis of obesity-related ovulatory dysfunction and hormone-sensitive carcinomas.

► DEFINITION AND MEASUREMENT OF OBESITY

Current guidelines for overweight and obesity are based on body mass index (BMI), which is weight in kilograms (kg) divided by height in meters (m) squared. The National Heart, Lung, and Blood Institute has established BMI cutoff points for overweight and three categories of obesity: A BMI of 25.0 to 29.9 kg/m^2 indicates *overweight;* a BMI of 30.0 to 34.9 kg/m^2 indi-

cates *obesity class I;* a BMI of 35.0 to 39.9 kg/m^2 indicates *obesity class II;* and a BMI of 40 kg/m^2 or greater indicates *obesity class III,* or *extreme obesity.*[1]

Determination of adiposity by direct measurement of total-body fat is difficult, usually requiring autopsy analysis. However, several indirect measurements, ranging from simple to sophisticated, have utility in research and clinical practice.[2]

1. *Anthropometric measurements* have the highest clinical utility. Although relatively simple to assess, they are less accurate than more sophisticated techniques. Height, weight, skinfold thickness, and body or limb circumferences and diameters have been correlated with body fat content. BMI, weight/height^2 in kilograms and meters, respectively (see above), is the measure on which the current National Institutes of Health (NIH) body weight guidelines are based.[1] Although relatively accurate on a population basis, BMI can over- or underestimate adiposity on an individual basis, particularly in individuals who have substantially more or less muscle mass than the average person. Measurement of subcutaneous skinfold thickness is also useful

clinically, although there are a number of problems with this technique, including selection of an appropriate instrument, selection of a site(s) for measurement, and observer reproducibility. There is no single skinfold measurement that is a reliable index of total body fat for both men and women, and usually a combination of sites must be assessed. However, even the most comprehensive skinfold assessment reflects only subcutaneous fat and does not estimate visceral or intramuscular fat, which may be critical components of total-body fat.

2. *Dilution techniques* involve the ingestion or injection of a known quantity of stable or radioactive isotope or other substance that, after equilibration, allows an estimation of total-body water, total-body potassium, or fat cell mass.

3. *Body density* can be estimated from body volume, which is obtained either by submersion into a water tank or by air-displacement plethysmography.[3] Body fat content is derived from body density using equations validated for this purpose. The equations make assumptions regarding the average densities of fat and fat-free mass.

4. *Dual-energy x-ray absorptiometry (DEXA),* originally developed for the diagnosis of osteoporosis, has become a useful tool for determining whole-body or regional composition. DEXA relies on the principle that soft tissue versus bone and fat versus fat-free soft tissue will cause differential attenuation of two intensities of x-ray beams as they pass through the body.

5. *Computed tomographic (CT) scanning and magnetic resonance imaging (MRI).* Single- or multiple-slice CT scanning or MRI, in conjunction with appropriate imaging software, can be used to quantify adipose or other tissue in two-dimensional images.

Prevalence of Obesity

Using BMI data from the most recent National Health and Nutrition Examination Survey (NHANES, 1999–2000), Flegal and colleagues[4] reported that the age-adjusted prevalence of obesity in the U.S. was 30.5 percent, up from 22.9 percent in the previous survey (1988–1994). Likewise, the prevalence of overweight increased from 55.9 to 64.5 percent over this time period, as did the prevalence of extreme obesity (BMI ≥ 40 kg/m^2, 2.9 to 4.7 percent). The changes were more or less parallel for all gender and ethnic groups and across all ages. Among women, non-Hispanic blacks showed the highest prevalence of both obesity and overweight, with approximately 50 percent of women age 40 years and older being obese and approximately 80 percent being overweight. Among Mexican-American women age 40 years and older, approximately 41 to 48 percent were obese, depending on age, and approximately 77 to 79 percent were overweight. The comparable figures for non-Hispanic white women age 40 years and older were approximately 33 to 34 percent obese and approximately 61 to 65 percent overweight.

Body Fat Distribution

Obesity is not a homogeneous condition but may occur in several topographic patterns: *upper-body, central,* or *android obesity; lower-body, peripheral,* or *gynoid obesity;* and *intraabdominal* or *visceral obesity.* In addition, fat can be stored in intramuscular and intramyocellular spaces. Upper-body obesity is associated more closely with metabolic disturbances than is lower-body obesity. Similarly, women with upper-body obesity are more prone to reproductive abnormalities than those with lower-body obesity, as evidenced by a lower frequency of ovulatory cycles (17.5 versus 35.2 percent).[5] The best measure of upper-body obesity is waist circumference; individuals with a waist circumference above 100 cm are at increased risk for metabolic abnormalities.[6]

The negative health effects of upper-body obesity have, in recent years, been attributed primarily to intraabdominal or visceral adipose tissue, in contrast to simply the presence of subcutaneous abdominal fat. Visceral fat is associated with insulin resistance, hyperinsulinemia, high triglyceride level, low high-density lipoprotein (HDL) cholesterol level, high apolipoprotein B level, small low-density lipoprotein (LDL) particle size, and high LDL particle density.[7] Relative to other depots, visceral fat is more sensitive to lipolytic stimuli and less sensitive to the antilipolytic effects of insulin. Because of this ability to readily mobilize free fatty acids, visceral fat may increase hepatic exposure to lipids, resulting in decreased insulin extraction, increased glucose production, and increased triglyceride production.

However, recent research has revealed that both total obesity and visceral obesity are associated with accumulation of lipid in skeletal muscle.[8,9] Lipid infiltration of skeletal muscle, both between and within the muscle fibers or myocytes, is associated with insulin resistance and dyslipidemia both clinically and in animal models. Intramyocellular triglyceride accumulation in particular has been correlated repeatedly with metabolic disturbance. Fatty acid metabolites, such as fatty acyl-CoA, diacylglyceride, and ceramide, are thought to interfere with insulin signaling by increasing intracellular concentrations of protein kinase C.[10] Protein kinase C promotes insulin resistance by blocking the tyrosine phosphorylation of insulin receptor substrates, an early step in insulin signaling. Thus intramuscular lipid, with its negative effects on metabolism, may be the mechanism through which obesity produces skeletal muscle insulin resistance. At this time, the relative contributions of subcutaneous, visceral, intramuscular, and intramyocellular lipid accumulation to the metabolic complications associated with obesity have not been entirely clarified.

The physiologic cause of abdominal/visceral obesity is not clear but may be endocrine in origin. Several perturbations of gonadal and adrenal hormone production have been linked to abdominal/visceral fat deposition. Among women, excess endogenous androgens[11] and administration of exogenous androgens[12,13] are associated with abdominal/visceral fat deposition. Paradoxically, among men, testosterone administration decreases, rather than increases, visceral fat.[14] Estrogens, possibly in conjunction with progesterone, promote fat deposition in the gluteofemoral area, leading to the characteristic gynoid fat distribution in obese, cyclic, premenopausal women. Upper body obesity in women is observed in individuals with depressed ovarian estrogen production/action, such as smokers[15] and postmenopausal women (see "Obesity and Menopause" below). Because many cases of female androgen excess are associated with estrogen and/or progesterone deficiency, the role of relatively low ovarian steroid hormones in promoting abdominal/visceral fat deposition cannot be discounted. The association between androgens and abdominal adiposity is not robust,[16] and in prospective analyses, low, rather than high, total testosterone concentration predicted deposition of upper body fat in postmenopausal women; bioavailable testosterone was not related to a change in the waist-hip ratio.[17] Taken together, data suggest that, among women, hyperandrogenicity occurs either secondary to or in conjunction with the development of upper body obesity but is unlikely to be a causal factor.

Racial Differences

At any given level of total-body fat, African-American women have less visceral fat and more subcutaneous abdominal fat than Caucasian women.[18,19] In addition, African-American women have higher insulin levels and are more insulin resistant than Caucasian women, if evenly matched for total-body fat and/or visceral fat.[20,21]

From an endocrine and metabolic perspective, observations made in Caucasian populations do not always apply to African-Americans. For example, among obese postmenopausal women, African-Americans and Caucasians had similar sex hormone–binding globulin (SHBG) and free testosterone concentrations, but African-Americans had 35 percent higher leptin concentrations, 34 percent higher fasting insulin concentrations, and a 39 percent greater insulin response to a glucose load.[22] SHBG was inversely correlated with BMI, waist circumference, visceral fat, and the insulin response to a glucose load and positively correlated with HDL cholesterol among Caucasians but not African-Americans (Fig. 14-1). Among Caucasian women, the association between SHBG and insulin area-under-the-curve disappeared after adjusting for visceral fat, suggesting that greater visceral fat accrual among Caucasian women was responsible for elevated insulin and associated suppression of SHBG.

With weight loss, overweight premenopausal Caucasian women lose more visceral fat and less subcutaneous abdominal fat than BMI-matched African-American women.[23] Nonethe-

less, the improvement in insulin sensitivity and lipids with weight loss does not differ with race, suggesting a differential effect of individual adipose tissue depots on risk factors in black and white women.

▶ ANDROGEN METABOLISM IN OBESITY

Circulating Androgen Concentrations in Obesity

In most studies of adults or adolescents with eumenorrheic obesity, circulating total andro-

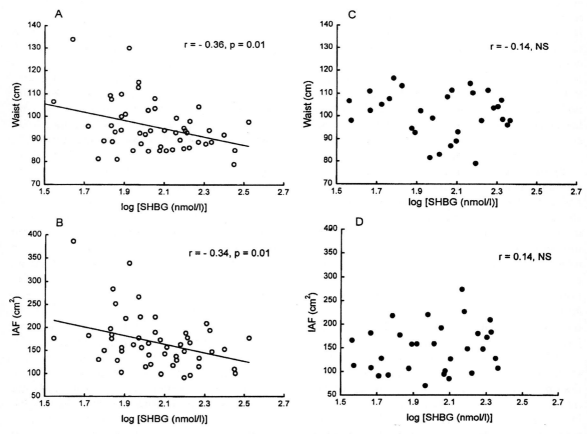

Figure 14-1 Relationship between waist circumference and SHBG concentration *(A, C)* and between intraabdominal fat (IAF) and SHBG *(B, D)* in Caucasian (○) and African-American (●) women. *(Used, with permission, from Berman et al.[22])*

gen levels do not differ from and actually may be lower than those of normal-weight controls.[24–29] Serum dehydroepiandrosterone sulfate (DHEAS) levels were reported to be lower among 217 obese women compared with normal-weight women and to be correlated with testosterone (T), androstenedione (A), and 24-hour urinary cortisol concentrations.[30]

Unbound, or bioavailable, T may be increased in otherwise euandrogenic obesity.[25] Evans and colleaguse[31] noted that BMI and waist-hip ratio correlated inversely with SHBG levels and directly with the proportion of free T. Higher free T levels were observed in obese eumenorrheic nonhirsute women despite a similar waist-hip ratio to nonobese controls, suggesting that the increase in free T is associated more closely with total rather than abdominal obesity.[32] Wajchenberg and colleagues[33] observed higher total and free T levels in obese eumenorrheic nonhirsute women. While some other studies have not confirmed the increase in free T levels in obese premenopausal[26] and postmenopausal[34] women, such a finding is consistent with the lower SHBG binding activity noted in obese subjects (discussed below).

In summary, it appears that circulating levels of plasma total androgens do not vary significantly with weight and, in fact, may be slightly lower in overweight subjects. However, because of an obesity-related decrease in the circulating level of SHBG, the percentage of free T may be somewhat elevated, in particular in those women with upper body fat distribution.

Androgen Production and Clearance in Obesity

Samojlik and colleagues[24] reported a higher metabolic clearance rate (MCR), as well as production rate (PR), of T, dihydrotestosterone (DHT), and 3α-androstanediol (3α-diol) in obese eumenorrheic women when compared with normal-weight subjects. The MCR of T was 1256 ± 145 and 740 ± 40 L/d in obese and normal-weight women, respectively. Be-

cause serum androgen levels were the same or slightly lower, the calculated production rates of T, DHT, and 3α-diol were 1.5- to 3-fold higher in obese subjects. This obesity-related increase in MCR and PR also was reported for A and dehydroepiandrosterone (DHEA).[35] Both BMI and waist-hip ratio correlated with the MCR of A and DHEA and with the PR of A. The PR of DHEA did not appear to be associated with the waist-hip ratio. The etiology of the obesity-related increase in androgen MCR is not clear but may relate to both decreased SHBG concentration and increased sequestration by adipose tissue. T and DHT are bound by SHBG in the circulation.[36] This carrier protein has a high affinity for these steroids but a low carrying capacity. As will be discussed later, the circulating levels of SHBG decrease with obesity, probably secondary to hyperinsulinemia. As SHBG levels decrease, the MCR of T increases, probably due to the increase in unbound T available for hepatic extraction and clearance.[37] Because A, DHEA, and DHEAS are not bound significantly by SHBG, variations in the concentration of this carrier protein with obesity do not explain their increased MCR. The increased clearance of these and other androgens may reflect adipose tissue sequestration or metabolism.

Fat tissue is able to sequester various steroids, including androgens, probably secondary to their lipid solubility. The observation that clearance of T, A, and estradiol (E_2) correlated with body weight in women infused with radiolabeled hormones may support the importance of adipose tissue sequestration as a significant component of clearance.[38] Most steroid hormones appear to be preferentially concentrated within human adipocytes rather than in plasma[39] (Table 14-1). Only cortisol is not significantly stored in fat tissue. Since the volume of fat in obese subjects is much larger than their intravascular space, and because tissue steroid concentrations are two- to thirteenfold higher than those in plasma, the steroid pool of severely obese subjects is far greater than that of normal-weight individuals.

▶ **TABLE 14-1:** STEROID CONCENTRATION
RATIOS: HUMAN ADIPOSE TISSUE
TO PERIPHERAL BLOOD

Steroid*	Adipose Tissue/Serum Ratio†
Cortisol	0.4 ± 0.7
DHEA	13.2 ± 4.4
Androstenedione	7.7 ± 3.4
Testosterone	7.0 ± 3.0
Estronet Estradiol	2.2 ± 1.5
Progesterone	6.3 ± 7.0
17-hydroxyprogesterone	4.0 ± 2.5

*For abbreviations see text.
†Mean ± standard error
Modified, with permission, from Feher and Bodrogi.[39]

In addition to serving as a reservoir, fat tissue can be the site of steroid metabolism. Androgens can be irreversibly aromatized to estrogens or converted to other androgens, a reversible process.[40] Between 1 and 5 percent of circulating A is converted to estrone (E_1) in women.[40–42] Peripheral aromatization is responsible for a large fraction of androgen clearance and will be discussed further in the section on estrogen metabolism and obesity.

Ovarian Function in Obesity

There is no evidence that ovarian enzymatic function is altered in euandrogenic obesity. However, the hyperinsulinemia that accompanies obesity may affect ovarian steroidogenesis in certain predisposed individuals and could be partly responsible for the hyperandrogenism associated with some cases of obesity. High levels of insulin stimulate androgen production in vivo, and insulin augments responsiveness to luteinizing hormone (LH) in vitro, indirectly stimulating steroidogenesis and androgen production.[43,44] Reduction of insulin with metformin reduced ovarian cytochrome P450C17α activity in obese women with polycystic ovary syndrome (PCOS).[45] Treated women showed

decreases in insulin area under the curve during an oral glucose tolerance test, basal serum 17α-hydroxyprogesterone and LH levels, and leuprolide-stimulated 17α-hydroxyprogesterone. Similarly, treatment of women with PCOS and an average BMI of approximately 35 to 38 kg/m^2 with the insulin-sensitizing agent troglitizone resulted in an increase in SHBG, a decrease in free T, improvement in most indices of insulin secretion/action, a decrease in hirsutism, and an increase in ovulation.[46] Insulin may stimulate ovarian steroid production through either the insulin or insulin-like growth factor I (IGF-I) receptors because both are present in the ovary.

Cortisol Dynamics in Obesity

Plasma cortisol concentrations are normal or slightly reduced in obesity despite an accelerated PR and MCR.[47,48] An increase in the urinary excretion of 17-hydroxycorticosteroids among obese individuals has been reported; however, normalization for body surface area and lean body mass reduced or eliminated the obesity-related difference in some cases. Urinary free cortisol is reported to be elevated in women with central obesity. Circulating concentrations of cortisol-binding globulin were reported not to differ in obese versus normal-weight women. Responsiveness to adrenocorticotropic hormone (ACTH) and corticotropin-releasing hormone (CRH) are normal in simple obesity but appear elevated in individuals with abdominal obesity; such enhanced adrenocortical function may lead to an increase in adrenal androgen production as well.

Weight Loss and Androgen Metabolism

If the alterations in androgen metabolism noted in obesity are due to the excess body fat, normalization of the metabolic aberration should be observed following weight loss. Most studies

▶ **TABLE 14-2:** SUMMARY OF CHANGES IN ANDROGEN METABOLISM WITH EUMENORRHEIC OBESITY AND WEIGHT LOSS

	Concentration†	Clearance†	Production†	Weight Loss
Total testosterone	Unchanged or slightly lower	Elevated	Elevated	No change
Free testosterone	Elevated	—	—	Decrease
Androstenedione	Decreased	Elevated	Elevated	Increase
DHEAS	Decreased	—	—	—
DHEA	—	Elevated	Elevated	—
SHBG	Decreased	—	Decreased	Increase

*For abbreviations, see text.
†Obese versus normal weight.

have not reported a difference in total T levels between normal and obese females and consequently do not report any change with weight loss (6.5 to 18 kg).[27,49,50] However, results may differ with massively obese women, among whom androgens may be elevated.[51] Kim and colleagues[50] reported a decrease in free T levels following weight reduction that depended on the degree of weight loss and starting body mass; total T did not change.

Weight loss has been associated with an increase in A among obese patients with depressed baseline hormone concentrations.[27,52] However, among massively obese women who displayed higher baseline A concentrations, weight loss resulted in a decrease in A.[51] Jakubowicz and Nestler[53] reported no change in total or free T or A but a 45 percent increase in DHEAS with a change in BMI from 32.2 ± 1.2 to 29.9 ± 1.1 kg/m^2 in obese eumenorrheic women; however, subjects were not weight-stable when tested. Because SHBG increased significantly in these subjects, either T production increased or clearance decreased in order for free T concentration to remain unchanged (Table 14-2).

▶ ESTROGEN METABOLISM IN OBESITY

Excess body fat leads to alterations in estrogen metabolism, which, in turn, may affect the hypothalamic-pituitary-ovarian axis and lead to ovulatory dysfunction. Functional hyperestrogenism in obesity also has been associated with an increased risk of breast and endometrial carcinoma.

Estrogen Plasma Concentrations in Obesity

The production of estrogen and its precursors, including A and T, decreases with age and menopause.[54] In reviewing estrogen metabolism in eumenorrheic obesity, premenopausal and postmenopausal patients need to be considered separately. In premenopausal women, Trichopoulos and colleagues[55] did not observe a difference in spot urinary E_1 and E_2 concentrations in women of varying weights. Other investigators have noted that the circulating levels of total E_1 and E_2 were not different between obese and normal-weight premenopausal eumenorrheic women[26,56] or were slightly lower in obese women.[27] In an attempt to eliminate the variability of single plasma measurements, the serum levels of E_1 and E_2 were assayed every 20 minutes for 24 hours, and no significant difference was observed between normal-weight and obese women.[25,57] Eumenorrheic obese women demonstrate lower circulating SHBG levels,[31] suggesting that the free fraction of circulating E_2 may be higher in obesity. Nonetheless, Dunaif and colleagues[26] were unable to confirm this.

In contrast to premenopausal individuals, in postmenopausal women, serum levels of E_1 and A are mildly correlated with the degree of obesity and fat mass.[58] Free E_2 concentration was higher in more obese postmenopausal women, and body size correlated positively with total and free E_2 concentration.[59] E_1 and E_2 circulating concentrations progressively decrease with age in postmenopausal females, and this drop begins 4 to 5 years earlier in obese women compared with normal-weight controls.[58]

These data suggest that the circulating levels of E_1 and total and/or free E_2 are slightly higher in obese postmenopausal women, presumably due to peripheral aromatization. In contrast, such increments in peripheral estrogen production among premenopausal women are overshadowed by ovarian estrogen production, although free E_2 may be slightly elevated.

Peripheral Production of Estrogens in Obesity

West and colleagues[60] first reported the aromatization of T to estrogens in castrated adrenalectomized women. The aromatization of A to E_1 by human adipose tissue has been demonstrated in vitro[61] and in vivo in premenopausal[40,42] and in postmenopausal[41] women. Aromatase activity is detected primarily in the stroma of adipose tissue and not in intact adipocytes.[62] Although adipose tissue is a significant source of aromatase activity in women, Longcope and colleagues[63] noted that muscle accounts for 25 to 30 percent of total peripheral aromatization, and adipose tissue accounts for only 10 to 15 percent in men. The liver and other organs account for the remaining portion of extragonadal aromatization. Nevertheless, the rate of peripheral A-to-E_1 conversion is clearly correlated with body weight in premenopausal[42] and postmenopausal[41] women (Fig. 14-2) and is greater in postmenopausal versus premenopausal women.[64]

A is the major substrate for peripheral estrogen formation, with 0.74 percent being aro-

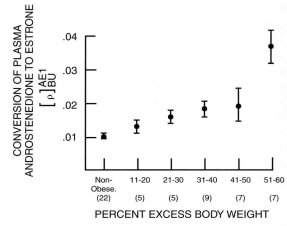

Figure 14-2 The extent of conversion of plasma androstenedione to estrone as a function of the percent excess body weight in ovulatory and anovulatory young women. The bars represent the standard error of the mean for each group. The numbers in parentheses represent the number of patients in that group. *(Reproduced, with permission, from Edman and MacDonald,[42] p. 456.)*

matized. Only 0.15 percent of T is converted to E_2, although this may become clinically significant because this estrogen is much more potent than E_1. Longcope and colleagues[41] reported a significant association between body weight and the conversion of T to E_2. DHEA contributes very little to circulating estrogens via A, with only 0.05 percent being converted.[65]

The interconversion of E_1 to E_2 has been demonstrated in vivo[66] and in vitro[67] in adipose tissue. The conversion of E_1 to E_2 is approximately 5 percent, whereas 15 percent of E_2 is converted back to E_1 in premenopausal women.[66] Adipose tissue 17β-hydroxysteroid dehydrogenase activity (measured by the conversion of E_1 to E_2) was higher in premenopausal than in postmenopausal women, and all females had a greater activity than males.[67] The conversion of E_1 to E_2 also was greater in omental than in subcutaneous abdominal fat and was noncompetitively inhibited by DHEA and DHEAS. The significance of this finding is not clear, but it appears that circulating adrenal androgens may influence peripheral estrogen metabolism. Although estrogen interconversion is observed in adipose tissue in vitro, Longcope and colleagues[41] were not able to demonstrate an association between body fat and interconversion rates in vivo.

The catabolism of estrogens may also be altered in obesity. Normal estrogen metabolism begins with E_2 that is subsequently oxidized to E_1. E_1 is metabolized to estriol (E_3) via the 16α-hydroxylation pathway or to catechol-estrogens via C_2 hydroxylation. Schneider and colleagues[68] reported that obesity was associated with a decrease in C_2 hydroxylation and little alteration in 16α-hydroxylation activity. These metabolic alterations can result in a higher E_3-to-catechol-estrogen ratio. Since E_3 has significantly more estrogenic activity than 2-hydroxy-estrone (a catechol-estrogen), the altered estrogen metabolism may contribute to the functional hyperestrogenism noted in obesity. Notwithstanding these metabolic disturbances, E_3 probably contributes little to the overall estrogenic activity of normal premenopausal women regardless of weight.[69]

Estrogens are not only a passive by-product of obesity but also can promote adipose tissue proliferation. 17β-Estradiol, but not 17α-estradiol, induced the replication and proliferation of adipocyte precursors in vitro. This growth stimulation was noted at physiologic concentrations of 17β-estradiol[70] (Table 14-3).

▶ SEX HORMONE–BINDING GLOBULIN IN OBESITY

Sex hormone–binding globulin (SHBG) is a circulating α-globulin produced by the liver that binds, in a high-affinity but low-capacity fashion, many of the circulating sex steroids.[71] Some of these steroids also are bound by albumin and other less well-described carrier proteins.

Traditionally, only the hormone fraction not bound to a carrier protein (the *free* fraction) has been considered available for tissue action. More recently, the albumin-bound fraction of sex steroids also appears to be available for tissue interaction. Using a rat brain perfusion model, Pardridge[36] have demonstrated that albumin-bound steroid is readily transported into the brain substance, whereas antibody- or SHBG-bound hormone is not. Tissue utilization of albumin-bound steroid depends on how closely the tissue-capillary transit time approximates the half-time of the hormone-protein dissociation rate. Tissues with high capillary transit time (e.g., liver, ± 5 seconds) will "strip" the steroid from albumin better than organs with short transit times (e.g., brain, ± 1 second).

The percentage of E_2 not bound to SHBG or albumin is 2 to 3 percent in normal women, whereas unbound T constitutes 1.5 to 2 percent of the total, as determined by in vitro experiments.[72] Alterations in SHBG levels have a profound impact on the metabolism and action

▶ **TABLE 14-3:** SUMMARY OF CHANGES IN ESTROGEN METABOLISM IN EUMENORRHEIC PRE- AND POSTMENOPAUSAL WOMEN WITH SIMPLE OBESITY

	Premenopausal		Postmenopausal	
	Concentration*	Production*	Concentration*	Production*
Estrone	No change	Increased	Elevated	Increased
Estradiol	No change	Slight increase	Elevated	Slight increase
Free estradiol	May be elevated	—	Elevated	—

*Obese versus normal weight.

of bound steroids. A decrease in SHBG plasma concentration is associated with an increase in the MCR and free fraction of T^{37} and E_2.[73] Furthermore, the blood conversion rates of T to A and T to DHT are positively correlated with the free T fraction but are independent of total plasma T.[37,74]

Circulating SHBG concentrations are influenced by a number of factors, including estrogens, androgens, and insulin. It is known that the administration of exogenous estrogen, particularly orally, leads to increased hepatic production of SHBG.[75] Androgens decrease, glucocorticoids may inhibit, and thyroid hormones increase SHBG levels in normal subjects.[72]

SHBG levels appear to be relatively sensitive to circulating androgens and estrogens throughout life, although other factors are clearly involved. Prior to puberty, there are no sexual differences in the levels of SHBG. At puberty, plasma SHBG concentrations decrease slightly in females and markedly in males.[72] However, this decrease is likely due to the increase in insulin observed at this time,[76] with increased androgen production further decreasing SHBG production in males. In the normal female population, SHBG is not correlated with androgen levels,[77] and there does not appear to be any consistent change in SHBG with age in postmenopausal woman.[72]

Obesity is clearly associated with lower SHBG levels in otherwise normal women.[25,27,56] The mechanism by which obesity decreases the production of SHBG is likely via elevated insulin. In vitro[78] and in vivo,[79] insulin decreases SHBG production, and circulating SHBG concentrations are inversely related to insulin in healthy women.[80] In obese hyperandrogenic women[81] and in women with PCOS,[82] a reduction in insulin was associated with an increase in SHBG and a decrease in free T. In premenopausal women of various body weights, percentage free T correlated directly with fasting insulin and the insulin response to an oral glucose tolerance test.[31] Both insulin secretory pulse frequency[83]

and fasting insulin concentration[80] have been associated with SHBG concentration.

Most investigators report an increase in SHBG plasma concentrations following weight reduction,[51,52] and the extent of the rise in SHBG correlates linearly with the amount of weight loss.[50] It appears that energy deficit has a synergistic effect with weight reduction in increasing SHBG levels.[49] Women who were fasting and who had lost an average of 20 kg had higher SHBG levels than subjects who had lost an average of 25 kg but were not fasting.

Summary

Obesity lowers the plasma concentration of SHBG by decreasing hepatic production, an effect that may be secondary to elevated insulin. The drop in circulating SHBG leads to greater levels in the unbound fraction of free E_2, T, and other sex steroids. As SHBG levels are reduced, the MCR for both E_2 and T subsequently increases, and the conversions of T to DHT and T to A increase. Weight reduction serves to normalize the SHBG plasma concentrations.

▶ INSULIN/GLUCOSE HOMEOSTASIS IN SIMPLE OBESITY

Insulin Concentrations in Simple Obesity

It is generally agreed that most obese women have an increased resistance to insulin-stimulated glucose uptake.[84] Although fasting glucose plasma levels are similar in obese and nonobese nondiabetic women, both fasting and postchallenge insulin concentrations are higher among obese women. The insulin resistance noted in most obese subjects may occur secondary to infiltration of skeletal muscle with lipid, as discussed earlier (see "Body Fat Distribution" above). Abnormalities in insulin/

glucose homeostasis resolve on weight reduction[85] and may be related to depletion of intramyocellular triglyceride.[86]

Effects of Androgens on Insulin Action

Obesity, especially abdominal obesity, is a risk factor for development of type 2 diabetes in women.[87] Although cause-and-effect relationships have not been fully established, the possibility exists that disturbances in androgen metabolism could play a role. Androgen excess in women is associated both with abdominal obesity and insulin resistance, a precursor to type 2 diabetes. Furthermore, women with type 2 diabetes were found to be hyperandrogenic, having high circulating free T secondary to depressed SHBG.[88] Thus the possibility exists that androgen excess may contribute to the pathogenesis of type 2 diabetes either directly, through promoting insulin resistance, or indirectly, through promoting abdominal fat deposition.

Studies with rats have shown that administration of T causes a suite of responses similar to those observed in women with abdominal obesity. T-treated female rats became insulin-resistant and developed a type of muscle morphology characterized by a relatively higher proportion of insulin-insensitive type IIb (fast twitch) fibers, relatively low capillarization, reduced glycogen synthase activity, and a reduced proportion of insulin-sensitive glycogen synthase.[89] Similarly, treatment of women with T reduces indices of glucose utilization, indicative of insulin resistance.[90] In both cross-sectional clinical studies and experimental mouse research, greater circulating concentrations of T are associated with lower concentrations of adiponectin, an adiocyte-derived protein that is associated with greater insulin sensitivity.[91] Thus both clinical and experimental observations support the hypothesis that obesity-related disturbances in androgen metabolism may be involved in the pathogenesis of type 2 diabetes, a disease commonly observed in obese women.

Effects of Insulin on Androgen Production and Clearance

The relationship of insulin and androgens has received considerable attention in the study of hyperandrogenic patients.[92,93] Nevertheless, the insulin/androgen relationship in obese eumenorrheic subjects is not clear. With a decrease in insulin induced by weight loss and negative energy balance, women with PCOS showed significant decreases in basal and leuprolide-stimulated 17α-hydroxyprogesterone and total and free T.[53] However, these changes were not observed among control obese women with normal menses despite a similar decrease in insulin; rather, control women showed increases in SHBG and DHEAS. It has been concluded from this study that obese women with PCOS differed from obese ovulatory women in sensitivity to insulin-mediated perturbations in ovarian cytochrome P450C17α activity and resulting T production.

Experimental administration of insulin is reported to increase A in obese and nonobese ovulatory women,[94] decrease DHEAS in nonobese ovulatory women,[95] and have no effect on T.[94,95] In vitro, insulin stimulates both A and T secretion from cultured theca cells through action at the insulin receptor.[92]

Both clearance and production of DHEA were strongly and positively correlated with insulin in healthy obese and nonobese women.[96]

Summary

Simple obesity is associated with hyperinsulinemia and insulin resistance that resolve with weight loss. Abdominal obesity is associated with both insulin resistance and elevated circulating androgens. Experimentally, administration of T increases insulin resistance, and administration of insulin increases A and T secretion. The extent to which the association between insulin resistance and elevated androgens is due to insulin stimulation of androgen production as opposed to androgen stimulation of insulin resistance is not clear.

► GROWTH HORMONE/INSULIN-LIKE GROWTH FACTOR AXIS IN OBESITY

Growth Hormone

Obesity is associated with decreased secretion[97] and increased clearance[98] of growth hormone (GH), resulting in depressed serum concentrations of GH. Low GH appears to be a consequence rather than a cause of obesity because weight loss restores normal GH levels.[99] The precise mechanism through which obesity alters GH release is not known but may be related to associated elevation in insulin. Insulin suppresses hepatic production of insulin-like growth factor (IGF)–binding protein 1 (IGFBP-1),[100] thus increasing free IGF-I and IGF bioavailability. Negative-feedback action of IGF-I on somatostatin-containing hypothalamic neurons may then depress pituitary GH release.

The clinical implications of depressed GH for reproductive function are not known. However, studies showing that the ovary is targeted by GH and is a site of GH reception and action have led some investigators to propose labeling GH a gonadotropin.[101] In the human ovary, GH stimulated E_2 synthesis both independently and in synergy with follicle-stimulating hormone (FSH).[102] Human GH both stimulated progesterone synthesis in human luteinized granulosa cells and enhanced the ability of low, generally ineffective concentrations of human chorionic gonadotropin (hCG) to stimulate progesterone production.[103] Additionally, GH treatment facilitates gonadotropin-induced ovulation in vivo in patients with amenorrhea and anovulatory infertility.[104] It is probably more accurate to consider GH a fa-

cilitator of gonadotropin action (a *cogonadotropin*) because most of its effects depend on the concurrent presence of physiologic gonadotropin concentrations. If GH has a role in normal ovarian physiology, the possibility exists that obesity-related changes in GH status could affect reproductive function.

Insulin-Like Growth Factors

Circulating IGF-I (formerly somatomedin-C) is derived largely from hepatic production, and is stimulated by GH. Serum IGF-I (of hepatic origin) has mitogenic effects on muscle and perhaps other tissues. IGF-I and IGF-II also are produced in the ovary, where they may affect steroidogenesis. In vitro studies have indicated that IGF-I stimulates aromatase activity[105] and estradiol secretion[106] both independently and in response to FSH. It also increases the expression of LH receptors[107] and stimulates LH-induced androgen synthesis in cultured thecal-interstitial cells from rats.[108] Both IGF-I and IGF-II stimulate LH-induced androgen synthesis in cultured thecal cells from euandrogenic women[109] (Fig. 14-3).

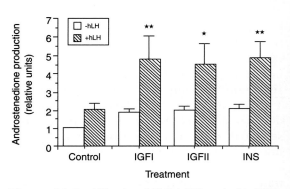

Figure 14-3 Effects of IGF-I (30 ng/mL), IGF-II (30 ng/mL), and insulin (30 ng/mL) in the presence and absence of LH on androstenedione production in thecal cell monolayers established from euandrogenic women. (*Reproduced, with permission, from Nahum, Thong, and Hillier,[109] pp 75–81.*)

The effect of obesity on serum IGF levels and on IGF action is not clear. Obese individuals are reported to have elevated,[110] depressed,[99] or unchanged[110] levels of IGF-I. Discrepant observations may derive from differences in both the type of obesity assessed (simple versus visceral) and the method of assessing IGF-I (total versus free). Visceral fat, but not adiposity per se, was associated with depressed levels of total IGF-I.[111] Both types of obesity are associated, to some degree, with elevated insulin. As mentioned earlier, insulin suppresses IGFBP-1 production, thereby increasing bioavailable IGF-I. Additionally, insulin acting at the IGF-I receptor[112] may further augment events normally mediated by IGF-I.

Summary

Obesity decreases circulating GH and is likely to affect IGF action at some level; secondary to obesity-related elevations in insulin, the ovary or adrenal may be exposed to increased circulating free IGFs or to increased insulin binding of IGF-I receptors. Changes in GH or IGF action at the level of the ovary or adrenal could affect steroidogenesis.

▶ OBESITY-RELATED HORMONES

Letpin

The hormone leptin is synthesized in and secreted from adipocytes of white adipose tissue. Circulating leptin concentrations are proportionate to adiposity, with more obese individuals having higher concentrations. In addition, leptin concentrations fluctuate with energy balance,[113] independent of changes in body weight or body fat content. Thus leptin serves as an endocrine signal of caloric status. Although leptin-deficient mice are obese, there is little evidence that leptin plays a role in the etiology of obesity in normal animal models or humans.

Leptin's ability to reflect energy balance suggests that it may serve as the link between nutritional status and reproduction. Food deprivation, caloric restriction, and high levels of physical activity can result in delayed puberty, suppressed ovulatory cycles, altered reproductive behavior, and altered gonadotropin secretion in animals and humans.[114] Treatment of normal prepubertal mice with leptin accelerates maturation of the reproductive tract, results in earlier onset of puberty, and advances age at first reproduction. Clinically, available evidence suggests that leptin may participate in the timing of puberty and in mediating the pathologic responses of the reproductive system to both under- and overnutrition.[115] Leptin's role in puberty appears to be largely permissive, although a 1 ng/mL increment in serum leptin is associated with a 1-month advance in menarche. In the few documented cases of human leptin deficiency or leptin receptor mutation, pubertal development failed to occur. Low leptin levels are observed in cases of anorexia nervosa and functional hypothalamic amenorrhea, as well as in elite athletes, and may serve as signal to the hypothalamus of energy deficit.

The known association of obesity with anovulation and follicular atresia suggests a link between excessive body fat and reproductive dysfunction. Thus several recent studies have been conducted to test the hypothesis that excessive leptin production has pathologic consequences. Brzechffa and colleagues[116] examined circulating leptin concentration in women with PCOS versus BMI-matched healthy controls. They found that 29 percent of women with PCOS, but none of the controls, had levels of leptin above the 99 percent prediction interval for BMI, suggesting that leptin production may be abnormally regulated in women with PCOS. However, these results were not confirmed in subsequent investigations.[115] In vitro data have suggested that high concentrations of leptin, such as occur in obesity, may interfere with normal hormonal stimulation of ovarian estradiol production.[115] However, in vivo data failed to support the hypothesis that obesity-mediated elevation in serum leptin impairs estradiol secretion.[117] Among both women with PCOS and healthy women, lower follicular fluid leptin concentration predicted successful pregnancy following in vitro fertilization or gamete intrafallopian transfer.[115]

A sharp increase in leptin occurs during the second and third trimesters of pregnancy, suggesting that leptin plays a role in maternal energy partitioning. Due to its ability to promote lipid oxidation, leptin may allow the maternal system to preferentially use lipid as a fuel, making glucose available to the fetus. However, the positive energy balance associated with pregnancy may be sufficient to explain the observation of elevated leptin among pregnant women.

In summary, leptin is likely to play a permissive role in the onset of puberty. The excessive leptin associated with obesity may impair reproductive function at the level of the ovary but does not appear to be responsible for the development of PCOS. The low leptin levels associated with energy deficit may contribute to amenorrhea through action at the hypothalamus. High leptin during pregnancy may play a role in maternal substrate partitioning, ensuring sufficient glucose transport to the fetal system. The hypothesized effects of leptin on reproductive endocrinology are illustrated in Figure 14-4, which indicates stimulatory effects centrally and inhibitory effects at the ovary.

Ghrelin

The newly discovered hormone ghrelin is a gastric peptide implicated in the control of food intake and energy balance.[118] When administered to animals or humans, ghrelin increases food intake, impedes lipid utilization, and promotes adipose tissue deposition.[119] Ghrelin binding has been detected in the human ovary.[120]

Due to ghrelin's association with both energy homeostasis and reproduction, its potential involvement in the pathogenesis of PCOS was investigated in two studies. In the first, women with PCOS had lower circulating concentrations of ghrelin than weight-matched controls.[121] In both groups, ghrelin concentration was inversely correlated with A concentration. However, ghrelin concentration was correlated with insulin sensitivity only among the PCOS group. In contrast, in a second study, ghrelin was not found to differ in PCOS versus control subjects, and no associations between circulating ghrelin levels and concentrations of several reproductive and metabolic hormones were observed within the PCOS group.[122] Thus additional research is needed to determine if ghrelin has a role in the reproductive dysfunction associated with PCOS.

Adiponectin

Adiponectin is a newly discovered protein hormone secreted by adipocytes.[123] Paradoxically, circulating adiponectin concentrations are inversely related to obesity and insulin resistance and are lower in individuals with type 2 diabetes.[124] Adiponectin has an insulin-sensitizing effect on peripheral tissues.[125]

Cytokines

Circulating concentrations of the cytokines interleukin 6 (IL-6), IL-18, C-reactive protein (CRP), and tumor necrosis factor α (TNF-α) are elevated in obese individuals.[126] Although IL-6 and TNF-α are synthesized by adipose tissue,[127] CRP is synthesized by and secreted from the liver[128]; the link between CRP and obesity may occur secondary to the obesity-related elevations in insulin[129] or IL-6.[128] Elevations in cytokines normalize on weight loss.[126,130]

Elevated cytokines are associated with several negative health outcomes. Increased TNF-α may promote insulin resistance[131] and has been observed to impair follicular development[132]; circulating CRP is positively and independently associated with cardiovascular

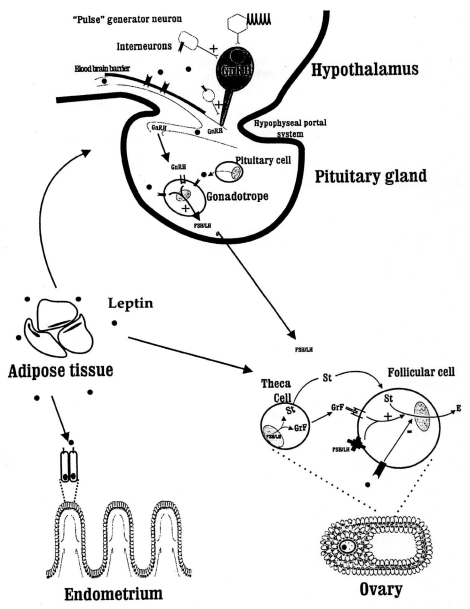

Figure 14-4 Schematic diagram illustrating the interaction of leptin with the hypothalamic-pituitary-gonadal axis and endometrium. Stimulatory effects are indicated at the hypothalamus, whereas inhibitory effects are indicated at the ovary. See text and ref. 115 for additional discussion. St = steroid precursors; GrF = growth factors; E = estrogens. *(Reproduced, with permission, from Moschos, Chan, and Mantzoros,[115] p 433.)*

disease[133] and insulin resistance[134] and is correlated with several components of the insulin resistance syndrome.[134] Women with PCOS have elevated levels of CRP,[129] presumably due to the combination of obesity and insulin resistance/hyperinsulinemia. Thus elevated cytokine levels may contribute to the increase in risk for cardiovascular disease, type 2 diabetes, and infertility in this group.

▶ GONADOTROPIN SECRETION IN OBESITY

Comparing premenopausal obese women with normal-weight subjects of the same age, most investigators have noted no difference in the basal or 24-hour LH and FSH plasma concentrations[25,26] or secretory dynamics,[135] whereas some have observed a decrease in basal[27] and 24-hour mean concentrations[136] and a decrease in the LH/FSH ratio.[29] No significant difference in LH pulsatility has been observed between normal-weight and obese premenopausal women.[25] No abnormality in the LH and FSH response to the intravenous administration of gonadotropin-releasing hormone (GnRH)/thyrotropin-releasing hormone (TRH)[56],or to GnRH alone[26] was observed in eumenorrheic obese women. Obese ovulatory women have higher A levels than nonobese women, indicating that obesity may result in hyperandrogenism, even when ovulation is not affected.[137] FSH and LH circulating levels are similar in obese and normal-weight perimenopausal and postmenopausal women. Although the perimenopausal rise in FSH is reported to occur 3 to 4 years earlier in overweight subjects,[52] menopause may be delayed.[138]

Weight reduction does not appear to have a great influence on premenopausal basal LH and FSH circulating levels.[27,51] The response of gonadotropins to GnRH was reported to be the same in obese subjects before and after weight reduction.[136] Weight loss in postmenopausal females appears to increase FSH,[49,52] with LH having a similar but less marked trend.[49] Short-term fasting led to the excretion of large quantities of urinary gonadotropins in obese postmenopausal women, although the serum concentrations of LH and FSH did not change.[139] The increased urinary concentration of gonadotropins was attributed to an energy-deficit-induced inability of the renal proximal tubular cells to reabsorb and metabolize small proteins, including gonadotropins.

In general, eumenorrheic obesity does not appear to be associated with gross alterations in gonadotropin levels or their hypothalamic-pituitary control. Weight reduction may increase FSH levels slightly in obese postmenopausal women, although it has little effect on premenopausal circulating levels.

▶ PROLACTIN IN EUMENORRHEIC OBESITY

The effect of obesity on prolactin (PRL) secretion is heterogeneous; in some cases, obesity is associated with an impaired PRL response to exogenous stimuli, a dampening of the normal circadian rhythm, and a delay in the nocturnal rise.[140] These perturbations may be mediated by insulin and generally resolve with weight loss. The interindividual variability in the obesity-PRL relationship may be due to the fat pattern; individuals with central obesity are more likely to show perturbations in PRL secretion than those with simple obesity. Altered PRL secretion in obesity may be a marker for a disturbance in the hypothalamic-pituitary system involving dopaminergic or seratoninergic tone. Obese women do not demonstrate any significant difference in baseline or 24-hour PRL concentrations.[25]

▶ CLINICAL IMPLICATIONS OF OBESITY

The various endocrinologic aberrations associated with obesity in females result in a number of clinical problems.

Obesity and Pubertal Development

Juvenile obesity is associated with an earlier age at menarche.[138] Furthermore, the peripubertal, and possibly the prepubertal, onset of obesity is associated with a higher risk of menstrual irregularities and oligoovulation.

Obese girls exhibit accelerated rates of linear growth and skeletal maturation, changes that may be due to higher circulating concentrations of insulin and IGF-I and lower IGFBP-1 (despite lower levels of GH[110]). As discussed above (see "Growth Hormone/Insulin-Like Growth Factor Axis in Obesity"), these hormones affect ovarian steroidogenesis in vitro and possibly in vivo and therefore potentially could affect normal pubertal events.

The hyperinsulinemia associated with childhood obesity may play a role in peripubertal ovulatory disturbances. Hyperinsulinemia was more prevalent in postpubertal females who had experienced premature pubarche or who were hyperandrogenic than in control girls and was positively correlated with the free androgen index.[141,142] Insulin sensitivity, often a cause of hyperinsulinemia, was inversely correlated with obesity. As discussed earlier, insulin may augment ovarian androgen production via specific receptors or via IGF-I receptors. Whether insulin and obesity-related elevations in insulin are involved in the early phases of reproductive dysfunction remains to be determined. However, this possibility is supported by the observation that ovarian volume and androgen production were associated with insulin concentration in adolescent girls with hyperandrogenism.[143]

Androgen status tracks from childhood to adulthood and is related to fertility; higher serum androgen concentrations were associated with lower fertility.[144] Thus aberrations in androgen production during puberty due to obesity or related metabolic complications may have long-lasting effects on reproductive function.

Oligoovulation and Obesity

Obesity is clearly associated with ovulatory disturbances. One of the most common causes of oligoovulation is PCOS, a heterogeneous disorder characterized by hyperandrogenism and chronic oligoovulation.[145] PCOS affects 5 to 7 percent of women of reproductive age. In addition to reproductive abnormalities, women with PCOS commonly have features of the metabolic syndrome, including upper body obesity, insulin resistance, and elevated circulating insulin levels.[92,93] The incidence of obesity among patients with PCOS is approximately 50 percent, and a history of weight gain often precedes development of the syndrome. Thus it has been suggested that obesity is involved in the pathogenesis of PCOS. This hypothesis is further bolstered by the observation that with weight loss patients often resume normal menstrual cycles and are able to become pregnant.

Obesity is likely to exacerbate PCOS by way of increasing insulin resistance and circulating concentrations of insulin. Among PCOS patients, serum insulin concentration has been correlated with concentrations of T, free T, and A. Weight loss and associated improvements in metabolic and reproductive outcomes are associated with a reduction in insulin, an increase in SHBG, and a decrease in free T. Addition of insulin-sensitizing agents to a weight-loss regime can further improve clinical outcomes.

Obesity also may affect the severity of the syndrome. Hirsutism, which is a common feature of PCOS, is more likely to be observed in obese than in lean patients. Likewise, obese PCOS patients have more severe menstrual abnormalities and anovulation.

Obesity and the Development of Hormone-Sensitive Carcinoma

Obesity is a risk factor for a number of cancers, including endometrial cancer.[146] The risk appears to increase with the degree of excess weight and may reach up to twenty-fold higher in premenopausal women with a BMI of 30 kg/m² or greater.[147] The incidence of breast cancer also appears to be higher in obese women.[148] Early menarche, common in obese girls, is a risk factor for breast cancer,[149] perhaps due to early exposure to estrogens or progesterone.

Several mechanisms have been postulated to account for the association between obesity and the development of hormone-sensitive carcinomas. Dietary fat has been implicated as a possible cause due to epidemiologic and experimental observations of an association between fat intake and breast/mammary cancer.[150] Greater energy intake was significantly associated with risk for endometrial cancer, independent of BMI, in a Norwegian cohort; lesser physical activity tended to be associated with risk (P = 0.06 for trend).[151]

More prevalent is the hypothesis that stresses the association between the endocrinologic alterations of obesity and cancer risk (Fig. 14-5). The risk for endometrial cancer is related to exposure to unopposed estrogen. Thus, prior to menopause, the increase in risk of endometrial cancer with obesity may be associated with the increased frequency of anovulatory menstrual cycles and associated decrease in exposure to progesterone.[147] The importance of obesity to breast cancer risk appears to be stronger in postmenopausal women.[152] Prior to menopause, obesity actually may have a "protective" effect against the development of breast cancer. The different relationships between obesity and cancer risk with reproductive status may reflect different etiologies of the disease. In premenopausal women, peripheral production of relatively weak estrogens may interfere with the action of estradiol (or other agonists) at the level of the receptor. Alternatively, obese premenopausal women may produce less progesterone,[152] also a stimulator of breast tissue growth. In postmenopausal women, in whom endogenous estrogens are normally very low, peripheral production of estrogens may stimulate growth of estrogen-sensitive tissue. In addition, free or bioavailable estrogen may be increased due to the obesity-related decrease in SHBG; this is particularly true in cases of central obesity.

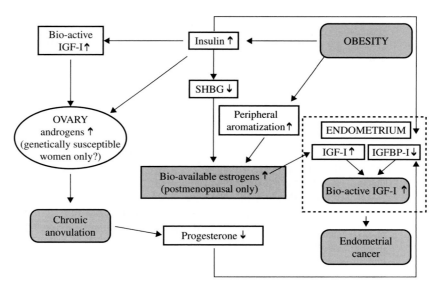

Figure 14-5 Endogenous hormones and endometrial cancer development. *(Used, with permission, from Kaaks et al.[146])*

Obesity-related increases in insulin also may play a role. Insulin has been implicated in risk for endometrial cancer through two potential mechanisms.[146] First, an insulin-mediated decrease in IGFBP-1 would increase free IGF-I, which is mitogenic. In addition, insulin itself is mitogenic. Second, insulin stimulation of ovarian androgen production would decrease the frequency of ovulatory menstrual cycles, thereby increasing exposure of the endometrium to unopposed estrogen.

The adipocyte-derived hormone adiponectin was linked to endometrial cancer in a case-control study involving Greek women.[153] Among women younger than 65 years, a 1 standard deviation increase in adiponectin was associated with a greater than 50 percent reduction in the risk for endometrial cancer, independent and BMI and other hormonal and nonhormonal risk factors. Although the physiologic basis for this relationship is not known, the insulin resistance associated with low adiponectin levels may be involved.

Recent evidence suggests that fat distribution, rather than obesity per se, may affect cancer risk. Central adiposity is associated with greater risk of postmenopausal breast cancer,[152] possibly due to the presence of greater visceral fat. Women with breast cancer had greater visceral fat, as assessed with CT scanning, than did control women matched for age, weight, and waist circumference.[154] The relative risk for breast cancer increased with increasing visceral-to-total fat ratio and decreasing subcutaneous abdominal-to-visceral fat ratio. Since visceral obesity is associated with insulin resistance and hyperinsulinemia, the association between visceral obesity and breast cancer may be secondary to insulin action. Breast tissue growth may be stimulated either directly by insulin or by the increase in free IGF-I that may occur with insulin-mediated suppression of IGFBP-1. Alternatively, the insulin-induced suppression of SHBG may increase circulating bioavailable estrogens, which, in turn, could promote the growth of estrogen-sensitive tissue.[155]

Obesity and Menopause

Obesity may affect menopause and post-menopausal symptomatology. Sherman and colleagues[138] noted that obesity was associated with a later age at menopause. Campagnoli and colleagues,[156] studying women from a geriatric center, noted that overweight women seemed to suffer less "somatic" symptoms, such as hot flashes, than normal-weight individuals, independent of their socioeconomic level. In contrast, "psychic" (anxiety, depression, irritability, crying spells) problems seemed to be more frequent and incapacitating in severely obese women of all socioeconomic classes and minimally obese women in the lower socioeconomic group. However, other studies have not confirmed these results,[157] and some studies have reported an increase in hot flashes among obese menopausal women.[158] Peripheral production of estrogens may contribute to differences in symptomology between overweight and normal-weight women.

It appears that menopause aggravates the metabolic disturbances already present in overweight subjects, including lipid and glucose regulation.[157] Furthermore, with the onset of menopause, the plasma level of T fell in normal-weight women, whereas it increased in overweight women. While obesity in menopause may be associated with an aggravation of the lipid and glucose tolerance profile, overweight women are at less risk for the development of osteoporosis after menopause.[159] Differences in bone mineral density between obese and normal-weight women are observable prior to menopause.

Menopause may affect both the amount and distribution of adipose tissue deposited. Cross-sectional analysis of body composition in pre- and postmenopausal women with DEXA indicated that total and upper body fat were greater and lower body fat was lesser in the postmenopausal group.[160] Data obtained with CT scanning suggest that the increase in upper body fat seen in postmenopausal women is visceral.[161] The increase in visceral fat with menopause may be associated with the increased risk for insulin resistance, dyslipidemia, and associated diseases seen in older women.

A growing literature suggests that hormone-replacement therapy may prevent or reverse the effects of menopause on adiposity and fat distribution. Interventional or longitudinal studies in general reported that women who used estrogen or combined estrogen-progestin therapy either lost body fat or gained less total and/or abdominal fat or body weight over the study period relative to the placebo group.[162,163] However, results varied with regimen; transdermal estrogen users, similar to placebo users, showed a gain in body fat that was primarily in the trunk area.[164] Estrogen use did not prevent the loss of lean mass unless combined with an androgenic progestin.[162] In women treated with androgens, lean mass was maintained or gained, but effects on adiposity were variable.[164–166] The lipid profile was improved by estradiol treatment and was not adversely affected by treatment with T implants.[165] In contrast, several relatively short-term interventions reported that hormone-replacement therapy either did not affect body composition or fat distribution[167] or increased rather than decreased adiposity.[168–169]

In summary, the menopause transition is associated with a gain in total body fat, a loss of fat-free mass, and a shift to an abdominal fat distribution. Most longitudinal studies indicate that estrogen replacement therapy, with or without a progestin, may prevent the increases in total and central adiposity; however, results are variable and may depend on the nature of the estrogen used and the mode of administration. Estrogen therapy, by minimizing central adiposity, may indirectly improve the lipid profile. Loss of fat-free mass may be minimized by inclusion of a progestin with androgenic effects in the regimen. Androgen treatment has beneficial effects on fat-free mass and does not appear to have a negative effect on lipids. The effect of exogenous androgens on abdominal adiposity appears to depend on the regimen used.

KEY POINTS

1. Female obesity is associated with a suppression of SHBG, an increase in free T, and increases in both the production and clearance rates of a number of androgens. The suppression of SHBG occurs secondary to an increase in insulin, which is related to an obesity-mediated increase in insulin resistance.

2. GH is lower in obese women, but total and free IGF-I are not altered in a consistent manner. IGFBP-1 is lower in obesity secondary to elevated circulating insulin.

3. Simple obesity is not associated with alterations in gonadotropin or prolactin concentrations.

4. Adipose tissue aromatization of androgens may increase circulating estrogens in postmenopausal women.

5. Levels of leptin, produced in human adipose tissue, are higher in obese women. Leptin appears to stimulate reproductive function centrally but to impair it at the level of the ovary.

6. Upper body/visceral obesity is associated with greater metabolic perturbation than generalized obesity due, at least in part, to a greater degree of insulin resistance and hyperinsulinemia. Accumulation of lipid within the muscle cell may explain the association between obesity and skeletal muscle resistance to insulin-stimulated glucose uptake.

7. Obesity is associated with earlier menarche and increased risk for oligoovulation, PCOS, endometrial cancer, and following menopause, breast cancer.

8. Menopause occurs later in obese women, with fewer somatic symptoms and less risk for osteoporosis. Both total and abdominal fat increase around the time of menopause,

perhaps contributing to the hyperlipidemia/dyslipidemia and glucose intolerance of aging. Effects of menopause on body composition and fat distribution may be prevented/reversed by hormone-replacement therapy.

▶ ACKNOWLEDGMENTS

Supported in part by the Clinical Nutrition Research Unit of the University of Alabama at Birmingham and NIDDK Grant No. R01DK58278.

REFERENCES

1. National Heart Lung and Blood Institute. *Clinical Guidelines on the Identification, Evaluation, and Treatment of Overweight and Obesity in Adults: Executive Summary*. Washington: National Institutes of Health, 1998:vii–xiii.
2. Roche AF, Heymsfield SB, Lohman TG. *Human Body Composition*. Champaign, IL: Human Kinetics, 1996.
3. Dempster P, Aikens S. A new air displacement method for the determination of human body composition. *Med Sci Sports Exerc* 1995;27:1692.
4. Flegal KM, Carroll MD, Ogden CL, Johnson CL. Prevalence and trends in obesity among US adults, 1999–2000. *JAMA* 2002;288:1723.
5. Moran C, Hernandez E, Ruiz JE, et al. Upper body obesity and hyperinsulinemia are associated with annovulation. *Gynecol Obstet Invest* 1999;47:1.
6. Pouliot MC, Despres JP, Lemieux S, et al. Waist circumference and abdominal sagittal diameter: Best simple anthropometric indexes of abdominal visceral adipose tissue accumulation and related cardiovascular risk in men and women. *Am J Cardiol* 1994;73:460.
7. Despres JP. Health consequences of visceral obesity. *Ann Med* 2001;33:534.
8. Kelley DE. Skeletal muscle triglycerides: An aspect of regional adiposity and insulin resistance. *Ann NY Acad Sci* 2002;967:135.
9. Sinha R, Dufour S, Peterson KF, et al. Assessment of skeletal muscle triglyceride content by ^{1}H nuclear magnetic resonance spectroscopy in lean and obese adolescents. *Diabetes* 2002;51:1022.
10. Shulman GI. Cellular mechanisms of insulin resistance. *J Clin Invest* 2000;106:171.
11. Ivandic A, Prpic-Krizevac I, Bozic D, et al. Insulin resistance and androgens in healthy women with different body fat distributions. *Wien Klin Wochenschr* 2002;114:321.
12. Lovejoy JC, Bray GA, Bourgeois MO, et al. Exogenous androgens influence body composition and regional body fat distribution in obese postmenopausal women: A clinical research center study. *J Clin Endocrinol Metab* 1996; 81:2198.
13. Elbers JMH, Asschemen H, Seidell JC, Gooren LJG. Effects of sex steroid hormones on regional fat depots as assessed by magnetic resonance imaging in transsexuals. *Am J Physiol* 1999;276:E317–E325.
14. Marin P, Holmang S, Gustafsson C, et al. Androgen treatment of abdominally obese men. *Obes Res* 1993;1:245.
15. Daniel M, Martin AD, Faiman C. Sex hormones and adipose tissue distribution in premenopausal cigarette smokers. *Int J Obes* 1992; 16:245.
16. Pasquali R, Casimirri F, Cantobelli S, et al. Insulin and androgen relationships with abdominal body fat distribution in women with and without hyperandrogenism. *Horm Res* 1993;39:179.
17. Goodman-Gruen D, Barrett-Connor E. Total but not bioavailable testosterone is a predictor of central adiposity in postmenopausal women. *Int J Obes* 1995;19:293.
18. Conway JM, Yanovski SZ, Avila NA, Hubbard VS. Visceral adipose tissue differences in black and white women. *Am J Clin Nutr* 1995;61:765.
19. Kanaley JA, Giannopoulou I, Tillapaugh-Fay G, et al. Racial differences in subcutaneous and visceral fat distribution in postmenopausal black and white women. *Metabolism* 2003; 52:186.
20. Lovejoy JC, de la Bretonne JA, Klemperer M, Tulley R. Abdominal fat distribution and metabolic risk factors: Effects of race. *Metabolism* 1996;45:1119.
21. Karter AJ, Mayer-Davis EJ, Selby JV, et al. Insulin sensitivity and abdominal obesity in African-American, Hispanic, and non-Hispanic white men and women. *Diabetes* 1996;45:1547.

22. Berman DM, Rodrigues LM, Nicklas BJ, et al. Racial disparities in metabolism, central obesity, and sex-hormone binding globulin in postmenopausal women. *J Clin Endocrinol Metab* 2001;86:97.

23. Gower BA, Weinsier RL, Jordan JM, et al. Effects of weight loss on changes in insulin sensitivity and lipid concentrations in premenopausal African-American and Caucasian women. *Am J Clin Nutr* 2002;76:923.

24. Samojlik E, Kirschner MA, Silber D, et al. Elevated production and metabolic clearance rates of androgens in morbidly obese women. *J Clin Endocrinol Metab* 1984;59:949

25. Zhang YW, Stern B, Rebar RW. Endocrine comparison of obese menstruating and amenorrheic women. *J Clin Endocrinol Metab* 1984; 58:1077.

26. Dunaif A, Mandeli J, Fluhr H, Dobrjanski A. The impact of obesity and chronic hyperinsulinemia on gonadotropin release and gonadal steroid secretion in the polycystic ovary syndrome. *J Clin Endocrinol Metab* 1988;66: 131.

27. Grenman S, Ronnemaa T, Irjala K, et al. Sex steroid, gonadotropin, cortisol, and prolactin levels in healthy, massively obese women: correlation with abdominal fat cell size and effect of weight reduction. *J Clin Endocrinol Metab* 1986;63:1257.

28. Kaufman ED, Mosman J, Sutton M, et al. Characterization of basal estrogen and androgen levels and gonadotropin release patterns in the obese adolescent female. *J Pediatr* 1981;98:990.

29. Bergh HJ, Gennarelli G, Wide L. The independent effects of polycystic ovary syndrome and obesity on serum concentrations of gonadotropins and sex steroids in premenopausal women. *Clin Endocrinol* 1994;41:473.

30. Maccario M, Mazza E, Ramunni J, et al. Relationship between dehydroepiandrosterone-sulfate and anthropometric, metabolic and hormonal variables in a large cohort of obese women. *Clin Endocrinol* 1999;50:595.

31. Evans DJ, Hoffman RG, Kalkhoff RK, Kissebah AH. Relationship of androgenic activity to body fat topography, fat cell morphology, and metabolic aberrations in premenopausal women. *J Clin Endocrinol Metab* 1983;57:304.

32. Azziz R, Zacur HA, Parker CRJ, et al. Effect of obesity on the response to acute adrenocorticotropin stimulation in eumenorrheic women. *Fertil Steril* 1991;56:427.

33. Wajchenberg BL, Marcondes JAM, Mathor MB, et al. Free testosterone levels during the menstrual cycle in obese versus normal women. *Fertil Steril* 1989;51:535.

34. Brody S, Carlstron K, Lagrelius A, et al. Serum sex hormone–binding globulin (SHBG), testosterone/SHBG index, endometrial pathology and bone mineral density in postmenopausal women. *Acta Obstet Gynaecol Scand* 1987;66: 357.

35. Kurtz BR, Givens JR, Komindr S, et al. Maintenance of normal circulating levels of delta-4-androstenedione and deydroeipandrosterone in simple obesity despite increased metabolic clearance rates: Evidence for a servo-control mechanism. *J Clin Endocrinol Metab* 1987;64: 1261.

36. Pardridge WM. Transport of protein-bound hormones into tissues in vivo. *Endocr Rev* 1981;2: 103, 1981

37. Vermeulen A, Ando S. Metabolic clearance rate and interconversion of androgens and the influence of the free androgen fraction. *J Clin Endocrinol Metab* 1979;48:320.

38. Longcope C, Baker S. Androgen and estrogen dynamics: relationship with age, weight, and menopausal status. *J Clin Endocrinol Metab* 1993;76:601.

39. Feher T, Bodrogi L. A comparitive study of steroid concentrations in human adipose tissue and peripheral circulation. *Clin Chim Acta* 1982; 126:135.

40. Longcope C, Kato T, Horton R. Conversion of blood androgens to estrogens in normal adult men and women. *J Clin Invest* 1969;48:2191.

41. Longcope C, Baker R, Johnston CCJ. Androgen and estrogen metabolism: relationship to obesity. *Metabolism* 1986;35:235.

42. Edman CD, MacDonald TC. Effect of obesity on conversion of plasma androstenedione to estrone in ovulatory and anovulatory young women. *J Obstet Gynecol* 1978;130:456.

43. Bergh C, Carlsson B, Olssonn JH, et al. Regulation of androgen production in cultured human thecal cells by insulin-like growth factor I and insulin. *Fertil Steril* 1993;59:323.

44. Poretsky L, Piper B. Insulin resistance, hypersecretion of LH, and a dual-defect hypothesis for the pathogenesis of polycystic ovary syndrome. *Obstet Gynecol* 1994;84:613.

45. Nestler JE, Jakubowicz DJ. Decreases in ovarian cytochrome P450C17-alpha activity and serum free testerone after reduction of insulin secretion in polycystic ovary syndrome. *N Engl J Med* 1996;335:617.

46. Azziz R, Ehrmann DA, Legro RS, et al. for the PCOS/Troglitizone Study Group. Troglitizone improves ovulation and hirsutism in the polycystic ovary syndrome: A multicenter, double-blind, placebo-controlled trial. *J Clin Endocrinol Metab* 2001;86:1626.

47. Bjorntorp P, Rosmond R. Obesity and cortisol. *Nutrition* 2000;16:924.

48. Chalew S, Nagel H, Shore S. The hypothalamic-pituitary-adrenal axis in obesity. *Obes Res* 1995; 3:371.

49. O'Dea JPK, Wieland RG, Hallberg MC, et al. Effect of dietary weight loss on sex steroid binding, sex steroids and gonadotropins in obese postmenopausal women. *J Lab Clin Med* 1979;93:1004.

50. Kim MH, Friedman CI, Barrows H, Rosenfield RL. Serum androgen concentrations in the massively obese reproductive woman: Their response to weight loss. *Trans Am Gynecol Obstet Soc* 1982;1:26.

51. Kopelman PG, White N, Pilkington TRE, Jeffcoate SL. The effect of weight loss on steroid secretion and binding in massively obese women. *Clin Endocrinol* 1981;14:113.

52. Klinga K, von Holst TH, Runnebaum B. Serum concentrations of FSH, oestradiol, oestrone and androstenedione in normal and obese women. *Maturitas* 1982;4:9.

53. Jakubowicz DJ, Nestler JE. 17α-Hydroxyprogesterone responses to leuprolide and serum androgens in obese women with and without polycystic ovary syndrome after dietary weight loss. *J Clin Endocrinol Metab* 1997;82:556.

54. Judd HL. Hormonal dynamics associated with the menopause. *J Clin Obstet Gynecol* 1976;19:775.

55. Trichopoulos D, Polychronopoulou A, Brown J, MacMahon B. Obesity, serum cholesterol, and estrogens in premenopausal women. *Oncology* 1983;40:227.

56. Kopelman PG, Pinkington TRE, White N, Jeffcoate SL. Abnormal sex steroid secretion and binding in massively obese women. *Clin Endocrinol* 1980;12:363.

57. Zumoff B, Strain GW, Kream J, et al. Obese young men have elevated plasma estrogen levels but obese premenopausal women do not. *Metabolism* 1981;30:1011.

58. Klinga K, von Holst TH, Runnebaum B. Influence of severe obesity on peripheral hormone concentrations in pre- and postmenopausal women. *Eur J Obstet Gynecol Reprod Biol* 1983; 15:103.

59. Davidson BJ, Gambone JC, Lagasse LV, et al. Free estradiol in postmenopausal women with and without endometrial cancer. *J Clin Endocrinol Metab* 1981;52:404.

60. West CD, Damast BL, Sarro SD, Pearson OH. Conversion of testosterone to estrogen in castrated, adrenalectomized human females. *J Biol Chem* 1956;218:409.

61. Nimrod A, Ryan KJ. Aromatization of androgens by human abdominal and breast fat tissue. *J Clin Endocrinol Metab* 1975;40:367.

62. Ackerman GE, Smith ME, Mendelson CR, et al. Aromatization of androstenedione by human adipose tissue stromal cells in monolayer culture. *J Clin Endocrinol Metab* 1981;53:412.

63. Longcope C, Pratt JH, Schneider SH, Fineberg SE. Aromatization of androgens by muscle and adipose tissue in vivo. *J Clin Endocrinol Metab* 1978;46:146.

64. MacDonald PC, Edman CD, Hemsell DL, et al. Effect of obesity on conversion of plasma androstenedione to estrone in postmenopausal women with and without endometrial cancer. *Am J Obstet Gynecol* 1978;130:448.

65. Hemsell DL, Grodin JM, Brenner PF, et al. Plasma precursors of estrogen: II. Correlation of the extent of conversion of plasma androstenedione to estrone with age. *J Clin Endocrinol Metab* 1974;38:476.

66. Longcope C, Layne DS, Tait JF. Metabolic clearance rates and interconversions of estrone and 17β-estradiol in normal males and females. *J Clin Invest* 1968;47:93.

67. Deslypere JP, Verdonck L, Vermulen A. Fat tissue: A steroid reservoir and site of steroid metabolism. *J Clin Endocrinol Metab* 1987;61:564.

68. Schneider J, Bradlow HL, Strain GW, et al. Effects of obesity on estradiol metabolism: decreased formation of nonuterotropic metabolites. *J Clin Endocrinol Metab* 1983;56:973.

69. Flood C, Pratt JH, Longcope C. The metabolic clearance and blood production rates of estriol

in normal, nonpregnant women. *J Clin Endocrinol Metab* 1976;42:1.

70. Roncari DAK, Van RLR. Promotion of human adipocyte precursor replication by 17β-estradiol in culture. *J Clin Invest* 1977;62:503.

71. Kato T, Horton R. Studies of testerone binding globulin. *J Clin Endocrinol Metab* 1968;28:1160.

72. Anderson DC. Sex-hormone-binding globulin. *Clin Endocrinol* 1974;3:69.

73. Nisker JA, Hammond GL, Davidson BJ, et al. Serum sex hormone–binding globulin capacity and the percentage of free estradiol in postmenopausal women with and without endometrial carcinoma. *Am J Obstet Gynecol* 1980;138:638.

74. Vermeulen A, Verdonck L, Van Der Straeten M, Orie N. Capacity of the testosterone-binding globulin in human plasma and influence of specific binding of testosterone on its metabolic clearance rate. *J Clin Endocrinol Metab* 1969;28:1470.

75. Levrant SG, Barnes RB. Pharmacology of estrogens, in Lobo RA (ed), *Treatment of the Postmenopausal Woman: Basic and Clinical Aspects.* New York: Raven Press, 1994; pp 57–68.

76. Holly JM, Smith CP, Dunger DB, et al. Relationship between the pubertal fall in sex hormone–binding globulin and insulin-like growth factor binding protein I: A synchronized approach to pubertal development. *Clin Endocrinol* 1989;31: 277.

77. Pugeat M, Crave JC, Elmidani M, et al. Pathophysiology of sex hormone–binding globulin (SHBG): Relation to insulin. *J Steroid Biochem Mol Biol* 1991;40:841.

78. Plymate SR, Matej LA, Jones RE, Friedel KE. Inhibition of sex hormone–binding globulin production in the human hepatoma (HepG2) cell line by insulin and prolactin. *J Clin Endocrinol Metab* 1988;66:460.

79. Fendri S, Arlot S, Marcelli JM, et al. Relationship between insulin sensitivity and circulating sex hormone binding–globulin levels in hyperandrogenic obese women. *Int J Obes* 1994;18:755.

80. Preziosi P, Barrett-Connor E, Papoz L, et al. Interrelation between plasma sex hormone–binding globulin and plasma insulin in healthy adult women: The Telecom Study. *J Clin Endocrinol Metab* 1993;76:283.

81. Nestler JE, Powers LP, Matt DW, et al. A direct effect of hyperinsulinemia on serum sex hormone–binding globulin levels in obese women with the polycystic ovary syndrome. *J Clin Endocrinol Metab* 1991;72:83.

82. Dunaif A, Scott D, Finegood D, et al. The insulin-sensitizing agent trogliatazone improves metabolic and reproductive abnormalities in the polycystic ovary syndrome. *J Clin Endocrinol Metab* 1996;81:3299.

83. Peiris AN, Stagner JI, Plymate SR, et al. Relationship of insulin secretory pulses to sex hormone–binding globulin in normal men. *J Clin Endocrinol Metab* 1993;76:279.

84. Pagano G, Cassader M, Bozzo C, et al. Insulin resistance in human obesity: in vivo studies by "insulin clamping" and in vitro by insulin binding and biologic activity on isolated adipocytes, in Enzi G, Grepaldi G, Pozza G, Renold AE (eds), *Obesity: Pathogenesis and Treatment,* Serono Symposium, Vol 28. New York: Academic Press, 1981; pp 175–183.

85. Olefsky JM, Reaven JM, Farquhar JW. Effects of weight reduction in obesity. *J Clin Invest* 1974; 53:64.

86. Greco AV, Mingrone G, Giancaterini A, et al. Insulin resistance in morbid obesity: Reversal with intramyocellular fat depletion. *Diabetes* 2002;51:144.

87. Lungren H, Bengtsson C, Blohme G, Ladipus L. Adiposity and adipose tissue distribution in relation to incidence of diabetes in women: Results from a prospective population study in Goteborg, Sweden. *Int J Obes* 1989;13:413.

88. Bjorntorp P. Androgens, the metabolic syndrome, and non-insulin-dependent diabetes mellitus. *Ann NY Acad Sci.* 1993;676:242.

89. Holmang A, Svedberg J, Jennische E, Bjorntorp P. Effects of testosterone on muscle insulin sensitivity and morphology in female rats. *Am J Physiol* 1990;259:E555–E560.

90. Livingstone C, Collison M. Sex steroids and insulin resistance. *Clin Sci* 2002;102:151.

91. Nishizawa H, Shimomura I, Kishida K, et al. Androgens decrease plasma adiponectin, an insulin-sensitizing adipocyte-derived protein. *Diabetes* 2002;51:2734.

92. Franks S, Gilling-Smith C, Watson H, Willis D. Insulin action in the normal and polycystic ovary. *Endocrinol Metab Clin North Am* 1999; 28:361.

93. Gambineri A, Pelusi C, Vicennati V, et al. Obesity and the polycystic ovary sundrome. *Int J Obes* 2002;26:883.

94. Stuart CA, Prince MJ, Peters MJ, Meyer WJI. Hyperinsulinemia and hyperandrogenemia: In vivo androgen response to insulin infusion. *Obstet Gynecol* 1987;69:921.

95. Nestler JE, Clore JN, Strauss JF, Blackard WG. Effects of hyperinsulinemia on serum testosterone, progesterone, dehydroepiandrosterone sulfate, and cortisol levels in normal women and in a woman with hyperandrogenism, insulin resistance and acanthosis nigricans. *J Clin Endocrinol Metab* 1987;64:180.

96. Farah MJ, Givens JR, Kitbchi AE. Bimodal correlation between the circulating insulin level and the production rate of dehydroepiandrosterone: Positive correlation in controls and negative correlation in the polycystic ovary sydrome with acanthosis nigricans. *J Clin Endocrinol Metab* 1990;70:1075.

97. Veldhuis JD, Liem AY, South S, et al. Differential impact of age, sex steroid hormones, and obesity on basal versus pulsatile growth hormone secretion in men as assessed in an ultrasensitive chemiluminescence assay. *J Clin Endocrinol Metab* 1995;80:3209.

98. Dubey AK, Hanukoglu A, Hansen BC, Kowarski AA. Metabolic clearance rates of synthetic human growth hormone in lean and obese males rhesus monkeys. *J Clin Endocrinol Metab* 1988;67:1064.

99. Rasmussen MH, Hvidberg A, Juul A, et al. Massive weight loss restores 24-hour growth hormone release profiles and serum insulin-like growth factor I levels in obese subjects. *J Clin Endocrinol Metab* 1995;80:1407.

100. Conover CA, Lee PDK, Kanaley JA, et al. Insulation regulation of insulin-like growth factor binding protein 1 in obese and nonobese humans. *J Clin Endocrinol Metab* 1992;74:1355.

101. Katz E, Ricciarelli E, Adashi EY. The potential relevance of growth hormone to female reproductive physiology and pathophysiology. *Fertil Steril* 1993;59:8.

102. Mason HD, Martkaninen H, Beard RW, et al. Direct gonadotrophic effect of growth hormone on oestradiol production by human granulosa cells. *J Endocrinol* 1990;126:R1–R4.

103. Lanzone A, Di S, Castellani R, et al. Human growth hormone enhances progesterone production by human luteal cells in vitro: Evidence of a synergistic effect with human chorionic gonadotropin. *Fertil Steril* 1990;57:92.

104. Homburg R, West C, Ostergaard H, Jacobs HS. Combined growth hormone and gonadotropin treatment for ovulation induction in patients with non-responsive ovaries. *Gynecol Endocrinol* 1991;5:33.

105. Erickson G, Gabriel GV, Magoffin D. Insulin-like growth factor I regulates aromatase activity in human granulosa cells and granulosa luteal cells of polycystic ovaries. *J Clin Endocrinol Metab* 1989;69:716.

106. Mason HD, Margara R, Winston RML, et al. Insulin-like growth factor I (IGF-I) inhibits production and IGF-binding protein 1 while stimulating estradiol secretion in granulosa cells from normal and polycystic human ovaries. *J Clin Endocrinol Metab* 1993;76:1275.

107. Cara JF, Fan J, Azzarello J, Rosenfield RL. Insulin-like growth factor I enhances luteinizing hormone binding to rat ovarian theca-interstitial cells. *J Clin Invest* 1990;86:560.

108. Cara JF, Rosenfield RL. Insulin-like growth factor I and insulin potentiate luteinizing hormone–induced androgen synthesis by rat ovarian theca-interstitial cells. *Endocrinology* 1988;123:733.

109. Nahum R, Thong KJ, Hillier SG. Metabolic regulation of androgen production by human thecal cells in vitro. *Hum Reprod* 1995;10:75.

110. Vanderschueren-Lodeweyckx M. The effect of simple obesity on growth and growth hormone. *Horm Res* 1993;40:23.

111. Rasmussen MH, Frystyk J, Anderson T, et al. The impact of obesity, fat distribution, and energy restriction on insulin-like growth factor I (IGF-I), IGF-binding protein 3, insulin, and growth hormone. *Metabolism* 1994;43:315.

112. Ehrmann DA, Barnes RB, Rosenfield RL. Polycystic ovary syndrome as a form of functional ovarian hyperandrogenism due to dysregulation of androgen secretion. *Endocr Rev* 1995;16:322.

113. Considine RV, Shinha MK, Heiman ML, et al. Serum immunoreactive leptin concentrations in normal weight and obese humans. *N Engl J Med* 1996;334:292.

114. Wade GN, Schneider JE, Li H. Control of fertility by metabolic cues. *Am J Physiol* 1996;270: E1–E19.

115. Moschos S, Chan JL, Mantzoros CS. Leptin and reproduction: A review. *Fertil Steril* 2002;77:433.

116. Brzechffa PR, Jakimiuk AJ, Agarwal SK, et al. Serum immunoreactive leptin concentrations in

women with polycystic ovary syndrome. *J Clin Endocrinol Metab* 1996;81:4166.

117. Urbancsek J, Fedorcsak P, Klinga K, et al. Impact of obesity and leptin levels on the secretion of estradiol, inhibin A and inhibin B during ovarian stimulation with gonadotropins. *Gynecol Endocrinol* 2002;16:285.

118. Wren AM, Seal LJ, Cohen MA, et al. Ghrelin enhances appetite and increases food intake in humans. *J Clin Endocrinol Metab* 2001;86:5992.

119. Ukkola O, Poykko S. Ghrelin, growth and obesity. *Ann Med* 2002;34:102.

120. Papotti M, Ghe C, Cassoni P, et al. Growth hormone secretagogue binding sites in peripheral human tissues. *J Clin Endocrinol Metab* 2000;85:3803.

121. Pagotto U, Gambineri A, Vicennati V, et al. Plasma ghrelin, obesity, and the polycystic ovary syndrome: Correlation with insulin resistance and androgen levels. *J Clin Endocrinol Metab* 2002;87:5625.

122. Orio F Jr, Lucida P, Palomba S, et al. Circulating ghrelin concentrations in the polycystic ovary syndrome. *J Clin Endocrinol Metab* 2003;88:942.

123. Scherer PE, Williams S, Fogliano M, et al. A novel serum protein similar to C1q, produced exclusively in adipocytes. *J Biol Chem* 1995;270:26746.

124. Weyer C, Funahashi T, Tanaka S, et al. Hypoadiponectinemia in obesity and type 2 diabetes: Close association with insulin resistance and hyperinsulinemia. *J Clin Endocrinol Metab* 2001;86:1930.

125. Beltowski J. Adiponectin and resistin: New hormones of white adipose tissue. *Med Sci Monit* 2003;9:RA55–RA61.

126. Esposito K, Pontillo A, Di Palo C, et al. Effect of weight loss and lifestyle changes on vascular inflammatory markers in obese women: A randomized trial. *JAMA* 2003;289:1799.

127. Fruhbeck G, Gomez-Ambrosi J, Muruzabal FJ, Burrell MA. The adipocyte: a model for integration of endocrine and metabolic signaling in energy metabolism regulation. *Am J Physiol* 2001;280:E827–E847.

128. Yudkin JS, Kumari M, Humphries SE, et al. Inflammation, obesity, stress, and coronary heart disease: Is interleukin 6 the link? *Atherosclerosis* 2000;148:209.

129. Kelly CCJ, Lyall H, Petrie JR, et al. Low-grade chronic inflammation in women with polycystic ovary syndrome. *J Clin Endocrinol Metab* 2001;86:2455.

130. Tchernof A, Nolan A, Sites C, et al. Weight loss reduces C-reactive protein levels in obese postmenopausal women. *Circulation* 2002;105:564.

131. Hotamisligil GS, Peraldi P, Budavari A, et al. IRS-1-mediated inhibition of insulin receptor tyrosine kinase activity in tumor necrosis factor alpha and obesity-induced insulin resistance. *Science* 1996;271:665.

132. Cianci A, Calogero AE, Palumbo MA, et al. Relationship between tumor necrosis factor and sex steroid concentrations in the follicular fluid of women with immunological infertility. *Hum Reprod* 1996;11:265.

133. Ridker PM, Rifai N, Rose L, et al. Comparison of C-reactive protein and low-density lipoprotein cholesterol levels in the prediction of first cardiovascular events. *N Engl J Med* 2002;347:1557.

134. Festa A, D'Augostino RJ, Howard G, et al. Chronic subclinical inflammation as part of the insulin resistance syndrome: The Insulin Resistance Atherosclerosis Study (IRIS). *Circulation* 2000;102:42.

135. Arroyo A, Laughlin GA, Morales AJ, Yen SSC. Inappropriate gonadotropin secretion in polycystic ovary syndrome: Influence of adiposity. *J Clin Endocrinol Metab* 1997;82:3728.

136. Zumoff B, Strain GW, Kream J, et al.. Subnormal 24-hour mean plasma LH concentration and elevated plasma FSH/LH ratio in obese premenopausal women. *J Reprod Med* 1983;28:843.

137. Unzer SRM, dos Santos JE, Moreira AC, et al. Alterations in plasma gonadotropin and sex steroid levels in obese ovulatory and chronically anovulatory women. *J Reprod Med* 1995;40:516.

138. Sherman B, Wallace R, Bean JA, Schlabaugh L. Relationship of body weight to menarcheal and menopausal age: Implications for breast cancer risk. *J Clin Endocrinol Metab* 1981;52:488.

139. Beitins IZ, Shah A, O'Loughlin K, et al. The effects of fasting on serum and urinary gonadotropins in obese postmenopausal women. *J Clin Endocrinol Metab* 1980;51:26.

140. Kopelman PG. Physiopathology of prolactin secretion in obesity. *Int J Obes* 2000;24:S104–S108.

141. Ibanez L, Potau N, Georgopoulos N, et al. Growth hormone, insulin-like growth factor I axis, and insulin secretion in hyperandrogenic adolescents. *Fertil Steril* 1995;64:1113.

142. Ibanez L, Potau N, Zampolli M, et al. Hyperinsulinemia in postpubertal girls with a history of premature pubarch and functional ovarian hyperandrogenism. *J Clin Endocrinol Metab* 1996; 81:1237.

143. Apter D, Butzow T, Laughlin GA, Yen SSC. Metabolic features of polycystic ovary syndrome are found in adolescent girls with hyperandrogenism. *J Clin Endocrinol Metab* 1995; 80:2966.

144. Apter D, Vihko R. Endocrine determinants of fertility: Serum androgen concentrations during follow-up of adolescents into the third decade of life. *J Clin Endocrinol Metab* 1990;71:970.

145. Franks S. Polycystic ovary syndrome. *N Engl J Med* 1995;333:853.

146. Kaaks R, Lukanova A, Kurzer MS. Obesity, endogenous hormones, and endometrial cancer risk: a synthetic review. *Cancer Epidemiol Biomark Prevent* 2002;11:1531.

147. Key TJ, Allen NE, Verkasalo PK, Banks E. Energy balance and cancer: the role of sex hormones. *Proc Nutr Soc* 2001;60:81.

148. Paffenbarger RSJ, Kampert JB, Chang HG. Characteristics that predict risk of breast cancer before and after the menopause. *Am J Epidemiol* 1980;112:258.

149. Lipworth L. Epidemiology of breast cancer. *Eur J Cancer Prev* 1990;4:7.

150. Howe GR, Hirohata T, Hislop TG, et al. Dietary factors and risk of breast cancer: combined analysis of 12 case-controlled studies. *J Natl Cancer Inst* 1990;82:561.

151. Furberg A-S, Thune I. Metabolic abnormalities (hypertension, hyperglycemia and overweight), lifestyle (high energy intake and physical inactivity) and endometrial cancer risk in a Norwegian cohort. *Int J Cancer* 2003;104:669.

152. Ballard-Barbash R. Anthropometry and breast cancer. *Cancer* 1994;74:1090.

153. Petridou E, Mantzoros C, Dessypris N, et al. Plasma adiponectin concentrations in relation to endometrial cancer: A case-control study in Greece. *J Clin Endocrinol Metab* 2003;88:993.

154. Schapira DV, Clark RA, Wolff PA, et al. Visceral obesity and breast cancer risk. *Cancer* 1994;74: 632.

155. Toniolo PG, Levitz M, Zeleniuch-Jacquotte A, et al. A prospective study of endogenous estrogens and breast cancer in postmenopausal women. *J Natl Cancer Inst* 1995;87:190.

156. Campagnoli C, Morra G, Belforte P, et al. Climacteric symptoms according to body weight in women of different socio-economic groups. *Maturitas* 1981;3:279.

157. Bottiglioni F, Aloysio D, Nicolett G, et al. Physiopathological aspects of body overweight in the female climacteric. *Maturitas* 1984;5: 153.

158. Garai J. Hepatic dysfunction in development of menopausal hot flushes? *Med Hypoth* 2002;58: 535.

159. Slemenda CW, Hui SL, Longcope C, et al. Predictors of bone mass in perimenopausal women: A prospective study of clinical data using photon absorptiometry. *Ann Intern Med* 1990;112:96.

160. Ley CJ, Lees B, Stevenson JC. Sex- and menopause-associated changes in body-fat distribution. *Am J Clin Nutr* 1992;55:950.

161. Toth MJ, Tchernof A, Sites CK, Poehlman ET. Effect of menopausal status on body composition and abdominal fat distribution. *Int J Obes* 2000;24:226.

162. Sorensen MB, Rosenfalck AM, Hojgaard L, Ottesen B. Obesity and sarcopenia after menopause are reversed by sex hormone replacement therapy. *Obes Res* 2001;9:622.

163. Gambacciani M, Ciaponi M, Cappagli B, et al. Prospective evaluation of body weight and body fat distribution in early postmenopausal women with and without hormonal replacement therapy. *Maturitas* 2001;39:125.

164. Hanggi W, Lippuner K, Jaeger P, et al. Differential impact of conventional oral or transdermal hormone replacement therapy or tibolone on body composition in postmenopausal women. *Clin Endocrinol* 1998;48:691.

165. Davis SR, Walker KZ, Strauss BJ. Effects of estradiol with and without testosterone on body composition and relationships with lipids in postmenopausal women. *Menopause* 2000;7: 395.

166. Gruber DM, Sator MO, Kirchengast S, et al. Effect of percutaneous androgen replacement therapy on body composition and body weight in postmenopausal women. *Maturitas* 1998;29: 253.

167. Munzer T, Marman M, Hess P, et al. Effects of GH and/or sex steroid administration on abdominal subcutaneous and visceral fat in healthy aged women and men. *J Clin Endocrinol Metab* 2001;86:3604.

168. O'Sullivan AJ, Crampton LJ, Freund J, Ho KY. The route of estrogen replacement therapy confers divergent effects on substrate oxidation and body composition in postmenopausal women. *J Clin Invest* 1998;102:1035.

169. Lwin R, Oster R, Darnell BE, et al. The effect of oral estrogen on postprandial lipid oxidation, fat mass, and lean body mass in postmenopausal women. *Obes Res* 2003;11(suppl): A50.

Infertility

CHAPTER 15

Diagnostic Evaluation and Treatment of the Infertile Couple

WENDY Y. CHANG, SANJAY K. AGARWAL, AND RICARDO AZZIZ

Fertility is defined as the ability of an individual to conceive and bear offspring. *Infertility* is the state of diminished or impaired capacity to do so. These definitions incorrectly imply a dichotomous state in which one is either fertile or infertile. Infertility is not an absolute or irreversible condition but rather a continuous clinical spectrum.[1] A better means of estimating the probability of conception uses the concept of fecundability. *Fecundability* is the probability of achieving a pregnancy in one menstrual cycle. In healthy, young couples, cycle fecundability has been estimated at 20 to 25 percent.[2] *Fecundity* is the probability of achieving a pregnancy that results in a live birth during one menstrual cycle. Fecundabilty and fecundity enable the quantitative analysis of fertility potential in patients presenting with different clinical characteristics.

▶ DEFINITION AND EPIDEMIOLOGY OF INFERTILITY

The clinical definition of infertility is the inability to conceive after 12 months of frequent, unprotected coitus. This definition is appealing from both historical and statistical perspectives.[3] It is based in part on large, retrospective studies including that of Guttmacher in 1956,[4] who studied 5574 women in the United Kingdom and in the United States engaging in unprotected intercourse and conceiving between 1946 and 1956. Of these women, 50 percent conceived within 3 months, 72 percent within 6 months, and 85 percent within 1 year. These results were consistent with those of a previous study by Tietze and colleagues in 1950,[5] who reported that the probability of conception was related to the age of the couple and the duration and frequency of coitus. Tietze found that in normal, healthy couples, 25 percent conceived after 1 month, 70 percent after 6 months, and 90 percent after 1 year.

These empirical findings are consistent with probability estimates using the fecundability concept. The cumulative probability of conception F within a particular number of months N can be calculated as follows[1]:

$$F = 1 - (1 - f)^N$$

Assuming fecundability f of 0.25, then the cumulative probability of pregnancy after one calendar year is 98 percent. The likelihood of possessing normal fecundability and not conceiving after 1 year is only 2 percent. Thus, using the 1-year interval in defining infertility is both historically and statistically relevant. However, determining the timing of evaluating and treating infertility always should be tempered by clinical judgment. One should not defer evaluation of couples presenting after less than 1 year of failure to conceive if there are clear metabolic and endocrinologic derangements to be addressed. Advancing maternal age, oligo-ovulation, and a history of surgical sterilization are only a few examples.

The prevalence of infertility is difficult to estimate because both the numerator (the number of infertile couples) and the denominator (the number of couples "at risk" for pregnancy) of the equation can vary significantly depending on the definitions being used.[2,3] Infertility data in the United States are derived from the National Survey of Family Growth, conducted by the National Center for Health Statistics. Data were compiled by interviewing representative cohorts of over 10,000 women. Despite increased public awareness and use of infertility therapies, the prevalence of infertility, de-fined as the inability to conceive after 12 months of frequent, unprotected intercourse among reproductive aged nulliparous women, has remained stable at 13.3 percent in 1965, 13.9 percent in 1982, 13.7 percent in 1988, and 13.5 percent in 1995.[6–9]

Social and demographic changes may have an impact on the epidemiology of infertility and use of infertility therapies. For example, in the United States, the trend to delay child-bearing has resulted in women attempting to conceive when of older reproductive age. This has resulted in a significant increase in the percentage of women with primary infertility. In 1995 more than one-half of infertile women had never conceived previously, whereas in 1965 only one in six infertile women were nulligravidas.[7,8] The prevalence of infertility is not significantly different across ethnic and racial groups, although medical resources for infertility treatment are used more frequently by patients in higher socioeconomic groups and with more extensive educational backgrounds.[7,8]

▶ ETIOLOGY OF INFERTILITY

Pregnancy represents the successful and timely completion of an elaborate series of physiologic events: ovulation of a competent oocyte, production of competent sperm, juxtaposition of oocyte and sperm in the reproductive tract, production of a viable embryo, embryo transport into the uterine cavity, and embryo implantation into the endometrium (Fig. 15-1). Any disruption in these essential steps can result in diminished fertility. A number of disorders can be associated with reduced fertility. Due to limitations in our own understanding and the complexity of human infertility, it is often difficult to distinguish whether these disease states are causal or associated factors. In addition, more than one factor may be contributing to infertility in a particular couple.

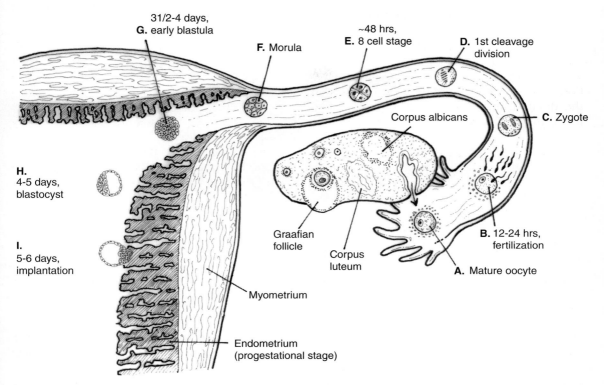

Figure 15-1   Schematic diagram depicting basic aspects of conception: viable gametes, juxtaposition of gametes, transport, and implantation of embryo   *(Used, with permission, from Barbieri.[1])*

Regardless, conditions that influence fecundability can be divided into four major categories:

1. Abnormalities in ovulation and oocyte production
2. Abnormalities of female reproductive tract transport, including cervical, uterine, tubal, and peritoneal factors
3. Abnormalities in sperm production
4. Unexplained or other conditions

Relative Incidence of Primary Infertility Diagnoses

The relative incidence of infertility etiologies varies depending on the population studied. Tabulating the frequency with which a particular factor is associated with infertility enables a rough estimation of that factor's relative social importance. Overall, the male and female partners contribute evenly to infertility, with some degree of male factor implicated in 40 percent of cases.[10] In a review of 21 published reports including over 14,000 infertile couples, Collins and colleagues[11] reported the distribution of primary diagnoses associated with infertility (Fig. 15-2). The contribution of each etiology largely has remained stable over time. Male factor comprises the sole diagnosis in approximately 25 percent of infertility cases. When the etiology of infertility is ascribed to the female partner, ovulatory and tubal factors contribute to the majority of cases (Table 15-1).

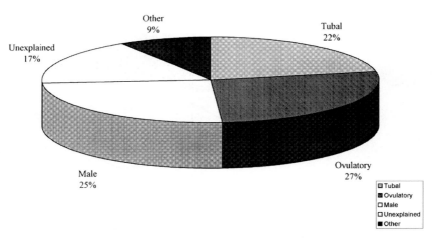

Primary Clinical Diagnoses in Infertile Couples

Figure 15-2 Distribution of primary clinical diagnoses in infertile couples evaluated from the 1980s to the 1990s. *(Adapted, with permission, from Barbieri.[1])*

The percentage of couples with unexplained infertility, in which no discernible cause can be identified, depends on the stringency of the evaluation. In most large, retrospective studies, unexplained infertility is diagnosed in 15 to 20 percent of couples. Other etiologies, including endometriosis, are diagnosed in 9 percent of couples.

▶ INITIAL CONSULTATION

Taking a Focused Medical History

The first infertility visit is the most critical one. Both partners should be present during this

visit to underscore the concept that infertility is a problem to be surmounted by the couple. This encounter will yield significant historical cues that guide the infertility evaluation, determine the pace of evaluation and treatment, and allow the physician an opportunity to assess and guide patient expectations. It also marks an excellent opportunity for patient education. Having the couple complete a health history questionnaire prior to the first visit will enable the physician to focus on relevant issues. A thorough medical, surgical, and family history should be elicited from both. Relevant occupational exposures should be discussed. The history of the male partner should be thorough enough to determine the need for immediate urologic referral (Table 15-2).

A complete history and review of systems should be elicited from the female partner. This includes questions regarding the age of menarche, menstrual pattern, contraception use, gravidity, and parity. A history of galactorrhea, thyroid abnormality, or other endocrine and metabolic derangements would warrant further evaluation. Risk factors such as previous episodes of sexually transmitted disease, pelvic

▶ TABLE 15-1: CAUSES OF FEMALE FACTOR INFERTILITY AND THEIR PREVALENCE

Ovulatory/ovarian dysfunction	30–40%
Tubal/peritoneal	30–40%
Unexplained	10–15%
Miscellaneous	10–15%

From Yao M, Schust D. Infertility, in Novak's Gynecology, 13th ed.[6]

▶ **TABLE 15-2:** THE INFERTILITY HISTORY IN THE MALE PARTNER

Developmental History
- Testicular descent
- Pubertal development
- Growth of facial and body hair
- Change in or loss of body hair pattern

Significant Past Medical History
- Include questions regarding sinopulmonary symptoms

History of Infections
- Sexually transmitted diseases
- Mumps/orchitis
- Genitourinary tract infections

Injury or Surgery of the Genital Tract

Sexual History
- Prior fertility
- Libido
- Intercourse frequency
- Nature and duration of sexual dysfunction

Lifestyle Issues
- Alcohol consumption
- Recreational drug use
- Anabolic steroid use

inflammatory disease, appendicitis, and abdominal or pelvic surgery would heighten suspicion for tubal disease. A complete history also indicates when additional evaluation is needed. A history of cyclic pelvic pain or pelvic inflammatory disease may prompt earlier laparoscopy. A history of hirsutism and oligomenorrhea would dictate additional endocrinologic evaluation.

Taking a complete medical history from both partners also increases patient comfort when discussing the coital history. The interviewer always should include questions regarding coital frequency and sexual dysfunction to screen for simple and easily treated fertility problems. We review the "fertile window" to help couples understand that conception is possible with intercourse from approximately 5 days before ovulation through the day of ovulation.[12,13] Couples practicing infre-

quent intercourse should be advised to increase to at least twice-weekly coitus. Many couples are uncertain or incorrectly counseled regarding optimal timing of intercourse. In couples with normal fertility and no male factor, daily intercourse during the 6 days of the fertile window is superior to less frequent intercourse because each act raises the probability of conception.[13] Although sperm concentrations become lower with increasing coital frequency, this decrease does not reduce the cumulative conception benefit of daily intercourse in those with normal semen parameters.[12,13] Common myths regarding coital position and fertility should be dispelled because they are unsupported or unexamined in the medical literature. The couple should be instructed to avoid any oil-based or spermicidal lubricants. A history of dyspareunia or sexual dysfunction warrants full evaluation and treatment.

Physical Examination of the Female Patient

The female patient should be examined at the initial visit. The patient's vital signs, height, and weight should be recorded. The patient's body habitus and hair distribution should be noted. Dermatologic abnormalities such as acne, alopecia, hirsutism, acanthosis nigricans, or abdominal striae, which may suggest androgen excess, insulin resistance, or Cushing's syndrome, should be noted. Particular attention should be paid to the thyroid because both clinical and subclinical thyroid diseases are common in women of reproductive age and can result in diminished fertility. A breast and pelvic examination should be performed. The patient should have documentation of cervical cytology within a year of starting any hormonal treatment. A careful bimanual and rectovaginal examination will yield valuable information on the size and contour of the uterus and adnexa and reveal any uterosacral nodularity consistent with endometriosis. The direction and depth of the uterine cavity and the presence of possible cervical stenosis should be assessed with a sterile catheter in patients considering artificial insemination or assisted reproductive techniques.

► OVERVIEW OF INFERTILITY TESTING

The goals of the infertility evaluation are manifold: (1) to determine the etiology of infertility in an expedient fashion, (2) to define appropriate treatment protocols, (3) to predict realistic success rates for treatment, and (4) to educate the couple on their infertility etiologies.[14] The primary diagnostic evaluation represents the first-line testing and should be broad and noninvasive (Table 15-3). This should include a semen analysis as a general screen of male fertility potential, either a serum luteal phase progesterone determination or basal

body chart to document ovulation, and a hysterosalpingogram for examination of reproductive tract patency. Due to the high prevalence of clinical and subclinical thyroid dysfunction in women during their reproductive years and their potential effects on fertility, we also check thyroid-stimulating hormone (TSH) levels if a test has not been done within the past year.[15–17] A baseline day 3 follicle-stimulating hormone (FSH) level, and possibly an estradiol level, should be determined in women 35 years of age and older to document ovarian reserve. If any abnormality is found during this evaluation, or if the clinical history is highly suggestive, then additional secondary tests may be indicated (Table 15-4). The clinician must balance the need for diagnostic certainty with the delay in treatment while evaluation is in progress. In addition, one must contemplate carefully the risks associated with any diagnostic procedure for a condition that is not life-threatening and occurring within a healthy individual.

► TABLE 15-3: PRIMARY EVALUATION OF THE INFERTILE COUPLE

Thorough History
- Including duration of infertility, previous infertility evaluation, pubertal development, menstrual function, sexual activity, dyspareunia, dysmenorrhea, pelvic pain, obstetric history, previous surgeries, risk factors for pelvic infection, medications, and history of weight loss/gain, excess hair growth, hot/cold intolerance, hot flashes, fatigue.

Documentation of Ovulation
- Menstrual history or, if eumenorrheic, basal body temperature
  and/or
- Midluteal progesterone level

Documentation of Female Reproductive Tract Patency
- Hysterosalpingogram

Documentation of Sperm Production
- Semen analysis

Diagnosis of Ovulatory Defects

Disorders of ovulation and oocyte production are among the most common causes of female infertility, found in approximately 40 percent of such individuals.[6] Diagnosis is facilitated by the menstrual history, which is an effective screening tool for assessing ovulation. Normal menstrual cycle length in reproductive-age women varies from 25 to 35 days, with most women reporting intercycle intervals of 27 to 31 days. Oligomenorrhea and menometrorrhagia imply ovulatory dysfunction and reduced fertility. Amenorrhea likely signifies anovulation. Conversely, regular, predictable menses associated with moliminal symptoms almost always represent regular ovulation.[6,18] We routinely assess ovulatory status in women with menstrual cycle lengths deviating from 25 to 35 days. Although pregnancy and retrieval of an oocyte from the reproductive tract remain the only absolute evidence for ovulation,[19,20] a number of clinical and laboratory findings can

▶ **TABLE 15-4:** SECONDARY EVALUATION OF THE INFERTILE COUPLE*

Monitoring of Ovulatory Function
- Monitoring of urinary LH surge

Serial Transvaginal Sonography

Evaluation of Cervical Function
- Postcoital test

Evaluation of Ovarian Reserve
- Day 3 FSH and estradiol level *or*
- Clomiphene challenge test

Evaluation of Female Reproductive Tract
- Laparoscopy
  -Hysteroscopy
- Transvaginal hydrolaparoscopy, salpingoscopy

Documentation of Sperm Production and Function
- Sperm chromatin structure assay
- Antisperm antibodies

Recurrent Pregnancy Loss
- Test for thrombophilias, antiphospholipid antibodies
- Thyroid function/autoantibodies
- Karyotype in both partners
- Evaluation for chronic disease

Preimplantation Genetic Diagnosis

Parental Genetic/Chromosomal Evaluation

Additional Endocrinologic Evaluation
- Serum androgen levels
- Testing for insulin resistance/glucose intolerance
- Thyroid function
- Prolactin

*Many of the tests will be dictated by the patient history and abnormalities identified on the primary evaluation.

help to confirm, predict, or assess the quality of ovulation.

Basal Body Temperature

The most cost-effective and least invasive test to confirm ovulation is the basal body temper-ature (BBT). Any oral thermometer can be used, although the basal body thermometer is easier to read and more precise in the tem-perature range of interest. The patient is in-structed to take the morning temperature be-fore rising from bed, eating, or drinking. For most women, BBT ranges from 97 to 98°F dur-ing the follicular phase. Luteal-phase tempera-tures are usually 0.5 to 1.0°F higher due to the presence of progesterone, a thermogenic hor-mone secreted by the corpus luteum. A bipha-sic pattern (Fig. 15-3) is almost always indica-tive of ovulation.[21] Patients with biphasic patterns can be counseled to perform daily coitus during the 6-day fertile window.

However, the role of BBT in infertility eval-uation is limited. BBT charts sometimes can be difficult to obtain and to interpret. The charts can only estimate the presumed day of ovula-tion retrospectively, which likely occurs 1 day before the temperature elevation. While the rise in BBT corresponds to serum progesterone levels of 4 ng/mL or greater,[21] it is not reliable in predicting the timing of ovulation.[22] In ad-dition, a small percentage of women exhibit monophasic BBT charts despite alternate doc-umentation of ovulation. Thus, while a bipha-sic chart almost always confirms ovulation, pa-tients with monophasic charts may require further testing to determine ovulatory status.

Midluteal Serum Progesterone

A more definitive means of confirming ovula-tion is the midluteal serum progesterone level. The normal follicular-phase serum proges-terone level is usually <2 ng/mL (<6 nmol/L). After ovulation, however, progesterone is se-creted by the corpus luteum in a fluctuating manner, with levels ranging between 6 and 25 ng/mL (19 and 80 nmol/L). In the European Society of Human Reproduction and Embryol-ogy (ESHRE) Capri Workshop Group's review of optimal infertility tests and treatments,[23] serum progesterone levels were determined to be the best test for confirming ovulation. The test is typically performed 18 to 24 days after the start of menses. However, variation in cycle

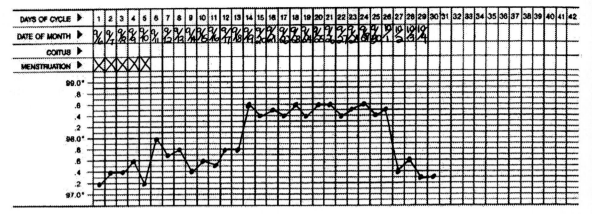

Figure 15-3 Basal body temperature chart demonstrating biphasic pattern consistent with ovulation.

length may result in inappropriate timing of the test and underestimation of ovulatory function.[24] Thus a single low value does not reliably diagnose abnormal ovulation or luteal phase. In addition, an absolute cutoff to define ovulatory progesterone levels is not well defined and is subject to interlaboratory variation. However, serum progesterone levels >4 to 6 ng/mL generally are accepted as indicative of ovulation.[24] Hull and colleagues[25] have suggested that an adequate midluteal progesterone level should exceed 9.4 ng/mL (30 nmol/L). Since progesterone levels exceeding this level were associated with higher per-cycle pregnancy rates. These investigators proposed that the higher cutoff value may be most relevant in clomiphene- or gonadotropin-treated cycles, in which multiple follicles may contribute to the total serum progesterone level.

Luteinizing Hormone (LH) Assays

The onset of the LH surge preceeds ovulation by approximately 34 to 36 h. The peak in serum LH levels preceeds ovulation by 10 to 12 h.[23] Documentation of elevated LH levels has been used as an indirect predictor of ovulation. Test kits for urinary LH surge are widely available to patients and can serve both diagnostic and therapeutic purposes. The LH surges in urine and serum have been shown to have excellent correlation

in a study of 75 normal and stimulated menstrual cycles.[26] Standard urine test kits provide colorimetric assays that become positive once urinary LH levels exceed a certain threshold. Patients are advised initially to begin testing several days before ovulation is anticipated. Ovulation is presumed to occur the day after the urinary LH surge but may vary with kit sensitivity. Patients should be cautioned that variations in renal clearance of LH and patient skill with the test can affect the sensitivity of the assay. However, with ideal use, urine LH surge assays predict ovulation with up to 100 percent sensitivity and 96 percent accuracy.[24]

Endometrial Biopsy

The endometrium exhibits characteristic progressive changes under the effects of estrogen and progesterone. The finding of secretory endometrium on biopsy has been used in the past as an additional means of confirming ovulation. The procedure generally is performed 2 to 3 days prior to the anticipated onset of menses and interpreted based on histologic criteria.[27] This method also has been used to demonstrate luteal-phase defects and deficiencies in progesterone secretion or target tissue action. However, both intraobserver and interobserver variations in reading the specimens, as well as the common occurrence of the out-of-phase endometrium in normally fertile women, have shown this test of be of little use in the initial infertility evaluation.[28,29]

Ultrasonography

High-resolution transvaginal ultrasonography can be used throughout the cycle to monitor development of ovarian follicles. The preovulatory follicle reaches normally 22 to 25 mm in diameter.[1] Ovulation is evidenced by decreased follicular size, collapse of the developing follicle, and appearance of fluid in the cul de sac.[30–32] In a prospective study of 14 spontaneous and 17 clomiphene-induced cycles, subjects were monitored with daily transvaginal ultrasound, determination of serum LH and estradiol levels, and urinary LH determination using standard test kits.[33] Transvaginal ultrasound detected ovulation in all cycles. However, ultrasound monitoring has not been shown to improve pregnancy rates in unselected patients undergoing clomiphene citrate ovulation induction.[34] The expense and time-consuming nature of this modality have limited its application largely to the superovulation induction cycle

Detection of Luteal-Phase Deficiency

The diagnosis of luteal-phase deficiency (LPD) is currently controversial, and it is unclear whether this entity exists or contributes significantly to diminshed fertility. LPD is defined as impaired corpus luteum function or hormone production. LPD can be diagnosed by two separate endometrial biopsies documenting more than a 2-day discrepancy between actual cycle day and histologic day of endometrial development. Some investigators also have used sustained BBT elevation of at least 0.4°F above follicular-phase levels for 12 to 15 days as clinical evidence of an adequate luteal phase.[14] The putative cause of LPD is suggested to be reduced progesterone synthesis by the corpus luteum. A single midluteal-phase progesterone of <10 ng/mL or a sum of three random serum progesterone measurements of <30 ng/mL also has been used as part of the diagnosis to reflect decreased quality of corpus luteal func-

tion and low integrated progesterone levels during the luteal phase.[35]

More recent data indicate that the incidence of greater than a 2-day lag in endometrial maturity can be as high as 51 percent in regularly menstruating women of normal fertility.[36] This prevalence of out-of-phase endometrium is equivalent to rates quoted for infertile populations. This and other similar studies have questioned the validity of the LPD diagnosis. Furthermore, the benefit of treatment for LPD has not been established. Consequently, the routine endometrial biopsy for diagnosing LPD is no longer a component of the primary infertility evaluation.

Maternal Age and Diminished Ovarian Reserve

Age-Related Decline in Female Fertility

Female fertility is limited by the aging oocyte and follicle. The association between maternal age and diminished fecundability has been well documented. The classic study examining the effects of age on fertility is that of the Hutterites, a religious sect based in Montana, the Dakotas, and adjacent regions of Canada. The Hutterites represent a uniquely stable, healthy population that eschews contraception. Their communal living arrangement eliminates incentive to limit family size. Tietze[37] reported on the fertility rate of the Hutterites in 1957. He noted an infertility rate of 2.4 percent. Average maternal age at last pregnancy was 40.9 years. Fertility rate was noted to decline progressively with age: 11 percent of the women were infertile by age 34, 33 percent by age 40, and 87 percent by age 45.

This pattern has been observed throughout various ethnic and racial populations. In a study of cumulative pregnancy rates in women with azoospermic husbands using a donor insemination program,[38] 74 percent of the women younger than age 31 achieved pregnancy within 1 year. Pregnancy rates fell to 62 percent in women aged 31 to 35 years and to 54 percent in women older than age 35. This effect of maternal age on fertility or oocyte quality is corroborated by data from oocyte donation programs. When embryos resulting from oocytes donated by younger women are transferred into older women, pregnancy rates approximate those of the young donor population.[39] The high pregnancy rates resulting from younger donor oocytes remain constant with increasing recipient age up to 50 years old.

The age-related decline in fertility arises from the finite nature of the ovarian follicle, depletion of the oocyte pool, and likely diminished quality of remaining oocytes. The number of oocytes and follicles in the human ovary is fixed and peaks in utero, with an exponential decline after the second trimester. At birth, the number of follicles and oocytes is approximately 2 million, with a further drop to 250,000 at the completion of puberty. The ovary will ovulate, on average, 500 oocytes before menopause, with progressive follicular attrition each cycle due to atresia of nondominant follicles. Because the oocyte is arrested in prophase of meiosis I from early gestation to the time of ovulation, which can be half a century later, it is predisposed to meiotic mishaps resulting in chromosomal aneuploidy. Follicular meiotic competence decreases with age.[40] Recent studies also have suggested that, in addition to nuclear chromosomal anomalies, the aging oocyte also harbors progressive deletions in mitochondral DNA.[41] These and other factors may contribute not only to the age-related decrease in female fecundity but also to the increased risk of spontaneous abortion with increasing maternal age.[42] Recent prospective data in patients undergoing in vitro fertilization suggest that maternal age is the most important predictor of pregnancy rates.[43]

Early Follicular-Phase Serum FSH and Estradiol Levels

In addition to maternal age, basal FSH and estradiol levels also serve as an excellent indicator of ovarian reserve. Laboratory evaluation of ovarian reserve typically is done through follicular-phase FSH levels. Pituitary FSH secretion is normally under the feedback inhibition of inhibin and estradiol. With progressive follicular loss and decreased follicular inhibin suppression, average FSH levels rise. In addition, higher FSH levels are required to stimulate follicular growth. Serum FSH levels to determine ovarian reserve typically are determined on cycle day 3, when estradiol levels are low and should not exert additional suppression on FSH. An elevated day 3 serum FSH level is a good marker of depleted follicular pool and decreased fecundability. In a study examining 1478 consecutive in vitro fertilization (IVF) cycles,[44] basal FSH level was determined to be an excellent predictor for all cycle outcome variables including total and ongoing pregnancy rates. Women with day 3 FSH levels exceeding 15 mIU/mL had reduced pregnancy rates.

Elevations of day 3 serum estradiol concentrations also have been associated with poor pregnancy outcome after IVF.[45] High estradiol levels appear to reflect reduced oocyte numbers and premature follicular recruitment. Many IVF centers opt to cancel cycles in which serum FSH levels exceed 20 mIU/mL or serum estradiol levels exceed 100 pg/mL. Persistent elevations in these two values warrant consideration of oocyte donation.

Clomiphene Citrate Challenge Test

The clomiphene citrate challenge test (CCCT) has been advocated by some investigators as a more sensitive indicator of diminished ovarian reserve than elevated day 3 serum FSH or E_2 levels.[28] Clomiphene citrate is a nonsteroidal estrogen receptor modulator. By blocking the negative-feedback inhibition exerted by estradiol on pituitary FSH secretion, clomiphene theoretically unmasks diminished inhibin secretion. The patient is instructed to take clomiphene citrate 100 mg orally on cycle days 5 through 9. Serum FSH levels are sampled on days 3 and 10; FSH elevations on either day would indicate decreased ovarian reserve.

A number of studies have demonstrated that IVF patients with abnormal day 10 FSH levels on CCCTs required higher doses of medication for stimulation, experienced higher cycle cancelation rates, and achieved lower pregnancy rates than patients with normal CCCT results.[46,47] However, the value of the CCCT in the fertility evaluation has been contested by studies showing poor predictive value and reliability. An abnormal CCCT does not necessarily preclude pregnancy.[48] There can be significant intercycle variations within the same individual.[48,49] While the CCCT is not a component of the primary infertility investigation, it may be of benefit in predicting cycle outcomes in older women with normal day 3 FSH levels.

Diagnosis of Female Anatomic Factors in Infertility

Anatomic abnormalities comprise 30 to 40 percent of female infertility. Risk factors for tubal and peritoneal disease include previous pelvic inflammatory disease (PID), pelvic surgery, and endometriosis.[50–54] The risk of tubal infertility after a single bout of PID is 12 percent; this figure rises to 23 percent after a second episode and to 54 percent after three episodes.[55] However, more than 50 percent of women with documented tubal disease reported no identifiable risk factors.[56] The majority of these cases are presumed to result from prior subclinical chlamydial infection.[57,58]

Uterine abnormalities also have been associated with infertility and spontaneous abortion. Clinically relevant lesions include congenital uterine anomalies, anomalies resulting from in utero exposure to diethylstilbestrol (DES), and acquired abnormalities such as leiomyomata, polyps, and synechiae. The presence of endometriosis is the sole abnormality found on evaluation in approximately 4 percent of patients. Evaluation of reproductive tract morphology is therefore an integral aspect of any infertility evaluation.

Hysterosalpingography

Hysterosalpingography (HSG) should be the primary test for documenting uterine and tubal morphology.[23] The HSG should be performed under fluoroscopic visualization. A catheter device is placed into the cervical os; a 3- to 4-mL bolus of radiopaque contrast material is injected slowly to delineate the uterine cavity; then additional contrast material is injected for a total bolus of 10 to 20 mL to demonstrate tubal filling or obstruction. A minimum of two radiographic pictures are needed: an early film demonstrating uterine cavity filling and a subsequent film documenting tubal filling and peritoneal spill (see Fig. 21-2). To avoid potentially disrupting an ongoing pregnancy, the test should be performed before ovulation, between cycle days 3 through 8. Common side effects include vaginal spotting, uterine cramping, and a mild febrile reaction. Prophylactic administration of a nonsteroidal anti-inflammatory agent may reduce discomfort. In addition, HSG is associated with a 1 to 3 percent risk of postprocedural infection, especially in the setting of prior or current pelvic infection and preexisting tubal damage.[59] If the clinical suspicion for current or chronic infection is high, the HSG should be postponed until the patient has completed a course of antibiotics. However, universal administration of prophylactic antibiotics prior to HSG has not been shown to reduce the risk of postprocedure infection, although it is associated with decreased incidence of febrile morbidity.[60] Nevertheless, many clinicians prescribe oral doxycycline 100 mg twice a day for 3 to 5 days beginning the day before HSG.

In a large metaanalysis, HSG has been shown to have a 65 percent sensitivity and an 83 percent specificity for tubal obstruction.[61] Thus, while a normal HSG cannot reliably predict normal tubal function, it is reliable for detecting significant tubal pathology. Alternatively, HSG is not reliable for the detection of peritubal or peritoneal adhesions.[62] Thus further evaluation may be needed in the setting of both an abnormal HSG and a normal HSG in a high-risk individual. Overall, the HSG is a cost-effective screening tool in couples presenting with infertility.[23,63] HSG with oil-soluble contrast material may have therapeutic benefit as well, with numerous studies demonstrating enhanced pregnancy rates after the procedure.[64]

Ultrasonography

While HSG remains the screening modality of choice for the primary evaluation of infertility, ultrasonography has gained increasing importance in the detection of uterine abnormalities. Ultrasound is the modality of choice for evaluation of the endometrium, ovaries, and tubal structure. Sonohysterography has been shown to be superior to HSG in detecting uterine anomalies, identifying 90 percent of such abnormalities in infertile patients.[65] The incorporation of simple contrast material with ultrasound evaluation, enabling visualization of both uterine contour and tubal patency, likely will gain increasing application to the primary evaluation of infertility.[23]

Laparoscopy

Laparoscopy is considered the gold standard for the diagnosis of tubal and peritoneal pathology. It enables direct visualization of all pelvic organs and immediate treatment of adhesions and other disease. A laparoscopy is the logical "next step" in patients who fail to conceive despite a negative primary infertility evaluation or when intraabdominal pathology is suspected. This procedure usually is performed during the follicular phase to avoid disruption of an ongoing pregnancy or the corpus luteum.[14] Chromopertubation, the injection of dyes such as indigo carmine through the uterus and tubes, enables determination of tubal patency. In addition, laparoscopic ablation or resection of endometriotic lesions and lysis of adhesions have been shown to increase subsequent pregnancy rates in women with even minimal to mild endometriosis.[66]

However, due to its invasiveness, laparoscopy should be reserved for identifying and treating pathology and evaluating symptomatic or high-risk patients. Candidates include women with symptoms strongly suggestive of endometriosis or a history of pelvic surgery, appendicitis, PID, and those failing to conceive following ovulation induction with clomiphene or gonadotropins.[67] In asymptomatic and low-risk patients, laparoscopy did not increase cumulative conception rates over preliminary HSG.[68] However, there have been many advances in the evaluation and treatment of women with tubal and peritoneal disease (see Chap. 21).

Cervical Factor Infertility and the Postcoital Test

The postcoital test (PCT) was introduced to detect potentially deleterious effects of the cervical mucus on spermatozoa. The technique and interpretation of the PCT lack standardization.[14] The PCT usually is performed 2 to 18 h after intercourse during the 1 to 3 days preceding ovulation. A sample of cervical mucus is aspirated and examined macroscopically and microscopically. Normal findings include a positive fern pattern, a >5-cm spinnbarkeit, absence of leukocytes, and presence of at least five motile sperm per high-power field.[67]

In couples with no other detectable cause of infertility, a "normal" PCT was shown to be associated with shorter time to conception in a small, prospective observational study[25] and a higher probability of conception within in 1 year of evaluation in a larger, retrospective study.[69] However, a subsequent prospective, randomized controlled trial[70] and a systematic review have shown PCT to be of limited value. The PCT resulted in increased cost, patient evaluation, and treatment but did not boost cumulative pregnancy. From a practical standpoint, many couples treated for infertility will undergo intrauterine insemination, theoretically bypassing potential cervical factors. Thus, despite widespread use, the PCT is of limited utility, and many do not consider it a component of the primary infertility evaluation. However, the PCT may be of diagnostic benefit in couples presenting with otherwise unexplained infertility or in women with previous cervical surgery or ablation who do not wish to undergo artificial insemination.

Diagnosis of Abnormalities in the Male Factor

Abnormalities of the male factor is diagnosed in 25 to 40 percent of couples presenting for infertility evaluation (Table 15-5). The causes and relative frequency of male infertility can be divided into four main groups: hypothalamic-pituitary disease, testicular disease, posttesticular disorders, and nonclassifiable.[71] Until recently, no specific etiology for male infertility could be found in up to 40 percent of cases. However, two major advances have contributed to improved understanding of male factor infertility: elucidation of Y chromosome microdeletions and identification of a genetic basis for congenital bilateral absence of the vas deferens (CBAVD).[72] The scope of male infertility evaluation has broadened to include the history, physical examination, semen analysis, and genetic or endocrinologic testing when indicated.

Semen Analysis

Although plagued by controversy regarding the proper range of "normal" values, semen analysis is an inexpensive and noninvasive test that has long been the cornerstone of male fertility assessment. The basic semen analysis measures seminal volume, pH, liquefaction time, sperm concentration, sperm motility and morphology, and microscopic debris and agglutination. Additional measurements, depending on the laboratory, include white cell count and fructose levels. The World Health Organization (WHO) has suggested normal values, which serve as general guidelines for evaluation (Table 15-6). Pronounced abnormalities in the semen analy-

▶ **TABLE 15-5:** CAUSES OF MALE INFERTILITY

Hypothalamic-pituitary disease (secondary hypogonadism)	1–2%
Testicular disease (primary hypogonadism)	30–40%
Posttesticular defects	10–20%
Nonclassifiable	40–50%

▶ **TABLE 15-6:** NORMAL VALUES FOR SEMEN ANALYSIS

Volume	>2.0 mL
Sperm concentration	>20 million/mL
Motility	>50%
Morphology	>30% normal forms

From World Health Organization. Laboratory Manual for the Examination of Human Semen and Sperm-Cervical Interaction. Cambridge, England: Cambridge University Press, 1992.

sis warrant referral to a urologist, preferably with special training in reproduction, for further evaluation.

SEMEN SPECIMEN COLLECTION

The semen specimen ideally should be collected after 2 to 7 days of abstinence. A masturbated sample collected in the physician's office is preferred, although specimens collected at home or in silicone condoms without chemical additives are acceptable if delivered to the laboratory within an hour of collection. Due to inherent, potentially pronounced variability of semen samples, at least two samples collected 1 to 2 weeks apart should be analyzed.

SEMEN VOLUME

Normal semen volume ranges between 2 and 5 mL. A low volume in the setting of severe oligospermia or azoospermia suggests genital tract obstruction, such as CBAVD, and seminal vesicle or ejaculatory duct obstruction. The former is diagnosed on physical examination and by low seminal pH; the latter, by the sonographic finding of dilated seminal vesicles.

SPERM CONCENTRATION

Sperm concentration, measured by hemocytometer or other cell-counting chamber, is usually above 20 million/mL. However, men with lower counts can be fertile. In patients undergoing in vitro fertilization, a concentration of 10 million/mL or less can be acceptable.[73] Sperm agglutination, the microscopic finding of sperm clumping, is suggestive of autoimmunity and should be confirmed by tests for sperm surface antibodies.

SPERM MOTILITY

Sperm motility can be classified as rapid progressive, slow progressive, nonprogressive, and nonmotile. The WHO criteria state that at least 50 percent of spermatozoa should be motile, with at least 25 percent demonstrating rapid progressive motility.

SPERM MORPHOLOGY

In the past, morphologic criteria described by the WHO were based primarily on shape, with greater than 30 percent normal forms deemed acceptable. Stricter criteria for evaluating morphology on standard light microscopy, such as the Tygerberg classification developed by Kruger and Menkveld in 1986,[74] have since been proposed to include assessment of the entire spermatozoa: width, length, width ratio, area of the acrosome, and neck and tail defects. The Tygerberg criteria are advantageous because of their predictive value for fertilization and pregnancy rates in the IVF cycle.

WHITE BLOOD CELLS/LEUKOCYTE COUNT

Many laboratories include round cell counts as part of the semen analysis. These round cells may represent immature germ cells, neutrophils, or lymphocytes, which can be distinguished by the Endtz test, an immunoperoxidase staining test for leukocytes. More than 5 million round cells per milliliter or more than 1 million leukocytes per milliliter is regarded as abnormal by the WHO. An elevation in immature sperm cells may indicate defective spermatogenesis and is associated with poor prognosis for fertilization. Alternatively, an increased leukocyte count may be indicative of infection or inflammation and would warrant further evaluation and treatment.

Specialized Semen Analysis

While the following tests are not ordered routinely, they can be useful in specific circumstances.

REACTIVE OXYGEN SPECIES

Reactive oxygen species (ROS) and peroxidase can be released by leukocytes and abnormal sperm. These substances can cause lipid peroxidation of the sperm membrane and be detrimental to sperm motility.[75] However, detection of ROS in sperm is still considered investigational and is not used often in the infertility evaluation.[73]

SPERM AUTOANTIBODIES

Sperm autoantibodies are detected in the serum and seminal fluid in approximately 4–8 percent of subfertile men.[73] Antisperm antibodies also have been detected in cervical mucus. In men, a humoral response to sperm may result from disruption of the blood-testis barrier. Possible etiologies include trauma, testicular torsion, occlusion of the vas deferens, vasectomy reversal, and genital tract infection. High titers of sperm surface antibodies of the IgA and IgG classes are strongly negatively correlated with spontaneous pregnancy.[76] Sperm autoimmunity is suggested by agglutination in the initial semen analysis. Numerous assays are available for the detection of antisperm antibodies, but the immunobead test and the mixed agglutination-antiglobulin reaction (MAR) are performed most commonly. Antisperm antibodies are considered clinically relevant when they coat more than 50 percent of spermatozoa and when they prevent penetration of preovulatory cervical mucus and zona-free hamster oocytes.

COMPUTER-AIDED SPERM ANALYSIS (CASA)

Sperm kinematics is the quantitative measurement of sperm motion. Characteristics measured include sperm velocity, amplitude of lateral movement, frequency of change in sperm head direction, and other aspects of path trajectory.[77] Kinematic data can be useful in toxicology studies and in the evaluation of men with unexplained infertility.[78,79] Sperm function characteristics derived from CASA have been demonstrated to be predictive of fertility both in vitro and in vivo.[80–84]

Prognostic Value of Semen Analysis

Although the semen analysis provides descriptive and quantitative data, no single parameter is powerful enough to distinguish between fertile and infertile men. Nevertheless, some clinical correlates have been reported. In a prospective study of 430 couples followed after discontinuing contraception for six menstrual cycles or until pregnancy was achieved, the probability of pregnancy correlated with increasing sperm concentration up to 40 million/mL.[85] The percentage of sperm with normal morphology correlated strongly with the probability of achieving pregnancy independent of concentration. Alternatively, semen volume and sperm motility were of limited value in predicting pregnancy. IVF studies have demonstrated enhanced fertilization rates in patients with more than 14 percent normal morphology by the Tygerberg strict criteria.[86] Overall, the percentage of normal morphology has demonstrated the greatest discriminatory power.

Sperm Functional Assays

Sperm functional assays attempt to describe in vitro sperm function as an indication of in vivo function. While they are expensive and of questionable benefit in routine fertility evaluation, they may yield additional information in couples with unexplained infertility or when the semen analysis is indeterminate.

SPERM PENETRATION ASSAY (SPA)

Denuded hamster oocytes can be penetrated by the spermatozoa of many mammalian species, including humans. The sperm penetration assay (SPA), or zona-free hamster oocyte penetration test (HOPT), was introduced by the clinical andrology laboratory to measure the ability of sperm to capacitate, penetrate, undergo acrosome reaction, and fuse with the oocyte. Sperm from the patient and normal fertile controls are incubated with zona-free hamster eggs. The laboratory reports the percentage or number of eggs penetrated.

The assay was purported to be predictive of in vivo and in vitro fertilization.[87] However,

the false-positive rates range from 20 to 30 percent, whereas the false-negative rates can range from 0 to 100 percent.[73] The SPA has not been shown to discriminate between fertile and infertile men.[88] It is a technically difficult test and not currently a routine component of the infertility evaluation.

HUMAN ZONA PELLUCIDA–BINDING TEST

The hemizona assay and the competitive zona-binding assay assess the ability of sperm to bind human zona pellucida. In the competitive binding assay, zona from an oocyte with no prior exposure to sperm is incubated with control and test spermatozoa that are labeled with different fluorochromes. In the hemizona assay, zona is bissected and incubated with either control or test sperm. In both assays, the number of test spermatozoa bound is compared with the control. Both tests are predictive of IVF success.[89,71] However, since these assays are technically difficult and require human oocytes, they are performed only rarely to determine which couples undergoing IVF would benefit from intracytoplasmic sperm injection (ICSI).

ASSAYS OF SPERM DNA/CHROMATIN INTEGRITY

Normal sperm chromatin exhibits a low degree of binding capacity for fluorochromes and DNA dyes due to its compact, insoluble structure.[90] Assays using specific fluorochromes have been developed to identify subtle defects in sperm chromatin and DNA structure, identify nonviable spermatozoa, and provide threshold values that predict subfertility.

COMET ASSAY

The comet assay is a gel electrophoresis assay that detects spermatozoa with high levels of DNA strand breaks. Sperm DNA is suspended on a microscope slide in agarose gel and stained with a DNA-binding fluorescent dye. The sample is electrophoresed, and spermatozoa with high levels of strand breaks can be distinguished by greater migration toward the anode. The picture obtained resembles a "comet," with a brightly fluorescent head and a tail region which increases in length as DNA damage increases, hence the name. The comet assay is a sensitive measure of DNA damage.[91] However, consistent and clinically relevant threshholds for infertility have not yet been established. The assay also does not distinguish between samples from normozoospermic fertile and infertile men.

TUNEL ASSAY

The terminal deoxynucleotidyl transferase mediated dUTP Nick End Labeling (TUNEL) assay quantifies single- and double-stranded DNA breaks in sperm DNA. Labeled deoxyuridine triphosphate (dUTP) is incorporated into strand breaks by terminal deoxynucleotidyl transferase (TdT). The amount of dUTP incorporated is then measured by flow cytometry or fluorescent light microscopy. The percentage of sperm with DNA fragmentation on TUNEL assay was correlated with semen analysis parameters. A significant negative correlation was seen between the percentage of sperm with DNA fragmentation and subsequent IVF and ICSI fertilization rates.[92,93]

SPERM CHROMATIN STRUCTURE ASSAY

The sperm chromatin structure assay (SCSA) was first described in 1980. It is based on the premise that abnormal chromatin structure renders sperm DNA more susceptible to acid denaturation. Fresh or frozen semen samples can be processed. Semen is diluted, treated with acidic buffer, and stained with acridine orange, which stains intact double-stranded DNA green and denatured DNA red. The proportion of spermatozoa with native versus fragmented DNA is quantitated by flow cytometry.[90] The SCSA can differentiate between infertile and fertile men.[94] It is of prognostic value in assisted reproductive technology (ART). The probability of pregnancy is extremely low during any IVF or ICSI cycles in which the sperm show greater than 27 percent susceptibility to denaturation.[95]

Genetic Testing in the Male Partner

Diagnosis of male infertility has been improved through genetic and chromosomal analyses. Identification of mutations in the cystic fibrosis transmembrane conductance regulator (CFTR) gene has been a major advancement in uncovering the etiology of congenital bilateral absence of the vas deferens (CBAVD). When Caucasian patients presenting with infertility due to CBAVD were screened for CFTR mutations, the majority demonstrated mutations in one or both copies of the CFTR gene.[96] The majority of these men had no pulmonary symptoms of cystic fibrosis (see Chap. 5).

Another genetic basis for male factor infertility was discovered with the identification of Y chromosome microdeletions. The observation that some men with azoospermia possessed small Y chromosomes led to the identification of long arm (Yq) microdeletions clustered in three main loci of the azoospermic factor (AZF) region, designated as AZFa, AZFb, and AZFc.[96] It is now known that 15 percent of infertile men who previously had been diagnosed with idiopathic oligospermia possess these microdeletions.[97,98] However, these deletions are rare in men with sperm concentrations over 5 million/mL.[96]

The application of ICSI technology now enables men with severe oligospermia and azoospermia to father children. However, the potential transmission of genetic defects must be considered. Although Y chromosomal microdeletions are largely de novo, men with such deletions who undergo ART can propagate these deletions, and potential infertility, to their sons.[99] To minimize the risk of transmitting cystic fibrosis to the offspring of men with CBAVD, the female partner should be tested for the common mutations in the CFTR gene. Excluding a common CFTR mutation in the female significantly reduces the risk of conceiving a child with cystic fibrosis or CBAVD. See

Chapter 16 for additional discussion of genetic testing in the male partner.[96]

Endocrine Evaluation of the Male Partner

Measurements of serum testosterone, LH, and FSH are the cornerstones of endocrine evaluation in the male infertility patient. Measurement of serum total testosterone is usually sufficient for initial screening. An additional measurement of serum free testosterone levels may be informative in men with borderline total testosterone values. In men with abnormally low testosterone levels, checking the serum LH and FSH concentrations gives additional information regarding possible etiologies of male hypogonadism. A low testosterone level in the setting of high serum LH and FSH concentrations indicates primary hypogonadism; low testosterone and low gonadotropins suggest secondary hypogonadism. Men who appear well androgenized but have low sperm counts and low LH concentrations should be questioned for exogenous steroid abuse.[73] Serum prolactin should be measured in men with low testosterone levels and normal to low LH levels to exclude a pituitary adenoma.

Summary of the Male Infertility Evaluation

Semen analysis remains the primary investigation and determines the direction of the evaluation for the couple. In general, if the semen analysis is normal, the woman should be evaluated thoroughly. If the routine semen analysis is abnormal, it should be repeated in 2 to 3 months. Severe oligospermia (<5 million/mL) or azoospermia on repeat semen analysis should prompt basal serum FSH, LH, and testosterone measurements. If the endocrine results are normal in the azoospermic patient, a postejaculatory urine sample should be tested for evidence of retrograde ejaculation and obstructive azoospermia. Low seminal fluid volume and pH suggest CBAVD. This diagnosis is supported by low or absent semen fructose be-

cause the seminal vesicles are usually absent in this condition. Men with oligospermia and normal serum hormone concentrations also should be evaluated for possible varicocele, antisperm antibodies, and reproductive tract infection before the diagnosis of idiopathic male infertility is entertained. Finally, a genetic evaluation can be performed in specialized centers. A karyotype and test for AZF deletions is indicated in men with severely impaired sperm production.[23] When a genetic or chromosomal abnormality is detected, the patient should undergo genetic counseling before treatment with ICSI. See Chapter 16 for additional discussion of treatment options in male infertility.

▶ TREATMENT OF OVULATORY INFERTILITY

Classes of Ovulatory Dysfunction

Ovulatory defects can be classified into four classes based on WHO definitions. These classes suggest different etiologies and, consequently, different optimal treatment approaches.[100,101]

Class I: Hypogonadotropic hypogonadism. Hypogonadotropic hypogonadal patients comprise 5 to 10 percent of anovuatory women. These patients have low serum FSH and estradiol levels. This category includes women with hypothalamic amenorrhea, stress-related amenorrhea, anorexia nervosa, and Kallmann's syndrome. These women will respond to gonadotropin therapy for ovulation induction.

Class II: Eugonadotropic hypogonadism. Patients are eugonadotropic, normoestrogenic, but anovulatory and constitute the majority of anovulatory women evaluated (60 to 85 percent). They exhibit normal FSH and estradiol levels. This category includes women with the polycystic ovary syndrome (PCOS), among other disorders. These women respond to most ovulatory agents.

Class III: Hypergonadotropic hypogonadism. These patients account for 10 to 30 percent of women evaluated for anovulation. These patients tend to be amenorrheic and hypoestrogenic, a category that includes all variants of ovarian failure and ovarian resistance syndromes. These patients will not respond to ovulation induction but are candidates for oocyte donation.

Class IV: Hyperprolactinemic anovulation. Even though this is the fourth group, practitioners tend not to use the class IV label. Hyperprolactinemia contributes to 5 to 10 percent of women with anovulation. Gonadotropin secretion is inhibited by elevated prolactin levels. Women in this category with no obvious etiology for hyperprolactinemia (such as neuroleptic drug use or hypothyroidism) should undergo a head CT scan or magnetic resonance imaging (MRI). These patients respond well to medications that lower prolactin secretion.

Pharmacologic Agents for Ovulation Induction

The armamentarium in ovulation induction consists of a basic set of medical or surgical maneuvers, but treatment regimens depend on the goal of therapy. The goal of ovulation induction is the formation of a single dominant follicle and ovulation of one oocyte per cycle in a woman who has not been ovulating regularly. Treatment is tailored to avoid ovulation of more than two oocytes to decrease the risk of multiple gestations and ovarian hyperstimulation. In contrast, the goal of superovulation, or controlled ovarian hyperstimulation (COH), is to cause the release of more than one egg per cycle to increase the overall probability of conception. See Chapter 17 for additional discussion of ovulation induction for the treatment of the anovulatory patient.

Ovulation Induction with Clomiphene Citrate

Clomiphene is an orally active nonsteroidal agent with weak estrogenic effects. It modulates hypothalamic function by occupying estrogen receptors for prolonged periods, altering the concentration of estrogen receptors, and reducing the estrogen signaling process. In essence, it blocks the negative-feedback effects of circulating estrogen. In normally cycling women, clomiphene causes increased FSH and LH pulse frequency. In anovulatory women, clomiphene stimulates increased gonadotropin pulse amplitude. Regardless, circulating levels of LH and FSH rise, stimulating the development and ovulation of one or more oocytes. Clomiphene citrate (CC) is indicated in the treatment of women with WHO class II oligoovulation and anovulation. Women with WHO class I and class III ovulatory dysfunction tend to have little or no response to clomiphene.

Clomiphene treatment begins on the third to fifth days of the cycle at an initial dose of 50 mg/d for a total of 5 d. The dose can be increased by 50-mg increments to a maximum of 250 mg/d. The lowest effective dose can be administered for three to four cycles before the patient is considered a clomiphene failure. The LH surge generally occurs 5 to 12 d after the last clomiphene pill is ingested. Clomiphene responders therefore are counseled to perform timed intercourse every other day beginning 4 to 5 d after the last dose. Intensive monitoring of the clomiphene patient is not necessary. Ultrasound and urinary LH testing have not been shown to significantly increase pregnancy rates.[34] It may be useful, however, to confirm ovulation at least in the initial treatment cycle by measuring progesterone levels on days 22 to 24 of the cycle.

Using clomiphene treatment, ovulation is induced in 80 percent of well-selected patients,[102] and approximately 40 percent conceive.[103] Approximately 70 percent of these patients will be ovulatory after three treatment cycles. A systematic review of randomized trials comparing the efficacy of clomiphene versus placebo in women with oligoovulatory infertility demonstrated a statistically significant increase in the pregnancy rate [odds ratio (OR) 3.41; 95 percent confidence interval 4.23–9.48] per treatment cycle in women who received clomiphene.[104] In couples with unexplained infertility, the combination of intrauterine insemination (IUI) with clomiphene treatment was shown to increase the pregnancy rate from 3.3 percent in the placebo group to 9.5 percent in the CC-IUI group.[105]

There is approximately a 10 percent multiple-pregnancy rate, almost exclusively consisting of twins (9 percent), and rarely triplet (0.3 percent) gestations, with this treatment. Clomiphene has not been associated with an increased risk of ectopic pregnancy[106] or congenital malformations.[107] Side effects include vasomotor instability (10 percent), abdominal distension and discomfort (6 percent), breast discomfort (2 percent), nausea and vomiting (2 percent), visual symptoms (1.5 percent), and headaches (1.3 percent). The risk of ovarian hyperstimulation syndrome is less than 1 percent.

Ovulation Induction with Gonadotropins

Human menopausal (hMG) and recombinant gonadotropins are available for ovulation and superovulation induction. They are appropriate for both WHO class I and II patients. These commercial preparations are available in ampules containing 75 IU of medication. Various treatment protocols have been devised, largely based on stimulating the ovary with hMG or urinary or recombinant FSH for 7 to 14 d at a usual starting dose of 75 to 150 IU/d beginning on days 2 to 4 of the cycle. The patient is evaluated 4 to 7 d later, and treatment is adjusted based on the response of follicular development and circulating estradiol levels. When estradiol and follicle size indicate adequate follicular development (i.e., 1 to 2 follicles reaching 16 to 20 mm in diameter and an estradiol level >800 pg/mL but <2000 pg/mL), ovulation is triggered with a single injection of 5000 to 10,000 units of human chorionic gonadotropin (hCG).

The ovarian response is monitored closely to determine the optimal day for triggering ovulation and to detect early signs of ovarian hyperstimulation. Serum estradiol levels are useful to determine degree of follicular response and predict the risk for ovarian hyperstimulation. Stimulation should be discontinued and hCG withheld if more than three large follicles >15 mm are noted or if the serum estradiol level exceeds 2000 pg/mL in patients whose primary goal is ovulation induction.

Cumulative pregnancy rates of 45 to 90 percent[108,109] have been reported in women with normogonadotropic anovulation and hypothalamic amenorrhea after six treatment cycles.[108] Risks include increased incidence of ectopic pregnancy, a multiple-pregnancy rate of approximately 26 percent, and a rate of serious ovarian hyperstimulation syndrome (OHSS) of 1 to 2 percent.

Ovulation Induction in the PCOS Patient

Polycystic ovary syndrome (PCOS) is the most common cause of ovulatory infertility,[9] occurring in approximately 4 to 6 percent of reproductive-age women.[110–112] The diagnosis is based on evidence of: (1) oligoovulation, (2) hyperandrogenemia or clinical hyperandrogenism, and (3) exclusion of other common etiologies such as 21-hydroxylase (21-OH)–deficient nonclassic adrenal hyperplasia (NCAH), androgen-secreting tumors, Cushing's syndrome, and thyroid or prolactin abnormality. Up to 50 percent of women with PCOS are obese. Weight loss should be a primary goal in the obese PCOS patient desiring fertility. Increasing body mass index (BMI) is significantly correlated with increased serum testosterone levels, hirsutism, and infertility. Loss of even 5 to 10 percent of initial weight is associated with significant improvements in hyperandrogenemia and hyperinsulinemia. In addition, weight loss of 10 kg or greater is associated with restoration of spontaneous ovulation and pregnancy in 90 and 30 percent of patients, respectively.[113] Currently, the first line of therapy for ovulation induction is clomiphene citrate.

INSULIN SENSITIZERS IN THE PCOS PATIENT

Insulin resistance is seen in 50 to 70 percent of women with PCOS, whether lean or obese.[114,115] The use of insulin-sensitizing agents in these patients has gained increasing acceptance in the ovulation-induction regimen. Metformin is an orally active biguanide agent that enhances peripheral insulin sensitivity and inhibits hepatic gluconeogenesis. Metformin has been shown to significantly enhance menstrual cyclicity, hyperandrogenemia, hyperinsulinemia, and insulin sensitivity in insulin-resistant women with PCOS.[116] In overweight (BMI >28 kg/m^2) PCOS patients who had failed previously to ovulate on clomiphene, 500 mg metformin taken three times a day resulted in return of spontaneous ovulations in 34 percent; the addition of clomiphene citrate to this regimen resulted in 89 percent ovulation rates, compared with 8 percent in obese PCOS women treated with clomiphene alone.[117] Metformin is a relatively safe medication with limited side effects. Gastrointestinal complaints are the primary side effect seen in patients, i.e., nausea or vomiting (up to 25 percent), diarrhea (10 to 53 percent), and flatulence (12 percent). Neuromuscular complaints (9 percent), headaches (6 percent), impaired vitamin B_{12} metabolism (7 percent), and very rare cases of lactic acidosis have been reported. Metformin should be avoided in patients with impaired renal and hepatic function.

Similar studies on troglitazone, an insulin sensitizer of the thiazolidinedione class, have demonstrated improvements in androgen and insulin profiles and increased rates of spontaneous ovulation in obese PCOS patients.[118,119] However, troglitazone was withdrawn from the market due to an increased risk of fulminant hepatic failure. Other thiazolidinediones used in treating diabetes, such as pioglitazone and rosig-litazone, have been been shown to improve menstrual cyclicity, ovulatory rate, and insulin sensitivity in small preliminary studies.[120–123]

SURGICAL METHODS OF OVULATION INDUCTION IN THE PCOS PATIENT

Medical ovulation induction in the PCOS patient can be problematic. PCOS patients tend to exhibit extremes in clinical response: absence of follicular development or florid polyfollicular response and elevated risk of ovarian hyperstimulation syndrome. Surgical treatment of PCOS with ovarian wedge resection was associated with subsequent pregnancy in the original report by Stein and Leventhal[124] but was largely abandoned due to the significant risk of postoperative adhesions.[125] Recently, laparoscopic ovarian "drilling" by laser or diathermy has been shown to result in a high rate of subsequent spontaneous ovulation and conception. In a review of 15 controlled trials examining ovulation induction in infertile PCOS patients, cumulative pregnancy and spontaneous abortion rates were found to be comparable to those with gonadotropin therapy for ovulation induction.[126] In addition, multiple-pregnancy rates were significantly lower in women who conceived after ovarian drilling. However, adhesion rates of 20 to 70 percent have been reported after either electrocautery or laser drilling.[127,128] In addition, surgical ovulation induction is associated with inherent anesthetic and surgical risks, as well as the the potential for premature ovarian failure. We therefore recommend that ovarian drilling for ovulation induction in PCOS patients be reserved for the clomiphene-resistant patient who is unable or unwilling to proceed to gonadotropins.

Ovarian Hyperstimulation Syndrome (OHSS)

The ovarian hyperstimulation syndrome is a potentially life-threatening complication of ovulation and superovulation induction. It encompasses a clinical spectrum ranging from mild, with nausea and abdominal bloating with mildly enlarged ovaries, to severe, with massive ascites and ovarian enlargement associated with hemoconcentration, renal failure, hypovolemic shock, and thromboembolic episodes.[129] The incidence of OHSS after gonadotropin ovulation induction ranges from 7 (mild) to 4.2 percent (severe).[6]

The pathogenesis of OHSS is not fully understood, but it appears to stem from increased capillary permeability resulting from the release of vasoactive substances in response to ovarian stimulation. Symptoms may be exacerbated by hCG administration and the onset of pregnancy. Management of moderate and severe OHSS includes hospitalization, supportive care (monitoring, hydration, therapeutic paracentesis for abdominal and respiratory discomfort), and thromboembolism prophylaxis.[129] Prophylactic maneuvers include withholding hCG until symptoms remit ("coasting") and deferring embryo transfer and cryopreserving embryos in IVF patients. All women undergoing ovulation induction should be educated about the signs and symptoms of OHSS and instructed to contact their physician immediately should such symptoms arise.

▶ TREATMENT OF TUBAL FACTOR INFERTILITY

Tubal factor infertility is implicated in 30 to 40 percent of infertile couples. Treatment options for tubal disease are covered in Chap. 21 and include: (1) correction of proximal, distal, or complex tubal disease, (2) correction of periadnexal disease, and (3) correction of iatrogenic abnormalities (such as tubal sterilization).[6]

Although improvements in ART and embryo culture conditions increasingly have replaced surgical correction in tubal infertility, basic principles of tubal reconstruction remain essential. Microsurgical technique should be used: minimal tissue handling and trauma, good hemostasis, and use of small, nonreactive suture material when absolutely necessary. The laparoscopic approach should be favored when feasible. Careful attention should be paid to adhesion prevention. In general, surgical treatment for tubal infertility is most successful when disease is localized to the distal tube.[1] Poor prognostic factors for pregnancy following tubal surgery include tubal diameter exceeding 20 mm, dense pelvic adhesions, ovarian adhesions, lack of visible fimbriae, advanced age in the female partner, and increasing duration of infertility.[130] Chapter 21 details further the treatment of tubal infertility.

▶ TREATMENT OF THE INFERTILE MALE

Male subfertility is detected in up to 50 percent of infertile couples.[131] Almost half of men examined for subfertility will be diagnosed with a potentially reversible defect, such as endocrinopathy, varicocele, and ductal obstruction. Treatment in these conditions may result in pregnancy rates of 70, 40, and 35 percent of these patients, respectively.[132] In addition, the introduction of ICSI has enabled conception in couples who otherwise would have been referred for donor insemination or adoption.

Secondary Male Infertility/Hypogonadotropic Hypogonadism

When hypogonadotropic hypogonadism results from hyperprolactinemia, fertility often can be restored by decreasing prolactin secretion. Treatment depends on the etiology of the hyperprolactinemia. If the condition is medically induced, consideration should be given to discontinuing the responsible medication, if feasible. Hyperprolactinemia resulting from lactotroph hypertrophy or adenoma can be treated with a dopamine agonist, such as bromocriptine, cabergoline, or pergolide.[73] Normalization of serum prolactin and testosterone levels usually is accompanied by restoration of the sperm count 3 to 6 months later. Patients with hyperprolactinemia due to a macroadenoma can have permanent damage to the gonadotrophs due to mass effect from the lesion, and normalization of hyperprolactinemia may not be sufficient to restore testosterone levels and spermatogenesis. If improvement is not seen within 6 months, these men should be started on gonadotropin treatment.

Hypogonadotropic hypogonadism due to hypothalamic and pituitary disease can be treated with gonadotropin therapy. Treatment usually begins with hCG, which exerts biologic effects similar to that of LH, at doses of 1500 to 2000 IU subcutaneously or intramuscularly three times a day. The dose of hCG can be adjusted based on symptoms, semen parameters, and serum testosterone levels.[73] Patients who remain severly oligospermic or azoospermic after more than 6 months of hCG treatment should have exogenous gonadotropin added to their regimen. Human urinary menopausal gonadotropin (hMG) traditionally was given at doses of 37.5 to 75 IU three times a week until pregnancy occurred. Recombinant gonadotropins are now increasingly and successfully replacing human-derived products. Gonadotropin therapy results in good-quality spermatogenesis, and pregnancy frequently occurs with sperm concentrations of less than 20 million/mL.[73] Men with hypothalamic disease also can be treated with GnRH delivered in an intravenous or pulsatile subcutaneous manner. However, the need for a portable pump with attached catheter and needle renders this treatment inconvenient for long-term use.

Primary Hypogonadism/Testicular Disease

The most common cause of gonadal failure in men is Klinefelter's syndrome (47,XXY).[1] There is currently no effective treatment for sterility resulting from Klinefelter's syndrome. However, there have been reports of pregnancies initiated by Klinefelter patients. A small case series of seven men with nonmosaic Klinefelter syndrome

treated with ICSI resulted in one successful pregnancy.[133] Donor insemination remains a viable option for these couples. Other conditions associated with testicular failure include mumps orchitis and severe cryptorchidism.

Obstructive Abnormalities/Posttesticular Disease

Patients with obstructive abnormalities can be treated with surgery or ART techniques. Obstruction of the epididymis can be repaired surgically through reanastomosis procedures. Success rates depend on operator skill, site of reanastomosis, and duration of obstruction.[73] Reappearance of sperm can be seen in up to 85 percent of patients; success is highest when obstruction is due to prior vasectomy and lower with other causes such as CBAVD or after infection. Ejaculatory duct obstruction can be corrected with transurethral resection; this can result in improved semen quality and pregnancy rates.[73] Several ART techniques have emerged to facilitate sperm retrieval. These include microsurgical epididymal sperm aspiration (MESA) and either open biopsy or fine-needle testicular sperm aspiration (TESA).

Varicocele

A varicocele is the dilatation in the pampiniform plexus of the scrotum. In a WHO study of over 9000 men, varicocele was detected in 11 percent of men with normal semen parameters and 25 percent of men with abnormal parameters on semen analysis.[134] The link between male infertility and varicocele has been ascribed to increased testicular temperature, impaired clearance of metabolites and toxins, hypoxia, and stasis.[73] For many years, the management of varicocele and ensuing fecundity was controversial. However, in 1997, the WHO published the results of a large, prospective, multicenter clinical trial comparing immediate versus delayed (1 year later) varicocele ligation.[135] The results showed a 35 percent cumulative pregnancy rate in the immediate-operation group versus 17 percent in the delayed group. Despite flaws in the study, these results and that of smaller studies suggest that ligation should be considered in infertile men with large varicoceles.

Intrauterine Insemination (IUI)

The artificial insemination procedure has evolved considerably. Historically, insemination of whole semen had been performed when sperm delivery via coitus was not possible. However, due to the high potential for reaction to prostaglandins, bacteria, and proteins in whole semen, this has been replaced largely by the use of washed sperm for intrauterine insemination (IUI). IUI consists of washing the semen specimen in culture medium, resuspending the sperm in a small aliquot of medium, and injecting the sperm into the endometrial cavity through a catheter traversing the cervical canal. IUI requires at least 1 million total sperm be inseminated because lower counts rarely lead to pregnancy.[136]

IUI has been practiced widely as an empirical treatment for male factor infertility and as a means to bypass defects in sperm–cervical mucus interaction. However, in two large, randomized, controlled trials of couples presenting with oligoasthenospermia and infertility, IUI alone was not shown to improve pregnancy rates above those achieved through timed intercourse.[137,138] However, a subsequent review that pooled data from six randomized, controlled studies demonstrated that IUI alone significantly increased the probability of conception in couples with male factor infertility. All included trials used either Percoll or swim-up techniques for sperm preparation.[139]

The practice of IUI has broadened considerably in the setting of female ovulation induction with clomiphene citrate or gonadotropins. In a prospective, randomized study sponsored by the National Institutes of Health (NIH), IUI with and without gonadotropin superovulation induction was demonstrated to significantly increase pregnancy rates in couples with unexplained infertility or endometriosis in the female partner.[140] The combination of clomiphene plus IUI also was shown to increase pregnancy rates significantly from 3.3 to 9.5 percent in couples with unexplained infertility or surgically corrected endometriosis.[105]

Intracytoplasmic Sperm Injection (ICSI)

ICSI is a micromanipulation technique injecting a single sperm into the cytoplasm of a mature oocyte.[141] The introduction of this technology in 1992 revolutionized the treatment of male infertility.[142] The procedure requires that oocytes be retrieved, usually resulting from controlled ovarian hyperstimulation. The oocyte is then stripped of the cumulus mass and corona radiata and immobilized in a droplet of medium. A single sperm is injected directly through the zona pellucida and oolema into the ooplasm (Fig. 15-4).

ICSI has improved the prognosis for men with severe semen abnormalities and even azoospermia. Indications for ICSI include all male factor infertility and cases where standard treatment options are limited by: (1) fewer than 2 million total motile spermatozoa per ejaculate, (2) prior fertilization failure with IVF, (3) infertility associated with antisperm antibodies, (4) greater than 95 percent abnormal sperm morphology, and (5) specific spermatozoa defects impairing spermatozoa-oocyte interaction. Overall fertilization rates in ICSI are approximately 40 to 70 percent.[143] These results are independent of the origin of the spermatozoa or cause of azoospermia.

Approximately 30 percent of ICSI cycles result in a live birth.[144] Infertile couples with male factor as the primary etiology should seek ART treatment in centers offering ICSI. Although ICSI

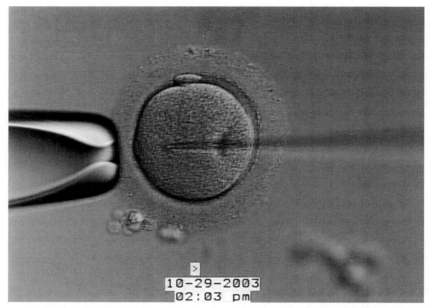

Figure 15-4 Intracytoplasmic sperm injection (ICSI). Insertion of pipette into oolemma and sperm injection. *(Photomicrograph courtesy of Dr. David Hill.)*

has not been shown to increase the incidence of major congenital defects above that of standard IVF, patients should be counseled regarding the potential transmission of genetic abnormalities, such as chromosomal abnormalities and Y chromosome microdeletions (see also Chap. 5).[143,145] Male offspring conceived through ICSI are at risk for inherit spermatogenic defects. In addition, recent reports suggest an increased incidence of imprinting disorders such as Angelman syndrome.[146,147] See Chapter 16 for additional discussion of treatment options in male infertility.

▶ TREATMENT OF UNEXPLAINED INFERTILITY

In up to 17 percent of couples, no specific etiology for infertility can be determined despite thorough evaluation. Before the diagnosis of unexplained infertility can be made, the evaluation must include documentation of ovulation and ovarian reserve, tubal patency, and semen analysis, usually including a laporoscopic evaluation of the pelvis. Expectant management in these couples is associated with a 1 to 3 percent per cycle pregnancy rate and should be reserved for couples in which the female partner is younger than 32 years of age. Lifestyle changes in the female partner, such as smoking cessation, reduction of alcohol and caffeine intake, and weight normalization, may improve fertility.[148] Couples with unexplained infertility and low coital frequency should be counseled to increase frequency to at least twice a week, with greater frequency during the fertile window. In a retrospective analysis of 45 studies in couples with unexplained infertility, the combined clinical pregnancy rates per initiated cycle were as follows: 1.3 to 4.1 percent with no treatment, 3.8 percent with IUI, 5.6 percent with clomiphene alone, 8.3 percent with clomiphene plus IUI, 7.7 percent with hMG, 17.1 percent with hMG plus IUI, and 20.7 percent with IVF.[149] The estimated cost

► **TABLE 15-7:** ESTIMATED PER-CYCLE COST AND PREGNANCY RATES FOR TREATMENT OF UNEXPLAINED INFERTILITY

Intervention	Cost per Cycle (US Dollars)	Pregnancy Rate per Cycle
Expectant	<$50	1–3%
Clomiphene citrate	$100	4–6%
Intrauterine insemination (IUI)	$300	4–6%
Clomiphene plus IUI	$400	7–9%
Gonadotropin injections	$2000	4–10%
Gonadotropic plus IUI	$2300	9–16%
In vitro fertilization	≥$8000	20–40%

Adapted with permission from Barbieri, 2003[148].

per pregnancy achieved increased with higher-technology treatments: $10,000 for clomiphene plus IUI, $17,000 for hMG plus IUI, and $50,000 for IVF. Treatment options should progress in a stepwise fashion (Table 15-7), beginning with low-cost, noninvasive procedures (lifestyle changes, IUI, clomiphene citrate) before progressing to high-cost and high-intensity treatments (gonadotropin superovulation induction, IVF).[1] See Chapter 18 for additional discussion of treatment options in the couple with unexplained infertility.

► ASSISTED REPRODUCTIVE TECHNOLOGY (ART)

Assisted reproductive technology encompasses all techniques involving the manipulation of gametes, zygotes, and embryos and will be covered indepth in subsequent chapters. Available procedures include gamete intrafallopian transfer (GIFT), zygote intrafallopian transfer (ZIFT), IVF, and ICSI. In the year 2000, more than 99,000 ART cycles were initiated, resulting in over 25,000 live births.[144]

IVF involves the retrieval of oocytes (usually after a controlled ovarian hyperstimulation regimen), fertilization of recovered oocytes with spermatozoa in vitro, culture of embryos in the laboratory, and transfer of embryos to the uterus. Current indications for IVF include fallopian tube occlusion or disease, severe pelvic disease, failed tubal reconstruction, endometriosis, unexplained infertility, and male factor infertility. Pregnancy rates after IVF are variable and subject to sample-size limitations, selection bias, and lack of standardization.[45] However, national and clinic-specific data from the national IVF registry are published annually by the Centers for Disease Control and Prevention (CDC) in the United States. Cumulative live-birth rates per embryo transfer have increased progressively during the past 5 years from 28 to 32 percent.[144] IVF treatment confers the highest per-cycle pregnancy rate within the shortest duration of treatment. However, IVF is associated with the highest degree of invasiveness and a high risk for multiple gestations (approximately 32 percent twins and 5 percent higher-order gestations). Nevertheless, IVF has assumed a central role in the treatment of infertility. Improvements in technique and accessibility continue to enhance fertility outcomes and further our understanding of all aspects of reproduction (see Chap. 21).

► LIFESTYLE AND ENVIRONMENTAL FACTORS

Lifestyle and environment exposures potentially can alter male and female reproductive tissues and thereby impair fertility.[150] Many studies have demonstrated that cigarette smoking has a significant negative effect on reproductive efficiency.[151,152] Smoking has been associated with impaired cervical mucus production, altered tubal ciliary transport, diminished spermatogenesis, decreased estradiol production, and reduced fecundability.[153] In patients undergoing IVF, smoking is associated with increased rates of spontaneous miscarriage and reduced chance of successful term pregnancy. In addition, cytogenetic analysis of oocytes retrieved from women who were heavy, light, or passive smokers and nonsmokers demonstrated that the incidence of oocyte diploidy, reflecting meiotic immaturity, correlated positively with amount of cigarette smoke exposure.[154] In couples desiring fertility, both partners should be counseled to stop smoking.

Alcohol consumption may have a threshold effect on infertility.[150] Harmful drinking patterns have been defined as heavy routine drinking (two or more drinks per day) and binge drinking (five or more drinks at one time). Heavy or frequent alcohol consumption in women has been associated with increased rates of menstrual abnormality, spontaneous abortion, and teratogenic effects, including fetal alcohol syndrome.[150] While heavy alcohol use in men has been associated erectile dysfunction and even with testicular atrophy,[155] heavy drinking has not been associated with diminished male fecundability or poor semen quality.[150]

The correlation between alcohol consumption and time to conception or waiting time to pregnancy is controversial. A European multicenter study of over 4000 couples demonstrated an increased waiting time in women consuming 8 or more drinks per week compared with nondrinkers.[156] A Danish study of self-reported data from 39,612 women showed no difference in waiting time in nulliparous women with moderate or high alcohol intake compared with nondrinkers. However, parous women consuming more than 14 drinks per week showed a nonsignificant trend to longer waiting time. Low levels of alcohol intake (fewer than 5 drinks per week) has not consistently shown to reduce female fecundability.[150] However, in a prospective study following 423 couples planning their first pregnancy, alcohol consumption by the woman was associated with a dose-dependent decrease in fecundability, even with light consumption of 1 to 5 drinks per week.[157] While the impact of alcohol on fecundability is not entirely clear, it is reasonable to encourage couples trying to conceive to limit or avoid alcohol consumption.[150]

The effect of caffeine consumption on fertility suggests a similar dose-dependent effect. While light caffeine consumption has not been associated with reduced fecundability,[158,159] the data on heavy caffeine intake suggests reduced fecundability and longer delay to achieve pregnancy. In a retrospective study of 1430 parous women, consumption of more than 300 mg caffeine per day was significantly associated with increased delay before conception.[159] A subsequent retrospective, multicenter study demonstrated that women with high caffeine consumption (exceeding 500 mg caffeine per day) had a significantly longer delay before achieving pregnancy.[160] In general, we counsel women with infertility to limit their caffeine consumption to <300 mg/d and ideally to less than 100 mg/d.

Every aspect of the infertility evaluation is potentially associated with emotional and psychological stress for the couple. While the incidence of psychopathology is not increased over that of fertile controls,[161] both male and female infertility patients demonstrated increased emotional distress.[14,162] The infertility evaluation, treatment process, and negative outcomes certainly can exert additional pressure on patients, potentially exacerbating preexisting psychiatric illness. In addition, a prospective study of over 150 women undergoing ART treatment demonstrated that higher levels of baseline acute and chronic stress were associated with negative outcomes in numbers of embryos retrieved and livebirth rates.[163] All couples experiencing infertility should be counseled on the psychological resources available: staff psychologists, counselors, and support groups. They should be especially encouraged to seek psychological support at the start of treatment, when psychiatric issues become manifest, after unsuccessful treatment, and with pregnancy loss.[14] In our practice, we find that the support of a clinical psychologist specializing in infertility patients can be an invaluable aid to our patients.

KEY POINTS

1. The clinical definition of infertility is the inability to conceive after 12 months of frequent, unprotected coitus. However, in certain populations (such as advanced maternal age or suspected endocrinopathy), it is not advisable to wait an entire year before evaluation and treatment is begun.

2. Male and female partners contribute equally to the etiology of infertility.

3. Both partners should be present at the initial infertility evaluation to enable adequate review of medical and reproductive histories.

4. Primary diagnostic evaluation of the infertile couple should be broad and noninvasive and includes semen analysis, documentation of ovulation, and assessment of female genital tract patency.

5. Women over the age of 35 should be assessed for ovarian reserve with baseline day 3 FSH and estradiol testing.

6. HSG is the best initial test to screen for female reproductive tract patency.

7. An elevation of the midluteal serum progesterone level is a sensitive and effective method to document ovulatory cycles.

8. Detection of the urinary LH surge is a sensitive indicator of the serum LH surge and predicts probable ovulation.

9. All male partners should undergo semen analysis on at least two separate occasions. If the semen analysis is abnormal, it should be repeated.

10. Men with severe oligospermia and azoospermia should be counseled regarding karyotypic and genetic evaluation to rule out a *CFTR* mutation and Y chromosome microdeletions. When a genetic or chromosomal abnormality is found, genetic counseling is recommended before proceeding to ICSI.

11. The diagnosis of unexplained infertility can be inferred only after the couple has completed a thorough infertility evaluation that includes a minimum of semen analysis, documentation of ovulatory status and ovarian reserve, a test of female reproductive tract patency and laparoscopic evaluation of the pelvis.

12. Treatment of unexplained infertility should be tailored based on efficacy, safety, cost, female age and ovarian reserve, and immediate reproductive goals. Treatment may begin with low-cost and low-invasiveness procedures, such as clomiphene and PUI, before progressing to more expensive and invasive modalities.

13. Treatment for WHO class I and II ovulatory infertility should be individualized based in patient age and the nature of ovulatory dysfunction. Options include ovulation induction with clomiphene citrate (class II) or human menopausal and recombinant gonadotropins (classes I and II).

14. IVF is the treatment modality associated with the greatest per-cycle pregnancy rate in the shortest duration of treatment. However, IVF is also associated with the greatest cost and invasiveness.

REFERENCES

1. Barbieri RL. Infertility, in Yen SS, Jaffe RB, Barbieri RL (eds), *Reproductive Endocrinology,* 4th ed. Philadelphia: Saunders, 1999; pp 562–593.
2. Cramer DW, Walker AM, Schiff I. Statistical methods in evaluating the outcome of infertility therapy. *Fertil Steril* 1979;32:80–86.

3. Guzick DS. Evaluation of the infertile couple. *UpToDate Online* 2004 *(http://www.uptodate. com)*.

4. Guttmacher AF. Factors affecting normal expectancy of conception. *JAMA* 1956;161:855–860.

5. Tietze C, Guttmacher AF, Rubin S. Time required for conception in 1727 planned pregnancies. *Fertil Steril* 1950;1:338–346.

6. Yao M., Schust D. Infertility in Berek J (ed.), in *Novak's Gynecology* 13th ed. Philadelphia: Lippincott, Williams & Wilkins, 2002; pp 973–1066.

7. Chandra A, Mosher WD. The demography of infertility and the use of medical care for infertility. *Infert Reprod Med Clin North Am* 1994; 5:283–296.

8. Abma JC, Chandra A, Mosher WD, et al. Fertility, family planning and women's health: New data from the 1995 National Survey of Family Growth. *Vital Health Stat* 1997;19:1–114.

9. Hull MG, Galzner CM, Kelly NJ, et al. Population study of causes, treatment and outcome of infertility. *Br Med J* 1985;91:1693–1697.

10. Mosher WD, Pratt WF. The demography of infertility in the United States, in Asch RH, Studd JW (eds), *Annual Progress in Reproductive Medicine*. Pearl River, NJ: Parthenon, 1993; pp 37–43.

11. Collins JA, So Y, Wilson EH, et al. Clinical factors affecting pregnancy rates among infertile couples. *Can Med Assoc J* 1984;130:269–273.

12. Wilcox AJ, Weinberg CR, Baird DD. Timing of sexual intercourse in relation to ovulation: Effects on probability of conception, survival of the pregnancy, and sex of the baby. *N Engl J Med* 1995;333:1517–1521.

13. Stanford JB, White GL, Hatasaka H. Timing intercourse to achieve pregnancy: Current evidence. *Obstet Gynecol* 2002;100:1333–1341.

14. Bradshaw K, Carr B. Modern diagnostic evaluation of the infertile couple, *in* Blackwell RE, Carr BR (eds), *Textbook of Reproductive Medicine*. New York: McGraw-Hill, 1998; pp 533–548.

15. Tunbridge WM, Evered DC, Hall R, et al. The spectrum of thyroid disease in a community: The Whickham survey. *Clin Endocrinol (Oxf)* 1977;7:481–493.

16. Vanderpump MP, Tunbridge WM. Epidemiology and prevention of clinical and subclinical hypothyroidism. *Thyroid* 2002;12:839–847.

17. Cramer DW, Sluss PM, Powers RD, et al. Serum prolactin and TSH in an in vitro fertilization population: Is there a link between fertilization and thyroid function? *J Assist Reprod Genet* 2003;20:210–215.

18. Malcolm CE, Cumming DC. Does anovulation exist in eumenorrheic women? *Obstet Gynecol* 2003;102:317–318.

19. Noyes RW, Clewe TH, Bonney WA, et al. Searches for ova in the human uterus and tubes: Review, clinical methodology and summary of findings. *Am J Obstet Gynecol* 1966;96:157–167.

20. Clewe TH, Morgenstern LL, Nyoes RW, et al. Searches for ova in the human uterus and tubes: II. Clinical and laboratory data on nine successful searches for human ova. *Am J Obstet Gynecol* 1971;109:313–334.

21. Moghissi KS. Ovulation detection. *Reprod Endocrinol* 1992;21:39–55.

22. Grinsted J, Jacobsen JD, Grinsted L, et al. Prediction of ovulation. *Fertil Steril* 1989;52:388–393.

23. Crosignani PG, Rubin BL. Optimal use of infertility diagnostic tests and treatments. The ESHRE Capri Workshop Group. *Hum Reprod* 2000;15:723–723.

24. Guermandi E, Vegett W, Bianchi MM, et al. Reliability of ovulation tests in infertile women. *Obstet Gynecol* 2001;97:92–96.

25. Hull GM, Savage PE, Bromham DR, et al. The value of a single serum progesterone measurement in the midluteal phase: A criterion of a potentially fertile cycle ("ovulation") derived from treated and untreated conception cycles. *Fertil Steril* 1982;37:355–360.

26. Elkind-Hirsch K, Goldzieher JW, Gibbons WE, et al. Evaluation of the OvuStick urinary luteinizing hormone kit in normal and stimulated menstrual cycles. *Obstet Gynecol* 1986;67:450–453.

27. Noyes RW, Hertig AT, Rock J. Dating the endometrial biopsy. *Am J Obstet Gynecol* 1975;122:262–263.

28. Scott RT, Snyder RR, Bagnall J, Reed KD, et al. Evaluation of the impact of intraobserver variability on endometrial dating and the diagnosis of luteal phase defects. *Fertil Steril* 1993;60:652–657.

29. Balasch J, Fabregues F, Creus M, et al. The usefulness of endometrial biopsy for luteal phase evaluation in infertility. *Hum Reprod* 1992;7:973–977.

30. Marinho AL, Sallan HN, Goessens LK, et al. Real time pelvic ultrasonography during the periovulatory period of patients attending an artificial insemination clinic. *Fertil Steril* 1982;37: 633–638.

31. Leader A, Wiseman D, Taylor PJ. The prediction of ovulation: A comparison of the basal body temperature graph, cervical mucus score, and real-time pelvic ultrasonography. *Fertil Steril* 1985;43:385–388.

32. Ecochard R, Marret H, Rabilloud M, et al. Sensitivity and specificity of ultrasound indices of ovulation in spontaneous cycles. *Eur J Obstet Gynecol* 2000;91:59–64.

33. Vermesh M, Kletzky OA, Davajan V, et al. Monitoring techniques to predict and detect ovulation. *Fertil Steril* 1987;47:259–264.

34. Smith YR, Randolph JF, Christman GM, et al. Comparison of low-technology and high-technology monitoring of clomiphene citrate ovulation induction. *Fertil Steril* 1998;70:165–168.

35. Jordan J, Craig K, Clifton D, Soules MR. Luteal phase defect: The sensitivity and specificity of diagnostic methods in common clinical use. *Fertil Steril* 1994;62:54–62.

36. Davis OK, Berkeley AS, Naus GJ, et al. The incidence of luteal phase defect in normal, fertile women, determined by serial endometrial biopsies. *Fertil Steril* 1989;51:582–586.

37. Tietze C. Reproductive span and rate of reproduction among Hutterite women. *Fertil Steril* 1957;8:89–97.

38. Navot D, Drews MR, Bergh PA, et al. Age-related decline in female fertility is not due to diminished capacity of the uterus to sustain embryo implantation. *Fertil Steril* 1994;61:97–101.

39. Sauer MV, Paulson RJ, Lobo RA. Reversing the natural decline in human fertility: An extended trial of oocyte donation to women with advanced reproductive age. *JAMA* 1992;268:1275–1279.

40. McGee EA, Hsueh AJ. Initial and cyclic recruitment of ovarian follicles. *Endocr Rev* 2000;21: 200–214.

41. Keefe DL, Niven-Fairchild T, Powell S, Buradagunta S. Mitochondrial deoxyribonucleic acid deletions in oocytes and reproductive aging in women. *Fertil Steril* 1995;64:577–583.

42. Warburton D. Reproductive loss: How much is preventable? *N Engl J Med* 1987;316:158–160.

43. Van Rooij IA, Bancsi LF, Broekmans FJ, et al. Women older than 40 years of age and those with elevated follicle-stimulating hormone levels differ in poor response rate and embryo quality in in vitro fertilization. *Fertil Steril* 2003;79:482–488.

44. Toner JP, Philput CB, Jones GS, Muasher SJ. Basal follicle-stimulating hormone level is a better predictor of in vitro fertilization performance than age. *Fertil Steril* 1991;55:784–791.

45. Paulsen R. In vitro fertilization. *UpToDate Online,* Oct. 3, 2003 *(http://www.uptodate.com).*

46. Csemiczky G, Harlin J, Fried G. Predictive power of clomiphene citrate challenge test for failure of in vitro fertilization treatment. *Acta Obstet Gynaecol Scand* 2002;81:954–961.

47. Van der Stege JG, van der Linden PJ. Useful predictors of ovarian stimulation response in women undergoing in vitro fertilization. *Gynecol Obstet Invest* 2001;52:43–46.

48. Rebar RW. Practical evaluation of hormonal status, in Yen SS, Jaffe RB, Barbieri RL (eds), *Reproductive Endocrinology,* 4th ed. Philadelphia: Saunders, 1999:709–747.

49. Hannoun A, Abu Musa A, Awwad J, et al. Clomiphene citrate challenge test: cycle to cycle variability of cycle day 10 follicle stimulating hormone level. *Clin Exp Obstet Gynecol* 1998;25:155–156.

50. Westrom L. Incidence, prevalence and trends of acute pelvic inflammatory disease and its consequences in industrialized countries. *Am J Obstet Gynecol* 1980;138:880.

51. Thonneau P, Quesnot S, Ducot B, et al. Risk factors for female and male infertility: Results of a case-control study. *Hum Reprod* 1992;7: 55–58.

52. Grodstein F, Goldman MB, Cramer DW. Relation of tubal infertility to history of sexually transmitted diseases. *Am J Epidemiol* 1993;137: 577–584.

53. Bahamondes L, Bueno JG, Hardy E, et al. Identification of main risk factors for tubal infertility. *Fertil Steril* 1994;61:478–482.

54. Westrom LV. Sexually transmitted diseases and infertility. *Sex Transm Dis* 1994;21:S32–37.

55. Lalos O. Risk factors for tubal infertility among infertile and fertile women. *Eur J Obstet Gynecol Reprod Biol* 1998;29:129–136.

56. Rosenfel DL, Seidman SM, Bronson RA, Scholl GM. Unsuspected chronic pelvic inflammatory disease in the infertile female. *Fertil Steril* 1983; 39:44–48.

57. Eckert LO, Hawes SE, Wolner-Hanssen P, et al. Prevalence and correlates of antibody to chlamydial heat shock protein in women attending sexually transmitted disease clinics and women with confirmed pelvic inflammatory disease. *J Infect Dis* 1997;175:1453–1458.

58. Mol BW, Dijkman B, Wertheim P, et al. *Chlamydia* antibody titers in the diagnosis of tubal pathology: A meta-analysis. *Fertil Steril* 1997;67:1031–1037.

59. Forsey JP, Caul EO, Paul ID, Hull MG. *Chlamydia trachomatis,* tubal disease, and the incidence of symptomatic and asymptomatic infection following hysterosalpingography. *Hum Reprod* 1990;5:444–447.

60. Stumpf PG, March CM. Febrile morbidity following hysterosalpingography: Identification of risk factors and recommendations for prophylaxis. *Fertil Steril* 1980;33:487–492.

61. Swart P, Mol B,WJ, van der Veen F, et al. The accuracy of hysterosalpingography and the diagnosis of tubal pathology: A meta-analysis. *Fertil Steril* 1995;64:486–491.

62. Tuveng JM, Vold I, Jerve F, et al. Hysterosalpingography: Value in estimating tubal function, and risk of infectious complications. *Act Eur Fertil* 1985;16:125–128.

63. Mol BW, Collins JA, Van Der Veen F, Bossuyt PM. Cost-effectiveness of hysterosalpingography, laparoscopy, and chlamydia antibody testing in subfertile couples. *Fertil Steril* 75;3:571–580.

64. Watson A, Van der Kerckhove P, Lilford R, et al. A meta-analysis of the therapeutic role of oil soluble contrast media at hysterosalpingography: A surprising result? *Fertil Steril* 1994;61:470–477.

65. Alantas C, Aksoy E, Akarsu C, et al. Evaluation of intrauterine abnormalities in infertile patients by sonohysterography. *Hum Reprod* 1997;12:487–490.

66. Marcoux S, Maheux R, Berube S, et al. Laparoscopic surgery in infertile women with minimal or mild endometriosis. *N Engl J Med* 1997;337:217–222.

67. Guzick DS. Evaluation of the infertile couple. *UpToDate Online* 2004 *(http://www.uptodate.com).*

68. Belisle S, Collins JA. The value of laparoscopy among infertile women with tubal patency. *J Soc Obstet Gynecol Can* 1996;18:326–336.

69. Eimers JM, te Velde ER, Gerritse R, et al. The validity of the postcoital test for estimating the probability of conceiving. *Am J Obstet Gynecol* 1994;171:65–70.

70. Oei SG, Helmerhorst FM, Bloemenkamp KW, et al. Effectiveness of the postcoital test: Randomised controlled trial. *Br Med J* 1998;317:502–505.

71. Swerdloff RS, Wang C. Causes of male infertility. *UpToDate Online,* 2004 *(http: //www.uptodate. com).*

72. de Kretser DM. Male infertility. Lancet 1997;349:787–790.

73. Swerdloff RS, Wang C. Evaluation of male infertility. *UpToDate Online,* 2004 *(http://www. uptodate.com).*

74. Kruger TF, Menkveld R, Lombard CJ, et al. Sperm morphologic features as a prognostic factor in in vitro fertilization. *Fertil Steril* 1986;46:1118–1123.

75. Aitken RJ. The role of free oxygen radicals and sperm function. *Int J Androl* 1989;12:95–97.

76. Abshagen K, Behre HM, Cooper TG, Nieschlag E. The influence of sperm surface antibodies on spontaneous pregnancy rates. *Fertil Steril* 1998;70:355–356.

77. Mortimer S. CASA: Practical aspects. *J Androl* 2000;21:515–524.

78. Davis RO, Katz DF. Computer-aided sperm analysis: Technology at a crossroads. *Fertil Steril* 1993;59:953–955.

79. Farrell PB, Foote RH, Zinaman MJ. Motility and other characteristics of human sperm can be measured by computer-assisted sperm analysis of samples stained with Heochst 33342. *Fertil Steril* 1996;66:446–453.

80. Chan SY, Wang C, Ng M, et al. Evaluation of computerized analysis of sperm movement characteristics and differential sperm tail swelling patterns in predicting human sperm in vitro fertilizing capacity. *J Androl* 1989;10:133–138.

81. Liu DY, Clarke GN, Baker HW. Relationship between sperm motility assessed with the Hamilton-Thorn motility analyzer and fertilization rates in vitro. *J Androl* 1991;12:231–239.

82. Barratt CLR, Tomlinson MN, Cooke ID. Prognostic significance of computerized motility analysis for in vivo fertility. *Fertil Steril* 1993;60:520–525.

83. Macleod IC, Irvine DS. Ther predictive value of computer-assisted semen analysis in the con-

text of a donor insemination programme. *Hum Reprod* 1995;10:580–586.

84. Krause W. Computer-assisted semen analysis systems: Comparison with routine evaluation and prognostic value in male fertility and assisted reproduction. *Hum Reprod* 1995:10(suppl):60–66.

85. Bonde JP, Ernst E, Jensen TK, et al. Relation between semen quality and fertility: A population-based study of 430 first-pregnancy planners. *Lancet* 1998;352:1172–1177.

86. Kruger TF, Acost AA, Simmons KF, et al. Predictive value of abnormal sperm morphology in in vitro fertilization. *Fertil Steril* 1988;49:112–117.

87. ESHRE Andrology Special Interest Group. Consensus workshop on advanced diagnostic andrology techniques. *Hum Reprod* 1996;11:1463–1479.

88. Mao C, Grimes DA. The sperm penetration assay: Can it discriminate between fertile and infertile men? *Am J Obstet Gynecol* 1988;159:279–286.

89. Oehninger S, Franken DR, Sayed E, et al. Sperm function assays and their predictive value for fertilization outcome in IVF therapy: A meta-analysis. *Hum Reprod Update* 2000;6:160–168.

90. Evenson DP, Larson KL, Jost LK. Sperm chromatin structure assay: Its clinical use for detecting sperm DNA fragmentation in male infertility and comparisons with other techniques. *J Androl* 2002;23:25–43.

91. Irvine DS, Twigg JP, Gordon EL, et al. DNA integrity in human spermatozoa: Relationships with semen quality. *J Androl* 2000;21:33–44.

92. Lopes S, Sun JG, Jurisicova A, et al. Sperm deoxyribonucleic acid fragmentation is increased in poor-quality semen samples and correlates with failed fertilization in intracytoplasmic sperm injection. *Fertil Steril* 1998;69:528–532.

93. Host E, Lindenberg S, Smidt-Jensen S. DNA strand breaks in human spermatozoa: Correlation with fertilization in vitro in oligozoospermic men and in men with unexplained infertility. *Acta Obstet Gynaecol Scand* 2000;79: 559–563.

94. Evenson DP, Jost LK, Marshall D, et al. Utility of the sperm chromatin structure assay as a diagnostic and prognostic tool in the human fertility clinic. *Hum Reprod* 1999;14:1039–1049.

95. Larson KL, De Jonge CJ, Barnes AM, et al. Relationship of assisted reproductive technique (ART) outcomes with sperm chromatin integrity and maturity as measured by the sperm chromatin structure assay (SCSA). *Hum Reprod* 2000;14:1717–1722.

96. De Kretser DM, Baker HWG. Infertility in men: Recent advances and continuing controversies. *J Clin Endocrinol Metab* 1999;84:3443–3450.

97. Bhasin S, MaK, de Kretser DM. Y chromosome microdeletions and male infertility. *Ann Med* 1997;29:261–263.

98. Kremer JA, Tuerlings JH, Meuleman EF et al. Microdeletions of the Y chromosome and intracytoplasmic sperm infjection: From gene to clinic. *Hum Reprod* 1997;12:687–691.

99. Page DC, Silber S, Brown LG. Men with infertility caused by AZFc deletion can produce sons by intracytoplasmic sperm injection, but are likely to trasmit the deletion and infertility. *Hum Reprod* 1999;14:1722–1726.

100. World Health Organization. *WHO Manual for the Standardized Investigation and Diagnosis of the Infertile Couple.* Cambridge, England: Cambridge University Press, 1993; pp 1–102.

101. ESHRE Capri Workshop Group. Anovulatory infertility. *Hum Reprod* 1995;10:1549–1553.

102. Gorlitsky GA, Kase NG, Speroff L. Ovulation and pregnancy rates with clomiphene citrate. *Obstet Gynecol* 1978;51:265–269.

103. Imani B, Eijkemans MJ, te Velde ER, et al. Predictors of chances to conceive in ovulatory patients during clomiphene citrate induciton of ovulation in normgonadotropic oligoamenorrheic infertility. *J Clin Endocrinol Metabl* 1999;84:1617–1622.

104. Hughes E, Collins J, Vanderkerckhove P. Clomiphene citrate for ovulation induction in women with oligomenorrhoea. *Cochrane Database Sys Rev* 2004;(2):CD000087.

105. Deaton JL, Gibson M, Blackmer KM, et al. A randomized, controlled trial of clomiphene citrate and intrauterine insemination in couples with unexplained infertility or surgically corrected endometriosis. *Fertil Steril* 1990;54:1083–1088.

106. Dickey RP, Matis R, Olar TT, et al. The occurrence of ectopic pregnancy with and without clomiphene citrate use in assisted and nonassisted reproductive technology. *J In Vitro Fert Embryo Transf* 1989;6:294–297.

107. Kurachi K, Aono T, Minagawa J, Miyake A. Congenital malformations of newborn infants after clomiphene-induced ovulation. *Fertil Steril* 1983;40:187–189.

108. Speroff L. Infertility, in Speroff L, Glass RH, Kase NG (eds), *Clinical Gynecologic Endocrinology and Infertility,* 6th ed. Philadelphia: Lippincott Williams & Wilkins, 1999; pp 1013–1042.

109. White DM, Polson DW, Kiddy D, et al. Induciton of ovulation with low-dose gonadotropins in polycystic ovary syndrome: An analysis of 109 pregnancies in 225 women. *J Clin Endocrinol Metab* 1996;81:3821–3824.

110. Knochenhauer ES, Key TJ, Kahsar-Miller M, et al. Prevalence of the polycystic ovary syndrome in unselected black and white women of the southeastern United States: A prospective study. *J Clin Endocrinol Metab* 1998;83:3078–3082.

111. Diamanti-Kandarakis, E, Kouli, CR, Bergiele, AT, et al. A survey of the polycystic ovary syndrome in the Greek island of Lesbos: Hormonal and metabolic profile. *J Clin Endocrinol Metab* 1999;84:4006–4011.

112. Asuncion M, Calvo RM, San Millan JL, et al. A prospective study of the prevalence of the polycystic ovary syndrome in unselected Caucasian women from Spain. *J Clin Endocrinol Metab* 2000;85:2434–2438.

113. Clark AM, Thornely B, Tomlinson L, et al. Weight loss in obese infertile women results in improvement in reproductive outcome for all forms of fertility treatment. *Hum Reprod* 1998; 13:1502–1505.

114. Dunaif A. Insulin resistance and the polycystic ovary syndrome: Mechanism and implications for pathogenesis. *Endocr Rev* 1997;18:774–800.

115. Ovalle F, Azziz R. Insulin resistance, polycystic ovary syndrome, and type 2 diabetes mellitus. *Fertil Steril* 2002;77:1095–1105.

116. Moghetti P, Castello R, Negri C, et al. Metformin effects on clinical features, endocrine and metabolic profiles, and insulin sensitivity in polycystic ovary syndrome: A randomized, double-blind, placebo-controlled 6-month trial, followed by open, long-term clinical evaluation. *J Clin Endocrinol Metab* 2000;85:139–146.

117. Nestler JE, Jakubowicz DJ, Evans WS, et al. Effects of metformin on spontaneous and clomiphene-induced ovualtion in the polycystic ovary syndrome. *N Engl J Med* 1998;338: 1876–1880.

118. Haesgawa I, Murakawa H, Suzuki M, et al. Effect of troglitazone on endocrine and ovulatory performance in women with insulin-resistance-related polycystic ovary syndrome. *Fertil Steril* 1999;71:323–327.

119. Dunaif A, Scott D, Finegood D, et al. The insulin-sensitizing agent troglitazone improves metabolic and reproductive abnormalities in the polycystic ovary syndrome. *J Clin Endocrin Metab* 1996;81:3299–3306.

120. Glueck CJ, Moreira A, Goldenberg N, et al. Pioglitazone and metformin in obese women with polycystic ovary syndrome not optimally responsive to metformin. *Hum Reprod* 2003;18: 1618–1625.

121. Romualdi D, Guido M, Giuliani M, et al. Selective effects of pioglitazone on insulin and androgen abnormalities in normo- and hyperinsulinaemic obese patients with polycystic ovary syndrome. *Hum Reprod* 2003;18:1210–1218.

122. Shobokshi A, Shaarawy M. Correction of insulin resistance and hyperandrogenism in polycystic ovary syndrome by combined rosiglitazone and clomiphene citrate therapy. *J Soc Gynecol Invest* 2003;10:99–104.

123. Ghazeeri G, Kutteh WH, Bryer-Ash M, et al. Effect of rosiglitazone on spontaneous and clomiphene citrate–induced ovulation in women with polycystic ovary syndrome. *Fertil Steril* 2003;79:562–566.

124. Stein IF, Leventhal ML. Amenorrhea associated with bilateral polycystic ovaries. *Am J Obstet Gynecol* 1935;29:181–182.

125. Portuondo JA, Melchor JC, Neyro JL, Alegre A. Periovarian adhesions following ovarian wedge resection or laparoscopic biopsy. *Endoscopy* 1984;16:14–16.

126. Fraquhar C, Vandekerckhove P, Lilford R. Laparoscopic "drilling" by diathermy or laser for ovulation induction in anovulatory polycystic ovary syndrome. *Cochrane Database Syst Rev* 2001;4:CD001122.

127. Naether OG, Baukloh V, Fischer R, Kowalczyk T. Long-term followup in 206 infertility patients with polycystic ovary syndrome after laparoscopic electrocautery of the ovarian surface. *Hum Reprod* 1994;9:2342–2349.

128. Pirwany I, Tulandi T. Laparoscopic treatment of polycystic ovaries: Is it time to relinquish the procedure? *Fertil Steril* 2003;80:241–251.

129. Whelan JG, Vlahos NF. The ovarian hyperstimulation syndrome. *Fertil Steril* 2000;73:883–896.

130. Schlaff WD, Hassiakos DK, Damewood MD, Rock JA. Neosalpinogostomy for distal tubal obtruction: Prognostic factors and impact of surgical technique. *Fertil Steril* 1990;54:984–990.

131. Sigman M. Assisted reproductive techniques and male infertiliy. *Urol Clin North Am* 1994;21:505–515.

132. Sandlow JA, Donovan JF. The infertile couple (letter). *N Engl J Med* 1994;330:1154–1155.

133. Reubinoff BE, Abeliovich D, Werner M, et al. A birth in nonmosaic Klinefelter's syndrome after testicular fine needle aspiration, intracytoplasmic sperm injection and preimplantation genetic diagnosis. *Hum Reprod* 1998;13:1887–1892.

134. WHO Scientific Group Report. *Recent Advances in Medically Assisted Conception*. WHO Technical Report Series 820. Geneva: World Health Organization, 1992. pp 1–111.

135. Hargreave TB. Varicocele: Overview and commentary on the results of the World Health Organization Varicocele Trial. in Waites GMH, Frick J, Baker GHW (eds), *Current Advances in Andrology*. Austria: Monduzzi, 1997:31–44.

136. Nulsen JC, Walsh S, Dumez S, Metzger DA. A randomized and longitudinal study of human menopausal gonadotropin with intrauterine insemination in the treatment of infertility. *Obstet Gynecol* 1993;82:780–786.

137. Hughes EG, Collins JP, Garner PR. Homologous artificial insemination for oligoasthenospermia: A randomized controlled study for comparing intracervical and intrauterine insemination. *Fertil Steril* 1987;48:278–281.

138. Ho J, Poon I, Chan S, Wang C. Intrauterine insemination is not useful in oligoasthenospermia. *Fertil Steril* 1989;51:682–684.

139. Cohlen BJ, Vandekeeckhove P, te Velde ER, Habbema JDF. Timed intercourse versus intrauterine insemination with or without ovarian hyperstimulation for subfertility in men. *Cochrane Database Sys Rev* 2003;3.

140. Guzick DS, Carson SA, Coutifaris C, et al. Efficacy of superovulation and intrauterine insemination in the treatment of infertility. *N Engl J Med* 1999;340:177–183.

141. Palermo G, Joris H, De P, et al. Pregnancies after intracytoplasmic injection of single spermatozoa into an oocyte. *Lancet* 1992;340:17–18.

142. Khorram O, Patrizio P, Wang C, Swedloff R. Reproductive technologies for male infertility. *J Clin Endocrinol Metab* 2001;86:2372–2379.

143. Miller JE, Smith TT. The effect of intracytoplasmic sperm injection and semen parameters on blastocyst development in vitro. *Hum Reprod* 2001;16:918–924.

144. CDC/NCCDPHP. *2001 Assisted Reproductive Technologies Success Rates*. Reproductive Health Information Source; *www.cdc.gov/nccdphp/drh/art.htm*.

145. Chang PL, Sauer MV, Brown S. Y chromosome microdeletion in a father and his four infertile sons. *Hum Reprod* 1999;14:2689–2694.

146. Cox GF, Burger J, Lip V, et al. Intracytoplasmic sperm injection may increase the risk of imprinting defects. *Am J Hum Genet* 2002;71:162–164.

147. Orstavik KH, Eiklid K, van der Hagen CB, et al. Another case of imprinting defect in a girl with Angelman syndrome who was conceived by intracytoplasmic semen injection. *Am J Hum Genet* 2003;72:218–219.

148. Barbieri RL. Treatment of unexplained infertility. *UpToDate Online*, 2004 (*http://www.uptodate.com*).

149. Guzik DS, Sullivan MW, Adamson GD, et al. Efficacy of treatment for unexplained infertility. *Fertil Steril* 1998;70:207–213.

150. Hruska KS, Furth PA, Seifer DB, et al. Environmental factors in infertility. Clin *Obstet Gynecol* 2000;43:821–829.

151. Olsen J, Rachootin P, Schiodt AV, Damsbo N. Tobacco use, alcohol consumption and infertility. *Int J Epidemiol* 1983;12:179–184.

152. Hughes EG, Brennan BG. Does cigarette smoking impair natural or assisted fecundity? *Fertil Steril* 1996;66:679–689.

153. Buster JE. Diagnostic evaluation of the infertile couple, in Stenchever M (ed), *Atlas of Clinical Gynecology and Reproductive Endocrinology*. Philadelphia: Current Medicine, 1999:9.2–9.18.

154. Zenzes MT, Wang P, Casper RF. Cigarette smoking may affect meiotic maturation of human oocytes. *Hum Reprod* 1995;10:3213–3217.

155. Anderson RA, Willis BR, Oswald C, Zaneveld LJ. Ethanol-induced male infertility: Impairment of spermatozoa. *J Pharmacol Exp Ther* 1983;225:479–486.

156. Olsen J, Bolumar F, Boldsen J, Bisanti L. Does moderate alcohol intake reduce fecundability? A European multicenter study on infertility and subfecundity. European Study Group on Infertility and Subfecundity. *Alcohol Clin Exp Res* 1997;21:206–212.

157. Jensen TK, Hjollund NH, Henriksen TB, et al. Does moderate alcohol consumption affect fertility? Follow-up study among couples planning first pregnancy. *Br Med J* 1998;22:505–510.

158. Curtis KM, Savitz DA, Arbuckle TE. Efefct of cigarette smoking, caffeine consumption and alcohol intake on fecundability. *Am J Epidemiol* 1997;146:32–41.

159. Stanton CK, Gray RH. Effects of caffeine consumption on delayed conception. *Am J Epidemiol* 1995;142:1322–1329.

160. Bolumar F, Olsen J, Rebagliato M, Bisanti L. Caffeine intake and delayed conception: A European multicenter study on infertility and subfecundity. European Study Group on Infertility and Subfecundity. *Am J Epidemiol* 1997;145:324–334.

161. Wilson JF, Kopitzke EJ. Stress and infertility. *Curr Womens Health Rep* 2002:2:194–199.

162. Conrad R, Schilling G, Langenbuch M, et al. Alexithymia in male infertility. *Hum Reprod* 2001;16:587–592.

163. Klonoff-Cohen H, Chu E, Natarajan L, Sieber W. A prospective study of stress among women undergoing in vitro fertilization or gamete intrafallopian transfer. *Fertil Steril* 2001;76:675–687.

CHAPTER 16

Male Infertility: Diagnosis and Treatment

Peter N. Kolettis

The field of male infertility is changing rapidly. Our understanding of some of the most severe forms of male factor infertility, such as nonobstructive azoospermia (NOA) and congenital bilateral absence of the vas deferens (CBAVD), has improved greatly secondary to advances in molecular genetics. Better empirical therapies, such as in vitro fertilization (IVF) with intracytoplasmic sperm injection (ICSI), can now help some couples with even the most severe male factor infertility conceive.[1] The cost and potential complications of assisted reproductive techniques (ARTs), however, should limit their use as first-line therapy and reinforce the importance of helping couples to conceive naturally by treating correctable conditions when present.[2–4]

The main purpose of the male infertility evaluation is to diagnose and treat correctable problems. This can allow a couple to conceive by the most natural, most cost-effective, and least invasive means. In addition, the evaluation may uncover either significant underlying medical or genetic pathology that is the cause of the infertility or incidental pathology that could affect the patient or his potential offspring. Finally, patients simply may desire information about their condition, even if it is not correctable, as a way of reassuring them they did not cause the problem themselves.

Of the 15 percent of couples with infertility, male factors are present in about 30 to 40 percent of cases.[5] A screening evaluation should be performed if a couple is unable to conceive after 1 year of unprotected intercourse. The evaluation can be initiated sooner if a man requests it or if known potential male or female factors, such as age over 35, are present. The initial screening evaluation includes a reproductive history and two semen analyses, ideally performed 1 month apart. A full evaluation (complete medical and reproductive history, physical examination by a male reproductive specialist, and two semen analyses) is recommended if the initial evaluation reveals an abnormal reproductive history or semen analysis.[6]

▶ EVALUATION

The complete evaluation of an infertile man consists of a medical history and physical examination and two semen analyses. Further evaluation can be carried out as indicated. In most cases, the evaluation can be completed in one or two office visits.

History

The male infertility specialist may be the first practitioner to interview the couple. Therefore, he or she should screen for risk factors for potential female factor infertility and initiate a referral, as well as perform the male factor evaluation. However, the couple still also should have a consultation with a female reproductive specialist. Any condition that affects reproductive or sexual function could impede the establishment of a pregnancy. The age of the partners, duration of unprotected intercourse, and previous pregnancies and fertility treatments should be noted. Documenting the sexual history is critical. The couple should be asked about the frequency and timing of intercourse, as well as the regularity of menstrual cycles. Because sperm can survive 48 h in the female reproductive tract, the optimal timing of intercourse is every day or every other day around the time of ovulation.[7] Sexual dysfunction should be addressed and treated. Erectile dysfunction (ED) and ejaculatory dysfunction can be signs of an underlying medical illness, such as vascular disease or diabetes mellitus. Further evaluation for these conditions should be carried out as indicated.

Specific questioning should be directed at identifying conditions such as cryptorchidism, spermatic cord torsion, previous inguinal or scrotal surgeries, or exposures to gonadotoxins that could affect fertility potential. It should be kept in mind that any general insult or illness can impair sperm production. Because a cycle of sperm production requires about 74 days, it may take 1 to 3 months to see any impact on the semen analysis. Similarly, improvement of a patient's semen analysis after an illness also may not be seen immediately. The critical features of the history are summarized in Table 16-1.[5]

Physical Examination

A thorough physical examination can reveal clues about the underlying cause of infertility.

▶ **TABLE 16-1:** EVALUATION OF MALE INFERTILITY: HISTORY[5]

- Age of partners
- Duration of infertility/duration of unprotected intercourse
- Previous pregnancies and outcomes
- Previous fertility treatments
- Sexual history
  - Frequency and timing of intercourse
  - Problems with ejaculation
  - Erectile dysfunction
- Conditions affecting the testes or reproductive function
  - Torsion
  - Mumps
  - Cryptorchidism
  - Inguinal or scrotal surgeries
  - Bladder neck or prostate surgery
  - Treatment for malignancy
- Urinary tract problems
  - Voiding dysfunction
  - Urinary tract infections (UTIs)
- Exposures
  - Occupational (chemical, radiation)
  - Heat
- Drugs
  - Alcohol
  - Alkylating agents
  - Allopurinol
  - Anabolic steroids
  - Cimetidine
  - Cocaine
  - Colchicine
  - Cyclosporine
  - Erythromycin
  - Gentamicin
  - Marijuana
  - Neomycin
  - Nitrofurantoin
  - Spironolactone
  - Sulfasalazine
  - Tetracyclines

The degree of virilization and hair distribution may suggest an underlying endocrine disorder, such as androgen deficiency. The head and neck, pulmonary, and cardiac examinations are important for assessing the overall health of the patient. The examiner may note unreported abdominal or inguinal scars that can be important clues to understanding the patient's condition.

The primary focus of the examination for infertility is the genitourinary examination. The size and position of the urethral meatus should be noted because severe hypospadias could impair deposition of sperm in the proximal vagina. The size and consistency of the testes should be assessed. A normal testis is at least 20 cc. A noticeably smaller or softer testis is indicative of testis atrophy. Careful palpation for testis masses is critical because a man with a testis tumor can present with infertility.[8,9]

Examination for a varicocele should be carried out with the patient in the standing position. The examiner should examine the spermatic cord for palpably or visibly distended veins. Varicoceles are graded based on the degree of distension/ease of detection: grade 1 (palpable with Valsalva maneuver only), grade 2 (palpable without Valsalva maneuver), and grade 3 (visible through the skin).

The presence of the vas deferens also should be confirmed. Absence of one or both vasa has significant implications for the patient and necessitates further evaluation (see below).[10–15] Epididymal abnormalities such as induration or fullness also can provide important clues, such as potential obstruction.[16] Vasal and epididymal anomalies frequently coexist because of their common embryologic origin. For example, men with CBAVD commonly have atresia of a significant portion of the epididymis as well. As couples delay pursuing parenthood, men at risk for prostate cancer may be evaluated for infertility. Thus abnormalities of the prostate, such as induration or nodules, should be evaluated with transrectal ultrasound (TRUS) and prostate biopsies to rule out prostate cancer. Enlarged seminal vesicles or a midline cyst also may be palpated on rectal examination and should prompt evaluation for ejaculatory duct obstruction with TRUS.[17–20] The critical features of the physical examination are summarized in Table 16-2.

▶ **TABLE 16-2:** EVALUATION OF MALE INFERTILITY: PHYSICAL EXAMINATION

- General examination (degree of virilization, hair distribution, gynecomastia, head, neck, pulmonary, cardiac, extremities)
- Genitourinary examination
  - Abdominal masses, hernias, unreported inguinal scars
  - Size and position of urethral meatus
  - Size, consistency of testes, presence of masses
  - Presence of vas deferens
  - Epididymis, irregularity or induration
  - Presence of varicocele
  - Prostate and seminal vesicles, nodules, irregularity, or masses

Laboratory Evaluation

Semen Analysis

The cornerstone of the laboratory evaluation for male infertility is the semen analysis. Two or more analyses should be collected by masturbation in nonspermatotoxic containers after 2 to 3 days' abstinence and analyzed within 1 h of collection. The semen analysis is not a fertility test but rather a test of fertility potential. The parameters that are usually measured include semen volume, semen pH, concentration, motility, and morphology. Additional testing can include viability and assays for white blood cells and antisperm antibodies. When interpreting a semen analysis, one must be careful not to equate "normal" with "fertile" or "abnormal" with "infertile." If a man has motile sperm in the semen, then he is potentially fertile. In general, the chance for pregnancy correlates with the total motile sperm count.[21,22] As a result, the term *reference values* rather than *normal values* is now preferred. Reference values for semen variables are summarized in Table 16-3.[23]

If a man is found to be azoospermic, i.e., no sperm are seen in the semen, the next step is centrifugation and resuspension of the pellet

▶ **TABLE 16-3:** REFERENCE VALUES OF SEMEN VARIABLES

Volume	$\geq$2 mL
pH	$\geq$7.2
Sperm concentration (per mL)	$\geq$20 $\times 10^6$
Motility	$\geq$50% motile (grades a + b) or 25% or more with progressive motility (grade a) within 60 minutes of ejaculation
Morphology	*
Viability	50% or more live
White blood cells	$<1 \times 10^6$
Immunobead test	$<$50% motile sperm with heads bound

*Multicenter trials are underway, but previous data suggest that the fertilization rate in vitro decreases if there are less than 15 percent normal-shaped sperm, as defined by the WHO manual.
From WHO criteria.[23]

with subsequent repeat microscopic examination. With this simple test, identification of any sperm whatsoever rules out complete ductal obstruction. If a man is azoospermic and has a semen volume of less than 1 mL, then a postejaculatory urine sample should be obtained and analyzed.[5] Typically, a man with sperm in his postejaculatory urine sample, however, also would have sperm present in the antegrade sample (if he can produce an antegrade ejaculate). See Chapter 15 for additional discussion of semen analysis.

Leukocytospermia, the presence of white blood cells (WBCs) in the semen, is a controversial topic. Round cells, representing either leukocytes or immature sperm, may be noted on a semen analysis. Special staining, such as the myeloperoxidase stain or Endtz test, is required to differentiate between these two types of cells.[5,24] If more than 1 million WBCs per milliliter are identified, then treatment for genital tract infection is reasonable. Possible antibiotic regimens include doxycycline (100 mg bid) or a quinolone for 2 weeks. In addition, more frequent ejaculation may help to clear the leukocytospermia as well.[25] The rationale for treatment is that WBCs can produce reactive oxygen species (ROS) that can impair sperm function, and many practitioners would be reluctant to perform an insemination if WBCs are present. On the other hand, WBCs simply may be an incidental finding, and small amounts of ROS probably are physiologic and critical for sperm function.[26] It should be remembered, though, that many men will be asymptomatic and not truly have genital tract infection and that leukocytospermia can resolve spontaneously as well.[27,28]

Antisperm Antibodies

Antisperm antibodies may be a contributing factor to infertility in as many as 10 percent of men, although their significance in many cases is not completely clear. For example, antisperm antibodies are common after vasectomy, but a large percentage of men can establish a pregnancy after a vasectomy reversal.[29,30] Other conditions, in addition to vasectomy, in which a violation of the blood-testis barrier may have occurred, such as testis biopsy, spermatic cord torsion, and trauma, can be associated with antisperm antibodies.[29] It is probably reasonable to pursue further evaluation for antisperm antibodies when there is profoundly decreased motility or marked agglutination of sperm.[24]

The measurement and treatment of antisperm antibodies are also controversial. Only IgG and IgA in the semen bound to the sperm head or midpiece are thought to be clinically significant. Many tests are available to detect seminal antisperm antibodies, and each has its shortcomings. One of the most popular methods to diagnose antisperm antibodies is the immunobead test.[24,29] Treatment of men felt to have significant antisperm antibodies includes sperm washing and intrauterine insemination (IUI), corticosteroid treatment, and IVF with ICSI. With regard to steroid treatment, several protocols have been proposed with varying results.[29,31] Immunologic infertility is probably one of the best indications for ICSI, and as a result, medical treatment has become less popular. It also should be kept in mind that aseptic necrosis of the hip, a catastrophic complication of steroid treatment, has been reported during steroid therapy for antisperm antibodies.[29]

Sperm Function Testing

A semen analysis does not evaluate sperm function. As a result, tests have been devised that are designed to assess some but not all functional properties of sperm. All are to some degree artificial measures of sperm function and therefore can be difficult to interpret. Results and interpretation also can vary from center to center, depending on its expertise with the different tests. Indications for sperm function testing vary but include infertility with a "normal" semen analysis or as a way to predict fertilization in vitro.[24]

Some of the commonly used sperm function tests include the mannose-binding test, the hemizona assay, the sperm penetration assay, and the acrosome reaction test. The purpose of the mannose-binding assay is to examine the patterns of mannose binding expressed on sperm. Mannose, a sugar, is important for sperm recognition of the zona pellucida of the oocyte. The assay is carried out by placing capacitated, washed sperm with fluorescein isothiocyanate–conjugated mannosylated bovine serum albumin and examining the patterns of mannose-binding sites. The result is expressed as a percentage and compared with a known fertile donor.[32,33] In the hemizona assay, patient and donor (control) sperm are incubated separately with bisected human oocytes. The hemizona index is equal to the number of patient sperm bound divided by the number of control sperm bound $\times$ 100.[24,32]

The sperm penetration assay is performed by incubating capacitated sperm with zona-free hamster oocytes. The percentage of oocytes penetrated is measured. In theory, more oocytes will be penetrated by sperm or more sperm will penetrate each oocyte from fertile rather than infertile men.[5,32] To perform the acrosome test, special staining methods or monoclonal antibody–coated beads or other means can be used to induce the acrosome reaction. The percentage of sperm that are then able to undergo the acrosome reaction is calculated and compared with a known standard.[24,34,35] See Chapter 15 for additional discussion of sperm function assays.

Endocrine Testing

Correctable endocrinopathies are rare causes of male infertility. The most common endocrine abnormality detected during a male infertility evaluation is an elevated serum follicle-stimulating hormone (FSH) level. This indicates testicular failure, which is not a correctable condition. Not all men require an endocrine evaluation. By limiting endocrine testing to men with a sperm concentration of less than 10 million/mL, the expense of the evaluation can be reduced, and the chance of missing a correctable endocrinopathy is remote.[36] When indicated, a screening endocrine evaluation consisting of serum FSH and testosterone (T) determinations can be performed. If the FSH concentration is elevated, no further endocrine evaluation is required. If the serum T concentration is low, then a serum luteinizing hormone (LH) level should be checked. A prolactin level also can be checked, particularly if the patient notes decreased libido. Low FSH, LH, and T concentrations suggest hypogonadotropic hypogonadism. High FSH, normal LH, and normal T concentrations suggest spermatogenic failure, and high FSH, high LH, and low T concentrations suggest testicular failure. If the prolactin level is high, then magnetic resonance imaging (MRI) of the pituitary should be performed to rule out a pituitary adenoma.[5,36]

Genetic Testing

Genetic abnormalities are associated with some of the more severe forms of male infertility.

Many of the cases of male infertility previously labeled as "idiopathic" ultimately may have an underlying genetic cause. While genetic abnormalities are not correctable, they can have an impact on the health of offspring, and therefore, appropriate genetic counseling is required. The three most common genetic tests performed during a male infertility evaluation are a karyotype, Y chromosome microdeletion analysis, and cystic fibrosis (CF) mutation testing.

KARYOTYPE

Azoospermic and severely oligospermic men should undergo karyotype testing. When these men are tested, 13.7 percent of azoospermic men and 4.6 percent of severely oligospermic men will have an abnormal karyotype. In azoospermic men, sex chromosomal abnormalities, such as Klinefelter's syndrome (47,XXY), predominate, whereas autosomal abnormalities predominate in severely oligospermic men.[37] Klinefelter's syndrome is seen in about 1 in 500 of the general male population, in about 1 to 2 percent of infertile men, and in about 7 to 13 percent of azoospermic men. The primary features include azoospermia with small, firm testes and an elevated serum FSH concentration.[38] Classically, these men also have been felt to possess other secondary characteristics and are described as tall, undervirilized, with gynecomastia, and intellectually deficient. Recently, this stereotype of a Klinefelter's patient has been challenged because many men with Klinefelter's syndrome lack some or all of these secondary features.[39]

Y CHROMOSOME MICRODELETION ANALYSIS

If a patient with azoospermia or severe oligospermia has a normal karyotype, then he should be offered Y chromosome microdeletion testing. In 1976, Tiepolo and Zuffardi first noted deletions of the distal portion of band q11 on the Y chromosome, termed the *azoospermia factor* (AZF), in six azoospermic men.[40] With current testing, about 15 percent of men with nonobstructive azoospermia (no sperm in the semen secondary to decreased sperm production) and a smaller percentage of men with severe oligospermia will have microdeletions of the Y chromosome.[41,42] In addition to providing information for diagnosis, this testing also can have an impact on treatment. In nonobstructive azoospermia, the type of deletion can be predictive of successful sperm retrieval with testicular sperm extraction (TESE). Men with deletions of the AZFa or AZFb region do not have sperm successfully retrieved, whereas the majority of men with AZFc deletions will have sperm retrieved successfully.[42,43] In addition, it has been shown that men who undergo ICSI with Y chromosome microdeletions can pass these abnormalities to offspring.[44]

CF MUTATION TESTING

CF is the most common lethal autosomal recessive disorder in northern European Caucasians, occurring in about 1 in 2500. It is characterized by chronic respiratory infections, exocrine pancreas insufficiency, and wolffian duct anomalies. The carrier frequency is about 1 in 25.[45] Nearly all men with clinical CF have CBAVD. This represents the most severe end of a phenotypic spectrum associated with CF mutations. CBAVD also can exist as an isolated defect with no other clinical signs of CF. Approximately 1.4 percent of azoospermic men have CBAVD, and about 70 percent of men with CBAVD are carriers for CF.[12,45] The most common combinations that result in CBAVD are a compound heterozygote for CF or a combination of a CF mutation and the intron 8 5T splice variant. Therefore, testing the man and his partner for CF mutations and the 5T variant is required for counseling patients about their risk of having a child with CF and CBAVD.[46] Unilateral absence of the vas is also associated with CF mutations, usually with a contralateral vas that is present and palpable but obstructed distal to the scrotum.[13,15]

Testis Biopsy

A testis biopsy is indicated in men with azoospermia and at least one palpable vas deferens.[47–50] Except in cases of vasectomy or most cases of CBAVD, a testis biopsy is required to document obstruction. In the era of IVF/ICSI, both diagnosis and treatment usually can be accomplished at a single setting. The biopsy can be performed and analyzed intraoperatively. If sufficient numbers of sperm are noted to suggest obstruction, then microsurgical reconstruction also can be performed.[51] If the degree of sperm production is not consistent with obstruction, then further biopsies can be performed. In either case, if sperm are noted, they can be cryopreserved. Pathologic review is performed to document the pattern of sperm production and to rule out underlying pathology such as intratubular germ cell neoplasia, which is found in 0.4 to 1.1 percent of infertile men.[47]

An open biopsy can be performed through a small scrotal incision with local, regional, or general anesthesia. The intratesticular arterial anatomy has been described by Jarow. To avoid injury to significant branches of the testicular artery, the biopsies should be performed in either the medial or lateral aspect of the upper pole of the testis.[52] Bilateral biopsies are indicated if there is significant size discrepancy between the two testes or if sperm retrieval is not successful with the first side. The tissue for pathologic examination should be placed in a fixative, such as Bouin's, that does not distort the testicular architecture. The classification system of Levin is useful to describe the pattern of spermatogenesis.[53] In an azoospermic patient, more than 20 mature spermatids per round tubule would be consistent with a sperm concentration of 10 million/mL.[54] A testis biopsy also can be performed percutaneously, although fewer tubules are obtained, making diagnosis more difficult in some cases.[55] The evaluation of management of azoospermia is summarized in Figure 16-1.

► TREATMENT

In general, correctable causes of infertility, when present, should be treated. Table 16-4 lists the causes found in a male infertility clinic. From this table it is evident that more than one-half of the men evaluated for infertility have a potentially correctable problem. The first section on treatment will be devoted to correctable causes.

Gonadotoxic Medications

Gonadotoxic medications are listed in Table 16-1. Some of these medications, such as sulfasalazine and cimetidine, appear to have reversible effects on spermatogenesis, so withdrawing them can result in increased sperm concentration. Anabolic steroids, which have received significant media attention because of apparent increased use by athletes, usually have reversible effects on spermatogenesis. These drugs inhibit gonadotropin secretion by the pituitary and as a result suppress spermatogenesis. After withdrawal of the medication, hypogonadism usually resolves after a few months. Unfortunately, some patients have irreversible azoospermia after steroid use. Consequently, patients should be questioned about steroid use and the medication stopped immediately with periodic reevaluation thereafter.[5]

Varicocele

A *varicocele* is defined as dilated veins of the pampiniform plexus of the spermatic cord. It is the most commonly identified abnormality in men evaluated for infertility. About 30 to 40 percent of men seen in an infertility clinic are diagnosed with a varicocele, but about 15 to 20 percent of men in the general public also may have a varicocele. Varicoceles are believed to exert their deleterious effects by elevating scrotal temperature, although other mechanisms also could be involved.[56] There is some evidence that a varicocele can cause a progressive decline in semen parameters and fertility.[57–59] Nonetheless, not all men with a varicocele are infertile. A World Health Organization

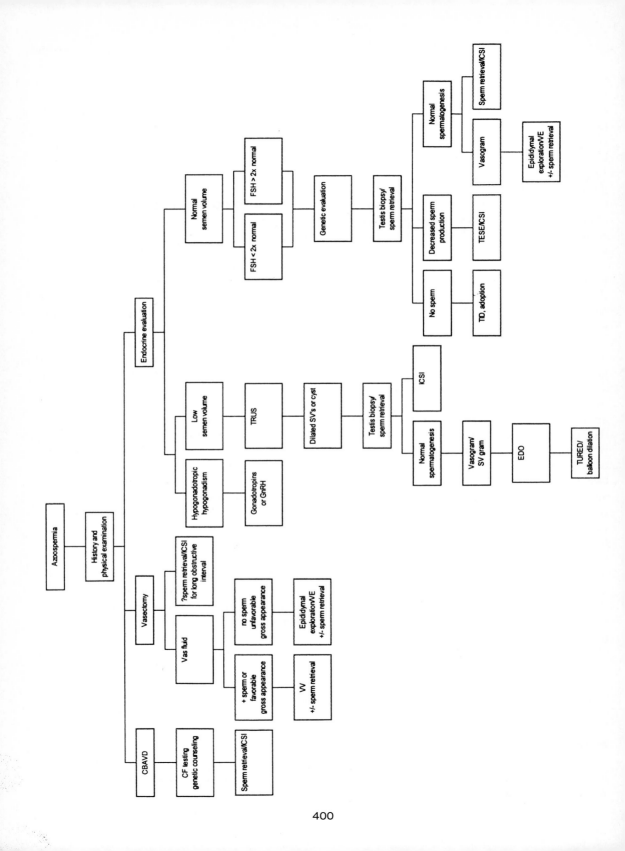

▶ **TABLE 16-4:** DIAGNOSES IN A MALE INFERTILITY CLINIC

Cause	Percent
Varicocele	42.2
Idiopathic	22.7
Obstruction	14.3
Normal/female factor	7.9
Cryptorchidism	3.4
Immunologic	2.6
Ejaculatory dysfunction	1.3
Testicular failure	1.3
Drug/radiation	1.1
Endocrinologic	1.1
Infection	0.9
Sexual dysfunction	0.3
Systemic disease	0.3
Sertoli cell only	0.2
Ultrastructural defect	0.2
Genetic	0.1
Testis cancer	0.1

Used with permission from Sigman M, Lipshultz LI, Howards SS. Evaluation of the subfertile male, in Lipshultz LI, Howards SS (eds), Infertility in the Male, 3d ed. St. Louis: Mosby, 1997:189.

(WHO) report in 1992, however, concluded that varicocele is associated with impaired testicular function and infertility.[60] Early research suggested that the detrimental effects of the varicocele were independent of varicocele size. More recent research, however, suggests that larger varicoceles have a greater detrimental effect than small varicoceles.[61] This raises doubts about the significance of the subclinical varicocele, one that is detected only by imaging techniques such as ultrasound. As a result, many fertility specialists would not treat a subclinical varicocele.

Varicocele correction can be performed as an outpatient procedure, either surgically or nonsurgically, with minimal morbidity. The nonsurgical approach is performed with angiographic embolization.[62] Surgical approaches include inguinal, subinguinal, or high-ligation/retroperitoneal routes. All have their advantages and disadvantages. The more distal (closer to the testis) the operation is performed, the more complex the anatomy and the more veins that are encountered. In general, optical magnification is required and is particularly helpful to identify all veins and to preserve the artery and lymphatics. An approach that has gained increasing popularity recently is the subinguinal microsurgical approach. More veins are encountered with this approach, but morbidity is less because the external oblique fascia is not opened.[63,64]

Not all men with a varicocele are infertile, and not all men benefit from varicocele correction. Furthermore, predicting which patients will benefit and the degree of expected improvement in semen parameters after varicocele correction is not possible. Thus there is controversy about whether a varicocele actually causes infertility and whether varicocele correction is beneficial. Most studies examining success rates after varicocele correction are uncontrolled. Reviews examining outcomes after varicocele correction have demonstrated that about 65 percent of men will improve their semen parameters and about 40 percent will establish a pregnancy.[65,66] One review of controlled studies demonstrated a 33 percent pregnancy rate with varicocele correction.[67] As expected, the pregnancy rate after varicocele correction for men with severely depressed sperm concentrations or azoospermia is less

Figure 16-1 Evaluation and management of azoospermia. (CBAVD = congenital bilateral absence of the vas deferens; CF = cysticfibrosis; ICSI = intracytoplasmic sperm injection; VV = vasovasostomy; VE = vasoepididymostomy; GnRH = gonadotropin-releasing hormone; TRUS = transrectal ultrasound; SVs = seminal vesicles; EDO = ejaculatory duct obstruction; TURED = transurethral resection of the ejaculatory ducts; FSH = follicle-stimulating hormone; TID = therapeutic insemination with donor sperm; TESE = testicular sperm extraction.) *(Used, with permission, from Kolettis PN. The evaluation and management of the azoospermic patient. J Androl 2002;23:294.)*

than for other men.[68–70] Two prospective, randomized studies have been performed, and both have demonstrated improvement in semen parameters.[71,72] One of these demonstrated an improvement in pregnancy rates.[71] Of note, two reports have demonstrated that varicocele repair is more cost effective than IVF as treatment for varicocele-related infertility.[67,73]

Obstruction

Vasectomy-Induced Obstruction

Vasovasostomy (VV) can correct vasal obstruction after vasectomy with patency and pregnancy rates of 75 to 93 percent and 46 to 82 percent, respectively[74–80] (see Table 16-5). Secondary epididymal obstruction can occur after vasectomy, particularly after longer obstructive intervals, and requires vasoepididymostomy (VE) for correction.[81] Patency and pregnancy rates range from 48 to 85 percent and 31 to 56 percent, respectively[82–88] (Table 16-6). It can take up to 6 to 12 months for sperm to appear after VV and VE, respectively.[83] The average time to achieve pregnancy after vasectomy reversal is 1 year.[74] Newer intussusception techniques for VE may result in earlier patency.[89,90] Couples with vasectomy-induced obstruction also can establish a pregnancy with sperm re-trieval and ICSI. Pregnancy rates with vasectomy reversal generally are superior to sperm retrieval and a single cycle of ICSI unless the obstructive interval is at least 15 and possibly 20 years.[74,91,92] In addition, vasectomy reversal is more cost effective and does not increase the risk of multiple births.[93,94]

Other Correctable Obstructions

Epididymal obstruction also can be idiopathic or congenital or occur secondary to infection or trauma. Typical features of a patient with epididymal obstruction are azoospermia with normal-size testes, normal FSH level, and induration or fullness of the epididymis.[16,95,96] As with epididymal obstruction secondary to vasectomy, it can be corrected with microsurgery (Table 16-6).

Ejaculatory Duct Obstruction

Ejaculatory duct obstruction is a rare cause of infertility. Men with low-volume (<1 mL) azoospermia, a normal FSH concentration, and at least one palpable vas deferens should have TRUS to evaluate for ejaculatory duct obstruction. Traditionally, this entity has been treated with transurethral resection of the ejaculatory ducts (TURED).[17–19] Alternatively, balloon dilation of the ejaculatory ducts can be performed.[20]

► **TABLE 16-5:** RESULTS OF MICROSURGICAL VASOVASOSTOMY

Authors	Year	No. of Patients	Patency Rate	Pregnancy Rate
Cos et al.[75]	1983	87	75% (66/87)	46% (32/69)
Requeda et al.[79]	1983	47	80% (38/47)	46% (18/39)
Owen and Kapila[78]	1984	475	93% (439/475)	82% (390/475)
Lee[77]	1986	324	90% (292/324)	51% (165/324)
Silber*[80]	1989	282	91% (258/282)	81% (228/282)
Belker et al.[74]	1991	1247	86% (865/1012)	52% (421/808)
Fox[76]	1994	103	84% (86/103)	48% (31/64)
Total		2565	88% (2044/2330)	62% (1285/2061)

*Excluding 44 patients with no sperm in the vasal fluid. Patency and pregnancy rates for the study population of 326 patients were 79 and 70 percent, respectively.

Used with permission from Kolettis PN. The evaluation and management of the azoospermic patient. *J Androl* 2002;23:297.

▶ **TABLE 16-6:** RESULTS OF MICROSURGICAL VASOEPIDIDYMOSTOMY

Authors	Year	No. of Patients	Patency Rate	Pregnancy Rate
Fogdestam et al.[82]	1986	41	85% (35/41)	37% (15/41)
Silber[81]	1989	190	77% (146/190)	49% (94/190)
Schlegel et al.[85]	1993	91	70% (64/90)	27% (25/91)
Thomas et al.[95]	1993	153	76% (116/153)	42% (64/153)
Matsuda et al.[84]	1994	26	81% (21/26)	38% (10/26)
Jarow et al.[83]	1997	131	67% (71/131)	27% (36/131)
Takihara[87]	1998	14	71% (10/14)	29% (4/14)
Kim et al.[96]	1998	43	81% (35/43)	37% (16/43)
Total		689	72% (498/689)	38% (264/689)

Note: Where not explicitly stated in the respective manuscripts, number of patent or pregnant patients were calculated by multiplying the published percentage by the total number of patients.

Used with permission from Kolettis PN. The evaluation and management of the azoospermic patient. *J Androl* 2002;23:298.

Ejaculatory Dysfunction

Ejaculatory dysfunction consists of failure of emission (fluid is not deposited in the posterior urethra) and retrograde ejaculation (semen flows backward into the bladder). Conditions associated with ejaculatory dysfunction include bladder neck or prostate surgery, retroperitoneal surgery with disruption of lumbar sympathetics, diabetes mellitus, spinal cord injury, and α-blockers (usually used to treat lower urinary tract symptoms).[97] Withdrawal of the α blocker should restore antegrade ejaculation. In spinal cord-injured men who are anejaculatory, pharmacologic treatment is unlikely to be beneficial. These men will require treatment with penile vibratory stimulation (PVS) and, if this is unsuccessful, electroejaculation (EEJ).[98]

The first step in treatment of the other forms of ejaculatory dysfunction is a trial of sympathomimetics such as pseudoephedrine (60 mg tid) beginning 3 days prior to a semen analysis. If this is unsuccessful, then PVS and then EEJ are required.[97] Sensate men require anesthesia for EEJ. Urinary alkalinization is useful and may improve the numbers of motile sperm retrieved from the postejaculatory urine, whether obtained after masturbation, PVS, or EEJ. If sperm cannot be obtained with any of these means, then testicular sperm extraction (TESE) can be employed. Testicular sperm must be used with ICSI. Sperm obtained by other means can be used with IUI or IVF. The total motile sperm count obtained dictates which technique is appropriate.[99]

Hypogonadotropic Hypogonadism

The most common correctable endocrinopathy associated with infertility is hypogonadotropic hypogonadism.[34] These men typically present with azoospermia, low or undetectable gonadotropin levels, low T levels, small testes, and signs of deficient virilization. Pituitary imaging should be performed first to rule out a pituitary mass lesion. If this is negative, then gonadotropin therapy is begun. Initially, human chorionic gonadotropin (hCG) is given until the serum T concentration is in the normal range. Then FSH or human menopausal gonadotropin (hMG) is administered, and follow-up endocrine profiles and semen analyses are obtained at regular intervals. It can take a year or longer for semen parameters to improve significantly, but these men can establish pregnancies with subnormal sperm concentrations.[100]

If no correctable underlying problem exists, then the couple may pursue treatment with ARTs. These powerful techniques can circumvent even the most severe forms of male infertility as long as viable sperm are available. Some examples of ARTs in the treatment of male factor infertility are outlined below.

CBAVD

Prior to IVF, men with CBAVD were considered sterile. With the introduction of ICSI, pregnancy rates improved significantly and are similar to those of couples undergoing IVF with no male factors.[50,101] In patients with this and other forms of obstructive azoospermia, sperm can be retrieved from the testis or epididymis, either open or percutaneously.[102,103]

Oligoteratozoospermia (OAT)

Couples in which the male partner has impaired semen parameters such as OAT can be treated with IUI or IVF. Indications for IVF include female factors such as tubal disease and severe male factor (total motile sperm count less than 5 or 10 million).[99]

Nonobstructive Azoospermia (NOA)

TESE and ICSI have allowed men with NOA to have their own biologic children, where previously it was not possible.[104–108] TESE involves extracting sperm from testis tissue removed with either an open or percutaneous biopsy. In general, sperm retrieval rates in NOA are higher with open biopsy techniques because of improved sampling, although success with percutaneous techniques also has been reported.[109–111] Predicting successful sperm retrieval is difficult and is independent of such factors as testicular size and FSH level.[112–114] Pregnancies with TESE/ICSI have been reported for men with nonmosaic Klinefelter's syndrome.[115] Two innovative techniques that can improve the chances for successful sperm re-

trieval are microdissection and fine-needle mapping.[116,117] Some men with NOA may not wish to pursue the preceding treatment possibilities and may opt for either adoption or donor insemination.

Empirical Medical Therapy

If couples do not wish to pursue ARTs, they may pursue empirical medical therapy. Traditionally, the most common form of empirical medical therapy has been some form of hormonal manipulation. Empirical T supplementation should be avoided because this will suppress gonadotropin secretion by the pituitary and actually decrease sperm production. Unfortunately, some men will remain permanently azoospermic after taking T.[118]

One medication commonly used for empirical medical treatment is clomiphene citrate. By interfering with the normal negative-feedback mechanism, this drug raises serum FSH and T levels. There may be a subpopulation of men who improve their sperm concentration, but controlled studies have not demonstrated any benefit. Men with an elevated FSH concentration are unlikely to increase their sperm concentration with clomiphene citrate.[119] Side effects include breast tenderness and increased aggressiveness. A typical regimen is 50 mg three times a week with repeat semen analysis and FSH, and T level determinations after 5 weeks. The medication is continued for 3 to 6 months, and the patient is followed with semen analyses, FSH and T determinations, and physical examinations. If there is significant worsening of the semen parameters, or if the hormone levels are more than 1½ times normal, the medication should be stopped.[24]

Another form of empirical medical therapy involves the use of aromatase inhibitors, such as testolactone. It is hypothesized that an abnormal T-to-estradiol (E) ratio can impair fertility and that normalization of this parameter could improve semen parameters and ultimately fertility. In one study, a group of men with abnormal T-to-E ratios were treated with oral testolactone. After treatment, improved sperm concentration and motility was noted. This study suggests that this form of therapy may be beneficial, and a randomized, controlled trial could be done to assess its efficacy more definitively.[120]

KEY POINTS

1. Infertility affects 15 percent of couples. Male factors are involved in about one-half of these couples.

2. The main purpose of the male infertility evaluation is to diagnose and treat correctable problems. In addition, the evaluation may uncover either significant underlying medical or genetic pathology that is the cause of the infertility or incidental pathology that could affect the patient or his potential offspring. Finally, patients simply may desire information about their condition, even if it is not correctable, as a way of reassuring them that they did not cause the problem themselves.

3. Evaluation of the infertile male consists of a complete medical history and physical examination and two semen analyses. An endocrine evaluation generally is not necessary if the sperm concentration is >10 million/mL. If endocrine testing is indicated, then serum FSH and T determinations are the initial recommended tests.

4. About one-half of male factor infertility has a potentially correctable cause. The most common correctable causes are varicocele and obstruction. Where a correctable male factor exists, it is generally more cost-effective to treat this correctable factor than to proceed directly to the use of ARTs.

5. The most common identifiable abnormality detected in a male infertility evaluation is a varicocele. The evidence for benefit with varicocele correction is mixed. Patients with severely impaired semen quality probably benefit less with varicocele correction. In general, about two-thirds of men will improve their semen quality, and 40 percent can establish a pregnancy after varicocele correction.

6. Azoospermia can be classified as either obstructive or nonobstructive. Nonobstructive azoospermia is not correctable, but in some cases sperm can be retrieved from the testis and used with ICSI. Obstructive azoospermia is correctable in many instances, such as after a vasectomy. Except in cases of prolonged obstructive intervals (>15 or possibly 20 years), microsurgical reconstruction generally is superior to and more cost effective than sperm retrieval with a single cycle of IVF/ICSI. Other forms of obstructive azoospermia, such as CBAVD, are not correctable. In these cases, sperm can be retrieved and used with ICSI.

7. Some of the more severe forms of male factor infertility have an underlying genetic basis. In these instances, appropriate genetic counseling is required.

REFERENCES

1. Palermo G, Joris H, Devroey P, Van Steirteghem AC. Pregnancies after intracytoplasmic injection of single spermatozoon into an oocyte. *Lancet* 1992;340:17–18.
2. Callahan TL, Hall JE, Ettner SL, et al. The economic impact of multiple-gestation pregnancies and the contribution of assisted-reproduction techniques to their incidence. *N Engl J Med* 1994;331:244–249.
3. Neumann PJ, Gharib SD, Weinstein MC. The cost of a successful delivery with in vitro fertilization. *N Engl J Med* 1994;331:239–243.
4. Schenker JG, Ezra Y. Complications of assisted reproductive techniques. *Fertil Steril* 1994;61:411–422.
5. Sigman M, Lipshultz LI, Howards SS. Evaluation of the subfertile male, in Lipshultz LI,

Howards SS (eds), *Infertility in the Male,* 3d ed. St Louis: Mosby, 1997; pp 173–193.

6. Jarow JP, Sharlip ID, Belker AM, et al. Best practice policies for male infertility. *J Urol* 2002;167:2138–2144.

7. Wilcox AJ, Weinberg CR, Baird DD. Timing of sexual intercourse in relation to ovulation: Effects on the probability of conception, survival of the pregnancy, and sex of the baby. *N Engl J Med* 1995;333:1517–1521.

8. Honig SC, Lipshultz LI, Jarow J: Significant medical pathology uncovered by a comprehensive male infertility evaluation. *Fertil Steril* 1994;62:1028–1034.

9. Kolettis PN Sabanegh ES. Significant medical pathology discovered during a male infertility evaluation. *J Urol* 2001;166:178–180.

10. Klapproth HJ, Young IS. Vasectomy, vas ligation and vas occlusion. *Urology* 1973;1:292–300.

11. Donohue RE, Fauver E. Unilateral absence of the vas deferens: A useful clinical sign. *JAMA* 1989;261:1180–1182.

12. Anguiano A, Oates RD, Amos JA, et al. Congenital bilateral absence of the vas deferens: A primarily genital form of cystic fibrosis. *JAMA* 1992;267:1794–1797.

13. Mickle J, Milunsky A, Amos JA, et al. Congenital unilateral absence of the vas deferens: A heterogeneous disorder with two distinct subpopulations based upon aetiology and mutational status of the cystic fibrosis gene. *Hum Reprod* 1995;10:1728–1735.

14. Schlegel PN, Shin, D, Goldstein, M. Urogenital anomalies in men with congenital absence of the vas deferens. *J Urol* 1996;155:1644–1648.

15. Kolettis PN, Sandlow JI. Clinical and genetic features of patients with congenital unilateral absence of the vas deferens. *Urology* 2002;60:1073–1076.

16. Kolettis PN. Is physical examination useful in predicting epididymal obstruction? *Urology* 2001;57:1138–1140.

17. Goluboff ET, Stifelman MD, Fisch H. Ejaculatory duct obstruction in the infertile male *Urology* 1995;45:925–931.

18. Meacham RB, Hellerstein DK, Lipshultz LI. Evaluation and treatment of ejaculatory duct obstruction in the infertile male. *Fertil Steril* 1993;59:393–397.

19. Pryor JP, Hendry WF. Ejaculatory duct obstruction in subfertile males: analysis of 87 patients. *Fertil Steril* 1991;56:725–730.

20. Schlegel PN. Management of ejaculatory duct obstruction, in Lipshultz LI, Howards SS (eds), *Infertility in the Male,* 3d ed. St Louis: Mosby, 1997; pp 385–394.

21. Schoysman R, Gerris J. Twelve-year follow-up study of pregnancy rates in 1291 couples with idiopathically impaired male infertility. *Acta Eur Fertil* 1983;14:51–56.

22. Guzick DS, Overstreet JW, Factor-Litvak P, et al. National Cooperative Reproductive Medicine Network: Sperm morphology, motility, and concentration in fertile and infertile men. *N Engl J Med* 2001;345:1388–1393.

23. World Health Organization. Reference values of semen variables, in *Who Laboratory Manual for the Examination of Human Semen and Sperm–Cervical Mucus Interaction,* 4th ed. Cambridge, England: Cambridge University Press, 1999:60–61.

24. Kolettis PN, Thomas AJ. Andrology, in Ransom SB, Dombrowski MP, McNeeley SG, et al (eds), *Practical Strategies in Obstetrics and Gynecology.* Philadelphia: Saunders, 1999; pp 629–640.

25. Yamamoto M, Hibi H, Katsuno S, et al. Antibiotic and ejaculation treatments improve resolution rate of leukocytospermia in infertile men with prostatitis. *Nagoya J Med Sci* 1995;58:41–45.

26. Aitken RJ, Baker HWG. Seminal leukocytes: passengers, terrorists or good Samaritans? *Hum Reprod* 1995;10:1736–1739.

27. Wolff H. The biologic significance of white blood cells in semen. *Fertil Steril* 1995;63:1143–1157.

28. Yanushpolsky EH, Politch JA, Hill JA, et al. Antibiotic therapy and leukocytospermia: A prospective, randomized, controlled study. *Fertil Steril* 1995;63:142–147.

29. Turek PJ. Immunopathology and infertility, in Lipshultz LI, Howards SS (eds), *Infertility in the Male.* St Louis: Mosby, 1997; pp 305–325.

30. Thomas AJ, Pontes JE, Rose NR, et al. Microsurgical vasovasostomy: Immunologic consequences and subsequent fertility. *Fertil Steril* 1981:35:447–450.

31. Haas GG. Antibody-mediated causes of male infertility. *Urol Clin North Am* 1987:14:539–550.

32. Tripp BM, Gagnon C. Advanced sperm fertiity tests, in Lipshultz LI, Howards SS (eds), *Infertility in the Male.* St Louis: Mosby, 1997; pp 194–209.

31. Benoff S, Cooper GW, Hurley I, et al. Human sperm fertilizing potential in vitro is correlated

with differential expression of a head-specific mannose-ligand receptor. *Fertil Steril* 1993;59: 854–862.

32. Henkel R, Muller C, Miska W, et al. Determination of the acrosome reaction in human spermatozoa is predictive of fertilization in vitro. *Hum Reprod* 1993;8:2128–2132.

33. Ohashi K, Saji F, Kato M, et al. Acrobeads test: a new diagnositc test for assessment of the fertilizing capacity of human spermatozoa. *Fertil Steril* 1995:63:625–630.

34. Sigman M, Jarow JP. Endocrine evaluation of infertile men. *Urology* 1997;50:659–664.

37. Van Asssche E, Bonduelle M, Tournaye H, et al. Cytogenetics of infertile men. *Hum Reprod* 1996;11(suppl 4):1–26.

38. Mak V, Jarvi KA. The genetics of male infertility. *J Urol* 1996;156:1245–1257.

39. Damani MN, Anglade RE, Oates. Are all men with Klinefelter's syndrome created equally? *Fertil Steril* 2001;76(3 suppl 1):S98–S99.

40. Tiepolo L, Zuffardi O. Localization of factors controlling spermatogenesis in the nonfluorescent portion of the human Y chromosome long arm. *Hum Genet* 1976;34:119–124.

41. Reijo R, Lee TY, Salo P, et al. Diverse spermatogenic defects in humans caused by Y chromosome deletions encompassing a novel RNA-binding protein gene. *Nature Genet.* 1995;10: 383–393.

42. Brandell RA, Mielnik A, Liotta D, et al. AZFb deletions predict the absence of spermatozoa with testicular sperm extraction: Preliminary report of a prognostic genetic test. *Hum Reprod* 1998;13:2812–2815.

43. Hopps CV, Mielnik A, Goldstein M, et al. Sperm retrieval in infertile men wih AZF deletion. *J Urol* 2003;169(4 suppl):449.

44. Page DC, Silber S, Brown LG. Men with infertility caused by AZFc deletion can produce sons by intracytoplasmic sperm injection, but are likely to transmit the deletion and infertility. *Hum Reprod* 1999;14:1722–1726.

45. Jaffe T, Oates RD. Genetic aspects of infertility, in Lipshultz LI, Howards SS (eds), *Infertility in the Male*. St Louis: Mosby, 1997; p 280.

46. Lissens W, Mercier B, Tournaye H, et al. Cystic fibrosis and infertility caused by congenital bilateral absence of the vas deferens and related clinical entities. *Hum Reprod* 1996; 11(suppl 4:)55–80.

47. Coburn M, Kim ED, Wheeler TM. Testicular biopsy in male infertility evaluation, in Lip-

shultz LI, Howards SS (eds), *Infertility in the Male,* 3d ed. St Louis: Mosby, 1997; pp 219–248.

48. Nagler HM Thomas AJ Jr. Testicular biopsy and vasography in the evaluation of male infertility. *Urol Clin North Am* 1987;14:167–176.

49. Jarow JP. Evaluation and treatment of the azoospermic patient. *Curr Prob Urol* 1992; Jan–Feb:4–30.

50. Kolettis PN. The evaluation and management of the azoospermic patient. *J Androl* 2002;23: 293–305.

51. Belker AM, Sherins RJ, Dennison-Lagos L. Simple, rapid staining method for immediate intraoperative examination of testicular biopsies. *J Androl* 1996;17:420–426.

52. Jarow JP. Clinical significance of intratesticular arterial anatomy. *J Urol* 1991;145:777–779.

53. Silber SJ, Rodriguez-Rigau LJ. Quantitative analysis of testicle biopsy: Determination of partial obstruction and prediction of sperm count after surgery for obstruction. *Fertil Steril* 1981;4:480–485.

54. Harrington TG, Schauer D, Gilbert BR. Percutaneous testis biopsy: An alternative to open testicular biopsy in the evaluation of the subfertile man. *J Urol* 1996;156:1647–1651.

55. Levin HS. Nonneoplastic diseases of the testis, in Sternberg S (ed), *Diagnostic Surgical Pathology,* 3d ed. Philadelphia: Lippincott, Williams & Wilkins, 1999; pp 1943–1971.

56. Jarow JP. Effects of varicocele on male fertility. *Hum Reprod Update* 2001;7:59–64.

57. Gorelick JI, Goldstein M. Loss of fertility in men with varicocele. *Fertil Steril* 1993;59: 613–616.

58. Chehval MJ, Purcell MH. Deterioration of semen parameters over time in men with untreated varicocele: Evidence of progressive testicular damage. *Fertil Steril* 1992;57:174–177.

59. Witt MA, Lipshultz LI. Varicocele: A progressive or static lesion? *Urology* 1993;42:541–543.

60. World Health Organization. The influence of varicocele on parameters of fertility in a large group of men presenting to infertility clinics. *Fertil Steril* 1992:57:1289–1293.

61. Steckel J, Dicker AP, Goldstein M. Relationship between varicocele size and response to varicocelectomy. *J Urol* 1993;149:769–771.

62. Dewire DM, Thomas AJ, Falk RM, et al. Clinical outcome and cost comparison of percutaneous embolization and surgical ligation of varicocele. *J Androl* 1994:15:38S–42S.

63. Marmar JL, Kim Y. Subinguinal microsurgical varicocelectomy: A technical critique and statistical analysis of semen and pregnancy data. *J Urol* 1994;152:1127–1132.

64. Nagler HM, Luntz RK, Martinis FG. Varicocele, in Lipshultz LI, Howards SS (eds), *Infertility in the Male*, 3d ed. St Louis, Mosby, 1997; pp 336–359.

65. Pryor JL, Howards SS. Varicocele. *Urol Clin North Am* 1987;14:499–513.

66. Schlesinger MH, Wilets IF, Nagler HM. Treatment outcome after varicocelectomy: A critical analysis. *Urol Clin North Am* 1994;21:517–529.

67. Schlegel PN. Is assisted reproduction the optimal treatment for varicocele-associated male infertility? A cost-effectiveness analysis. *Urology* 1997;49:83–90.

68. Matthews GJ, Matthews ED, Goldstein M. Induction of spermatogenesis and achievement of pregnancy after microsurgical varicocelectomy in men with azoospermia and severe oligoasthenospermia. *Fertil Steril* 1998;70:71–75.

69. Kim ED, Leibman BB, Grinblat DM, et al. Varicocele repair improves semen parameters in azoospermic men with spermatogenic failure. *J Urol* 1999;162:737–740.

70. Matkov TG, Zenni M, Sandlow J, et al. Preoperative semen analysis as a predictor of seminal improvement following varicocelectomy. *Fertil Steril* 2001;75:63–68.

71. Madgar I, Weissenberg R, Lunenfeld B, et al. Controlled trial of high spermatic vein ligation for varicocele in infertile men. *Fertil Steril* 1995;63:120–124.

72. Nieschlag E, Hertle L, Fischedick A, et al. Update on treatment of varicocele: Counseling as effective as occlusion of the vena spermatica. *Hum Reprod* 1998;13:2147–2150.

73. Penson DF, Paltiel AD, Krumholz HM, et al. The cost-effectiveness of treatment for varicocele related infertility. *J Urol* 2002;168:2490–2494.

74. Belker AM, Thomas AJ Jr, Fuchs EF, et al. Results of 1469 microsurgical vasectomy reversals by the Vasovasostomy Study Group. *J Urol* 1991;145:505–511.

75. Cos LR, Valvo JR, Davis RS, Cockett AT. Vasovasostomy: Current state of the art. *Urology* 1983;22:567–575.

76. Fox M. Vasectomy reversal-microsurgery for best results. *Br J Urol* 1994;73:449–453.

77. Lee HY. A 20-year experience with vasovasostomy. *J Urol* 1986;136:413–415.

78. Owen E, Kapila H. Vasectomy reversal Review of 475 microsurgical vasovasostomies. *Med J Aust* 1984;140:398–400.

79. Requeda E. Fertilizing capacity and sperm antibodies in vasovasostomized men. *Fertil Steril* 1983;39:197–203.

80. Silber SJ. Pregnancy after vasovasostomy for vasectomy reversal: A study of factors affecting long-term return of fertility in 282 patients followed for 10 years. *Hum Reprod* 1989;4:318–322.

81. Silber SJ. Epididymal extravasation following vasectomy as a cause for failure of vasectomy reversal. *Fertil Steril* 1979;31:309–315.

82. Fogdestam I, Fall M, Nilsson S. Microsurgical vasoepididymostomy in the treatment of occlusive azoospermia. *Fertil Steril* 1986;46(5):925–929.

83. Jarow JP, Sigman M, Buch JP, Oates RD. Delayed appearance of sperm after end-to-side vasoepididymostomy. *J Urol* 1995;153:1156–1158.

84. Matsuda T, Horii Y, Muguruma K, et al. Microsurgical vasoepididymostomy for obstructive azoospermia: Factors affecting postoperative fertility. *Eur Urol* 1994;26:322–326.

85. Schlegel PN, Goldstein M. Microsurgical vasoepididymostomy: refinements and results *J Urol* 1993;150:1165–1168.

86. Silber SJ. Results of microsurgical vasoepididymostomy: Role of epididymis in sperm maturation. *Hum Reprod* 1989;4:298–303.

87. Takihara H. The treatment of obstructive azoospermia in male infertility-past present and future. *Urology* 1998;51(suppl 5A):150–155.

88. Thomas AJ, Howards SS. Microsurgical treatment of male infertility, in Lipshultz LI, Howards SS (eds), *Infertility in the Male*, 3d ed. St Louis: Mosby, 1997; pp 371–384.

89. Berger RE. Triangulation end to side vasoepididymostomy. *J Urol* 1998;159:1951–1953.

90. Marmar JL. Modified vasoepididymostomy with simultaneous double needle placement, tubulotomy, and tubular invagination. *J Urol* 2000;163:483–486.

91. Fuchs EF, Burt R. Vasectomy reversal performed 15 years or more after vasectomy: Correlation of pregnancy outcome with partner age and with pregnancy results of in vitro fertilization with intracytoplasmic sperm injection. *Fertil Steril* 2002;77:516–519.

92. Kolettis PN, Sabanegh ES, D'Amico AM, et al. Outcomes for vasectomy reversal performed

after obstructive intervals of at least ten years. *Urology* 2002;60:885–888.

93. Kolettis PN, Thomas AJ Jr. Vasoepididymostomy for vasectomy reversal: A critical assessment in the era of intracytoplasmic sperm injection. *J Urol* 1997;158:467–470.

94. Pavlovich CP, Schlegel PN. Fertility options after vasectomy: A cost-effectiveness analysis. *Fertil Steril* 1997;67:133–141.

95. Thomas AJ Jr. Vasoepididymostomy. *Urol Clin North Am* 1987;14:527–538.

96. Kim ED, Winkel E, Orejuela F, Lipshultz LI. Pathological epididymal obstruction unrelated to vasectomy: Results with microsurgical reconstruction. *J Urol* 1998;160:2078–2080.

97. Shaban SF, Seaman EK, Lipshultz LI. Treatment of abnormalities of ejaculation, in Lipshultz LI, Howards SS (eds), *Infertility in the Male,* 3d ed. St Louis: Mosby, 1997; pp 423–438.

98. Ohl DA, Bennett CJ, McCabe M, et al. Predictors of success in electroejaculation of spinal cord injured men. *J Urol* 1989;142:1483–1486.

99. Dickey RP, Pyrzak R, Lu PY, et al. Comparison of the sperm quality necessary for successful intrauterine insemination with World Health Organization threshold values for normal sperm. *Fertil Steril* 1999;71:684–689.

100. Burgues S, Calderon MD. Subcutaneous self-administration of highly purified follicle stimulating hormone and human chorionic gonadotrophin for the treatment of male hypogonadotropic hypogonadism. Spanish Collaborative Group on Male Hypogonadotropic Hypogonadism. *Hum Reprod* 1997;12: 980–986.

101. Tournaye H, Devroey P, Liu J, et al. Microsurgical epididymal sperm aspiration and intracytoplasmic sperm injection: A new effective approach to infertility as a result of congenital bilateral absence of the vas deferens. *Fertil Steril* 1994;61:1045–1051.

102. Sheynkin YR, Ye Z, Menendez S, et al. Controlled comparison of percutaneous and microsurgical sperm retrieval in men with obstructive azoospermia. *Hum Reprod* 1998;13: 3086–3089.

103. Craft IL, Khalifa Y, Boulos A, et al. Factors influencing the outcome of in-vitro fertilization with percutaneous aspirated epididymal spermatozoa and intracytoplasmic sperm injection in azoospermic men. *Hum Reprod* 1995;10: 1791–1794.

104. Devroey P, Liu J, Nagy Z, et al. Pregnancies after testicular sperm extraction and intracytoplasmic sperm injection in non-obstructive azoospermia. *Hum Reprod* 1995;10:1457–1460.

105. Gil-Salom M, Romero J, Minguez Y, et al. Testicular sperm extraction and intracytoplasmic sperm injection: A chance of fertility in nonobstructive azoospermia. *J Urol* 1998;160: 2063–2067.

106. Kahraman S, Ozgur S, Alatas C, et al. Fertility with testicular sperm extraction and intracytoplasmic sperm injection in nonobstructive azoospermic men. *Hum Reprod* 1996;11: 756–760.

107. Oates RD, Mulhall J, Burgess C, et al. Fertilization and pregnancy using intentionally cryopreserved testicular tissue as the sperm source for intracytoplasmic sperm injection in 10 men with non-obstructive azoospermia. *Hum Reprod* 1997;12:734–739.

108. Palermo GD, Schlegel PN, Hariprashad JJ, et al. Fertilization and pregnancy outcome with intracytoplasmic sperm injection for azoospermic men. *Hum Reprod* 1999;14:741–748.

109. Friedler S, Raziel A, Strassburger D, et al. Testicular sperm retrieval by percutaneous fine needle sperm aspiration compared with testicular sperm extraction by open biopsy in men with nonobstructive azoospermia. *Hum Reprod* 1997;12:1488–1493.

110. Ezeh UI, Moore HD, Cooke ID. A prospective study of multiple needle biopsies versus a single open biopsy for testicular sperm extraction in men with nonobstructive azoospermia. *Hum Reprod* 1998;13:3075–3080.

111. Lewin A, Reubinoff B, Porat-Katz A, et al. Testicular fine needle aspiration: The alternative method for sperm retrieval in nonobstructive azoospermia. *Hum Reprod* 1999;14:1785–1790.

112. Ezeh UI, Taub NA, Moore HD, et al. Establishment of predictive variables associated with testicular sperm retrieval in men with nonostructive azoospermia. *Hum Reprod* 1999;14: 1005–1012.

113. Su LM, Palermo GD, Goldstein M, et al. Testicular sperm extraction with intracytoplasmic sperm injection for nonobstructive azoospermia: Testicular histology can predict success of sperm retrieval. *J Urol* 1999;161:112–116.

114. Tournaye H, Verheyen G, Nagy P, et al. Are there any predictive factors for successful testicular

sperm recovery in azoospermic patients? *Hum Reprod* 1997;12:80–86.

115. Palermo GD, Schlegel PN, Sillis ES, et al. Births after intracytoplasmic sperm injection of sperm obtained by testicular extraction from men with nonmosaic Klinefelter's syndrome. *N Engl J Med* 1999;338:588–590.

116. Schlegel PN. Testicular sperm extraction: microdissection improves sperm yield with minimal tissue excision. *Hum Reprod* 1999;14:131–135.

117. Turek PJ, Givens CR, Schriock ED, et al. Testis sperm extraction and intracytoplasmic sperm injection guided by prior fine-needle aspiration mapping in patients with nonobstructive azoospermia. *Fertil Steril* 1999;71:552–557.

118. Turek PJ, Williams RH, Gilbaugh JH, et al. The reversibility of anabolic steroid-induced azoospermia. *J Urol* 1995;153:1628–1630.

119. Jarow JP. Nonsurgical therapy of male infertility: Empirical therapy, in Lipshultz LI, Howards SS (eds), *Infertility in the Male,* 3d ed. St Louis: Mosby, 1997; pp 410–422.

120. Pavlovich CP, King P, Goldstein M, et al. Evidence of a treatable endocrinopathy in infertile men. *J Urol* 2001;165:837–841.

CHAPTER 17

Ovulation Induction for Anovulatory Women

SEJAL P. DHARIA AND RICHARD E. BLACKWELL

Ovulation induction was used initially to treat women with oligomenorrhea, amenorrhea, and irregular ovulation. Ten to fifteen percent of women suffer with ovulatory dysfunction. In recent years, the medications and role for ovulation induction have expanded to include women who are ovulatory but have unexplained infertility or subfertility to recruit multiple follicles for assisted reproductive techniques (ARTs).

▶ CANDIDATES FOR OVULATION INDUCTION

Ovulatory disorders are classified according to the World Health Organization (WHO). The WHO categorizes three groups of ovulatory dysfunction based on the type of abnormality. Group I includes patients with hypothalamic-pituitary hypofunction, which is represented by patients with amenorrhea related to stress, eating disorders, and strenuous exercise. Kallmann's syndrome [related to an absent migration of gonadotropin-releasing hormone (GnRH) progenitor cells] and isolated gonadotropin deficiency also are included in this group.

The second category (WHO group II) encompasses patients who have hypothalamic-pituitary-ovarian dysregulation. These patients have eugonadotropic ovarian dysfunction with varying degrees of anovulation and oligomenorrhea. Patients in group II can have polycystic ovarian syndrome, hyperthecosis, or the HAIRAN syndrome (*h*irsutism, *a*novulation, *i*nsulin *r*esistance, and *a*canthosis *n*igricans).

The last category, WHO group III, consists of those patients with end-organ deficiency or resistance. These patients have hypergonadotropic hypogonadism and include those with premature ovarian failure or ovarian resistance. Typically, these patients respond poorly to efforts at ovulation induction.

Ovulation induction also can be used for other indications (see Table 17-1), including unexplained infertility (see Chap. 18), subfertility from endometriosis (see Chap. 20), and ARTs (see Chap. 22). In this chapter the focus is on ovulatory dysfunction.

▶ PREREQUISITES FOR OVULATION INDUCTION

The induction of ovulation is initiated after underlying etiologies are identified and addressed through an infertility workup. Each couple will have a complete history and

▶ **TABLE 17-1:** INDICATIONS FOR
OVULATION INDUCTION

Type I
Type II
Type III
Others • Failed clomiphene therapy • Endometriosis • Unexplained infertility • Assisted reproductive techniques (IVF, GIFT, ZIFT, oocyte donation)

physical examination. The history documents ovulatory disturbances through either the lack of menstrual cycles or cycle lengths of less than 26 or greater than 32 days. The history also can uncover signs and symptoms of endocrinopathies, such as hirsutism, virilization, galactorrhea, or changes associated with hypoestrogenism. The importance of collecting these data cannot be overstated because the onset of symptoms, the severity, and any prior therapy often will dictate the choice of ovulation-inducing agent. A genetic component that affects fertility is unveiled through the presence of a family history of infertility or ovarian or adrenal disease. On physical examination, the patient's blood pressure, pulse, and weight may give a hint as to the etiology of disease, such as adrenal hyperplasia, thyroid disease, or obesity. Evaluating the skin for the presence of acanthosis nigricans, discolored striae, or changes in hypo-hyperpigmentation, respectively, may suggest insulin resistance, ectopic adrenocorticotropic hormone (ACTH) production, and estrogen status. The breast examination should focus on galactorrhea, often associated with hyperprolactinemia. Key components to the head and neck evaluation include testing for thyromegaly and visual changes such as bilateral temporal hemianopsia, which suggests a pituitary mass lesion. Finally, the genitourinary examination should evaluate the cer-

vical os and the quality of its mucus, the uterine contour and adnexa to rule out the presence of a tumor or myomas that may affect the uterine cavity.

The diagnostic evaluation of infertility seeks to demonstrate the presence of competent sperm, competent egg growth, and a patent, receptive reproductive tract. The first stage of testing requires a semen analysis to rule out an occult male factor, which is present 40 percent of the time in patients with infertility.[1]

The next stage of testing determines the presence of anovulation and its etiology. The basal body temperature chart may be used to accomplish this task. A woman's temperature is charted every morning before arising from the start of one menses to the start of another using a thermometer measured out in tenths. An increase in the basal body temperature of 0.5-1.0 degree suggests ovulation and is sustained for the duration of the luteal phase. This test is inexpensive but labor-intensive for the patient, and in up to 20 percent of cases, the basal body temperature may be monophasic in the presence of ovulation (measured by other means).[2]

A second method to determine ovulation uses a luteinizing hormone (LH) urinary assay. This kit is used between days 10 and 16 (because the majority of patients will ovulate in this time window). The LH surge occurs in the morning, and the LH kit will be most accurate in the midafternoon to early evening. The accuracy of the test varies by the brand, but this is an expensive method to document ovulation (and it is more precise than a basal body temperature chart). Other methods that can detect ovulation include the measurement of a midluteal progesterone concentration (with an absolute value greater than 3 ng/mL), the presence of a mature follicle (1.6 to 2.2 m) at midcycle, the presence of a corpus luteum, peritoneal free fluid around the time of ovulation, or an endometrial biopsy (around cycle day 25), which is less popular today because it is more invasive than the other methods.

The third stage in evaluation of an infertile couple is the postcoital test. An abnormality suggests an occult male factor or a cervical factor. The test is performed the morning after the onset of the LH surge. The couple is instructed to have intercourse 4 to 6 hours prior to the test. A sample of cervical mucus is obtained, evaluated for the spinnbarkheit (8 to 10 cm) and the number and quality of directionally motile sperm (10 to 15) under a microscope. The accuracy and efficacy of this test remains controversial.

Stages 4 and 5 encompass imaging of the reproductive tract through a hysterosalpingogram (HSG) or a laparoscopy/hysteroscopy, respectively, which will rule out an anatomic abnormality. HSGs are performed in conjunction with radiology and use either an oil- or water-based dye. The oil-based dye defines the uterine cavity more accurately, whereas water-based dyes define the tubal anatomy more clearly. There is some evidence that the HSG performed with oil-based dye increases the pregnancy rate, although the physiology is not understood. Laparoscopy/hysteroscopy (stages 4, 5), performed after empirical therapy, will reveal pathology in 80 percent of patients. Saline-infusion sonography has been popularized recently, but its ability to define tubal anatomy is not conclusive. Thus it cannot be recommended at this juncture.

Other testing to identify the etiology of anovulation includes measurement of serum prolactin, thyroid-stimulating hormone (TSH), and follicle-stimulating hormone (FSH). If the patient presents with hirsutism (discussed further in Chap. 13), laboratory evaluation of serum 17-hydroxyprogesterone (17-OHP), dehydroepiandrosterone sulfate (DHEAS), total testosterone, free testosterone, and sex hormone–binding globulin will help to exclude adrenal and ovarian disease or pathology in the production or metabolism of testosterone.

▶ MANAGEMENT OF THE PATIENT WITH AN OVULATORY DISORDER

Treatment of Patients in WHO Group I (Hypothalamic-Pituitary Hypofunction)

Euprolactinemic Patient

Patients in WHO group I with euprolactinemia have hypothalamic dysfunction and encompass patients with Kallmann's syndrome and patients with stress- or weight loss–induced anovulation. If the patient is markedly underweight, attempts to increase her caloric intake until ideal body weight is achieved should be made in conjunction with a dietician. Patients usually resume ovulation once sufficient weight is acquired. If ovulation is not achieved, clomiphene citrate can be administered, although most women will not respond to this therapy[2] and are excellent candidates for gonadotropins.[3] Studies have shown that a mixture of LH and FSH produces optimal results.[4] Pulsatile [GnRH] can also be utilized (see Table 17-2.)

Hyperprolactinemic Patient

The incidence of hyperprolactinemia is presumed to be 30 percent in patients with menstrual irregularities. The mechanism of anovulation is mediated by dopamine inhibition of GnRH in the hypothalamus. Once the etiology of hyperprolactinemia is identified and

▶ **TABLE 17-2:** TREATMENT FOR WHO GROUP I OVULATORY DYSFUNCTION

Hypothalamic Pituitary Hypofunction   • LH/FSH-containing gonadotropins   • Gonadotropin-releasing hormone (pulsatile)   **Hypothalamic-Pituitary Hypofunction with Hyperprolactinemia**   • Dopamine agonists   • Clomiphene/gonadotropins

addressed, the primary treatment of choice is a dopamine agonist, with which more than 85 percent of patients will regain ovulatory function. In women who cannot tolerate or have failed to ovulate with a dopamine agonist, gonadotropins and, in some rare cases, clomiphene are used to induce ovulation.

Treatment of Patients in WHO Group II (Eugonadotropic Anovulation)

Hyperandrogenic Patient

The hyperandrogenic anovulatory patient is defined as having either clinical evidence of hyperandrogenism or laboratory evidence of hyperandrogenemia in the presence of anovulation according to the 1990 National Institutes of Health (NIH) Consensus Conference. The first step is to identify the underlying etiology and to rule out a malignancy, which must be treated surgically. If the pathology is a result of elevated adrenal androgens, suppression through glucocorticoids may result in ovulation. First described in patients with congenital adrenal hyperplasia, glucocorticoid therapy (either 5.0 to 7.5 mg prednisone or 0.5 mg dexamethasone) blunts the adrenal contribution of circulating androgens and diminishes the androgen level in the microenvironment of the follicle. Prednisone restores ovulatory function[5] and should be maintained until documentation of pregnancy.[6]

Patients with Chronic Anovulation

Patients who suffer from chronic anovulation may have a normal or elevated (>2:1) LH/FSH ratio. Regardless, clomiphene citrate is the drug of choice in the therapy of these patients. If these patients are part of the polycystic ovarian syndrome (PCOS) spectrum, with or without insulin resistance, treatment with an insulin sensitizer (i.e., metformin) may be an option either alone or in conjunction with clomiphene citrate. Gonadotropin therapy is reserved for patients who do not ovulate or conceive after

▶ **TABLE 17-3:** TREATMENT FOR WHO GROUP II OVULATORY DYSFUNCTION

Hypothalamic-Pituitary Dysfunction
• Initially treat with clomiphene citrate in incremental doses each cycle until ovulation is achieved
• If fails clomiphene, move to gonadotropins (FSH-containing)
• With premature LH surges in each cycle -GnRH agonist -GnRH antagonist
• With insulin resistance -Insulin sensitizer
• Elevated adrenal androgens -Glucocorticoids

a defined period with clomiphene (four to six ovulatory cycles) (see Table 17-3).

Treatment of Patients in WHO Group III (Hypergonadotropic Hypogonadism)

A persistent measurement of serum FSH concentration above 40 mIU/mL indicates ovarian resistance (normal cohort of primordial follicles) or ovarian failure (absence or depletion of primordial follicles). Regardless of the etiology, the prognosis for spontaneous pregnancy is poor. However, pregnancy may occur if serum gonadotropins return to normal spontaneously. Sporadic pregnancies also have occurred in women on cyclic hormone replacement therapy. Occasionally, patients will respond to high-dose gonadotropin therapy; however, ovulation induction is almost always unsuccessful in producing a pregnancy in women with elevated FSH concentrations and therefore is not recommended. These patients are best served by egg-donation treatment (see Table 17-4).

Others

Endometriosis is a disease that usually is associated with a degree of subfertility related to

▶ **TABLE 17-4:** TREATMENT FOR WHO GROUP III OVULATORY DYSFUNCTION

Hypergonadotropic Hypogonadism
• Gonadotropins rarely work
• Sporadic pregnancies resulted from cyclic replacement therapy
• If no spontaneous pregnancy, recommend oocyte donation

both structural and immunologic factors. Although these patients probably do not have a major ovulatory dysfunction, three randomized, controlled trials have evaluated the induction of ovulation for increasing fertility in women with endometriosis. Ovulation induction plus intrauterine insemination in two of three studies demonstrated a threefold increase in fertility as compared with controls.[7] Another recently incorporated indication for controlled ovarian hyperstimulation is unexplained infertility, in which the use of ovulation induction and intrauterine insemination has shown a statistically significant increase in pregnancy rates as compared with controls.[8]

▶ OVULATION-INDUCTION AGENTS

Commonly used ovulation-induction agents include clomiphene citrate, human menopausal gonadotropins, urinary FSH, recombinant FSH, recombinant FSH/LH, GnRH agonists, GnRH antagonists, and pulsatile GnRH. Each of these agents will be discussed separately (see Table 17-5 for brand names).

Clomiphene Citrate

Introduced in 1956, clomiphene citrate entered clinical trials as early as 1960 and by 1967 received Food and Drug Administration (FDA) approval for ovulation induction. Clomiphene citrate can be used alone or in conjunction with other medications (e.g., dexamethasone, metformin, bromocriptine, or gonadotropins) to increase its efficacy.

Pharmacology

Structurally, clomiphene citrate is a triphenylethylene derivative composed of a racemic mixture of two stereochemical isomers, *trans* and *cis*. These two isomers were renamed to *enclomiphene* and *zuclomiphene citrate*, respectively, and the more active component of the two isomers appears to be zuclomiphene.[9] Clomiphene citrate is well absorbed orally and is metabolized by the liver to inactive metabolites. Clomiphene citrate has a half-life of approximately 5 days. The main route of excretion is through the feces, although small amounts are found in urine.

Mechanism of Action

Clomiphene citrate acts as both an agonist and an antagonist, competitively binding to the hypothalamic and pituitary estrogen receptors, displacing endogenous estrogen, removing the feedback inhibition, stimulating the release of gonadotropins, and promoting follicular growth.[6] This mechanism of action is demonstrated indirectly in humans through an elevation in LH pulse frequency after administration of clomiphene citrate.[10]

Indications

The primary indication of clomiphene citrate is in the eugonadotropic, euprolactinemic, euthyroid anovulatory patient. These patients typically have abundant circulating estrogen, may develop endometrial irregularities, and therefore respond to the local antiestrogenic qualities of clomiphene.[11] In fact, women with hypogonadotropic hypogonadism usually are poor candidates for ovulation induction with clomiphene citrate. The one exception may be the patient with low-level hyperprolactinemic anovulation, who will benefit from clomiphene citrate with a dopamine agonist. Clomiphene also has been used in the management of unexplained infertility, subfertility resulting from endometriosis, and minimally in ARTs. Women

▶ **TABLE 17-5:** TABLE TITLE ?????????

• **Ovulation Induction Agents with Commonly Used Brand Names:**	
—Clomiphene Citrate	*Clomid, Serophene*
—Human Menopausal Gonadotropins	*Pergonal, Repronex Humegon*
—Highly purified Urinary FSH	*Fertinex, Bravelle*
—Urinary hCG	*Novarel, Pregnyl, Profasi*
—Recombinant FSH	*Follistim, Gonal-F*
—Recombinant hCG	*Ovidrel*
—GnRH Agonist	*Lupron*
—GnRH Antagonists	*Cetrotide, Antagon*

who fall into WHO group III, with hypergonadotropic hypogonadism, also will respond poorly to clomiphene because they already have elevated gonadotropins, but no response can be elicited from the ovary.

Contraindications and Side Effects

Clomiphene citrate has a relatively wide margin of safety compared with most therapeutic agents, so there are a limited number of contraindications.

Ovarian cysts. Clomiphene stimulates follicular growth and in the presence of ovarian cysts can increase their size further. Although rare, this can lead to massive ovarian enlargement or torsion. Most cysts resolve spontaneously within one or two cycles,[6] after which clomiphene citrate can be reinitiated.

Pregnancy. Although an obvious contraindication, the impact of clomiphene on early human gestation is unknown because it has not been associated with an increased incidence of congenital anomalies. However, testing after each clomiphene citrate cycle with no spontaneous menses will prevent this occurrence.[11]

Liver disease. Since clomiphene citrate is metabolized through the liver, the presence of liver disease or dysfunction is a contraindication to its use.

Visual problems. Visual disturbances occur in 2 percent of cycles and include blurring of vision or scotomata. The physiology of these symptoms is unknown, but they usually disappear in a few days to 2 weeks once the medication is discontinued.[6]

Other adverse effects. Hot flushes occur in 10 percent of patients and are related to the antiestrogenic properties of clomiphene citrate. Once the medication is discontinued, the symptoms will resolve. Other reported symptoms include mood swings, depression, headaches (1 percent), nausea and breast tenderness (2 percent), and dryness and loss of hair (0.3 percent). These also will resolve after discontinuation of clomiphene citrate.[3] Complications such as ovarian hyperstimulation and multiple pregnancy and the long-term risk of malignancy will be addressed at the end of this chapter.

Method of Administration

Clomiphene citrate is usually initiated on days 2 through 5 after a spontaneous or induced menses and is continued for 5 days. The initial dose should be 50 mg. Lack of a response ideally should be determined at the end of a single treatment cycle, allowing an incremental increase during the next cycle. The maximal dose ranges from 200 to 250 mg, although 50 percent of pregnancies will occur at a dose of 50 mg and another 20 percent at 100 mg.[13] Once an ovulatory dosage is obtained, there is no benefit from increasing the dose; in fact, the antiestrogenic properties of clomiphene may make it disadvantageous. This ovulatory dose should be continued for four to six cycles. Approximately 80 percent of patients who were previously anovulatory will ovulate on clomiphene citrate, although only 40 percent achieve a live birth.[14] This discrepancy may be attributed to either underlying infertility factors or the antiestrogenic effect of clomiphene.

Monitoring of the patient on clomiphene citrate is minimal. The first requirement is to document ovulation. As discussed earlier, this can be done through the use of a basal body temperature chart (see Fig. 17-1). Basal body temperature is monitored for the full cycle or an abbreviated time period from the last dose of clomiphene until a temperature rise sustained over 3 days or the onset of the next menses.[11] Another more commonly employed method is to obtain a midluteal progesterone level (cycle days 22 to 23). Ideally, this will

correlate with the peak progesterone production about 1 week after ovulation.[15] At this time the value will exceed 10 ng/mL. The levels of progesterone may be higher in stimulated cycles as compared with spontaneous ovulation because multiple follicles may be mature and luteinized. A measurement of urinary LH concentration also can document ovulation. Clomiphene citrate ingestion induces the release of large amounts of LH, and LH testing may yield false-positive results. For this reason, testing should be initiated 2 days after the last dose of clomiphene citrate.[5]

In patients in whom clomiphene citrate alone does not elicit ovulation, an alternative is to provide prolonged regimens of clomiphene

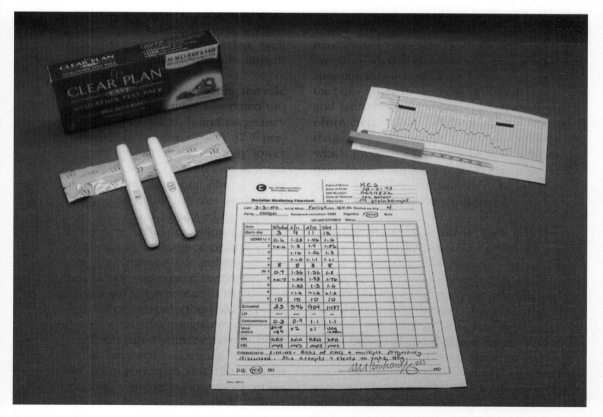

Figure 17-1 Methods used to detect ovulation. Basal body temperature charting requires patient motivation and may be monophasic in up to 20 percent of patients who undergo ovulation. The LH urinary assay is more specific and expensive and can be falsely positive in the presence of endogenous/exogenous LH.

citrate (daily from days 5 through 13). Ovulation rates in patients who fail the traditional regimen are 60 percent, with a conception rate of 38 percent.[16] Others, however, have not confirmed these results. Another alternative form of management described by O'Herlihy and colleagues is to administer clomiphene and incrementally increase the dose until an appropriate rise in estradiol concentration is noted.[17]

In patients who fail to ovulate using the traditional clomiphene regimen, human chorionic gonadotropin (hCG) can be added to trigger ovulation. Clomiphene is administered in the traditional manner. On cycle day 14 or 15, a transvaginal ultrasound is performed, and in the presence of a mature lead follicle (18 to 20 mm), hCG can be administered (10,000 IU subcutaneously). This should stimulate ovulation 36 h after administration.[18]

These forms of management are most effective in the anovulatory WHO group II patients, who are eugonadotropic and euestrogenic. It is important to choose a regimen efficiently and not to prolong clomiphene therapy because 75 percent of women will ovulate in the first three ovulatory cycles.[19]

Clomiphene citrate can be combined with other medications (e.g., dopamine agonists, glucocorticoids, or gonadotropins), or these medications can be used alone to improve ovulatory capability.

Dopamine Agonists

The most commonly prescribed and well-studied dopamine agonist is bromocriptine mesylate (Parlodel), which is a semisynthetic product derived from a family of ergot alkaloids or ergopeptines.

Mechanism of Action
A dopamine agonist, this drug exerts a direct effect at the level of the pituitary, competing with dopamine for binding sites (D1 and D2) to the anterior pituitary. It inhibits the release and synthesis of prolactin at the level of the lactotroph but also at the level of the tuberoinfundibular neurons in the hypothalamus.

Indications
The drug is used to treat patients with a prolactin-secreting adenoma or idiopathic hyperprolactinemia.

Administration
The oral dose is 1.25 to 20 mg/d, although the typical dose is 2.5 mg twice daily (as a comparison, in Parkinson disease, the average dose may be as high as 140 to 160 mg/d). The drug's effect on prolactin levels is rapid and can be reassessed after 1 to 2 weeks. Ovulatory function will return to 80 to 90 percent of patients once they are optimized on bromocriptine, usually within one to two cycles.[20] Although bromocriptine usually is discontinued as soon as pregnancy is established, teratogenic effects have not been described.[3]

Contraindications
Dopamine agonists should be discontinued in the face of uncontrolled hypertension or hypersensitivity to ergot derivatives.

Adverse Effects
In some patients, bromocriptine may induce nausea, vomiting, headaches, nasal congestion, and postural hypotension, causing more than 5 percent of patients to discontinue the drug.[6] For patients who cannot tolerate bromocriptine orally, vaginal administration can be used, although side effects are similar. An alternative is cabergoline (Dostinex), a pure D2 receptor agonist. Cabergoline has a long half-life and is administered once or twice weekly. Multiple studies have shown equal efficacy of cabergoline and bromocriptine with <50 percent of the side effects.[21] Rarely, patients may experience nausea and vomiting with cabergoline therapy; these patients may be treated with intravaginal cabergoline.[22] Permax (Pergolide), not approved for the use in ovulation induction, has been shown to achieve euprolactinemia in a small number of studies.[23]

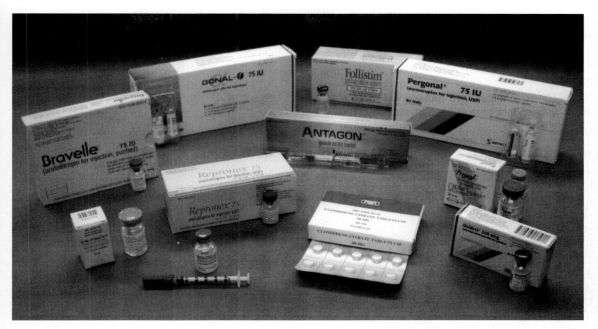

Figure 17-2 A sample of the variety of medications available for ovulation induction or as adjuncts. The syringe in front is used for subcutaneous administration.

Glucocorticoids

Indication

Suppression of excessive androgen secretion by glucocorticoid administration was first described in patients with congenital adrenal hyperplasia.[24] Raj and colleagues found that their PCOS patients with elevated adrenal androgen production had ovulation rates of 17 percent while on clomiphene. Sixty-five percent of the remaining anovulatory women subsequently ovulated when placed on prednisone alone.[25] In another study, Rodriguez-Rigau restored ovulatory activity with glucocorticoids in 91 percent of patients with anovulation.[26]

Indication

Glucocorticoids are a treatment option for anovulatory patients with an adrenal component to their disease.

Mechanism of Action

Glucocorticoids blunt the nighttime peak of ACTH secretion and subsequently the contribution of adrenal androgens to the ovary. In addition to its adrenal effects, glucocorticoid treatment partially inhibits ovarian androgen secretion.[27]

Administration

To maximize suppression, prednisone 5.0 to 7.5 mg or dexamethasone 0.5 mg should be given as a single or split dose, with the majority of the drug being given at night. When administered in classic (adult) onset congenital adrenal hyperplasia, the required dosage may vary. Customization of the dosage requirement will require measurement of the precursor hormone 17-OHP, or if there are concerns of adrenal suppression, a random 8 A.M. cortisol determination can be done. If ovulatory function does not resume with glucocorticoids, then clomiphene citrate can be used as an adjunct. Lobo and colleagues showed that the addition of clomiphene citrate to dexamethasone when DHEAS levels were >2700 ng/mL induced ovulation in 50 percent of patients.[28] Glucocorticoids do not appear to increase the incidence of fetal developmental anomalies in neonates whose mothers were treated with prednisone.[29]

Contraindications

Contraindications include hypersensitivity to glucocorticoids and systemic fungal infections. There are many side effects with chronic use.

Insulin Sensitizers

Metformin hydrochloride (Glucophage) is an oral antihyperglycemic agent used in the management of type 2 diabetes mellitus and in group II anovulatory patients with insulin resistance.

Mechanism of Action

In diabetic patients, metformin decreases hepatic gluconeogenesis and increases the peripheral uptake of glucose.

Administration

Most studies or case reports of metformin have shown an increase in menstrual cyclicity, ovulatory function, and fertility when administered as 500 mg three to four times daily. Doses can be increased incrementally from 500 mg once a day up to a total of 2000 mg daily.[30] Combining the results of nine uncontrolled studies, metformin was shown to restore regular menses in 62 percent of patients with oligomenorrhea or amenorrhea and was more effective in achieving ovulation as compared with placebo in five uncontrolled studies.[31] The only exception, according to one study, may be in women with morbid obesity (BMI approached 40 kg/m^2).[32] Metformin can be used as an adjunct to clomiphene citrate in patients who do not ovulate with clomiphene citrate alone and was found to improve the rates of both ovulation and pregnancy.[33] However, Nestler and colleagues in one study demonstrated that metformin was more efficacious than clomiphene in terms of ovulation induction.[31] The efficacy of metformin alone is being addressed through a Reproductive Medicine Network Study currently underway.

Adverse Effects

Metformin produces dose-related gastrointestinal side effects that often subside over time; however, it is prudent to start with a low dose, followed by a gradual increase over 3 to 4 weeks. Also, it is important for patients taking metformin to consume a low-carbohydrate diet, which will further minimize gastrointestinal symptoms. Liver function tests should be evaluated both prior to the administration and periodically while a patient is on metformin.

Metformin also has been used with gonadotropins in two small studies that demonstrated no improvement in number of dominant follicles, estradiol concentrations, or pregnancy rates,[31] although more studies are needed to evaluate this issue.

Thiazolidinediones (e.g., Troglitazone, Rosiglitazone, Pioglitazone), an alternative group of insulin-sensitizing agents, have all been shown to induce ovulation.[30] However, Troglitazone was taken off the market in March of 2000 for its association with liver disease. Nevertheless, studies on the other thiazolidinediones appear promising.

A third alternative is D-Chiro-Inositol, an insulin-sensitizing drug not yet commercially available, which was demonstrated to increase the frequency of ovulation,[34] by Nestler et al.

Gonadotropins

The first gonadotropins were derived from the pituitaries of human cadavers and used to induce ovulation in amenorrheic women. The therapy was successful but expensive, and it was a laborious endeavor requiring the processing of multiple pituitary glands. Simultaneously, gonadotropins were semipurified from the urine of menopausal women by Brono Lunenfeld, who also subsequently reported the first human pregnancy from human menopausal gonadotropins.

Indications

Gonadotropins are used for anovulatory infertility, oligoovulation resistant to clomiphene citrate, WHO group I (hypothalamic hypofunction), and controlled ovarian hyperstimulation for in vitro fertilization or gamete intrafallopian tubal transfer. Ovulatory rates in WHO group I patients without hyperprolactinemia and group II patients who have failed treatment with clomiphene are much higher with the use of gonadotropins (90 to 95 percent).

Contraindications

Untreated hyperprolactinemia and ovarian failure are contraindications to therapy, as discussed earlier. Patients with uncontrolled thyroid, adrenal dysfunction, or pituitary tumors should not use gonadotropins until their primary disease is treated. Ovarian cysts and abnormal vaginal bleeding of unknown origin are also contraindications to gonadotropin therapy. Since gonadotropins require close monitoring and strict compliance, contraindications also include lack of appropriate monitoring capability, patient cooperation, or trained personnel.

Physiology

FSH binds to the granulosa cells and through a cyclic AMP-mediated second-messenger system that induces the aromatase enzyme, increases granulosa cell number, and induces LH receptors. Gonadotropins will promote follicle growth and maturation and in most cases will require an additional injection of hCG to induce ovulation and luteinization. FSH is responsible for the initiation of follicle growth. Although controversial, there is some evidence that LH is required for maintenance of folliculogenesis (two-cell hypothesis).

Clinical Management

The traditional step-up protocol uses between 2 and 8 ampules per day starting on day 4 of the menstrual cycle. This will be continued daily until the serum estradiol level reaches between 500 and 1500 pg/mL (in general) and follicle size by ultrasound reaches 16 to 18 mm in mean diameter. Follicular growth is linear initially and then exponential, at a rate of 2 mm per day. If there is no response, the dosage can be increased, but it should be maintained once estradiol begins to rise and the follicles begin to expand. A second form of gonadotropin management is the step-down protocol. The patient is started on 2 ampules of FSH. Subsequently, the dose is decreased to 1.5 ampules and then again decreased to 1 ampule 3 days later. This management promotes monofollicular growth and prevents multiple pregnancy. No mention is made of pregnancy rates, although theoretically they would be lower.[35] Once the follicles are mature, a single injection (5000 or 10,000 IU) of hCG is given 24 h after the last injection of gonadotropins to achieve ovulation. Only one injection is needed because hCG remains detectable in the serum for up to 10 days. In some cases of an exuberant hormonal response to gonadotropins, "coasting" is recommended, or withholding gonadotropins for a defined period of time, in order to minimize the chance of ovarian hyperstimulation syndrome. However, there is insufficient data to determine if coasting is an effective strategy, and at this time it cannot be recommended.[36]

Clomiphene citrate and gonadotropins also can be combined for ovulation induction. Clomiphene is given initially for 5 days, after which gonadotropins are started at a dose of 2 ampules. Once a lead follicle is mature, hCG is administered to induce ovulation. This method will produce lower pregnancy rates as compared with gonadotropins alone and in the face of gonadotropin availability should not be recommended.

Method of Administration

The medications (urinary-derived gonadotropins) were marketed originally for intramuscular use because these preparations contained relatively high amounts of urinary proteins, and subcutaneous administration may induce adverse local reactions. However, multiple studies show that both urinary-derived preparations of FSH or FSH/LH[38] and recombinant gonadotropins have the same pharmacokinetics after either subcutaneous or intramuscular injection.[37]

Results

The majority of pregnancies will occur in the first four to six cycles of therapy. Success varies with the form of therapy. The pregnancy rate for patients with hypothalamic-pituitary anovulation is high, with a cumulative pregnancy rate of 91 percent using menotropins. Patients with WHO group II ovulatory dysfunction attain pregnancy rates of 21 to 40 percent per cycle using a purified FSH gonadotropin. In these patients, LH supplementation typically is not given because most patients have a high endogenous level of LH secretion.[6]

Menotropins

Menopausal gonadotropins are glycoproteins derived from the urine of postmenopausal women. Urinary gonadotropins are made by taking bulk urine from menopausal donors and employing chromatography to remove some of the very high- and low-molecular-weight impurities from the solution. The remaining solution has a combination of FSH and LH, plus a large number of urinary proteins (i.e., cytokines, growth factors, transferrins, and other proteins). This solution is referred to as *menotropins*. Menotropins are supplied in ampules as lyophilized powder containing 75 or 150 IU of FSH and LH.

Urofollitropins

Purification of these menotropins resulted in the production of urofollitropin. Antibodies to hCG are placed on a chromatography column, and the close relationship of hCG to LH allows LH to selectively bind to hCG antibodies. This produces an LH-specific immunoaffinity column in which LH is retained on the column and most urinary proteins are filtered out, leaving a gonadotropin composed almost entirely FSH.

Highly Purified Preparations of FSH

Once urofollitropins were developed, these were then highly purified. A column was created with monoclonal antibodies to FSH. The urinary solution passed through the column, and the LH and urinary proteins were removed. The FSH that was retained on the column was eluted, leaving a product more than 90 percent pure as compared with urofollitropins, which were 2 percent pure.

Recombinant Preparation of FSH or FSH/LH

The most recent form of gonadotropins produced is recombinant human FSH and FSH/LH. They are made in mammalian cells (currently used are Chinese hamster ovaries) and are similar to urofollitropin preparations in terms of bioactivity, half-lives, and maximum concentrations.[39] In terms of ovulation, pregnancy rates, and the rate of miscarriage, there were no differences in four randomized, controlled trials between recombinant FSH and urinary FSH.[40] There are certain advantages of recombinant FSH as compared with the urinary form. First, under controlled manufacturing, there is reduced interbatch variability compared with purification of enormous quantities of heterogeneous urine. Because they are such a pure product, these medications can be given subcutaneously. Also, the supply is unlimited, and because these agents are not derived from a human source, there is no risk of contamination. The only possible disadvantage is the increased cost of the product.[41]

Gonadotropin-Releasing Hormone

Sequenced and synthesized in the sheep by Guillemin and colleagues and in the pig by Schally and colleagues, GnRH was identified as a therapeutic option for women with WHO group I anovulation. GnRH was administered in a pulsatile fashion with an ideal time interval of 60–90 minutes, as presented by Knobil and colleagues. They found that a continuous infusion of GnRH suppressed gonadotropin production but that a pulsatile release would restore normal ovulatory function.[42]

Method of Administration

GnRH is available as a powder that is soluble in aqueous solution. The optimal method of administration can be either intravenous or subcutaneous. Subcutaneously, GnRH can be administered with a programmable pulsatile infusion pump at 10 to 20 μg/pulse.

Indication

The most common indication for GnRH therapy is as noted earlier—WHO group I patients with euprolactinemia.

Clinical Management

Minimal monitoring is required because endogenous control mechanisms are in effect, but the luteal phase needs to be supported either with the GnRH pump or exogenous progesterone.[11]

Results

Results of GnRH therapy demonstrate ovulatory rates of 90 percent and pregnancy rates of from 25 to 30 percent per ovulatory cycle.[3] Use of GnRH is a valuable alternative, although it is diminishing in popularity secondary to the maintenance required by the physician and the patient.

Surgical Therapy

Surgical ovulation induction is effective in patients with WHO group II ovulatory dysfunction who have failed first-line therapy with clomiphene citrate. Traditionally, surgical resection involved bilateral ovarian wedge resection, in which the ovarian volume was reduced significantly through a laparotomy incision. This resulted in temporary resumption of ovulation with pregnancy rates of 60 to 70 percent but also created significant postoperative adhesions.[43] Evolution of surgical ovulation induction turned to laparoscopically assisted ovarian puncture, which includes multiple ovarian punch biopsies, ovarian electrocauterization, laser vaporization, or photocoagulation.[44] Early reports with ovarian electrocautery in patients with PCOS resulted in ovulation rates of 70 to 97 percent (based on body weight) and an average pregnancy rate of 84 percent.[45] Similar results were obtained with laser fulguration.[46] Adhesion formation is still a potential complication, although less than with ovarian wedge resection, and in 199 PCOS patients treated with ovarian electrocautery, 19.5 percent developed de novo adhesion formation, as determined by a second-look laparoscopic procedure.[47] Other complications include compromise to the ovarian vascular supply, which can result in loss of ovarian function, and even premature ovarian failure.[44]

Surgical therapy is thought to reduce the stromal mass or disrupt the parenchymal blood supply and therefore temporarily reduce ovarian androgen production (androstenedione and testosterone). Studies have shown that laparoscopic ovarian puncture resulted in higher pregnancy and ovulation rates as compared with patients with ovarian wedge resection and suggest that a diminution in volume may not be the only reason for a reduction in ovarian androgens.[48]

Surgical therapy in the management of PCOS patients has a dominant role and is comparable with gonadotropins (both human menopausal gonadotropins and pure FSH) in terms of pregnancy and ovulatory rates.[49]

▶ GONADOTROPIN AGONISTS AND ANTAGONISTS

Initially, before the advent of GnRH agonist therapy, 10 to 25 percent of cycles were canceled due to premature luteinization. The use of GnRH agonists allowed clinicians to induce a state to prevent the premature LH surge and decrease the percentage of canceled cycles. This has become standard therapy for ARTs procedures. Synthetic agonists and antagonists of GnRH were developed to inhibit the secretion of LH and FSH. There are four regimens that use GnRH agonists administered in conjunction with exogenous gonadotropins. The first is called the *long protocol* and consists of a GnRH agonist administered in the midluteal phase of the preceding cycle and continued until hCG administration. This regimen appears to produce a greater number of prevoulatory follicles, embryos, and increased pregnancy rates over the use of gonadotropins alone. A second alternative is the *short protocol,* which consists of initiating the GnRH agonist early in the follicular phase concomitantly with the exogenous gonadotropins and stopping it on the day of hCG administration. GnRH agonists also can be given during the luteal phase only; however, very limited data are available to review this method. The last method begins the GnRH agonist with the gonadotropins but stops them after 3 days. Data are also limited with use of this approach.[50]

First-generation GnRH antagonists were water-insoluble and induced a significant release of histamine. However, this is circumvented in the third-generation medications used currently.

Results

Trials comparing the agonists to the antagonists have shown that GnRH antagonists require a shorter duration of treatment, decreased frequency of injections, and a lower dose of gonadotropins. Disadvantages include a learning curve associated with scheduling patients and the perception that the pregnancy rates are lower. Fertilization rates appear identical, but the total number of embryos obtained with the antagonist is lower. Estradiol levels with the use of an antagonist are inversely related to dosage.[4]

Clinical Management

Clinically, these patients are started on gonadotropins on cycle day 2. From cycle day 7, when a premature LH surge may occur, the GnRH antagonist is administered subcutaneously in a daily fashion until induction of ovulation with hCG. The daily dose of the antagonist can range from 0.25 to 3 mg. Below a dose of 0.1 mg there is no protection from premature LH surges.[51] Two protocols have been used. The first is the traditional approach, as mentioned earlier, and the second gives a single injection of 3 mg of the antagonist on day 8 or 9 (when follicular diameter is greater than 14 mm or E_2 per follicle equals 150 to 200 pg/mL). This is effective for 96 h, after which, if ovulation is not induced, 0.25 mg can be given every day until ovulation. Patients who are treated with an antagonist should be maintained on progesterone supplementation.[51]

► COMPLICATIONS

Ovulation-induction regimens demand a well-controlled environment in view of the potential complications that occur before and during pregnancy. One complication is ovarian hyperstimulation syndrome (OHSS), which is seen in its mild form in 5 to 10 percent of the cycles (50 percent of pregnancy cycles), moderate form in 3 to 4 percent, and severe form in 0.1 to 0.2 percent of cycles.[52] This syndrome is heterogeneous in its clinical and laboratory presentation. The presentation can be explained by the immediate increase in capillary permeability modulated by the regulatory compounds secreted by the granulosa cell, which result in a shift of fluids from the intravascular compartment into the intervascular space and into the peritoneal and pleural cavities. Hemodynamically, these patients are dehydrated, with decreased renal perfusion and excretion, impaired liver function, respiratory distress, thromboembolic phenomena, and hemoconcentration.

There are three types of ovarian hyperstimulation, as alluded to earlier. There is a mild form, also known as *chemical hyperstimulation,* that presents with ovaries <5 cm in diameter,[53] abdominal pain, and no ascites. Physical findings include bilateral ovarian enlargement. Occasionally, a cyst may rupture or undergo torsion.

Moderate hyperstimulation results in ovaries <10 cm in diameter (see Fig. 17-3A, B); gastrointestinal symptoms such as nausea, vomiting, and diarrhea are present.[53] Weight gain and ascites can be found on physical examination. Most patients will develop OHSS within 10 days of hCG administration. In conception cycles, the symptoms may disappear much later. In nonconception cycles, the symptoms typically disappear by the onset of menses. However, these patients have residual ovarian cysts and usually skip an ovulation-induction cycle to allow for resolution of the ovarian cysts.

Severe OHSS is a serious, life-threatening complication. Ovaries are greater than 10 cm. There may be hydrothorax and tension ascites with subsequent pressure on the inferior vena cava, which will decrease cardiac output. Patients also may develop thromboses from dehydration, heptocellular changes. and prerenal failure secondary to impaired perfusion.

There are several risk factors associated with OHSS: young age (<35 years), low body weight, polycystic-like ovaries, pregnancy, hCG luteal supplementation, high serum estradiol concentration, and multiple follicles (>35).[53] Treatment includes close observation, cautious hydration, prevention of thromboembolic phenomena, and prevention of ovarian torsion or hemorrhage through avoidance of vaginal manipulation. Moderate OHSS requires close observation, but in most instances, hospitalization can be avoided. Patients with severe disease require immediate hospitalization and treatment. The outcome is optimistic. Schenker and colleagues showed a 73.2 percent pregnancy rate among those patients with severe OHSS.[54] OHSS can be minimized through close monitoring of follicle size and number and estradiol values.[54]

A second complication is multiple pregnancy. In the last decade, the significant increase in the incidence of multiple births may be attributed to the increased use of ARTs. The incidence of twins with the use of clomiphene citrate is 10 percent and triplets or other higher order multiples approximately 1 percent.[55] Treatment with gonadotropins increases the risk of multiple pregnancy to approximately 25 percent (17 percent twins and 3 to 6 percent higher-order multiples). With ARTs, according to the 1999 Society for Assisted Reproductive Technology (SART) data, there is a 30 percent multiple-pregnancy rate (24 percent twins and 6 percent higher-order multiples). With an increase in the incidence of multiple pregnancy, there is an increase in maternal and perinatal morbidity and mortality.[55] The most common perinatal complication is prematurity, whereas the most common maternal complication is maternal hypertension in patients with multiple gestation. Other maternal complications include iron deficiency, increased operative delivery, uterine rupture, and preterm labor. In terms of neonatal morbidity, there is an increase in premature rupture of the membranes, intrauterine growth retardation, and prematurity with multiple pregnancies as compared with singletons.[55] Prevention is the most important means of decreasing the morbidity of multiple gestations.

A recent issue brought to the forefront of media attention is the use of fertility drugs and the association with ovarian cancer. Several epidemiologic studies have suggested a possible relationship between subfertility and/or fertility therapy and ovarian cancer. Since subfertile populations have lower pregnancy rates than the general population, and low parity is an important risk factor for ovarian cancer, risk estimates are difficult to interpret. In general, the most common type of ovarian cancer is epithelial, although granulosa cell and others have been reported. There was no clear association of the type of subfertility with an increased risk of ovarian cancer because the studies were of limited power. In terms of the types of fertility drugs and the incidence of ovarian cancer, all but one study showed no convincing evidence of a positive association. A large metaanalysis has shown that the incidence of tumors of low malignant potential is similar to that of invasive

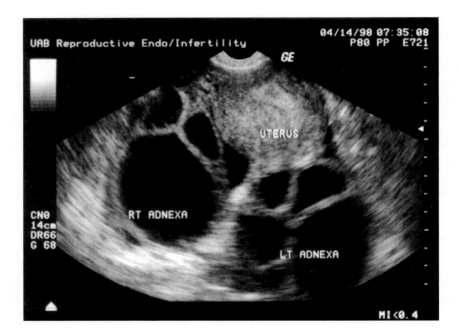

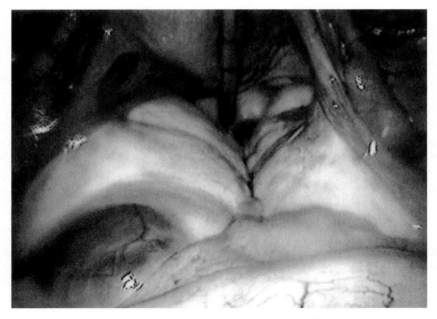

Figure 17-3   Complications of ovulation induction, include OHSS as shown by ovarian enlargement in addition to a constellation of symptoms.

tumors. The risk of nonepithelial ovarian cancer is even less clear. In summary, an association between fertility drugs and ovarian malignancies has not been clearly demonstrated. The risk of other cancers such as breast, melanoma, and thyroid also has not been proven convincingly with respect to fertility medications.[56]

KEY POINTS

1. Ovulation induction was created to treat ovulation dysfunction as categorized by the WHO classification. The indications have now expanded to include unexplained infertility, subfertility from endometriosis, and ARTs.

2. A prerequisite to ovulation induction is an infertility workup, which should include semen analysis, determination of ovulation (basal body temperature charting, LH urinary assay, transvaginal ultrasound, midluteal progesterone, or endometrial biopsy), a postcoital test, and a normal reproductive tract (hysterosalpingogram or laparoscopy/hysteroscopy).

3. Management of ovulatory disorders depends on the diagnosis. WHO group I patients with hyperprolactinemia should be treated with a dopamine agonist or, rarely, clomiphene. Patients in WHO group I with euprolactinemia benefit from both LH/FSH-containing gonadotropins.

4. Patients in WHO group II derive ovulatory success from clomiphene and, if clomiphene-resistant, gonadotropins. These patients, especially if they are insulin-resistant, may benefit from having an insulin sensitizer added to the regimen or used alone. Patients with hyperandrogenism, more specifically, elevated adrenal androgens, will benefit from glucocorticoids used alone or as a supplement to clomiphene.

5. Patients in WHO group III may ovulate sporadically on cyclic hormone replacement therapy and may achieve pregnancy during a normal period of gonadotropins. These patients usually respond poorly to ovulation induction and benefit from egg donation therapy.

6. Clomiphene citrate is a selective estrogen receptor modulator that increases follicular recruitment and ovulatory rates. Clomiphene can be administered in doses of 50 mg per cycle and increased up to 250 mg until ovulation is achieved. Seventy-five percent of clomiphene pregnancies occur at dosages of 50 to 100 mg and in the first three cycles.

7. Clomiphene citrate can be combined with dopamine agonists, glucocorticoids, or insulin sensitizers to increase ovulatory rates and pregnancy.

8. Gonadotropins provide FSH and/or LH to directly stimulate the granulosa cells of the ovary. Gonadotropins are given at doses of 2 to 8 ampules for 5 days with subsequent management based on estradiol levels and transvaginal ultrasounds until the lead follicle reaches 16 to 18 mm, at which point, hCG is required to stimulate ovulation. There are three different types of gonadotropin preparations. There is urinary FSH/LH (menotropins), urinary FSH (urofollitropins), and recombinant FSH or FSH/LH (recombinant gonadotropins).

9. GnRH provided in a pulsatile fashion of 60 to 90 minutes (ideal interval) can be used effectively in patients with hypogonadotropic euprolactinemic hypogonadism to stimulate ovulation (90 percent of patients will ovulate with this method). The only disadvantage is maintenance of the pump.

10. GnRH agonists and GnRH antagonists can be used to prevent a premature LH surge during ovulation induction in selected patients.

> 11. Complications of ovulation induction include multiple gestation and ovarian hyperstimulation syndrome. The purported risk of ovarian cancer remains to be proven.

REFERENCES

1. Collins JA. Unexplained infertility. In Keye WR, Chang RJ, Rebar RW, Soules MR. *Infertility: Evaluation and Treatment.* Philadelphia, WB Saunders. 1995; pp 249–262.

2. Blackwell RE. The infertility workup and diagnosis. *J Reprod Med* 1989;34:81–85.

3. Blacker CM. Hyperprolactinemia. Evaluation and management., *Endocrinol Metab Clin North Am* 1992; 21(1):105–124.

4. Gordon K. Gonadotropin-releasing hormone antagonist: Implications for oocyte quality and uterine receptivity. *Annals NY Acad Sci* 2001; 943:49–54.

5. March CM. Ovulation induction. *J Reprod Med* 1993;38(5):335–346.

6. Derman SG, Adashi EY. Induction of ovulation. *Comprehensive Therapy* 1995;21(10):583–589.

7. Olive DL, Pritts EA. Treatment of endometriosis. *N Engl J Med* 2001;345(4):266–275.

8. Glazener CM, Coulson C, Lambert PA, et al. Clomiphene treatment for women with unexplained infertility: Placebo-controlled study of hormonal responses and conception rates. *Gynecol Endocrinol* 1990;4(2):75–83.

9. Charles D, Klein T, Lunn SF, et al. Clinical and endocrinological studies with the isomeric components of clomiphene citrate. *J Obstet Gynaecol Br Commonw* 1969;76(12):1100–1110.

10. Baier H, Taubert H-D. Effect of clomiphene upon plasma FSH-activity and hypothalamic FSH-RF content in ovariectomized estrogen-progesterone blocked rats. *Endocrinology* 1969;84:946–949.

11. Kennedy JL, Adashi EY. Ovulation induction. *Obstet Gynecol Clin North Am* 1987;14(4):831–864.

12. Vollenhoven BJ, Healy DL. Short- and long-term effects of ovulation induction. *Endocrinol Metab Clin North Am* 1998;27(4):903–914.

13. Gysler M, Marsh CM, Mishell DR, et al. A decade's experience with an individualized clomiphene treatment regimen including its effect on the postcoital test. *Fertil Steril* 1982;37(2):168–174

14. Imani B, Eijkemans MJ, te Velde ER, Habbema JD, Fauser BC. A nomogram to predict the probability of live birth after clomiphene citrate induction of ovulation in normogonadotropic oligoamenorrheic infertility. *Fertil Steril* 2002;77:91–97.

15. Israel R, Mishell DR Jr, Stone SC, Thorneycroft LH, Moyer DL. Single luteal phase serum progesterone assay as an indicator of ovulation. *Am J Obstet Gynecol* 1972;112(8):1043–1046.

16. Lobo RA, Granger LR, Davajan V, et al. An extended regimen of clomiphene citrate in women unresponsive to standard therapy. *Fertil Steril* 1982;37(6):762–766.

17. O'Herlihy C, Pepperell RJ, Brown JB, Smith MA, Sandri L, McBain JC. Incremental clomiphene therapy: A new method for treating persistent anovulation. *Obstet Gynecol* 1981;58(5): 535–542.

18. Wolf LJ. Ovulation induction. *Clin Obstet Gynecol* 2000;43(4):902–915.

19. Gorlistsky GA, Kase NG, Speroff L. Ovulation and pregnancy rates with clomiphene citrate. *Obstet Gynecol* 1978;51(3):265–269.

20. Molitch ME. Disorders of prolactin secretion. *Endocrinol Metab Clin* 2001;30(3):1–20.

21. Ciccarelli E, Giusti M, Miola C, Potenzoni F, Sghedoni D, Camanni F, Giordano G. Effectiveness and tolerability of long-term treatment with cabergoline, a new long lasting ergoline derivative in hyperprolactinemic patients. *J Clin Endocrinol Metab* 1989;69(4):725–728.

22. Motta T, de Vincentiis S, Marchini M, Colombo N, D'Alberton A. Vaginal cabergoline in the treatment of hyperprolactinemic patients intolerant to oral dopaminergics. *Fertil Steril* 1996;65(2):440–442.

23. Freda PU, Andreadis CI, Khandji AG, Khoury M, Bruce JN, Jacobs TP, Wardlaw SL. Long-term treatment of prolactin secreting macroadenomas with pergolide. *J Clin Endocrinol Metab* 2000;85(1):8–13.

24. Orr FR. Glucocorticoids in the treatment of endocrine disorders. *Appl Ther* 1967;9(3):257–258.

25. Raj SG, Thompson JE, Berger MJ, Taymor ML. Clinical aspects of polycystic ovary syndrome. *Obstet Gynecol* 1977;49(5):552–556.

26. Rodriguez-Rigau LV, Smith KD, Tcholakian RK, Steinberger E. Effect of prednisone on plasma testosterone levels and on duration of the

phases of the menstrual cycles in hyperandrogenic women. *Fertil Steril* 1979;32(4):408–413.

27. Janata J, Starka L. Effect of cortisol on the production of ovarian androgens. *J Endocrinol* 1964;29:93–94.

28. Lobo RA, Paul W, March C, Granger L. Kletzky OA. Clomiphene and dexamethasone in women unresponsive to clomiphene alone. *Obstet Gynecol* 1982;60(4):497–501.

29. Lee F, Nelson N, Faiman C, Choi NW, Reyes FI. Low-dose corticoid therapy for anovulation: Effect upon fetal weight. *Obstet Gynecol* 1982; 60(3):314–317.

30. Nestler JE, Stovall D, Akhter N, Iuomo MJ, Jakubowicz DJ. Strategies for the use of insulin-sensitizing drugs to treat infertility in women with polycystic ovary syndrome. *Fertil Steril* 2002;77(2):209–215.

31. Nestler JE, Jakubowicz DJ, Evans WS, Pasquali R. Effects of metformin on spontaneous and clomiphene-induced ovulation in the polycystic ovary syndrome. *N Engl J Med* 1998;338(26): 1876–1880.

32. Ehrmann DA, Cavaghan MK, Imperial J, Sturis J, Rosenfield RL, Polonsky KS. Effects of metformin on insulin secretion, insulin action, and ovarian steroidogenesis in women in polycystic ovary syndrome. *J Clin Endocrinol Metab* 1997;82(2):524–530.

33. Costello MF, Eden JA. A systematic review of the reproductive system effects of metformin in patients with polycystic ovary syndrome. *Fertil Steril* 2003;79(1):1–13.

34. Nestler JE, Jakubowicz DJ, Reamer P, Gunn R, Allan G. Ovulatory and metabolic effects of D-chiro-inositol in the polycystic ovary syndrome. *N Engl J Med* 1999;340(17):1314–1320.

35. Macklon NS, Fauser BCJM. Gonadotropin therapy for the treatment of anovulation and for ovarian hyperstimulation for IVF. *Mol Cell Endocrinol* 2002;186(2):159–161.

36. Cochrane Database of Systemic Reviews. "Coasting" (withholding gonadotropins) for preventing ovarian hyperstimulation syndrome. 2002; Issue 4(1).

37. Voortman G, Mannaerts BM, Huisman JAM. A dose proportionality study of subcutaneously and intramuscularly administered recombinant human follicle-stimulating hormone (follistim/ puregon) in health female volunteers. *Fertil Steril* 2000;73(6):1187–1193.

38. Nichols J, Knochenhauer E, Fein SH, Nardi RV, Marshall DC, and the Repronex SC Ovulation Induction Study Group. Subcutaneously administered Repronex in oligoovulatory female patients undergoing ovulation induction is as effective and well tolerated as intramuscular human menopausal gonadotropin treatment. *Fertil Steril* 2001;76(1):58–66.

39. Gast MJ. Evolution of clinical agents for ovulation induction. *Am J Obstet Gynecol* 1995;172(2), Part 2:753–759.

40. Cochrane Database of Systemic Reviews. Recombinant FSH versus urinary gonadotropins or recombinant FSH for ovulation induction in subfertility associated with polycystic ovary syndrome. 2002; Issue 4(1).

41. Balen AH, Hayden CJ, Rutherford AJ. Clinical efficacy of recombinant gonadotropins. *Hum Reprod* 1999;14(6):1411–1417.

42. Olive DL. The role of gonadotropins in ovulation induction. *Am J Obstet Gynecol* 1995;172(2): 759–765.

43. Adashi EY, Rock JA, Guzick D, Wentz AC, Jones GS, Jones HW Jr. Fertility following bilateral ovarian wedge resection: A critical analysis of 90 consecutive cases of the polycystic ovarian syndrome. *Fertil Steril* 1981;36(3):320–325.

44. Gurgan T, Yarali H, Urman B. Laparoscopic treatment of polycystic ovarian disease. *Hum Reprod* 1994;9(4):573–577.

45. Gjonnaess H. Ovarian electrocautery in the treatment of women with polycystic ovary syndrome (PCOS): Factors affecting the results. *Acta Obstet Gynecol Scand* 1994;73(5):407–412.

46. Daniell JF, Miller W. Polycystic ovaries treated by laparoscopic laser vaporization. *Fertil Steril* 1989;51(2):232–236.

47. Naether OG, Fischer R. Adhesion formation after laparoscopic electrocoagulation of the ovarian surface in polycystic ovary patients. *Fertil Steril* 1993;60(1):95–98.

48. Alborzi S, Khodaee R, Parsanejad ME. Ovarian size and response to laparoscopic ovarian electro-cauterization in polycystic ovarian disease. *Int J Gynaecol Obstet* 2001;74(3):269–274.

49. Abdel Gadir A, Mowafi RS, Alnaser HM, Alrashid AH, Alonezi OM, Shaw RW. Ovarian electrocautery versus human menopausal gonadotrophins and pure follicle-stimulating

hormone therapy in the treatment of patients with polycystic ovarian disease. *Clin Endocrinol* 1990;33(5):585–592.

50. Filicori M, Cognigni GE, Arnone R, Carbone F, Falbo A, Tabarelli C, et al. Role of different GnRH agonist regimens in pituitary suppression and the outcome of controlled ovarian hyperstimulation. *Hum Reprod* 1996; 11(Suppl 3): 123–132.

51. Felberbaum RE, Ludwig M, Diedrich K. Clinical application of GnRH antagonists. *Mol Cell Endocrinol* 2000;166(1):9–14.

52. Schenker JG, Ezra Y. Complications of assisted reproductive techniques. *Fertil Steril* 1994;61(3): 411–422.

53. Navot D, Rebou A, Birkenfeld A, Rabninowitz R, Brzezinski A, Margalioth EJ. Risk factors and prognostic variables in the ovarian hyperstimulation syndrome. *Am J Obstet Gynecol* 1988; 159(1):210–215.

54. Schenker JG. Clinical aspects of ovarian hyperstimulation syndrome. *Eur J Obstet Gynecol Reprod Biol* 1999;85(1):13–20.

55. ESHRE Capri Workshop Group. Multiple gestation pregnancy. *Hum Reprod* 2000;15(8):1856–1864.

56. Klip H, Burger CW, Kenemans P, Van Leeuwen FE. Cancer risk associated with subfertility and ovulation induction: A review. *Cancer Causes Control* 2000;11(4):319–344.

CHAPTER 18

Unexplained Infertility

DEBORAH MANZI-SMITH AND WILLIAM D. SCHLAFF

Unexplained infertility is the diagnosis of exclusion given to infertile couples who have had a complete infertility evaluation with no abnormal findings. The reported prevalence of unexplained infertility ranges from 6 to 58 percent,[1] with the average incidence being reported as 15 percent.[2] This variation in the reported prevalence is mostly attributed to the differences in the definition of unexplained infertility used by medical professionals, the evaluation process that is considered "complete," and the interpretation of test results.

Thus far there is no agreement in the medical community regarding which tests make up a standard infertility evaluation, nor are there standard protocols for management of unexplained infertility. Differences in the interpretation of research data, in addition to the lack of prospective, randomized trials, account for this variability in the diagnosis and treatment of unexplained infertility. This chapter will present the best available clinical evidence regarding the diagnosis and treatment of unexplained infertility.

▶ DIAGNOSIS OF UNEXPLAINED INFERTILITY

In order to make the diagnosis of unexplained infertility, a complete infertility evaluation should be performed. There are multiple tests available for determining the cause of infertility; however, there is no consensus on which tests are essential before reaching the diagnosis of "unexplained" infertility.

Classically, infertility testing has included a semen analysis, postcoital test (PCT), an assessment of ovulation, a hysterosalpingogram (HSG), antisperm antibody testing, and a laparoscopy.[3] More recently, the widespread use of all these tests has fallen out of favor mostly because of the lack of clinical evidence to support their continued use. In 1992, the American Fertility Society (now known as the American Society for Reproductive Medicine, or ASRM) and the World Health Organization (WHO) recommended that infertile women be evaluated in five areas. These organizations described the complete basic workup as: (1) a semen analysis, (2) assessment of ovulation, (3) evaluation of the uterine cavity and tubes, (4) the postcoital test, and (5) a laparoscopy[4] (Table 18-1). In the same year, the European Society of Human Reproduction and Embryology (ESHRE) grouped the basic infertility tests into three categories (Table 18-2). ESHRE's groups for infertility testing are based on the prognostic utility of these tests.[5] The ESHRE classification was updated in 1996 and 2000.[6,7] For the purpose of this chapter, the basic workup will be defined minimally as a good history and physical examination, HSG, semen analysis, and documentation of ovulation, unless otherwise

▶ **TABLE 18-1:** AMERICAN FERTILITY SOCIETY DIAGNOSIS OF UNEXPLAINED INFERTILITY (ASRM 1992)

1. Evidence of ovulation by basal body temperature and/or midluteal phase serum progesterone
2. Normal semen parameters
3. Normal sperm-mucus interaction with a postcoital test
4. Normal uterus and tubes by hysterosalpingogram (HSG)
5. Normal pelvic anatomy as demonstrated by laparoscopy to evaluate the pelvic structures (hysteroscopy not required)

specified. Only studies that used this evaluation as the minimum for basic infertility testing to diagnose patients with unexplained infertility will be discussed unless otherwise noted.

▶ **TABLE 18-2:** ESHRE WORKSHOP ON UNEXPLAINED INFERTILITY

Category 1: Tests with Established Correlation to Pregnancy
1. Semen analysis
2. Documentation of tubal patency (HSG, laparoscopy)
3. Midluteal phase progesterone for documentation of ovulation

Category 2: Tests Not Consistently Correlated with Pregnancy
1. Zona-free hamster egg penetration assay
2. Postcoital test (PCT)
3. Antisperm antibody testing

Category 3: Tests that Do Not Correlate with Pregnancy
1. Endometrial biopsy for dating
2. Varicocele assessment
3. Chlamydia testing

Note: The 1996 and 2000 European Society of Human Reproduction and Embryology (ESHRE) Capri workshops concluded that a midluteal phase progesterone was the best test for confirming ovulation and that the primary investigation of the uterus and tubes should be the HSG.

▶ CONTROVERSIAL ISSUES IN INFERTILITY TESTING: VALIDITY AND CLINICAL UTILITY

Even among large organizations there is significant variability in the tests defined as part of a basic infertility workup. The role and importance of the PCT, antisperm antibody determination, and laparoscopy as a mandatory part of the basic infertility workup are controversial.

Laparoscopy

Pelvic pathology of the female reproductive tract is often a cause of infertility. Complete evaluation for the presence of adhesions and endometriosis involves invasive surgical techniques. Laparoscopy traditionally has been included as a mandatory step in the basic infertility evaluation to rule out pelvic disease. In an evaluation of 24 cases of "unexplained infertility," Drake and colleagues found abnormal laparoscopic findings in 75 percent of patients (46 percent had endometriosis and 29 percent had peritubal adhesions). In 1977, these authors concluded that laparoscopy should be a mandatory step in an otherwise negative workup for infertility.[8] Since that time, laparoscopy traditionally has been considered an important diagnostic procedure in the evaluation of the infertile couple and considered complementary to the HSG. The superiority of laparoscopy over HSG has been demonstrated in many studies for evaluating peritubal adhesions and endometriosis.[4,9,10] However, in light of a normal HSG, the "mandatory" need for laparoscopy has been questioned recently by fertility specialists.[5,6,11] It has been estimated that using laparoscopy as a standard test of tubal function would reduce the incidence of unexplained infertility from 10 to 3.5 percent.[8] Gleicher argued that in cases of a negative history for pelvic disease, normal examination, and normal HSG, the probability of finding clinically relevant disease was low.[12] He additionally stated that in order to perform a cost-effective evaluation, gynecologists should perform laparoscopies on an as-needed basis. Fatum and colleagues agreed with Gliecher's opinion[13] and went on to state that patients with unexplained infertility and a negative history for pelvic disease should be offered three to six cycles of ovulation induction with intrauterine insemination (IUI) as the next course of therapy rather than a laparoscopy.

It is now typical that infertility specialists will take a detailed history (question the patient for evidence of pelvic inflammatory disease, sexually transmitted diseases, dyspareunia, and dysmenorrhea), perform a detailed examination using the single-digit technique described by Ripps and colleagues,[14,15] and perform an HSG. If the history and testing are normal, most reproductive endocrinologists will forego the laparoscopy and proceed with ovarian hyperstimulation with IUI.

Postcoital Test (PCT)

The postcoital test has been considered part of the basic infertility workup for over 100 years.[16] For several years now, the role of PCT has been questioned widely. In fact, the ASRM considers the PCT part of the standard infertility evaluation, but the ESHRE considers the PCT a category 2 test (not consistently correlated with pregnancy; see Tables 18-1 and 18-2). Its utility has been limited by the fact that there is no universally agreed on normal values, and there are significant controversies around treatment protocols for abnormal results. In a review of

the literature evaluating the benefit of the PCT, many of the studies validating its use have design flaws. These flaws include the use of infertile couples with various infertility diagnoses, no attempt to correlate the PCT results with subsequent pregnancy rates, and failure to compare PCT results between fertile and infertile populations.[1,16–20] Despite these problems, a few studies warrant mentioning.[1,16,17,19,20,21] In a study by Collins and colleagues, the authors found no differences in subsequent pregnancy rates among groups undergoing a PCT having no sperm, no motile sperm, 1 to 5 motile sperm, 6 to 10 motile sperm, and greater than 11 motile sperm per high-power field (HPF) on the PCT.[21] These results question the utility of the PCT in predicting infertility and subsequent pregnancy rates. In a study evaluating only fertile couples, Kovacs and colleagues found that 20 percent of fertile couples had either no sperm or less than 1 sperm per HPF on the PCT. This is about the same incidence of abnormal PCTs that is found in the infertile population.[17] These results further question the prognostic ability of the PCT. However, as shown in Table 18-3, significant differences in pregnancy rates were noted between the patients with normal and abnormal PCT results. Additionally, it is important to note that the results of the PCT seldom make a difference in the clinical management of the infertile couple. Many physicians feel that the widespread use of IUI has made the PCT merely an academic exercise because treatment of the infertile couple is the same regardless of the results of the PCT. These findings make it difficult to justify the PCT as an essential part of an infertility evaluation.

▶ **TABLE 18-3:** POSTCOITAL TEST

	Normal		Abnormal	
Author	Number of Cycles	% Pregnant	Number of Cycles	% Pregnant
Hull[1]	295	13.9%	406	2.7%
Portuondo[19]	176	34.7%	87	11.5%
Skaf[20]	38	60.5%	12	8.3%

Antisperm Antibody Testing

Numerous methods are available to detect sperm antibodies. The mixed antiglobulin reaction (MAR) and the immunobead test are the two most commonly used methods. Both these assays allow for direct assessment of antibody interaction with sperm surface antigens.

The sperm MAR is performed by mixing semen, human IgG–coated latex particles, and IgG antiserum on a microscope slide. If antibodies are present in the sperm, the latex particles will bind in the sperm and the antisera and cause clumping. The immunobead test uses latex beads coated with antibodies against human IgG, IgM, and IgA. For the direct assay, washed sperm are mixed with beads on a glass slide. Results are recorded according to type of immunoglobulin bound and the location of the bead binding. The immunobead test also can be used to "indirectly" test serum, seminal plasma, follicular fluid, or cervical mucus for the presence of antibodies.

The World Health Organization (WHO) laboratory manual states that the immunobead test is considered positive when 20 percent or more of motile sperm are bound, with 50 percent or more sperm binding considered to be clinically significant.[22] Additionally, the location of the immunobead binding has been shown to reflect sperm function in vitro. Antibodies that bind to the head region may interfere with gamete interaction. Immunobead binding restricted to the tail tip is not considered clinically significant.

Approximately 10 percent of male partners in infertile couples will have some degree of autoimmunity to sperm surface antigens.[23,24] Haas and colleagues[25] evaluated sera from 624 men and women with unexplained infertility and have found that 7 percent of the men had antisperm antibodies.

Review of retrospective and prospective analyses of pregnancy rates for couples with sperm antibodies questions the prognostic value of antisperm antibody screening for the diagnosis of infertility. Some studies have reported a significant association between antibody presence in male partners and spontaneous pregnancy rates, whereas others have not found an effect of antibodies on pregnancy rates.[25–30] The inconclusive and inconsistent results of these studies can be attributed to the presence of heterogeneous antibodies, the varying degree of their ability to impair fertility, and varying antibody titers.[23–30] It is now recognized that not all sperm antibodies impair fertilization. In addition, low levels of sperm antibodies have been shown to have poor prognostic value in predicting fertility.[29] Therefore, diagnosing someone as having antisperm antibodies in general does not have a clear prognostic significance.

Testing for sperm antibodies may help to explain the cause of infertility in some men, particularly those who have had vasectomy reversals, testicular trauma, or surgery. The results of the testing, however, seldom make a difference in clinical management of the couple. The reason is that sperm antibodies may result in a state of subfertility but rarely produce absolute infertility in couples. In addition, there are no proven treatments for this condition. Immunosuppressive therapy with corticosteroids has been suggested as treatment for men with antibodies. Whether fertility is improved by this method is unclear.[30] Washing sperm to get rid of antibodies is usually unsuccessful because of the high affinity of the antibody-antigen bond, although washing may prevent sperm agglutination. Most clinicians empirically use assisted reproductive techniques (ARTs), including IUI and in vitro fertilization (IVF) for treating couples with antisperm antibodies. Therefore, treatment options are the same as those for couples with otherwise unexplained infertility. In other words, the test outcome does not often change the recommended therapy. The prognosis for couples with these treatments (IUI and IVF) does not seem to be altered by the presence of sperm antibodies.[30]

► MORE ADVANCED TESTS FOR INFERTILITY

Various markers of subfertility have been described in the literature, some of which may be used in clinical practice. Over the past decade, there has been great interest in the evaluation of embryo implantation and ovarian reserve. Subtle changes in the oocyte quality (as reflected by ovarian reserve) or the endometrium may be the cause of unexplained infertility.

Tests Evaluating Endometrial Function

Li and colleagues examined the endometrial expression of the *HOXA-10* gene in normal fertile women and in women with unexplained infertility.[31] These authors found a higher incidence of aberrant *HOXA-10* expression in patients with unexplained infertility. The study suggested that altered development of the endometrium at a molecular level may contribute to the etiology of infertility.

A second study evaluating the role of the endometrium in unexplained infertility was described by Lessey and colleagues.[32] They compared in-phase and out-of-phase biopsies plus β-3 integrin levels in the endometrium of fertile control women with those of women with unexplained infertility. A significant reduction was found in β-3 integrins in the unexplained infertility group. It is important to note that both infertile women with out-of-phase and in-phase biopsies demonstrated this abnormal pattern of β-3 expression. It also was noted that atypical endometriosis occurred more frequently in women with in-phase endometrium who lacked β-3 integrins.[32]

Tests of Ovarian Reserve (Day 3 FSH or CCCT)

Some form of ovarian reserve screening has been a part of the patient evaluation for most patients with infertility since description of the benefit of a day 3 follicle-stimulating hormone (FSH) concentration in predicting IVF success.[33] Although most women with abnormal ovarian function could be identified by cycle day 3 FSH and estradiol determinations alone, the use of the clomiphene citrate challenge test (CCCT) has improved the ability to detect patients with subtle ovarian dysfunction.

Ovarian reserve screening using the CCCT was first described by Navot and colleagues[34] in 1987 as a means to assess pregnancy potential. Since its original description, numerous studies have validated its use.[33–36] The CCCT has been used to predict which patients will respond poorly to gonadotropin stimulation for IUI or IVF cycles. In general, about 10 percent of infertile women will have an abnormal CCCT. As expected, only 3 percent of women younger than 30 years of age and 26 percent of women 40 years of age or older will have an abnormal CCCT. Interestingly, 38 percent of women with unexplained infertility (basic workup plus a PCT, prolactin level, thyroid-stimulating hormone (TSH) determination, evaluation for luteal-phase defects, and laparoscopy) were found to have an abnormal CCCT result.[36] Scott and colleagues, in their prospective analysis of the CCCT, concluded that significantly more women with the diagnosis of unexplained infertility and a normal CCCT became pregnant than women with unexplained infertility and an abnormal CCCT. Therefore, a CCCT may help to predict which patients with unexplained infertility will respond to therapy.[36]

► MANAGEMENT OF UNEXPLAINED INFERTILITY

Unexplained infertility is a common clinical problem for which there is no standard treatment protocol. Very few randomized clinical trials are available to assess the benefit of treatment, and treatment plans are often empirical. The definition of unexplained infertility, investigation protocols, and inclusion criteria vary among clinical trials in patients with unexplained infertility. Some studies include only patients under 38 years of age, whereas other studies do not report age limits.[37] Some studies include couples with mild male factor infertility[84] and minimal endometriosis.[37–39] This variability among studies makes it difficulty to interpret data, and therefore, most of the data presented will be limited by small sample size.

Expectant Management

Spontaneous conception in couples with unexplained infertility is well documented.[40–44] A cumulative live birth rate of 33 percent at 36 months was estimated from a Canadian study,[45] and a study performed in the Netherlands suggested a live birth rate of 60 percent at 36 months without treatment.[46] The reported cumulative pregnancy rate without treatment varies in the literature and is based on the length of infertility, age of the female partner, and whether this is primary or secondary infertility.

Lenton and colleagues studied 80 untreated couples with primary unexplained infertility of at least 2 years' duration.[42] It was found that after a basic evaluation (plus a laparoscopy with no abnormal findings), 43 percent of couples conceived before the study was completed. The maximum study length was 8 years. Conceptions occurred at a rate of about 10 percent per year for the first 2 years and then 5 percent per year after that. Women with secondary infertility seemed to fare better, with a cumulative pregnancy rate of 89 percent after 7 years of study. In patients with secondary infertility, there was a spontaneous pregnancy rate of 18 percent per year for the first 5 years then 10 percent per year, thereafter.[42]

Age of the female partner also plays a role in predicting the spontaneous pregnancy rates in patients with unexplained infertility. In a multicenter trial of 470 couples with unexplained infertility (diagnosis made by basic evaluation plus laparoscopy), it was found that the age of the infertile female and length of infertility affected the prognosis.[40] In this multicenter evaluation, the average age of those obtaining pregnancy was 29.5 years, and the average age of those not obtaining pregnancy was 30.4 years. The cumulative pregnancy rate was 42 percent in women younger than 30 years of age and 31 percent in women older than 30 years of age. In this study it was noted that if the duration of infertility was less than 36 months, the pregnancy rate was 46 percent over the next 7 years compared with 27 percent in couples with greater than 36 months of infertility.[40]

Options for the Active Management of Unexplained Infertility

Obviously, the exact etiology of unexplained infertility remains unknown. Unexplained infertility most likely represents a broad range of defects in folliculogenesis, gamete development, fertilization, and embryo implantation. Due to the decreased reproductive capacity in couples with unexplained infertility, options to increase the number of gametes available for fertilization have been considered good treatment options.

A number of studies have sought to evaluate the use of ovulation induction with or without IUI in the treatment of unexplained infertility. Most of these studies were not randomized. Below is a summary of the current data available on the use of ovulation induction with or without IUI for the treatment of unexplained infertility (Table 18.4).

Ovulation Induction without Intrauterine Insemination (IUI)
Clomiphene Citrate without IUI
Several trials have been published evaluating the benefit of clomiphene citrate (CC) in the treatment of unexplained infertility.[38,47–52] Fisch

► **TABLE 18-4:** RESULTS OF DIFFERENT RANDOMIZED, CONTROLLED TRIALS COMPARING hMG/INTRAUTERINE INSEMINATION VERSUS hMG/TIMED INTERCOURSE

Study	hMG/IUI		hMG/Intercourse	
	Preg/Cycle	Cycle Fecundity	Preg/Cycle	Cycle Fecundity
Melis	22/123	0.18	23/126	0.18
Chung 1995	24/110	0.22	10/130	0.08
Gregoriou 1995	19/74	0.26	6/67	0.09
Zikopoulos 1993	6/40	0.15	5/45	0.11
Karlstrom 1993	3/15	0.20	3/24	0.13
Evans 1991	2/16	0.13	1/26	0.04
Crosignani 1991	55/241	0.23	9/106	0.09
Martinez 1991	3/40	0.08	2/37	0.05
Martinez 1990	2/14	0.14	0/11	0.00
Doyle 1991	1/13	0.08	1/17	0.09
Arcaini 1996	22/116	0.19	12/127	0.09
Nan 1994	11/127	0.09	4/122	0.03
Total	**170/929**	**0.18**	**76/838**	**0.09**

and colleagues evaluated the use of CC, human chorionic gonadotropin (hCG), and intercourse in the treatment of primary unexplained infertility.[51] A significant improvement in pregnancy rates was found in 36 patients in the randomized trial. It is important to note in this trial that there were no pregnancies in the control (placebo) group. Hughes and colleagues, in a review of the literature,[47] found that CC alone was slightly superior to no treatment in patients with unexplained infertility. The absolute treatment effect was small and may not be clinically significant. However, when counseling patients regarding the effectiveness of clomiphene, it is important to remember that the baseline cycle fecundity is 1 to 2 percent for patients with unexplained infertility without therapy, and the cycle fecundity with CC/intercourse would be enhanced to 2 percent.[48,50] This low pregnancy rate dramatically limits the role of CC/intercourse in the treatment of unexplained infertility.

HUMAN MENOPAUSAL GONADOTROPIN (HMG) WITHOUT IUI

Gonadotropins have been used for years for the treatment of unexplained infertility.[53] It is felt that ovarian stimulation increases the number of preovulatory follicles and may correct subtle ovulatory dysfunction. In a randomized, controlled trial of various therapies for the treatment of unexplained infertility, Guzick and colleagues reported a pregnancy rate of 7.7 percent per cycle in the hMG/intercourse group compared with a 17.1 percent rate in hMG/IUI groups. The lower pregnancy rate in the hMG-alone group suggests that IUI may be beneficial for patients with unexplained infertility[48] (Table 18.4).

Intrauterine Insemination with or without Ovulatory Agents

IUI ALONE

For many years, IUI has been used widely as a treatment option for couples with unexplained infertility. Its effectiveness has been debated heavily. In natural cycles (without the use of ovulation-induction agents), it has been reported that IUI does not improve the probability of conception in patients with unexplained infertility when compared with timed intercourse.[54] It is therefore not a good treatment option for couples with unexplained infertility.

CC/IUI

Although IUI alone does not improve pregnancy rates, when controlled ovarian hyperstimulation (COH) is added to the protocol, it appears to significantly improve the chance of conception.[48] Arici and colleagues compared CC/hCG/IUI with spontaneous, unstimulated cycle/ovulation predictor kit–timed IUI. A twofold increase in pregnancy rates was found with the addition of CC.[49] Deaton and colleagues, in a randomized, controlled trial, treated patients with unexplained infertility or surgically treated endometriosis. This study used CC (50 mg) and used hCG when the lead follicle was 18 mm, followed by IUI at 36 h after hCG. A significant benefit to CC/IUI was reported. In the 148 CC/IUI-treated cycles, the cycle fecundity was 9.5 percent, compared with 3.3 percent in 150 untreated couples.[38] Martinez and colleagues in a randomized, prospective fashion compared four different treatment protocols for patients with unexplained infertility. The groups were: (1) CC with a lutenizing hormone (LH) kit–timed IUI, (2) CC with timed intercourse, (3) IUI in a spontaneous unstimulated cycle, and (4) timed intercourse (control). Cycle fecundity was 14 percent in the CC/IUI group, 3 percent in the CC/intercourse group, 9 percent in the IUI group, and 0 percent in the control group. The findings confirmed that CC/IUI improved pregnancy rates over CC or IUI alone.[50] Based on a review of the subject, it appears that patients with unexplained infertility undergoing CC/IUI therapy should be quoted an approximate pregnancy rate of 8 to 12 percent per cycle.

It is important to note that the age of the patient may play a role in the success of CC/IUI therapy. Agarwal and colleagues found a significantly lower pregnancy rate per cycle in women over the age of 35 using CC/IUI therapy. Additionally, this study also found that 96 percent of pregnancies occurred in the first four cycles (up to six cycles were studied); therefore, CC/IUI should be limited to four cycles.[55]

An important study to mention when discussing CC/IUI therapy is a study by Deaton and colleagues. A comparison was made between the pregnancy rate in patients treated with CC and those patients using IUI. This study evaluated the difference between using LH testing (ovulation predictor kit) and ultrasound monitoring with hCG to time the insemination. There was no difference in the pregnancy rate between these two groups.[56] Therefore, it may be more cost effective and less invasive to use LH testing to time inseminations in this group of patients.

Gonadotropins with IUI

Many reports in the literature support the effectiveness of hMG/IUI in the treatment of unexplained infertility.[57–59] Unfortunately, most of the studies evaluating the benefit are uncontrolled and retrospective.

Simon and colleagues treated 87 couples with unexplained infertility and reported a cumulative pregnancy rate of 34 percent after 446 total cycles.[57] Nielsen and colleagues performed a randomized study comparing IUI in a natural cycle timed by LH kit with hMG/IUI in 119 couples. They found a cycle fecundity rate of 19.3 percent for couples with unexplained infertility treated with hMG/IUI compared with 2.4 percent in those treated with IUI alone.[58] In an uncontrolled study, Dodson and colleagues reported a 19 percent pregnancy rate per cycle in patients with unexplained infertility using hMG/IUI therapy.[59] In a retrospective analysis of patients with unexplained infertility of greater than 4 years' duration, Aboulghar and colleagues found significant improvement in cumulative pregnancy rates with hMG/IUI therapy. In this review, patients were treated with hMG/IUI for one to three cycles. A total of 268 couples underwent 463 hMG/IUI cycles compared with 112 couples who did not have treatment. Cycle fecundity in the hMG/IUI group was 20 percent, with a cumulative pregnancy rate of 34.7 percent. This rate was significantly higher than the 8.9 percent cumulative pregnancy rate in the untreated group[60] (Table 18.5).

Interestingly, there are two large studies comparing the use of hMG/IUI with a GnRH

▶ **TABLE 18-5:** THE RESULTS OF DIFFERENT RANDOMIZED, CONTROLLED TRIALS
COMPARING hMG/IUI VERSUS IUI

Study	hMG/IUI		IUI Alone	
	Preg/Cycle	Cycle Fecundity	Preg/Cycle	Cycle Fecundity
Cohlen (1998)	21/153	0.14	13/155	0.08
Martinez (1990)	2/14	0.14	2/10	0.20
Nielsen (1993)	7/54	0.13	1/41	0.02
Guzick (1999)	76/231	0.33	42/234	0.18

agonist (GnRH-a)–downregulated hMG/IUI cycle in patients with infertility.[61,62] In a retrospective study, Gagliardi and colleagues found a higher pregnancy rate in the GnRH-downregulated group.[61] However, Manzi and colleagues, in a randomized, prospective trial, found similar pregnancy rates between these groups but a significantly higher live birth rate in the GnRH-downregulated group.[62] The findings by Manzi and colleagues were confirmed by other studies,[59–61] but not all,[63–65] It may be that for select populations with subtle ovulatory defects there may be an advantage to the addition of the GnRH-a to improve the live birth rate.[62,66]

In Vitro Fertilization (IVF)

IVF is a widely used treatment for unexplained infertility. With increasing awareness of the role of expectant management and the benefits of less invasive procedures (e.g., IUI), it is extremely important to evaluate the role of IVF in the treatment of couples with unexplained infertility. Despite being empirical and expensive, IVF is considered to be an effective treatment option. IVF also may play a diagnostic role in couples with unexplained infertility by recognizing fertilization failure and poor embryo quality.

IVF versus Expectant Management

Soliman and colleagues evaluated the pregnancy rate from a single cycle of IVF with expectant management of 6 months' duration in patients with unexplained infertility.[67] The study found that the pregnancy rate for expectant management was slightly higher than a single IVF cycle; however, these rates were not

significantly different. This study is limited by its small sample size ($n = 14$ expectant management, $n = 21$ IVF). Additionally, since the time of this study (over 10 years ago), IVF pregnancy rates have improved dramatically. The lack of statistical difference may not be true at present with the current IVF success rates.

IVF versus IUI Alone or COH/IUI

Goverde and colleagues compared the use of IVF with IUI and COH/IUI in couples with unexplained infertility.[37] This study included patients with minimal endometriosis and mild male factor infertility. The age of the female partner in this prospective trial was not discussed. No significant differences were found in the cumulative live birth rate per couple after 6 months between these three treatment options, although the pregnancy rate per cycle was significantly higher in the IVF group than in the IUI and COH/IUI groups (12.2 versus 7.4 versus 8.7 percent, respectively). This was most likely due to the fact that couples in the IVF group were more likely to abandon treatment before six cycles (42 percent dropout rate versus 15 and 16 percent, respectively for the IUI and COH/IUI groups) when compared with the IUI groups. Therefore, at the end of 6 months, regardless of the number of cycles of therapy completed, the cumulative pregnancy rates were similar between groups. It is important to note, however, that the cost per pregnancy was significantly lower in the IUI groups (IVF $14,679 versus IUI $4511 to $5710). This study also was limited by its small sample size (54 couples for IUI and 59 couples for IVF).

GIFT VERSUS HMG/IUI FOR UNEXPLAINED INFERTILITY

There are six trials that evaluate gamete intrafallopian transfer (GIFT) versus hMG/IUI in the treatment of unexplained infertility. It should be noted that none of these studies has sufficient power or confidence.[68–71] The data from these articles, however, suggest that there is no difference in pregnancy rate per couple between these two options.

IVF OR HMG/IUI VERSUS EXPECTANT MANAGEMENT

In a metaanalysis of 22 reported studies on hMG/IUI and IVF, Peterson and colleagues found higher pregnancy rates in the treated groups when compared with expectant management.[72]

IVF VERSUS GIFT

Tanbo and colleagues compared pregnancy rates in women with unexplained infertility using GIFT versus IVF. A significantly higher pregnancy rate was found with IVF compared with GIFT.[39] The study also included patients with mild male factor infertility and minimal endometriosis. Other studies[68,70] have not shown this benefit, but these studies favored IVF because it was the least invasive of the two procedures.[73] Therefore, it seems that GIFT has a limited role in the treatment of unexplained infertility.

SUMMARY OF IVF DATA

Probably the best review of the efficacy and cost effectiveness of the various therapies was published by the members of the Reproductive Medicine Network in 1998. In a retrospective analysis of 45 studies on the subject, a pregnancy rate per initiated cycle of 1.3 to 4.1 percent was found with no treatment, 3.8 percent with IUI alone, 5.6 percent with CC and intercourse, 8.3 percent with CC/IUI, 7.7 percent with hMG and intercourse, 17.1 percent with hMG/IUI, 20.7 percent with IVF, and 27 percent with GIFT. It has been concluded that CC/IUI is a cost-effective first-line treatment for unexplained infertility and that if this treatment fails to result in pregnancy, patients should be offered hMG/IUI[48] (Table 18.6).

▶ **TABLE 18-6:** EFFICACY OF VARIOUS TREATMENT OPTIONS FOR UNEXPLAINED INFERTILITY

Treatment	Pregnancy Rate
No treatment	1.3%–4.1%
IUI alone	3.8%
CC/intercourse	5.6%
CC/IUI	8.3%
hMG/intercourse	7.7%
hMG/IUI	17.1%
IVF	20.7%
GIFT	27%

From Fertil Steril 1998;70(2):207–213.

Abbreviations: IUI = intrauterine insemination; CC = clomiphene citrate; hMG = human menopausal gonadotropin; IVF = in vitro fertilization; GIFT = gamete intrafallopian transfer.

The existing data appear insufficient to suggest that IVF is more effective than other treatment options available for unexplained infertility. Adverse events such as ovarian hyperstimulation syndrome (OHSS) and multiple pregnancy, in addition to cost, must be taken into consideration when IVF is considered as a treatment option. Until further evidence is available, IVF should not be considered a first-line treatment option in patients with unexplained infertility and should be reserved for those who fail COH with IUI.

FERTILIZATION FAILURE IN UNEXPLAINED INFERTILITY

Fertilization failure or lower-than-expected fertilization rates at the time of IVF as a cause of infertility have been well documented in couples with unexplained infertility.[74–77] Despite the lower-than-normal fertilization rates, cleavage rates and implantation rates are similar.[76,77] In a well-controlled, prospective study of this subject, Aboulghar and colleagues[76] performed IVF and intracytoplasmic sperm injection (ICSI) on sibling oocytes of 22 patients with unexplained infertility. There was a total failure of fertilization in the IVF group in 5 of 22 patients

(22.7 percent) and in 0 percent in the ICSI group. Gurgan and colleagues confirmed this finding in their study of 157 IVF cycles,[77] with failure of fertilization in 11.4 percent of couples and no failure of fertilization with ICSI. Patients with unexplained infertility who are proceeding to IVF should be counseled about the benefits of ICSI.

Fallopian Tube Sperm Perfusion (FSP)

FSP is described as another method of intrauterine insemination.[78] With FSP, a large volume of sperm suspension (4 mL) is injected to reach the tubes via the cervix by transcervical insemination. Several studies have reported higher pregnancy rates with this technique compared with the traditional IUI.[78–81] In a prospective, randomized study, Mamas demonstrated a cycle fecundity of 12 percent with hMG/traditional IUI compared with 26 percent with hMG/FSP.[79] Trout and Kemmann confirmed these results.[80] However, it is important to note that there are several prospective, randomized trials that show no benefit to FSP when compared with traditional IUI.[81,82] Secondary to this, most infertility programs still perform the traditional IUI.

Tubal Flushing

Couples with the diagnosis of unexplained infertility may benefit from a tubal flushing procedure. In an evaluation of this technique, Nugent and colleagues randomized couples to tubal flushing with an oil-soluble medium (Lipiodol) or no therapy. There was a significantly higher pregnancy rate in the Lipiodol group.[83] It has been well established in the past that the use of an oil-based media for HSG improves pregnancy rates for patients with normal fallopian tubes.[84] The risks associated with using an oil-based medium led to abandonment of this therapy by most practitioners.

Alternative Medical Therapies

Many different medical therapies have been studied for the treatment of unexplained infertility, the majority of which lack sufficient evidence to support their use. The use of bromocriptine has been studied, and it has not been shown to improve pregnancy rates in women with unexplained infertility.[85] Similarly, Danazol has been evaluated. A Cochrane review of the studies examining the benefit of Danazol in the treatment of unexplained infertility showed no benefit.[86]

► OBSTETRIC OUTCOME

Infertility and the use of ART have been thought to increase the risk of poor pregnancy outcome.[87,88] This is especially true when multiple pregnancies are factored in. In some poorly controlled studies evaluating women with unexplained infertility treated with ART, it was found that women with unexplained infertility had a higher risk of intrauterine growth retardation (IUGR)[87] and low-birth-weight babies[88] when compared with fertile controls or women with unexplained infertility conceiving spontaneously. Some practitioners have guessed that infertility treatment may lead to placental insufficiency.[87–89] However, in a well-controlled trial by Isaksson and colleagues, no differences were noted in gestational duration, major congenital anomalies, perinatal mortality, or mean birth weight in women with unexplained infertility using fertility therapy compared with spontaneous pregnancies.[88,89] These data refute the finding that unexplained infertility is associated with a poor pregnancy outcome.

► CONCLUSION

Unexplained infertility is a difficult problem for both the infertile couple and their physician. As research advances and we better understand the molecular/genetic mechanisms involved in ovulation, fertilization, and embryo implantation, undoubtedly we will find more subtle causes of infertility. Fortunately, the current strategies used for the treatment of unexplained infertility work fairly well and probably will limit the practicability of more esoteric testing to academic use.

KEY POINTS

1. Unexplained infertility is a diagnosis of exclusion given to infertile couples who have had a complete infertility evaluation with no abnormal findings.

2. The incidence of unexplained infertility is approximately 15 percent.

3. Spontaneous conception without treatment is well documented for couples with unexplained infertility. Conceptions occur at a rate of about 10 percent per year during the first 2 years and then 5 percent per year after that in couples with primary infertility. In couples with secondary infertility, conceptions occur at a rate of 18 percent per year for the first 5 years then 10 percent per year thereafter.

4. Options for active management include CC/IUI, hMG/IUI, and IVF. COH/IUI appears to improve pregnancy rates significantly over treatment options using COH with intercourse.

5. Consideration should be given to the use of ICSI in patients undergoing IVF with the diagnosis of unexplained infertility. High rates of fertilization failure are seen in this group of patients, especially those failing to conceive with COH/IUI.

REFERENCES

1. Hull MGR, Savage PE, Bromham DR. Prognostic value of the postcoital test: A prospective study based on time-specific conception rates. *Br J Obstet Gynnaecol* 1982;89:299.

2. Templeton P. The incidence, characteristics, and prognosis of patients whose infertility is unexplained. *Fertil Steril* 1982;37:175–182.

3. Lobo RA. Unexplained infertility. *J Reprod Med* 1993;38:241.

4. Rowe PJ, Comhaire FH, Hargreave TB, et al. *WHO Manual for the Standardized Investigation of the Infertile Couple*. Cambridge, England: Cambridge University Press, 1993.

5. Crosignani PG, Collin J, Cooke ID, et al. Recommendations of the ESHRE workshop on unexplained infertility, Anacapri, August 28–29, 1992. *Hum Reprod* 1992;8:977.

6. ESHRE Capri Workshop. Guidelines to the prevalence, diagnosis, treatment, and management of infertility. *Hum Reprod* 1996;11:1775.

7. Crosignani PG, Ruben BL. Optimal use of infertility diagnostic tests and treatments. *Hum Reprod* 2000;15:723.

8. Drake T, Tredway D, Buchanan G, et al. Unexplained infertility: A reappraisal. *Obset Gynecol* 1977;50:644.

9. Ragah R, McHugo JM, Obhrai M. The role of HSG in modern gynecological practice. *Br J Radiol* 1992;65:849.

10. Henig I, Prough SG, Cheatwood M, Delong E. Hysterosalpingography, laparoscopy, and hysteroscopy in infertility: A comparative study. *J Reprod Med* 1991;36:573.

11. Tanahatoe SJ, Hompes PG, Lambalk CB. Investigation of the infertile couple: Should diagnostic laparoscopy be performed in the infertility workup program in patients undergoing intrauterine insemination. *Hum Reprod* 2003; 18:8.

12. Gleicher N. Cost-effective infertility care. *Hum Reprod Update* 2000;6:190.

13. Fatum M, Laufer N, Simon A. Investigation of the infertile couple: Should diagnostic laparoscopy be performed after normal hysterosalpingography in treating infertility suspected to be of unknown origin. *Hum Reprod* 2002; 17:1.

14. Ripps BA, Martin DC. Correlation of focal pelvic tenderness with implant dimension and stage of endometriosis. *J Reprod Med* 1992;37:620.

15. Ripps BA, Martin DC. Endometriosis and chronic pelvic pain. *Obstet Gynecol Clin North Am* 1993;20:709.

16. Speert H. *Obstetrics and Gynecology Milestones Illustrated*. New York: Parthenon, 1996.

17. Kovac GT, Newman GB, Henson GL. The postcoital test: What is normal. *BMJ* 1978;1:818.

18. Jette NT, Glass RM. Prognostic value of the postcoital test. *Fertil Steril* 1972;23:29.

19. Portuondo JA, Echanojauregui AD, Herran C, Agustin A. Prognostic value of postcoital test in unexplained infertility. *Int J Fertil* 1982;27:184.

20. Skaf RA, Kemmann E. Postcoital testing in women during menotrophin therapy. *Fertil Steril* 1982;37:514.

21. Collins JA, So Y, Wilson EH, et al. The post-coital test as a predictor of pregnancy among 355 infertile couples. *Fertil Steril* 1984;41:703.

22. World Health Organization. *WHO Laboratory Manual for the Examination of Human Semen and Sperm–Cervical Mucus Interaction,* 3d ed. New York: Cambridge University Press; 1992; pp 3–27.

23. Pattinson HA, Mortimer D. Prevalence of sperm surface antibodies in the male partners of infertile couples as determined by immunobead screening. *Fertil Steril* 1987;48:466.

24. Mandelbaum SL, Diamond MP, DeCherney AH. Relationship of antibodies to sperm head to etiology of infertility in patients undergoing in vitro fertilization/embryo transfer. *Am J Reprod Immunol* 1989;19:3.

25. Hass GG, Cines DB, Schrieber AD. Immunologic infertility: identification of patients with antisperm antibodies. *N Engl J Med* 1980;303:722.

26. Bronson R, Cooper G, Rosenfeld D. Sperm antibodies: Their role in infertility. *Fertil Steril* 1984;42:171.

27. Snow K, Ball BG. Characterization of human sperm antigens and antisperm antibodies in infertile patients. *Fertil Steril* 1992;58:1011.

28. Matson PL, Junk SM, Spittle JW, Yovich JL. Effect of antispermatozoal antibodies in seminal plasma upon spermatozoal function. *Int J Androl* 1998;11:101.

29. Barratt CLR, Dunphy BC, McLeod I, Cooke ID. The poor prognosis value of low to moderate levels of sperm surface-bound antibodies. *Hum Reprod* 1992;7:95.

30. Marshburn PB, Kutteh WH. The role of antisperm antibodies in infertility. *Fertil Steril* 1994;61:799.

31. Li H, Chen S, Xing F. Expression of *HOXA10* gene in human endometrium and its relationship with unexplained infertility. *Chin J Obstet Gynecol* 2002;37:30.

32. Lessey BA, Castelbaum AJ, Sawin SW, et al. Integrins as markers of uterine receptivity in women with primary unexplained infertility. *Fertil Steril* 1998;63:535.

33. Toner JP, Philput CB, Jones GC, Mausher SJ. Basal follicle stimulating hormone level is a better predictor of in vitro fertilization performance than age. *Fertil Steril* 1991;55:784.

34. Navot D, Rosenwaks Z, Margalioth EJ. Prognostic assessment of female fecundity. *Lancet* 1987;2:645.

35. Tanbo T, Dale PO, Lunde O, et al. Prediction of response to controlled ovarian hyperstimulation: A comparison of basal and clomiphene citrate stimulated follicle-stimulating hormone levels. *Fertil Steril* 1992;57:819.

36. Scott RT Jr, Leonardi MR, Hofmann GE, et al. A prospective evaluation of clomiphene citrate challenge test screening of the general infertility population. *Obstet Gynecol* 1993;82:539.

37. Goverde AJ, McDonnell J, Vermeiden JPW, et al. Intrauterine insemination or in vitro fertilization in idiopathic subfertility and male subfertility: A randomized trial and cost-effectiveness analysis. *Lancet* 2000;355:13.

38. Deaton GB, Nakajima ST, Badger GJ, Brumstead JR. A randomized, controlled trial of CC/IUI in couples with unexplained infertility or surgically corrected endometriosis. *Fertil Steril* 1990;54:1083.

39. Tanbo T, Dale PO, Abyholm T. Assisted fertilization in infertile women with patent fallopian tubes: A comparison of in vitro fertilization, gamete intrafallopian transfer and tubal embryo stage transfer. *Hum Reprod* 1990;36:266.

40. Collins J, Rowe T. Age of the female partner is a prognostic factor in prolonged unexplained infertility: A multicenter study. *Fertil Steril* 1989;52:15.

41. Berube S, Marcoux S, Langeoun M, et al. Fecundity of infertile women with minimal or mild endometriosis and women with unexplained infertility. *Fertil Steril* 1998;69:1034.

42. Lenton E, Weston G, Cook I. Long-term followup of the apparently normal couple with a complaint of infertility. *Fertil Steril* 1977;28:913.

43. Dunphy BC, Kay R, Barratt CLR, Cooke ID. Female age, the length of involuntary infertility prior to investigations and fertility outcome. *Hum Reprod* 1989;4:527.

44. Daly D. Treatment validation of ultrasound-defined abnormal follicular dynamics as a cause of infertility. *Fertil Steril* 1989;51:51.

45. Collins JA, Burrows FA, Willian AR. The prognosis for live birth among untreated infertile couples. *Fertil Steril* 1995;64:22.

46. Snick HKA, Snick TS, Evers JUH, Collins JA. The spontaneous pregnancy prognosis in untreated subfertile couples: The Walcheren

Primary Care Study. *Hum Reprod* 1997;12:1582.

47. Hughes E, Collins J, Vandekerckhove P. Clomiphene citrate for unexplained infertility in women. *Cochrane Database Syst Rev* 2003.

48. Guzick DS, Sullivan MS, Adamson D, et al. Efficacy of treatment for unexplained infertility. *Fertil Steril* 1998;70:207.

49. Arici A, Byrd W, Bradshaw K, et al. Evaluation of CC and hCG treatment: A prospective, randomized crossover study during IUI cycles. *Fertil Steril* 1994;61:314.

50. Martinez A, Bernardus K, Voorhorst F, et al. Intrauterine insemination does and CC does not improve fecundity in couples with infertility due to male or idiopathic factors: A prospective, randomized, controlled study. *Fertil Steril* 1990;53:847.

51. Fisch P, Casper RF, Brown SE, et al. Unexplained infertility: Evaluation of treatment with clomiphene citrate and human chorionic gonadotropin. *Fertil Steril* 1989;51:828.

52. Glagener CMA, Coulson C, Lambert PA, et al. Clomiphene treatment for women with unexplained infertility. *Gynecol Endocrinol* 1990;4:75.

53. Wang CF, Gemzill C. Pregnancy following treatment with human gonadotropins in primary unexplained infertility. *Acta Obset Gynaecol Scand* 1979;58:141.

54. Cohen B. Intrauterine insemination and controlled ovarian hyperstimulation, in Templeton A, Cook I, O'Brien S (eds), *Evidence-Based Fertility Treatments*. London RCOG Press, 1999; pp 205–216.

55. Agarwal SK, Buyalos RP. Clomiphene citrate with intrauterine insemination: Is it effective therapy in women above the age of 35 years? *Fertil Steril* 1996;65:759.

56. Deaton JL, Clark RR, Pittaway DE, et al. Clomiphene citrate ovulation induction in combination with a timed intrauterine insemination: The value of urinary LH versus human chorionic gonadotropin timing. *Fertil Steril* 1997;68:43.

57. Simon A, Avidan B, Mordel N, et al. The value of menotrophin treatment for unexplained infertility prior to an in vitro fertilization attempt. *Hum Reprod* 1991;6:222.

58. Nielsen JC, Walsh S, Dumeg S, Metzgar DA. A randomized and longitudinal study of human menopausal gonadotropins with intrauterine insemination in the treatment of infertility. *Obset Gynecol* 1993;82:780.

59. Dodson WC, Whitesiders DB, Hughes CL, et al. Superovulation with intrauterine insemination in the treatment of infertility: A possible alternative to gamete intrafallopian transfer and in vitro fertilization. *Fertil Steril* 1987;48:441.

60. Aboulghar MA, Mansour RT, Serour GI, et al. Ovarian superstimulation and intrauterine insemination for the treatment of unexplained infertility. *Fertil Steril* 1993;60:303.

61. Gagliardi CL, Emmi AM, Weiss G, Schmidt CL. GnRH-a improves the efficiency of COH/IUI. *Fertil Steril* 1991;55:393.

62. Manzi DL, Dumez S, Scott LB, Nulsen JC. Selective utilization of leuprolide acetate in women undergoing superovulation with intrauterine insemination results in significant improvement in pregnancy outcome. *Fertil Steril* 1995;63:866.

63. Dodson WC, Walmer DK, Hughes CL, et al. Adjunctive leuprolide therapy does not improve cycle fecundity in controlled ovarian hyperstimulation and intrauterine insemination of subfertile women. *Obstet Gynecol* 1991;78:187.

64. Sengokee K, Tamale K, Takaoka U, et al. A randomized, prospective study of gonadotrophin with or without GnRH-a for treatment of unexplained infertility. *Hum Reprod* 1994;9:1043.

65. Karlstrom DO, Berght, Lundkuist O. Addition of GnRH-a and two inseminations with husband's sperm do not improve the pregnancy rate in superovulated cycles. *Acta Obset Gynaecol Scand* 2000;79:37.

66. Younis JS, Haddad S, Matilsky, et al. Premature luteinization: Could it be an early manifestation of low ovarian reserve? *Fertil Steril* 1998;59:461.

67. Soliman S, Daya S, Collin J, Jarrell J. A randomized trial of in vitro fertilization versus conventional treatment for infertility. *Fertil Steril* 1993;59:1239.

68. Crosignani PG, Walters DE, Soliani A. The ESHRE multicentre trial on the treatment of unexplained infertility: A preliminary report. *Hum Reprod* 1991;6:953.

69. Murdoch AP, Harris M, Mahroo M, et al. Gamete intrafallopian transfer (GIFT) compared with intrauterine insemination in the treatment of unexplained infertility. *Br J Obstet Gynaecol* 1991;98:1107.

70. Mills MS, Eddowes HA, Cahill DJ. A prospective, controlled study of in vitro fertilization, gamete intrafallopian transfer and intrauterine insemination combined with superovulation. *Hum Reprod* 1991;7:490.

71. Iffland CA, Rerd W, Am SON, et al. A within patient comparison between superovulation IUI using husband washed spermatozoa and gamete intrafallopian transfer in unexplained infertility. *Eur J Obstet Gynecol Reprod Biol* 1991; 39:181.

72. Peterson CM, Hatasaka HH, Jones KP, et al. Ovulation induction with gonadotropins and IUI compared with in vitro fertilization and no therapy: A prospective, nonrandomized, cohort study and meta-analysis. *Fertil Steril* 1994;62: 535.

73. Ranieri M, Beckett VA, Marchants S, et al. Gamete intrafallopian transfer or in vitro fertilization after failed ovarian stimulation and intrauterine insemination in unexplained infertility. *Hum Reprod* 1995;10:2023.

74. MacKenna AL, Zegars-Hochschild F, Fernandez EO, et al. Fertilization rate in couples with unexplained infertility. *Hum Reprod* 1992;7:233.

75. Trounson AO, Lecton JF, Wood C, et al. The investigation of idiopathic infertility by in vitro fertilization. *Fertil Steril* 1980;34:431.

76. Aboulghar MA, Mansour G, Serour GI, et al. Intracytoplasmic sperm injection and conventional in vitro fertilization for sibling oocytes in cases of unexplained infertility and borderline semen. *J Assoc Reprod Genet* 1996;13:38.

77. Gurgan T, Urman B, Yanali H, Kisnisci HA. The results of in vitro fertilization–embryo transfer in couples with unexplained infertility failing to conceive with superovulation and intrauterine insemination. *Fertil Steril* 1995;64:93.

78. Kahn JA, Sunde A, Von During V, et al. Intrauterine insemination. *Ann NY Acad Sci* 1991; 626:452.

79. Mamas L. Higher pregnancy rates with a simple method for fallopian tube sperm perfusion, using the cervical clamp double nut bivalve speculum in the treatment of unexplained infertility: A prospective, randomized study. *Hum Reprod* 1996;11:2618.

80. Trout SW, Kemmann E. Fallopian sperm perfusion versus intrauterine insemination: A randomized, controlled trial and metaanalysis of the literature. *Fertil Steril* 1999;71:881.

81. Nuojua-Iluttunene S, Tuomivaara L, Juntunen K, et al. Comparison of fallopian tube sperm perfusion with IUI in the treatment of infertility. *Fertil Steril* 1997;67:939.

82. El Sadek MM, Amer MK, Abdel Malak G. Questioning the efficacy of fallopian tube sperm perfusion. *Hum Reprod* 1998;13:3053.

83. Nugent D, Watson AJ, Kellick SR, et al. A randomized, controlled trial of tubal flushing with Lipiodol for unexplained infertility. *Fertil Steril* 2002;77:173.

84. Vandekerckhove P, Watson A, Luford R, et al. Oil-soluble versus water-soluble media for assessing tubal patency with HSG or laparoscopy in subfertile women. *Cochrane Database Syst Rev* 2003.

85. Hughes CJ, Vandekerckhove P. Bromocryptine for unexplained subfertility in women. *Cochrane Database Syst Rev* 2003.

86. Hughes TG, Vandekerckhove P. Danazol for unexplained infertility. *Cochrane Database Syst Rev* 2003.

87. Wang JX, Clark AM, Kirby CA, et al. The obstetric outcome of singleton pregnancies following in vitro fertilization/gamete intrafallopian transfer. *Hum Reprod* 1994;9:141.

88. Isaksson R, Tiitinen A. Obstetric outcome in patients with unexplained infertility: Comparison of treatment related and spontaneous pregnancies. *Acta Obstet Gynaecol Scand* 1998;77: 849.

89. Isaksson R, Gissler M, Tiitinen A. Obstetric outcome among women with unexplained infertility after IVF: A matched case-control study. *Hum Reprod* 2002;17:1755.

CHAPTER 19

Uterine Diseases

Yinka Oyelese and Craig A. Winkel

Disorders of the uterus are a major cause of ill health and distress that not infrequently lead women to seek the attention of a gynecologist. This is reflected in the fact that some 600,000 hysterectomies are performed each year in the United States, making extirpation of the uterus second only to cesarean section as the most frequently performed major surgical procedure.[1] The word *hysteria* derives from *hysteros,* the Greek word meaning "uterus," reflecting the belief of ancient civilizations that this relatively small muscular organ was responsible for women's whims, moods, and passions. It is now generally accepted that the uterus serves no significant biologic role apart from serving as a residence for the developing fetus. As such, when uterine pathology occurs in women of reproductive age, therapy frequently must be directed at restoration or preservation of fertility.

Diseases of the uterus may be congenital or acquired and not infrequently result in abnormalities of the menstrual cycle, pelvic pain, infertility, or pregnancy wastage. Tumors of the uterus may grow to a considerable size, leading to problems related to mass effect. This chapter presents a practical approach to the clinical problems that result from pathologic conditions of the uterus that may affect fertility potential. Relevant normal physiology and then pathophysiology are first discussed, followed by the methods of diagnosis. Finally, management options and outcomes are presented, including recent developments in the therapies for management of uterine diseases.

▶ DEVELOPMENTAL ABNORMALITIES

Embryology of the Müllerian Ducts

Congenital anomalies of the uterus resulting from arrested or defective development of the müllerian ducts are the most common malformations of the reproductive system.[2] Some knowledge of the embryologic development of the müllerian system is crucial to understanding the defects that occur and to guiding the gynecologist in making appropriate therapeutic decisions (Fig. 19-1). The müllerian ducts are formed between the fifth and sixth weeks of embryonic life.[3] They run longitudinally, cephalad to caudad, and lie in close proximity to the more well-developed wolffian ducts. An important anatomic landmark is the insertion of the ligamentum inguinale, destined to become the round ligament, into the urogenital cord, thus dividing the müllerian ducts into two segments. The segments above this insertion remain separate and become the fallopian tubes; the segments below this insertion move

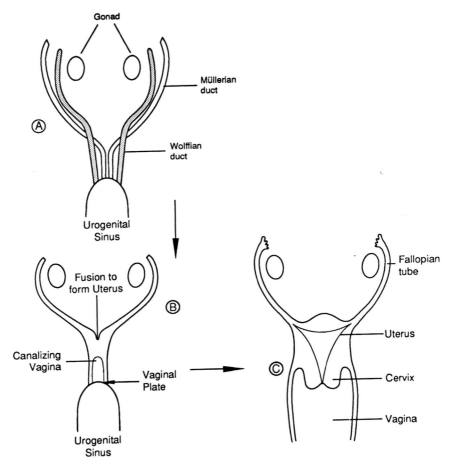

Figure 19-1 Embryology of the müllerian system.

medially, will fuse eventually, and form the uterus and upper portion of the vagina. During the twelfth to fourteenth weeks of embryonic life, the medial walls between the adjacent and parallel lower segments of the two fused müllerian ducts begin to disintegrate from below upward. What remains is a lumen that begins to form at the cervical region and gradually migrates upward until the uterus is formed fully. At the same time that this sequence of events is occurring, the urinary system is developing in close anatomic proximity (Table 19-1).

Keeping these developmental processes in mind, the clinician should have little difficulty in understanding the resulting uterine anomalies based on the time at which an aberration occurs. Unilateral or bilateral failure of formation of the müllerian duct(s) may occur anytime during the first 4 weeks of development (Fig. 19-2), whereas uterus didelphys or duplicated uterus and vagina may occur between 8 and 10 weeks as a result of failure of the müllerian ducts to fuse (Fig. 19-3). The formation of a bicornuate uterus, septated uterus, subseptated uterus, or arcuate uterus may occur between the twelfth and sixteenth weeks of gestational age as a result of failure of the mechanism of canalization to continue cephalad

▶ **TABLE 19-1:** TIMING OF DEVELOPMENT OF GENITAL AND URINARY SYSTEMS

Week	Crown-Rump Length (mm)	Genital	Urinary
4	5	—	Wolffian ducts reach cloaca, urethral buds form
5	8	—	Ureters, pelvis forming, kidneys move to lumbar region
6	12	Müllerian ducts form	Nephrogenesis, urorectal septum forming
7	17	—	Collecting tubules form, urorectal septum complete
8	23	Müllerian ducts cross medially to wolffian ducts	—
	28	Müllerian ducts meet in the midline below insertion of the ligamentum inguinale	—
	35	Müllerian ducts join urogenital sinus	—
10	40	Wolffian ducts degenerate	Kidney secretes
12	56	Uterine horns fused, canalization at cervix	—
	66	Canalization continues upward, vaginal wall forming	Urethral orifices appear
16	112	Uterus and vagina complete	

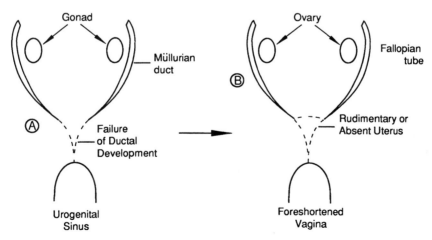

Figure 19-2 Müllerian anomalies that result from failure of development during the first 4 weeks of embryonic life.

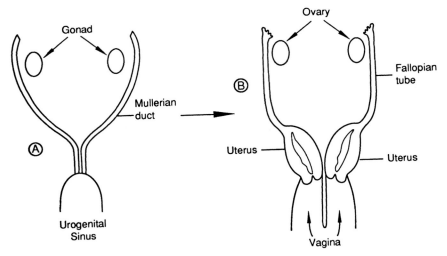

Figure 19-3 Müllerian anomalies that result from failure of fusion of the müllerian ducts.

from the cervix to the fundus. Finally, it is possible also to observe asymmetric alterations in müllerian duct development and the uterine defects that may ensue. For instance, complete or incomplete arrest of the development of a unilateral müllerian duct may result in the formation of a bicornuate uterus or a unicornuate uterus with an accessory, rudimentary horn

(Figs. 19-4 and 19-5). More uncommonly, anomalies occur that do not seem to follow any one specific area of dysfunction during the developmental processes.[4,5] It has been proposed that a minor mesonephric defect may induce an isolated müllerian defect, much in the same way that Gruenwald suggested that mesonephric defects may induce wolffian abnormalities.[6]

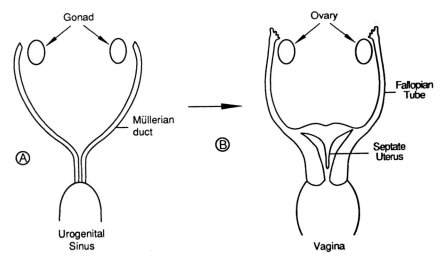

Figure 19-4 Failure to canalize during the final stages of müllerian development may result in the formation of a uterine septum.

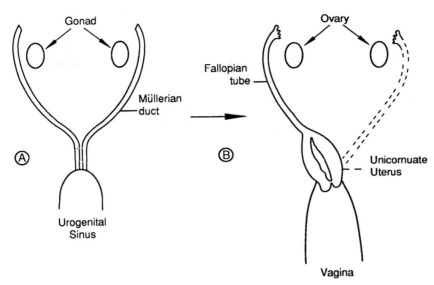

Figure 19-5 Incomplete arrest of development of one müllerian duct may result in the formation of a unicornuate uterus with or without a remnant of the contralateral uterine horn.

Congenital Anomalies of the Uterus

The true incidence of congenital müllerian anomalies, of which uterine malformations constitute the majority, is unknown.[7] Most cases are diagnosed during evaluation for infertility, pelvic pain, recurrent miscarriage, or recurrent preterm labor; in the absence of symptoms, most anomalies go undiagnosed. Since up to 57 percent of women with uterine defects have successful fertility and pregnancy, the true incidence of congenital müllerian defects may be significantly understated. Simon and colleagues found uterine anomalies in 3.2 percent of 679

fertile women undergoing laparoscopic tubal sterilization.[8] Nahum determined that the prevalence of uterine anomalies in the general population was 1 in 201 women (0.5 percent).[7] Uterine anomalies were identified in 1 in 594 fertile women (0.17 percent) compared with 1 in 29 (3.5 percent) infertile women. Distribution of these anomalies between subtypes is given in Table 19-2. Differences in percentages are attributable to the diagnostic methods used; the majority of double uteri diagnosed on hysterosalpingography (HSG) as bicornuate are, in fact, septate.[9] When the diagnoses are accurate, the septate uterus appears to be the most

▶ **TABLE 19-2:** DISTRIBUTION OF SUBTYPES OF UTERINE ANOMALIES

Type of Anomaly	Percent (Acien)[12]	Percent (Grimbizis)[17]	Percent (Nahum)[7]
Bicornuate	46	26	39
Septate	22	34.9	34
Didelphic	11	8.4	11
Arcuate	15	18.3	7
Unicornuate	4.5	9.6	5
Hypoplastic/others	4	2.9	4

common uterine anomaly.[10] A summary of the American Fertility Society classification for müllerian anomalies is provided in Table 19-3.[11] There is consensus that more severe uterine developmental defects are associated with a high incidence of reproductive complications, including spontaneous abortion, failed first-trimester pregnancy termination, malpresentation (Fig. 19-6), premature labor and delivery, and low birth weight.[12–17] Acien found that only 53 percent of pregnancies in women with uterine malformations ended with a child surviving more than 7 days, compared with 89 percent in women with a normal uterus.[12] It appears, however, that uterine anomalies only rarely result in infertility, although very early miscarriage may be misconstrued as infertility. Acien reported an infertility rate of only 6 percent in infertile women with uterine anomalies who had no other explanation for their inability to conceive.[12] The incidence of infertility in one series of women with these disorders was 9.6 percent, a value little different from the 10 percent incidence of infertility estimated for the general population.[13] The mechanism(s) by which uterine anomalies result in reproductive failure are not clear. Reduced uterine capacity and failure to compensate adequately for the growing fetus may be implicated, as well as distortion of the uterine cavity.[10] These factors may lead to increased intrauterine pressure and relative cervical incompetence.[10] Uterine septa are poorly vascularized, leading to sub-

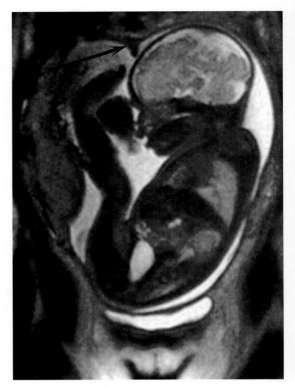

Figure 19-6 Breech fetus in a septate uterus. Septum is indicated by an arrow. *(Courtesy Dr. Reena Jha.)*

optimal implantation and placentation.[10] Luteal phase dysfunction may occur more frequently in women with a malformed uterus because of altered blood supply to the endometrium.[13] It also has been suggested that faulty müllerian development may be associated with defective formation of estrogen and progesterone receptors within internal reproductive tissues.[18]

Common Uterine Anomalies

Septate Uterus

The septate uterus is the most common uterine malformation and the one with the poorest pregnancy outcomes.[10,15] A septate uterus arises due to nonresorption of the midline sep-

▶ **TABLE 19-3:** AMERICAN FERTILITY SOCIETY CLASSIFICATION OF MÜLLERIAN ANOMALIES

Class	Type of Anomaly
I	Hypoplasia/agenesis
II	Unicornuate uterus
III	Didelphyic uterus
IV	Bicornuate uterus
V	Septate uterus
VI	Arcuate uterus
VII	DES drug-related

tum, an aberration that occurs at 12 to 16 weeks of intrauterine life. The septum may be partial or complete. Spontaneous miscarriage rates have been estimated at greater than 60 percent, with live births occurring in only 6 to 28 percent of pregnancies.[15] Pregnancies also may be complicated by malpresentation (see Fig. 19-6), preterm labor, and intrauterine growth restriction. Pregnancy loss may be secondary to poor vascularization of the septum and endometrial atrophy that results in poor placentation.[15] The septum consists of fibroelastic tissue[19] and connective tissue.[20] Dabrirashrafi and colleagues[21] biospied uterine septa and found mostly myometrium, raising the possibility that pregnancy loss was secondary to increased and uncoordinated contractions or poor decidualization and placentation. The presence of a septum alone is not an indication for surgery. When a septum is found in association with recurrent pregnancy loss, however, surgery should be considered.

Bicornuate Uterus

Unless adequate methods to assess uterine morphology are employed, most uteri thought to be bicornuate are, in fact, septate. In one study when laparoscopy is performed on women thought to have a bicornuate uterus on the basis of HSG, the diagnosis was changed to septate uteri in 38 of 39.[9] Most women with a bicornuate uterus have a normal pregnancy.[10] A bicornuate uterus, nonetheless, is associated with increased rates of spontaneous abortion, malpresentation, recurrent midtrimester loss, and premature delivery.[10] Importantly, obstetric outcomes seem to improve with each subsequent pregnancy, possibly as a result of stretching of the myometrium and improved vascularization.[10] Thus it is difficult to evaluate the success of surgical correction. It is questionable, therefore, whether young women with recurrent pregnancy loss and a bicornuate uterus should undergo a corrective surgical procedure. For the older woman with a history of pregnancy wastage, however, metroplasty may be considered early.

Uterus Didelphys/Unicornuate Uterus

These malformations are relatively uncommon.[10,22] Most reports focus primarily on obstructive symptoms due to associated rudimentary uterine horns or vaginal malformations. These anomalies occasionally are diagnosed during investigation for pelvic pain or a pelvic mass. Uterus didelphys is a condition in which there are two separate uterine bodies, each with its own fallopian tube and cervix (Fig. 19-7), and almost invariably associated with a longitudinal vaginal septum. This vaginal septum may cause dyspareunia. Associated renal anomalies, including absent, hypoplastic, pelvic, or horseshoe kidneys, are common.[23] Li and colleagues found renal agenesis in 13 of 16 women with didelphic uteri who had magnetic resonance imaging (MRI).[23] Uterus didelphys has little impact on fertility, and surgical correction is not indicated.[10] The primary indication for surgery is evidence of obstruction. In most cases, correction consists of excision of the rudimentary horn. Pregnancy may occur in a rudimentary horn and may lead to rupture. Both the unicornuate uterus and the didelphic uterus are associated with poor pregnancy outcomes, with spontaneous abortion rates of 44 and 36 percent, respectively, and term delivery rates of 44 and 45 percent, respectively.[10,22,24,25] The cause is diminished capacity of the abnormal uterus.

Uterine Anomalies Due to in Utero Exposure to Diethylstilbestrol

A discussion of congenital anomalies of the müllerian system would be incomplete without mention in utero exposure to diethylstilbestrol (DES) or other synthetic estrogens. Smith suggested in 1948 that treatment with DES, a synthetic nonsteroidal estrogen first synthesized in 1938, reduced complications of pregnancy, namely, spontaneous abortion, premature delivery, pregnancy-induced hypertension, and fetal death in utero.[26] These benefits were refuted in 1953.[27] In 1980, Kaufman and colleagues reported the association between intrauterine exposure to DES and upper genital

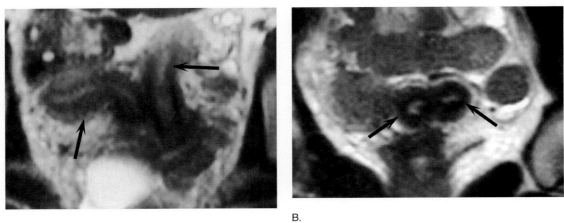

A.

B.

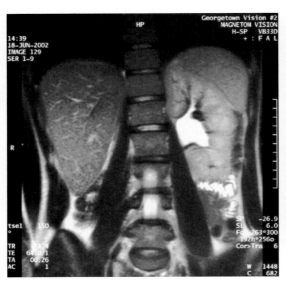

C.

D.

Figure 19-7 *A.* MRI of a uterus didelphys. The two separate uteri can be seen *(arrows)*. *B.* Two separate cervices are demonstrated *(arrows)*. *C.* MRI of the abdomen in the same patient showing an absent right kidney. The left kidney can be seen.   *(Courtesy Dr. Reena Jha.)* *D–H.* (A patient with uterus didelphys, blind hemivagina and ipsilateral renal agenesis.) *D.* A cross-sectional (transverse section) MRI revealing both uteri (RU, LU), a small right vagina (RV) and large distended left vagina (LV). S, septum. *E.* A cross-sectional MRI revealing the association of the bladder (B) with the left vagina (LV) and right vagina (RV). *F.* Longitudinal MRI revealing the bladder (B), left uterus (LU), and cervic (C), and the communication with the left vagina (LV). *G.* An intravenous pyelogram (IVP) demonstrating absence of the left kidney and ureter. *H.* Laparoscopic view of the uterus didelphys with left (LU) and right (RU) uteri.   *(From Carr BB and Blackwell RE. Study Guide for Textbook of Reproductive Medicine 2nd ed. Appleton & Lange, Stamford, CT. 1998; pp 132–138.*

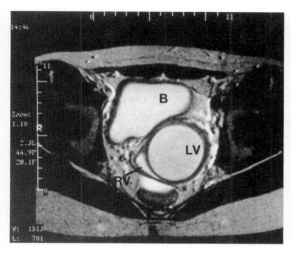

E.

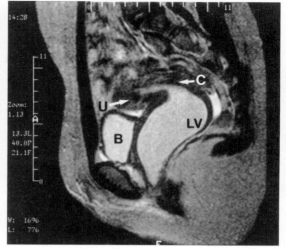

F.

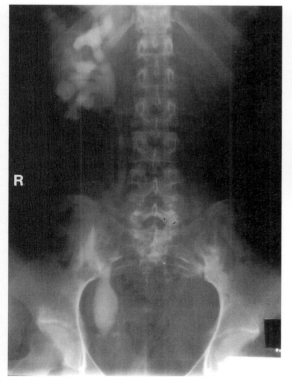

G.

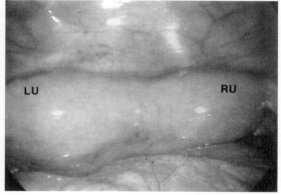

H.

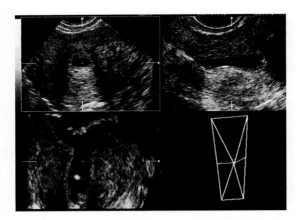

Figure 19-8 Three-dimensional sonogram of a T-shaped uterus. *(Courtesy Dr. Stephen Lincoln.)*

tract lesions that include constrictions within the uterine body, hypoplasia of the uterus, and formation of a T-shaped uterus[28] (Fig. 19-8). Furthermore, there is an association between in utero DES exposure, infertility, and reproductive failure.[29–34] Included in the role of the National Cooperative Diethylstilbestrol Adenosis (DESAD) Project was an attempt to compare fertility rates among DES-exposed women with those of nonexposed controls. Initial analysis revealed no differences in pregnancy rates between the two groups of women[29] or among women in a similar study undertaken in southern California.[30] However, infertility rates of up to 30 percent have been reported among women exposed to DES.[31–34] Kaufman recently published data indicating no third-generation carry-over effect of DES.[35] While there is considerable disagreement as to whether or not DES exposure is linked closely with infertility, there is also disagreement as to whether women exposed in utero to DES are at significant risk for poor pregnancy outcome. While etiologic factors remain to be elucidated, alterations in uterine blood supply, diminished uterine volume and capacitance, and defective uterine or cervical connective tissues have been suggested as possible causative factors. The presence of a hypoplastic or T-shaped uterus

seems to predispose to a particularly poor reproductive outcome. Pregnancy outcomes appear to improve with each subsequent pregnancy.

Diagnosis

Most congenital uterine malformations are found during investigation for infertility, recurrent miscarriage, or recurrent preterm labor. Bimanual vaginal examination is of very limited value in detecting uterine anomalies. A uterine congenital malformation should be suspected when a cervical or vaginal anomaly is found. A longitudinal vaginal septum should lead to a suspicion of a uterus didelphys. To make a definitive diagnosis, some invasive or imaging procedure is required.

The diagnostic tools available to the clinician for the purpose of demonstrating a uterine anomaly include two- and three-dimensional sonography, sonohysterography, HSG, MRI, laparoscopy, and hysteroscopy. To make an accurate diagnosis, both the uterine cavity and the external uterine fundal contour need to be defined. Frequently, techniques such as HSG or two-dimensional sonography will diagnose a "double uterus." These modalities are poor in differentiating between the various types of uterine duplication mainly because they cannot reliably define the outer fundal contour of the uterus.[36] Accurate differentiation is crucial because a bicornuate uterus is uncommonly associated with a poor obstetric outcome, whereas a septate uterus is. Furthermore, septa are readily amenable to hysteroscopic resection. In most cases the clinician will find the application of a combination of techniques most useful in making an accurate diagnosis.

Hysterosalpingography
HSG is very sensitive in identifying abnormalities of the uterine cavity (Figs. 19-9 and 19-10). One cannot distinguish, however, between a bicornuate and a septate uterus on the basis of an HSG alone.[36] Thus, as a rule, direct

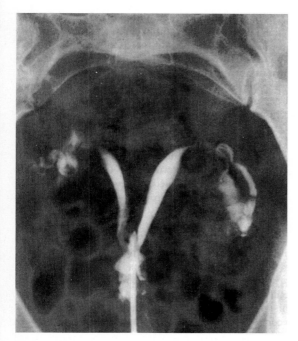

Figure 19-9 Hysterosalpingogram demonstrating a bicornuate uterus. *(Courtesy Dr. S. Karasick.)*

visualization with laparoscopy is required in addition to HSG. HSG is invasive, causes significant patient discomfort, involves the use of ionizing radiation, and carries risks of infection, uterine perforation, and allergic response to the contrast material.

Sonography

Because ultrasound is the most readily available imaging technique, it plays a key role in the detection of congenital uterine anomalies.[37] A high index of suspicion and good sonographic skills are required. Detecting uterine malformations is particularly difficult in the nongravid state. Early in pregnancy, when a gestation sac is visible in one uterine horn and decidualization occurs in the opposite uterine horn, a bicornuate or septate uterus may be readily identified (Fig. 19-11). In the more advanced pregnancy, uterine anomalies may be easily mistaken for ectopic pregnancy or uter-

ine leiomyomata. To diagnose a congenital uterine abnormality during pregnancy, sonography should be performed ideally in the first trimester.[38] The sonographic features most indicative of a midline uterine anomaly are best demonstrated on a high transverse image through the uterine fundus (see Fig. 19-11). Conventional two-dimensional sonography is sensitive in detecting uterine malformations; however, distinguishing between the different anomalies is often difficult or impossible.[39,40]

Three-Dimensional Sonography

Three-dimensional sonography allows presentation of scanned images in different orthogonal planes and permits precise spatial reconstruction of the uterus.[39–42] Thus both the

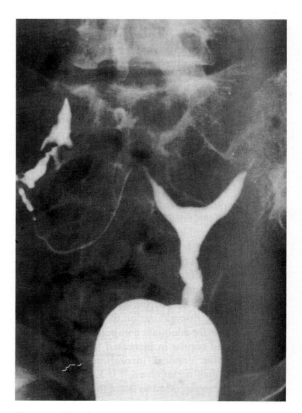

Figure 19-10 Hysterosalpingogram demonstrating a septate uterus. *(Courtesy Dr. S. Karasick.)*

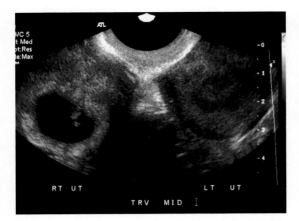

Figure 19-11 Transvaginal sonogram of a bicornuate uterus. The right horn contains a gestational sac. *(Courtesy Dr. Reena Jha.)*

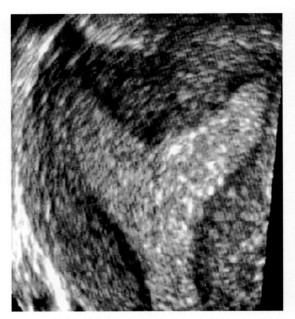

Figure 19-12 Three-dimensional sonogram of a septate uterus with a short, incomplete septum dividing the upper aspect of the uterine cavity. *(Courtesy Dr. Davor Jurkovic.)*

uterine cavity and the uterine fundal contour can be appreciated.[39–42] Jurkovic and colleagues compared two- and three-dimensional sonography in women with previous HSG.[39] Three-dimensional ultrasound had a 100 percent sensitivity and specificity for a normal uterus, arcuate uterus, and uteri with a major congenital malformations compared with a sensitivity of 67 to 88 percent and specificity of 94 to 95 percent on two-dimensional sonography. The most useful plane for distinguishing a uterine anomaly is the transverse section from the fundus to the cervix, allowing assessment of the fundal contour and the entire length of a septum if one is present (Figs. 19-12 through 19-15). Three-dimensional sonography has the advantages of being noninvasive and reproducible.[43]

Sonohysterography

The instillation of fluid into the endometrial cavity at the time of sonography allows more thorough evaluation of the uterine cavity. Some operators have found this a reliable method for differentiating uterine anomalies.[44,45] Alborzi and colleagues argued that sonohysterography eliminated the need for laparoscopy.[44] Like sonography, however, sonohysterography cannot always reliably demonstrate the uterine fundal contour.

Magnetic Resonance Imaging

MRI is noninvasive and allows evaluation of both the uterine cavity and the external fundal contour.[46–49] Thus it may reliably distinguish between the septate and bicornuate uterus (Figs. 19-7 and 19-16). In addition, MRI is useful in assessing the urinary tract[23] (see Fig. 19-7C). Two basic patterns on MRI are demonstrated in patients with uterine anomalies. With the bicornuate uterus, two high-signal areas (endometrium) are surrounded by a low-signal junctional zone, and the separation increases as the fundus is approached. With the septate uterus, only a low-intensity zone separates the cavities, and this is lost moving away from the fundus (Fig. 19-17). MRI is arguably the imaging modality of choice for the diagnosis and assessment of müllerian anomalies.[50] MRI is underutilized in gynecologic imaging.[50] The reasons include misconceptions about cost, lack of adequate training and expertise, and ignorance about the role of MRI.[51]

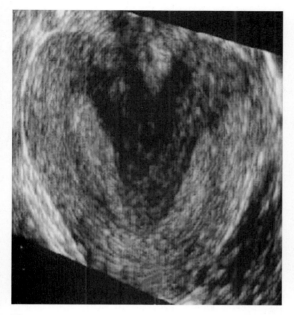

Figure 19-13 Three-dimensional sonographic image of a bicornuate uterus. There are two horns and the indentation in the uterine fundus is clearly shown. *(Courtesy Dr. Davor Jurkovic.)*

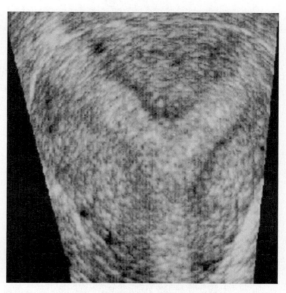

Figure 19-15 Septate uterus with a deep septum extending toward the middle of the uterine cavity. *(Courtesy Dr. Davor Jurkovic.)*

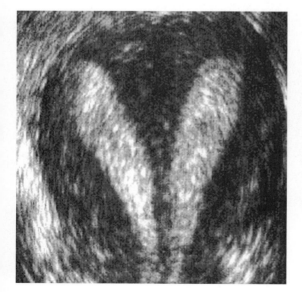

Figure 19-14 Three-dimensional sonogram of a uterus with a complete septum. *(Courtesy Dr. Davor Jurkovic.)*

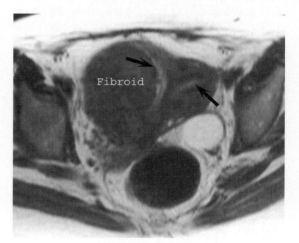

Fibroid

Figure 19-16 MRI demonstrating a septate uterus. The cavity is divided into two *(arrows)* by a thick, long septum. There is a leiomyoma on the right. The fundus is not indented, making it clear that this is not a bicornuate uterus. *(Courtesy Dr. Reena Jha.)*

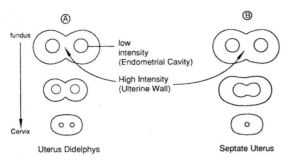

Figure 19-17 Patterns observed upon MRI of the uterus in a woman with a bicornuate uterus versus a septate uterus.

Hysteroscopy and Laparoscopy

The combination of laparoscopy and hysteroscopy is considered the gold standard for evaluation of congenital uterine malformations. Hysteroscopy allows evaluation of the uterine cavity, but it does not adequately assess the external fundal contour. To distinguish between the various uterine anomalies, simultaneous laparoscopy is required. An advantage of the hysteroscopic approach to diagnosis is the ability to simultaneously surgically correct the uterine defect. Hysteroscopy also allows the surgeon to evaluate the uterus for conditions that may appear on HSG to be congenital defects, such as intrauterine synechiae and uterine leiomyomata. Hysteroscopy, however, is associated with risks that include perforation, hemorrhage, infection, fluid overload, and electrolyte imbalance, whereas laparoscopy, apart from anesthetic risks, may result in injury to vessels or abdominal viscera.

Treatment

There is little disagreement that surgical correction is the only effective therapy for the patient with a congenital uterine anomaly. Before undertaking a surgical procedure to correct such a defect, however, there are a number of prerequisites. First, the surgeon must have a thorough understanding of the embryologic defect that resulted in the anomaly to ensure

selection of the appropriate surgical technique. Second, it is essential that all other potential causes of either infertility or recurrent pregnancy loss have been excluded. As such, assessment of male factors, endocrine function, luteal-phase function, and other anatomic factors such as the condition of the fallopian tubes must be accurate and complete. Third, thorough evaluation of the urinary tract should be performed[23] (see Fig. 19-7C). Fourth, before attempting any surgical procedure, the surgeon should discuss with the patient the potential outcome of surgical therapy compared with the results likely to occur without surgery.

In the past, it was not uncommon to treat all cases of double uterus in a similar fashion, by performing abdominal metroplasty. The different anomalies have different obstetric prognoses.[10,12,15] The septate uterus can be treated easily, effectively, and safely by hysteroscopic resection.[15,52–55] Recent advances in technology have led to improved hysteroscopic equipment, modification of the resectoscope, and the appearance of laser equipment of wavelengths that allow for operation in a liquid environment. Hysteroscopy for the septate uterus has rendered the traditional method of transabdominal metroplasty obsolete.[15] The hysteroscopic approach to septal resection avoids a laparotomy incision and reduces the potential for the formation of intraabdominal adhesions that may result in subsequent infertility or chronic pelvic pain.[15,52–55] It is also associated with shorter hospitalization time and postoperative recovery period and minimizes the risk of uterine rupture in a subsequent pregnancy.[52–55] Hysteroscopic resection is best performed with simultaneous laparoscopy; this helps to accurately differentiate between a septate and a bicornuate uterus, reduces the risk of perforation of the uterine wall and injury to adjacent structures, and allows evaluation and treatment of coexisting tubal or adnexal pathology.[15]

The term *excision* is a misnomer; all that is required is incision of the septum because spontaneous retraction normally occurs.[15,53]

The septum is visualized hysteroscopically and is incised midway between the anterior and posterior uterine walls from the cervical aspect upward. Hysteroscopic incision of the septum may be accomplished with microscissors, a resectoscope with a wire loop, or various fiberoptic laser modalities.[15,52–55] Preoperative endometrial thinning with agents such as danazol, progestins, or gonadotropin-releasing hormone (GnRH) analogues is not essential but may be of some benefit when there is a wide or complete septum.[15] The procedure is best performed in the follicular phase of the cycle when the endometrium is thin, the risk of bleeding is reduced, and visibility is best. Some surgeons advocate insertion of an intrauterine contraceptive device or an inflatable balloon following metroplasty or septal resection to separate uterine surfaces and prevent intrauterine adhesions during the healing process.[53] Vercellini and colleagues compared women who had intrauterine devices (IUDs) inserted postoperatively with women who did not and found no postoperative intrauterine adhesions in either group.[56] While it is generally recommended that patients receive postoperative treatment with estrogen to promote endometrial growth and reduce the formation of intrauterine adhesions at the site of the septal incisions, Dabirashrafi and colleagues found no benefit of such therapy.[57]

Abdominal Metroplasty

Abdominal metroplasty is performed less frequently than in the past because the septate uterus can be managed hysteroscopically. Metroplasty is reserved primarily for the woman with bicornuate or didelphic uterus, but it is rarely required. A brief description of the techniques for abdominal metroplasty follows.

For a woman with a bicornuate or didelphic uterus, the Strassman procedure is the appropriate technique.[58] It is not generally recommended that a divided cervix be unified because this may lead to incompetence. In brief, an incision is made in the fundus of the uterus between the round ligaments. The rea-

sons for a transverse incision are: (1) reduced blood loss, (2) minimal loss of tissue, (3) the resulting single cavity fully restores the normal intrauterine volume, and (4) converting the transverse incision into an anteroposterior suture line ensures that the raw surfaces of the endometrium are not approximated during healing, thus avoiding formation of intrauterine adhesions. Thereafter, the partition between the two uterine cavities is incised, creating a single space. The incision is closed in an anteroposterior direction (Fig. 19-18).

In the past, most surgeons employed either the Jones technique or the Tompkins technique for removal of an intrauterine septum. The Jones technique involves removal of a wedge of myometrium that includes the septum.[59] A wedge-shaped incision in the anteroposterior direction is made in the fundus of the uterus incorporating the septum. The wedge of tissue

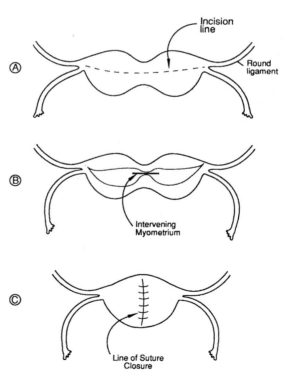

Figure 19-18 Technique for performance of the Strassman metroplasty.

is removed, and the incision is closed in layers in the same anteroposterior direction. The first layer incorporates the endometrium and is an interrupted layer. The second layer in the closure is an interrupted layer approximating the myometrium. The last layer is an inverted running stitch to approximate the serosa (Fig. 19-19).

The Tompkins technique, on the other hand, avoids the removal of any myometrium, thus theoretically retaining maximal size of the uterine cavity following surgical correction.[60] This technique is commenced by making a single anteroposterior incision in the fundus of the uterus directly over the midline septum and extending this incision through the lower extent of the septum. The septum is sharply incised on either side without removal of any tissue. The single incision is then closed in layers in a manner similar to that described for the Jones technique. It should be noted that the first layer of suture that

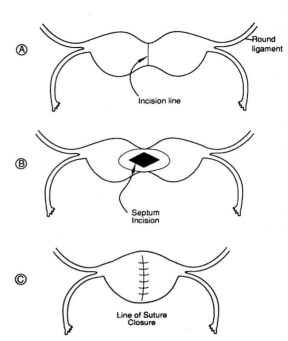

Figure 19-20 Technique for the performance of the Tompkins metroplasty.

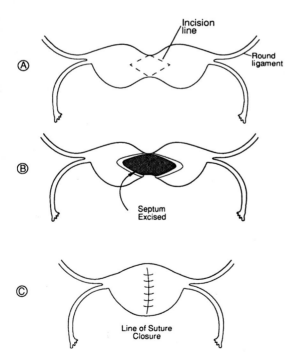

Figure 19-19 Technique for the performance of the Jones metroplasty.

incorporates the endometrium includes also the edges of the cut septum (Fig. 19-20).

The main difficulties encountered while performing abdominal metroplasty by any of the techniques are bleeding from myometrium (the septum, because of its recognizably diminished blood supply, bleeds very little) and postoperative adhesion formation. The use of a tourniquet around the lower uterine segment may temporarily reduce blood flow through the uterine fundus. In addition, injection of the site of the anticipated uterine incision with a dilute solution of Pitressin (usually 20 IU Pitressin diluted in 10 to 50 mL of normal saline) is effective in inducing vasoconstriction of the microvessels, thus reducing intraoperative blood loss. Of course, neither technique replaces good surgical hemostasis. Finally, following completion of the uterine closure, application of an adhesion barrier to the incision site may reduce the adherence of bowel and omentum to the healing uterine scar.

Surgical therapy for DES uterine defects appears to be of limited value. Attempts at enlarging the uterine cavity by "shaving" of the myometrium under hysteroscopic visualization have not met with success. However, Katz and colleagues suggest that women with a T-shaped uterus may benefit from hysteroscopic metroplasty.[61]

Pregnancy in a rudimentary horn is likely to result in rupture during pregnancy, and diagnosis of this condition prior to conception is extremely unlikely. If such a diagnosis were made, surgical extirpation of the rudimentary horn might be indicated. At the present time, surgical therapy to improve reproductive outcome or potential appears not to be effective for women with conditions that result from müllerian agenesis.

Results of Treatment

The absence of randomized, controlled trials (RCTs) of various therapeutic approaches to uterine malformation produces a number of problems in assessing the efficacy of these procedures. Most series have been retrospective and include small numbers. Furthermore, different anomalies frequently have been lumped together. Finally, few studies correct for the presence or absence of additional factors that may affect fertility or subsequent maintenance of pregnancy. Fedele found posthysteroscopic metroplasty cumulative pregnancy rates at 36 months of 89 and 80 percent for women with a complete septum and women with a partial septum, respectively.[62] The cumulative live birth rate at 36 months was 39 percent in women with infertility and 62 percent in women with miscarriages, suggesting that outcomes differ based on the indication for metroplasty.[62] Homer and colleagues summarized the results of 16 retrospective studies and found that postmetroplasty outcomes were favorable, with pregnancy rates of 80 percent and miscarriage rates of only 15 percent.[15] Rock and Jones reported the results of their extensive ex-

perience with surgical correction in women with uterine malformation. Successful pregnancy occurred in 59 percent of women with a duplicated uterus with conservative management alone.[63] On the other hand, surgical therapy improved pregnancy success rates to 71 and 81 percent, respectively, depending on whether there was an associated extrauterine abnormality.[63]

Hysteroscopically directed techniques are associated with much less perioperative morbidity and appear to provide successful pregnancy rates that are similar to those obtained following conventional surgical methods (73 to 82 percent).[15] Results with various hysteroscopic methods (laser, resectoscope, sharp incision) are similar.[15,64] Uterine rupture has been reported following hysteroscopic metroplasty[65–67] regardless of technique.

▶ ACQUIRED ABNORMALITIES

Uterine Leiomyomas

Uterine leiomyomas, or fibroids, are the most common pelvic tumors in women.[68] Their incidence varies widely depending on the method of diagnosis used. They generally are said to occur in approximately 25 percent of women of childbearing age.[68] In necropsy specimens in premenopausal women, leiomyomas were found in 77 percent.[69]

The term *fibroid* is a misnomer; these tumors are actually composed of smooth muscle. They cause compression of surrounding tissue, resulting in a pseudocapsule. Fibroids are believed to originate directly from the myometrium but also may derive from mesenchymal cells of coelomic origin. Townsend demonstrated that each of the cells that comprise a given leiomyoma is of an identical glucose-6-phosphate dehydrogenase subtype, whereas the cells of two different leiomyomas in the same woman may be of different enzyme subtypes, strongly suggesting that each leiomyoma arises from a single aberrant cell.[70]

It is generally accepted that hormones play a crucial role in the pathogenesis of uterine leiomyomas; leiomyomas tend to arise only during the reproductive years and rarely develop before puberty or after menopause. Furthermore, they may grow dramatically during pregnancy when there are elevated levels of estrogens and progesterone. Fibroids also typically regress spontaneously and progressively following natural or artificial menopause. The plasma concentrations of estradiol in women with leiomyomas are no higher than those of women without leiomyomas[71]; however, there are more estrogen receptors in the cells of leiomyomas than in normal myometrium,[72–74] and the metabolism of estradiol to estrone is greater in leiomyoma cells than in normal myometrium.[75] While there also is evidence that human growth hormone and human chorionic somatotropin act synergistically with estrogen to stimulate the growth of uterine leiomyomas in laboratory animals,[76] there are no data to support such actions of these hormones in humans. Finally, it has been proposed that growth factors may explain the various rates of growth of different leiomyomas within the uterus of a given woman.

Leiomyomas within the uterine wall are called *intramural fibroids*. *Submucosal leiomyomas* lie just below the endometrium and often protrude into the uterine cavity. Buttram has recommended use of the term *intracavitary leiomyoma* so that true submucosal fibroids may be differentiated from intramural leiomyomas that protrude into the endometrial cavity.[77] The term *subserosal leiomyoma* is used to describe one protruding on the external (serosal) surface of the uterus. Fibroids that develop a stalk are called *pedunculated fibroids*. When a pedunculated fibroid takes its blood supply from a secondary source and loses its connection with the uterus, the term *parasitic fibroid* is used. Fibroids also may arise in the cervix and the broad ligament. Fibroids vary greatly in size, ranging from seedlings to tumors that extend to the xiphisternum. We recently removed a 72-lb fibroid from a woman whose preoperative weight was 141 pounds. The largest fibroid on record weighed 63.6 kg (140.2 lb).[78]

It is estimated that between 20 and 50 percent of women will experience symptoms directly attributable to leiomyomas.[68] The severity of the symptoms appears to be related primarily to the size and location of the leiomyomas. Among the symptoms reported are menorrhagia and abnormal uterine bleeding, pelvic pain and pressure, reduced urinary bladder capacity, constipation, and reproductive dysfunction. Proposed mechanisms for abnormal uterine bleeding from leiomyomas include increased endometrial surface area, ulceration of the endometrium overlying a submucosal leiomyoma, increased uterine vascularity and blood flow, and interference with normal uterine contractility. While it is commonly taught that leiomyomas frequently are the cause of abnormal uterine bleeding, there are data in the medical literature supportive of a different view. It is true that menorrhagia may be linked frequently with the presence of leiomyomas, but in up to 48 percent of women no such bleeding is observed. One should not expect a pedunculated fundal or subserous leiomyoma to be associated with abnormal bleeding, whereas a submucous location more likely would lead to such signs. Jacobson and Enzer reported no abnormal bleeding in 41 percent of women with submucous leiomyomas.[79] Suffice it to say that the presence of leiomyomas alone is not predictive of the incidence of abnormal uterine bleeding. Furthermore, even if leiomyomas are present, a search for other causes of abnormal bleeding is prudent. Polycythemia[80,81] and a pseudo-Meigs syndrome with ascites and pleural effusion[82] have been reported in a small percentage of women with leiomyomas; the mechanisms involved remain unclear.

Infertility

Controversy continues regarding the role of uterine leiomyomas in the etiology of infertility.[83,84] If leiomyomas interfere with fertility, it is most likely by mechanical means. Perhaps by interference with sperm or ovum transport; large leiomyomas may obstruct the endocervix or tubal ostia. They also may distort pelvic anatomy sufficiently to interfere with the normal anatomic relationship between fallopian tube and ovary. Uterine contractility may be abnormal, leading to impaired gamete transport.[68,85,86] In fact, Coutinho and Maia hypothesized that the action of prostaglandins derived from seminal plasma, which induce rhythmic uterine contractions, thus facilitating transuterine sperm transport, is hampered by the presence of large uterine leiomyomas.[86] Large posterior leiomyomas may alter the normal relationship between the cervical os and the vaginal pool of semen by elevating the cervix into an anterior position behind the symphysis pubis. Finally, leiomyomas may interfere with endometrial blood supply, potentially impeding implantation.[87]

Stovall and coworkers, investigating the role of myomas on conception rates in women undergoing in vitro fertilization, found pregnancy rate of 37.4 percent compared with 52.7 percent in matched controls.[88] Significantly lower implantation and pregnancy rates in women with submucosal and intramural fibroids were reported compared with patients with subserosal or no myomas.[89] Improved conception rates have been reported following myomectomy. Vercellini and colleagues reviewed 24 trials between 1982 and 1996 and found improved success after myomectomy in 9 prospective studies of 57 percent.[90] Li and colleagues found a postmyomectomy conception rate of 57 percent, with a pregnancy loss rate of 60 percent, compared with 24 percent prior to surgery.[91] Bulletti and colleagues compared spontaneous conception in infertile women with and without myomas in whom other causes of infertility had been excluded.[92] Those who underwent laparoscopic myomectomy had higher delivery rates (42 percent) than those who did not (11 percent). Infertile women who had myomectomy had higher delivery rates

than infertile women without myomas (25 percent). Finally, Pritts, in a review of myomas and infertility, found that when women with submucosal myomas underwent myomectomy, pregnancy rates were increased compared with infertile controls [RR 1.72; 95 percent confidence interval (CI) 1.13–2.58].[84] While the results of most of these studies suggest a beneficial effect of myomectomy, they must be taken with caution because a percentage women undergoing infertility investigation will conceive spontaneously. To date, there have been no randomized, controlled studies examining the role of myomectomy in infertility.

Pregnancy Wastage

Leiomyomas are found in 1 to 4 percent of pregnancies. It is widely accepted that these tumors are associated with early pregnancy bleeding, spontaneous abortion, premature uterine contractions, preterm delivery, fibroid degeneration and pain, malpresentation, placental abruption, obstructed labor, and postpartum hemorrhage.[93–97] While the exact mechanisms by which myomas cause spontaneous abortion remain to be defined, it is likely the result of impaired endometrial function. Deligdish and Loewenthal reported atrophy of endometrial glands and stroma, presumably the result of pressure and/or diminished blood flow, overlying or opposite the leiomyoma.[86] At the margin of the leiomyoma, on the other hand, hyperplastic glands were observed, possibly secondary to increased vascularity and thus increased hormone delivery. The endometrium at distant sites appeared to function normally. Farrer-Brown and colleagues found venous dilatation in endometrium overlying as well as adjacent to leiomyoma, presumably resulting from vascular obstruction by the leiomyoma.[98] It is possible that these changes result in atrophy of the endometrium directly over submucous leiomyomas, leading to disordered placentation and early pregnancy wastage. It appears that the location of a myoma in relationship to the placenta is more important than the size of the fibroid.[95,96]

Several mechanisms have been invoked to explain the apparent increase in incidence of spontaneous pregnancy loss and uterine irritability associated with uterine leiomyomas. Spontaneous miscarriage is more likely if implantation occurs over a submucosal leiomyoma.[95,96] Multiple submucous leiomyomas may interfere with fetal enlargement or limit compliance of the uterus as it must expand to accommodate the enlarging fetus. It also has been suggested, but without scientific documentation, that inadequate blood flow to rapidly enlarging leiomyomas within the pregnant uterus results in spontaneous degeneration. The inflammatory response to degeneration is likely associated with increased eicosanoid production that results in decidual activation, myometrial contractibility, preterm labor, and abdominal pain. Whether a similar but less dramatic occurrence results in increased uterine irritability remains to be determined. Finally, uterine leiomyomas may lead to fetal malpresentation because of mechanical limitation to intrauterine change in fetal position.

Strobelt and co-workers performed sonograms every 2 to 4 weeks on pregnant women known to have fibroids before pregnancy and found that the majority of fibroids 5 cm or less in diameter could no longer be seen during pregnancy, whereas most myomas greater than 5 cm in diameter remained stable or decreased in size.[99] Multiple myomas were less likely to disappear than solitary myomas.

Diagnosis

Bimanual Examination and Sonography

The diagnosis of uterine leiomyomas is made most often by bimanual palpation, which reveals an enlarged, irregular, firm uterus. There is a strong correlation between bimanual palpation and sonography in estimation of the size of a fibroid uterus.[100] Uterine enlargement at times may be difficult to appreciate, particularly in the obese or tense patient. Also, fibroids may be impossible to distinguish from some other pelvic mass. Thus it is not unwise to perform sonography on women who have a pelvic mass suspected to be a fibroid uterus or on women in whom body habitus precludes thorough pelvic bimanual examination. Sonography is reasonably sensitive for the diagnosis of fibroids and may distinguish between a fibroid uterus and pathologic ovarian enlargement. It also allows objective assessment of fibroid growth. While sonography is relatively inexpensive, readily available, and generally easy to perform, there are limitations in its ability to accurately define the location, size, and number of leiomyomas. Any solid mass may appear to have the appearance of a leiomyoma on sonographic scanning.[101] Furthermore, determination of the exact location of a leiomyoma within the uterus may be difficult even with today's high-resolution technology. For these reasons, computed tomography (CT) scans and MRI are used in the evaluation of women suspected of having leiomyomas.[101,102]

Hysterosalpingography

HSG in the evaluation of women with uterine myomas is only of value in the investigation of infertility. If leiomyomas are large, or if multiple leiomyomas are present, one would expect to observe some distortion of the uterine cavity. While there is no argument that HSG may allow for elucidation of a submucous or pedunculated intracavitary leiomyoma, a striking relationship between preoperative distortion of the uterine cavity and subsequent postoperative outcome has not been observed.[103]

Other Sonographic Techniques

Sonohysterography allows for highly accurate detection and evaluation of submucosal leiomyomas.[104,105] Becker demonstrated that this technique yielded more information than transvaginal sonography alone.[104] This may be important in determining the appropriate surgical approach because submucosal leiomyomas are readily removed hysteroscopically. Three-dimensional sonography also has been used recently for evaluation of uterine anatomy, allowing evaluation of the relationships between myomas, myometrium, and endometrial cavity.[39] Again, this may facilitate the surgeon's selection of the most appropriate surgical approach.

Magnetic Resonance Imaging

MRI is the most precise imaging technique for demonstrating leiomyomas. It has the advantages of accurately depicting the number of leiomyomas and their exact location (Fig. 19-21), especially relative to the endometrial cavity, as well as in differentiating between leiomyomas and adenomyosis.[106,107]

Treatment

Indications

Indications for treatment of leiomyomas are listed in Table 19-4. A strong desire to retain fertility potential is the most common reason for choosing myomectomy as opposed to hys-

▶ **TABLE 19-4:** INDICATIONS FOR TREATMENT OF LEIOMYOMAS

- Severe menorrhagia
- Pelvic pressure or pain
- Hydronephrosis
- Bowel or bladder dysfunction
- Rapid growth/suspicion of malignancy
- Large size
- Recurrent miscarriage
- Infertility*

*Rarely an indication; other causes of infertility must be excluded first.

terectomy. The presence of leiomyomas alone, however, in the absence of symptoms or complaints is not an acceptable indication for surgical intervention. It was taught previously that uterine size greater than corresponding to 12 weeks of gestation alone was an indication for hysterectomy even in the absence of symptoms. This view is not widely held in contemporary gynecologic practice. A recent study, we found that women with a uterus of less than 12 weeks' size who underwent myomectomy were more likely to require further surgery than women with a uterus of 12 weeks' or greater size.[108] Several retrospective studies have suggested that fertility improves following myomectomy in infertility patients with myomas.[88–92] It is our opinion that myomectomy should be considered an appropriate therapy for fertility only in women in whom tubal occlusion is believed to be secondary to the location of the leiomyoma or as a final possibility in a woman with large (10 cm or more) leiomyomas in whom other causes of infertility have been excluded. Most important, such women should be counseled extensively regarding the relatively low rate of improvement in fertility associated with myomectomy, the risks of surgery, and the other options available in her pursuit of fertility.

Most clinicians agree that large myomas are associated with an increased incidence of early pregnancy wastage, preterm labor, and other obstetric complications. Furthermore, a review

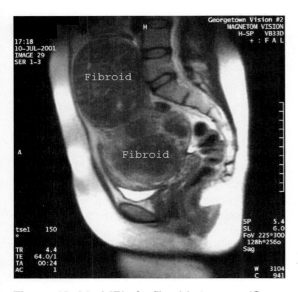

Figure 19-21   MRI of a fibroid uterus.   *(Courtesy Dr. Reena Jha.)*

of the literature is suggestive of an improvement in the rate of fetal salvage following myomectomy that varies between 4 and 47 percent.[68] It appears that improved fetal salvage following myomectomy is greatest when previous history of recurrent loss can be attributed primarily to the presence of uterine leiomyomas.

Leiomyosarcomas are rare.[109] Some pathologists feel that these malignant tumors arise de novo and not secondarily from benign leiomyomas. Parker and colleagues found that the incidence of leiomyosarcoma (0.23 percent) did not justify the concept of increased risk of uterine sarcoma in women with "rapidly growing" leiomyomas.[109] Hannigan and Gomez reported that 40 percent of patients proven histologically to have a sarcoma appeared to have a simple leiomyoma on gross inspection.[110] For this reason, if the primary indication for surgery is rapid enlargement, myomectomy may be inappropriate.

Medical Therapy

Until recently, the only options for the treatment of fibroids were surgical. Both hysterectomy and myomectomy carry significant morbidity and require inpatient hospitalization and significant recovery time. Moreover, hysterectomy removes any chance of further childbearing; myomectomy, while preserving fertility, is associated with reduced conception rates and carries the risk of uterine rupture in subsequent pregnancies. Thus a search for alternative methods of treatment is ongoing. Because uterine leiomyomas have been shown to be sensitive to hormones, most forms of medical therapy have been directed at either counteraction of the effects of estrogen or reduction in estrogen production.

Early studies suggested that treatment with progestational agents led to degeneration of uterine leiomyomas.[111] The effect of progestins was found to be unpredictable at low doses, and the side effects associated with therapy with large doses of progestins are intolerable. The recent introduction of long-acting GnRH analogues for the treatment of women with uterine leiomyomas is a significant advance. Treatment with GnRH creates a pseudomenopausal state.[112] With the withdrawal of estrogen, estrogen-dependent leiomyomas can be expected to regress.

Filicori and colleagues first reported treatment with GnRH analogues for uterine leiomyomas.[113] Subsequently, other authors found similar results.[114] Most investigators, including ourselves, have found that treatment with GnRH analogues reduces the size of uterine leiomyomas by 40 to 50 percent.[114–116] The maximal effect is achieved after 3 months of therapy. Reduction in size of both the leiomyomatous mass and the normal myometrium occurs due to reduction in cell size rather than an actual reduction in cell number.

Uterine leiomyomas begin to increase in size within 2 to 3 months following cessation of therapy with GnRH analogues. Twelve months after cessation of therapy, the leiomyomas attain a size similar to that observed prior to the commencement of therapy.[116] Until recently, GnRH analogues were used for a maximum of 6 months. For these reasons, therapy with GnRH analogues in patients with uterine leiomyomas primarily has been as an adjunct to surgical therapy. However, intermittent GnRH therapy in 6-month cycles has proven beneficial in the nonsurgical management of women with fibroids.[117] Add-back therapy with estrogen and progestin may prevent osteoporosis, allowing for longer durations of therapy.[118] GnRH analogues may have an important role in delaying the need for surgery in perimenopausal women with uterine leiomyomas in anticipation of the hypoestrogenic state expected at the time of menopause.[114,119] Treatment with these drugs also is of potential benefit in creating a state of amenorrhea in woman who develop anemia secondary to heavy and persistent uterine bleeding associated with leiomyomas.[120] This allows natural erythropoiesis sufficient time to restore a normal hemoglobin concentration prior to surgical therapy, thereby avoiding blood transfusion.[114] Finally, therapy with GnRH analogues for a few months preceding surgery may be beneficial even in the patient about to undergo hysterectomy. Such therapy may lead to a reduction of uterine volume sufficient to allow for a vaginal as opposed to an abdominal approach to hysterectomy or allow a transverse abdominal incision instead of a midline one.[114]

Because progesterone is implicated in the growth of leiomyomas, some interest has focused on therapy with the antiprogesterone mifepristone (RU-486). Murphy and colleagues studied mifepristone as a therapy for leiomyomas.[121] A recent study has indicated that mifepristone therapy in a dose of 5 to 10 mg daily leads to reduction in fibroid size as well as regression of symptoms.[122] Further studies are required. Treatment of women with leiomyomas with danazol, a synthetic androgen, also has been investigated.[123] While there was the suggestion of some benefit, this drug has considerable side effects that preclude its widespread use for this indication.

Finally, a word about the combined oral contraceptive pill (OCP) in women with leiomyomas. The OCP is not contraindicated in women with leiomyomas. Friedman and Thomas found that in most women with leiomyomas, low-dose OCPs led to reduced menstrual flow without leading to an increase in fibroid size.[124.]

Surgical Therapy

Myomectomy, surgical removal of leiomyomas, is performed primarily for women who desire further childbearing. It is a more difficult procedure than hysterectomy and is associated with greater risk of complications. It may be performed by laparotomy, laparoscopy, or under hysteroscopy. The procedure for hysteroscopic myomectomy typically is performed with the resectoscope. Pretreatment with a GnRH analogue is beneficial only if the uterine size is consistent with that of a 14- to 16-week size or greater. Myomectomy, when the uterine size is less than 14 weeks, is not significantly easier or associated with less blood loss following medical pretreatment than without pretreat-

ment. While the concept of removing fibroids laparoscopically is attractive, it is our opinion that leiomyomas that can be removed satisfactorily by this technique probably are of such a size and location as to have little clinical significance.

At laparotomy, the most important principles of multiple or single myomectomy include gentle handling of tissues, appropriate selection of incision site, and atraumatic repair to limit subsequent adhesion formation. Excessive intraoperative blood loss and postoperative adhesion formation are the principal difficulties to be avoided. Various techniques for myomectomy have been described. It is our opinion that the following technique allows the best chance of success with a minimum of complications.

Initially, it is necessary to select an appropriate site to incise the uterine serosa. An anterior incision is less likely to adhere to bowel, omentum, tubes, or ovaries than a posterior one.[125] It is important to avoid making multiple uterine incisions so as to reduce the risk of postoperative adhesion formation. As such, the uterine incision should be made in such a location as to afford removal of the maximal numbers of leiomyomas through a single incision. Prior to making the incision, the serosa and underlying leiomyomas are injected with a solution of vasopressin (20 IU Pitressin in 10 to 50 mL of normal saline) to reduce bleeding at the incision site.[126] To limit blood loss, other operators have advocated use of a Penrose drain torniquet at the level of the internal os and temporary clamping of the infundibulopelvic ligaments. A randomized, controlled trial has demonstrated that vasopressin is more effective than tourniquet in preventing blood loss.[126] The incision is made through the myometrium down to the pseudocapsule of the leiomyoma. Since the majority of blood vessels tend to be compressed to the sides of the leiomyoma, avoidance of blunt dissection reduces the amount of bleeding associated with extirpation of the leiomyoma. For these reasons, the leiomyoma is grasped with a tenaculum or Lahey thyroid clamp and elevated. The capsular tissue is thus placed under tension. Using either a contact neodymium:YAG laser, a KTP laser, an electrocautery needle, or a scalpel, a gentle, shallow incision is made across the adventitial tissue, allowing the vessels to retract under tension or with gentle pressure without cutting across the vessels themselves. Once the leiomyoma is removed, any large vessels in the resulting cavity are ligated individually. The cavity is closed in layers using an absorbable suture material, making sure not to leave potential spaces for subsequent fluid or blood collection. The serosa is closed employing a running baseball-stitch technique to invert the edges and to expose minimal suture material to the peritoneal cavity. After meticulous hemostasis is obtained, we routinely place a sheet of Interceed (Johnson & Johnson, New Brunswick, NJ), an absorbable anti-adhesion formation barrier, over the incision site.

Laparoscopic myomectomy, first described by Semm in 1979,[127] has generated considerable interest and controversy.[128] It is generally not recommended for women with three or more leiomyomas or for leiomyomas greater than 6 to 10 cm in diameter.[128] Preoperative use of GnRH analogues reduces total uterine and fibroid volume prior to surgery.[114] While one study has shown a beneficial effect on intraoperative blood loss and operative time,[129] another has indicated a detrimental effect.[130]

The technique for performing laparoscopic myomectomy follows the general principles already described. The serosa overlying the leiomyoma is injected with a dilute solution of Pitressin and then incised with an electrocautery needle, a laser, or scissors following blanching and coagulation of the surface with an endocoagulator or some other coagulation device. Excessive electrocautery may lead to necrosis, poor healing, and uterine dehiscence in subsequent pregnancy.[128] The leiomyoma is dissected free of the surrounding myometrium and removed. Small fibroids may be removed from the peritoneal cavity through the laparoscopy port. Larger leiomyomas require mor-

cellation or a posterior colpotomy for extirpation. The remaining cavity should be irrigated and any bleeding sites cauterized. The myometrium is sutured tightly closed with several layers of absorbable suture. The serosa should then be approximated with a fine absorbable suture. Needless to say, laparoscopic myomectomy should only be performed by a surgeon experienced and competent in laparoscopic suturing.[128]

Laparoscopic myolysis coagulates the blood supply to the myoma, leading to shrinkage. This is performed with electrocautery, a laser, or by cryotherapy. The procedure carries the risk of postoperative adhesions and poor uterine wall integrity. Cryomyolysis involves freezing of the leiomyomas using specialized liquid nitrogen probes; this technique remains under investigation.

Uterine Artery Embolization

The use of uterine artery embolization (UAE) in obstetrics and gynecology was first reported in 1979 when the procedure was used to control postpartum hemorrhage.[131] Subsequently, Ravina and coworkers found that UAE performed prior to myomectomy for the purpose of reduction of intraoperative blood loss led to diminution in fibroid and uterine volume and a significant improvement in symptoms.[132] Enthusiasm for the procedure has increased, and greater than 30,000 of these procedures have been performed worldwide.[133] UAE causes ischemic infarction of fibroids, while the uterus continues to receive blood supply from collateral circulation. The procedure offers the advantages of a short hospital stay, quick recovery, minimal blood loss, uterine conservation, and avoidance of general anesthesia and surgical morbidity.[134] It also may be associated with reduced overall costs when compared with hysterectomy or myomectomy.[135]

PATIENT SELECTION

The main indication for UAE is symptomatic uterine fibroids unresponsive to medical therapy in a woman who desires to preserve her uterus. UAE also may be performed on women

▶ **TABLE 19-5:** CONTRAINDICATIONS TO UTERINE ARTERY EMBOLIZATION (UAE)

- Pregnancy
- Submucous fibroids
- Desire for future fertility
- Allergy to contrast material
- Malignancy
- Unexplained abnormal bleeding
- Pelvic infection

who are poor surgical candidates. Symptoms for which UAE is performed include abnormal uterine bleeding, urinary frequency, large abdominopelvic masses, pelvic pressure, and abdominal or pelvic pain. Malignancy, endometrial hyperplasia, or pregnancy as the cause of the symptoms should be excluded. UAE generally is not recommended for submucosal fibroids because these are readily and more effectively treated by hysteroscopic resection. Because data on the safety of pregnancy following UAE are limited, a desire for future childbearing is considered by most to be a relative contraindication to UAE. Contraindications are listed in Table 19-5.

TECHNIQUE

Uterine artery embolization is performed under fluoroscopic guidance by an interventional radiologist. Unilateral or bilateral femoral artery puncture is performed. Following selective catheterization of one uterine artery, the embolizing agent is injected until flow through the uterine artery ceases. Embolization of the contralateral uterine artery is then performed. Polyvinyl alcohol (PVA) particles or tris-acryl gelatin microspheres are the most commonly used occluding agents, with typical particle sizes ranging from 300 to 710 μm. Other occluding agents include steel coils or absorbable gelatin sponges. The procedure is carried out with antibiotic coverage and usually under local or regional anesthetic.

It is usual for the patient to experience moderate to severe crampy abdominal pain following UAE. This is typically managed with intravenous patient-controlled narcotic analgesia and nonsteroidal anti-inflammatory agents. Occasionally, epidural anesthesia may be necessary. Spies and colleagues found that the degree of postprocedural pain could not be predicted based on baseline uterine or fibroid volume, nor could the severity of pain predict outcome.[136] Most patients are admitted for 24 hours after UAE.

RESULTS

UAE generally has been associated with favorable results[138–140] (Table 19-6). The mean

▶ **TABLE 19-6:** RESULTS OF UTERINE ARTERY EMBOLIZATION FOR LEIOMYOMAS

Investigator	Number	Improvement in Bleeding	Improvement in Other Symptoms	Mean % Reduction in Dominant Fibroid Volume	Mean % Reduction in Uterine Volume	Percent Patient Satisfaction
Walker & Pelage[138]	400	84%	79%	64 67 (median)	53 54 (median)	97
Spies et al.[139]	200	90%	91%	58	38	92
Pron et al.[137]	538	83%	77/86%	33 42 (median)	27 35 (median)	91
Ravina et al.[140]	286	86%	N/A	60%	N/A	N/A

reported improvement in symptoms is 87 percent, with a mean reduction in fibroid volume of 46 percent. Satisfaction rates are high. In a randomized, controlled study comparing UAE with hysterectomy for the management of women with fibroids and abnormal uterine bleeding, Pinto and colleagues reported 86 percent clinical success with UAE and a mean hospital stay 4.14 days.[141] Ten percent of UAE patients had mild complications compared with 20 percent of those who had a hysterectomy. It has been concluded that UAE is a safe and effective alternative to hysterectomy. Broder and colleagues, comparing long-term outcomes following UAE with abdominal myomectomy, found similar satisfaction rates and high success rates with both procedures.[142] Women who underwent UAE were more likely to have further invasive management for their fibroids.

COMPLICATIONS

Complications of UAE are listed in Table 19-7; major complications are rare. Spies and coworkers, reporting on 400 cases, found a serious complication rate of 1.25 percent.[143] There have been two reported deaths following UAE, one due to sepsis and multiorgan failure and the other due to pulmonary embolism. Postembolization syndrome occurs in approximately 15 percent of women undergoing the procedure and consists of fever, pain, and leukocytosis.

PREGNANCY AFTER UAE

Goldberg and colleagues reviewed the world literature on outcomes of pregnancies following UAE in the treatment of uterine fibroids and found increased rates of spontaneous abortion, malpresentation, premature delivery, cesarean delivery, and postpartum hemorrhage among these women.[150] Concerns remain about the risk of uterine rupture, placental insufficiency, and placenta accreta.

CAUSES OF FAILURE

Spies reviewed causes of failure of UAE.[151] These were (1) failure of the operator to suc-

▶ **TABLE 19-7:** COMPLICATIONS OF UTERINE ARTERY EMBOLIZATION

- Pain
- Postembolization syndrome
- Infection/sepsis
- Infarction of nontarget organs[148]
- Allergic/anaphylactic reactions to contrast material
- Contrast-induced renal failure
- Arterial perforation
- Fibroid sloughing/prolapse through cervix
- Endometritis
- Total uterine necrosis[147]
- Premature ovarian failure[145]
- Sexual dysfunction/anorgasmia
- Groin hematoma
- Bowel obstruction[146]
- Arterial thrombosis
- Pulmonary embolism
- Death (4 cases reported)

cessfully catheterize one or both uterine arteries, (2) collateral circulation to the fibroid, (3) clumping of the occluding agent, leading to a false impression of successful embolization, and (4) spasm of the uterine arteries, causing delivery of less than optimal amounts of the embolic agent.

Asherman Syndrome

Fritsch in 1894 first described intrauterine adhesions in a woman who developed amenorrhea following postpartum curettage.[152] Subsequently, in 1948, Asherman published his classic article in which he described eight cases of intrauterine adhesions; the condition came to bear his name.[153] Intrauterine adhesions most frequently follow vigorous postpartum curettage of the uterine cavity that results in partial or total removal of endometrium and exposure of the underlying myometrium.[154,155] In the healing process, the anterior and posterior walls of the uterus become adherent to each other, leading to partial or total obliteration of the uterine cavity with resulting amenorrhea or reduced menstrual flow. Concomitant infection may be implicated. Asherman syndrome (amenorrhea traumatica) also may develop following curettage for an incomplete abortion or following myomectomy or hysteroscopic surgery.[155] The condition has been observed with some frequency in countries with a high incidence of endometrial tuberculosis.[152]

Diagnosis

The diagnosis of intrauterine adhesions is suggested by amenorrhea or hypomenorrhea that follows postpartum or postabortal dilatation and curettage. Because the ovaries are unaffected, hormonal parameters are normal, and cyclic ovulation occurs. Thus patients frequently continue to experience cyclic somatic symptoms and premenstrual molimina associated with normal ovarian function. The diagnosis can be confirmed by HSG or hysteroscopy.[152] Sonography and hysterosonography do not appear to be reliable techniques for evaluation of the uterus for intrauterine adhesions. HSG can be accomplished usually even if the adhesions extend to the internal cervical os (Fig. 19-22). Once the uterus is sounded, instillation of contrast material outlines filling defects within the uterine cavity. The defects may be minimal or extensive and result in failure to demonstrate tubal patency. Hysteroscopic evaluation frequently is more accurate than radio-graphic studies, especially when the degree of intrauterine adhesion formation is minimal and involves only the lateral aspects of the uterine cavity or the lower uterine segment. MRI has been proposed as a method of diagnosing the condition but is expensive and is no more accurate than hysteroscopy.[152]

Treatment

Prior to the advent of hysteroscopic surgery, blind endometrial curettage followed by insertion of an intrauterine device to separate opposing intrauterine surfaces was the standard therapy.[152] Hysteroscopic lysis of adhesions is the treatment of choice for women with intrauterine adhesions.[152,154,156] Adhesiolysis can

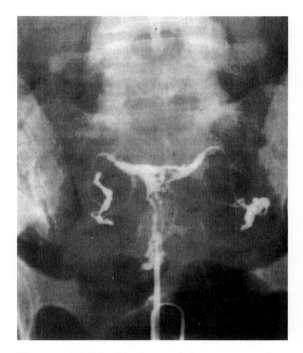

Figure 19-22 Hysterosalpingogram of a woman with Asherman syndrome. *(Courtesy Dr. S. Karasick.)*

be accomplished employing a variety of flexible or rigid scissors, a resectoscope, electrosurgery, or laser. Following the procedure, an intrauterine device or a small balloon catheter should be inserted into the uterine cavity to ensure separation of the opposing walls. In addition, the patient should be treated with estrogen to stimulate endometrial reepithelialization.[152]

Results of Treatment

Uterine curettage is somewhat effective. Most patients experience resumption of menses, and over 90 percent demonstrate restoration of the uterine cavity on the basis of subsequent HSG. Subsequent pregnancy rates are 20 to 25 percent. Using a hysteroscopic approach, on the other hand, pregnancy rates of 40 to 70 percent have been achieved.[152] Subsequent pregnancies should be monitored closely for evidence of abnormal placentation, intrauterine growth restriction, and uteroplacental insufficiency.

Uterine Infection

Under ordinary circumstances, the endometrium and uterine cavity are sterile. Following childbirth, spontaneous or therapeutic abortion, or surgical invasion of the endometrial cavity, endometritis may occur as a result of inoculation of bacteria into the cavity. Ascending infection from the cervix with organisms such as *Neisseria gonorrhoeae* and *Actinomyces israelii* also can result in endometritis. Actinomyctic colonization of the endometrium is not uncommon, occurring in 3 percent of women with intrauterine contraceptive devices.[157]

More indolent infection with *Chlamydia trachomatis* also has been recognized as a potential cause of infertility because this pathogen may alter endometrial function and result in tubal occlusion or peritubal adhesion formation. If an acute endometrial infection is suspected, appropriate cultures should be taken and therapy with appropriate broad-spectrum antibiotics commenced. Chronic endometritis is a subject of very limited discussion in the medical literature but one of potential significance in the woman who presents with a complaint of infertility. The most common cause of chronic endometrial infection is tuberculosis, which is rare in developed countries. In underdeveloped countries, the incidence of pelvic tuberculosis is much higher. Indeed, in India, tuberculosis is involved in nearly 15 percent of women with a complaint of primary amenorrhea.

If nontuberculous chronic endometritis is suspected, cultures should be obtained, and broad-spectrum antibiotics should be administered. After antibiotic therapy has been instituted, a gentle uterine curettage may be effective in eliminating the bulk of the infected endometrium. Care should be taken not to curette the endometrial cavity too vigorously to prevent the development of intrauterine adhesions. Thereafter, treatment with estrogen (conjugated estrogen, 2.5 to 10 mg orally daily, or the equivalent) is recommended for 1 to 2 months to induce regeneration of healthy endometrium. Although most cases of actinomycotic colonization of the endometrium associated with IUDs are asymptomatic, severe infections have been reported. Therefore, it may be wise to remove the IUD and treat the patient.

Adenomyosis

Bird defined *adenomyosis* as "the benign invasion of endometrium into the myometrium, producing a diffusely enlarged uterus which microscopically exhibits ectopic, non-neoplastic endometrial glands and stroma surrounded by hypertrophic and hyperplastic myometrium."[158] While the condition shares some similarity in symptomatology with endometriosis (lower abdominal pain, dysmenorrhea, and dyspareunia), it is clear that the two are very different conditions that are found in the same patient only 20 percent or less of the time.[159] Adenomyosis is derived from aberrant endometrial glands that arise in the basalis layer of the endometrium. As a consequence of the abnormal nature of these glands, the normal proliferative and secretory changes associated with the cyclic ovarian hormone production are not observed in adenomyosis. The pathogenesis and true incidence of adenomyosis remain unknown. It is generally believed that this condition occurs most frequently in older and multiparous women, implicating parturition in its etiology.[160] Adenomyosis is diagnosed as an incidental finding by the pathologist during histologic examination of the hysterectomy specimen.[160] Older women have hysterectomies performed with greater frequency. Most studies reporting the incidence of adenomyosis on hysterectomy specimens do not correct for the numbers of hysterectomies performed in each age group.[160] When 200 consecutive hysterectomy specimens were examined, adenomyosis was found in 31 percent.[158] When further blocks of tissue were examined, 61 further cases were found, raising the incidence to 61.5 percent. Adenomyosis has been found in 50 to 53.7 percent of cadavers.[160]

It has been suggested that adenomyosis results from the expansion of spaces between myometrial fibers and resulting insinuation or trapping of endometrial elements during parturition. Serial histologic specimens confirm continuity between glandular elements of adenomyosis and the basal layer of the endometrium. Thus adenomyosis is the result of direct extension of the endometrium. For an unknown reason, there is disruption of the endometrial-myometrial interface.[161] This disruption may be related to pregnancy termination.[162] At first, the stromal elements and then the glandular gradually grow into the myometrium. Elevated concentrations of estrogen stimulate growth of the basal layer of endometrium along the planes of least resistance, which commonly follow alongside lymphatic and vascular channels. The most common histologic pattern is a diffuse one that involves both the anterior and posterior walls of the uterus. Occasionally, it is possible also to observe a more localized form of the disease, an adenomyoma, often mistaken for a leiomyoma, in which the areas of ectopic endometrium may be encapsulated.[158]

Most women with adenomyosis are asymptomatic or experience only minor symptoms that do not lead to evaluation. Women with symptomatic adenomyosis are typically in their forties and present with heavy, painful periods. Examination reveals a symmetrically enlarged, boggy, tender uterus. These findings are especially pronounced immediately prior to the onset of menses. Most patients attribute the increase in dysmenorrhea and menstrual flow to the aging process.

Some imaging techniques are useful occasionally in the detection of adenomyosis. HSG may detect a pattern of "spiculation" at the interface of dye and endometrium suggestive of adenomyosis.[163] In addition, "lollipop" diverticuli (collections of dye separated by radiolucency from the endometrial cavity) also have been described.[164] Transvaginal sonography is a useful tool providing that the adenomyosis is significant enough to result in the development of anechoic areas in the myometrium.[165] At present, MRI is the diagnostic modality of choice.[166] MRI is as accurate as surgery in making the diagnosis and may distinguish leiomyomas from adenomyosis.[166]

As mentioned previously, it is unusual for the endometrial glands and stroma of adenomyosis to undergo the cyclic changes of the normal endometrium. Indeed, it has even been suggested that there is a relative deficiency of progesterone and estrogen receptors in the adenomyomatous cells compared with endometrial cells. This deficiency may explain the apparent diminished response of this tissue to ovarian hormones, as well as to exogenous hormonal therapy. The standard criterion for the diagnosis of adenomyosis on the basis of histologic examination is the demonstration of endometrial glands and stroma more than one low-power field (2.5 mm) from the basalis layer of the endometrium. The glands exhibit an inactive or proliferative pattern, although cystic hyperplasia and a secretory pattern have been described. Interestingly, the presence of endometrial tissue appears to have a mitogenic action on the surrounding myometrium because there is often associated hyperplasia and hypertrophy of individual muscle fibers adjacent to the adenomyosis implants.

Treatment

The definitive treatment for adenomyosis is hysterectomy. The condition can only be diagnosed accurately by pathologic examination of the surgically removed uterus. Various other therapies have been attempted with very limited success. Prostaglandin synthetase inhibitors may lead to reduced symptoms of pain and bleeding, especially if therapy is commenced 1 to 2 days before the expected onset of menses. IUDs containing danazol[167] and levonorgestrel[168] have been used with moderate success. Experiments on the mouse model suggest that bromocriptine[169] and RU-486, an antiprogestational agent,[170] may have a suppressive effect on adenomyosis. Hormonal manipulation has not met with success, although the use of progestin-dominant oral contraceptives or cyclic administration of strong progestins with the intent of suppressing pituitary function and thus limiting ovarian estrogen production has had limited benefit. Several investigators have suggested GnRH agonists as a means of reducing estrogenic stimulation.[171] On the other hand, our experience with this form of therapy has not been overly positive. It may be that the relative lack of ability of the adenomyosis cells to respond to hormones limits the usefulness of these forms of therapy. For these reasons, hysterectomy is the most successful form of therapy. It should be emphasized, however, that the accuracy of making the diagnosis of adenomyosis prior to hysterectomy depends in large part on the index of suspicion of the clinician. Other potential causes of the symptoms should be eliminated preoperatively.

▶ ABNORMAL UTERINE BLEEDING (AUB)

In the woman of reproductive age, abnormal bleeding may be anovulatory or ovulatory. In most cases of anovulatory bleeding, the causes are hormonal, whereas most cases of abnormal bleeding in ovulatory women have an organic etiology. It is important to distinguish between the two because their management differs significantly.

Anovulatory Abnormal Uterine Bleeding

Failure of ovulation, from whatever cause, leads to disruption in the normal pattern of uterine bleeding. If estrogen action is unopposed or fails to be interrupted by the action of progesterone, endometrial growth continues unabated and results in endometrial hyperplasia, irregular shedding, and AUB.[172] Anovulation occurs most commonly at the extremes of reproductive life. Common causes in women of reproductive age include polycystic ovarian disease, hyperprolactinemia, stress, thyroid dysfunction, and weight loss.

Diagnosis

A history of regular, cyclic, and predictable menstrual periods makes a diagnosis of anovulation unlikely. Laboratory and imaging investigations may be necessary to determine the cause of anovulation; endometrial sampling may be indicated to eliminate the possibility of an endometrial malignancy. It should be emphasized that endometrial curettage is, under these circumstances, a diagnostic rather than a therapeutic procedure.

Treatment

Intermittent treatment with oral progestins such as medroxyprogesterone acetate, 5 to 10 mg/d for 5 to 10 days per month, or norethindrone acetate, 5 mg/d for 5 to 10 days per month, or cyclic combined oral contraceptives will result in orderly endometrial sloughing and restoration of regular menstrual bleeding. Occasionally, the anovulatory woman fails to produce adequate quantities of estrogen to maintain endometrial integrity. This results in endometrial atrophy and may lead to AUB. A search for an endocrine etiology for anovulation should be conducted. Histologic examination of the endometrium is likely to reveal endometrial atrophy. In such women, intermittent treatment with progestin only leads to exacerbation of the atrophic changes and likely will result in increased rather than decreased uterine bleeding. These women may be treated with cyclic oral contraceptives or with oral estrogen (conjugated estrogen, 0.625 to 1.25 mg or the equivalent daily) and progestin (medroxyprogesterone acetate, 5 to 10 mg or the equivalent daily) in a sequential manner. Such regimens will result in regular endometrial sloughing and eliminate AUB.

Abnormal Uterine Bleeding in the Ovulatory Woman

AUB in ovulatory women usually results from an organic lesion within the endometrial cavity. These include submucosal leiomyomas, polyps, neoplasia, and adenomyosis. Without treatment of the lesion, hormonal therapy is likely to be of temporary benfit. When abnormal bleeding recurs despite hormonal therapy, a search for an organic lesion should be undertaken.

Diagnosis

Sonography, HSG, and hysteroscopy are useful tools. Dilation and curettage as a rule should be performed with simultaneous hysteroscopy because lesions such as polyps otherwise may go undetected. Sonohysterography will aid in detecting intracavitary lesions such as submucosal leiomyomas and polyps. HSG may reveal an intrauterine "filling defect" but is less useful in differentiating between a polyp, carcinoma, or a submucosal leiomyoma.

Hysteroscopy

Hysteroscopy, which allows for direct visualization of the uterine cavity, is the ideal technique for evaluation of intrauterine pathology.[173] Operative hysteroscopy also allows the opportunity for simultaneous therapeutic management. Diagnostic hysteroscopy may be performed as an outpatient procedure under suitable analgesia with or without light anesthesia and is an effective and accurate technique in identifying a causes of abnormal bleeding. Therapeutic hysteroscopy is usually performed employing a liquid medium for distension of the endometrial cavity. Carbon dioxide as a distension medium has limited use for therapeutic hysteroscopy because even a small amount of intrauterine bleeding will very quickly obscure the operative field.

The technique for hysteroscopy varies, depending on the operator's experience. Briefly, under general anesthesia or with the combined use of intravenous analgesia and local anesthesia, the cervix is dilated sufficiently to accommodate an operating hysteroscope. Following introduction of the distension medium, visualization of the entire endometrial cavity is carried out, and the offending lesion is removed.

Lesions Found on Hysteroscopy

1. *Endometrial polyps.* The incidence of endometrial polyps varies from 9 to 40 percent. Usually benign, polyps may be single or multiple and can appear at virtually any age after puberty. The tissue type may vary from adenomatous to adenomyomatous, fibrous, or telangiectasic. In the postmenopausal woman, 15 percent of endometrial polyps are cancerous.[174] Telangectasia in an endometrial polyp is a rare occurrence. Polypectomy may be performed by grasping the individual polyp at the base with a pair of rigid or flexible scissors or biopsy forceps, thereafter excising the polyp by pulling it loose from its attachment.

2. *Submucosal leiomyomas.* Submucous myomas may cause intermenstrual spotting or bleeding as a result of ulceration or poor vascularization of the overlying endometrial layer. Leiomyomas <3 cm in size may be treated by sharp dissection with scissors, a wire loop of a resectoscope, or a fibreoptic laser, all with good success.[175–177] If depth of penetration of the leiomyoma into the myometrium is questionable, it may be appropriate to perform hysteroscopic resection under laparoscopic control to avoid inadvertent myometrial perforation and injury to intraabdominal structures. When a larger leiomyoma is visualized, it is preferable to employ a urologic resectoscope with its heavier wire loop. This technique involves the curettage of fragments from the central portion of the leiomyoma. As this is accomplished, the natural tendency of normal myometrium to contract will cause the remaining myomatous tissue to bulge into the uterine cavity. In this way, the leiomyoma can be shaved down to the pseudocapsule. Large tumors can take a considerable amount of

time to remove in this manner, with the risk of fluid overload. When resecting large leiomyomas, concomitant laparoscopy may be prudent.

3. *Carcinoma*. Rarely, carcinoma may be found on hysteroscpy in a woman of reproductive age. Most commonly, this is in a woman on unopposed estrogen therapy. Discussion of endometrial carcinoma is beyond the scope of this chapter.

Medical Treatment of Ovulatory Abnormal Uterine Bleeding

Various therapies have been used for treating women with menorrhagia. The combined oral contraceptive pill, primarily by the effect of progestins on the endometrium, may reduce menstrual flow by as much as 50 percent. The antifibrinolytic tranexamic acid has been used widely in Europe. A Cochrane meta-analysis shows this is an effective therapy for heavy menstrual bleeding.[178] Nonsteroidal antiinflammatory drugs act by inhibition of the prosta-glandin pathway and significantly reduce menstrual flow.[179] Finally, the levonorgestrel-containing intrauterine system Mirena™, presumably by its effect on the endometrium, reduces menstrual flow by up to 90 percent.[180] Comparison with endometrial ablation reveals similar rates of reduction in menstrual flow and patient satisfaction.[180]

Endometrial Ablation

The quest for less invasive alternatives to hysterectomy in women in whom no uterine pathology is found has led to the development of several therapeutic modalities. In the past, most of these were based on the observation that Asherman syndrome frequently resulted in amenorrhea. Thus procedures and techniques were developed with the goal of artificially inducing Asherman syndrome. These included the introduction of such chemicals as paraformaldehyde, methylcyanacrylate, ocalic acid, and quinacrine into the uterine cavity. Other therapies employed were intracavitary insertion of radium, direct application of superheated steam, and cryocoagulation. Needless to say, all these carried considerable risks and side effects, and most met only limited success.

In 1981, Goldrath and colleagues first described hysteroscopic photovaporization of the endometrium using the neodymium-YAG laser.[181] Shortly thereafter, the urologic resectoscope was modified and used to perform transcervical resection of the endometrium (TCRE).[182] In 1989, Vancaille reported rollerball electrosurgical ablation of the endometrium.[183] Since then, TCRE has become widely used for AUB. Compared with hysterectomy, these techniques aim at reduced operative morbidity, shorter hospitalization and recovery time, and reduced costs to hospital and society.

Technique

These procedures are performed hysteroscopically under general or regional anesthesia. A nonionic, low-viscosity fluid is used for uterine distension. Pretreatment with an endometrial thinning agent such as danazol (800 mg/d) or a GnRH agonist is effective in inducing endometrial atrophy resulting in easier, more efficient, and more effective surgery and improved short-term success rates.[184] The goal is to vaporize the endometrium to a depth of 0.2 to 0.4 cm, a depth sufficient to eliminate the regenerative layer of basal endometrium. Prior to the procedure, endometrial hyperplasia or neoplasia must be excluded as the cause of the abnormal bleeding.

Results

About 50 percent of women will experience amenorrhea following endometrial ablation. Of the 50 percent who continue to have menses, about half experience hypomenorrhea and only half continue to have regular menses. A meta-analysis comparing endometrial ablation and resection with hysterectomy found reduced operative morbidity and shorter hospitalization and recovery time with the ablation techniques.[185] Patients undergoing hysterectomy reported greater satisfaction and improvement in symptoms. Women who underwent ablation were more likely to require further surgical procedures for their symptoms.

Complications

The MISTLETOE study, a prospective study of 10,686 women in the United Kingdom, studied the frequency of complications of endometrial resection and ablation.[186] There was low morbidity, with early and late complication rates of 0.77 to 1.51 and 1.25 to 4.58 percent, respectively. Two directly related deaths were reported. There was a lower incidence of complications with laser and rollerball ablations than with TCRE. Preoperative use of endometrial thinning agents was not associated with fewer complications. Procedures performed on fibroid uteri were more likely to result in hemorrhage. Uterine perforation was less likely to complicate surgery performed by more experienced operators, but operator experience had no impact on the incidence of operative hemorrhage. Other complications are listed in Table 19-8. Fluid overload, the most common intraoperative complication, can be prevented by meticulous attention to input and output of the distension medium. Immediate postoperative bleeding results from unroofing of venous sinuses and may be managed by inserting a Foley catheter with a 30-mL balloon within the uterine cavity. The balloon should be inflated just until bleeding stops and may be left in

▶ **TABLE 19-8:** COMPLICATIONS OF ENDOMETRIAL ABLATION

- Fluid overload
- Uterine perforation
- Hemorrhage
- Infection
- Fluid embolism
- Gas embolism
- Thermal injury to adjacent viscera
- Hematometrium

place for 6 to 24 h. Necrosis involving the primary uterine vessels may result in profound delayed bleeding necessitating hysterectomy. Because the cervical branch of the uterine artery enters the uterus approximately 4 cm from the external os, it is recommended that endometrial ablation should not be carried down the lower uterine segment below this point.

Long-Term Complications

Occasionally, remaining isolated pockets of active endometrium have resulted in hematometrium. Rarely, the development of adenocarcinoma in the remaining endometrium has been reported.[187] Of concern is the possibility that malignancy may go undetected because of lack of subsequent uterine bleeding. Pregnancy after endometrial ablation has been described.[188] There is considerable risk of placenta accreta, uteroplacental insufficiency, and uterine rupture.[188]

Second-Generation Procedures

The techniques of TCRE and ablation are a viable, effective, and less invasive alternative to hysterectomy.[185] However, these procedures usually require general anesthetia and some skill in hysteroscopy. To overcome these limitations, several new techniques for endometrial destruction have been developed.[189,190] These techniques aim at minimal demands on operator skill and training, reduced operating time, and reduced complications. Generally, they can be performed under local anesthesia in an outpatient setting.

The Hydro ThermAblator (HTA)™

The Hydro ThermAblator (HTA; Boston Scientific Corporation, Teterboro, NJ) uses normal saline heated to 90°C to produce endomyotrial necrosis to a depth of 2 to 4 mm.[190] The system consists of a control unit with a microprocessor that controls the temperature, inflow, and outflow. A sheathed 3-mm hysteroscope is inserted through the cervix into the uterus, and the heated saline is circulated in the uterine cavity for 10 minutes. Intrauterine pressure is maintained between 35 and 50 mmHg. According to the manufacturer, this prevents leakage of the heated fluid through the fallopian tubes into the peritoneal cavity because leakage requires an intrauterine pressure in excess of 70 mmHg. A 1-minute cooling cycle precedes withdrawal of the hysteroscope. Following this therapy, amenorrhea was reported in 46 percent, hypomenorrhea in 16 percent, eumenorrhea in 16 percent, and no change in 22 percent of women at 6 months of follow-up.[190]

The Novasure Impedance-Controlled Endometrial Ablation System™

The Novasure device (Novacept, Palo Alto, CA), according to the manufacturer, requires only 90 seconds to completely destroy the endometrium; hysteroscopy is unnecessary. The procedure can be performed at any time in the menstrual cycle and does not need endometrial pretreatment.[191] The device uses bipolar energy, which is dispersed via a gold-plated, porous, disposable metallic mesh that expands into a fan shape to conform to the uterine cavity. A tabletop power generator and microprocessor control the treatment cycle. The radiofrequency generator delivers power up to 180 W at 500 kHz; the technique produces tissue desiccation to a depth of 4.0 to 4.5 mm and 2.0 to 2.9 mm in the uterine body and cornual region, respectively. Prior to activating the device, the uterine cavity is measured, and the uterine length and width are keyed into the controller, which then calculates the optimal power output necessary to ablate the endometrium. The device is designed to check uterine wall integrity prior to its activation, thereby detecting any uterine perforation. Contraindications include submucosal fibroids and uteruses less than 4 cm or greater than 10 cm in length. The amenorrhea rate at 12 months is 36 percent, with a 91 percent success rate.[191]

The Thermachoice Uterine Balloon Therapy System™

The Thermachoice™ balloon (Gynecare, Inc, Somerville, NJ, an Ethicon company) uses a soft silicone balloon that is inserted through the cervix into the uterine cavity.[192,193] The balloon is attached to a control unit, which displays the temperature of the fluid, the intrauterine pressure, and the treatment time. Sterile fluid (5% dextrose) heated to 87°C is circulated through the balloon for 8 minutes at pressures between 160 and 180 mmHg. The balloon expands, conforming to the uterine cavity. When the treatment cycle is completed, the balloon is deflated and removed from the uterine cavity. The treated uterine lining sloughs off over the next 7 to 10 days. Results are similar to those achieved with rollerball ablation. A similar device, the Cavaterm system, is available in Europe. Short-term results achieved with this system are similar to those following Nd:YAG laser endometrial ablation.[194]

The Her Option™ Uterine Cryoablation Therapy System

The Her Option™ device (CryoGen, Inc., San Diego, CA) destroys the endometrium by application of extreme cold and produces 9 to 12 mm of tissue destruction.[195] The device uses a proprietary compressed-gas mixture to generate temperatures of less than −100°C. A 5.5-mm "cryoprobe" is inserted into the uterus, requiring little or no cervical dilation; only the tip of the probe gets cold. A disposable sheath with a metallic tip to facilitate thermal conduction covers the probe. The cryoprobe is attached to a portable console that contains a compact compressor. Sonographic monitoring is essential to provide a safe area between the "cryozone" and the serosal surface of the uterus. This technique has the disadvantage of requiring sonography.

The Radiofrequency Thermal Balloon

The radiofrequency balloon is not currently available in the United States. This device consists of an expandable Silastic balloon with 12 electrodes mounted on its surface.[190] The balloon is inflated with 10 to 15 mL of air to bring the electrodes into contact with the endometrial surface. Radiofrequency heats these electrodes to a surface temperature of 70 to 75°C, with a slightly lower temperature in the cornual region in order to avoid extrauterine thermal injury. The cervix must be dilated prior to the procedure. The treatment cycle lasts 4 minutes. Data submitted to the FDA indicate a 40 percent 3- and 6-month postablation amenorrhea rate for this device.

Microwave Endometrial Ablation

The Microwave Endometrial Ablation™ (MEA) device (Microsulis Americas, Boca Raton, FL) has been used extensively in Europe and was introduced in the United States in 2003.[196] This device uses microwave energy at a frequency of 9.2 GHz to produce tissue desiccation to a depth of 6 mm. The MEA applicator is a one-piece reusable instrument that is inserted through the cervix into the uterine cavity until its tip reaches the fundus. The surgeon uses a foot switch to control power to the applicator. Microwave energy emanates semiradially from the applicator tip and is absorbed by the surrounding endometrial tissue. The control unit displays the treatment temperature. The applicator is moved slowly from side to side in the fundal area until intrauterine temperature reaches 70 to 80°C. Treatment is continued with side-to-side movements while the surgeon withdraws the applicator from the uterine cavity, all the while maintaining the treatment temperature. The treatment cycle averages 3 minutes for anormal-sized uterus. When the applicator tip reaches the cervix, the microwave energy is deactivated and the applicator is fully withdrawn. Success rates are similar to those achieved with TCRE, although in one study patient satisfaction with microwave endometrial ablation was slightly higher (79 percent) than that following TCRE (67 percent).[197]

Laser Interstitial Hyperthermy

This device (Gynelase, ESC Medical Systems, Norwood, MA) uses Nd:YAG laser energy to achieve global endometrial ablation [endometrial laser intrauterine thermal therapy (ELITT)].[190] The device uses a three-fiber instrument that, when introduced into the uterus, develops a triangular configuration conforming to the uterine cavity. Hysteroscopy is not required. The treatment destroys the entire endometrium and an additional 10 to 35 mm of adjacent myometrium. Treatment time is 5 to 7 min. Amenorrhea rates at 1-year follow-up were 71 percent. The device is currently not available in the United States.

Comparison of Results of First- and Second-Generation Endometrial Ablation Techniques

A Cochrane database meta-analysis comparing these so-called second-generation ablation techniques with the first-generation techniques of TCRE and ablation found that second-generation techniques were as effective in reducing heavy menstrual flow as first-generation methods.[189] Second-generation techniques took less time to perform and were more likely to be performed under local anesthesia. The second-generation techniques were associated more often with equipment failure.

▶ SUMMARY

Diseases of the uterus not infrequently lead women to seek gynecologic care. This chapter provides a review of developmental processes that give rise to the normal and abnormal uterus. Contemporary methods of diagnosis, investigation, and management of uterine diseases have been presented. Exciting advances in technology have made possible effective nonsurgical and minimally invasive therapies for most uterine disorders. The restoration or preservation of fertility is the goal of therapy in most women of childbearing age. It is hoped that the information presented in this chapter will prove to be of significant value to the clinician in caring for women.

KEY POINTS

1. The most common malformations of the female reproductive system are congenital abnormalities of the uterus that result from arrested or defective development of the müllerian duct.

2. MRI appears to be the imaging modality of choice for the diagnosis and assessment of müllerian anomalies because it allows for accurate distinction between septate and bicornuate uterus while simultaneously allowing for evaluation of the urinary tract.

3. The presence of a uterine septum has been associated with increased risk of spontaneous miscarriage as well as fetal malpresentation. Surgical correction of the uterine septum, most appropriately accomplished by hysteroscopic incision, is indicated, however, only when there is evidence of pregnancy wastage rather than when the abnormality is identified in an asymptomatic woman or a woman without a history of previous pregnancy loss.

4. Abdominal metroplasty is rarely indicated because uterine septa can be managed by the hysteroscopic approach. When a bicornuate uterus is identified and thought to be causative in previous pregnancy loss or premature delivery, the Strassman procedure is the appropriate technique.

5. Between 20 and 50 percent of women will experience symptoms related to uterine leiomyomas, and the severity of symptoms appears to be related primarily to size and location. Whereas leiomyomas have been associated with abnormal uterine bleed-

ing, pelvic pressure, symptoms related to compression of pelvic organs, and early pregnancy loss, these tumors are infrequently related directly to infertility.

6. Myomectomy appears to improve pregnancy rates and reduce pregnancy loss when the leiomyomas are located submucosally. Myomectomy performed for removal of tumors located at sites other than submucosal remains controversial because there are no randomized, prospective, controlled trials that demonstrate significant improvement in fertility or pregnancy outcomes following myomectomy.

7. MRI is the most precise imaging technique for demonstrating size and location of uterine leiomyomas.

8. Leiomyosarcomas are rare tumors that arise de novo rather than following malignant degeneration of leiomyomas, and many leiomyosarcomas have the appearance of a benign tumor on gross inspection.

9. Many medications such as GnRH agonists and the antiprogesterone mifepristone have been used successfully for the medical management of uterine leiomyomas. Oral contraceptives, long said to mimic pregnancy, are not contraindicated in women with uterine leiomyomas.

10. Uterine artery embolization is recognized as an appropriate technique for the management of women with uterine leiomyomas who are desirous of uterine preservation and for women who are believed to be poor surgical candidates. The impact of uterine artery embolization, however, on subsequent pregnancies has not been studied prospectively, and desire for future pregnancy should remain a relative contraindication to this procedure.

11. Hysteroscopic lysis of adhesions is the treatment of choice for the management of women with intrauterine synechiae (Ash-

erman syndrome). Following hysteroscopic therapy, there may be an increased incidence of uterine rupture and invasive placentation.

12. MRI appears to be the diagnostic modality of choice in identification of adenomyosis.

13. Under most circumstances, abnormal uterine bleeding in women who are ovulatory is likely due to organic lesion(s) within the uterus. While hormonal therapy for the management of such women may be temporarily effective, hysteroscopic evaluation and therapy is the approach of choice.

14. Techniques for permanent destruction of the endometrium for the management of abnormal uterine bleeding are not required to induce amenorrhea to be considered successful by the patient.

15. Second-generation techniques for transcervical resection of the endometrium (TCRE) include a variety of devices such as the Hydrothermal Ablator, Novasure, Thermachoice, and Her Option and are as effective in reducing heavy menstrual flow as the first-generation (rollerball and laser) techniques. Second-generation techniques, however, typically take less time to perform and can be performed under local anesthesia.

REFERENCES

1. Farquhar CM, Steiner CA. Hysterectomy rates in the United States, 1990–1997. *Obstet Gynecol* 2000;99:229–234.

2. Green LK, Harris RE. Uterine anomalies: Frequency of diagnosis and associated obstetric complications. *Obstet Gynecol* 1976;47:427–429.

3. Jarcho J. Malformations of the uterus: Review of the subject, including embryology, comparative anatomy, diagnosis and report of cases. *Am J Surg* 1946;106.

4. Candiani M, Busacca M, Natale A, Sambruni I. Bicervical uterus and septate vagina: Report of a previously undescribed müllerian anomaly. *Hum Reprod* 1996;11:218–219.

5. Wai CY, Zekam N, Sanz LE. Septate uterus with double cervix and longitudinal vaginal septum: A case report. *J Reprod Med* 2001;46(6):613–617.

6. Gruenwald P. The relation of the growing müllerian duct to the wolffian duct and its importance for the genesis of malformations. *Anat Rec* 1941;81:1.

7. Nahum GG. Uterine anomalies: How common are they, and what is their distribution among subtypes? *J Reprod Med* 1998;43:877–887.

8. Simon C, Martinez L, Pardo F, et al. Müllerian defects in women with normal reproductive outcome. *Fertil Steril* 1991;56:1192–1193.

9. Buttram VC, Gibbons WE. Müllerian anomalies: A proposed classification (an analysis of 144 cases). *Fertil Steril* 1979;32:40–46.

10. Goldberg JM, Falcone T. Müllerian anomalies: Reproduction, diagnosis, and treatment, in Gidwani G, Falcone T (eds), *Congenital Malformations of the Female Genital Tract*. Philadelphia: Lippincott Williams & Wilkins, 1999:Chap 11.

11. The American Fertility Society. The American Fertility Society classifications of adnexal adhesions, distal tubal occlusion, tubal occlusion secondary to tubal ligation, tubal pregnancies, müllerian anomalies and intrauterine adhesions. *Fertil Steril* 1988;49:944–955.

12. Acien P. Reproductive performance of women with uterine malformations. *Hum Reprod* 1993; 8:122–126.

13. Jones HW. Reproductive impairment and the malformed uterus. *Fertil Steril* 1981;36:137–148.

14. Jermy K, Oyelese O, Bourne T. Uterine anomalies and failed surgical termination of pregnancy: The role of routine preoperative transvaginal sonography. *Ultrasound Obstet Gynecol* 1999;14:431–433.

15. Homer HA, Li T-C, Cooke ID. The septate uterus: A review of management and clinical outcome. *Fertil Steril* 2000;73:1–14.

16. Raga F, Bauset C, Remohi J, et al. Reproductive impact of congenital uterine anomalies. *Hum Reprod* 1997;12:2277–2281.

17. Grimbizis GF, Camus M, Tarlatzis BC, et al. Clinical implications of uterine malformations and hysteroscopic treatment results. *Hum Reprod* Update 2001;7:161–174.

18. Hein P, Stolte T, Esker T. The motility of the non-pregnant congenitally malformed uterus. *Eur J Obstet Gynecol* 1974;4:51

19. March CM. Hysteroscopy as an aid to diagnosis in female infertility. *Clin Obstet Gynecol* 1983;26:302–312.

20. Fayez JA. Comparison between abdominal and hysteroscopic metroplasty. *Obstet Gynecol* 1986; 68:399–403.

21. Dabirashrafi H, Bahadori M, Mohammad K, et al. Septate uterus: New idea on the histologic features of the septum in this abnormal uterus. *Am J Obstet Gynecol* 1995;172:105–107.

22. Andrews MC, Jones HW. Impaired reproductive performance of the unicornuate uterus: Intrauterine growth retardation, infertility, and recurrent abortion in five cases. *Am J Obstet Gynecol* 1982;144:173–176.

23. Li S, Qayyum A, Coakley FV, Hricak H. Association of renal agenesis and mullerian duct anomalies. *J Comput Assist Tomogr* 2000;24: 829–834.

24. Moutos DM, Damewood MD, Schlaff WD, Rock JA. A comparison of the reproductive outcome between women with a unicornuate uterus and women with a didelphic uterus. *Fertil Steril* 1992;58:88–93.

25. Fedele L, Zamberletti D, Vercellini P, et al. Reproductive performance of women with a unicornuate uterus. *Fertil Steril* 1987;47;416–419.

26. Smith OW. Diethylstilbestrol in the prevention and treatment of complications of pregnancy. *Am J Obstet Gynecol* 1948;56:821–834.

27. Dieckmann WJ, Davis ME, Rynkiewicz LM, Pottinger RE. Does the administration of diethylstilbestrol during pregnancy have therapeutic value? *Am J Obstet Gynecol* 1953;66:1062–1081.

28. Kaufman RH, Adam E, Burder GL, Gerthoffer E. Upper genital tract changes and pregnancy outcome in offspring exposed in utero to diethylstilbestrol. *Am J Obstet Gynecol* 1980;137: 299–308.

29. Barnes AB, Colton T, Gundersen J, et al. Fertility and outcome of pregnancy in women exposed in utero to diethylstilbestrol. *N Engl J Med* 1980;302:609–613.

30. Cousins L, Karp W, Lacey C, Lucas WE. Reproductive outcome of women exposed to diethylstilbestrol in utero. *Obstet Gynecol* 1980;56: 70–76.

31. Schmidt G, Fowler WC Jr, Talbert LM, Edelman DA. Reproductive history of women exposed to diethylstilbestrol in utero. *Fertil Steril* 1980; 33:21–24.

32. Herbst AL, Hubby MM, Blough RR, Azizi F. A comparison of pregnancy experience in DES-exposed and DES-unexposed daughters. *J Reprod Med* 1980;24:62–69.

33. Palmer JR, Hatch EE, Rao RS, et al. Infertility among women exposed prenatally to diethylstilbestrol. *Am J Epidemiol* 2001;154:316–321.

34. Kaufman RH, Adam E, Hatch EE,. et al. Continued follow-up of pregnancy outcomes in diethylstilbestrol-exposed offspring. *Obstet Gynecol* 2000;96:483–489.

35. Kaufman RH. Findings in offspring of women exposed in utero to diethylstilbestrol. *Obstet Gynecol* 2002;99:197–200.

36. Reuter KL, Daly DC, Cohen SM. Septate versus bicornuate uteri: errors in imaging diagnosis. *Radiology* 1989;172:749–752.

37. Jurkovic D, Gruboeck K, Tailor A, Nicolaides KH. Ultrasound screening for congenital uterine anomalies. *Br J Obstet Gynaecol* 1997;104: 1320–1321.

38. Pennes DR, Bowerman RA, Silver TM. Congenital uterine anomalies and associated pregnancies: Findings and pitfalls of sonographic diagnosis. *J Ultrasound Med* 1985;4:531

39. Jurkovic D, Geipel A, Gruboeck K, et al. Three-dimensional ultrasound for the assessment of uterine anatomy and detection of congenital anomalies: Comparison with hysterosalpingography and two-dimensional ultrasonography. *Ultrasound Obstet Gynecol* 1995;5:233–237.

40. Raga F, Bonilla-Musoles F, Blanes J, Osborne NG. Congenital müllerian anomalies: Diagnostic accuracy of three-dimensional ultrasound. *Fertil Steril* 1996;65:523–528.

41. Woelfer B, Salim R, Banerjee S,. et al. Reproductive outcomes in women with congenital uterine anomalies detected by three-dimensional ultrasound screening. *Obstet Gynecol* 2001;98: 1099–1103.

42. Wu MH, Hsu CC, Huang KE. Detection of congenital mullerian duct anomalies using three-dimensional ultrasound. *J Clin Ultrasound* 1997; 25:487–492.

43. Salim R, Woelfer B, Backos M, et al. Reproducibility of three-dimensional ultrasound diagnosis of congenital uterine anomalies. *Ultrasound Obstet Gynecol* 2003;21:578–582.

44. Alborzi S, Dehbashi S, Parsanezhad ME. Differential diagnosis of septate and bicornuate uterus by sonohysterography eliminates the

need for laparoscopy. *Fertil Steril* 2002;78: 176–178.

45. Soares SR, Barbosa dos Reis MM, Camargos AF. Diagnostic accuracy of sonohysterography, transvaginal sonography, and hysterosalpingography in patients with uterine cavity diseases. *Fertil Steril* 2000;73:406–411.

46. Minto CL, Hollings N, Hall-Craggs M, Creighton S. Magnetic resonance imaging in the assessment of complex müllerian anomalies. *Br J Obstet Gynaecol* 2001;108:791–797.

47. Pellerito JS, McCarthy SM, Doyle MB, et al. Diagnosis of uterine anomalies: Relative accuracy of MR imaging, endovaginal sonography, and hysterosalpingography. *Radiology* 1992;183:795–800.

48. Carrington BM, Hricak H, Nuruddin RN, et al. Müllerian duct anomalies: MR imaging evaluation. *Radiology* 1990;176:715–720

49. Fielding JR. MR imaging of müllerian anomalies: Impact on therapy. *AJR* 1996;167:1491–1495.

50. Mitchell CS, Goske MJ, Applegate K. Imaging of müllerian anomalies, in Gidwani G, Falcone T (eds), *Congenital Malformations of the Female Genital Tract*. Philadelphia: Lippincott Williams & Wilkins 1999:Chap 4.

51. Hricak H. Widespread use of MRI in gynecology: a myth or reality. *Abdom Imag* 1997;22:597–601.

52. Choe JK, Baggish MS. Hysteroscopic treatment of septate uterus with neodymium-YAG laser. *Fertil Steril* 1992;57:81–84.

53. Israel R, March CM. Hysteroscopic incision of the septate uterus. *Am J Obstet Gynecol* 1984; 149:66–73.

54. Cararach M, Penella J, Ubeda A, Labastida R. Hysteroscopic resection of the septate uterus: Scissors versus resectoscope. *Hum Reprod* 1994; 9:87–97.

55. Daly DC, Walters CA, Soto-Albors CE, Riddick CH. Hysteroscopic metroplasty: Surgical techniques and obstetric outcome. *Fertil Steril* 1983; 39:623–628.

56. Vercellini P, Fedele L, Arcaini L, et al. Value of intrauterine device insertion and estrogen administration after hysteroscopic metroplasty. *J Reprod Med* 1989;34:447–450.

57. Dabirashrafi H, Mohammad K, Alavi M, et al. Is estrogen necessary after hysteroscopic incision of the uterine septum? *J Am Assoc Gynecol Laparosc* 1996;3:623–625.

58. Strassman EO. Fertility and unification of the double uterus. *Fertil Steril* 1966;2:165.

59. Jones HW Jr, Jones GE. Double uterus as an etiological factor in repeated abortion: Indications for surgical repair. *Am J Obstet Gynecol* 1953;65:325–339.

60. Tompkins P. Comments on the bicornuate uterus and training. *Surg Clin North Am* 1962; 42:1049–1062.

61. Katz Z, Ben-Arie A, Lurie S, et al. Beneficial effect of hysteroscopic metroplasty on the reproductive outcome in a "T-shaped" uterus. *Gynecol Obstet Invest* 1996;41:41–43.

62. Fedele L, Arcaini L, Parazzini F, et al. Reproductive prognosis after hysteroscopic resection in 102 women: Life-table analysis. *Fertil Steril* 1993;59:768–772.

63. Rock J, Jones HW. The clinical management of the double uterus. *Fertil Steril* 1977;28:789–806.

64. Vercellini P, Vendola N, Colombo A, et al. Hysteroscopic metroplasty with resectoscope or microscissors for the correction of septate uterus. *Surg Gynecol Obstet* 1993;176:439–442.

65. Conturso R, Redaelli L, Pasini A, Tenore A. Spontaneous uterine rupture with amniotic sac protrusion at 28 weeks subsequent to previous hysteroscopic metroplasty. *Eur J Obstet Gynecol Reprod Biol* 2003;107:98–100.

66. Lobaugh ML, Bammel BM, Duke D, Webster BW. Uterine rupture during pregnancy in a patient with a history of hysteroscopic metroplasty. *Obstet Gynecol* 1994;83:838–840.

67. Angell NF, Tan Domingo J, Siddiqi N. Uterine rupture at term after uncomplicated hysteroscopic metroplasty. *Obstet Gynecol* 2002;100: 1098–1099.

68. Buttram VC, Reiter RC. Uterine leiomyomata: Etiology, symptomatology, and management. *Fertil Steril* 1981;36:433–445.

69. Cranmer SF, Patel A. The frequency of uterine leiomyomas. *Am J Clin Pathol* 1990;94:435–438.

70. Townsend DE, Sparkes RS, Baluda MC, McClelland G. Unicellualr histogenesis of uterine leiomyomas as determined by electrophoresis of glucose-6-phosphate dehydrogenase. *Am J Obstet Gynecol* 1970;107:1168–1173.

71. Spellacy WN, LeMaire WJ, Buhl WC, et al. Plasma growth hormone and estradiol levels in women with uterine myomas. *Obstet Gynecol* 1972;40:829–834.

72. Puuka MJ, Kontula KK, Kauppila AJI, et al. Estrogen receptor in human myoma tissue. *Mol Cell Endocrinol* 1976;6:35–44.

73. Tamaya T, Motoyama T, Ohono Y, et al. Estradiol-17β-progesterone and 5α-dihydrotestosterone receptors of uterine myometrium and myoma in the human subject. *J Steroid Biochem* 1979;10:615–622.

74. Pollow K, Geilfuss J, Boquoi E, Pollow B. Estrogen and progesterone binding proteins in normal human myometrium and leiomyoma tissue. *J Clin Chem Clin Biochem* 1978;16:503–511.

75. Pollow K, Sinnecker G, Boquoi E, Pollow B. In vitro conversion of estradiol-17β into estrone in normal human myometrium and leiomyoma. *J Clin Chem Clin Biochem* 1978;16:493–502.

76. Grattarola R, Li CH. Effect of growth hormone and its combination with estradiol-17β on the uterus of hypophysectomized and hypophysectomized-ovariectomized rats. *Clin Endocrinol* 1959;65: 802.

77. Buttram VC, Snables MC. Indications for myomectomy. *Semin Reprod Endocrinol* 1992;10:378–389.

78. Hunt SH. Fibroid weighing one hundred and forty pounds. *Am J Obstet Gynecol* 1888;21:62–63.

79. Jacobson FJ, Enzer N. Uterine myomas and the endometrium: Study of the mechanism of bleeding. *Obstet Gynecol* 1956;7:206.

80. Clark CL, Wilson TO, Witzig TE. Giant uterine fibromyoma producing secondary polycythemia. *Obstet Gynecol* 1994;84:722–724.

81. LevGur M, Levie MD. The myomatous erythrocytosis syndrome: A review. *Obstet Gynecol* 1995;86:1026–1030

82. Migishima F, Jobo T, Hata H, et al. Uterine leiomyoma causing massive ascites and left pleural effusion with elevated CA 125: A case report. *J Obstet Gynaecol Res* 2000;26:283–287.

83. Donnez J, Jadoul P. What are the implications of myomas on fertility? A need for a debate? *Hum Reprod* 2002;17:1424–1430.

84. Pritts EA. Fibroids and infertility: A systematic review of the evidence. *Obstet Gynecol Surv* 2001;56:483–491.

85. Hunt JE, Wallach EE. Uterine factor in infertility: An overview. *Clin Gynecol* 1974;17:44–64.

86. Coutinho EM, Maia HS. The contractile response of the human uterus, fallopian tubes, and ovary to prostaglandins in vivo. *Fertil Steril* 1971;22:539–543.

87. Deligdish L, Loewenthal M. Endometrial changes associated with myomata of the uterus. *J Clin Pathol* 1970;23:676–680.

88. Stovall DW, Parrish SB, Van Voorhis BJ, et al. Uterine leiomyomas reduce the efficacy of assisted reproduction cycles: Results of a matched follow-up study. *Hum Reprod* 1998;13:192–197.

89. Eldar-Geva T, Meagher S, Healy DL, et al. Effect of intramural, subserosal, and submucosal uterine fibroids on the outcome of assisted reproductive technology treatment. *Fertil Steril* 1998;70:687–691.

90. Vercellini P, Maddalena S, De Giorgi O, et al. Abdominal myomectomy for infertility: A comprehensive review. *Hum Reprod* 1998;13:873–879.

91. Li TC, Mortimer R, Cooke ID. Myomectomy: A retrospective study to examine reproductive performance before and after surgery. *Hum Reprod* 1999;14:1735–1740.

92. Bulletti C, De Ziegler D, Polli V, Flamigni C. The role of leiomyomas in infertility. *J Am Assoc Gynecol Laparosc* 1999;6:441–445.

93. Coronado GD, Marshall LM, Schwartz SM. Complications in pregnancy, labor, and delivery with leiomyomas: A population-based study. *Obstet Gynecol* 2000;95:764–769.

94. Benson CB, Chow JS, Chang-Lee W, et al. Outcome of pregnancies in women with uterine leiomyomas identified by sonography in the first trimester. *J Clin Ultrasound* 2001;29:261–264.

95. Exacoustos C, Rosati P. Ultrasound diagnosis of uterine myomas and complications in pregnancy. *Obstet Gynecol* 1993;82:881–882.

96. Vergani P, Ghidini A, Strobelt N, et al. Do uterine leiomyomas influence pregnancy outcome? *Am J Perinatol* 1994;11:356–358.

97. Koike T, Minakami H, Kosuge S, et al. Uterine leiomyoma in pregnancy: Its influence on obstetric performance. *J Obstet Gynecol Res* 1999;25:309–313.

98. Farrer-Brown G, Beilby JO, Tarbit MH. Venous changes in the endometrium of myomatous uteri. *Obstet Gynecol* 1971;38:743–751.

99. Strobelt N, Ghidini A, Cavallone M, et al. Natural history of uterine leiomyomas in pregnancy. *J Ultrasound Med* 1994;13:399–401

100. Cantuaria GH, Angioli R, Frost L, et al. Comparison of bimanual examination with ultrasound examination before hysterectomy for uterine leiomyoma. *Obstet Gynecol* 1998;92:109–112.

101. Weinreb JC, Barkoff ND, Megibow A, De-mopoulos R. The value of MR imaging in dis-tinguishing leiomyomas from other solid pelvic masses when sonography is indeterminate. *AJR* 1990;154:295–299.

102. Karasick S, Lev-Toaff AS, Toaff ME. Imaging of uterine leiomyomas. *AJR* 1992;158:799–805

103. Babaknia A, Rock JA, Jones HW Jr. Pregnancy success following abdominal myomectomy for infertility. *Fertil Steril* 1978;30:644–647.

104. Becker E Jr, Lev-Toaff AS, Kaufman EP, et al. The added value of transvaginal sonohysterog-raphy over transvaginal sonography alone in women with known or suspected leiomyoma. *J Ultrasound Med* 2002;21:237–247.

105. Cicinelli E, Romano F, Anastasio PS, et al. Transab-dominal sonohysterography, transvaginal sonog-raphy, and hysteroscopy in the evaluation of submucous myomas. *Obstet Gynecol* 1995;85: 42–47.

106. Bazot M, Salem C, Frey I, Darai E. Imaging of myomas: is preoperative MRI useful? *Gynecol Obstet Fertil* 2002;30:711–716 (in French).

107. Murase E, Siegelman ES, Outwater EK, et al. Uterine leiomyomas: Histopathologic features, MR imaging findings, differential diagnosis, and treatment. *Radiographics* 1999;19:1179–1197.

109. Stewart EA, Faur AV, Wise LA, et al. Predictors of subsequent surgery for uterine leiomyomata after abdominal myomectomy. *Obstet Gynecol* 2002;99:426–432.

109. Parker WH, Fu YS, Berek JS. Uterine sarcoma in patients operated on for presumed uterine leiomyoma and rapidly growing leiomyoma. *Obstet Gynecol* 1994;83:414–418.

110. Hannigan EV, Gomez LG. Uterine leiomyosar-coma. *Am J Obstet Gynecol* 1979;134:557–564.

111. Goldzieher JW, Maqueo M, Ricaud L, et al. In-duction of degenerative changes in uterine my-omas by high-dosage progestin therapy. *Am J Obstet Gynecol* 1966;96:1078–1087.

112. Knobil E. The neuroendocrine control of the menstrual cycle. *Recent Prog Horm Res* 1980;36: 53–88

113. Filicori M, Hall DA, Loughlin JS, et al. A con-servative approach to the management of uter-ine leiomyoma: pituitary desensitization by a luteinizing hormone–releasing hormone ana-logue. *Am J Obstet Gynecol* 1983;147:726–727

114. Lethaby A, Vollenhoven B, Sowter M. Efficacy of preoperative gonadotrophin hormone–releasing analogues for women with uterine fi-broids undergoing hysterectomy or myomec-tomy: A systematic review. *Br J Obstet Gynaecol* 2002;109:1097–1108.

115. Coddington CC, Collins RL, Shawker TH, et al. Long-acting gonadotropin hormone–releasing hormone analogue used to treat uteri. *Fertil Steril* 1986;45:624–629.

116. Letterie GS, Coddington CC, Winkel CA, et al. Efficacy of a gonadotropin-releasing hormone agonist in the treatment of uterine leiomyomata: Long-term follow-up. *Fertil Steril* 1989;51:951–956.

117. Scialli AR, Levi AJ. Intermittent leuprolide ac-etate for the nonsurgical management of women with leiomyomata uteri. *Fertil Steril* 2000;74:540–546.

118. Thomas EJ. Add-back therapy for long-term use in dysfunctional uterine bleeding and uterine fi-broids. *Br J Obstet Gynaecol* 1996;103(suppl 14): 18–21.

119. Parazzini F, Bortolotti A, Chiantera V, et al. Goserelin acetate to avoid hysterectomy in premenopausal women with fibroids requiring surgery. *Eur J Obstet Gynecol Reprod Biol* 1999; 87:31–33.

120. Stovall TG, Muneyyirci-Delale O, Summitt RL Jr, Scialli AR. GnRH agonist and iron versus placebo and iron in the anemic patient before surgery for leiomyomas: A randomized, con-trolled trial. Leuprolide Acetate Study Group. *Obstet Gynecol* 1995;86:65–71.

121. Murphy AA, Kettel LM, Morales AJ, et al. Re-gression of uterine leiomyomata in response to the antiprogesterone RU-486. *J Clin Endocrinol Metab* 1993;76:513–517.

122. Eisinger SH, Meldrum S, Fiscella K, et al. Low-dose mifepristone for uterine leiomyomata. *Ob-stet Gynecol* 2003;101:243–250.

123. De Leo V, La Marca A, Morgante G. Short-term treatment of uterine fibromyomas with dana-zol. *Gynecol Obstet Invest* 1999;47:258–262.

124. Friedman AJ, Thomas PP. Does low-dose com-bination oral contraceptive use affect uterine size or menstrual flow in premenopausal women with leiomyomas? *Obstet Gynecol* 1995; 85:631–635.

125. Tulandi T, Murray C, Guralnick M. Adhesion formation and reproductive outcome after my-omectomy and second-look laparoscopy. *Ob-stet Gynecol* 1993;82:213–215.

126. Fletcher H, Frederick J, Hardie M, Simeon D. A randomized comparison of vasopressin and torniquet as hemostatic agents during myomectomy. *Obstet Gynecol* 1996;87:1014–1018.

127. Semm K. New methods of pelviscopy (gynecologic laparoscopy) for myomectomy, ovariectomy, tubectomy, and adenectomy. *Endoscopy* 1979;11:85–93.

128. Milad MP, Sankpal RS. Laparoscopic approaches to uterine leiomyomas. *Clin Obstet Gynecol* 2001; 44:401–411.

129. Zullo F, Pellicano M, De Stefano R, et al. A prospective, randomized study to evaluate leuprolide acetate treatment before laparoscopic myomectomy: efficacy and ultrasonographic predictors. *Am J Obstet Gynecol* 1998;178:108–112.

130. Campo S, Garcea N. Laparoscopic myomectomy in premenopausal women with and without preoperative treatment using gonadotrophin-releasing hormone analogues. *Hum Reprod* 1999; 14:44–48.

131. Heaston DK, Mineau DE, Brown BJ, Miller FJ Jr. Transcatheter arterial embolization for control of persistent massive puerperal hemorrhage after bilateral surgical hypogastric artery ligation. *AJR* 1979;133:152–154.

132. Ravina JH, Herbreteau D, Ciraru-Vigneron N, et al. Arterial embolisation to treat uterine myomata. *Lancet* 1995;346:671–672.

133. Goldberg J, Pereira L, Mude-Nochumson H. Uterine artery embolization for symptomatic fibroids: Pros and cons. *ObG management* 2003;15:69–79.

134. Goodwin SC, Wong GCH. Uterine artery embolization for uterine fibroids: A radiologist's perspective. *Clin Obstet Gynecol* 2001;44:412–424.

135. Baker CM. Winkel CA, Subramanian S, Spies JB. Estimated costs for uterine artery embolization and abdominal myomectomy for uterine leiomyomata: A comparative study at a single institution. *J Vasc Intervent Radiol* 2002;13:1207–1210.

136. Roth AR, Spies JB, Walsh SM, et al. Pain after uterine artery embolization for leiomyomata: Can its severity be predicted and does severity predict outcome? *J Vasc Intervent Radiol* 2000; 11:1047–1152.

137. Pron G, Bennett J, Common A, et al. The Ontario Uterine Fibroid Embolization Trial: 2. Uterine fibroid reduction and symptom relief after uterine artery embolization for fibroids. *Fertil Steril* 200;79:120–127.

138. Walker WJ, Pelage JP. Uterine artery embolisation for symptomatic fibroids: Clinical results in 400 women with imaging follow up. *Br J Obstet Gynaecol* 2002;109:1262–1272.

139. Spies JB, Ascher SA, Roth AR, et al. Uterine artery embolization for leiomyomata. *Obstet Gynecol* 2001;98:29–34

140. Ravina JH, Aymard A, Ciraru-Vigneron N, et al. Arterial embolization of uterine myoma: Results apropos of 286 cases. *J Gynecol Obstet Biol Reprod (Paris)* 2000;29:272–275 (in French).

141. Pinto I, Chimeno P, Romo A, et al. Uterine fibroids: Uterine artery embolization versus hysterectomy for treatment. A prospective, randomized, and controlled clincal trial. *Radiology* 2003;226:425–431.

142. Broder MS, Goodwin S, Chen G, et al. Comparison of long-term outcomes of myomectomy and uterine artery embolization. *Obstet Gynecol* 2002;100:864–868.

143. Spies JB, Spector A, Roth AR, et al. Complications after uterine artery embolization for leiomyomas. *Obstet Gynecol* 2002;100:873–880.

144. Vashisht A, Studd JWW, Carey AH, et al. Fibroid embolisation: A technique not without significant complications. *Br J Obstet Gynaecol* 2000;107:1166–1170.

145. Tropeano G, Litwicka K, Di Srasti C, et al. Associated with endometrial atrophy after uterine artery embolization for symptomatic uterine fibroids. *Fertil Steril* 2003;79:132–135.

146. Payne JF, Haney AF. Serious complications of uterine artery embolization for conservative treatment of fibroids. *Fertil Steril* 2003;79:128–131.

147. McLucas B, Sostrin S. Uterine necrosis after uterine artery embolization for leiomyoma. *Obstet Gynecol* 2002;100:1357–1358.

148. Yeagley TJ, Goldberg J, Klein TA, Bonn J. Labial necrosis after uterine artery embolization for leiomyomata. *Obstet Gynecol* 2002;100:881–882.

149. Pron G, Mocarski E, Cohen M, et al. Hysterectomy for complications after uterine artery embolization for leiomyoma: Results of a Canadian multicenter clinical trial. *J Am Assoc Gynecol Laparosc* 2003;10:99–106.

150. Goldberg J, Pereira L, Berghella V. Pregnancy after uterine artery embolization. *Obstet Gynecol* 2002;100:869–872.

151. Spies JB. Uterine artery embolization for fibroids: Understanding the technical causes of failure. *J Vasc Intervent Radiol* 2003;14:11–14.

152. Al-Inany H. Intrauterine adhesions. *Acta Obstet Gynaecol Scand* 2001;80:986–993.

153. Asherman JG. Amenorrhoea traumatica. *J Obstet Gynaecol Br Emp* 1948;55:23–30.

154. Schenker JG, Margalioth EJ. Intrauterine adhesions: An updated appraisal. *Fertil Steril* 1982; 37:593–610.

155. Westendorp IC, Ankum WM, Mol BW, Vonk J. Prevalence of Asherman's syndrome after secondary removal of placental remnants or a repeat curettage for incomplete abortion. *Hum Reprod* 1998;13:3347–3350.

156. Capella-Allouc S, Morsad F, Rongieres-Bertrand C, et al. Hysteroscopic treatment of severe Asherman's syndrome and subsequent fertility. *Hum Reprod* 1999;14:1230–1233.

157. Aubert JM, Gobeaux-Castadot MJ, Boria MC. Actinomyces in the endometrium of IUD users. *Contraception* 1980;21:577–583.

158. Bird CC, McElin TW, Manalo-Estrella P. The elusive adenomyosis of the uterus—revisited. *Am J Obstet Gynecol* 1972;112:583–593.

159. Emge LA. The elusive adenomyosis of the uterus. *Am J Obstet Gynecol* 1962;83:1541.

160. Matalliotakis IM, Kourtis AI, Panidis DK. Adenomyosis. *Obstet Gynecol Clin North Am* 2003; 30:63–82.

161. Duwela AS, Perera MA, Aiqing L, Fraser IS. Endometrial-myometrial interface: Relationship to adenomyosis and changes in pregnancy. *Obstet Gynecol Surv* 2000;55:390–400.

162. Levgur M, Abadi MA, Tucker A. Adenomyosis: symptoms, histology, and pregnancy terminations. *Obstet Gynecol* 2000;95:688–691.

163. Marshak RH, Eliasoph J. The roentgen findings in adenomyosis. *Am J Obstet Gynecol* 1955;64:846.

164. Wolf DM, Spataro RF. The current state of hysterosalpingography. *Radiographics* 1988;8:1041.

165. Fedele L, Bianchi S, Dorta M, et al. Transvaginal sonography in the diagnosis of diffuse adenomyosis. *Fertil Steril* 1992;58:94–97.

166. Arnold LL, Ascher SM, Schruefer JJ, Simon JA. The nonsurgical diagnosis of adenomyosis. *Obstet Gynecol* 1995;86:461–465.

167. Tamaoka Y, Orikasa H, Sumi Y, et al. Direct effect of danazol on endometrial hyperplasia in adenomyotic women: Treatment with danazol-containing intrauterine device. *Hum Cell* 2000; 13:127–133.

168. Fedele L, Bianchi S, Raffaelli R, et al. Treatment of adenomyosis-associated menorrhagia with a levonorgestrel-releasing intrauterine device. *Fertil Steril* 1997;68:426–429.

169. Nagasawa H, Mori T. Stimulation of mammary tumorigenesis and suppression of uterine adenomyosis by temporary inhibition of pituitary prolactin secretion during youth in mice (41492). *Proc Soc Exp Biol Med* 1982;171:164–167.

170. Nagasawa H, Aoki M, Mori T, et al. Stimulation of mammary tumorigenesis and inhibition of uterine adenomyosis by suppressed progesterone effects in SHN mice. *Anticancer Res* 1989;9:827–832.

171. Grow DR, Filer RB. Treatment of adenomyosis with long-term GnRH analogues: A case report. *Obstet Gynecol* 1991;78:538–539.

172. Smith DC, Prentice RL, Bauermeister DE. Endometrial carcinoma: Histopathology, survival, and exogenous estrogens. *Gynecol Obstet Invest* 1981;12:169–179.

173. Valle RF, Sciarra JJ. Current status of hysteroscopy in gynecologic practice. *Fertil Steril* 1979;32:619–632.

174. Peterson W, Novak E. Endometrial polyps. *Obstet Gynecol* 1956;8:40.

175. Emanuel MH, Wamsteker K, Hart AA, et al. Long-term results of hysteroscopic myomectomy for abnormal uterine bleeding. *Obstet Gynecol* 1999;93:743–748.

176. Gimpelson RJ. Hysteroscopic treatment of the patient with intracavitary pathology (myomectomy/polypectomy). *Obstet Gynecol Clin North Am* 2000;27:327–337.

177. Glasser MH. Endometrial ablation and hysteroscopic myomectomy by electrosurgical vaporization. *J Am Assoc Gynecol Laparosc* 1997;4:369–374.

178. Lethaby A, Farquhar C, Cooke I. Antifibrinolytics for heavy menstrual bleeding. *Cochrane Database Syst Rev* 2000;4:CD000249

179. Lethaby A, Augood C, Duckitt K. Nonsteroidal anti-inflammatory drugs for heavy menstrual bleeding. *Cochrane Database Syst Rev* 2002;1:CD000400.

180. Lethaby AE, Cooke I, Rees M. Progesterone/progestogen-releasing intrauterine systems versus either placebo or any other medication for

heavy menstrual bleeding. *Cochrane Database Syst Rev* 2000;2:CD002126.

181. Goldrath MH, Fuller TA, Segal S. Laser photovaporization of endometrium for the treatment of menorrhagia. *Am J Obstet Gynecol* 1981;140: 14–19.

182. DeCherney AH, Diamond MP, Lavy G, Polan ML. Endometrial ablation for intractable uterine bleeding: Hysteroscopic resection. *Obstet Gynecol* 1987;70:668–670.

183. Vancaillie TG. Electrocoagulation of the endometrium with the ball-end resectoscope. *Obstet Gynecol* 1989;74:425–427.

184. Sowter MC, Lethaby A, Singla AA. Preoperative endometrial thinning agents before endometrial destruction for heavy menstrual bleeding. *Cochrane Database Syst Rev* 2002;3:CD001124.

185. Lethaby A, Shepperd S, Cooke I, Farquhar C. Endometrial resection and ablation versus hysterectomy for heavy menstrual bleeding. *Cochrane Database Syst Rev* 2000;2:CD000329.

186. Overton C, Hargreaves J, Maresh M. A national survey of the complications of endometrial destruction for menstrual disorders: The MISTLETOE study. *Br J Obstet Gynaecol* 1997;104: 1351–1359.

187. Brooks-Carter GN, Killackey MA, Neuwirth RS. Adenocarcinoma of the endometrium after endometrial ablation. *Obstet Gynecol* 2000;96:836– 837.

188. Pugh CP, Crane JM, Hogan TG. Successful intrauterine pregnancy after endometrial ablation. *J Am Assoc Gynecol Laparosc* 2000;7:391–394.

189. Lethaby A, Hickey M. Endometrial destruction techniques for heavy menstrual bleeding: A Cochrane review. *Hum Reprod* 2002;17:2795– 2806.

190. Roy KH, Mattox JH. Advances in endometrial ablation. *Obstet Gynecol Surv* 2002;57:789–802.

191. Gallinat A, Nugent W. Novasure impedance-controlled system for endometrial ablation. *J Am Assoc Gynecol Laprosc* 2002;9:283–289.

192. Vilos GA, Aletebi FA, Eskandar MA. Endometrial thermal balloon ablation with the ThermaChoice system: Effect of intrauterine pressure and duration of treatment. *J Am Assoc Gynecol Laparosc* 2000;7:325–329.

193. Loffer FD. Three-year comparison of thermal balloon and rollerball ablation in treatment of menorrhagia. *J Am Assoc Gynecol Laparosc* 2001; 8:48–54.

194. Hawe J, Abbott J, Hunter D, et al. A randomised, controlled trial comparing the Cavaterm endometrial ablation system with the Nd:YAG laser for the treatment of dysfunctional uterine bleeding. *Br J Obstet Gynaecol* 2003;110: 350–357.

195. Duleba AJ, Heppard MC, Soderstrom RM, Townsend DE. A randomized study comparing endometrial cryoablation and rollerball electroablation for treatment of dysfunctional uterine bleeding. *J Am Assoc Gynecol Laparosc* 2003;10:17–26.

196. Milligan MP, Etokowo G, Kanumuru S, Mannifold N. Microwave endometrial ablation: Patients' experiences in the first 3 months following treatment. *J Obstet Gynaecol* 2002;22: 201–204.

197. Cooper KG, Bain C, Parkin DE. Comparison of microwave endometrial ablation and transcervical resection of the endometrium for treatment of heavy menstrual loss: A randomised trial. *Lancet* 1999;354:1859–1861.

CHAPTER 20

Endometriosis

NEAL G. MAHUTTE AND AYDIN ARICI

Endometriosis is characterized by the presence of ectopic endometrial tissue. Endometriosis occurs most frequently on the ovaries, utero-sacral ligaments, pelvic sidewalls, and posterior cul-de-sac. Although not all women are symptomatic, complications of endometriosis are believed to result from cyclic bleeding into surrounding tissues that results in inflammation, scarring, and adhesions. Endometriosis is found in up to 60 percent of women with dysmenorrhea and 40 to 50 percent of reproductive-age women with pelvic pain or deep dyspareunia.[1] Endometriosis is also encountered frequently in women undergoing evaluation for infertility.

Endometriosis is an estrogen-dependent disease. Although the presence of steroid hormone receptors in endometriotic tissue is variable, all commonly used medical treatments for endometriosis derive their efficacy by inducing amenorrhea via suppression or opposition of estrogen action. Estrogen dependency also explains why endometriosis is very rare after menopause. When such cases are encountered, peripheral conversion of androgens to estrogens or exogenous steroid administration is usually the root cause.

▶ DIAGNOSIS OF ENDOMETRIOSIS

Endometriosis is defined as the presence and proliferation of endometrial tissue outside the uterus. Peritoneal implants may appear white, red, clear, or bluish black. Because of variability in the appearance of endometriosis, reliance solely on visual inspection or clinical symptomatology is unreliable. Whenever possible, surgical impressions should be confirmed by histologic findings before the diagnosis of endometriosis is assumed. Typical blue-black powder-burn nodules correlate with histology in 75 to 90 percent of patients.[2,3] However, endometriosis may manifest in a myriad of other ways.[4] These so-called atypical lesions may be overlooked easily and do not always correlate with strict histologic criteria for endometriosis (Table 20-1).

Misdiagnosis of endometriosis also may result from overreliance on strict gold standard histologic criteria. Surgical specimens from obvious endometriotic lesions do not always meet histologic criteria, whereas biopsy of visually normal-appearing peritoneum in asymptomatic, fertile women occasionally may demonstrate all the histologic elements for endometriosis.[3,5]

▶ **TABLE 20-1:** CORRELATION BETWEEN LESION APPEARANCE AND STRICT HISTOLOGIC CRITERIA FOR ENDOMETRIOSIS

	Likelihood of Histologic Diagnosis of Endometriosis[2–4]
Typical Implant	
• Classic blue-black powder burn	75–90%
Atypical Implants	
• Red, flamelike lesion	60–80%
• White opacified peritoneum	60–80%
• Glandular	67%
• Subovarian adhesions	20–50%
• Yellow-brown peritoneum	47%
• Circular peritoneal defects	12–45%
Completely Normal Peritoneum	6–13%

At the present time, the diagnosis of endometriosis is best when clinical manifestations, visual findings at the time of surgery, and tissue findings on histology are all correlated.

Minimally Invasive Techniques for Endometriosis Diagnosis

The costs and risks of surgery have stimulated interest in less invasive methods for the detection of endometriosis. One method investigated extensively is serum CA-125.[6] Serum CA-125 is elevated in 50 to 80 percent of untreated women with moderate to severe endometriosis but only 10 to 30 percent of women with minimal to mild disease.[7–9] Because of this disparity and the lack of specificity of serum CA-125, it is not a reliable marker for endometriosis. However, there may be a role for CA-125 in monitoring response to treatment and reactivation of disease in women known to have an elevated serum CA-125 concentration prior to therapy.[9–12]

The performance of ultrasonography and magnetic resonance imaging (MRI) in the detection of endometriosis also has been well characterized.[13] Neither modality is very reliable for peritoneal endometriosis, but both are excellent for endometriomas. When visualized ultrasonographically, a endometrioma appears as a persistent, thick-walled cystic ovarian mass with fine, diffuse homogeneous echoes. Occasionally, endometriomas may be septated or fluid-filled. In a study of almost 1000 women, the sensitivity and specificity of transvaginal ultrasound in the diagnosis of endometriomas were 87 and 99 percent, respectively.[14] MRI offers similar accuracy in the identification of endometriomas but also may detect deep peritoneal implants.[15] Endometriosis lesions typically are hyperintense on T_1-weighted images and hypointense on T_2-weighted images. MRI sensitivities of 61 to 71 percent and specificities of 60 to 98 percent for the detection of endometriosis have been reported.[16–19]

Endometrial biopsy specimens also may be used to detect endometriosis. Several studies have shown that aromatase P450 is expressed in the eutopic endometrium of women with endometriosis but not in disease-free controls.[20,21] Aromatase P450 also may be expressed in the eutopic endometrium of women with other hormone-dependent disorders such as leiomyomata, adenomyosis, and tubal disease. Given these potential confounding factors, the sensitivity and specificity of endometrial aromatase P450 gene expression for endometriosis are approximately 80 and 60 percent, respectively.[22]

In the coming years, use of genomic and proteomic technology is likely to yield an abundance of novel diagnostic markers for endometriosis. It will be important to ensure that these tests are applicable to the broad, diverse population of reproductive-age women not simply small study samples of women with and without endometriosis. In each case, the timing of sampling in relation to the menstrual cycle, the presence of other pelvic pathology, and the influence of medications are but a few of the potential confounding factors that will need to be addressed.

► CLASSIFICATION OF ENDOMETRIOSIS

Over the last 80 years, a plethora of staging/scoring systems have been proposed for women with endometriosis. The purpose of such systems is to allow uniform reporting of results, provide prognostic information for patients, and facilitate research. The current standard for staging endometriosis is the revised classification of the American Society for Reproductive Medicine.[23] This classification divides endometriosis into four stages (minimal, mild, moderate, and severe) based on the total score from a weighted point system. Points are assigned based on the size and depth of endometriotic lesions, as well as the extent of pelvic adhesions.

One of the major problems with such classification algorithms is their reliance on arbitrary scoring assignments. The scoring systems are prone to significant inter- and intraobserver variation and are not based on empirical data.[24] For example, complete obliteration of the posterior cul-de-sac is assigned a score of 20, whereas partial obliteration of the cul-de-sac is assigned a score of 4 even though there is no evidence that one is five times worse than the other. Such problems may explain at least in part why there is so little correlation between endometriosis staging scores and clinical manifestations such as pain or infertility.[25,26]

► PATHOGENESIS OF ENDOMETRIOSIS

In the 1920s, John Sampson of Albany, New York, proposed that endometriosis results from seeding of the peritoneal cavity by refluxed endometrial tissue.[27] Sampson's theory of retrograde menstruation is supported by a variety of observations (Table 20-2). Although implantation of exfoliated endometrial cells remains the most widely accepted theory for the development of endometriosis, Sampson's theory cannot explain all cases. For example, endometriosis occasionally may occur at distant sites, such as the lung or brain. These cases are believed to result from lymphovascular spread of endometrial tissue. Other examples may result from coelomic metaplasia.[28] Coelomic

► **TABLE 20-2:** OBSERVATIONS SUPPORTING SAMPSON'S THEORY FOR THE PATHOGENESIS OF ENDOMETRIOSIS

- Distribution of endometriosis implants occurs in the dependent portions of the pelvis.[233,234]
- Existence of retrograde menstruation is well documented.
- Endometrial debris from menstrual effluent can grow in tissue culture.[235]
- Human endometrial tissue can adhere to peritoneal tissue.[236]
- In animal models, menstrual endometrium transposed to the peritoneal cavity may cause endometriosis.[237]
- There is a very high incidence of endometriosis in women who have müllerian anomalies with outflow tract obstruction.[238]
- There is an association of endometriosis with risk factors such as increased menstrual flow, frequent menstruation, and early menarche.[239,240]
- There is frequently tubal patency despite the presence of extensive pelvic disease.

metaplasia is believed to be responsible for the development of endometriosis in men who receive exogenous estrogen treatment.[29,30] Coelomic metaplasia also may explain cases of endometriosis in perimenarchal teenage girls.[31,32]

Genetics of Endometriosis

Because retrograde menstruation occurs in almost all women but only a minority develops endometriosis, genetic and immune factors have been invoked to explain differences in individual susceptibility to the disease. Studies in monozygotic twins have shown that 75 percent or more are concordant for the development of endometriosis.[33,34] Other studies examining the risk of endometriosis in women with a first-degree relative with endometriosis have reported concordance rates of 4 to 7 percent.[35–38] This recurrence risk is compatible with a polygenic/multifactorial mode of inheritance. Given that the control group in these studies was reported to have endometriosis in only 1 to 2 percent of cases, the relative risk of endometriosis in women with a first-degree relative with endometriosis would appear to be elevated two- to sevenfold. It should be noted, however, that estimates of the incidence of endometriosis in first-degree relatives were based on responses to questionnaires, not surgical findings with histologic confirmation.

Immunology of Endometriosis

Endometriosis is associated with changes in both cell-mediated and humoral immunity (Table 20-3). The peritoneal fluid of women with endometriosis contains increased numbers of activated macrophages.[39–41] Macrophages normally play a key role in first-line host defense mechanisms, but in women with endometriosis, their function appears to be altered from an inhibitory to a facilitatory role.[42] For example, although monocytes from fertile women significantly sup-

▶ **TABLE 20-3:** IMMUNE ALTERATIONS IN ENDOMETRIOSIS

Increased Macrophage Number and Activity
- Increased angiogenic factors
- Increased endometrial growth factors
- Increased chemotactic factors

Increased Production of Inflammatory Cytokines

Decreased Cell-Mediated Immunity
- Decreased natural killer cell responsiveness to ectopic endometrial cells
- Decreased T-cell responsiveness to ectopic endometrial cells

Increased Humoral Immune Responses
- Increased B-cell activity
- Increased immunoglobulins and complement proteins

press endometrial cell proliferation, monocytes from women with endometriosis enhance endometrial cell proliferation.[43] Concomitantly, there is a decline in natural killer (NK) cell cytotoxicity toward endometrial cells.[41,44,45] Both sera and peritoneal fluid from women with endometriosis have been shown to reduce NK cell cytotoxicity, and NK cell cytotoxicity has been inversely correlated with the stage of endometriosis.[46–48]

Inflammatory cytokines appear to be key mediators of the development and progression of endometriosis (Table 20-4). A good example is interleukin 8 (IL-8).[49] IL-8 is be produced by a variety of cell types, including macrophages and endometrial cells. IL-8 is markedly expressed in vivo by both endometrial glands and stromal cells, and expression is highest in the late secretory and early proliferative phases of the cycle, the time when retrograde menstruation occurs.[50,51] IL-8 stimulates the adhesion of endometrial stromal cells to fibronectin in a concentration-dependent manner, suggesting a potential role for IL-8 in the initial attachment of endometrial cells to the peritoneal

▶ **TABLE 20-4:** INFLAMMATORY CYTOKINES MEDIATING ANGIOGENESIS, ENDOMETRIAL CELL PROLIFERATION, AND RECRUITMENT OF INFLAMMATORY CELLS

Angiogenesis
- VEGF, IL-8, IL-15, IL-18, leptin, MIF, FGF, PDGF

Endometrial Cell Proliferation
- IL-8, PDGF, MDGF, EGF, TGF-β, leptin

Recruitment of Inflammatory Cells
- IL-8, MCP-1, MIF, RANTES

Abbreviations: VEGF = vascular endothelial growth factor; IL = interleukin; MIF = macrophage migration inhibitory factor; FGF = fibroblast growth factor; PDGF = platelet-derived growth factor; MDGF = macrophage-derived growth factor; EGF = epidermal growth factor; TGF-β = transforming factor β; MCP-1 = monocyte chemoattractant protein 1; RANTES = regulated on activation, normal T-cell expressed and secreted.

▶ **TABLE 20-5:** CRITICAL STEPS IN THE PATHOGENESIS OF PERITONEAL ENDOMETRIOSIS AFTER RETROGRADE MENSTRUATION

- Attachment of endometrial cells to the peritoneal surface
- Endometrial cell invasion into the mesothelium
- Angiogenesis around nascent endometriosis implants
- Endometrial cell proliferation
- Recruitment of inflammatory cells that subserve the implant

surface.[52] IL-8 also has been shown to upregulate matrix metalloproteinases, factors believed to play a key role in endometrial cell invasion of the extracellular matrix.

A key condition for the survival and growth of nascent endometriosis implants is the establishment of a blood supply. Active endometriosis implants are markedly vascularized. Important mediators of local angiogenesis include vascular endothelial growth factor (VEGF), macrophage migration inhibitory factor (MIF), and IL-8.[53,54] In vitro, IL-8 also increases endometrial stromal cell proliferation in a concentration-dependent manner, and anti-IL-8 antibody inhibits endometrial stromal proliferation.[55] Finally, IL-8 exerts chemotactic activity on neutrophils and macrophages and inhibits neutrophil apoptosis even in the presence of Fas engagement.[56]

Another important cytokine appears to be MIF.[57] Macrophages, lymphocytes, and ectopic endometrial cells are all capable of producing MIF. MIF is a potent mitogenic factor for endothelial cells and is named for its ability to activate and inhibit macrophage migration. Thus MIF both induces angiogenesis and helps re-

tain macrophages in the area of the implant, thus augmenting the local accumulation of other cytokines and growth factors. Finally, in some tissues MIF has been shown to reduce NK cell cytotoxicity, a role that has yet to be investigated in women with endometriosis.[58,59]

Critical Steps in the Development of Endometriosis after Retrograde Menstruation

Five critical steps have been postulated to explain the development of endometriosis after retrograde menstruation (Table 20-5). The two initial steps are attachment of endometrial cells to the peritoneal surface and invasion of these cells into the mesothelium. Angiogenesis around the nascent implant, endometrial cellular proliferation, and recruitment of inflammatory cells subservient to the implant then become important. It would appear that endometriotic tissues, local immune cells, and inflammatory cytokines mediate each of these steps.

▶ ENDOMETRIOSIS-ASSOCIATED PAIN

Endometriosis-associated pain is among the most challenging conditions in gynecologic practice. Careful evaluation of the patient is paramount to maximize the chance of therapeutic success and minimize the possibility of misdiagnosis. Particular attention should be given to past surgical and medical treatments in planning future management. If the diagnosis of endometriosis is not well established, consideration should be given to laparoscopic evaluation. While a number of medical treatments can effectively suppress endometriosis, they generally have no effect on other potential causes of pelvic pain such as adhesions, adnexal cysts, interstitial cystitis, or inflammatory bowel disease.

It is well established that there is no correlation between pain symptomology and the number of endometriotic lesions.[25,60] In a classic study, Fedele demonstrated that the incidences of dysmenorrhea (70 to 80 percent), dyspareunia (30 percent), and pelvic pain (40 percent) were no different in a group of 68 women with stage I to II endometriosis compared with a group of 92 women with stage III to IV endometriosis. There may be better correlation between pain symptomology and the depth of endometriotic lesions.[25,61,62]

Medical Management of Endometriosis-Associated Pain

The ability of medical therapies to relieve endometriosis-associated pain is related to their capacity to induce amenorrhea.[63] Most hormonal therapies currently used in the treatment of endometriosis-associated pain do this effectively and are equipotent in terms of inducing lesion regression and reducing pain scores.[64–66] The choice of which treatment to use depends primarily on side effects and cost. Progestins generally are the least expensive option, whereas gonadotropin-releasing hormone (GnRH) agonists with immediate add-back therapy offer the most benign side-effect profile (Table 20-6). Considerable effort should be made to anticipate medication side effects and, whenever possible, to mitigate them. For example, use of a progestin-releasing intrauterine device (IUD) decreases the likelihood of systemic side effects from progestins, and initiating a GnRH agonist with immediate add-back therapy significantly reduces the frequency and severity of GnRH agonist–induced vasomotor symptoms.

Oral Contraceptives

Oral contraceptives are used widely in the initial management of endometriosis-associated pain. Oral contraceptives generally are inexpensive, well tolerated, and effective in both reducing and regulating menstrual flow. Despite these attributes, there is a paucity of data critically examining the use of oral contraceptives in women with endometriosis.[67] In a prospective, randomized trial, oral contraceptives were shown to be effective in the treatment of dysmenorrhea, dyspareunia, and pelvic

▶ **TABLE 20-6:** SIDE EFFECTS AND COSTS OF EQUIPOTENT MEDICAL TREATMENTS FOR ENDOMETRIOSIS[66,77,78,82,89,95,96,109,112,241]

	Danazol	Progestins	GnRH Agonists	GnRH Agonists with Add-Back
Hot flashes	50%	—	90%	50%
Acne, oily skin	50%	20%	—	—
Weight gain	50%	50%	—	—
Breakthrough bleeding	40%	70%	25%	25%
Mood changes	20%	10%	10%	10%
Monthly cost (U.S. dollars)	$450	$20–140	$600	$630

Note: Cost estimates are taken from the *Yale Physician Pharmacy,* June 2003.

pain.[68] However, the relief of dysmenorrhea and dyspareunia after 6 months of therapy was less pronounced than in women receiving a GnRH agonist.

Women with endometriosis should use low-dose monophasic oral contraceptives continuously, starting a new pack every 21 days. This method provides constant progestin-mediated suppression of endometrial growth and often induces amenorrhea. Satisfaction rates of 60 to 70 percent have been reported with minimal side effects.[69]

If a 3-month trial of continuous oral contraceptives and a nonsteroidal anti-inflammatory drug (NSAID) is ineffective, then more aggressive hormonal therapy is warranted. There is no evidence that switching from one oral contraceptive or one NSAID to another is beneficial in this setting.

Danazol

Danazol derives its efficacy from its capacity to produce a high-androgen/low-estrogen environment.[70–73] This hormonal profile induces endometrial atrophy both within the uterus and at ectopic sites.[74,75] Danazol also suppresses the midcycle surge of luteinizing hormone (LH) and follicle-stimulating hormone (FSH).[76] As a result, most women using high-dose danazol experience amenorrhea.

Danazol 600 mg/d has been compared favorably with placebo in two small prospective, randomized trials.[77,78] This finding was in keeping with earlier cohort studies reporting symptomatic improvements in 80 to 90 percent of women using danazol 600 to 800 mg/d.[79–81] Not surprisingly, women who develop amenorrhea have the highest response rates.[80] Over the last decade, the use of danazol in North America has been greatly curtailed due to its high cost and significant side-effect profile. Up to 80 percent of women using danazol 600 to 800 mg/d experience major androgenic side effects.[82] For this reason, lower doses of danazol (in the range of 50 to 200 mg qd) have been investigated.[80,83–86] Participants in these studies have reported fewer side effects. However,

most of them continued to menstruate on these dosages, and clinical efficacy rates were between 50 and 75 percent. Because danazol is a potential teratogen, it is important to stress the need for a barrier form of contraception with this therapy.

Progestins

Progestins are as effective as danazol in the treatment of endometriosis-associated pain.[77,78,87–89] The best described is oral medroxyprogesterone acetate (Provera) in doses of 50 to 100 mg/d. An alternate route to oral progestins is intramuscular depot medroxyprogesterone acetate (Depoprovera). Depoprovera is inexpensive, and within 6 to 12 months, most women develop amenorrhea. With high-dose progestins, both eutopic and ectopic endometrial tissue undergoes atrophic changes. Initially, this may lead to breakthrough bleeding. Other side effects include fluid retention, weight gain, breast tenderness, and mood changes.[77,87]

The levonorgestrel-releasing IUD may be an effective alternative to systemic progestins for women with endometriosis-associated pain. Because progestin levels are concentrated locally within the pelvis, therapeutic efficacy can be maximized while minimizing side effects. Recently, two small studies have investigated its potential in women with endometriosis-associated pain.[90,91] Both studies reported excellent patient satisfaction rates (85 to 95 percent) and significant reductions in pain scores. The levonorgestrel IUD may be particularly appropriate for women with endometriosis of the rectovaginal septum.[91]

Gonadotropin-Releasing Hormone (GnRH) Agonists

Depot GnRH agonists are used widely in the treatment of endometriosis-associated pain. After an initial gonadotropin flare, they induce pituitary downregulation and hypoestrogenism.[92] There is no therapeutic advantage of one GnRH agonist over another.[93,94] Two randomized, placebo-controlled, double-blind trials have demonstrated significant improvements in pain with the use of GnRH agonists compared with placebo.[95,96] In one study, 77 percent of the participants assigned to placebo withdrew because of worsening pain, whereas 94 percent of the women assigned the GnRH agonist were satisfied with the treatment.[95] Numerous randomized trials have compared the efficacy of GnRH agonists with that of danazol.[97–108] In every case, GnRH agonists and danazol were equivalent at reducing pain.

Side effects of GnRH agonists are related to hypoestrogenism. Between 80 and 90 percent of women experience hot flashes.[95,109] GnRH agonists also have adverse effects on bone density and lipid profiles. The average loss of bone density after a 6-month course of a GnRH agonist is 4 to 6 percent. Although most women regain any losses in bone density when the treatment is stopped, the use of a GnRH agonist without add-back therapy is limited to a maximum of 6 months. Add-back therapy relies on the hierarchy of end-organ responses to estrogen. The threshold estrogen level that accompanies hot flashes and bone loss usually is lower than the threshold estrogen level that stimulates endometriosis implants.[110] Thus one may add back sufficient amounts of estrogen to alleviate hypoestrogenic side effects without compromising the efficacy of the GnRH agonist. Simple add-back regimens that have been proven to preserve bone density for up to 1 year of continuous GnRH agonist use include norethindrone acetate 5 mg/d, with or without 0.625 mg conjugated equine estrogen.[111,112] Numerous studies have demonstrated equivalent clinical efficacy between GnRH agonists used alone and GnRH agonists combined with immediate add-back therapy.[112–116] The immediate introduction of add-back therapy does not compromise pain relief but does significantly reduce vasomotor symptoms and bone loss.

Other Medical Treatments

The antiprogestin RU-486 (mifepristone) has potential applications for women with en-

dometriosis because it inhibits ovulation and disrupts endometrial integrity. In small, open-label cohort studies, mifepristone doses between 50 and 100 mg/d induced amenorrhea (without hypoestrogenism) and lowered pain scores.[117,118] Nevertheless, to date, mifepristone has not been used widely for the treatment of endometriosis-associated pain. Although not available in the United States, gestrinone has been used successfully in Europe. Gestrinone is derived from a 19-nortestosterone steroid nucleus and bears many similarities to danazol. Gestrinone has both antiestrogen and antiprogesterone effects on the endometrium. Like danazol, it results in endometrial atrophy and amenorrhea.[119] Several large, randomized trials have demonstrated equivalent efficacy for gestrinone (2.5 mg twice a week) compared with either danazol[120,121] or a GnRH agonist.[122,123] The side effects of gestrinone are also similar to those of danazol (i.e., acne, hirsutism, hot flashes).

Future Medical Treatments

Among the most promising novel strategies for the treatment of endometriosis are aromatase inhibitors and immune system modulators. Aromatase converts C_{19} androgens to estrogens. Although normal endometrium does not express aromatase, endometriosis implants have this capacity and thus may generate the fuel that sustains their existence. Local estrogen also stimulates prostaglandin E_2, which, in turn, stimulates aromatase activity, creating a positive-feedback loop within the lesions.[124] Complicating matters, deficient 17β-hydroxysteroid dehydrogenase in endometriosis implants impairs inactivation of estradiol to estrone.[125] Clinical trials are currently in progress to assess if aromatase inhibitors will benefit premenopausal women with endometriosis. Studies in animal models have shown promise, with near-total resolution of endometriotic nodules.[126] Aromatase inhibitors are already the treatment of choice in postmenopausal women because estrogen in these women is predominantly derived from the peripheral conversion of androgens.[127]

Immune system modulators provide another potential treatment approach. Endometriosis is characterized by amplified secretion of cytokines and growth factors. Among these is tumor necrosis factor α (TNF-α). In animals, pentoxifylline (an anti-TNF therapy) has been shown to reverse endometriosis-associated infertility and induce lesion regression.[128,129] A small pilot study in women with endometriosis-associated infertility also suggested benefit.[130] As our understanding of the pathophysiology of endometriosis improves, one anticipates greater interest in potential applications of immune system modulators to women with endometriosis.

Longevity of Medical Treatment Effects

Between 80 and 90 percent of women treated with current medical treatments experience reductions in pain and decreases in endometriotic implants. However, there is a widely held belief that hormonal therapies result in permanent destruction of endometriosis implants. On the contrary, evidence suggests that endometriosis implants often resume functioning after cessation of treatment.[96,131] A prospective study comparing danazol with GnRH agonists reported that only 4 to 18 percent of biopsies from previously identified endometriotic lesions demonstrated complete resolution of endometriosis.[97] In short, hormonal treatment is suppressive therapy, not extirpative therapy.[132]

The length of time to recurrence of pain after cessation of medical therapy is variable. Recurrence rates between 30 and 70 percent have been reported.[79,80,83,84,95,101,109,133] The mean length of time to symptom recurrence generally is between 6 and 18 months.[83,95,101,133,134]

Suggested Approach to Medical Treatment

Typically, continuous low-dose oral contraceptives and NSAIDs are first-line therapy because of their mild side effects and low cost (Table 20-7). If adequate relief is not obtained, one should consider progestins (oral, intramuscu-

▶ **TABLE 20-7:** RECOMMENDED APPROACH TO THE TREATMENT OF ENDOMETRIOSIS-ASSOCIATED PAIN

First line: Continuous low-dose monophasic oral contraceptive with nonsteroidal anti-inflammatories
Second line: Progestins (oral, depo, or IUD)
Third line: GnRH agonist with immediate add-back therapy
Fourth line: Repeat surgery, followed by 1, 2, or 3

lar, or IUD) or a GnRH agonist with immediate add-back therapy. Progestins are less expensive, but GnRH agonists with add-back may be better tolerated. If none of these medications proves beneficial, or if side effects prove intolerable, then surgery is indicated for analgesic value and to reconfirm the diagnosis.

Surgical Management of Endometriosis-Associated Pain

Surgical treatment of endometriosis-associated pain may be either conservative (fertility preserving) or definitive (removing the uterus and ovaries). In either case, an attempt should be made to excise or ablate all suspected areas of endometriosis. Excision of suspected implants has the advantage of allowing histologic confirmation and may avert incomplete treatment of lesions that are deceptively deep. Whereas in the past many surgeries were done by laparotomy, now most are performed laparoscopically. There is no difference in efficacy between the two types of surgery, but laparoscopy significantly shortens recovery times and is more cost-effective. The magnification and improved visualization attained via laparoscopy also may improve the detection and treatment of endometriotic lesions.

Benefits of conservative laparoscopic surgery in women with endometriosis-associated pain have been documented in a randomized, double-blind, placebo-controlled trial involving

63 women.[135] Visual analogue pain scores were significantly lower after 6 months, and these benefits continued up to 1 year.[136] The optimal conservative treatment strategy for endometriomas is somewhat controversial. Beretta and colleagues conducted a prospective, randomized trial in 64 women comparing fenestration and bipolar coagulation of the inner cyst wall with cystectomy.[137] Significantly lower rates of symptom recurrence were reported for women who underwent cystectomy. However, other surgeons have reported excellent patient satisfaction rates and significant reductions in pain scores using fenestration techniques.[138]

In women who no longer desire childbearing and in whom all other treatments have failed, definitive surgery may be appropriate. Traditionally, this has implied total abdominal hysterectomy and bilateral salpingo-oophorectomy, but less invasive approaches are now available using laparoscopy. The relative importance of hysterectomy versus bilateral oophorectomy has been the subject of some debate. In a retrospective analysis, the recurrence of pain and the need for reoperation were significantly higher in women who underwent hysterectomy alone versus women who underwent hysterectomy with bilateral oophorectomy.[139] Moreover, most of the women whose symptoms recurred after bilateral oophorectomy were on estrogen-replacement therapy. The risk of symptom recurrence with estrogen-replacement therapy (10 percent) does not appear to be lowered by delaying the initiation of replacement therapy for 6 weeks after surgery.[140] A better approach after bilateral oophorectomy may be the use of selective estrogen receptor modulators (SERMs) or bisphosphonates to prevent early-onset osteoporosis.[141]

Several adjunctive surgical procedures have been described for women with endometriosis-associated pain. These include laparoscopic uterosacral nerve ablation (LUNA) and presacral neurectomy. There is no compelling evidence that LUNA improves pain relief beyond that achieved by endometriosis surgery alone.[142] Conversely, presacral neurectomy has been reported in prospective clinical trials to benefit women with significant midline dysmenorrhea.[143,144] However, presacral neurectomy requires careful patient selection and considerable operative expertise. Proximity to the common iliac vessels can result in significant intraoperative bleeding, and postoperative complications include gastrointestinal and urinary disorders.

Role of Medical Treatments after Conservative Surgery for Endometriosis-Associated Pain

Several studies have shown that a 3-month course of postoperative medical treatment (e.g., danazol, GnRH agonists) does not delay the recurrence of endometriosis-associated pain.[145–147] However, other studies have clearly demonstrated that postoperative therapies continued for 6 months or more extend pain relief and reduce the need for future surgery.[78,86,134,148] Given the risks of surgery and the frequency with which endometriosis-associated pain recurs, it would seem prudent to administer medical therapy postoperatively, assuming that treatment is well tolerated.

▶ ENDOMETRIOSIS-ASSOCIATED INFERTILITY

The association between endometriosis and infertility is controversial. Although advanced stages of endometriosis may manifest easily recognizable infertility factors, such as tubal distortion/obstruction, the mechanisms underlying reproductive dysfunction in women with minimal or mild endometriosis are less clear. Some of the difficulties in understanding the true relationship between endometriosis and infertility derive from poor study designs, small numbers of participants, and nonstandardized criteria for subject selection. Another significant problem is that many studies do not factor the impact of prior surgical treatments, such as cystectomy/oophorectomy, into their analysis.

Does Minimal to Mild Endometriosis Cause Infertility?

Both clinical research and basic science research have been hampered by the lack of an accurate, minimally invasive diagnostic test for endometriosis. Because of this, the true prevalence of endometriosis in women of reproductive age is unknown. Our epidemiologic data are derived primarily from three different surgical sources—women undergoing tubal ligation, women with pelvic pain, and women with infertility. The reported incidence of endometriosis in women undergoing laparoscopy for the evaluation of infertility is 20 to 50 percent, with most women having minimal to mild disease.[149–152] These figures traditionally have been compared with those of women undergoing tubal ligation, where endometriosis is typically found in 1 to 5 percent of cases. This gross disparity in prevalence between the two groups is one of the foundations of the idea that minimal to mild endometriosis causes infertility.

Other core evidence for a relationship between minimal to mild endometriosis and infertility is derived from animal models and donor insemination cycles. In mice and rabbits, the injection of peritoneal fluid from women with endometriosis lowers implantation rates.[153,154] Similarly, surgical implantation of endometrial tissue into the peritoneal cavity of rats and rabbits lowers fecundity rates.[153,155–157] In human studies, some, but not all, investigators have reported reduced fecundity rates in women with endometriosis undergoing donor insemination.[158–161]

This evidence is opposed by questions regarding the true prevalence of endometriosis in reproductive-age women. Fertile women undergoing tubal ligation are not an ideal control group. Many of these women are recently postpartum and/or discontinuing hormonal contraceptive therapies. In either case, the hormonal milieu would be expected to suppress endometriosis development. Compounding matters, a detection bias between performance of a tubal ligation and the more thorough evaluation of a woman with infertility may lead to underreporting of endometriosis in control populations. Recently, a study accounted for these potential confounding factors by comparing the incidence of endometriosis in women with unexplained infertility with the incidence of endometriosis in women whose partners had azoospermia.[162] Endometriosis was found in 35 percent of infertile women whose partner had a normal semen analysis ($n = 750$) and in 32 percent of women whose cause for infertility was entirely explainable by the partner's lack of sperm ($n = 150$). Other factors against endometriosis as a cause of infertility include the lack of correlation between endometriosis staging and fertility, the inability of hormonal-suppressive therapies to improve natural conception rates, and the observation that endometriosis detected in women with infertility may improve spontaneously or even resolve completely on second-look laparoscopy.[25,26,163]

Potential Mechanisms for Endometriosis-Associated Infertility

Aside from cases of tubal obstruction/distortion, virtually every other aspect of reproduction in women with endometriosis has been investigated and purported to be impaired.[164] Generally, the reported reproductive defects may be classified into four categories (Table 20-8). These include the inflammatory milieu and defects in oocyte quality, fertilization, and implantation.

Oocyte Quality
Several studies have demonstrated decreased ovarian reserve in women with endometriosis.[165–167] Independent of age, increasing stages of endometriosis have been associated with progressive loss of ovarian reserve.[168–171] However, what is unclear from these data is whether the decline in ovarian reserve is a direct consequence of advanced endometriosis or an iatrogenic sequela of prior surgical interventions.

Recently, it has been suggested that granulosa cell impairments may have a detrimental

▶ **TABLE 20-8:** POTENTIAL FACTORS MEDIATING ENDOMETRIOSIS-ASSOCIATED INFERTILITY

Compromised Oocyte Quality
- Decreased ovarian reserve
- Increased granulosa cell apoptosis
- Altered follicular fluid

Impaired Fertilization
- Increased sperm phagocytosis
- Decreased sperm motility
- Impaired binding sperm to the zona pellucida

Inflammatory Factors in the Peritoneal Fluid
- Embryotoxicity
- Inhibition of fertilization

Implantation Defects
- Decreased integrin $\alpha_v\beta_3$ and LIF
- Decreased *HOX-A10* expression

impact on folliculogenesis in women with endometriosis. Granulosa cells from women with moderate to severe endometriosis demonstrate higher rates of apoptosis than cells obtained from women undergoing in vitro fertilization (IVF) for other reasons.[172] Granulosa cell apoptotic bodies have been shown to predict oocyte quality,[173] and the incidence of apoptotic bodies increases with increasing stages of endometriosis.[169]

Follicular fluid composition is also altered in women with endometriosis. TNF-α and IL-6 levels are elevated, whereas VEGF levels are decreased.[174] Additionally, granulosa cell production of inflammatory cytokines such as IL-1β and IL-8 is increased in women with endometriosis.[175] Follicular fluid TNF-α levels have been correlated with poor-quality oocytes,[176] and it has been speculated that the cytokine-induced proinflammatory milieu may compromise oocyte/embryo quality.[177] If so, impairments in fertilization and implantation could be the result of defects during folliculogenesis.

Fertilization

Endometriosis has been associated with reduced fertilization rates in natural cycles.[178] Spermatozoa incubated in follicular fluid from women with endometriosis demonstrate lower zona binding than spermatozoa incubated in follicular fluid from women with tubal infertility.[179] Additionally, sperm exposed to peritoneal fluid from women with endometriosis perform poorly on zona-free hamster egg sperm penetration assays.[180]

Some,[181–183] but not all,[184,185] investigators have reported reduced fertilization rates in women with endometriosis undergoing IVF. In addition, several studies have suggested that there is an inverse correlation between endometriosis staging and fertilization rates.[186,187] Curiously, an analysis of 980 cases in which intracytoplasmic sperm injection (ICSI) was used for male infertility found no difference in fertilization rates among the 101 women with endometriosis.[166] Clearly, if endometriosis compromises fertilization, these data would suggest that ICSI may overcome this deficit.

Inflammatory Peritoneal Environment

Both serum and peritoneal fluid from infertile women with endometriosis are embryotoxic to two-cell mouse embryos.[188] Interestingly, in this study, serum and peritoneal fluid derived from fertile women with endometriosis or women with unexplained infertility did not demonstrate embryotoxicity. In addition, the presence of macrophages and antibodies in the peritoneal fluid of women with endometriosis may inhibit sperm function.[189–192] However, other investigators have been unable to document impairments in sperm function resulting from exposure to peritoneal fluid from infertile women with endometriosis.[193,194]

Implantation

Several studies have suggested impaired expression of molecular markers of endometrial receptivity in women with endometriosis. In murine models, peritoneal fluid from infertile women with endometriosis decreases implantation rates, as well as markers of endometrial receptivity such as integrin $\alpha_v\beta_3$ and leukemia inhibitory factor.[154] In addition, aberrant expression of *HOXA10* and *HOXA11,* homeobox genes essential for implantation, has been documented in midluteal endometrium of women with endometriosis.[195]

As mentioned previously, decreased implantation rates also could result from impaired oocyte/embryo quality. One method of separating oocyte quality from endometrial receptivity is with analysis of oocyte donation cycles. When oocytes originate from donors with endometriosis, reduced implantation rates and pregnancy rates have been reported.[196] However, when only the oocyte recipient has endometriosis, implantation rates and pregnancy outcomes are normal.[196] This finding was confirmed recently in a study in which oocytes from healthy donors were shared between recipients with and without moderate to severe endometriosis.[197] Oocyte recipients with stage III to IV endometriosis had the same implantation rates as controls. Further confirmation comes from a retrospective analysis of 239 oocyte recipients demonstrating no adverse effects on implantation rates, even when recipients were subdivided by stage of endometriosis.[198] However, it may be prudent to consider the differences between natural cycles and recipient cycles. It is possible that subtle impairments in uterine receptivity relevant to natural cycles may be overcome by the pretreatment of recipients with GnRH agonists and the use of very high quality oocytes.

Traditional Approaches to Fertility Management in Endometriosis

Given the ability of medical treatments to suppress endometriosis, can they be used to enhance fertility in women with endometriosis? Numerous controlled clinical trials have examined the effects of progestins, danazol, and GnRH agonists in women with endometriosis-associated infertility.[199–202] Individually, none of these trials showed a significant benefit, and a metaanalysis of the studies confirms no improvement in the odds ratio of natural conception after the use of hormonal-suppressive therapies.[203] Moreover, studies comparing danazol with other hormonal-suppressive therapies find no advantage of one treatment over another.[101,103,104,107,108,204–206] Possible explanations for the lack of efficacy of hormonal-suppressive treatments in women attempting natural conception include delayed return to ovulatory cycles and rapid recurrence of endometriosis implants with cessation of treatment. Alternatively, the lack of benefit may reflect lack of a causal relationship between endometriosis implants and infertility.

The role of surgical treatments for women with endometriosis-associated infertility also has been studied. Several metanalyses of nonrandomized cohort trials have suggested improved fecundity after surgical intervention.[207,208] However, the heterogeneous nature of the study designs makes interpretation of the results difficult. In women undergoing laparoscopic surgery for moderate to severe endometriosis, postoperative monthly fecundity rates between 2.1 and 3.3 percent have been reported.[209,210] To date, the best study of surgical therapy for women with minimal to mild endometriosis is the ENDO-CAN trial.[211] This multicenter study randomized 241 infertile women at the time of laparoscopy to no further treatment or surgical excision/ablation of endometriosis implants. Women randomized to surgical intervention had a significantly higher pregnancy rate (30.7 percent) than controls (17.7 percent) after 36 weeks of follow-up. The mean monthly fecundity rate also was improved from 2.4 to 4.7 percent. Unfortunately, a similar trial that enrolled 101 infertile women with minimal to mild endometriosis was unable to confirm an improvement in conception rates.[212] It would appear that any increase in monthly fecundity realized by women undergoing surgical treatment for endometriosis is marginal, at best.

Optimal Management of Infertility in Women with Endometriosis

Fertility treatments that offer more impressive improvements in monthly fecundity include controlled ovarian hyperstimulation and IVF. Three randomized, controlled trials have demonstrated benefits of fertility medications in women with endometriosis.[213–215] Controls in these studies attained monthly fecundity rates of 2 to 5 percent, whereas women undergoing superovulation with or without intrauterine insemination had monthly fecundity rates of 10 to 15 percent. Clearly, the per-cycle chance of pregnancy is higher with superovulation treatments compared with surgical interventions. However, this improvement is accompanied by the risks of multiple pregnancy and ovarian hyperstimulation syndrome.

IVF offers the highest per-cycle chance of pregnancy. In general, IVF is reserved for women with endometriosis who have failed surgical treatment and/or superovulation. In the United States, endometriosis accounts for approximately 15 percent of all women undergoing IVF treatment. It appears that the benefits of IVF in women with endometriosis derive from downregulation and the superabundance of oocytes obtained by controlled ovarian stimulation. This may allow for subtle defects in oocyte quality and fertilization to be overcome. Moreover, selection of a sufficient number of high-quality embryos for transfer may compensate for implantation impairments.

The impact of endometriosis on IVF outcomes is controversial.[216] A recent metaanalysis suggested that pregnancy rates for women with endometriosis undergoing IVF are almost 50 percent lower than for women undergoing IVF for other reasons.[217] However, this finding is not supported by data from the Society for Assisted Reproductive Technology (SART).[218,219] Considering virtually all the IVF cycles done in the United States in the years 1997 to 1999, there was no clinically significant difference in the per-cycle chance of pregnancy for women undergoing IVF for endometriosis compared with any other infertility diagnosis. Individually, none of the four largest studies comparing IVF outcomes in women with endometriosis to women with tubal disease found significant differences in per-cycle pregnancy rates.[181,184,220,221]

The beneficial role of GnRH agonists in IVF cycles should not be underestimated. At least six studies have suggested benefits for prolonged downregulation with GnRH agonists in women with endometriosis prior to beginning controlled ovarian hyperstimulation.[222–227] Whether this effect is due to better-quality oocytes or an enhanced implantation milieu is unclear, but the efficacy of a 3-month course of GnRH agonists prior to commencing controlled ovarian hyperstimulation was confirmed recently in a multicenter, prospective, randomized trial.[228]

Finally, the optimal management of endometriomas in women with infertility is controversial. To date, no prospective, randomized trials have compared surgical treatment with superovulation or IVF. Some, but not all, retrospective studies have suggested diminished ovarian responsiveness after surgical treatment.[229–232] In women with adnexal pain, it would appear that conservative ovarian surgery by a skilled operator is unlikely to significantly impair ovarian reserve. Conversely, proceeding directly to superovulation or IVF in women with asymptomatic endometriomas may reduce the time to achieve pregnancy, the costs of treatment, and the potential complications of laparoscopic surgery.

KEY POINTS

1. The definition of endometriosis relies on surgical visualization and histologic confirmation of ectopic endometrial glands and stroma.

2. The exact prevalence of endometriosis is unknown. However, endometriosis is commonly reported in 3 to 5 percent of women undergoing tubal ligation, 40 to 60 percent of women with pelvic pain, and 30 to 40 percent of women with infertility.

3. Current classifications of endometriosis cannot be used to predict the presence of pain or the outcome of fertility treatments.

4. Why endometriosis develops in some women but not others is unknown. One of the critical factors believed to determine the susceptibility to endometriosis is the host immune response.

5. Major alterations in the peritoneal fluid of women with endometriosis include increased macrophages and inflammatory cytokines and decreased NK cell cytotoxicity.

6. Accumulating evidence suggests that cytokines recondition local immune responses in women with endometriosis in a manner favorable to the survival and growth of ectopic endometrial implants.

7. The ability of medical therapies to relieve endometriosis-associated pain is related directly to their capacity to induce amenorrhea.

8. Danazol, progestins, and GnRH agonists (with or without add-back therapy) are of equivalent efficacy. The choice of which to use should be based on consideration of costs and side effects.

9. Effective conservative surgery for endometriosis-associated pain consists of excision/ablation of peritoneal implants and cystectomy for ovarian endometriotic cysts. In women desiring definitive surgery for endometriosis-associated pain, both ovaries should be removed.

10. Surgical treatments for endometriosis-associated infertility provide, at best, marginal improvement in monthly fecundity rates.

11. The success of superovulation and IVF relies on stimulating an ample number of preovulatory follicles in order to overcome potential deficits in oocyte quality, fertilization, and implantation.

12. The role of GnRH agonists in women with endometriosis-associated infertility is evolving. They do not enhance the chance of natural conception. However, a 2- to 3-month course may improve per-cycle pregnancy rates in women undergoing IVF.

REFERENCES

1. Eskenazi B, Warner M, Bonsignore L, et al. Validation study of nonsurgical diagnosis of endometriosis. *Fertil Steril* 2001;76:929.
2. Moen MH, Halvorsen TB. Histologic confirmation of endometriosis in different peritoneal lesions. *Acta Obstet Gynaecol Scand* 1992;71:337.
3. Nisolle M, Paindaveine B, Bourdon A, et al. Histologic study of peritoneal endometriosis in infertile women. *Fertil Steril* 1990;53:984.
4. Jansen RP, Russell P. Nonpigmented endometriosis: Clinical, laparoscopic, and pathologic definition. *Am J Obstet Gynecol* 1986;155:1154.
5. Balasch J, Creus M, Fabregues F, et al. Visible and nonvisible endometriosis at laparoscopy in fertile and infertile women and in patients with chronic pelvic pain: A prospective study. *Hum Reprod* 1996;11:387.
6. Mol BW, Bayram N, Lijmer JG, et al. The performance of CA-125 measurement in the detection of endometriosis: A metaanalysis. *Fertil Steril* 1998;70:1101.
7. Barbieri RL, Niloff JM, Bast RC Jr, et al. Elevated serum concentrations of CA-125 in patients with advanced endometriosis. *Fertil Steril* 1986;45:630.
8. Colacurci N, Fortunato N, De Franciscis P, et al. Relevance of CA-125 in the evaluation of endometriosis. *Clin Exp Obstet Gynecol* 1996;23:150.
9. Chen FP, Soong YK, Lee N, et al. The use of serum CA-125 as a marker for endometriosis in patients with dysmenorrhea for monitoring therapy and for recurrence of endometriosis. *Acta Obstet Gynaecol Scand* 1998;77:665.
10. Fraser IS, McCarron G, Markham R. Serum CA-125 levels in women with endometriosis. *Aust NZ J Obstet Gynaecol* 1989;29:416.

11. Takahashi K, Musa AA, Nagata H, et al. Serum CA-125 and 17β-estradiol in patients with external endometriosis on danazol. *Gynecol Obstet Invest* 1990;29:301.

12. Franssen AM, van der Heijden PF, Thomas CM, et al. On the origin and significance of serum CA-125 concentrations in 97 patients with endometriosis before, during, and after buserelin acetate, nafarelin, or danazol. *Fertil Steril* 1992;57:974.

13. Umaria N, Olliff JF. Imaging features of pelvic endometriosis. *Br J Radiol* 2001;74:556.

14. Dogan MM, Ugur M, Soysal SK, et al. Transvaginal sonographic diagnosis of ovarian endometrioma. *Int J Gynaecol Obstet* 1996;52:145.

15. Kinkel K, Chapron C, Balleyguier C, et al. Magnetic resonance imaging characteristics of deep endometriosis. *Hum Reprod* 1999;14:1080.

16. Zawin M, McCarthy S, Scoutt L, et al. Endometriosis: Appearance and detection at MR imaging. *Radiology* 1989;171:693.

17. Arrive L, Hricak H, Martin MC. Pelvic endometriosis: MR imaging. *Radiology* 1989;171:687.

18. Ha HK, Lim YT, Kim HS, et al. Diagnosis of pelvic endometriosis: Fat-suppressed T_1-weighted versus conventional MR images. *AJR* 1994;163:127.

19. Stratton P, Winkel C, Premkumar A, et al. Diagnostic accuracy of laparoscopy, magnetic resonance imaging, and histopathologic examination for the detection of endometriosis. *Fertil Steril* 2003;79:1078.

20. Noble LS, Simpson ER, Johns A, et al. Aromatase expression in endometriosis. *J Clin Endocrinol Metab* 1996;81:174.

21. Kitawaki J, Noguchi T, Amatsu T, et al. Expression of aromatase cytochrome P450 protein and messenger ribonucleic acid in human endometriotic and adenomyotic tissues but not in normal endometrium. *Biol Reprod* 1997;57:514.

22. Dheenadayalu K, Mak I, Gordts S, et al. Aromatase P450 messenger RNA expression in eutopic endometrium is not a specific marker for pelvic endometriosis. *Fertil Steril* 2002;78:825.

23. Medicine ASfR. Revised American Society for Reproductive Medicine classification of endometriosis: 1996. *Fertil Steril* 1997;67:817.

24. Hornstein MD, Gleason RE, Orav J, et al. The reproducibility of the revised American Fertility Society classification of endometriosis. *Fertil Steril* 1993;59:1015.

25. Fedele L, Parazzini F, Bianchi S, et al. Stage and localization of pelvic endometriosis and pain. *Fertil Steril* 1990;53:155.

26. Guzick DS, Silliman NP, Adamson GD, et al. Prediction of pregnancy in infertile women based on the American Society for Reproductive Medicine's revised classification of endometriosis. *Fertil Steril* 1997;67:822.

27. Sampson J. Peritoneal endometriosis due to the menstrual dissemination of endometrial tissue into the peritoneal cavity. *Am J Obstet Gynecol* 1927;14:422.

28. Suginami H. A reappraisal of the coelomic metaplasia theory by reviewing endometriosis occurring in unusual sites and instances. *Am J Obstet Gynecol* 1991;165:214.

29. Oliker AJ, Harris AE. Endometriosis of the bladder in a male patient. *J Urol* 1971;106:858.

30. Schrodt GR, Alcorn MO, Ibanez J. Endometriosis of the male urinary system: A case report. *J Urol* 1980;124:722.

31. Schifrin BS, Erez S, Moore JG. Teenage endometriosis. *Am J Obstet Gynecol* 1973;116:973.

32. El-Mahgoub S, Yaseen S. A positive proof for the theory of coelomic metaplasia. *Am J Obstet Gynecol* 1980;137:137.

33. Hadfield RM, Mardon HJ, Barlow DH, et al. Endometriosis in monozygotic twins. *Fertil Steril* 1997;68:941.

34. Moen MH. Endometriosis in monozygotic twins. *Acta Obstet Gynaecol Scand* 1994;73:59.

35. Simpson JL, Elias S, Malinak LR, et al. Heritable aspects of endometriosis: I. Genetic studies. *Am J Obstet Gynecol* 1980;137:327.

36. Lamb K, Hoffmann RG, Nichols TR. Family trait analysis: A case-control study of 43 women with endometriosis and their best friends. *Am J Obstet Gynecol* 1986;154:596.

37. Moen MH, Magnus P. The familial risk of endometriosis. *Acta Obstet Gynaecol Scand* 1993;72:560.

38. Stefansson H, Geirsson RT, Steinthorsdottir V, et al. Genetic factors contribute to the risk of developing endometriosis. *Hum Reprod* 2002;17:555.

39. Halme J, Becker S, Hammond MG, et al. Increased activation of pelvic macrophages in infertile women with mild endometriosis. *Am J Obstet Gynecol* 1983;145:333.

40. Zeller JM, Henig I, Radwanska E, et al. Enhancement of human monocyte and peritoneal

macrophage chemiluminescence activities in women with endometriosis. *Am J Reprod Immunol Microbiol* 1987;13:78.

41. Hill JA, Faris HM, Schiff I, et al. Characterization of leukocyte subpopulations in the peritoneal fluid of women with endometriosis. *Fertil Steril* 1988;50:216.

42. Dmowski WP, Gebel HM, Braun DP. The role of cell-mediated immunity in pathogenesis of endometriosis. *Acta Obstet Gynaecol Scand* Suppl 1994;159:7.

43. Braun DP, Muriana A, Gebel H, et al. Monocyte-mediated enhancement of endometrial cell proliferation in women with endometriosis. *Fertil Steril* 1994;61:78.

44. Oosterlynck DJ, Cornillie FJ, Waer M, et al. Women with endometriosis show a defect in natural killer activity resulting in a decreased cytotoxicity to autologous endometrium. *Fertil Steril* 1991;56:45.

45. Wilson TJ, Hertzog PJ, Angus D, et al. Decreased natural killer cell activity in endometriosis patients: Relationship to disease pathogenesis. *Fertil Steril* 1994;62:1086.

46. Oosterlynck DJ, Meuleman C, Waer M, et al. Immunosuppressive activity of peritoneal fluid in women with endometriosis. *Obstet Gynecol* 1993;82:206.

47. Kanzaki H, Wang HS, Kariya M, et al. Suppression of natural killer cell activity by sera from patients with endometriosis. *Am J Obstet Gynecol* 1992;167:257.

48. Ho HN, Chao KH, Chen HF, et al. Peritoneal natural killer cytotoxicity and CD25+ CD3+ lymphocyte subpopulation are decreased in women with stage III–IV endometriosis. *Hum Reprod* 1995;10:2671.

49. Arici A. Local cytokines in endometrial tissue: The role of interleukin-8 in the pathogenesis of endometriosis. *Ann NY Acad Sci* 2002;955:101.

50. Akoum A, Lawson C, McColl S, et al. Ectopic endometrial cells express high concentrations of interleukin 8 (IL-8) in vivo regardless of the menstrual cycle phase and respond to oestradiol by up-regulating IL-1-induced IL-8 expression in vitro. *Mol Hum Reprod* 2001;7:859.

51. Arici A, Seli E, Senturk LM, et al. Interleukin-8 in the human endometrium. *J Clin Endocrinol Metab* 1998;83:1783.

52. Garcia-Velasco JA, Arici A. Interleukin-8 stimulates the adhesion of endometrial stromal cells to fibronectin. *Fertil Steril* 1999;72:336.

53. McLaren J, Prentice A, Charnock-Jones DS, et al. Vascular endothelial growth factor is produced by peritoneal fluid macrophages in endometriosis and is regulated by ovarian steroids. *J Clin Invest* 1996;98:482.

54. Taylor RN, Lebovic DI, Mueller MD. Angiogenic factors in endometriosis. *Ann NY Acad Sci* 2002;955:89.

55. Arici A, Seli E, Zeyneloglu HB, et al. Interleukin-8 induces proliferation of endometrial stromal cells: A potential autocrine growth factor. *J Clin Endocrinol Metab* 1998;83:1201.

56. Kwak JY, Park SW, Kim KH, et al. Modulation of neutrophil apoptosis by plasma and peritoneal fluid from patients with advanced endometriosis. *Hum Reprod* 2002;17:595.

57. Kats R, Metz CN, Akoum A. Macrophage migration inhibitory factor is markedly expressed in active and early-stage endometriotic lesions. *J Clin Endocrinol Metab* 2002;87:883.

58. Apte RS, Sinha D, Mayhew E, et al. Cutting edge: Role of macrophage migration inhibitory factor in inhibiting NK cell activity and preserving immune privilege. *J Immunol* 1998;160:5693.

59. Repp AC, Mayhew ES, Apte S, et al. Human uveal melanoma cells produce macrophage migration-inhibitory factor to prevent lysis by NK cells. *J Immunol* 2000;165:710.

60. Vercellini P, Trespidi L, De Giorgi O, et al. Endometriosis and pelvic pain: Relation to disease stage and localization. *Fertil Steril* 1996;65:299.

61. Koninckx PR, Meuleman C, Demeyere S, et al. Suggestive evidence that pelvic endometriosis is a progressive disease, whereas deeply infiltrating endometriosis is associated with pelvic pain. *Fertil Steril* 1991;55:759.

62. Chapron C, Fauconnier A, Dubuisson JB, et al. Deep infiltrating endometriosis: Relation between severity of dysmenorrhea and extent of disease. *Hum Reprod* 2003;18:760.

63. Mahutte NG, Arici A. Medical management of endometriosis-associated pain. *Obstet Gynecol Clin North Am* 2003;30:133.

64. Olive DL, Pritts EA. The treatment of endometriosis: A review of the evidence. *Ann NY Acad Sci* 2002;955:360.

65. Child TJ, Tan SL. Endometriosis: Aetiology, pathogenesis and treatment. *Drugs* 2001;61:1735.

66. Prentice A, Deary AJ, Goldbeck-Wood S, et al. Gonadotrophin-releasing hormone analogues for pain associated with endometriosis. *Cochrane Database Syst Rev* 2000;CD000346.

67. Moore J, Kennedy S, Prentice A. Modern combined oral contraceptives for pain associated with endometriosis. *Cochrane Database Syst Rev* 2000;CD001019.

68. Vercellini P, Trespidi L, Colombo A, et al. A gonadotropin-releasing hormone agonist versus a low-dose oral contraceptive for pelvic pain associated with endometriosis. *Fertil Steril* 1993;60:75.

69. Vercellini P, De Giorgi O, Mosconi P, et al. Cyproterone acetate versus a continuous monophasic oral contraceptive in the treatment of recurrent pelvic pain after conservative surgery for symptomatic endometriosis. *Fertil Steril* 2002;77:52.

70. Selak V, Farquhar C, Prentice A, et al: Danazol for pelvic pain associated with endometriosis. *Cochrane Database Syst Rev* 2001;CD000068.

71. Telimaa S, Apter D, Reinila M, et al. Placebo-controlled comparison of hormonal and biochemical effects of danazol and high-dose medroxyprogesterone acetate. *Eur J Obstet Gynecol Reprod Biol* 1990;36:97.

72. Luciano AA, Hauser KS, Chapler FK, et al. Danazol: Endocrine consequences in healthy women. *Am J Obstet Gynecol* 1981;141:723.

73. Steingold KA, Lu JK, Judd HL, et al. Danazol inhibits steroidogenesis by the human ovary in vivo. *Fertil Steril* 1986;45:649.

74. Fedele L, Marchini M, Bianchi S, et al. Endometrial patterns during danazol and buserelin therapy for endometriosis: Comparative structural and ultrastructural study. *Obstet Gynecol* 1990;76:79.

75. Sakata M, Terakawa N, Mizutani T, et al. Effects of danazol, gonadotropin-releasing hormone agonist, and a combination of danazol and gonadotropin-releasing hormone agonist on experimental endometriosis. *Am J Obstet Gynecol* 1990;163:1679.

76. Barbieri RL, Ryan KJ. Danazol: Endocrine pharmacology and therapeutic applications. *Am J Obstet Gynecol* 1981;141:453.

77. Telimaa S, Puolakka J, Ronnberg L, et al. Placebo-controlled comparison of danazol and high-dose medroxyprogesterone acetate in the treatment of endometriosis. *Gynecol Endocrinol* 1987;1:13.

78. Telimaa S, Ronnberg L, Kauppila A. Placebo-controlled comparison of danazol and high-dose medroxyprogesterone acetate in the treatment of endometriosis after conservative surgery. *Gynecol Endocrinol* 1987;1:363.

79. Barbieri RL, Evans S, Kistner RW. Danazol in the treatment of endometriosis: Analysis of 100 cases with a 4-year follow-up. *Fertil Steril* 1982;37:737.

80. Moore EE, Harger JH, Rock JA, et al. Management of pelvic endometriosis with low-dose danazol. *Fertil Steril* 1981;36:15.

81. Buttram VC Jr, Reiter RC, Ward S. Treatment of endometriosis with danazol: Report of a 6-year prospective study. *Fertil Steril* 1985;43:353.

82. Selak V, Farquhar C, Prentice A, et al. Danazol for pelvic pain associated with endometriosis. *Cochrane Database Syst Rev* 2000;CD000068.

83. Biberoglu KO, Behrman SJ. Dosage aspects of danazol therapy in endometriosis: Short-term and long-term effectiveness. *Am J Obstet Gynecol* 1981;139:645.

84. Dmowski WP, Kapetanakis E, Scommegna A. Variable effects of danazol on endometriosis at 4 low-dose levels. *Obstet Gynecol* 1982;59:408.

85. Vercellini P, Trespidi L, Panazza S, et al. Very low dose danazol for relief of endometriosis-associated pelvic pain: A pilot study. *Fertil Steril* 1994;62:1136.

86. Morgante G, Ditto A, La Marca A, et al. Low-dose danazol after combined surgical and medical therapy reduces the incidence of pelvic pain in women with moderate and severe endometriosis. *Hum Reprod* 1999;14:2371.

87. Vercellini P, Cortesi I, Crosignani PG. Progestins for symptomatic endometriosis: A critical analysis of the evidence. *Fertil Steril* 1997;68:393.

88. Luciano AA, Turksoy RN, Carleo J. Evaluation of oral medroxyprogesterone acetate in the treatment of endometriosis. *Obstet Gynecol* 1988;72:323.

89. Prentice A, Deary AJ, Bland E. Progestagens and anti-progestagens for pain associated with endometriosis. *Cochrane Database Syst Rev* 2000;CD002122.

90. Vercellini P, Aimi G, Panazza S, et al. A levonorgestrel-releasing intrauterine system for

the treatment of dysmenorrhea associated with endometriosis: A pilot study. *Fertil Steril* 1999; 72:505.

91. Fedele L, Bianchi S, Zanconato G, et al. Use of a levonorgestrel-releasing intrauterine device in the treatment of rectovaginal endometriosis. *Fertil Steril* 2001;75:485.

92. Belchetz PE, Plant TM, Nakai Y, et al. Hypophysial responses to continuous and intermittent delivery of hypopthalamic gonadotropin-releasing hormone. *Science* 1978;202:631.

93. Agarwal SK, Hamrang C, Henzl MR, et al. Nafarelin versus leuprolide acetate depot for endometriosis: Changes in bone mineral density and vasomotor symptoms. Nafarelin Study Group. *J Reprod Med* 1997;42:413.

94. Bergqvist A. A comparative study of the acceptability and effect of goserelin and nafarelin on endometriosis. *Gynecol Endocrinol* 2000; 14:425.

95. Dlugi AM, Miller JD, Knittle J. Lupron depot (leuprolide acetate for depot suspension) in the treatment of endometriosis: A randomized, placebo-controlled, double-blind study. Lupron Study Group. *Fertil Steril* 1990;54:419.

96. Bergqvist A, Bergh T, Hogstrom L, et al. Effects of triptorelin versus placebo on the symptoms of endometriosis. *Fertil Steril* 1998;69:702.

97. Bulletti C, Flamigni C, Polli V, et al: The efficacy of drugs in the management of endometriosis. *J Am Assoc Gynecol Laparosc* 1996;3:495.

98. Cirkel U, Ochs H, Schneider HP. A randomized, comparative trial of triptorelin depot (D-Trp6-LHRH) and danazol in the treatment of endometriosis. *Eur J Obstet Gynecol Reprod Biol* 1995;59:61.

99. Adamson GD, Kwei L, Edgren RA. Pain of endometriosis: Effects of nafarelin and danazol therapy. *Int J Fertil Menopaus Stud* 1994;39:215.

100. Rock JA, Truglia JA, Caplan RJ. Zoladex (goserelin acetate implant) in the treatment of endometriosis: A randomized comparison with danazol. The Zoladex Endometriosis Study Group. *Obstet Gynecol* 1993;82:198.

101. Nafarelin European Endometriosis Trial Group (NEET). Nafarelin for endometriosis: A large-scale, danazol-controlled trial of efficacy and safety, with 1-year follow-up. *Fertil Steril* 1992; 57:514.

102. Wheeler JM, Knittle JD, Miller JD. Depot leuprolide versus danazol in treatment of women with symptomatic endometriosis: I. Efficacy results. *Am J Obstet Gynecol* 1992;167:1367.

103. Shaw RW. An open randomized comparative study of the effect of goserelin depot and danazol in the treatment of endometriosis. Zoladex Endometriosis Study Team. *Fertil Steril* 1992;58: 265.

104. Fraser IS, Shearman RP, Jansen RP, et al. A comparative treatment trial of endometriosis using the gonadotrophin-releasing hormone agonist, nafarelin, and the synthetic steroid, danazol. *Aust NZ J Obstet Gynaecol* 1991;31:158.

105. Shaw RW. Nafarelin in the treatment of pelvic pain caused by endometriosis. *Am J Obstet Gynecol* 1990;162:574.

106. Trabant H, Widdra W, de Looze S. Efficacy and safety of intranasal buserelin acetate in the treatment of endometriosis: A review of six clinical trials and comparison with danazol. *Prog Clin Biol Res* 1990;323:357.

107. Fedele L, Bianchi S, Arcaini L, et al. Buserelin versus danazol in the treatment of endometriosis-associated infertility. *Am J Obstet Gynecol* 1989; 161:871.

108. Henzl MR, Corson SL, Moghissi K, et al. Administration of nasal nafarelin as compared with oral danazol for endometriosis: A multicenter double-blind comparative clinical trial. *N Engl J Med* 1988;318:485.

109. Fedele L, Bianchi S, Bocciolone L, et al. Buserelin acetate in the treatment of pelvic pain associated with minimal and mild endometriosis: a controlled study. *Fertil Steril* 1993;59:516.

110. Barbieri RL. Hormone treatment of endometriosis: The estrogen threshold hypothesis. *Am J Obstet Gynecol* 1992;166:740.

111. Surrey ES, Hornstein MD. Prolonged GnRH agonist and add-back therapy for symptomatic endometriosis: Long-term follow-up. *Obstet Gynecol* 2002;99:709.

112. Hornstein MD, Surrey ES, Weisberg GW, et al. Leuprolide acetate depot and hormonal add-back in endometriosis: A 12-month study. Lupron Add-Back Study Group. *Obstet Gynecol* 1998;91:16.

113. Franke HR, van de Weijer PH, Pennings TM, et al. Gonadotropin-releasing hormone agonist plus "add-back" hormone replacement therapy for treatment of endometriosis: A prospective, randomized, placebo-controlled, double-blind trial. *Fertil Steril* 2000;74:534.

114. Gregoriou O, Konidaris S, Vitoratos N, et al. Gonadotropin-releasing hormone analogue plus hormone replacement therapy for the treatment of endometriosis: A randomized, controlled trial. *Int J Fertil Womens Med* 1997;42:406.

115. Kiilholma P, Tuimala R, Kivinen S, et al. Comparison of the gonadotropin-releasing hormone agonist goserelin acetate alone versus goserelin combined with estrogen-progestogen add-back therapy in the treatment of endometriosis. *Fertil Steril* 1995;64:903.

116. Kiesel L, Schweppe KW, Sillem M, et al. Should add-back therapy for endometriosis be deferred for optimal results? *Br J Obstet Gynaecol* 1996; 103:15.

117. Kettel LM, Murphy AA, Morales AJ, et al. Treatment of endometriosis with the antiprogesterone mifepristone (RU486). *Fertil Steril* 1996; 65:23.

118. Kettel LM, Murphy AA, Morales AJ, et al. Clinical efficacy of the antiprogesterone RU486 in the treatment of endometriosis and uterine fibroids. *Hum Reprod* 1994;9:116.

119. Marchini M, Fedele L, Bianchi S, et al. Endometrial patterns during therapy with danazol or gestrinone for endometriosis: Structural and ultrastructural study. *Hum Pathol* 1992; 23:51.

120. Halbe HW, Nakamura MS, Da Silveira GP, et al. Updating the clinical experience in endometriosis: The Brazilian perspective. *Br J Obstet Gynaecol* 1995;102:17.

121. Bromham DR, Booker MW, Rose GL, et al. Updating the clinical experience in endometriosis: The European perspective. *Br J Obstet Gynaecol* 1995;102:12.

122. Gestrinone Italian Study Group. Gestrinone versus a gonadotropin-releasing hormone agonist for the treatment of pelvic pain associated with endometriosis: A multicenter, randomized, double-blind study. *Fertil Steril* 1996;66:911.

123. Nieto A, Tacuri C, Serra M, et al. Long-term follow-up of endometriosis after two different therapies (Gestrinone and Buserelin). *Clin Exp Obstet Gynecol* 1996; 23:198.

124. Bulun SE, Zeitoun KM, Takayama K, et al. Molecular basis for treating endometriosis with aromatase inhibitors. *Hum Reprod Update* 2000; 6:413.

125. Bulun SE, Zeitoun KM, Takayama K, et al. Estrogen biosynthesis in endometriosis: Molecular basis and clinical relevance. *J Mol Endocrinol* 2000;25:35.

126. Fang Z, Yang S, Gurates B, et al. Genetic or enzymatic disruption of aromatase inhibits the growth of ectopic uterine tissue. *J Clin Endocrinol Metab* 2002;87:3460.

127. Takayama K, Zeitoun K, Gunby RT, et al. Treatment of severe postmenopausal endometriosis with an aromatase inhibitor. *Fertil Steril* 1998; 69:709.

128. Steinleitner A, Lambert H, Suarez M, et al. Immunomodulation in the treatment of endometriosis-associated subfertility: Use of pentoxifylline to reverse the inhibition of fertilization by surgically induced endometriosis in a rodent model. *Fertil Steril* 1991;56:975.

129. Nothnick WB, Curry TE, Vernon MW. Immunomodulation of rat endometriotic implant growth and protein production. *Am J Reprod Immunol* 1994;31:151.

130. Balasch J, Creus M, Fabregues F, et al. Pentoxifylline versus placebo in the treatment of infertility associated with minimal or mild endometriosis: A pilot randomized clinical trial. *Hum Reprod* 1997;12:2046.

131. Revelli A, Modotti M, Ansaldi C, et al. Recurrent endometriosis: A review of biological and clinical aspects. *Obstet Gynecol Surv* 1995; 50:747.

132. Brosens IA, Verleyen A, Cornillie F. The morphologic effect of short-term medical therapy of endometriosis. *Am J Obstet Gynecol* 1987;157: 1215.

133. Miller JD, Shaw RW, Casper RF, et al. Historical prospective cohort study of the recurrence of pain after discontinuation of treatment with danazol or a gonadotropin-releasing hormone agonist. *Fertil Steril* 1998;70:293.

134. Hornstein MD, Hemmings R, Yuzpe AA, et al. Use of nafarelin versus placebo after reductive laparoscopic surgery for endometriosis. *Fertil Steril* 1997;68:860.

135. Sutton CJ, Ewen SP, Whitelaw N, et al. Prospective, randomized, double-blind, controlled trial of laser laparoscopy in the treatment of pelvic pain associated with minimal, mild, and moderate endometriosis. *Fertil Steril* 1994;62: 696.

136. Sutton CJ, Pooley AS, Ewen SP, et al. Follow-up report on a randomized, controlled trial of laser laparoscopy in the treatment of pelvic

pain associated with minimal to moderate endometriosis. *Fertil Steril* 1997;68:1070.

137. Beretta P, Franchi M, Ghezzi F, et al. Randomized clinical trial of two laparoscopic treatments of endometriomas: Cystectomy versus drainage and coagulation. *Fertil Steril* 1998;70:1176.

138. Jones KD, Sutton C. Patient satisfaction and changes in pain scores after ablative laparoscopic surgery for stage III–IV endometriosis and endometriotic cysts. *Fertil Steril* 2003;79:1086.

139. Namnoum AB, Hickman TN, Goodman SB, et al. Incidence of symptom recurrence after hysterectomy for endometriosis. *Fertil Steril* 1995;64:898.

140. Hickman TN, Namnoum AB, Hinton EL, et al. Timing of estrogen replacement therapy following hysterectomy with oophorectomy for endometriosis. *Obstet Gynecol* 1998;91:673.

141. Evans A, Vollenhoven B, Healy D. Modern antioestrogens and the coming revolution in women's health care. *Aust NZ J Obstet Gynaecol* 1999;39:334.

142. Wilson ML, Farquhar CM, Sinclair OJ, et al. Surgical interruption of pelvic nerve pathways for primary and secondary dysmenorrhea. *Cochrane Database Syst Rev* 2000;CD001896.

143. Candiani GB, Fedele L, Vercellini P, et al. Presacral neurectomy for the treatment of pelvic pain associated with endometriosis: A controlled study. *Am J Obstet Gynecol* 1992;167:100.

144. Tjaden B, Schlaff WD, Kimball A, et al. The efficacy of presacral neurectomy for the relief of midline dysmenorrhea. *Obstet Gynecol* 1990;76:89.

145. Parazzini F, Fedele L, Busacca M, et al. Post-surgical medical treatment of advanced endometriosis: Results of a randomized clinical trial. *Am J Obstet Gynecol* 1994;171:1205.

146. Bianchi S, Busacca M, Agnoli B, et al. Effects of 3-month therapy with danazol after laparoscopic surgery for stage III/IV endometriosis: A randomized study. *Hum Reprod* 1999;14:1335.

147. Busacca M, Somigliana E, Bianchi S, et al. Postoperative GnRH analogue treatment after conservative surgery for symptomatic endometriosis stage III-IV: A randomized, controlled trial. *Hum Reprod* 2001;16:2399.

148. Vercellini P, Crosignani PG, Fadini R, et al. A gonadotropin-releasing hormone agonist compared with expectant management after conservative surgery for symptomatic endometriosis. *Br J Obstet Gynaecol* 1999;106:672.

149. Hasson HM. Incidence of endometriosis in diagnostic laparoscopy. *J Reprod Med* 1976;16:135.

150. Drake TS, Grunert GM. The unsuspected pelvic factor in the infertility investigation. *Fertil Steril* 1980;34:27.

151. Strathy JH, Molgaard CA, Coulam CB, et al. Endometriosis and infertility: A laparoscopic study of endometriosis among fertile and infertile women. *Fertil Steril* 1982;38:667.

152. Verkauf BS. Incidence, symptoms, and signs of endometriosis in fertile and infertile women. *J Fla Med Assoc* 1987;74:671.

153. Hahn DW, Carraher RP, Foldesy RG, et al. Experimental evidence for failure to implant as a mechanism of infertility associated with endometriosis. *Am J Obstet Gynecol* 1986;155:1109.

154. Illera MJ, Juan L, Stewart CL, et al. Effect of peritoneal fluid from women with endometriosis on implantation in the mouse model. *Fertil Steril* 2000;74:41.

155. Schenken RS, Asch RH. Surgical induction of endometriosis in the rabbit: Effects on fertility and concentrations of peritoneal fluid prostaglandins. *Fertil Steril* 1980;34:581.

156. Vernon MW, Wilson EA. Studies on the surgical induction of endometriosis in the rat. *Fertil Steril* 1985;44:684.

157. Barragan JC, Brotons J, Ruiz JA, et al. Experimentally induced endometriosis in rats: Effect on fertility and the effects of pregnancy and lactation on the ectopic endometrial tissue. *Fertil Steril* 1992;58:1215.

158. Jansen RP. Minimal endometriosis and reduced fecundability: Prospective evidence from an artificial insemination by donor program. *Fertil Steril* 1986;46:141.

159. Bordson BL, Ricci E, Dickey RP, et al. Comparison of fecundability with fresh and frozen semen in therapeutic donor insemination. *Fertil Steril* 1986;46:466.

160. Yeh J, Seibel MM. Artificial insemination with donor sperm: A review of 108 patients. *Obstet Gynecol* 1987;70:313.

161. Byrd W, Bradshaw K, Carr B, et al: A prospective, randomized study of pregnancy rates following intrauterine and intracervical insemination using frozen donor sperm. *Fertil Steril* 1990;53:521.

162. Matorras R, Rodriguez F, Pijoan JI, et al. Women who are not exposed to spermatozoa and infertile women have similar rates of stage I endometriosis. *Fertil Steril* 2001;76:923.

163. Harrison RF, Barry-Kinsella C. Efficacy of medroxyprogesterone treatment in infertile women with endometriosis: A prospective, randomized, placebo-controlled study. *Fertil Steril* 2000;74:24.

164. Mahutte NG, Arici A. New advances in the understanding of endometriosis related infertility. *J Reprod Immunol* 2002;55:73.

165. Chang MY, Chiang CH, Hsieh TT, et al. The influence of endometriosis on the success of gamete intrafallopian transfer (GIFT). *J Assist Reprod Genet* 1997;14:76.

166. Minguez Y, Rubio C, Bernal A, et al: The impact of endometriosis in couples undergoing intracytoplasmic sperm injection because of male infertility. *Hum Reprod* 1997;12:2282.

167. Dokras A, Habana A, Giraldo J, et al. Secretion of inhibin B during ovarian stimulation is decreased in infertile women with endometriosis. *Fertil Steril* 2000;74:35.

168. Hock DL, Sharafi K, Dagostino L, et al. Contribution of diminished ovarian reserve to hypofertility associated with endometriosis. *J Reprod Med* 2001;46:7.

169. Nakahara K, Saito H, Saito T, et al. Ovarian fecundity in patients with endometriosis can be estimated by the incidence of apoptotic bodies. *Fertil Steril* 1998;69:931.

170. Yanushpolsky EH, Best CL, Jackson KV, et al. Effects of endometriomas on ooccyte quality, embryo quality, and pregnancy rates in in vitro fertilization cycles: A prospective, case-controlled study. *J Assist Reprod Genet* 1998;15:193.

171. Al-Azemi M, Bernal AL, Steele J, et al. Ovarian response to repeated controlled stimulation in in-vitro fertilization cycles in patients with ovarian endometriosis. *Hum Reprod* 2000;15:72.

172. Toya M, Saito H, Ohta N, et al. Moderate and severe endometriosis is associated with alterations in the cell cycle of granulosa cells in patients undergoing in vitro fertilization and embryo transfer. *Fertil Steril* 2000;73:344.

173. Nakahara K, Saito H, Saito T, et al. The incidence of apoptotic bodies in membrana granulosa can predict prognosis of ova from patients participating in in vitro fertilization programs. *Fertil Steril* 1997;68:312.

174. Pellicer A, Albert C, Mercader A, et al. The follicular and endocrine environment in women with endometriosis: local and systemic cytokine production. *Fertil Steril* 1998;70:425.

175. Carlberg M, Nejaty J, Froysa B, et al. Elevated expression of tumor necrosis factor alpha in cultured granulosa cells from women with endometriosis. *Hum Reprod* 2000;15:1250.

176. Lee KS, Joo BS, Na YJ, et al. Relationships between concentrations of tumor necrosis factor-alpha and nitric oxide in follicular fluid and oocyte quality. *J Assist Reprod Genet* 2000;17: 222.

177. Pellicer A, Albert C, Garrido N, et al. The pathophysiology of endometriosis-associated infertility: follicular environment and embryo quality. *J Reprod Fertil Suppl* 2000;55:109.

178. Cahill DJ, Wardle PG, Maile LA, et al. Ovarian dysfunction in endometriosis-associated and unexplained infertility. *J Assist Reprod Genet* 1997;14:554.

179. Qiao J, Yeung WS, Yao YQ, et al. The effects of follicular fluid from patients with different indications for IVF treatment on the binding of human spermatozoa to the zona pellucida. *Hum Reprod* 1998;13:128.

180. Aeby TC, Huang T, Nakayama RT. The effect of peritoneal fluid from patients with endometriosis on human sperm function in vitro. *Am J Obstet Gynecol* 1996;174:1779.

181. Hull MG, Williams JA, Ray B, et al. The contribution of subtle oocyte or sperm dysfunction affecting fertilization in endometriosis-associated or unexplained infertility: A controlled comparison with tubal infertility and use of donor spermatozoa. *Hum Reprod* 1998;13:1825.

182. Bergendal A, Naffah S, Nagy C, et al. Outcome of IVF in patients with endometriosis in comparison with tubal-factor infertility. *J Assist Reprod Genet* 1998;15:530.

183. Harlow CR, Cahill DJ, Maile LA, et al. Reduced preovulatory granulosa cell steroidogenesis in women with endometriosis. *J Clin Endocrinol Metab* 1996;81:426.

184. Geber S, Paraschos T, Atkinson G, et al. Results of IVF in patients with endometriosis: The severity of the disease does not affect outcome, or the incidence of miscarriage. *Hum Reprod* 1995; 10:1507.

185. Arici A, Oral E, Bukulmez O, et al. The effect of endometriosis on implantation: Results from

the Yale University in vitro fertilization and embryo transfer program. *Fertil Steril* 1996;65:603.

186. Pal L, Shifren JL, Isaacson KB, et al. Impact of varying stages of endometriosis on the outcome of in vitro fertilization-embryo transfer. *J Assist Reprod Genet* 1998;15:27.

187. Azem F, Lessing JB, Geva E, et al. Patients with stages III and IV endometriosis have a poorer outcome of in vitro fertilization-embryo transfer than patients with tubal infertility. *Fertil Steril* 1999;72:1107.

188. Martinez-Roman S, Balasch J, Creus M, et al. Immunological factors in endometriosis-associated reproductive failure: Studies in fertile and infertile women with and without endometriosis. *Hum Reprod* 1997;12:1794.

189. Jha P, Farooq A, Agarwal N, et al. In vitro sperm phagocytosis by human peritoneal macrophages in endometriosis-associated infertility. *Am J Reprod Immunol* 1996;36:235.

190. Oral E, Arici A, Olive DL, et al. Peritoneal fluid from women with moderate or severe endometriosis inhibits sperm motility: The role of seminal fluid components. *Fertil Steril* 1996;66:787.

191. Pillai S, Rust PF, Howard L. Effects of antibodies to transferrin and α2-HS glycoprotein on in vitro sperm motion: Implications in infertility associated with endometriosis. *Am J Reprod Immunol* 1998;39:235.

192. Mathur SP. Autoimmunity in endometriosis: Relevance to infertility. *Am J Reprod Immunol* 2000;44:89.

193. Sharma RK, Wang Y, Falcone T, et al. Effect of peritoneal fluid from endometriosis patients on sperm motion characteristics and acrosome reaction. *Int J Fertil Womens Med* 1999;44:31.

194. Szczepanska M, Skrzypczak J, Kamieniczna M, et al. Antizona and antisperm antibodies in women with endometriosis and/or infertility. *Fertil Steril* 2001;75:97.

195. Taylor HS, Bagot C, Kardana A, et al. *HOX* gene expression is altered in the endometrium of women with endometriosis. *Hum Reprod* 1999;14:1328.

196. Simon C, Gutierrez A, Vidal A, et al. Outcome of patients with endometriosis in assisted reproduction: Results from in-vitro fertilization and oocyte donation. *Hum Reprod* 1994;9:725.

197. Diaz I, Navarro J, Blasco L, et al. Impact of stage III–IV endometriosis on recipients of sibling oocytes: Matched case-control study. *Fertil Steril* 2000;74:31.

198. Sung L, Mukherjee T, Takeshige T, et al. Endometriosis is not detrimental to embryo implantation in oocyte recipients. *J Assist Reprod Genet* 1997;14:152.

199. Thomas EJ, Cooke ID. Successful treatment of asymptomatic endometriosis: Does it benefit infertile women? *Br Med J (Clin Res Ed)* 1987;294:1117.

200. Telimaa S. Danazol and medroxyprogesterone acetate inefficacious in the treatment of infertility in endometriosis. *Fertil Steril* 1988;50:872.

201. Bayer SR, Seibel MM, Saffan DS, et al. Efficacy of danazol treatment for minimal endometriosis in infertile women: A prospective, randomized study. *J Reprod Med* 1988;33:179.

202. Fedele L, Parazzini F, Radici E, et al. Buserelin acetate versus expectant management in the treatment of infertility associated with minimal or mild endometriosis: A randomized clinical trial. *Am J Obstet Gynecol* 1992;166:1345.

203. Hughes E, Fedorkow D, Collins J, et al. Ovulation suppression for endometriosis. *Cochrane Database Syst Rev* 2000;CD000155.

204. Noble AD, Letchworth AT. Medical treatment of endometriosis: A comparative trial. *Postgrad Med J* 1979;55:37.

205. Fedele L, Bianchi S, Viezzoli T, et al. Gestrinone versus danazol in the treatment of endometriosis. *Fertil Steril* 1989;51:781.

206. Dmowski WP, Radwanska E, Binor Z, et al. Ovarian suppression induced with buserelin or danazol in the management of endometriosis: A randomized, comparative study. *Fertil Steril* 1898;51:395.

207. Hughes EG, Fedorkow DM, Collins JA. A quantitative overview of controlled trials in endometriosis-associated infertility. *Fertil Steril* 1993;59:963.

208. Adamson GD, Pasta DJ. Surgical treatment of endometriosis-associated infertility: Metaanalysis compared with survival analysis. *Am J Obstet Gynecol* 1994;171:1488.

209. Candiani GB, Vercellini P, Fedele L, et al. Conservative surgical treatment for severe endometriosis in infertile women: Are we making progress? *Obstet Gynecol Surv* 1991;46:490.

210. Busacca M, Bianchi S, Agnoli B, et al. Follow-up of laparoscopic treatment of stage III–IV

endometriosis. *J Am Assoc Gynecol Laparosc* 1999; 6:55.

211. Marcoux S, Maheux R, Berube S. Laparoscopic surgery in infertile women with minimal or mild endometriosis. Canadian Collaborative Group on Endometriosis. *N Engl J Med* 1997; 337:217.

212. Parazzini F. Ablation of lesions or no treatment in minimal–mild endometriosis in infertile women: A randomized trial. Gruppo Italiano per lo Studio dell'Endometriosi. *Hum Reprod* 1999;14:1332.

213. Deaton JL, Gibson M, Blackmer KM, et al. A randomized, controlled trial of clomiphene citrate and intrauterine insemination in couples with unexplained infertility or surgically corrected endometriosis. *Fertil Steril* 1990;54:1083.

214. Fedele L, Bianchi S, Marchini M, et al. Superovulation with human menopausal gonadotropins in the treatment of infertility associated with minimal or mild endometriosis: A controlled, randomized study. *Fertil Steril* 1992;58:28.

215. Tummon IS, Asher LJ, Martin JS, et al. Randomized, controlled trial of superovulation and insemination for infertility associated with minimal or mild endometriosis. *Fertil Steril* 1997; 68:8.

216. Mahutte NG, Arici A. Endometriosis and assisted reproductive technologies: are outcomes affected? *Curr Opin Obstet Gynecol* 2001;13:275.

217. Barnhart K, Dunsmoor-Su R, Coutifaris C. Effect of endometriosis on in vitro fertilization. *Fertil Steril* 2002;77:1148.

218. Assisted reproductive technology in the United States: 1999 results generated from the American Society for Reproductive Medicine/Society for Assisted Reproductive Technology Registry. *Fertil Steril* 2002;78:918.

219. Assisted reproductive technology in the United States: 1998 results generated from the American Society for Reproductive Medicine/Society for Assisted Reproductive Technology Registry. *Fertil Steril* 2002;77:18.

220. Olivennes F, Feldberg D, Liu HC, et al. Endometriosis: A stage by stage analysis—The role of in vitro fertilization. *Fertil Steril* 1995;64:392.

221. Tanbo T, Omland A, Dale PO, et al. In vitro fertilization/embryo transfer in unexplained infertility and minimal peritoneal endometriosis. *Acta Obstet Gynaecol Scand* 1995;74:539.

222. Dicker D, Goldman GA, Ashkenazi J, et al. The value of pretreatment with gonadotrophin-releasing hormone (GnRH) analogue in IVF-ET therapy of severe endometriosis. *Hum Reprod* 1990;5:418.

223. Nakamura K, Oosawa M, Kondou I, et al. Menotropin stimulation after prolonged gonadotropin releasing hormone agonist pretreatment for in vitro fertilization in patients with endometriosis. *J Assist Reprod Genet* 1999;113.

224. Marcus SF, Edwards RG. High rates of pregnancy after long-term down-regulation of women with severe endometriosis. *Am J Obstet Gynecol* 1994;171:812.

225. Kim CH, Cho YK, Mok JE. Simplified ultralong protocol of gonadotropin-releasing hormone agonist for ovulation induction with intrauterine insemination in patients with endometriosis. *Hum Reprod* 1996;11:398.

226. Damario MA, Moomjy M, Tortoriello D, et al. Delay of gonadotropin stimulation in patients receiving gonadotropin-releasing hormone agonist (GnRH-a) therapy permits increased clinic efficiency and may enhance in vitro fertilization (IVF) pregnancy rates. *Fertil Steril* 1997;68:1004.

227. Rickes D, Nickel I, Kropf S, et al. Increased pregnancy rates after ultralong postoperative therapy with gonadotropin-releasing hormone analogs in patients with endometriosis. *Fertil Steril* 2002;78:757.

228. Surrey ES, Silverberg KM, Surrey MW, et al. Effect of prolonged gonadotropin-releasing hormone agonist therapy on the outcome of in vitro fertilization-embryo transfer in patients with endometriosis. *Fertil Steril* 2002;78:699.

229. Loh FH, Tan AT, Kumar J, et al. Ovarian response after laparoscopic ovarian cystectomy for endometriotic cysts in 132 monitored cycles. *Fertil Steril* 1999;72:316.

230. Tinkanen H, Kujansuu E. In vitro fertilization in patients with ovarian endometriomas. *Acta Obstet Gynaecol Scand* 2000;79:119.

231. Marconi G, Vilela M, Quintana R, et al. Laparoscopic ovarian cystectomy of endometriomas does not affect the ovarian response to gonadotropin stimulation. *Fertil Steril* 2002;78:876.

232. Donnez J, Wyns C, Nisolle M. Does ovarian surgery for endometriomas impair the ovarian response to gonadotropin? *Fertil Steril* 2001; 76:662.

233. Jenkins S, Olive DL, Haney AF. Endometriosis: Pathogenetic implications of the anatomic distribution. *Obstet Gynecol* 1986;67:335.

234. Ishimura T, Masuzaki H. Peritoneal endometriosis: Endometrial tissue implantation as its primary etiologic mechanism. *Am J Obstet Gynecol* 1991;165:210.

235. Kruitwagen RF, Poels LG, Willemsen WN, et al. Endometrial epithelial cells in peritoneal fluid during the early follicular phase. *Fertil Steril* 1991;55:297.

236. Witz CA, Dechaud H, Montoya-Rodriguez IA, et al. An in vitro model to study the pathogenesis of the early endometriosis lesion. *Ann NY Acad Sci* 2002;955:296.

237. D'Hooghe TM, Bambra CS, Raeymaekers BM, et al. Intrapelvic injection of menstrual endometrium causes endometriosis in baboons *(Papio cynocephalus and Papio anubis)*. *Am J Obstet Gynecol* 1995;173:125.

238. Olive DL, Henderson DY. Endometriosis and mülerian anomalies. *Obstet Gynecol* 1987;69: 412.

239. Cramer DW, Wilson E, Stillman RJ, et al. The relation of endometriosis to menstrual characteristics, smoking, and exercise. *JAMA* 1986;255:1904.

240. Darrow SL, Vena JE, Batt RE, et al. Menstrual cycle characteristics and the risk of endometriosis. *Epidemiology* 1993;4:135.

241. Vercellini P, De Giorgi O, Oldani S, et al. Depot medroxyprogesterone acetate versus an oral contraceptive combined with very-low-dose danazol for long-term treatment of pelvic pain associated with endometriosis. *Am J Obstet Gynecol* 1996;175:396.

CHAPTER 21

Tubal Disorders

ASHIM KUMAR, SANJAY K. AGARWAL, AND RICARDO AZZIZ

Fallopian tube disease affects a sizable portion of women and leads to sequelae causing significant emotional distress and financial expenditure. Tubal pathology commonly presents to the reproductive endocrinologist as infertility or as ectopic gestation. The diagnostic procedures available range from a simple serum evaluation to surgical appraisal. Although the major treatment options continue to be surgical or assisted reproductive technology (ART) procedures, advances in ART techniques have shifted the fulcrum in the choice between surgery and in vitro fertilization.

► EPIDEMIOLOGY

Approximately one-third to one-fourth of all infertile women/couples are diagnosed with tubal disease in developed countries, with the number approaching two-thirds of infertile women in Africa.[1–3] The prevalence of tubal disease may be higher depending on how scrupulously the tubes are evaluated. Several studies have found significant numbers of women with tubal disease on laparoscopy after they had been declared normal by hysterosalpingography (HSG).[4,5]

Age, race, and lifestyle have been evaluated in their relation to tubal infertility. There is a trend toward increasing prevalence of tubal disease with age, although younger women had a statistically significant higher prevalence of severe disease than their older counterparts.[6] Sharara and McClamrock reported an increased incidence of tubal factor infertility in black women in an inner-city university-based in vitro fertilization (IVF) program relative to their white counterparts.[7] On a review of multiple lifestyle factors, only cigarette smoking and intrauterine device (IUD) use (especially the Dalkon shield) have been associated with tubal factor infertility.[8]

► TUBAL FUNCTION

The fallopian tubes develop from the müllerian ducts along with the uterus and the upper two-thirds of the vagina (see Chap. 7). The cephalad aspect gives rise to the infundibulum, and the caudal portion develops into the isthmic and intramural regions.[9] They are 7 to 14 cm in length and transport sperm toward the ovaries and the oocyte and embryo toward the uterus. This is accomplished through the beating action of cilia (toward the uterus) and peristaltic waves created by both inner circular and outer longitudinal muscular layers. Almost 70 percent of the cells of the epithelium are ciliated in the fertile woman.[10] Secretion of embryotrophic factors and removal of toxic metabolites are also functions of the tubal epithelium.[11] The tubal epithelium undergoes cyclic changes with the menstrual cycle with cytoplasmic extrusion during the secretory phase.[12]

The oviduct may be divided into four regions based on morphologic and anatomic differences. The infundibulum is approximately 1 cm in length and is important for ova pickup. The ampulla averages 5 to 8 cm in length, with a lumen that decreases from 1 cm adjacent to the infundibulum to 1 to 2 mm near the isthmus. Fertilization and early cleavage occur in the ampulla, which is the most common site of ectopic gestation (see Fig. 15-1). The isthmus extends to the uterus and is usually 2 to 3 cm in length. In the isthmus, the tubal musculature increases as the lumen continues to narrow. The intramural portion of the fallopian tube may be straight, curved, or tortuous.[13] The three layers of muscles are well defined and act as a sphincter to control the flow of sperm and embryo between the uterus and tube.[14]

Normal tubal function can be impaired through disruption of tubal function or patency. Agglutination or obliteration of the fimbria leads to poor ova retrieval. Denudation of the epithelium and its cilia results in poor transport of the gametes or the embryo. Obviously, physical obstruction, including mucus plugs, scarring, and surgical interruption, leads to a failure of transport. Subfertility can be a consequence of the toxic environment caused by intraluminal endometriosis or fluid (hydrosalpinx). Pelvic adhesions cause subfertility by interfering with ova pickup or tubal function.

▶ ETIOLOGY OF TUBAL DISEASE

A small number of common etiologies of tubal damage account for the majority of disease (Table 21-1). A singular theme underlies these instigators—inflammation. Both infectious and noninfectious causes can lead to an inflammatory response that results in functional or physical impairment of the fallopian tubes. Other

▶ **TABLE 21-1:** ETIOLOGY OF TUBAL FACTOR INFERTILITY

Infectious	Noninfectious
Pelvic Inflammatory Disease (PID)	Endometriosis
	Prior pelvic surgery
Tuberculosis	Congenital anomalies
Ruptured appendix	
Postoperative infections	Salpingitis isthmica nodosa
Septic abortion	

less common etiologies of tubal disease are congenital. These include diethylstilbestrol (DES) exposure and salpingitis isthmica nodosa (SIN). An iatrogenic etiology (e.g., tubal ligation) is not infrequently encountered by the reproductive specialist.

Much of the tubal factor infertility attributable to inflammation is mediated by adhesions. Pelvic adhesions are found to be the etiology of infertility in 15 to 20 percent of patients.[15] Pelvic adhesions may interfere directly with retrieval of the oocyte by the fimbria or may inhibit transfer of the gametes. Another possible mechanism of tubal factor infertility is the production of cytotoxic factors, including free radicals, by a chronic inflammatory response. Infection may lead to hydrosalpinx and peritubal adhesions, which may impair fertility. This may occur even during IVF or embryo transfer (ET), by mechanical "flushing" of the embryos from the uterus.[16] Lastly, there are studies implicating direct tubal mucosal damage as the cause of infertility specific to *Chlamydia trachomatis*.[17,18]

Infectious Etiologies

Pelvic inflammatory disease (PID) is the leading cause of tubal disease, including tubal factor infertility. PID has been clearly linked to tubal factor infertility and ectopic gestation.[19–21] Approximately 10 to 13 per 1000 women aged 15 to 39 years are diagnosed annually with acute PID, with the incidence increasing to 20 per 1000 in women aged 20 to 24 years.[20]

An increased incidence of tubal disease is reported commonly in women who have used IUDs. However, recent data indicate that the risk of tubal damage and infertility associated with IUD use has been overestimated, suggesting that the risk of salpingitis with an IUD versus that without an IUD is similar.[22] The lesser risk of tubal infection associated with IUD use currently may be a function of the evolution of the IUD over the past 20 years, such as the use of monofilament rather than braided thread for removal.

The risk of tubal damage increases with successive episodes of PID. In a study of 415 women with known PID, involuntary infertility due to tubal obstruction rate was 10, 31, and 75 percent after one, two, and three or more episodes of PID, respectively[19] (Table 21-2). A corollary study revealed an association between the severity of PID observed at laparoscopy and the rate of infertility, with live births of 90 percent following a mild episode, 82 percent with a moderate infection, and 57 percent with severe infection during 12 years of follow-up.[23]

Since most diagnoses of PID are based on clinical criteria and not confirmed by laparoscopy, a wide range of symptoms and signs is used by clinicians to reach such a diagnosis. Less than half the patients present with the classic symptoms of pain, fever, and lower gen-ital tract infection. Because of the substantial sequelae of a missed diagnosis versus the low risk of treatment, practitioners should have a low threshold to treat. The standards outlined by the Centers for Disease Control and Prevention (CDC) include a triad of minimal criteria necessary to diagnose PID: (1) cervical motion tenderness, (2) adnexal tenderness, and (3) lower abdominal tenderness.[24] The presence of leukorrhea, cervicitis, or leukocytosis is not required for the diagnosis of PID. Treatment should be broad spectrum and on an outpatient or inpatient basis as indicated.

C. trachomatis is the major pathogen in PID.[25] Other potential pathogens include *Neisseria gonorrhoeae, Mycoplasma hominis,* and endogenous aerobic or anaerobic bacteria. In underdeveloped nations, the high prevalence of tuberculosis makes it a frequent etiology of tubal factor infertility.[26] For example, on the Indian subcontinent, pelvic tuberculosis is responsible for approximately 40 percent of tubal infertility.[27]

Other infections inside the peritoneal cavity also can wreak havoc on tubal function. Trimbos-Kemper and colleagues documented that appendicitis complicated by perforation, a periappendiceal inflammatory mass, or an appendiceal abscess was associated with a significantly greater risk of tubal disease compared with patients having undergone an uncomplicated appendectomy or controls.[28]

▶ **TABLE 21-2:** PREGNANCY OUTCOME FOLLOWING PELVIC INFECTION IN RELATION TO NUMBER OF EPISODES OF ACUTE PID

	Episodes of Acute PID		
	One	Two	≥Three
Pregnant	217 (67.6%)	40 (57.1%)	6 (25.0%)
Not pregnant			
Voluntarily	56 (17.4%)	8 (11.4%)	0 (0%)
Involuntarily, tubal occlusion	32 (10.0%)	22 (31.4%)	18 (75.0%)
Involuntarily, other causes	16 (5.0%)	0 (0%)	0 (0%)
Total	321 (100%)	70 (100%)	24 (100%)

Adapted with permission from Westrom L. Effect of acute pelvic inflammatory disease on fertility. Am J Obstet Gynecol 1975;121(5):707–713.

These results were corroborated by Mueller and colleagues, who found that a history of a ruptured appendix was associated with a relative risk of tubal infertility of 4.8, whereas a history of simple appendectomy without rupture carried no excess risk in a cohort of 279 women.[29] Alternatively, other investigators have suggested that a history of ruptured appendix does not significantly elevate the risk of infertility.[30]

Postoperative infections after any procedure involving the peritoneal cavity also may lead to intrapelvic adhesions and disruption of the pelvic architecture.[31] The inflammatory process that ensues after peritonitis or abscess formation can cause peritubal or paraovarian adhesions that prevent ovum pickup or transport. In gynecologic surgery, postoperative infection rates range from 1 to 15 percent of procedures.[32]

Septic abortion is a clear risk factor for tubal factor infertility. Although the incidence of septic abortions has decreased significantly following legalization of elective termination of pregnancy in the United States, the incidence is on the rise in other parts of the world.[33] A history of infectious complications following any evacuation of products of conception should be elicited by the physician and, if present, should raise the possibility of tubal damage and direct the diagnostic evaluation.

Noninfectious Etiologies

Noninfectious inflammatory etiologies of tubal factor infertility include endometriosis and surgical damage. Endometriosis can cause tubal infertility principally through two mechanisms: putative production of toxic factors and adhesion formation[34] (see Chap. 20). There is little doubt that disruption of the normal pelvic architecture that is evident in patients with stage III or IV endometriosis impairs tubal function. However, even mild endometriosis can be associated with adhesion formation that may affect tubal performance. In addition, endometriosis has been reported inside the lumen of the oviduct and may lead to subfertility by similar mechanisms.[35]

A history of prior gynecologic surgery is a major risk factor for tubal factor infertility. The rate of de novo pelvic adhesion formation is approximately 75 percent following abdominal or pelvic surgery via laparotomy even with the use of microsurgical technique.[36,37] Ischemia or desiccation of the surgical site adds to the likelihood of adhesions. The use of laparoscopy may reduce the chances of de novo adhesions but does not preclude adhesion formation or re-formation at the surgical site. Use of adhesion barriers such as Interceed, Gore-Tex, or Intergel reduces adhesion formation by approximately 50 percent (see below).[37]

Congenital Anomalies

The prevalence of congenital anomalies of the fallopian tubes is relatively low because most müllerian anomalies are the result of fusion defects and therefore do not affect the fallopian tubes. However, in utero exposure to DES has been associated with various tubal abnormalities, such as short, tortuous tubes or shriveled fimbria with small ostia, leading to infertility.[38] The congenital versus infectious etiology of SIN is unresolved. It represents a disorder in which diverticula of the isthmic tubal mucosa extend into the muscularis up to the serosa (Fig. 21-1). It is progressive in nature and leads ultimately to tubal occlusion and infertility.[39] SIN is also associated with an increased risk of ectopic pregnancy.

Yablonski and colleagues reported on a series of 100 cesarean sections in previously infertile women compared with 100 cesarean sections in fertile women.[40] They found a significant increase in the incidence of tubal anomalies in previously infertile women, with accessory tubes encountered in 13 percent and accessory ostia in 10 percent of these patients. Congenital unilateral absence of a fallopian tube or agenesis of bilateral distal fallopian tubes also has been reported.[41] However, in a case series of six patients with apparently uni-

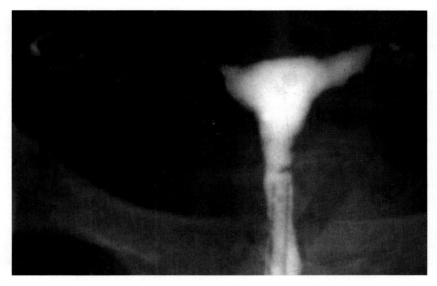

Figure 21-1 HSG film revealing salpingitis isthmica nodosa in right fallopian tube.

lateral absence of the tube and ovary, evidence or remnants of the missing ovary were observed in four.[42] These patients did not have concurrent anomalies of the uterus or urinary system. The investigators concluded that unilateral absence of the adnexa most likely resulted from prior torsion leading to necrosis and resorption rather than congenital absence.

▶ DIAGNOSIS

Consistent with any medical evaluation, a detailed history is imperative because the presence or absence of risk factors will guide the clinician in proper evaluation of the patient (Table 21-3). Overall assessment includes age, duration of infertility, and primary versus secondary infertility. In order to extract risk factors of an infectious

▶ **TABLE 21-3:** HISTORY AND PHYSICAL EXAMINATION IN PATIENTS AT RISK FOR POSSIBLE TUBAL DISEASE

History		
General	Infections	**Physical Examination**
Age	Age at first coitus	Cervical, uterine, or adnexal
Duration of infertility	Number of sexual partners	tenderness
Primary versus	History of IUD use	Uterine or ovarian fixation
secondary infertility	History of STDs or PID	Nodularity or tenderness along
Endometriosis	Complications after surgery,	the uterosacral ligaments
Dysmenorrhea	including D&C	Cervical cultures & wet prep
Dyspareunia	Prior gynecologic surgery	
History of DES	History of ruptured appendix	
exposure		

Abbreviations: D&C = dilatation and curettage; DES = diethylstilbestrol; STDs = sexually transmitted diseases; IUD = intrauterine device; PID = pelvic inflammatory disease.

etiology for tubal disease from the history, one should inquire about age at first coitus, number of sexual partners, history of IUD use, and history of sexually transmitted diseases (STDs) or PID.[43] For endometriosis, important symptoms include the presence of dysmenorrhea and/or dyspareunia. Surgical risk factors include a history of prior gynecologic surgery or appendectomy or the development of infectious complications after surgery, especially after dilatation and curettage (D&C) of a parous uterus.[44]

During the physical examination, cervical cultures for STDs and a wet prep for bacterial vaginosis should be done. Uterine, adnexal, or cervical motion tenderness should be sought. Tenderness or nodularity along the uterosacral ligaments on rectovaginal examination can suggest the presence of endometriosis. Endometriosis also may be manifest through a decreased mobility of the pelvic organs with fixation of the uterus or adnexa. Adnexal masses may be consistent with hydrosalpinx or endometriomas and warrant further investigation.

Chlamydial Serology

A number of investigators have advocated the use of chlamydial serology routinely in the evaluation of the infertile women as a surrogate for an HSG and/or laparoscopy or to provide information regarding the risk for tubal disease. In a cost-effectiveness analysis, Mol and colleagues advocated starting the diagnostic workup with chlamydial antibody testing (CAT) in infertile couples with good prognostic indicators.[45] This is consistent with previous data correlating *Chlamydia* antibody titers in serum with the presence of tubal infertility.[46] However, in a retrospective study evaluating the use of CAT as a screening tool for performing laparoscopy in infertile women, Johnson and colleagues concluded that selective laparoscopy in the routine evaluation of infertile couples based on CAT was not supported.[47]

Currently CAT is not used routinely in clinical practice. However, because there are multiple and developing algorithms for the evaluation of tubal disease, CAT should remain an option in the armamentarium of the diagnostician. It may be a useful test in patients who do not desire HSG or laparoscopy for fear of pain or surgical risks or for financial reasons. Whether used as a screening or a diagnostic tool, the positive predictive value of the test will depend on the prevalence of *Chlamydia* in the specific population studied—the higher the prevalence, the higher the predictive value.

Hysterosalpingogram

The HSG has been the traditional test for evaluating tubal status in the initial evaluation of the infertile women (Fig. 21-2). Significant advantages include its relative simplicity, ease of procedure, rapidity, and relatively low risk (Table 21-4). However, numerous investigators have questioned the accuracy of HSG in assessing tubal pathology.[48,49] A large metaanalysis of 20 studies with over 4000 patients estimated the sensitivity and specificity of HSG for tubal patency at 0.65 and 0.83, respectively.[50] Although its main purpose is to evaluate tubal patency, occasionally it can divulge additional information to the astute interpreter. Proximal versus distal obstruction can be elucidated easily, but evidence of other pathology, such as mucosal lesions from previous infections, tubal motility, tubal endometriosis, hydrosalpinx, SIN, adhesions, and tubal anomalies (e.g., accessory ostia), also can be detected by an HSG (Fig. 21-3).

Another advantage of HSG is that it may be of therapeutic value. Several Cochrane Database meta-analyses have evaluated fecundity following HSG. Johnson and colleagues conducted a review of eight randomized studies to determine the effect of an HSG on subsequent fertility and concluded that in terms of clinical practice "there is some evidence of effectiveness that tubal flushing with oil-soluble contrast media increases the odds of pregnancy versus no intervention."[51] In a review designed to evaluate oil-soluble contrast media (OSCM)

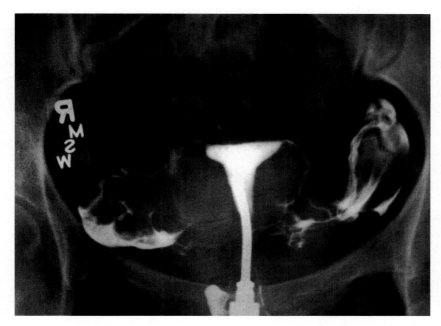

Figure 21-2 A normal HSG depicting a normal uterine cavity and bilaterally patent fallopian tubes. Mucosal folds are visible in the infundibular region. Lack of pooling of contrast material is evidence against adhesions.

versus water-soluble contrast media (WSCM), Vandekerckhove and colleagues noted that there was evidence to support the hypothesis that some cases of infertility may be due to proximal tubal plugs leading to proximal tubal occlusion and that flushing of the tubes with OSCM did increase pregnancy rates.[52] Although OSCM may improve fecundity, WSCM may be better tolerated by the patient and offers improved resolution. To obtain advantages of both, serial use of WSCM followed by OSCM has been recommended.[53]

Disadvantages to the use of HSG include limited information obtained regarding the status of the pelvis as a whole and difficulty distinguishing between tubal spasms and obstruction. Absolute contraindications to HSG include allergy to the contrast medium and current cervicitis or PID. Complications associated with HSG are allergic reaction to the medium, intravasation of the medium into the vasculature, and a 1 to 3 percent risk of postprocedure infectious peritonitis requiring hospitalization. To

decrease the risk of peritonitis subsequent to HSG, it is prudent to evaluate the patient for bacterial vaginosis or cervicitis prior to the procedure. Prophylactic use of antibiotics has been suggested, although there are little data to support its routine use. Use of nonsteroidal anti-inflammatory drugs (NSAIDs) prior to the procedure can improve patient comfort by inhibiting prostaglandin synthesis caused by distension of the uterus.

Laparoscopy with Chromopertubation

The gold standard for the evaluation of tubal pathology is laparoscopy with chromopertubation. However, there has been some controversy regarding the need for diagnostic laparoscopy in the infertile woman with a negative workup, i.e., a normal HSG. Several factors contradict the supposition that the diagnostic laparoscopy is unnecessary. The first is

▶ **TABLE 21-4:** HYSTEROSALPINGOGRAM (HSG) VERSUS LAPAROSCOPY

	HSG	**Laparoscopy**

Advantages	Simple
	Easy to perform
	Rapid
	Low risk
	Diagnose multiple intratubal
	  disease processes
	Modest therapeutic value
		Assesses intrapelvic disease
		Allows treatment of pathology
		  identified

Disadvantages	May not distinguish between tubal
	  spasms and obstruction
	Provides limited information on
	  intrapelvic disease
		Anesthesia required
		Increased risk
		Expensive

Contraindications	Allergy to contrast medium
	Cervicitis or pelvic inflammatory
	  disease (PID)
		Contraindications to anesthesia
		  or surgery

Complications	Infectious or chemical peritonitis
	Intravasation of contrast medium
		Anesthesia related
		Injury to intraabdominal organs
		  such as bowel, bladder, blood
		  vessels, or ureter

the poor sensitivity and specificity of HSG in the detection of tubal disease. The second is the fact that the history of the patient may not clearly denote the risk of tubal disease or other pelvic pathology such as endometriosis. Third, intrapelvic disease found during laparoscopy, such as adhesions or endometriosis, may aid the physician in formulating a management plan specific for the patient rather than relegating the patient's care to a preset algorithm.[54,55] Findings such as significant adhesive disease may lead a physician to forego needless cycles of ovulation induction and proceed directly to IVF.[56,57] Mild adhesive disease or endometriosis may be treated intraoperatively to increase fecundity.[58]

Patients requiring ovulation induction should be allowed to attempt conception for several cycles with clomiphene citrate and/or intrauterine insemination (IUI) after a normal HSG, with a diagnostic/operative laparoscopy performed prior to ovulation induction with gonadotropins.[54,59,60] The two procedures (HSG and laparoscopy with chromopertubation) should be viewed as complementary. However, if the patient has risk factors for in-

trapelvic disease, such as a history of PID, prior laparotomy, or a history of a ruptured appendix, laparoscopy may be performed sooner, perhaps with the initial workup.

Similar to HSG, laparoscopy should be performed during the follicular phase both to avoid disruption of an early pregnancy and to facilitate concomitant hysteroscopy, if necessary. Informed consent obtained from the patient should incorporate the potential need for indicated procedures should intrapelvic disease be found, such as lysis of adhesions, resection/ablation of endometriosis and endometriomas, fimbrioplasty, neosalpingostomy, or salpingectomy, and a thorough discussion of the risks of the procedure.

Transvaginal Hydrolaparoscopy

Transvaginal hydrolaparoscopy has been advocated in the diagnosis of tubal and intrapelvic pathology. The procedure involves insertion of a small-caliber endoscope through the vagina into the cul-de-sac. Normal saline is used as

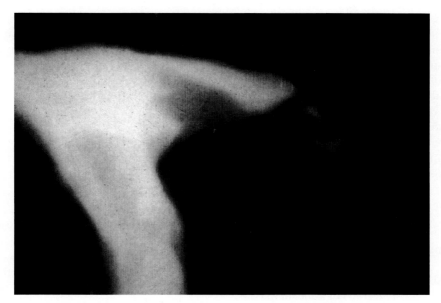

Figure 21-3   Intraluminal polyp was diagnosed within the left fallopian tube.

the distension medium. It offers some of the same advantages of traditional laparoscopy, with direct visualization of the viscera, along with potential additional benefits such as decreased anesthesia requirements.[61] However, these perceived advantages are offset by such disadvantages as the inability to manipulate viscera or to operate through the endoscope to correct any pathology discovered during the procedure. This procedure may be used in lieu of a diagnostic test such as HSG but should not be used in a patient who has risk factors for intrapelvic pathology and thus may require operative laparoscopy.

Endoscopic Evaluation of Tubal Mucosa

Two approaches used to assess the status of the tubal lumen and mucosa are falloposcopy and salpingoscopy. Falloposcopy uses a transcervical approach with hysteroscopic guidance to evaluate the entire fallopian tube with a fiberoptic microendoscope. The flexible falloposcope is placed through the tubal ostia and advanced over a guiding catheter. Continuous irrigation/distension allows for visualization of the tubal lumen in a retrograde fashion. The guiding catheter or the falloposcope may be used to recannulate obstructions, especially proximal tubal obstructions. Unfortunately, falloposcopy requires additional equipment (a falloposcope and its accessories) above the standard gynecologic endoscopic armamentarium and significant training and technical skill.[62] A large multicenter study revealed that less than 57 percent of patients undergoing the procedure received a full falloposcopic assessment.[63] Mucosal folds are normal findings, but adhesions, mucosal denudation (flat areas), and obstruction are pathologic findings. Falloposcopy has selected indications for diagnostic and therapeutic purposes, but its use is limited by technical difficulty and a high failure rate for completion of the procedure.[64] Therefore, falloposcopy is not used routinely for clinical purposes.

Salpingoscopy uses either a flexible or rigid salpingoscope inserted transfimbrially during laparoscopy. The salpingoscope is placed through a transabdominal ancillary port that allows for direct evaluation of the ampullary tubal epithelium. Salpingoscopic findings, such as intraluminal adhesions and epithelial denudation, have good prognostic value with respect to subsequent cumulative pregnancy rates.[65–67] Advantages of salpingoscopy are that the procedure is relatively easy to perform and minimal additional equipment is necessary. Its shortfalls are the limited length of the fallopian tube that can be visualized and the possibility that the procedure adds little to the information already gleaned from laparoscopic visualization of the fimbria.

Ultrasonography

Transvaginal ultrasonography has been used routinely to diagnose fibroids or adnexal masses, and recently, intrauterine space-occupying lesions also have been detected by sonohysterogram. With the transcervical injection of sonoopaque materials during ultrasonography, tubal patency can be evaluated with relative accuracy.[68] This procedure, termed *hysterosalpingocontrast sonography* (HyCoSy), has been advocated as a replacement for HSG as the initial procedure to evaluate tubal patency. A metaanalysis of three clinical studies with 986 women comparing HyCoSy and laparoscopy plus chromopertubation versus HSG and laparoscopy plus chromopertubation revealed false occlusion rates of 10.3 and 12.5 percent and false-positive (patency) rates of 6.7 and 11.2 percent, respectively. Ten percent of women experienced severe pain during HyCoSy, and 1.9 percent required treatment for adverse events such as vasovagal reaction or nausea.[69] Follow-up studies demonstrate similar results with no clear advantage for HyCoSy or HSG in terms of diagnosing tubal patency.[70] Both methodologies are equally capable of providing information on the condition of the endometrial cavity.[71] Advantages of HSG include better identification of specific tubal pathology such as tubal endometriosis or SIN, whereas the advantage of HyCoSy is

that it allows for assessment of the myometrium and adnexa. The initial diagnostic test of choice may be decided on availability, expertise, cost, and best fit for the patient. However, use of both HSG and HyCoSy in the same patient generally would be considered redundant.

Other Modalities

Several other modalities have been used or are now advocated for the evaluation of tubal disease and function. Tubal insufflation is a technique that evaluates tubal patency by passing carbon dioxide through the cervix and determining patency by auscultation of the abdomen for air or pressure changes of the carbon dioxide. Tubal insufflation is currently used minimally in clinical practice due to difficult interpretation of results leading to poor sensitivity and specificity.[72] A multicentered trial sponsored by the World Health Organization (WHO) concluded that "tubal insufflation should not be employed as a method of investigating tubal patency."[73] Tubal insufflation also has been associated with air embolus.

Radionuclide hysterosalpingography (RN-HSG) is purported to evaluate tubal function, specifically transport, in addition to patency. The procedure involves deposition of radioactively labeled human albumin microspheres in the vaginal fornix and cervical canal. Transport of the substance to the ovarian surface is then measured using a gamma camera.[74] Although initially promising test results were obtained, follow-up studies were unable to conclude that the procedure was capable of diagnosing tubal patency in a consistent manner.[75,76] RN-HSG is not in routine clinical use today.

▶ TREATMENT

Treatment options for tubal disease include surgery and IVF.

Surgical Options

Proximal Tubal Occlusion

Proximal tubal occlusion is present in 10 to 25 percent of women with tubal occlusion.[77] The surgical options available for repair include tubal resection and reanastomosis (macrosurgical or microsurgical), or tubal cannulation, performed either hysteroscopically or under fluoroscopy (Fig. 21-4). Microsurgical reanastomosis is superior to the macrosurgical technique, and subsequent pregnancy rates are reported to be greater than 50 percent.[78,79] In a study by Schill and colleagues, transhysteroscopic fallopian tube catheterization and recannulation was successful in achieving patency in 53 percent of tubes,[80] whereas Thurmond and colleagues reported success rates of 71 to 92 percent under fluoroscopic guidance.[81] Of note, hysteroscopic cannulation yielded higher pregnancy rates (40 to 50 percent) compared to fluoroscopic cannulation (30 percent).[82] Currently, the highest pregnancy rates occur after microsurgical anastomosis, although selected patients may be appropriate for the less invasive fluoroscopic or hysteroscopic procedures. The pregnancy rates following reanastomosis depend on the skill and experience of the surgeon.

Distal Tubal Occlusion

Distal tubal disease can be treated effectively through laparotomy or laparoscopy. The extent of tubal disease present is a good prognostic indicator of subsequent pregnancy rates.[83] With minimal disease present, pregnancy rates approach 80 percent, compared with 16 percent in those with severe tubal disease.[84] With such poor outcome in severe disease, surgical therapy should be reserved for those with mild to moderate damage. Oh conducted a study to evaluate three methods of laparoscopic neosalpingostomy.[85] Deagglutination with grasping forceps was superior to creating new ostia with scissors or an electrocoagulator in restoring fertility. Reocclusion rates approach 50 percent after surgical correction.

Bilateral neosalpingostomy for hydrosalpinx resulted in cumulative pregnancy rates of 20.5 percent during a 2-year follow-up.[86] Alternatively, IVF offers an approximately 30 percent pregnancy rate per cycle.[87] The presence of a hydrosalpinx impairs fertility even during IVF, possibly through mechanical flushing or release of embryotoxic factors. In patients undergoing IVF, disruption of the communication between the hydrosalpinx and the uterus by salpingectomy or proximal tubal interruption results in improved IVF pregnancy rates.[88,89] In women not undergoing IVF, the role of salpingostomy versus salpingectomy in those with a hydrosalpinx and a normal contralateral tube is less clear.

Tubal Anastomosis

Microsurgical tubal reanastomosis is an excellent option with good pregnancy rates in selected patients with prior tubal sterilization (Fig. 21-5). Newer techniques have been proposed with use of fewer sutures or staples; however, further research is necessary to validate these methods.[90,91] Live birth rates following

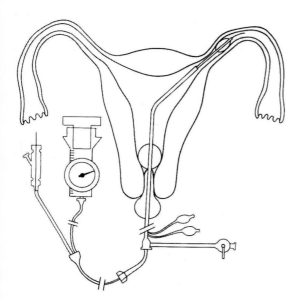

Figure 21-4 Schematic representation of transcervical tubal cannulation.

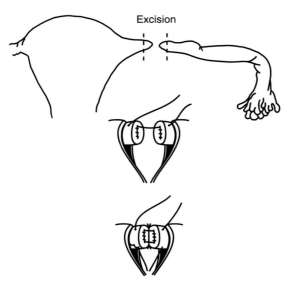

Excision

Figure 21-5 Microsurgical tubal reanastomosis.

microsurgical tubotubal anastomosis via laparotomy for reversal of sterilization vary from 50 to 80 percent[92] There is less experience with laparoscopic microsurgical reanastomosis, although pregnancy rates from 65 to 80 percent have been reported.[93,94]

Prior to microsurgical tubal reanastomosis the patient and partner (unless donor sperm is to be used) should be examined in regard to reproductive potential. The patient should have adequate ovarian reserve and be ovulatory, age being an important prognostic indicator of postoperative pregnancy rates.[95] Her partner's semen analysis should be reviewed; severe male factor would shift the management plan from surgery to IVF with intracytoplasmic sperm injection (ICSI). The preoperative evaluation also should assess for indicators of remaining length of fallopian tube, with higher pregnancy rates associated with increasing length of the fallopian tubes after anastomosis.[96] The operative note from the sterilization procedure should be reviewed, if possible. HSG can forewarn against poor outcome by estimating the length of the fallopian tube and identifying the site of occlusion.

Optimal results are achieved when the surgeon adheres to the principles of microsurgery, careful tissue handling, minimal damage to tissue (e.g., use of needle cautery), and avoiding desiccation of tissue. Costs may be relatively comparable between reanastomosis performed by laparoscopy or by laparotomy if the open procedure is done through a minilaparotomy on an outpatient basis. Recovery time may be less with laparoscopy. However, the main criterion determining the approach to tubotubal anastomosis should be the skill level of the surgeon.

Adhesion Prevention

Adhesions are formed after any type of inflammatory reaction. Peritubal adhesions can result from infection or surgical trauma. Microsurgical technique attempts to minimize the damage but does not prevent adhesions.[97] As the exudate from the inflammatory reaction resolves, inadequate fibrinolytic activity leads to deposits of fibrinous bands. With the accompanying release of cytokines, angiogenesis ensues, and fibroblasts migrate to the damaged tissue.[98] This causes persistence and occasional thickening of the adhesions.

Several agents have been used to prevent adhesion formation. Traditionally, fluid of various types has been instilled in the pelvic cavity prior to closure of the surgical incision to prevent de novo adhesions or adhesion reformation after lysis. Examples of such agents include normal saline/crystalloids, heparinized saline, Hyskon, and so on. Unfortunately, there is little evidence supporting the use of these substances in adhesion prevention.

Currently, three barrier membranes are used routinely to prevent adhesions. Each has its distinct advantages and disadvantages. Interceed is an absorbable oxidized cellulose product that is flexible and can be applied over the adnexa via laparotomy or laparoscopy. Several well-designed trials have shown it to be approximately 50 percent effective in decreasing adhesion formation/re-formation.[37,99] Disadvantages include the need for complete hemostasis and difficulty covering diffuse areas of tissue damage. Seprafilm is another absorbable barrier made from hyaluronic acid and carboxymethylcellulose. A prospective, randomized, multicenter study revealed that Seprafilm did reduce adhesions significantly compared with controls.[100] Disadvantages of Seprafilm stem from its poor flexibility; it cannot be used laparoscopically and is difficult to use in the adnexa.

Gore-Tex is a polytetrafluoroethylene material that may be sutured in place and acts as a physical barrier to adhesion formation with proven effectiveness in several prospective trials.[101,102] It is flexible and does not require complete hemostasis. However, it requires removal, usually laparoscopically, due to its nonabsorbability.

Obviously, the surgical site is at most risk for adhesions. However, frequently adhesions also can be found in adjacent areas, and diffuse adhesion prevention is necessary when multiple surgical sites are involved. To address these issues, several fluid adhesion-prevention products have been developed. Another advantage is ease of use during laparoscopy. Both Intergel and Sepracoat are hyaluronic acid products in a crystalloid solution. Randomized, prospective trials have shown both to be effective at reducing adhesion formation/re-formation.[103,104]

With the high likelihood of adhesion formation/re-formation after some gynecologic procedures (e.g., myomectomy) and the ready availability of preventative measures, adhesion barriers should be used routinely in gynecologic surgery to optimize fertility. The choice of product should be decided on an individualized basis as indicated.

Surgery versus IVF

With the continued improvements in IVF pregnancy rates (see Chap. 22), as well as parallel advances in endoscopy, the choice between surgery and IVF for tubal disease is not an easy one. A thorough evaluation coupled with the specific technical skill of the physician will help to guide the patient-physician team. In comparing IVF and tubal surgery, Penzias and DeCherney propose that the fecundability rate is the appropriate yardstick to compare the two treatment options.[105] The fecundability rate of an IVF cycle (20 percent) is much higher than that after tubal reanastomosis (2 to 4 percent). In addition, they calculated the cost per live birth to be greater with tubal surgery than with IVF ($17,000 versus $12,000).

Distinct advantages are present with each therapeutic option. Surgery offers a chance at several pregnancies, avoidance of ovarian hyperstimulation syndrome, and higher-order multiple gestations. It should be advocated for young patients with good prognostic indicators. Alternatively, IVF offers hope to those with more severe pelvic pathology. In general, in older patients and in those with multiple factors affecting fertility (such as tubal disease and male factor), the decision to proceed with IVF rather than surgery is appropriate.

KEY POINTS

1. One-fourth to one-third of all infertile couples are diagnosed with tubal disease. PID is the leading cause of tubal factor infertility, increasing with each episode of PID. Between 15 and 20 percent of tubal factor infertility is due to pelvic adhesions.

2. Fertilization and early cleavage occur in the ampulla, and it is the most common site of ectopic gestation. Pelvic adhesions, agglutination of the fimbria, obstruction of the tube, and denudation of the mucosa lead to subfertility.

3. Cigarette smoking and IUD use have been associated with tubal factor infertility. History of endometriosis, prior gynecologic surgery, ruptured appendix, postoperative infection of the pelvis, and septic abortion are risk factors for tubal factor infertility.

4. Congenital anomalies such as unilateral absence of fallopian tube, accessory tubal ostia, elongated fimbria-ovarica, or those caused by DES exposure are uncommon causes of infertility but are found more often in infertile women.

5. HSG is currently the procedure of choice in determining tubal patency. Sensitivity and specificity for HSG for tubal patency is 65 and 83 percent, respectively.

6. Laparoscopy with chromopertubation is the gold standard for evaluating tubal disease. One stratagem for appropriate timing of laparoscopy for infertility is after clomiphene citrate therapy but prior to gonadotropins.

7. Proximal tubal occlusion may be treated by microsurgical reanastomosis or recanulation by transcervical endoscopic or fluoroscopic guidance.

8. Surgery for distal occlusion should be reserved for those with mild disease. In a patient with hydrosalpinx planning to undergo IVF, the fallopian tube should be excised or interrupted prior to IVF.

9. In young women with good prognostic indicators, microsurgical tubal reanastomosis is preferable. However, in older patients or those with multiple factors contributing to infertility, IVF is the procedure of choice.

REFERENCES

1. Vayena E, Rowe PJ, Griffin PD. *Current Practices and Controversies in Assisted Reproduction.* Geneva: World Health Organization, 2002.
2. Serafini P, Batzofin J. Diagnosis of female infertility, a comprehensive approach. *J Reprod Med* 1989;34:29–40.
3. Stewart-Smythe GW, van Iddekinge B. Lessons learned from infertility investigation in the public sector. *S Afr Med J* 2003;93:141–143.
4. Tanahatoe SJ, Hompes PG, Lambalk CB. Accuracy of diagnostic laparoscopy in the infertility workup before intrauterine insemination. *Fertil Steril* 2003;79:361–366.
5. Coson SL, Cheng A, Gutmann JN. Laparoscopy in the "normal" infertile patient: A question revisited. *J Am Assoc Gynecol Laparosc* 2000;7: 317–324.
6. Miller JH, Weinberg RK, Canino NL, et al. The pattern of infertility diagnosis in women of advanced reproductive age. *Am J Obstet Gynecol* 1999;181:952–957.
7. Sharara FI, McClamrock HD. Differences in in vitro fertilization outcome between white and black women in an inner-city, university-based IVF program. *Fertil Steril* 2000;73:1170–1173.
8. Buck GM, Sever LE, Batt RE, Mendola P. Lifestyle factors and female infertility. *Epidemiology* 1997;8:435–441.
9. Ludwig KS. The Mayer-Rokitansky-Kuster syndrome: An analysis of its morphology and embryology. Part II. Embryology. *Arch Gynecol Obstet* 1998;262:27–42.
10. Eddy CA, Pauerstein CJ. Anatomy and physiology of the fallopian tube. *Clin Obstet Gynecol* 1980;23:1177–1193.
11. Herschlag A, Diamond MP, DeCherney AH. Tubal physiology: An appraisal. *Gynecol Surg* 1989;5:3–25.
12. Patek E, Nilsson L, Johannisson E. Scanning electron microscope study of the human fallopian tube: I. The proliferative and secretory stages. *Fertil Steril* 1972;23:459
13. Sweeny W. The interstitial portion of the uterine tube: Its gross anatomy, course, and length. *Obstet Gynecol* 1962;19:3–8
14. Vasen L. The intramural part of the fallopian tube. *Int J Fertil* 1959;4:309–314.
15. Drollette CM, Badawy SZ. Pathophysiology of pelvic adhesions: Modern trends in preventing infertility. *J Reprod Med* 1992;37:107–121.
16. Strandell A, Lindhard A. Why does hydrosalpinx reduce fertility? The importance of hydrosalpinx fluid. *Hum Reprod* 2002;17:1141–1145.
17. Ajonuma LC, Ng EH, Chan HC. New insights into the mechanism underlying hydrosalpinx fluid formation and its adverse effect on IVF outcome. *Hum Reprod Update* 2002;8:255–264.
18. Leng Z, Moore DE, Mueller BA, et al. Characterization of ciliary activity in distal fallopian biopsies of women with obstructive tubal infertility. *Hum Reprod* 1998;13:3121–3127.
19. Westrom L. Effect of acute pelvic inflammatory disease on fertility. *Am J Obstet Gynecol* 1975;121: 707–713.

20. Westrom L. Incidence, prevalence, and trends of acute pelvic inflammatory disease and its consequences in industrialized countries. *Am J Obstet Gynecol* 1980;138:880–892.

21. Westrom L, Joesoef R, Reynolds G, et al. Pelvic inflammatory disease and fertility: A cohort study of 1844 women with laparoscopically verified disease and 657 control women with normal laparoscopic results. *Sex Transm Dis* 1992;19:185–192.

22. Grimes DA. Intrauterine device and upper-genital-tract infection. *Lancet* 2000;356:1013–1019.

23. Lepine LA, Hillis SD, Marchbanks PA, et al. Severity of pelvic inflammatory disease as a predictor of the probability of live birth. *Am J Obstet Gynecol* 1998;178:977–981.

24. Workowski KA, Berman SM: CDC sexually transmitted disease treatment guidelines. *Clin Infect Dis* 2002;35:S135–137.

25. Westrom LV. *Chlamydia* and its effect on reproduction. *J Br Fertil Soc* 1996;1:23–30.

26. Sheikh HH. Infertility due to genital tuberculosis. *J Am Assoc Gynecol Laparosc* 1996;3:453–459.

27. Parikh FR, Nadkarni SG, Kamat SA, et al. Genital tuberculosis: A major pelvic factor causing infertility in Indian women. *Fertil Steril* 1997;67:497–500.

28. Trimbos-Kemper T, Trimbos B, van Hall E. Etiological factors in tubal infertility. *Fertil Steril* 1982;37:384–388.

29. Mueller BA, Daling JR, Moore DE, et al. Appendectomy and the risk of tubal infertility. *N Engl J Med* 1986;315:1506–1508.

30. Urbach DR, Marrett LD, Kung R, Cohen MM. Association of perforation of the appendix with female tubal infertility. *Am J Epidemiol* 2001;153:566–571.

31. Bahamondes L, Bueno JG, Hardy E, et al. Identification of main risk factors for tubal infertility. *Fertil Steril* 1994;61:478–482.

32. Evaldson GR, Frederici H, Jullig C, et al. Hospital-associated infections in obstetrics and gynecology: Effects of surveillance. *Acta Obstet Gynecol Scand* 1992;71:54–58.

33. Stubblefield PG, Grimes DA. Current concepts: Septic abortion. *New Engl J Med* 1994;331:310–314.

34. Santanam N, Murphy AA, Parthasarathy S. Macrophages, oxidation, and endometriosis. *Ann NY Acad Sci* 2002;955:183–198.

35. Donnez J, Casanas-Roux F. Histology: A prognostic factor in proximal tubal occlusion. *Eur J Obstet Gynecol Reprod Biol* 1988;29:33–38.

36. DeCherney AH, Mezer HC. The nature of post tuboplasty pelvic adhesions as determined by early and late laparoscopy. *Fertil Steril* 1984;41:643–646.

37. Azziz R. Microsurgery alone or with Interceed absorbable adhesion barrier for pelvic sidewall adhesion re-formation: The Interceed (TC7) adhesion barrier study group II. *Surg Gynecol Obstet* 1993;177:135–139.

38. DeCherney AH, Cholst I, Naftolin F. Structure and function of the fallopian tubes following exposure to diethylstilbestrol (DES) during gestation. *Fertil Steril* 1981;36:741–745.

39. Saracoglu FO, Mungan T, Tanzer F. Salpingitis isthmica nodosa in infertility and ectopic pregnancy. *Gynecol Obstet Invest* 1992;34:202–205.

40. Yablonski M, Sarge T, Wild RA. Subtle variations in tubal anatomy in infertile women. *Fertil Steril* 1990;54:455–458.

41. McBean JH, Brumsted JR. Pregnancy after laparoscopic neosalpingostomy in a patient with atresia of the distal fallopian tubes. *Fertil Steril* 1994;61:1163–1164.

42. Nissen ED, Kent DR, Nissen SE, Feldman BM. Unilateral tuboovarian autoamputation. *J Reprod Med* 1977;19:151–153.

43. Eschenbach DA. Epdiemiology and diagnosis of acute pelvic inflammatory disease. *Obstet Gynecol* 1980;55:142S–153S.

44. Forman RG, Robinson JN, Mehta Z, Barlow DH. Patient history as a simple predictor of pelvic pathology in subfertile women. *Hum Reprod* 1993;8:53–55.

45. Mol BW, Collins JA, Van Der Veen F, Bossuyt PM. Cost-effectiveness of hysterosalpingography, laparoscopy, and *Chlamydia* antibody testing in subfertile couples. *Fertil Steril* 2001;75:571–580.

46. Land JA, Evers JL. *Chlamydia* infection and subferility. *Best Pract Res Clin Obstet Gynaecol* 2002;16:901–912.

47. Johnson NP, Taylor K, Nadgir, K, et al. Can diagnostic laparoscopy be avoided in routine investigation for infertility? *Br J Obstet Gynaecol* 2000;108:127–128.

48. Adelusi B, al-Nuaim L, Makanjuola D, et al. Accuracy of hysterosalpingography and laparoscopic hydrotubation in diagnosis of tubal patency. *Fertil Steril* 1995;63:1016–1020.

49. Ismajovich B, Wexler S, Golan A, et al. The accuracy of hysterosalpingography versus laparoscopy in evaluation of infertile women. *Int J Gynaecol Obstet* 1986;24:9–12.

50. Swart P, Mol BW, van der Veen F, et al. The accuracy of hysterosalpingography in the diagnosis of tubal pathology: a meta-analysis. *Fertil Steril* 1995;64:486–491.

51. Johnson N, Vandekerckhove P, Watson A, et al. Tubal flushing for subfertility. *Cochrane Database Syst Rev* 2002;CD003718.

52. Vandekerckhove P, Watson A, Lilford R, et al. Oil-soluble versus water-soluble media for assessing tubal patency with hysterosalpingography or laparoscopy in subfertile women. *Cochrane Database Syst Rev* 2002;CD000092.

53. Steiner AZ, Meyer WR, Clark RL, Hartmann KE. Oil-soluble contrast during hysterosalpingography in women with proven tubal patency. *Obstet Gynecol* 2003;101:109–113.

54. Capelo FO, Kumar A, Steinkampf MP, Azziz R. Laparoscopic evaluation following failure to achieve pregnancy with clomiphene citrate ovulation induction. *Fertil Steril* 2003;80:1450–1453.

55. Al-Badawi IA, Fluker MR, Bebbington MW. Diagnostic laparoscopy in infertile women with normal hysterosalpingograms. *J Reprod Med* 1999;44:953–957.

56. Tanahatoe S, Hompes PG, Lambalk CB. Accuracy of diagnostic laparoscopy in the infertility workup before intrauterine insemination. *Fertil Steril* 2003;79:361–366.

57. Corson SL, Cheng A, Gutmann JN. Laparoscopy in the "normal" patient: a question revisited. *J Am Assoc Gynecol Laparosc* 2000;7:317–324.

58. Marcoux S, Maheux R, Berube S. Laparoscopic surgery in infertile women with minimal or mild endometriosis. Canadian Collaborative Group on Endometriosis. *N Engl J Med* 1997;337:217–222.

59. Opsahl MS, Miller B, Klein TA. The predictive value of hysterosalpingography for tubal and peritoneal infertility factors. *Fertil Steril* 1993;60:444–448.

60. Cundiff G, Carr BR, Marshburn PB. Infertile couples with a normal hysterosalpingogram: Reproductive outcome and its relationship to clinical and laparoscopic findings. *J Reprod Med* 1995;40:19–24.

61. Gordts S. Campo R, Puttemans P, et al. Investigation of the infertile couple: A one-stop outpatient endoscopy-based approach. *Hum Reprod* 2002;17:1684–1687.

62. Surrey ES. Microendoscopy of the human fallopian tube. *J Am Assoc Gynecol Laparosc* 1999;6:383–389.

63. Rimbach S, Bastert G, Wallwiener D. Technical results of falloposcopy for infertility diagnosis in a large multicentre study. *Hum Reprod* 2001;16:925–930.

64. Surrey ES. Microendoscopy of the human fallopian tube. *J Am Assoc Gynecol Laparosc* 1999;6:383–389.

65. Marana R, Catalano GF, Muzii L, et al. The prognostic role of salpingoscopy in laparoscopic tubal surgery. *Hum Reprod* 1999;14:2991–2995.

66. Heylen SM, Brosens IA, Puttemans PJ. Clinical value and cumulative pregnancy rates following rigid salpingoscopy during laparoscopy for infertility. *Hum Reprod* 1995;10:2913–2916.

67. Marana R, Muzii L, Rizzi M, dell'Acqua S, Mancuso S. Prognostic role of laparoscopic salpingoscopy of the only remaining tube after contralateral ectopic pregnancy. *Fertil Steril* 1995;63:303–306.

68. Boudghene FP, Bazot M, Robert Y, et al. Assessment of fallopian tube patency by HyCoSy: Comparison of a positive contrast agent with saline solution. *Ultrasound Obstet Gynecol* 2001;18:525–530.

69. Holz K, Becker R, Schurmann R. Ultrasound in the investigation of tubal patency: A meta-anlysis of three comparative studies of Echovist-200 including 1007 women. *Zentralb Gynakol* 1997;119:366–373.

70. Dijkman AB, Mol BW, van der Veen F, et al. Can hysterosalpingocontrast-sonography replace hysterosalpingography in the assessment of tubal subfterility? *Eur J Radiol* 2000;35:44–48.

71. Strandell A, Bourne T, Bergh C, et al. The assessment of endometrial pathology and tubal patency: A comparison between the use of ultrasonography and x-ray hysterosalpingography for the investigation of infertility patients. *Ultrasound Obstet Gynecol* 1999;14:200–204.

72. Portuondo JA, Echanojauregui AD, Pena Irala J, Calonge J. Triple evaluation of tubal patency. *Int J Fertil* 1980;25:307–310.

73. World Health Organization. Comparative trial of tubal insufflation, hysterosalpingography, and

laparosocopy with dye hydrotubation for assessment of tubal patency. *Fertil Steril* 1986;46:1101–1107.

74. Stone SC, McCalley M, Braunstein P, Egbert R. Radionuclide evaluation of tubal function. *Fertil Steril* 1985;43:757–760.

75. McQueen D, McKillop JH, Gray HW, et al. Investigation of tubal infertility by radionuclide migration. *Hum Reprod* 1991;6:529–532.

76. Lundberg S, Wramsby H, Bremmer S, et al. Radionuclide hysterosapingography does not distinguish between fertile women, before tubal sterilization, and infertile women. *Hum Reprod* 1997;12:275–278.

77. Novy MJ, Thurmond AS, Patton P, et al. Diagnosis of corneal obstruction by transcervidal fallopian tube cannulation *Fertil Steril* 1988;50:434–440.

78. Gomel V. Tubal reanastomosis by microsurgery. *Fertil Steril* 1977;28:59–65.

79. Diamond E. A comparison of gross and microsurgical techniques for the repair of cornual occlusion in infertility: A retrospective study, 1968–1978. *Fertil Steril* 1979;32:370–376.

80. Schill T, Bauer O, Felberbaum R, et al. Transcervical falloscopic dilatation of proximal tubal occlusion: Is there an indication? *Hum Reprod* 1999;14:137–144.

81. Thurmond AS, Machan LS, Maubon AJ. A review of selective salpingography and fallopian tube catheterization. *Radiographics* 2000;20:1759–1768.

82. Honore GM, Holden AE, Schenken RS. Pathophysiology and management of proximal tubal blockage. *Fertil Steril* 1999;71:785–795.

83. Rock JA, Katayama P, Martin EJ, et al. Factors influencing the success of neosalpingostomy techniques for distal fimbrial obstruction. *Obstet Gynecol* 1978;52:591–596.

84. Schlaff WD, Hassiakos DK, Damewood MD, Rock JA. Neosalpingostomy for distal obstruction: Prognostic factors and surgical technique. *Fertil Steril* 1990;54:984–990.

85. Oh ST. Tubal patency and conception rates with three methods of laparoscopic terminal neosalpingostomy. *J Am Assoc Gynecol Laparosc* 1996;3:519–523.

86. Milingos SD, Kallipolitis GK, Loutradis DC, et al. Laparoscopic treatment of hydrosalpinx: factors affecting pregnancy rate. *J Am Assoc Gynecol Laparosc* 2000;7:355–361.

87. Wright VC, Schieve LA, Reynolds MA, Jeng G. Assisted reproductive technology surveillance—United States, 2000. *MMWR Morb Mortal Wkly Rep* 2003;52:1–16.

88. Johnson NP, Mak W, Sowter MC. Laparoscopic salpingectomy for women with hydrosalpinges enhances the success of IVF: A Cochrane review. *Hum Reprod* 2002;17:543–548.

89. Stadtmauer LA, Riehl RM, Toma SK, Talbert LM. Cauterization of hydrosalpinges before in vitro fertilization is an effective surgical treatment associated with improved pregnancy rates. *Am J Obstet Gynecol* 2000;183:367–371.

90. Dubuisson JB, Chapron C. Single suture laparoscopic tubal reanastomosis. *Curr Opin Obstet Gynecol* 1998;10:307–313.

91. Stadtmauer L, Sauer M. Outpatient reversal of sterilization with laparoscopically placed titanium staples. *J Am Assoc Gynecol Laparosc* 1996;3:S47.

92. Gomel V. Reconstructive tubal surgery, in Rock JA, Thompson JD (eds), *Te Linde's Operative Gynecology*. Philadelphia: Lippincott Raven, 1997:575.

93. Koh CH, Janik GM. Laparoscopic microsurgery: current and future status. *Curr Opin Obstet Gynecol* 1999;11:401–407.

94. Bissonnette F, Lapensee L, Bouzayen R. Outpatient laparoscopic tubal anastomosis and subsequent fertility. *Fertil Steril* 1999;72:549–552.

95. Hanafi MM. Factors affecting the pregnancy rate after microsurgical reversal of tubal ligation. *Fertil Steril* 2003;80:434–440.

96. Silber SJ, Cohen R. Microsurgical reversal of female sterilization: The role of tubal length. *Fertil Steril* 1980;33:598–601.

97. Diamond MP, DeCherney AH. Pathogenesis of adhesion formation/re-formation: Application to reproductive pelvic surgery. *Microsurgery* 1987;8:103–107

98. Farquhar C, Vandekerckhove P, Watson A, et al. Barrier agents for preventing adhesions after surgery for subfertility. *Cochrane Database Syst Rev* 2002;4:1–34.

99. Nordic Adhesion Prevention Study Group. The efficacy of Interceed (TC7) for prevention of re-formation of postoperative adhesions on ovaries, fallopian tubes, and fimbriae in microsurgical oprations for fertility: A multicenter study. *Fertil Steril* 1995;63:709–714.

100. Diamond MP. Reduction of adhesions after uterine myomectomy by Seprafilm membrane (HAL-F): A blinded, prospective, randomized, multicenter clinical study. *Fertil Steril* 1996;66:904–910.

101. Haney AF, Hesla J, Hurst BS, et al. Expanded polytetrafluoroethylene (Gore-Tex Surgical Membrane) is superior to oxidized regenerated cellulose (Interceed TC7) in preventing adhesions. *Fertil Steril* 1995;63:1021–1026.

102. The Myomectomy Adhesions Multicenter Study Group. An expanded polytetrafluoroethylene barrier (Gore-Tex Surgical Membrane) reduces post-myomectomy adhesion formation. *Fertil Steril* 1995;63:491–493.

103. Diamond MP and the Sepracoat Adhesion Study Group. Reduction of de novo postsurgical adhesions by intraoperative precoating with Sepracoat (HAL-C) solution: A prospective, randomized, blinded, placebo-controlled multicenter study. *Fertil Steril* 1998;69:1067–1074.

104. Johns D. Reduction of postsurgical adhesions with Intergel adhesion prevention solution: A multicenter study of safety and efficacy after conservative gynecologic surgery. *Fertil Steril* 2001;76:595–604.

105. Penzias AS, DeCherney AH. Is there ever a role for tubal surgery? *Am J Obstet Gynecol* 1996;174:1218–1223.

CHAPTER 22

Assisted Reproductive Technology: Clinical Aspects

DAVID R. MELDRUM

► ASSISTED REPRODUCTIVE TECHNOLOGY (ART) PROCEDURES

In Vitro Fertilization–Embryo Transfer (IVF-ET)

IVF-ET involves the aspiration of an oocyte or oocytes from ovarian follicles, fertilization of resulting mature eggs, and transfer of embryos into the uterine cavity. In the year 1999, 64,000 cycles were done in the United States, with a mean delivery rate per oocyte retrieval of 29.4 percent.[1] All causes of infertility refractory to standard treatment except uterine causes can be treated by IVF-ET. This ART procedure has become the cornerstone of advanced infertility therapy and will be discussed at greater length in the remainder of this chapter.

Gamete Intrafallopian Transfer (GIFT)

GIFT involves the aspiration of mature oocytes from ovarian follicles and transfer of oocytes and sperm to the fallopian tube via laparoscopy. Because of its invasive nature and the need for an operating room, GIFT now accounts for only 9.5 percent of ART cycles.[1] GIFT is an excellent choice for women with a difficult embryo transfer, is particularly successful in cases of failed donor insemination,[2–4] in which case the fertilizing capacity of the sperm is high, and may be more successful in women of advanced age,[1] allowing the oocytes and embryos maximum exposure to in vivo conditions. GIFT requires at least one normal fallopian tube and has a reduced outcome with advanced male factor.[4] The laparoscopy offers additional diagnostic or even therapeutic opportunities that may be advantageous in specific circumstances. GIFT is the only ART procedure officially allowed by the Roman Catholic Church. The delivery rate per oocyte retrieval in 1999 was 27.9 percent, which is similar to IVF,[1] and controlled studies have shown success rates similar to IVF.[5] In the absence of specific indications, in most programs GIFT is not an advantage over IVF. Efforts to place gametes into the fallopian tube by ultrasound guidance or hysteroscopy have not been as successful in most hands.

Tubal Embryo Transfer (TET)

TET or zygote intrafallopian transfer (ZIFT) involves the placement of fertilized eggs (zygotes) or embryos into the fallopian tube. The delivery rate per oocyte retrieval in 1999 was 29.8 percent, which is similar to IVF,[1] and controlled

535

studies have also shown success rates similar to IVF.[6] TET has been reported to increase the success rate of thawed embryo transfer.[7] Since culture with various cell types can rescue poor-quality embryos, contact with the fallopian tube epithelium may provide a more optimal environment for the growth of frozen-thawed embryos.

As noted earlier, as IVF results have improved steadily, that procedure has become the procedure of choice for most couples. Success rates have more than doubled during the last 15 to 20 years. Table 22-1 outlines the factors most responsible for this dramatic development. This chapter will describe a holistic approach to optimizing IVF results through attention to detail throughout the entire process.

▶ **TABLE 22-1:** ADVANCES RESPONSIBLE FOR THE CURRENT LEVEL OF IVF SUCCESS AND HIGHER LEVELS ANTICIPATED IN THE FUTURE

1. Control of LH levels/activity through GnRH agonist, oral contraceptive pretreatment, GnRH antagonist, and LH add-back
2. Use of adjuncts such as low-dose aspirin and glucocorticoids (poor responders) and metformin (PCOS)
3. Resolution of interfering factors through antibiotics, removal of hydrosalpinges, and treatment of endometriosis
4. High rate of oocyte retrieval by transvaginal ultrasound guidance
5. Consistently good fertilization through use of ICSI when appropriate
6. Improved culture techniques, media, and embryo selection
7. Atraumatic embryo transfer, optimally with ultrasound guidance
8. Enhancement of implantation through assisted hatching, stress reduction, progesterone and estrogen support, and possibly pretreatment endometrial biopsy

See text for key to abbreviations.

▶ PATIENT PREPARATION

Lower-Level Treatment Completed

IVF-ET is expensive, has a substantial risk of multiple pregnancy, and may be associated with small increases in pregnancy complications and fetal abnormalities. Based on a thorough fertility evaluation, simpler, less invasive treatments and those with lesser risk of multiple pregnancy should be advised before recommending IVF-ET.

Health and Infections Screening

Both partners should be screened for human immunodeficiency virus (HIV) infection, hepatitis B and C infection, and syphilis so that appropriate treatment, informed consent, and protective measures (e.g., vaccination of the female partner and alerting the ART laboratory personnel) can be carried out. Health screening such as a Pap smear and mammogram should be up to date. Egg-donation recipients over age 45 should have a more thorough health evaluation, including a stress electrocardiogram (ECG), blood lipid panel, glucose tolerance test, chemistry panel, and chest x-ray when indicated.

Chlamydia and *ureaplasma* have been reported to affect implantation[8,9] and increase miscarriage rates.[10] Since these organisms can be present in the upper reproductive tract with negative cervical samples,[11] an empirical course of doxycycline for both partners is logical. Other benefits are treatment of unrecognized endometritis or bacterial colonization of the seminal fluid.

Ovarian Reserve Screening

Age,[1] day 3 follicle-stimulating hormone (FSH)[12] and estradiol concentrations,[13] and antral follicle count (AFC)[14,15] allow assessment of prognosis regarding the ART cycle outcomes, choice of the most appropriate stimulation, and in some cases a recommendation to use donor eggs. Because of between-cycle variability, more than one FSH measurement is helpful. An elevated level of FSH (over 10 to 12 mIU/mL in most current assays) predicts a poor prognosis, particularly in women over 40 years of age and in those with a low AFC. Multiple elevated levels of FSH predict a worse prognosis than a single abnormal value.[16] Low AFC and high FSH and high estradiol concentrations each predict an increased chance of cycle cancellation.[12–15] In some women, a clomiphene citrate challenge test[17] will reveal an abnormal day 10 FSH level in a patient whose day 3 FSH concentration was normal and takes less time than relying on multiple day 3 measurements.

Evaluation of the Uterus, Fallopian Tubes, and Pelvis

Uterine Defects

A high-resolution transvaginal ultrasound in the follicular phase together with hysterosalpingography (HSG) is often sufficient to evaluate the uterus. If these tests are not completely satisfactory, a sonohysterogram or hysteroscopy should be done. Polyps, synechiae, or a uterine septum should be treated before any ART procedure. Submucous myomas markedly reduce implantation[18] and should be resected by hysteroscopy or, if necessary, by laparotomy. Data on intramural myomas are mixed,[18–23] suggesting less impact and possibly more dependence on size and location (the definition of intramural versus submucosal myomas is not clear) and whether there is any distortion of the endometrial cavity. Subserosal fibroids do not appear to influence outcome.[18] Recently, a prospective, randomized study showed a marked and significant increase of implantation when endometrial biopsies were done in the cycle before IVF. The authors hypothesized that the healing reaction led to improved implantation through release of growth

factors.[24] Viable pregnancy is reduced by about 50 percent with a history of diethylstilbestrol (DES) exposure.[25] Outcome is particularly poor with constrictions or a T-shaped cavity but is normal when the cavity is merely small.[25]

Hydrosalpinx

The presence of a hydrosalpinx reduces IVF success by approximately 50 percent[26] as a result of both reduced implantation and increased miscarriage. Outcomes are normalized by salpingectomy[27] and by interruption of the proximal tube.[28] These measures also reduce ectopic pregnancy and serious infections that can occur with oocyte retrieval or embryo transfer in women with a hydrosalpinx. The impact may be less when the hydrosalpinx is not visible on transvaginal (TV) ultrasonography.[29] However, hydrosalpinges enlarge during stimulation[30] and may only become visible during the IVF cycle. The adverse effect of hydrosalpinx may be by a mechanical effect of fluid refluxing into the uterus and a toxic effect on embryos and endometrium. Endometrial biopsy has shown reduced or absent integrin and often a retarded endometrium in these patients.[31] It is not clear whether aspiration of the hydrosalpinx at the time of oocyte retrieval is beneficial. An endometrial biopsy for integrin may be helpful when surgery is contraindicated. Most IVF practitioners would agree that a hydrosalpinx generally should be removed or isolated from the uterus before IVF. This also may allow pregnancy without IVF if the other tube is functional.[32] The procedure logically should be done before any intrauterine manipulation, which could seed bacteria into the obstructed tube.

Endometriosis

Metaanalysis yielded an odds ratio of 0.56 for successful pregnancy with IVF in women with endometriosis.[33] Some publication bias is suspected because the U.S. IVF Registry has not shown such an effect.[1] Also, in some older studies included in the metaanalysis, oocyte yield was reduced because of difficult laparoscopic retrieval. However, in two recent randomized trials of 3 to 6 months of treatment with a gonadotropin-releasing hormone (GnRH) agonist, significant improvements were noted in IVF success immediately following medical treatment in women with stage III and IV endometriosis.[34,35] These studies indicate that active endometriosis may influence IVF success. There has been concern that prolonged suppression could reduce ovarian response, but in one study when a subcutaneous GnRH agonist was started 30 to 45 days after the third depot injection of agonist, the number of oocytes retrieved was the same as in the group without pretreatment.[34] Success with GIFT also has been reported to be lower in the presence of endometriosis.[36]

Preparation of the Patient with Polycystic Ovary Syndrome (PCOS)

Metformin, which reduces insulin and androgens in women with PCOS, improves the success of IVF by increasing fertilization and implantation rates.[37] Metformin also may reduce excessive response[38] and miscarriage.[39] It may be started before or with initiation of oral contraceptive pretreatment and generally is stopped with a positive pregnancy test.

Low-Dose Aspirin

A prospective, double-blind, placebo-controlled study has shown that 100 mg aspirin daily resulted in increased ovarian response, pregnancy, and delivery rates and increases in uterine and ovarian blood flow.[40] Since ovarian stromal blood flow correlates with ovarian response[41] and good blood supply of the follicle may improve oocyte function[42] and even chromosomal normality,[43] this adjunct should logically be assumed to improve success. Aspirin should be started before ovarian stimulation and continued daily through the entire cycle. With years of routine use, we

have not observed any effect on bleeding at the time of oocyte retrieval. The 24 h before oocyte retrieval may be the most sensitive period for the oocyte because most aneuploidy occurs during resumption of meiosis.

Mock Embryo Transfer

A rehearsal of the embryo transfer (ET) has been shown to improve IVF outcome by markedly reducing difficult transfers.[44] With the accumulating evidence of higher success rates using ultrasound-guided ET, the mock ET logically also should be done with ultrasound guidance. More accurate measurements of uterine depth are obtained, and the optimal choice of speculum and extent of bladder fullness can be planned. In the small percentage of women whose mock ET is difficult with proper uterine positioning and ultrasound guidance, cervical dilation[45] or even hysteroscopic resection of obstructing ridges[46] can be done and the mock ET repeated before initiating ovarian stimulation.

Preparation of the Male Partner

Semen Analysis Including Leukocytes and Strict Morphology

A complete semen analysis should include evaluation of the grade of motility and strict morphology because abnormalities may lead to low or failed fertilization with standard insemination of the oocytes.[47,48] Although a high insemination number in males with low strict morphology may increase fertilization, the implantation rate remains low,[48] probably due to the adverse effects of a large number of abnormal sperm on the culture environment. A specific stain for leukocytes will differentiate white blood cells from immature sperm forms. Urologic consultation and antibiotic treatment may lead to improvements in sperm function.[49]

Sperm Penetration Assay (SPA), Antisperm Antibodies (ASAs), and Sperm Chromatin Structure Assay (SCSA)

The SPA can be helpful in defining a male partner at risk for failed fertilization.[50] Since overnight incubation with test-yolk buffer (TYB) normalizes the SPA in most men with a low SPA and otherwise normal semen and TYB improves fertilization with IVF,[51] I have abandoned this test, routinely using TYB for all oocyte inseminations not accompanied by intracytoplasmic sperm injection (ICSI). Using a TYB specimen from the day before and the day of oocyte retrieval, failed fertilization has been rare. An ASA determination should be done in men with a history of genital trauma, surgery, or infection and should be considered for any couple with unexplained infertility. Newer tests to evaluate sperm DNA integrity (SCSA) may elucidate an

unrecognized lower prognosis with IVF.[52] SCSA has indicated that the method of sperm preparation for IVF is critical. Density-gradient centrifugation increases the number of sperm with nuclear integrity by 450 percent,[53] in addition to improving morphology and motility.

Choice of Oocyte Insemination or Intracytoplasmic Sperm Injection (ICSI)

In most IVF programs, ICSI is advised whenever a significant chance of low or failed fertilization is present. In some programs, ICSI is advised for all couples with unexplained infertility or for half their oocytes because of their increased chance of failed fertilization. ICSI is always required for surgically retrieved sperm. Figure 22-1 shows the ICSI procedure.

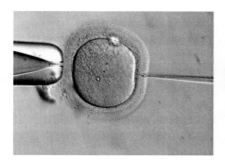
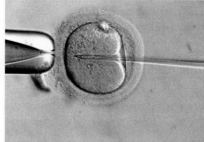
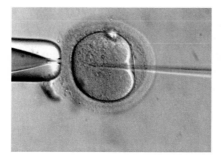

Figure 22-1 Intracytoplasmic sperm injection (ICSI). Note the sperm clearly seen in the end of the injection pipette and after being deposited into the cytoplasm *(arrows)*. *(Courtesy of Minda Hamilton.)*

Choice and Timing of Sperm Retrieval Technique

In obstructive azoospermia (OA), sperm can be retrieved by microsurgical epididymal sperm aspiration (MESA), which provides the largest number of sperm for cryopreservation for future cycles; by percutaneous epididymal sperm aspiration (PESA), which is less invasive but obtains fewer sperm; or by testicular sperm extraction (TESE) by needle aspiration or open biopsy. In nonobstructive azoospermia (NOA), an open testicular biopsy is usually done. Identification of tubules containing sperm can be facilitated by using microsurgical techniques, which also allows avoidance of testicular blood vessels and minimizes the amount of tissue removed. In one report, microsurgical technique increased the percentage of cases with sperm retrieval from 45 to 63 percent.[54] In NOA, repeat biopsy may not necessarily yield sperm for a further cycle, but the incidence is higher (80 versus 25 percent) if at least 6 months is allowed for the testicle to recover its function between biopsies.[55] Motility of testicular sperm in NOA is minimal and cannot be assured after cryopreservation. Motility of sperm in OA and particularly NOA increases over 24 to 48 hours of in vitro incubation, thus increasing the number of sperm available for oocyte insemination and for cryopreservation.[56]

Genetic Testing

Men with very low sperm density (<5 million/mL) should have a blood karyotype because of a low incidence of chromosomal anomalies.[57] Men with Kleinfelter's syndrome (XXY) have had TESE/ICSI, and most, but not all, conceptuses thus far reported have been normal.[58] All men with NOA should be offered testing for Y chromosome microdeletions, which can be passed to their male offspring, requiring ICSI for them to be fertile.[57] Both men with congenital absence of the vas deferens and their female partners should be tested for cystic fibrosis (CF)

mutations because of the high incidence of CF mutations in these males[57] and the chance that the CF mutation in the male is not part of the screening panel being used.

Sexual Dysfunction

Having a frozen backup specimen and sildenafil (Viagra) available for men with sexual dysfunction will reduce the risk of not having sperm to inseminate the oocytes.

Lifestyle Changes

Smoking by the female partner decreases oocyte yield and fertilization, lowers the success rate of IVF by about 50 percent,[59] and increases miscarriage. Therefore smoking must be stopped before and during the cycle. Smoking cessation by the male may improve sperm function.[60] Vitamin C has been shown to improve sperm quality[61] in smokers. Caffeine has effects on female fertility. A recent study suggested that the best outcome with IVF is achieved with 2 mg or less consumption per day (equivalent to one cup of decaffeinated coffee).[62] Alcohol, even in small amounts, has been linked to female infertility.[63] I advise no alcohol for the female and limited intake for the male partner.

Stress, anxiety, and depression have been linked to reduced IVF outcome,[64–66] and intervention has been shown to improve success.[67] Couples should choose a time of lowest possible stress for their cycle, with time off from work sometimes being the best option for stress reduction.

▶ OVARIAN PREPARATION

Unstimulated Cycle

Oocyte retrieval without ovarian stimulation has resulted in an ongoing pregnancy rate per transfer of 16 percent.[68] However, because of cycle cancellations due to a luteinizing hormone (LH) surge and reduced number of oocytes retrieved, the ongoing pregnancy rate per started cycle is only 7 percent.[68] One of the difficult problems is allowing full oocyte maturation because of the likelihood of an LH surge before human chorionic gonadotropin (hCG) administration. This problem may be overcome by using a GnRH antagonist with support of the follicle with human menopausal gonadotropin (hMG).[69] This approach was reported recently to yield a 17 percent delivery rate per oocyte retrieval.[70] Use of antagonist and development of techniques to achieve a very high retrieval rate could make the natural cycle an effective option, thus avoiding the risks of ovarian stimulation and multiple pregnancy.

Retrieval of immature oocytes and maturation in vitro have been applied successfully to women with PCOS, with a pregnancy rate per ET of 27 percent.[71] This laboratory-intensive technique is available in a very small number of centers worldwide and requires ICSI to achieve a good rate of fertilization. Because of the small number of babies born to date, this technique should be considered experimental.

Long GnRH Agonist Regimens

The use of a GnRH agonist markedly reduces cycle cancellation due to a premature LH surge or poor response, increases the number of oocytes and embryos, increases the number of oocytes available for cryopreservation, allows flexibility for timing of oocyte retrieval, and increases the pregnancy rate twofold compared with regimens not using a GnRH agonist.[72,73] For all these reasons, a GnRH agonist is used routinely by virtually all IVF practitioners. The "long protocol" is used most commonly, in which ovarian stimulation is begun only after ovarian function is suppressed.

GnRH agonists vary widely in potency, route of administration, and dose schedule, all of which influence the degree of gonadotropin suppression. The most common agonist used in the United States is leuprolide acetate, the full dose in normal women being 1.0 mg/d until ovarian suppression and then 0.5 mg/d until hCG administration.[72]

Midluteal Start

Starting the long GnRH agonist protocol in the midluteal phase reduces cyst formation by reducing the agonist phase of gonadotropin release.[74] Significantly more oocytes are obtained by starting at least 8 days after ovulation compared with starting in the early luteal phase.[75] In one study, starting the long protocol during the luteal phase resulted in a significantly higher pregnancy rate than starting in the early follicular phase.[76]

Oral Contraceptive Overlap

Pretreatment with an oral contraceptive (OC) further reduces cyst formation to essentially nil and results in an improved response to stimulation.[77] It is most commonly given as a 2- to 3-week course with overlapping GnRH agonist for 5 to 7 days. Varying the duration of OC minimizes menopausal side effects due to prolonging the GnRH agonist to achieve cycle programming. Figure 22-2 shows a typical OC-agonist long protocol.

Choice of Gonadotropin and Dose

Newer recombinant preparations of FSH (rFSH) have the advantage of high purity and consistency, subcutaneous administration, and avoidance of human-derived material. However, some women on full doses of GnRH agonist or a GnRH agonist with oral contraceptive overlap and some women on a GnRH antagonist, particularly with oral contraceptive pretreatment, have very low levels of LH. This lower exposure of LH to the maturing follicle has been associated with lower fertilization rates,[78,79] lower implantation rates,[80] and increased early fetal loss.[81]

Based on these findings, it is currently very common for rFSH to be used together with hMG to provide LH activity. Since most of the

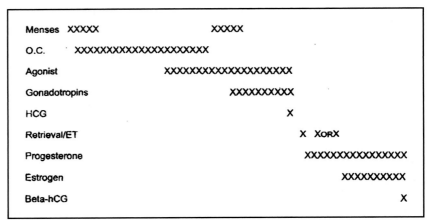

Figure 22-2 The sequence of medications and procedures in a typical oral contraceptive/GnRH agonist long protocol.

LH activity of hMG is derived from small amounts of hCG in the hMG (averaging approximately 10 units per vial), it has been suggested that 20 to 30 units of hCG (mini-hCG) could be used instead of hMG.[82] This tiny dose of hCG can be given subcutaneously with no reaction, mixed with the rFSH, and provides more consistent LH activity than hMG.[83,84]

The dose of gonadotropin must be individualized according to age, weight, day 3 FSH level, AFC, prior ovarian response, and presence of PCOS. For example, a normal-weight woman with PCOS on metformin or a young, thin non-PCOS patient with a normal FSH level and AFC would be given a dose of 150 IU or less per day, whereas a heavy patient with prior low response might be given 450 IU or more per day. In general, a higher initial dose tapering toward the time of hCG is more physiologic. Serum estradiol has been used commonly to aid in the timing of dose reduction. Increasing the gonadotropin dose after the first 5 days of ovarian stimulation is not helpful.[85]

Short or Flare Regimens

Flare protocols take advantage of the agonist phase of gonadotropin release from the pituitary with the initiation of GnRH agonist treatment before pituitary desensitization occurs, with the potential advantages of a shorter treatment time and lower total dose of gonadotropin. Disadvantages are lack of flexibility because treatment is started on cycle day 2, fewer follicles and oocytes,[86] and an apparent complete lack of flexibility in the timing of hCG. In one randomized study, a delay of only 1 day for hCG administration beyond 17 mm mean diameter resulted in dramatically reduced implantation rate.[87] It is possible that OC pretreatment could improve ovarian response by providing a more synchronous group of early antral follicles, as well as restoring flexibility by being able to vary the OC duration. Currently, flare regimens are used for a minority of ART stimulations.

GnRH Antagonist

Since GnRH antagonists can suppress gonadotropins within hours, they can be used in a very short course of daily injections confined to the time when follicle maturation is more advanced. A large dose-ranging study determined that 250 μg/d of ganirelix acetate is sufficient to prevent the LH surge and was the dose associated with the highest rate of implantation.[88] Lower doses provided less LH suppression and lower implantation rates. Higher doses dramatically lowered implantation, possibly related in part to marked suppression of LH. Since frozen embryos from those high-dose cycles implanted well, a direct effect of antagonist on the endometrium also has been suggested.

Large multicenter studies have been done to compare outcomes of GnRH antagonists against agonists. These studies together have shown small but significant decreases in ovarian response and implantation (odds ratio 0.79, confidence limits 0.63–0.99) compared with long GnRH agonist regimens.[89] These minor differences probably were due to inexperience, a lesser synchronization of follicles when ovarian stimulation was begun, the rigidity of research protocols, and excessive suppression of LH in some women.

Initially, many practitioners did not appreciate the profound suppression of endogenous gonadotropin that occurs with the antagonist, which results in a natural step-down of gonadotropin exposure to the follicles. In addition, with antagonist use estradiol rises more rapidly in the early phase of stimulation.[90] Consequently, practitioners would try to change the estradiol levels, firstly decreasing the level of FSH and then rapidly increasing the dose as estradiol levels dropped. Hence the gonadotropin dose should be maintained constant when antagonist is begun.

Second, the initiation of ovarian stimulation in the early follicular phase when dominant follicle selection is underway is a logical explanation for the lower ovarian response compared with GnRH agonist cycles, where stimulation is begun with a suppressed and more synchronous cohort of follicles. The use of OC pretreatment[91] will provide both flexibility and better synchrony. Based on recovery of gonadotropins after OC administration,[92] the fourth or fifth day after discontinuation of the OC has been used to start ovarian stimulation. I have used day 5 for women over age 35 or poor responders because recovery of gonadotropins is slower in older women.[93]

Third, since research protocol called for starting the antagonist on day 6 of stimulation rather than at a specific lead follicle diameter, this may have resulted in a much greater exposure of the endometrium to the antagonist in some women. Since a direct effect of the GnRH antagonist on implantation has been suggested,[94,95] the current trend of starting the antagonist at 14 mm lead follicle diameter should minimize any adverse endometrial effect.

Finally, although mean LH levels were identical in agonist and antagonist cycles,[90] there is approximately a 75 percent further suppression of LH after each dose of antagonist,[96] resulting in very low LH levels in many women. It is therefore currently popular to substitute hMG for part of the FSH when antagonist is started. Since recovery of LH suppression may not occur consistently on day 4 after stopping the OCs and LH levels remain lower, it is logical to use some hMG or to add mini-hCG from the beginning of ovarian stimulation in OC/antagonist cycles.

Poor-Responder Stimulation Protocols

Lower-Dose Long Agonist Protocol
An improved response in poor responders has been observed with a reduction of the dose of GnRH agonist used.[97] A common dose reduction with leuprolide acetate has been 0.5 mg until suppression followed by 0.25 mg until hCG.

Increased Gonadotropin Dose
An increase in the gonadotropin dose to 450 IU daily yields a modest increase in response. Most practitioners do not believe higher amounts are helpful except with high body weight.

Mini leuprolide Flare
Use of a very small dose of leuprolide acetate (40 μg twice daily) starting on the third day after discontinuing OC, followed by beginning ovarian stimulation on the third day of the mini-flare, increases the ovarian response compared with the long protocol.[98]

GnRH Antagonist

Use of a GnRH antagonist avoids the suppression of endogenous gonadotropin occurring with the long protocol. Experience suggests outcomes similar to the miniflare. OCs before treatment may provide improved synchrony. Since recovery of gonadotropin secretion is delayed in older women,[93] it is logical to delay initiating ovarian stimulation until day 5 after cessation of OCs (see above).

Glucocorticoids

Use of 1.0 mg dexamethasone has been reported in a large double-blind, placebo-controlled study to markedly reduce cycle cancellation, with a trend toward a higher pregnancy rate.[99] Interestingly, an equivalent dose of prednisolone has been reported to significantly increase the pregnancy rate of IVF cycles with a trend toward a better follicular response.[100]

Clomiphene/Gonadotropin

Clomiphene/gonadotropins have been used in poor responders with success.[101] An OC/prednisolone/clomiphene/gonadotropin protocol has been described recently that yields results similar to the long protocol in unselected women.[102]

GnRH Agonist Stop Protocols

In an uncontrolled study, a favorable outcome was reported in women considered likely to respond poorly to stimulation by stopping GnRH agonist at the start of stimulation.[103] Randomized studies, however, have not shown improved outcomes with this technique[104,105] with possibly some adverse effects.[104]

High-Responder Stimulation Protocols

Lower Gonadotropin Dose

A reduction in gonadotropin dose to 150 IU or even 112.5 IU per day is often sufficient to avoid an excessive response.

Long OC/High-Dose Leuprolide/Low-Dose Gonadotropin

Pretreatment with an OC for 25 days, with leuprolide overlapping at 1.0 mg/day, is effective in preventing an excessive response in most women.[106] For women with PCOS, metformin may further help in controlling the response.[38]

Coasting

Continuation of GnRH agonists without further gonadotropin administration (coasting) decreases but does not eliminate the risk of severe ovarian hyperstimulation syndrome (OHSS).[107–109] Coasting should be started when sufficient oocyte maturity has been achieved so that there are a good number of follicles that are relatively gonadotropin-independent (e.g., 16 to 18 mm). The estradiol will continue to rise then fall, with hCG being given when the estradiol level falls below 3000 pg/mL. Poor prognostic signs are coasting for more than 3 to 5 days and a marked fall in estradiol. These can be prevented by initiating gonadotropin dose reduction early so that the number of small follicles and the FSH level will not be excessive when coasting is begun.

Reduced hCG Dose

Most studies suggest that 5000 IU of hCG yields a fertilization rate equivalent to 10,000 IU, and the lower dose may reduce the risk of OHSS. However, it would be prudent to be sure that the interval from hCG to retrieval and the length of oocyte preincubation are adequate.

Freezing All Embryos

Since the most severe and prolonged cases of OHSS occur with conception, freezing all embryos will reduce but not eliminate the risk of severe OHSS in high responders. The outcome for pregnancy may be reduced compared with proceeding with a fresh transfer at the time of the cycle.[110]

► OOCYTE RETRIEVAL

hCG Dose and Interval

A dose of 10,000 units of hCG is customary to induce oocyte maturity prior to retrieval. Since the patient or her partner usually gives this critically important injection, instructions for preparation must be very specific. On the morning after administration, proper procedure should be confirmed. Every possible error in hCG administration has occurred, including giving only the diluent or purchasing an incompletely filled vial of hCG. Inadequate or insufficient hCG administration has been associated with the empty-follicle syndrome (see below). Oocyte retrieval is done most often at 35 to 36 hours after hCG injection. Since ovulation rarely occurs before 38 h in GnRH agonist cycles, this allows for flexibility in case of delays. However, with larger follicles, lower doses of agonist, and difficult retrievals, I have occasionally seen follicles collapse spontaneously when there was a delay in retrieval beyond 36 h.

Analgesia

Follicle aspiration generally is done with conscious sedation using a sedative and narcotic or more commonly recently with deep sedation using Propofol. Although studies have demonstrated the ability of Propofol to adversely affect the oocyte, large, highly successful programs have used it routinely and did not notice a change in success rates when it was instituted. However, it is a logical precaution to begin the Propofol only after all other preparations are complete, immediately before aspiration.

Vaginal Preparation

The vagina should be cleansed and rinsed thoroughly to reduce the chance of bacterial contamination of the oocyte culture. Povidone-iodine is used very commonly, but a well-designed study showed the critical importance of thoroughly removing the antiseptic prior to retrieval.[111] I use a mechanical and dilutional technique with phosphate-buffered saline, swabbing the vagina with five four-by-fours and irrigating the vaginal vault with at least 100 mL with a speculum in place, followed by four more soaks and finally a dry four-by-four.

Aspiration Procedure

A 16- or 17-gauge needle is used that has a very sharp tip. The needle should be handled carefully because even roughly placing it into a culture tube can blunt the tip. Disposable needles are used to avoid embryotoxicity. Rinsing of the needle prior to insertion ensures that any possible embryotoxic residue is removed and that the aspiration system is functioning normally. Aspiration pressure should not be excessive (generally not over 120 mmHg), as fracture of the zona pelicida can occur. Flushing of follicles has been shown overall not to increase oocyte yield.[112] My impression has been that large follicles that fold in with aspiration may benefit from flushing.

The needle is guided by ultrasound across the vaginal fornix into the center of each follicle, maintaining a good flow throughout the aspiration by rotating and positioning the needle tip, followed by a gentle curetting motion. The needle is passed into each successive follicle, withdrawing as necessary into previously aspirated follicles to direct the needle into other parts of the ovary. Often only a single vaginal puncture is required on each side. Maintaining a constant temperature of the oocyte is critical to prevent low temperature from damaging the meiotic spindle.

Difficult Retrievals

A mobile or high ovary can be repositioned manually by using a hand placed on the lower abdomen by an assistant. For a particularly mobile ovary, the uterus and attached ovary can be brought down by a tenaculum on the cervix.[113] An ovary lying in the cul-de-sac or behind the uterus often can be positioned up laterally by sweeping the ultrasound transducer across the posterior vaginal fornix or bimanually by the surgeon. An ovary that is adherent to the back of the uterine fundus can be aspirated across the uterus, occasionally even from the opposite side. This does not appear to influence the subsequent implantation rate.[114]

Endometriomas should be avoided, if possible, to prevent addition of embryotoxic material to the culture and, rarely, infection. If an endometrioma is entered, it should be aspirated completely to minimize infection and leakage. The needle and aspirating system should be flushed thoroughly before aspirating other follicles.

Empty-Follicle Syndrome

The lack of oocyte retrieval from an adequate number of mature follicles is usually due to low or absent hCG exposure to the follicle because one action of hCG is to loosen the oocyte-cumulus complex. The embryologist also may note very clear fluid with granulosa cells that are not luteinized. Serum levels of hCG and/or progesterone will be low. If an inadequate hCG injection is identified on the morning after hCG administration, it could be repeated that evening. If no oocytes are retrieved with a typical appearance of aspirated fluid, the aspiration can be halted, hCG administration repeated, and successful oocyte retrieval can be achieved by a second procedure.[115,116] even from previously aspirated follicles. Since in this circumstance pregnancies have occurred with frozen but not fresh transfer,[115,116] it appears that the endometrial advancement expected with 48 h of minor increases of circulating progesterone may be sufficient to close the window of implantation.

Complications

The incidence of pelvic infection following oocyte retrieval has been 0.2 to 0.3 percent[117,118] and should decrease with most hydrosalpinges now being removed. The incidence of significant bleeding is likewise very rare.[117,118] Rupture of an endometrioma can occur, with symptoms not becoming apparent until several hours after egg retrieval.[117] Infection of an endometrioma also has been reported.[119] Other rare complications reported are ureteral injury, massive retroperitoneal hematoma, and osteomyelitis of the sacrum.

▶ CLINICAL ASPECTS OF LABORATORY TECHNIQUE

Length of Culture and Embryo Selection

For many years the standard duration for culturing the retrieved oocytes was 48 h. This has evolved worldwide to 72 h to permit better selection of the best embryos for fresh transfer, and to allow for procedures such as assisted hatching (AH), which is best done close to when compaction is occurring, and preimplantation genetic diagnosis, which ideally is done at the eight-cell stage. Embryo selection can be based on pronuclear morphology[120] (Fig. 22-3), early cleavage to the two-cell stage,[121] and various morphologic characteristics of day 3 embryos (e.g., even cell division, lack of fragmentation and multinucleation, and signs of compaction; see Fig. 22-3). Development of media specific to the embryos' requirements during the two distinct 48-h periods following fertilization has made it possible to achieve high-quality blastocysts (see Fig. 22-3) with excellent implantation potential.[122] Transfer on day 5 allows further criteria of blastocyst morphology to be used for embryo selection, with transfer of two or even a single embryo. There have been no randomized studies using these

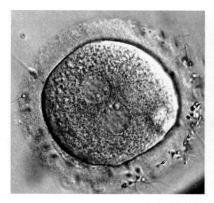
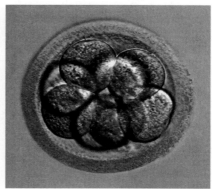
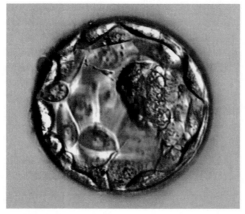

Figure 22-3   A fertilized oocyte showing the male and female pronuclei (note the nucleoli lined up in an ideal pattern), a high-grade eight-cell embryo (note the even blastomeres and absence of fragments), and a high-quality blastocyst (note the well-formed inner cell mass and trophectoderm.   *(Courtesy of Minda Hamilton and Lucinda Veeck.)*

various methods of embryo selection to determine whether one method is superior. There have been reports of increased monozygotic twinning with blastocyst culture,[123] which may decrease as better culture conditions improve the integrity of the inner cell mass.

Assisted Hatching (AH)

Following on the observation that thinning of the zona pelucida is one of the aspects of embryo morphology most predictive of implanta-

tion,[124] chemical and mechanical means have been used to create an artificial opening in the zona. Initial studies, had the data been analyzed by analysis of variance, demonstrated an overall benefit of AH with increasing age.[125] Subsequently, many conflicting studies have been published indicating that the procedure is highly technique-dependent. A recent meta-analysis calculated an odds ratio of 1.63 overall, with a greater benefit for older women and for those with prior ART procedure failures.[126] An increased incidence of monozygotic twinning also has been reported with AH.[127]

Preimplantation Genetic Diagnosis (PGD)

A wide variety of genetic disorders can be diagnosed on a single blastomere removed from the day 3 embryo.[128] The cell can be transported to a reference laboratory, and the result can be available for a day 5 transfer. The pregnancy rate has been similar, suggesting that the higher fertility of these couples offsets any negative effect of removing a blastomere. The blastomere also can be tested for aneuploidy by fluorescence in situ hybridization (FISH) so that only chromosomally normal conceptuses are replaced. An inherent limitation of aneuploidy testing is that 5 to 10 percent of normal conceptuses are discarded due to mitotic errors, although the rest of the embryo is normal. In selected older women with a good number of embryos, a highly experienced laboratory has reported increased implantation.[129]

▶ EMBRYO TRANSFER (ET)

Number of Embryos

Risk factors for multiple pregnancy are younger than 35 years of age, good ovarian response (over 10 to 12 mature follicles or oocytes), good embryo quality, extra embryos adequate for cryopreservation, and first or second IVF attempt. These factors have been used to devise guidelines for ET circulated by the American Society for Reproductive Medicine.[130] With these guidelines, most often only two embryos are transferred in women under age 35 (including donated oocytes) and three to four for those between the ages of 35 and 40 years. These guidelines have reduced the incidence of twins and triplets in the United States to about 30 and 4 percent, respectively. In many European countries, guidelines are more restrictive, with some advising single-embryo transfer in women at highest risk.

Timing of ET

Generally, ET is performed on day 3 following oocyte retrieval, at about the eight-cell embryo stage. However, a number of centers are advocating later transfers, generally on day 5 at the blastocyst stage, because of the potential higher implantation rate per embryo transferred. It has also been suggested that one reason for higher implantation rates with day 5 ET is the lower observed rate of spontaneous uterine contractions at that time compared with day 3.[131] In addition, the uterus does not provide a biochemical environment as suitable for early-cleavage embryos.[132]

Determinants of Successful ET

Traumatic or difficult ET has been correlated with reduced implantation, whether graded subjectively or using indicators such as blood on the catheter or at the cervix.[44,133] Reduced success also has been correlated with a higher frequency of uterine contractions at the time of transfer,[134] dilatation of the cervix,[135] and retention of embryos in the transfer catheter.[136] A continuous fluid column[137] and aspiration of mucus from the cervix[138] reduce expulsion of fluid and embryos. Touching the uterine fundus, which induces uterine contractions,[139] should be avoided. Traumatic transfer and transfer close to the fundus increase the risk of ectopic pregnancy.[140,141] Studies have reported a clear correlation of bacterial contamination of the transfer catheter with a lower pregnancy rate.[142,143] Even with transfer volumes as low as 40 μL, mock transfer using radiopaque dye or methylene blue has shown fluid entering the tubes or cervix.[138,144]

Ultrasound-Guided ET

Multiple randomized trials have shown a higher rate of implantation with ET performed under ultrasound guidance.[145–147] However, patients in the control groups of these studies usually did not have a full bladder, which itself has been shown to improve ET success.[148] The controls also did not consistently benefit from a verified measurement of uterine depth, and in some control groups the catheter was passed to the top of the fundus and withdrawn. The value of ultrasound-guided ET remains to be demonstrated.

Bladder Preparation

For each patient there is an extent of bladder fullness that is ideal for visualization and uterine position. I have the patient void 60 min before transfer and drink 15 oz of fluid over the 30 min before arriving and 15 oz over the 30 min waiting in the facility. Periodic scanning can help in gauging the ideal degree of bladder fullness. If overfilling occurs, patients usually can void a set amount and stop. Catheterization is also an effective way of ensuring the best conditions for ET. With a posterior uterus, visualization abdominally may be poor, in which case the bladder should be emptied completely.

Choice of Speculum

Choice of speculum type is important for good visualization and uterine positioning. In many cases a shorter speculum allows the cervix to come down toward the introitus and the uterus to thus align with the vaginal canal. Tipping the speculum blades forward often rotates the cervix forward and the uterine fundus back, aligning the anterior uterus with the vaginal canal. Tipping the speculum blades posteriorly does the opposite for the posterior uterus. Vaginal ultrasound can be used effectively with the posterior uterus or for the obese patient with poor visualization abdominally. With the speculum handle opened widely, a reasonably thin

vaginal probe can be used to guide the catheter to the proper depth.

ET Procedure

The cervix should be cleansed with culture medium, and mucus should be swabbed away and aspirated from the cervical os. Soft catheters such as the Wallace catheter can be passed by allowing them to follow the cervical canal. If resistance causes the catheter to bend, the outer sheath can be advanced over the catheter to increase the rigidity of a shorter extended portion of catheter. Ultrasound guidance often determines optimal repositioning of the uterus or angulation of the catheter for passage. If necessary, an obturator can be used for the outer sheath, making angulation possible in more difficult cases.

The catheter should be advanced to about 1.5 to 2.0 cm from the top of the fundus,[149] and the embryos should be expelled gently. If ultrasound guidance is not available, favorable results have been achieved by advancing the catheter to 0.5 to 1.0 cm less than the previously measured fundal depth. Since blind measurements may underestimate depth by the catheter tip abutting the uterine wall, and because the uterus grows during stimulation, I have seen instances when embryo deposition by blind measurement would have been at the internal os, as much as 4 to 5 cm below the top of the uterine cavity (Fig. 22-4). Commonly, the catheter is withdrawn slightly during expulsion of the transfer fluid. The volume of transfer fluid is usually kept to 20 to 30 μL. After ET, the transfer catheter should be inspected carefully microscopically for any retained embryos.

Posttransfer Activity

Few studies have addressed whether limiting activity after ET will improve results. Commonly,

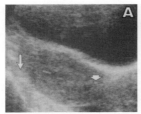
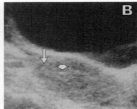
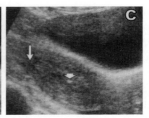

Figure 22-4 *A.* Catheter passed to 1.0 cm less than blind measurement is at internal os, 4.5 cm from top of endometrial cavity. *B.* Catheter advanced further to 1.5 cm from top of endometrial cavity. *C.* Air bubble after ET has moved down slightly to 2.3 cm from top of cavity (different patient).

patients rest in a head-down position for 30 min. I advise resting for an additional 2 days and then avoiding strenuous activity until pregnancy is confirmed. I have not had any instance of ovarian torsion using these precautions.

► LUTEAL PHASE SUPPORT

With GnRH agonist cycles, luteal support is necessary for optimal pregnancy rates because estradiol and progesterone concentrations begin a precipitous decline 8 days following hCG administration.[150] Progesterone generally is started 1 to 3 days after oocyte retrieval, with 25 to 50 mg intramuscularly daily or 200 mg micronized progesterone three times daily or 80 mg progesterone gel daily intravaginally.[150] Oral progesterone is ineffective because of extensive liver metabolism. hCG is effective[150] but increases the risk of OHSS. In addition, estrogen supplementation appears to improve implantation[150] because the estradiol level declines precipitously following hCG administration.

► FROZEN EMBRYO TRANSFER

In 1999, 12,005 frozen ETs resulted in a delivery rate of 18.6 percent per ET.[1] Thawed embryos are transferred most often in controlled hormone-replacement cycles. Hormone administration is similar to that described for egg donation below, except that GnRH agonist is not required.[151] Provided that estrogen is begun on day 1 of menses, follicular growth is inhibited. A transvaginal ultrasound is done after 14 days of estrogen administration to ensure an endometrial thickness of at least 9 mm. Counting the first day of progesterone as day 15, pronuclear embryos are thawed on day 16 and day 3 embryos on day 18. Timing of transfer is one day earlier per frozen than fresh embryos in an egg-donation recipient, thus allowing 24 hours for intrauterine recovery and reinitiation of cleavage of the frozen embryos. Recently, AH has been reported to be helpful to improve the implantation of frozen embryos because the zona hardens with freezing.[152]

► PREGNANCY FOLLOWING IVF-ET

Ultrasound Monitoring

The principal reasons for ultrasound monitoring of ART pregnancies are to assess whether a pregnancy is progressing normally, to diagnose ectopic or heterotopic pregnancy, and to determine whether twinning, particularly monozygotic, has occurred.

Ectopic and Heterotopic Pregnancy

The incidence of ectopic pregnancy has declined steadily form 4 to 2 percent of pregnancies[1,153] because of a higher proportion of nontubal cases, because hydrosalpinges are operated on before IVF, and because of better transfer technique. Cornual pregnancy can still occur after salpingectomy.[154] Also, ovarian and cervical pregnancies occur rarely. Heterotopic pregnancy occurs in less than 1 percent of pregnancies and is also becoming more rare. The intrauterine pregnancy generally proceeds normally after salpingectomy. With combined cornual and intrauterine pregnancy, potassium chloride injection into the ectopic gestational sac has been successful.

Hormone Support/Metformin

Estrogen is stopped at 6 weeks gestation and progesterone at 6 to 8 weeks or earlier if the serum progesterone concentration exceeds 60 ng/mL.[155] It also has been suggested that progesterone can be stopped routinely 2 weeks following ET.[156] For women with PCOS and a history of miscarriage, continuing metformin into pregnancy may reduce fetal loss.[39] However, most practitioners do not feel that there is sufficient experience with metformin in early pregnancy to make continuation routine.

Pregnancy Complications

Premature labor and intrauterine growth retardation are slightly increased with IVF-ET, even with singleton pregnancies.[157] There have been reports of increased risk for placenta previa, vaginal bleeding, hypertension requiring hospitalization, and cesarean births.[157] In one report, the fetal loss rate with chorion villous sampling was 3.7 percent in IVF/ICSI pregnancies versus 0.7 percent with amniocentesis.[158] Since placentation may not be entirely normal with IVF, amniocentesis may be a safer method of prenatal diagnosis.

Offspring of ART Procedures

Many reports have documented similar rates of congenital anomalies in IVF or ICSI pregnancies versus the control population.[159] However, in one report, a twofold increase was reported.[160] This could represent a publication bias or a statistical outlier because it does not fit with generally reported experience. Increases in both autosomal and sex chromosome anomalies have been reported with ICSI,[161] emphasizing the importance of doing karyotypes in men with severe oligospermia and following the recommendation for prenatal genetic testing for ICSI pregnancies. Developmental outcome of ICSI children has been reported to be normal,[162] although there have been recent reports of an increased risk for rare "imprinting" disorders that could be due to the effects of embryo culture.[163,164] Continued vigilance is required to evaluate outcomes of these relatively new technologies.

▶ OOCYTE DONATION (OD) AND SURROGACY

The delivery rates for donated oocytes using fresh and frozen embryo transfers for the year 1999 were 41.8 and 23.6 percent, respectively,[1] which are higher than routine IVF and are due almost entirely to the younger age of the oocyte donors. The delivery rate for gestational surrogacy was 33.6 percent, which is higher than for routine IVF because of the uniformly normal uterine factor.[1]

With OD, the donator of the oocytes signs a release of any rights regarding offspring. Legal precedents have established the genetic parents as the legal parents for gestational surrogacy in which the birth mother has no genetic link to the offspring. In some states such as California, the court can establish this before birth so that the birth certificate can list the contracting couple as the legal parents.

Recipient Preparation and Synchronization

Unless the recipient is clearly menopausal, a GnRH agonist is given to prevent ovarian activity from affecting implantation. Use of OCs and an overlapping agonist for both donor and recipient allows synchronization without prolonged menopausal symptoms during extended GnRH agonist suppression. The recipient is prepared with estrogen (oral estradiol 4–8 mg/d constantly or in increasing step-wise fashion; or transdermal estradiol 0.2–0.4 mg/d) for a minimum of 14 days. Progesterone is begun in the recipient on the day following hCG administration to the donor (progesterone in oil 50–100 mg/d IM; less commonly, Crinone® 90 mg once or twice per day, or progesterone suppositories 150–600 mg/d transvaginally), resulting in 3-day embryos being transferred on day 19, with day 15 being the first day of progesterone administration. Performance of a mock cycle in the recipient will ensure that the estrogen dose used will achieve an adequate endometrial thickness at the time of predicted transfer, therefore allowing for dose adjustments if necessary. Vaginal administration of estradiol has been reported to improve endometrial thickness that is refractory to standard doses of oral estrogen.[165] Endometrial biopsy is not done routinely by all programs because the impact of delayed glandular maturation is uncertain. Women with thin endometria due to previous radiation therapy may benefit from a prolonged course of pentoxyfylline/vitamin E.[166] This also has been used on women with premature ovarian failure resistant to standard hormone-replacement therapy.[167] Estrogen is continued until 8 to 10 weeks and progesterone until 10 to 12 weeks of pregnancy.

▶ SUMMARY

ART techniques require thorough preparation and testing of the infertile couple and ovarian stimulation carefully tailored to the ovarian status of the individual woman. Transvaginal ultrasound-guided retrieval is highly efficient and well suited to an office/outpatient environment. Refined techniques for embryo transfer, including ultrasound guidance, are important to optimal success. Oocyte donation and surrogacy are highly successful when required due to ovarian or uterine functional deficiencies. ART pregnancies are associated with a remarkably low rate of complications or abnormalities specific to the ART procedure, but differences from non-ART pregnancies emphasize the importance of using non-ART infertility treatments whenever appropriate. Preimplantation genetic diagnosis (PGD) will play an increasing role for couples wishing to avoid having an abnormal offspring or pregnancy termination. Finally, as techniques for embryo selection further improve, the risk of multiple pregnancy will continue to decrease by minimizing the number of embryos transferred.

KEY POINTS

1. Lower-level treatments should be completed before recommending IVF.

2. Hydrosalpinges should be removed or isolated from the uterus before IVF.

3. Medical treatment of endometriosis immediately before IVF may increase implantation.

4. Pretreatment with metformin should be considered for any woman with PCOS having IVF.

5. Most IVF stimulations are done using a midluteal agonist in a long protocol or with a GnRH antagonist. In both instances, OC pretreatment and supplementation of LH activity are advantageous.

6. Assisted hatching improves IVF outcomes, with greater benefits in older women and in those with prior IVF failure.

7. Ultrasound guidance has been associated with improved success of embryo transfer.

8. Both luteal progesterone and estrogen enhance implantation in GnRH agonist cycles.

REFERENCES

1. Society for Assisted Reproductive Technology and the American Society for Reproductive Medicine. Assisted reproductive technology in the United States: 1999 results generated from the American Society for Reproductive Medicine/Society for Assisted Reproductive Technology Registry. *Fertil Steril* 2002;78:918.

2. Cefalu E, Cittadini E, Balmaceda JP, et al. Successful gamete intrafallopian transfer following failed artificial insemination by donor: evidence for a defect in gamete transport? *Fertil Steril* 1988;50:279.

3. Formigli L, Coglitore MT, Roccio C, et al. One-hundred-and-six gamete intrafallopian transfer procedures with donor semen. *Hum Reprod* 1990;5:549.

4. Seracchioli R, Bafaro G, Bianchi L, et al. Influence of spermatozoa characteristics on gamete intra-fallopian transfer procedures: Analysis of results obtained utilizing normozoospermic, oligoasthenozoospermic and donor spermatozoa. *Hum Reprod* 1993;8:2098.

5. Tanbo T, Dale PO, Abyholm T. Assisted fertilization in infertile women with patent fallopian tubes: A comparison of in-vitro fertilization, gamete intra-fallopian transfer and tubal embryo stage transfer. *Hum Reprod* 1990;5:266.

6. Tournaye H, Devroey P, Camus M, et al. Zygote intrafallopian transfer or in vitro fertilization and embryo transfer for the treatment of male-factor infertility: A prospective, randomized trial. *Fertil Steril* 1992;58:344.

7. Van Voorhis BJ, Syrop CH, Vincent RD, et al. Tubal versus uterine transfer of cryopreserved embryos: A prospective, randomized trial. *Fertil Steril* 1995;63:578.

8. Rowland GF, Forsey T, Moss TR, et al. Failure of in vitro fertilization and embryo replacement following infection with *Chlamydia trachomatous*. *J In Vitro Fert Embryo Transfer* 1985;2:151.

9. Lunenfeld E, Shapiro BS, Sarov B, et al. The association between chlamydial-specific IgG and IgA antibodies and pregnancy outcome in an in vitro fertilization program. *J In Vitro Fert Embryo Transfer* 1989;6:222.

10. Licciardo F, Grifo JA, Rosenwaks Z, et al. Relation between antibodies to *Chlamydia trachomatis* and spontaneous abortion following in vitro fertilization. *J Assist Reprod Genet* 1992;9:207.

11. Shepard MK, Jones RB. Recovery of *Chlamydia trachomatis* from endometrial and fallopian tube biopsies in women with infertility of tubal origin. *Fertil Steril* 1989;52:232.

12. Muasher SE, Oehninger S, Simonetti S, et al. The value of basal and or stimulated serum gonadotropin levels in prediction of stimulation response and in vitro fertilization outcome. *Fertil Steril* 1998;50:298.

13. Frattarelli JL, Bergh PA, Drews MR, et al. Evaluation of basal estradiol levels in assisted reproductive technology cycles. *Fertil Steril* 2000;74:518.

14. Frattarelli JL, Lauria-Costa DF, Miller BT, et al. Basal antral follicle number and mean ovarian diameter predict cycle cancellation and ovarian responsiveness in assisted reproductive technology cycles. *Fertil Steril* 2000;74:512.

15. Bancsi LF, Broekmans FJ, Eijlmans MJ, et al. Predictors of poor ovarian response in in vitro fertilization: A prospective study comparing basal markers of ovarian reserve. *Fertil Steril* 2002;77:328.

16. Lass A, Gerrard A, Abusheikha N, et al. IVF performance of women who have fluctuating early follicular FSH levels. *J Assist Reprod Genet* 2000;17:566.

17. Scott RT, Leonardi MR, Hoffman GE, et al. A prospective evaluation of clomiphene citrate challenge test screening in the general infertility population. *Obstet Gynecol* 1993;82:539.

18. Eldar-Geva T, Meagher S, Healy DL, et al. Effect of intramural, subserosal and submucosal uterine fibroids on the outcome of assisted reproductive technology treatment. *Fertil Steril* 1998;70:687.

19. Check JH, Choe JK, Lee G, et al. The effect on IVF outcome of small intramural fibroids not compressing the uterine cavity as determined by a prospective matched control study. *Hum Reprod* 2002;17:1244.

20. Hart R, Khalaf Y, Yeong C-T, et al. A prospective, controlled study of the effect of intramural uterine fibroids on the outcome of assisted conception. *Hum Reprod* 2001;16:2411.

21. Stovall DW, Parrish SB, Van Voorhis BJ, et al. Uterine myomas reduce the efficacy of assisted

reproduction cycles: Results of a matched follow-up study. *Hum Reprod* 1998;13:192.

22. Ramzy AM, Saltar M, Amin Y, et al. Uterine myomata and outcome of assisted reproduction. *Hum Reprod* 1998;13:198.

23. Surrey ES, Lietz AK, Schoolcraft WB: Impact of intramural leiomyomata in patients with a normal endometrial cavity on in vitro fertilization–embryo transfer outcome. *Fertil Steril* 2001; 75:405.

24. Barash A, Dekel N, Fieldust S, et al. Local injury to the endometrium doubles the incidence of successful pregnancies in patients undergoing in vitro fertilization. *Fertil Steril* 2003;79: 1317.

25. Karande VC, Lester RG, Muasher SJ, et al. Are implantation and pregnancy outcome impaired in diethylstilbestrol-exposed women after in vitro fertilization and embryo transfer. *Fertil Steril* 1990;54:287.

26. Camus E, Poncelet C, Goffinet F, et al. Pregnancy rates after in-vitro fertilization in cases of tubal infertility with and without hydrosalpinx: A meta-analysis of published comparative studies. *Hum Reprod* 1999;14:1243.

27. Shelton KE, Butler L, Toner JP, et al. Salpingectomy improves the pregnancy rate in in-vitro fertilization patients with hydrosalpinx. *Hum Reprod* 1996;11:523.

28. Surrey ES, Schoolcraft WB. Laparoscopic management of hydrosalpinges before in vitro fertilization–embryo transfer: Salpingectomy versus proximal tubal occlusion. *Fertil Steril* 2001;75:612.

29. de Wit W, Gowrising CJ, Kuik DJ, et al. Only hydrosalpinges visible on ultrasound are associated with reduced implantation and pregnancy rates after in-vitro fertilization. *Hum Reprod* 1998;13:1696.

30. Hill GA, Herbert CM, Fleischer AC, et al. Enlargement of hydrosalpinges during ovarian stimulation protocols for in vitro fertilization and embryo replacement. *Fertil Steril* 1986;45: 883.

31. Meyer WR, Castelbaum AJ, Somkuti S, et al. Hydrosalpinges adversely affect markers of endometrial receptivity. *Hum Reprod* 1997;12: 1393.

32. McComb PF, Taylor RC. Pregnancy outcome after unilateral salpingostomy with a contralateral patent oviduct. *Fertil Steril* 2001;76:1278.

33. Barnhart K, Dunsmoor-Su R, Coutifaris C. Effect of endometriosis on in vitro fertilization. *Fertil Steril* 2002;77:1148.

34. Surrey ES, Silverberg KM, Surrey MW, et al. Effect of prolonged gonadotropin-releasing hormone agonist therapy on the outcome of in-vitro fertilization-embryo transfer in patients with endometriosis. *Fertil Steril* 2002;78:699.

35. Rickes D, Nickel I, Kropf S, Kleinstein J. Increased pregnancy rates after ultralong postoperative therapy with gonadotropin-releasing hormone analogs in patients with endometriosis. *Fertil Steril* 2002;78:757.

36. Guzick DS, Yao YA, Berga SL, et al. Endometriosis impairs the efficacy of gamete intrafallopian transfer: Results of a case-control study. *Fertil Steril* 1994;62: 1186.

37. Stadtmauer LA, Toma SK, Riehl RM, et al. Metformin treatment of patients with polycystic ovarian syndrome undergoing in vitro fertilization improves outcomes and is associated with modulation of the insulin-like growth factors. *Fertil Steril* 2001;75:505.

38. De Leo V, la Marca A, Ditto A, et al. Effects of metformin on gonadotropin-induced ovulation in women with polycystic ovary syndrome. *Fertil Steril* 1999;72:282.

39. Jakubowicz DJ, Ivorno MJ, Jakubowicz S, et al. Effects of metformin on early pregnancy loss in the polycystic ovary syndrome. *J Clin Endocrinol Metab* 2002;87:524.

40. Rubinstein M, Marazzi A, Polak de Fried E. Low-dose aspirin treatment improves ovarian responsiveness, uterine and ovarian blood flow velocity, implantation, and pregnancy rates in patients undergoing in vitro fertilization: A prospective, randomized, double-blind, placebo-controlled study. *Fertil Steril* 1999;71:825.

41. Popovic-Todorovic B, Loft A, Bredkjaeer HE, et al. A prospective study of predictive factors of ovarian response to "standard" IVF/ICSI patients treated with recombinant FSH: A suggestion for a recombinant FSH dosage normogram. *Hum Reprod* 2003;18:781.

42. Huey S, Abuhamad A, Barroso G, et al. Perifollicular blood flow Doppler indices, but not follicular O_2, pCO_2, or pH, predict oocyte developmental competence in in vitro fertilization. *Fertil Steril* 1999;72:707.

43. Hu Y, Betzendahl I, Cotvrindt R, et al. Effects of low O_2 and ageing on spindles with chro-

mosomes in mouse oocytes from pre-antral follicle culture. *Hum Reprod* 2001;16:737.

44. Mansour R, Aboulghar M, Serour G. Dummy embryo transfer: A technique that minimizes the problems of embryo transfer and improves the pregnancy rate in human in vitro fertilization. *Fertil Steril* 1990;54:678.

45. Abusheikha N, Lass A, Akagbosu F, et al. How useful is cervical dilation in patients with cervical stenosis who are participating in an in vitro fertilization-embryo transfer program? The Bourn Hall experience. *Fertil Steril* 1999;72:610.

46. Noyes N, Licciardi F, Grifo J, et al. In vitro fertilization outcome relative to embryo transfer difficulty: A novel approach to the forbidding cervix. *Fertil Steril* 1999;72:261.

47. Oehninger S, Acosta AA, Kruger T, et al. Failure of fertilization in in vitro fertilization: the "occult" male factor. *J In Vitro Fertil Embryo Transfer* 1988;5:181.

48. Grow DR, Oehninger S, Seltman HJ, et al. Sperm morphology as diagnosed by strict criteria: Probing the impact of teratozoospermia on fertilization rate and pregnancy outcome in a large in vitro fertilization population. *Fertil Steril* 1994;62:559.

49. Wolff H, Politch JA, Martinez A, et al. Leukocytospermia is associated with poor semen quality. *Fertil Steril* 1990;53:528.

50. Margalioth EJ, Navot D, Laufer N, et al. Correlation between the zona-free hamster egg sperm penetration assay and human in vitro fertilization. *Fertil Steril* 1986;45:665.

51. Katayama KP, Stehlik E, Roesler M, et al. Treatment of human spermatozoa with an egg yolk medium can enhance the outcome of in vitro fertilization. *Fertil Steril* 1989;52:1077.

52. Larson KL, De Jonge CJ, Barnes AM, et al. Sperm chromatin structure assay parameters as predictors of failed pregnancy following assisted reproductive procedures. *Hum Reprod* 2000;15:1717.

53. Tomlinson MJ, Moffatt O, Manicardi GC, et al. Interrelationships between seminal parameters and sperm nuclear DNA damage before and after density gradient centrifugation: Implications for assisted conception. *Hum Reprod* 2001;16:2160.

54. Schlegel PN: Testicular sperm extraction: Microdissection improves sperm yield with minimal tissue excision. *Hum Reprod* 1999;14:131.

55. Schlegel PN, Su LM. Physiologic consequences of testicular sperm extraction. *Hum Reprod* 1998;12:1688.

56. Wu B, Wong D, Dickstein S, et al. In vitro maturation of fresh and frozen-thawed testicular sperm to optimize ICSI in azoospermic patients. *Fertil Steril* 2003;79(suppl 2):S9.

57. Johnson MD. Genetic risks of intracytoplasmic sperm injection in the treatment of male infertility: Recommendations for genetic counseling and screening. *Fertil Steril* 1998;70:397.

58. Ron-El R, Strassburger D, Gelman-Kohan S, et al. A 47,XXY fetus conceived after ICSI of spermatozoa from a patient with non-mosaic Kleinefelter's syndrome. *Hum Reprod* 2000;15:1804.

59. Hughes EG, Yeo J, Claman P, et al. Cigarette smoking and the outcomes of in vitro fertilization: Measurement of effect size and levels of action. *Fertil Steril* 1994;62:807.

60. Vine MF, Tse CKJ, Hu P-C, et al. Cigarette smoking and semen quality. *Fertil Steril* 1996;65:835.

61. Dawson EB, Harris WA, Teter MC, et al. Effect of ascorbic acid supplementation on the sperm quality of smokers. *Fertil Steril* 1992;58:1034.

62. Klonoff-Cohen H, Bleha J, Lam-Kruglick P. A prospective study of the effects of female and male caffeine consumption on the reproductive endpoints of IVF and gamete intrafallopian transfer. *Hum Reprod* 2002;17:1746.

63. Hakim RB, Gray RH, Zacur H. Alcohol and caffeine consumption and decreased fertility. *Fertil Steril* 1998;70:632.

64. Sanders KA, Bruce NW. Psychosocial stress and treatment outcome following assistant reproductive technology. *Hum Reprod* 1999;14:1656.

65. Klonoff-Cohen H, Chu E, Natarajan L, et al. A prospective study of stress among women undergoing in vitro fertilization or gamete intrafallopian transfer. *Fertil Steril* 2001;76:675.

66. Smeenk JMJ, Verhaak CM, Eugster A, et al. The effect of anxiety and depression on the outcome of in-vitro fertilization. *Hum Reprod* 2001;16:1420.

67. Domar AD, Clapp D, Slawsby EA, et al. Impact of group psychological interventions on pregnancy rates in infertile women. *Fertil Steril* 2000;73:805.

68. Pelinck MJ, Hoek A, Simons AH, et al. Efficacy of natural cycle IVF: A review of the literature. *Hum Reprod Update* 2002;8:129.

69. Meldrum DR, Rivier J, Garzo G, et al. Successful pregnancies with unstimulated cycle oocyte donation using an antagonist of gonadotropin-releasing hormone. *Fertil Steril* 1994;61:556.

70. Rongieres-Bertrand C, Olivennes F, Righini C, et al. Revival of the natural cycle in in vitro fertilization with the use of a new gonadotropin-releasing hormone antagonist (Cetrorelix): A pilot study with minimal stimulation. *Hum Reprod* 1999;14:683.

71. Cha KY, Han SY, Chung HM, et al. Pregnancies and deliveries after in vitro maturation culture followed by in vitro fertilization and embryo transfer without stimulation in women with polycystic ovary syndrome. *Fertil Steril* 2000;73: 978.

72. Meldrum DR. GnRH agonists as adjuncts for in vitro fertilization. *Obstet Gynecol Surv* 1989;44: 314.

73. Hughes EG, Fedorkow DM, Daya S, et al. The routine use of gonadotropin-releasing hormone agonists prior to in vitro fertilization and gamete intrafallopian transfer: A meta-analysis of randomized, controlled trials. *Fertil Steril* 1992;58:988.

74. Meldrum DR, Wisot A, Hamilton F, et al. Timing of initiation and dose schedule of leuprolide influences the time course of ovarian suppression. *Fertil Steril* 1988;50:400.

75. Pellicer A, Simon C, Miro, F, et al. Ovarian response and outcome of in-vitro fertilization in patients treated with gonadotropin-releasing hormone analogues in different phases of the menstrual cycle. *Hum Reprod* 1989;4:285.

76. Urbancsek J, Witthaus E. Mid-luteal Buserelin is superior to early follicular phase Buserelin in combined gonadotropin-releasing hormone analogue and gonadotropin stimulation in in vitro fertilization. *Fertil Steril* 1996;65:966.

77. Biljan MM, Mahutte NG, Dean N, et al. Effects of pretreatment with an oral contraceptive on the time required to achieve pituitary suppression with gonadotropin-releasing hormone analogues and on subsequent implantation and pregnancy rates. *Fertil Steril* 1998;70:1063.

78. Westergaard LG, Erb K, Laursen S, et al. The effect of human menopausal gonadotropin and highly purified, urine-derived follicle-stimulating hormone on the outcome of in-vitro fertilization in down-regulated normogonadotrophic women. *Hum Reprod* 1996;11: 1209.

79. Soderstrom-Anttila V, Foudila F, Hovatta O. A randomized comparative study of highly purified follicle-stimulating hormone and human menopausal gonadotropin for ovarian hyperstimulation in an oocyte donation programme. *Hum Reprod* 1996;11:1864.

80. Gordon UD, Harrison RF, Fawzy M, et al. A randomized, prospective, assessor-blind evaluation of luteinizing hormone dosage and in vitro fertilization outcome. *Fertil Steril* 2001;75: 324.

81. Westergaard LG, Laursen SB, Andersen CY. Increased risk of early pregnancy loss by profound suppression of luteinizing hormone during ovarian stimulation in normogonadotropic women undergoing assisted reproduction. *Hum Reprod* 2000;15:1003.

82. Thompson KA, LaPolt PS, Rivier J, et al. Gonadotropin requirements of the developing follicle. *Fertil Steril* 1995;63:273.

83. Stone BA, Quinn K, Quinn P, et al. Responses of patients to different lots of human menopausal gonadotropins during controlled ovarian hyperstimulation. *Fertil Steril* 1989;52:745.

84. Stokman PGW, de Leeuw R, van Wijngaard HAGW, et al. Human chorionic gonadotropin in commercial human menopausal gonadotropin preparations. *Fertil Steril* 1993;60:175.

85. van Hooff MHA, Alberda AT, Huisman GJ, et al. Doubling the human menopausal gonadotropin dose in the course of an in vitro fertilization treatment cycle in low responders: A randomized study. *Hum Reprod* 1993;8:369.

86. San Ramon GA, Surrey ES, Judd HL, et al. A prospective, randomized comparison of luteal phase versus concurrent follicular phase initiation of gonadotropin-releasing hormone agonist for in vitro fertilization. *Fertil Steril* 1992;58: 744.

87. Clark L, Stanger J, Brinsmead M. Prolonged follicle stimulation decreases pregnancy rates after in vitro fertilization. *Fertil Steril* 1991;55: 1192.

88. The Ganirelix Dose-Finding Study Group. A double-blind, randomized, dose-finding study to assess the efficacy of the gonadotropin-releasing hormone antagonist ganirelix (Org 37462) to prevent premature luteinizing hormone surges in women undergoing ovarian stimulation with recombinant follicle-stimulating hormone (Puregon). *Hum Reprod* 1998;13: 3023.

89. Al-Inany H, Aboulghar M. GnRH antagonist in assisted reproduction: A Cochrane review. *Hum Reprod* 2002;17:874.

90. The North American Ganirelix Study Group. Efficacy and safety of ganirelix acetate versus leuprolide acetate in women undergoing controlled ovarian hyperstimulation. *Fertil Steril* 2001;75:38.

91. Meldrum D, Scott R, Levy MJ, et al. A pilot study to assess oral contraceptive pretreatment in women undergoing controlled ovarian hyperstimulation in ganirelix acetate cycles. *Fertil Steril* 2002;76(suppl 3):S176.

92. Van Heusden AM, Fauser BCJM. Activity of the pituitary ovarian axis in the pill-free interval during use of low-dose combined oral contraceptives. *Contraception* 1999;59:237.

93. Fitzgerald C, Elstein M, Spona J. Effect of age on the response of the hypothalamic pituitary-ovarian axis to a combined oral contraceptive. *Fertil Steril* 1999;71:1079.

94. Kol S. Embryo implantation and GnRH antagonists in ART: lower embryo implantation? *Hum Reprod* 2000;15:1881.

95. Hernandez ER. Embryo implantation and GnRH antagonists: Embryo implantation—the Rubicon for GnRH antagonists. *Hum Reprod* 2000; 15:1211.

96. Oberye JJL, Mannaerts BMJL, Huisman JAM, et al. Pharmacokinetic and pharmacodynamic characteristics of ganirelix (Antagon/Orgalutran): II. Dose proportionality and gonadotropin suppression after multiple doses of ganirelix in healthy female volunteers. *Fertil Steril* 1999;72:1006.

97. Feldberg D, Farhi J, Ashkenazi J, et al. Minidose gonadotropin-releasing hormone agonist is the treatment of choice in poor responders with high follicle-stimulating hormone levels. *Fertil Steril* 1994;62:343.

98. Schoolcraft W, Schlenker T, Gee M, et al. Improved controlled ovarian hyperstimulation in poor responders in vitro fertilization patients with a microdose follicle-stimulating hormone flare, growth hormone protocol. *Fertil Steril* 1997;67:93.

99. Keay SD, Lenton EA, Cooke ID, et al. Low-dose dexamethasone augments the ovarian response to exogenous gonadotropins leading to a reduction in cycle cancellation rate in a standard IVF programme. *Hum Reprod* 2001;16:1861.

100. Kemeter P, Feichtinger W. Prednisolone supplementation to clomid and/or gonadotropin stimulation for in-vitro fertilization: A prospective, randomized trial. *Hum Reprod* 1986;1:441.

101. Benadiva CA, Davis O, Kligman I, et al. Clomiphene citrate and hMG: An alternative stimulation protocol for selected failed in vitro fertilization patients. *J Assist Reprod Genet* 1995;12:8.

102. Weigert M, Krischker W, Pohl M, et al. Comparison of stimulation with clomiphene citrate in combination with recombinant follicle-stimulating hormone and recombinant luteinizing hormone to stimulation with a gonadotropin-releasing hormone agonist protocol: A prospective, randomized study. *Fertil Steril* 2002; 78:34.

103. Faber BM, Mayer J, Cox B. Cessation of gonadotropin-releasing hormone agonist therapy combined with high-dose gonadotropin stimulation yields favorable pregnancy results in low responders. *Fertil Steril* 1998;69:826.

104. Smitz J, Van Den Abbeel E, Bollen N, et al. The effect of gonadotropin-releasing hormone (GnRH) agonist in the follicular phase on in-vitro fertilization outcome in normo-ovulatory women. *Hum Reprod* 1992;7:1098.

105. Dirnfeld M, Fruchter O, Yshai D, et al. Cessation of gonadotropin-releasing hormone analogue (GnRH-a) upon down-regulation versus conventional long GnRH-a protocol in poor responders undergoing in vitro fertilization. *Fertil Steril* 1999;72:406.

106. Damario MA, Barmat L, Liu H-C, et al. Dual suppression with oral contraceptives and gonadotrophin releasing-hormone agonists improves in-vitro fertilization outcome in high responder patients. *Hum Reprod* 1997;12:2359.

107. Benadiva CA, Davis O, Kligman I, et al. Withholding gonadotropin administration is an effective alternative for the prevention of ovarian hyperstimulation syndrome. *Fertil Steril* 1997; 67:724.

108. Fluker MR, Hooper WM, Yuzpe AA. Withholding gonadotropins ("coasting") to minimize the risk of ovarian hyperstimulation during superovulation and in vitro fertilization-embryo transfer cycles. *Fertil Steril* 1999;71:294.

109. Tortoriello DV, McGovern PG, Colon JM, et al. "Coasting" does not adversely affect cycle outcome in a subset of highly responsive in vitro fertilization patients. *Fertil Steril* 1998;69:454.

110. Awonuga AO, Pittrof RJ, Zaidi J, et al. Elective cryopreservation of all embryos in women at risk of developing ovarian hyperstimulation syndrome may not prevent the condition but reduces the live birth rate. *J Assist Reprod Genet* 1996;13:401.

111. Van Os HC, Roozenburg BJ, Janssen-Caspers HAB, et al. Vaginal disinfection with povidone-iodine and the outcome of in-vitro fertilization. *Hum Reprod* 1992;7:349.

112. Tan SL, Waterstone J, Wren M, et al. A prospective, randomized study comparing aspiration only with aspiration and flushing for transvaginal ultrasound-directed oocyte recovery. *Fertil Steril* 1992;58:356.

113. Licciardi FL, Schwartz LB, Schmidt-Sarosi C. A tenaculum improves ovarian accessibility during difficult transvaginal follicular aspiration: A novel but simple technique. *Fertil Steril* 1995;63:677.

114. Wisanto A, Bollen N, Camus M, et al. Effect of transuterine puncture during transvaginal oocyte retrieval on the results of human in-vitro fertilization. *Hum Reprod* 1989;7:790.

115. Ubaldi F, Nagy Z, Janssenwillen C, et al. Ovulation by repeated human chorionic gonadotropin in "empty follicle syndrome" yields a twin pregnancy. *Hum Reprod* 1997;12:454.

116. Papier S, Lipowicz R, De Vincentiis S, et al. Pregnancy obtained by the transfer of frozen-thawed embryos originating from a rescued empty follicle syndrome cycle. *Fertil Steril* 2000;74:603.

117. Dicker D, Ashkenazi J, Feldburg D, et al. Severe abdominal complications after transvaginal ultrasonographically guided retrieval of oocytes for in vitro fertilization. *Fertil Steril* 1993;59:1313.

118. Bennett SJ, Waterstone JJ, Chevy WC, et al. Complications of transvaginal ultrasound-directed follicle aspiration: A review of 2670 consecutive procedures. *J Assist Reprod Genet* 1993;10:72.

119. Yaron Y, Peyser MR, Samuel D. Infected endometriotic cysts secondary to oocyte aspiration for in-vitro fertilization. *Hum Reprod* 1994;9:1759.

120. Tesarik J, Greco E. The probability of abnormal preimplantation development can be predicted by a single static observation on pronuclear stage morphology. *Hum Reprod* 1999;14:1318.

121. Sakkas D, Percival G, D'Arcy Y, et al. Assessment of early cleaving in vitro fertilized human embryos at the two-cell stage before transfer improves embryo selection. *Fertil Steril* 2001;76:1150.

122. Gardner DK, Schoolcraft WB, Wagley L, et al. A prospective, randomized trial of blastocyst culture and transfer in in-vitro fertilization. *Hum Reprod* 1998;13:3434.

123. Behr B, Fisch JD, Racowsky C, et al. Blastocyst-ET and monozygotic twinning. *J Assist Reprod Genet* 2000;17:349.

124. Cohen J, Inge KL, Suzman M, et al. Videocinematography of fresh and cryopreserved embryos: A retrospective analysis of embryonic morphology and implantation. *Fertil Steril* 1989;51:820.

125. Cohen J, Alikani M, Trowbridge J, et al. Implantation enhancement by selective assisted hatching using zona drilling of human embryos with poor prognosis. *Hum Reprod* 1992;7:685.

126. Edi-Osagie E, Hooper L, Seif MW. The impact of assisted hatching on live birth rates and outcomes of assisted conception: A systematic review. *Hum Reprod* 2003;18:1828.

127. Schieve LA, Meikle SF, Peterson HB, et al. Does assisted hatching pose a risk for monozygotic twinning in pregnancies conceived through in vitro fertilization? *Fertil Steril* 2000;74:288.

128. ESHRE PGD Consortium Steering Committee. ESHRE Preimplantation Genetic Diagnosis Consortium: Data collection III (May 2001). *Hum Reprod* 2002;17:233.

129. Munne S, Cohen J, Sable D. Preimplantation genetic diagnosis for advanced maternal age and other indications. *Fertil Steril* 2002;78:234.

130. American Society for Reproductive Medicine Practice Committee Report. *Guidelines on Number of Embryos Transferred*. Birmingham, AL: ASRM, November 1999.

131. Fanchin R, Ayoubi J-M, Righini C, et al. Uterine contractility decreases at the time of blastocyst transfers. *Hum Reprod* 2001;16:1115.

132. Gardner DK, Lane M, Calderon I, et al. Environment of the preimplantation embryo in vivo: Metabolite analysis of oviduct and uterine fluids and metabolism of cumulus cells. *Fertil Steril* 1996;65:349.

133. Spandorfer SD, Goldstein J, Navarro J, et al. Difficult embryo transfer has a negative impact on the outcome of in vitro fertilization. *Fertil Steril* 2003;79:654.

134. Fanchin R, Righini F, Oliveness R, et al. Uterine contractions at the time of embryo transfer alter pregnancy rates after in vitro fertilization. *Hum Reprod* 1998;13:1968.

135. Groutz A, Lessing JB, Wolf Y, et al. Cervical dilation during ovum pick-up in patients with cervical stenosis: Effect on pregnancy outcome in an in vitro fertilization-embryo transfer program. *Fertil Steril* 1997;67:909.

136. Visser D, Fourie F, Kruger H. Multiple attempts at embryo transfer: Effect on pregnancy outcome in an in vitro fertilization and embryo transfer program. *J Assist Reprod Genet* 1993; 10:37.

137. Poindexter AN, Thompson DJ, Gibbons WE, et al. Residual embryos in failed embryo transfer. *Fertil Steril* 1986;46:262.

138. Mansour RT, Abolughar MA, Serour GI, et al. Dummy embryo transfer using methylene blue due. *Hum Reprod* 1994;9:1257.

139. Lesney P, Killick SR, Tetlow RL, et al. Embryo transfer: Can we learn anything new from the observation of junctional zona contractions? *Hum Reprod* 1998;13:1540.

140. Yovich JL, Turner SR, Murphy AJ. Embryo transfer technique as a cause of ectopic pregnancies in in vitro fertilization. *Fertil Steril* 1985;44:318.

141. Nazari A, Askari HI, Check JH. Embryo transfer technique as a cause of ectopic pregnancy in in vitro fertilization. *Fertil Steril* 1993;60:919.

142. Fanchin R, Harmas A, Benaoudia F, et al. Microbial flora of the cervix assessed at the time of embryo transfer adversely affects in vitro fertilization outcome. *Fertil Steril* 1998;70:866.

143. Egbase PE, Al-Sharhan M, Al-Othman S, et al. Incidence of microbial growth from the tip of the embryo transfer catheter after embryo transfer in relation to clinical pregnancy rate follow in-vitro fertilization and embryo transfer. *Hum Reprod* 1996;11:1687.

144. Knutzen V, Stratton CJ, Sher G, et al. Mock embryo transfer in early luteal phase, the cycle before in vitro fertilization and embryo transfer: A descriptive study. *Fertil Steril* 1992;57:156.

145. Coroleu B, Carreras O, Veiga A, et al. Embryo transfer under ultrasound guidance improves pregnancy rates after in-vitro fertilization. *Hum Reprod* 2000;15:616.

146. Buckett WM. A meta-analysis of ultrasound-guided versus clinical touch embryo transfer. *Fertil Steril* 2003;80:1037.

147. Sallam HN, Sadek SS. Ultrasound-guided embryo transfer: A meta-analysis of randomized, controlled trials. *Fertil Steril* 2003;80:1042.

148. Lewin A, Schenker JG, Avrech O, et al. The role of uterine straightening by passive bladder distension before embryo transfer in IVF cycles. *J Assist Reprod Genet* 1997;14:32.

149. Coroleu G, Barri PN, Carreras O, et al. The influence of the depth of embryo replacement into the uterine cavity on implantation rates after IVF: A controlled, ultrasound-guided study. *Hum Reprod* 2002;17:341.

150. Pritts EA, Atwood AK. Luteal phase support in infertility treatment: A meta-analysis of the randomized trials. *Hum Reprod* 2002;17:2287.

151. de Ziegler D, Cornel C, Bergeron C, et al. Controlled preparation of the endometrium with exogenous estradiol and progesterone in women having functioning ovaries. *Fertil Steril* 1991;56:851.

152. Check JH, Hoover L, Nazari A, et al. The effect of assisted hatching on pregnancy rates after frozen embryo transfer. *Fertil Steril* 1996;65: 254.

153. Society for Assisted Reproductive Technology. In vitro fertilization–embryo transfer in the United States: 1988 results from the IVF-ET Registry. *Fertil Steril* 1990;53:13.

154. Agarwal SK, Wisot AL, Garzo, G, et al. Cornual pregnancies in patients with prior salpingectomy undergoing in vitro fertilization and embryo transfer. *Fertil Steril* 1996;65:659.

155. Stovall DW, Van Voorhis BJ, Sparks AET, et al. Selective early elimination of luteal support in assisted reproduction cycles using a gonadotropin-releasing hormone agonist during ovarian stimulation. *Fertil Steril* 1998;70:1056.

156. Schmidt KLT, Ziebe S, Popovic B, et al. Progesterone supplementation during early gestation after in vitro fertilization has no effect on the delivery rate. *Fertil Steril* 2001;75:337.

157. Tan SL, Doyle P, Campbell S, et al. Obstetric outcome of in vitro fertilization pregnancies compared with normally conceived pregnancies. *Am J Obstet Gynecol* 1992;167:778.

158. Kolibianakis E, Osmanagaoglu K, De Catte L, et al. Prenatal genetic testing by amniocentesis appears to result in a lower risk of fetal loss than chorionic villus sampling in singleton pregnancies achieved by intracytoplasmic sperm injection. *Fertil Steril* 2003;79:374.

159. Bonduelle M, Legein J, Buysse A, et al. Prospective follow-up of 423 children born after intracytoplasmic sperm injection. *Hum Reprod* 1996;11:1558.

160. Hansen M, Kurinczuk JJ, Bower C, et al. The risk of major defects after intracytoplasmic sperm injection and in vitro fertilization. *N Engl J Med* 2002;346:725.

161. Bonduelle M, Van Assche E, Joris H, et al. Prenatal testing in ICSI pregnancies: Incidence of chromosomal anomalies in 1586 karyotypes and relation to sperm parameters. *Hum Reprod* 2002;17:2600.

162. Bonduelle M, Ponjaert I, Van Steirteghem A, et al. Developmental outcome at 2 years of age for children born after ICSI compared with children born after IVF. *Hum Reprod* 2003;18:342.

163. De Baun MR, Niemitz EL, Feinberg AP. Association of in vitro fertilization with Beckwith-Wiedemann syndrome and epigenetic alterations of LIT1 and H19. *Am J Hum Genet* 2003; 72:156.

164. Orstavik KH, Eiklid K, van der Hagen CB, et al. Another case of imprinting defect in a girl with Angelman syndrome who was conceived by intracytoplasmic sperm injection. *Am J Hum Genet* 2003;72:218.

165. Tourgeman DE, Slater CC, Stanczyk FZ, et al. Endocrine and clinical effects of micronized estradiol administered vaginally or orally. *Fertil Steril* 2001;75:200.

166. Letur-Konirsch H, Guis F, Delanian S. Uterine restoration by irradiation sequelae regression with combined pentoxyfylline-tocopherol: A phase II study. *Fertil Steril* 2002;77:1219.

167. Letur-Konirsch H, Delanian S. Successful pregnancies after combined pentoxyfylline-tocopherol treatment in women with premature ovarian failure who are resistant to hormone replacement therapy. *Fertil Steril* 2003;79:439.

CHAPTER 23

Assisted Reproductive Technologies: Laboratory Aspects

JUERGEN LIEBERMANN AND MICHAEL J TUCKER

With human in vitro fertilization (IVF) laboratory technology well into its third decade, it is a good time to take stock of where we have been, are currently, and hope to go within the near future. What started out as a simple clinical scientific endeavor has now turned into a multi-million-dollar industry with profound and far-reaching ramifications both ethically and socially. It once was the case that IVF laboratory technologists were recruited mostly for their academic thirst and ability to handle confidently human gametes and embryos. Now the demands of increased turnover of patient cycles, escalating technology, and the constant threat of litigious consequences haunt the everyday pursuits of the clinical embryologist in the twenty-first century. Nevertheless, these are exciting times for embryologists with improved laboratory accreditation, management, and understanding of their role, and it is gratifying to be able to produce results from our labors at a rate nearly threefold what they were in terms of embryonic implantation 20 years ago (Tables 23-1 and 23-2). These levels of success have arisen from a combination of innovation, invention, consistency, and old-fashioned hard work. An ultimate goal is for the IVF laboratory to achieve routine selection of single human embryos for transfer with high potential for viability—all of which is achievable only in the context of the greater team that enables us to operate in possibly the only clinical specialty that requires such close and continuous cooperation between the clinical and scientific worlds.

► MICROMANIPULATION

Assisted Fertilization

Intracytoplasmic sperm injection (ICSI)[1] not only has become the insemination of choice for all cases of IVF where fertilization failure may occur, but it also may become the only form of insemination in vitro,[2,3] although others may strongly disagree.[4] Use of a laser to assist ICSI in cases of oocytes prone to rupture has been proposed; by predrilling the zona where the ICSI needle is to go, this seems to reduce egg degeneration.[5] This may be one area where the original technique of ICSI may

▶ **TABLE 23-1:** NON-DONOR-EGG RESULTS AT SHADY GROVE FERTILITY (2002)

	<35 Years	35–37 Years	38–40 Years	>40 Years	Overall
Cycles	749	508	490	197	1944
Eggs collected	654	420	378	149	1601
Transfers	633	400	369	148	1550
Pregnancies	370	198	141	44	753
PR/ET	58%	50%	38%	30%	49%
PR/EC	57%	47%	37%	30%	47%

be improved on. Nevertheless, ICSI remains a profoundly effective form of insemination in vitro for nearly all forms of male infertility where spermatozoa can be retrieved from testicular tissue,[6] if it is performed optimally, that is (see refs 7 and 8). A cloud still hangs over the invasive nature of ICSI and how it may have long-term implications for offspring. In some cases there is a clear need for preimplantation and prenatal screening of embryos/fetuses that arise when the severest forms of male factor sperm are used, e.g., in cases of congenital absence of the vas deferens linked to cystic fibrosis. Nevertheless, overall there appears little distinction to be made between the birth defects arising from conventional IVF and ICSI.[9] Bonduelle and colleagues[10] have established that there is little grounds to suspect a postzygotic (postfertilization, i.e., iatrogenic) impact on embryonic abnormalities as a result of the ICSI procedure and simply noted a relationship between higher rates of sex chromosome and autosomal structural anomalies and lower sperm counts and motility. Recently,

higher than anticipated incidences of imprinting defects seemingly linked with ICSI have raised concerns that, while not common, may indeed be a worrisome complication of the ICSI process, where it may interfere with the normal establishment of the maternal imprint in the oocyte or embryo.[11,12]

Spermatozoa do not need to be morphologically normal or even alive in the conventional sense to participate in embryo development; as long as they have intact genomes, they potentially can produce normal offspring.[13] Chromosomes within the first and second polar bodies can be used as substitutes for female pronuclei for the production of normal mouse offspring.[13] The nuclei of adult somatic cells can be used for production of animals. This procedure, involving introduction of cell nuclei into enucleated oocytes (genomic cloning), is rather inefficient at present. Many obstacles must be overcome before it may be accepted as a safe, novel method to produce scientifically, medically, or economically valuable animals. For human cloning, the prime

▶ **TABLE 23-2:** RECIPIENT/DONOR-EGG CYCLES AT SHADY GROVE FERTILITY

	2000	2001	2000+1	2002
Cycles	107	143	251	178
Percent canceled	16%	15%	16%	14%
Eggs collected	90	121	211	153
Transfers	88	121	209	153
Clinical PR/ET	56 (67%)	82 (68%)	141 (67%)	106 (69%)
Viable PR/EC	44 (49%)	71 (49%)	115 (55%)	101 (66%)

consideration must be the welfare of the child. Haploidization of somatic cell nuclei within enucleated eggs, followed by reconstitution of a diploid status with addition of a partner's gamete, may be considered a plausible and acceptable form of semireproductive cloning[14,15]; however, the same concerns that apply to all nuclear-transfer technologies apply here also.

Assisted Hatching

This technology continues to be applied with varying reports of effectiveness.[16,17] When undertaken with acidified Tyrode's medium to drill the zona pellucida, cell fragment removal has been carried out with some reported success.[18] Laser zona ablation[19] also may be used, as well as physical rupture of the zona with a glass needle.[20] Assisted hatching could be eliminated in its present forms and be replaced by whole-zona dissolution prior to blastocyst transfer.[21] The risk of exposure of the "naked" blastocyst and its trophectoderm to the enzyme pronase and its vulnerability during embryo transfer (ET) have to be weighed against the potential benefits of releasing the blastocyst from all zonal constraints during its preimplantation phase. As we learn more about the actual characteristics of zona pellucida behavior under the influence of the expanding blastocyst, we learn more about how this might correlate with the timing and potential of hatching.[22]

From personal experience,[23] we have found that there is a distinct difference in ongoing pregnancy and implantation rates between day 5 and day 6 transfers. The simplistic interpretation would be that day 6 transfers are suboptimal and best avoided. However, in fairness, the patients in this group generally were older and had undergone more repeat IVF cycles than the day 5 group. In an attempt to address these poorer outcomes, we now routinely undertake assisted hatching on all day 6 transfer cases following exposure of the blastocysts to 0.2 M sucrose; this shrinks the blastocyst away from the zona pellucida and so

minimizes the risk of damage to the trophectoderm during drilling (Fig. 23-1). A large hole can be drilled (40 μm) with little risk of disruption to the blastocyst, and commonly hatching is observed by the time of uterine ET. The noncontact laser is very convenient for this process, and the newer-generation instruments have minimal thermal impact on the embryo being drilled. The use of an erbium-ytrium-aluminum-garnet (YAG) laser, as proposed by Strohmer and Feichtinger,[24] was considered safe. This type of laser has a working wavelength that is sufficiently distant from the maximum absorption of DNA. As such, it is believed that it will not have a negative impact on the genetic structure of cells.[25] Its wavelength, however, is strongly absorbed by water, thus limiting this type of laser to contact mode only. Current laser systems use a 1.48-μm-diode laser beam. At this wavelength, absorption by the culture dish and culture medium is minimized, and there are no reported thermal or mutagenic effects in animal studies.[26] This type of laser is relatively cost-effective and can be adapted to currently used microscope systems. It also has the advantage of being able to function in a noncontact mode, which results in precise and consistent zona drilling.

Despite growing and successful clinical application of laser zona pellucida removal, is there enough accumulated data to warrant its widespread use? Malter and colleagues[27] have urged careful evaluation before clinical use because of "cryptic damage" observed following laser ablation in the mouse. In contrasting studies, the laser was found to be nontoxic, quick, and precise[28] and to pose no additional threat to cell viability or development in the mouse. Also, there have been numerous human studies that seem to suggest that there is relatively no risk in the application of laser zona drilling or thinning to human embryos.[19,29–32] Perhaps the major deterrent to implementation of a laser system in IVF laboratories is cost because it still remains a relatively expensive system to purchase. However, there is technically no need for any hydraulic micromanipulators. The

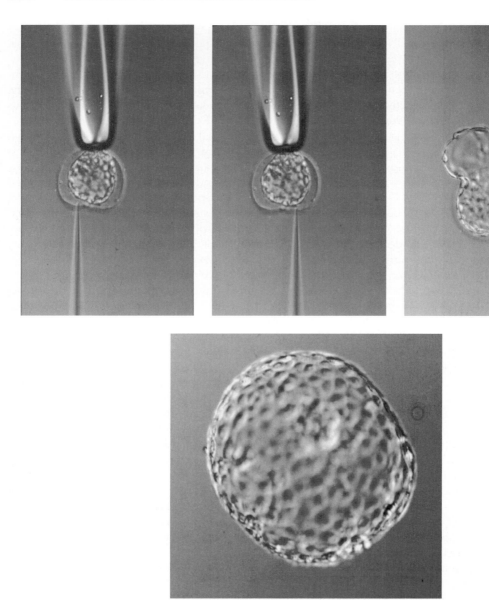

Figure 23-1 Assisted hatching of a day 6 human blastocyst using acidified Tyrode's medium and subsequent hatching of the blastocyst free from its zona pellucida.

properties of the laser are such that the embryo does not have to be held in place by a holding pipette. Since most lasers in use today operate in noncontact mode, there is no need for glass fibers or assisted-hatching needles.

Not to understate the technical issues involved, the embryo is placed on the microscope stage, the area to be ablated is focused, and a button is pushed. The hole in the zona pellucida is consistently and precisely achieved.

Laser zona drilling also may nicely facilitate human embryo biopsy. Immediately after hatching is performed, the biopsy can take place without first necessitating removal of the assisted-hatching pipette (if using acidified Tyrode's medium) and replacing with an embryo biopsy pipette. In the event the hole in the zona is not large enough, on-the-spot adjustments may be made with the laser. It is very likely that laser-assisted hatching may become the method of choice because it inherently reduces technical issues. In other words, it may standardize a very unstandardized process.[33]

We routinely undertake assisted hatching of all thawed embryos irrespective of the stage at which they are frozen. With blastocyst thawing, it is preferable to drill the zona before re-expansion, thus avoiding the need for sucrose shrinkage of the blastocyst. Potential viability of cryopreserved blastocysts generally is good, allowing for fewer numbers to be thawed and transferred in frozen embryo transfer (FET) cycles while achieving good success rates.

Embryo Biopsy

As the ability to obtain more and more feedback on the normality and viability of an embryo from one or two cells grows, clinical justification for this technology will grow apace. Currently, polar body biopsy from the oocyte[34] and blastomere biopsy from cleavage-stage embryos (Fig. 23-2) have been applied successfully to screen for embryo sex, aneuploidy, translocations, and single-gene-region disorders.[35-37] Trophectoderm biopsy from the blastocyst has yet to prove to be so popular an approach due mostly to the shorter period of time available between biopsy and the time of transfer, limiting the time available to run a diagnostic screen. Although this problem is countered in part by the greater number of cells available for removal. Coupling of laser zona ablation with biopsy[38,39] greatly facilitates removal of tissue from the embryo (see use of laser for assisted hatching). We are currently

routinely using the Hamilton Thorne laser system (Beverly, MA) to aid embryo biopsy, and besides the less apparent stress involved for the embryo, the actual operation time is approximately halved, thus reducing further the stress experienced by the embryo undergoing biopsy.[33]

The breadth of use of preimplantation genetic diagnosis (PGD) inexorably spreads,[40] and the reader is best referred to the European Society of Human Reproduction and Embryology (ESHRE) PGD consortium review, which gives a listing of all procedures reported to date from registered centers worldwide.[41] This report details all the uses to which PGD has been applied since 1989 with polymerase chain reaction (PCR) and fluorescent in situ hybridization (FISH) technologies and includes also some reporting on the use of these for "gender screening" of embryos. More recently, a statement from ESHRE[42] and two other authors[43,44] lays down a careful consideration of fundamental ethical principles, specific problems in cases of high genetic risk and aneuploidy screening, HLA typing, and embryo sexing in general. Limitations of current PGD technologies all arise from the very small amounts of material (one to two blastomeres, embryo cells) that are screened. Attempts to increase the number of chromosomes and ease of screening for structural anomalies through rehybridization and genome amplification techniques have been sought. Ultimately, however, it will take fundamentally new approaches to achieve the level of information about an individual embryo that is sought. Most likely this will involve DNA microarray technology that will score, for example, all 24 chromosomes and enable simultaneous resolution of any anomalous DNA in one screening test[45] and may conceivably even include markers for actual embryo metabolic status, although this last factor also may be monitored noninvasively.[46] The more information obtainable per cell removed will increase the justifiability of more routine embryo biopsy. Currently, the application of microarray technologies to mouse

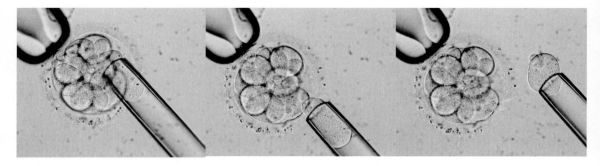

A.

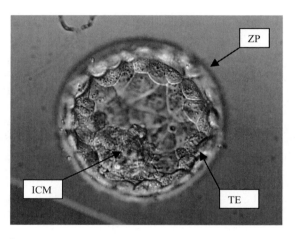

B.

Figure 23-2 *A.* Blastomere biopsy from cleavage-stage embryos. *B.* Fully expanded blasto-cysts on day 5 of development: healthy blastocyst with good morphology, grade 2AA. (ZP = zona pellucida; ICM = inner cell mass; TE = trophectoderm.)

embryology/genetics has been limited due to the unavailability of microarrays containing large numbers of embryonic genes and the gap between microgram quantities of RNA required by typical microarray methods and the minis-cule amounts of tissue available to researchers. An in situ–synthesized novel microarray has overcome many of these problems.[47] At least 98 percent of the probes contained in the mi-croarray correspond to clones in the publicly available collections, making cDNAs readily available for further experimentation on genes of interest. These characteristics, combined with the ability to profile very small samples, make this system a resource for stem cell and em-bryogenomics research.[47] Additionally, funda-mental questions about the protein profiles of the embryo also could be available, thus al-lowing actual screening of the metabolic nor-mality or otherwise of the embryo.[48]

▶ EXTENDED CULTURE

The beneficial effect of growth factors (also called *cytokines*) such as granulocyte-macrophage colony-stimulating factor (GM-CSF) has been examined in sequential-media systems.[49] The addition of GM-CSF increased the proportion of embryos that developed to the blastocyst stage from 30 to 76 percent. The developmental competence of these blastocysts, as assessed by hatching and attachment to extracellular matrix–coated culture dishes, also was improved by GM-CSF. The period in culture required for 50 percent of the total number of blastocysts to form was reduced by 14 hours, and blastocysts grown in GM-CSF were found to contain approximately 35 percent more cells, due primarily to an increase in the size of the inner cell mass. These data support a physiologic role of GM-CSF in promoting the development of the human embryos and suggest that addition of this cytokine to embryo culture media may improve the yield of implantation-competent blastocysts in human IVF programs.[49]

Not all human embryos form blastocysts according to a strict developmental timetable,[22] although there is clearly a relationship between rate of development and potential viability.[50] Rate of blastocyst development appears to be correlated with ultimate ability for blastocysts to hatch free from their zonae pellucidae.[22] It has been proposed that more slowly forming blastocysts may benefit from assisted hatching in order to compensate for their poorer potential to escape the zona pellucida[23] and thereby improve implantation presumably by both guaranteeing hatching and hastening contact of the trophectoderm with the endometrium following uterine ET. While intrinsic problems may exist with an embryo that is developmentally tardy, nevertheless, earlier hatching promoted by assisted hatching may compensate for asynchrony between the embryo and the endometrium ("window of implantation"). Consequently, assisted hatching may improve implantation by this mechanism. A report of a twin delivery following day 7 fresh transfer of blastocysts[51] should encourage cryopreservation of day 7 blastocysts. This would be with a view to achieving pregnancies from such embryos in thaw cycles. In this way, more slowly developing blastocysts may be accommodated at thawing by treating them as if they had formed on day 5. A report of successful day 7

blastocyst cryopreservation bodes well for more routine use of day 7 blastocysts.[52] However, it is essential to point out that assisted hatching is critical here to help these embryos to divest themselves of their zonae pellucidae and so improve their potential for implantation. This would then remain true whether the day 7 blastocysts were fresh or thawed.

Regardless of the issue of developmental speed, the main essence of blastocyst transfer versus earlier-stage transfer is to improve the discrimination of which embryos to select at the blastocyst transfer,[53] thus improving overall implantation and pregnancy rates (see Tables 23-1 and 23-2). The number of IVF cycles in a clinic that are undertaken using blastocyst ET may range from 0 to 100 percent. With relatively conservative use of extended culture in our own experience, where in the years 2000 through 2002 between 30 and 36 percent of all IVF cycles included fresh transfer of blastocysts (see Tables 23-1 and 23-2). These results have allowed a very healthy pregnancy rate to be maintained while reducing significantly the number of high-order multiples that used to arise from routine transfer of three or more embryos.

There remain strong concerns in some minds over the benefits or otherwise of blastocyst ET for reasons of suboptimal extended culture conditions and perceived inconsistency with blastocyst cryopreservation.[54] Therefore, many clinics choose to continue to undertake embryo transfer and cryopreservation at earlier stages. Ultimately, this view is short-sighted and inevitably slows the pace of discovery of how to improve extended in vitro culture. The goal should be to move toward single-embryo transfer at all reasonable costs, and this will happen most effectively with routine blastocyst ET and cryopreservation.

Blastocyst Scoring

Regardless of the relative environmental merits of in vivo or in vitro development, it is understood that approximately 120 hours (day 5) into development the healthy human embryo optimally should be at the blastocyst stage. At this time it should be comprised of some 50 to 200 cells, of which about 20 to 30 percent make up the inner cell mass (ICM), the remainder making up the trophectoderm (TE) (Fig. 23-3). Loss of the *zona pellucida* (ZP) occurs by about day 6, and thus the blastocyst, if viable, is ready to undergo implantation into the uterine *mucosa* (Fig. 23-4). Any assessment of blastocyst quality therefore must accommodate a measure of the three chief elements of the embryo at this stage: ICM, TE, and the ZP.[55,56] The presumed virtue of extended in vitro culture of the human embryo is the improved discrimination of potential viability based on morphology when compared with earlier embryo stage morphologic scoring (Fig. 23-5). This is very clear when making the change from routine day 3 transfers to the blastocyst stage.[53] Here some significant uncoupling of which embryos are graded as good quality on day 3 may occur in terms of their ultimate blastocyst formation and quality on day 5 or 6, when embryos are tracked individually. If any improvements are seen in terms of pregnancy rates with a shift to blastocyst transfer, it is solely through improved selection of embryos, not through intrinsic improvement of embryonic quality through extended culture. At this time the main drive to move to blastocyst transfer is to reduce the number of embryos transferred routinely in an attempt to reduce multiple implantation after IVF-ET therapy. It is the case that blastocyst quality is very much determined by the quality of the gametes from which it came,[57,58] tempered by the in vitro environment in which it was cultured. There currently are no clear or uncontroversial means by which we actually might improve embryo quality over that which might occur in vivo. Consequently, the only potential way for embryo quality to go in vitro is down. Thus we as clinical embryologists have a very real responsibility to "do no harm" while nurturing the preimplantation human embryo; conversely, extended culture is a real privilege that allows us access to study the complete preimplantation period of development in the human. This said, where do we stand with morphologic assessment of blastocysts as a measure of quality? We are very limited with respect to noninvasive tests of potential embryo viability. Cell biopsy is possible but remains a demanding though exciting area of embryo viability as-

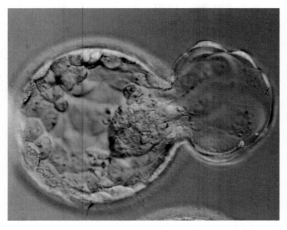
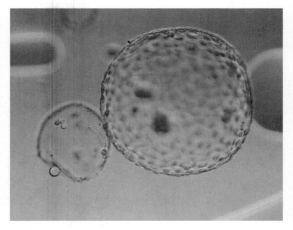

A.

B.

Figure 23-3 *A.* Fully expanded blastocysts on day 6 of development: healthy blastocyst with good morphology, grade 2AA. *B.* Unused blastocyst that was fully hatched by day 8.

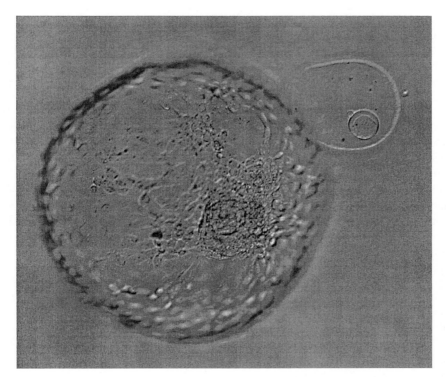

Figure 23-4 Fully expanded blastocysts comprised of over 200 cells that has totally hatched free from its zona pellucida, that can be seen to the upper right still containing a cellular fragment.

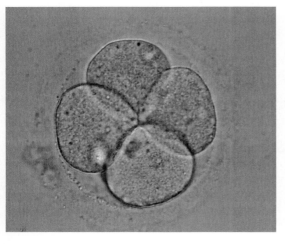

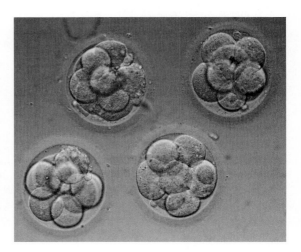

A.   B.

Figure 23-5 *A.* Grade 3 day 3 four-cell embryo with minimal fragmentation. This would be an excellent embryo on day 2 of development. *B.* Grade 1 day 3 eight-cell embryos with less than 5 percent fragmentation.

sessment that is distinctly invasive. Morphologic observation needs to be made sufficiently objective to be useful for intercenter comparison, and to this end, several systems have been developed to grade blastocyst morphology. As with early-stage embryonic development, the simple description of morphology would be rather "one dimensional" without factoring in rate of development. Therefore, for grading of blastocysts to be effective, it must take this into consideration because the passage of time clearly will have a profound impact on cell number relative to the number of cell cycles that the embryo has had time to undergo. This is also true of earlier embryo-stage assessment too. Dokras and colleagues[59] proposed a fairly simple approach to blastocyst grading that incorporates both morphology and rate of development. Its simplicity to some extent, however, compromises its usefulness because it does not allow sufficient flexibility of description. Gardner and Lane,[60] on the other hand, have suggested an approach to grading that is more comprehensive; and in addition it incorporates assessment of rate of development and independent comments on the ICM and TE. A modification of this system to accommodate a tradition of embryo quality scoring that has graded the best embryos with a low number is presented in Table 23-3. Figures 23-6 and 23-7 show a series of blastocysts with differing quality scores using this approach. Ultimately, though, by far the best morphologic assessments are based on photographic images themselves. While numeric and alphabetic scores can be ascribed, a permanent record of the actual image of a blastocyst linked with a photolibrary for embryo grading leaves little to the imagination (see,e.g., ref. 61). Therefore, storage of digital images for all patients will allow the most accurate record of embryos generated in an individual IVF cycle.

▶ **TABLE 23-3:** BLASTOCYST SCORING

Each blastocyst has an overall numerical score based on rate of development and expansion. Day 7 blastocysts always will run one number higher on the overall score (see Fig. 23-4)

Good	1. Fully expanded or hatching day 5
Adequate	2. Fully expanded or hatching day 6
	Moderate expansion day 5
Mediocre	3. Moderate expansion day 6
	Early cavitation day 5
Poor	4. Early cavitation day 6
	Morula day 5/6

• Add to this two alphabetic scores to grade   1. Inner cell mass
                                                2. Trophectoderm

Good	A. High cell number with good cell-cell adhesion
Mediocre	B. Lower cell number with poorer cell-cell attachment
Poor	C. No cells apparent (ICM); sparse, granular (degenerate?), and/or low cell number (trophectoderm)

Example: (1) Good-quality, well-expanded blastocyst on day 6 with good ICM, and good integrity of trophectoderm would be scored as 2AA.

(2) Fully expanded blastocyst on day 5 with nice trophectoderm but nonexistent ICM would be scored as 1CA.

Modified from Gardner and Lane.[60]

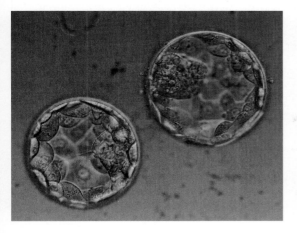

A.

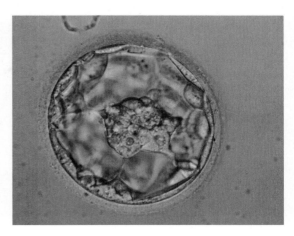

B.

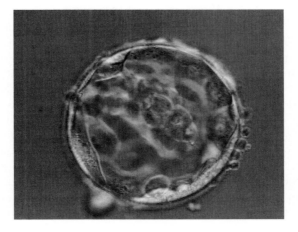

C.

Figure 23-6 *A.* Two fully expanded day 5 blastocysts, grade 1AA. *B.* Fully expanded day 5 blastocyst, grade 1AB. *C.* Fully expanded day 5 blastocyst with small ICM on the "back wall" of the TE, grade 1BB.

▶ NEW APPROACHES TO IN VITRO CULTURE

Historically, there have been three general ways of undertaking in vitro culture of human embryos: test tubes, open culture dishes, and microdroplets under mineral oil. Each approach has had or remains to have its advocates. We have carried out IVF in all three systems, and while all present certain advantages and dis-

advantages, it has to be said that the most realistically controllable system in our opinion is the last—the microdrop system under oil. The essence of all three of these systems remains the same, however, in that they all present a very static environment for the gametes and embryos to reside in. This has been countered to some extent by the recent evolution of the concept of sequential culture media for growth of embryos at different stages of

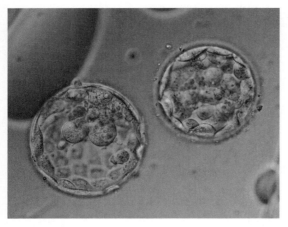

Figure 23-7 Two day 7 blastocysts, fully expanded, grade 3BA *(left),* and midexpanded with no ICM, grade 3CA *(right).*

development. This, in turn, has increased the realization that culture media themselves can become exhausted metabolically, and buildup of metabolic waste products over 24 to 48 h can have a significantly deleterious effect on embryo development. Therefore, the need to change out the culture medium routinely for fresh medium either of the same or different constitution has led to the thought that we really need to make in vitro culture systems more dynamic. By this is meant that with some change in approach the culture medium could

be supplied continuously and then removed from around the embryo, thus providing a more seamless transition through different culture medium types, with the added advantage that waste products are removed constantly with no potentially damaging buildup. This concept has been referred to as *microfluidic culture*[62] (Fig. 23-8).

► CYTOPLASMIC AND NUCLEAR TRANSFER

Cytoplasmic transfer has been applied in the clinical setting successfully[63]; nuclear transfer has not. Both technologies, in essence, attempt to address the same problem—that of reduced viability of embryos in certain poor-prognosis and older patients. Oocyte donation or indeed embryo donation can be used to overcome apparent or total inability to produce viable embryos for some couples. Cytoplasmic transfer, however, attempts to bolster egg and subsequent embryo quality through injection of donor-egg cytoplasm into a recipient's own eggs. The precise components of cytoplasm that achieve the "boost" given to the recipient egg are not completely clear but may involve the supply of healthier mitochondria, messenger RNA, and proteins.[64] While mitochondrial heteroplasmy has been proven to occur in

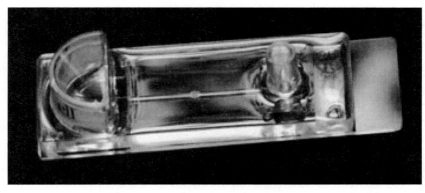

Figure 23-8 Dynamic cell culture system from Penetrating Innovations, Inc., Verona, WI, Vitæ-Cell. *(Adapted from Penetrating Innovations, Inc.)*

some of the offspring, it has not seemed to be problematic, combining apparently healthy mitochondrial DNA from two sources without the fear of mitochondrial DNA–related diseases.[64] Some disagreement exists as to the need for developmental synchrony between the two sources of cytoplasm, with some proposing the need for synchrony[65] between the mature recipient oocyte and the donor cytoplasm from mature oocytes only. Five infants, on the other hand, have been born following the partial donation of zygotic cytoplasm from tripronucleate eggs.[66] The problems of juxtaposing synchronous donor and recipient oocytes have been attempted to be resolved by use of frozen donor oocytes after thawing, and ooplasmic transfer has been reported with successful delivery of a twin following thawed ooplasmic donation.[67] Worldwide, using an ICSI-style sperm and donor cytoplasm technique, approximately 30 healthy babies have been born following partial cytoplasmic transfer.[64] As yet no births have been reported from the electrofusion of donor cytoplasts.

Compared with partial cytoplasmic transfer, nuclear transfer (NT) goes a step farther by replacing all the recipient's ooplasm with donor-egg cytoplasm (total cytoplasmic transfer). In this procedure, a donated germinal-vesicle-stage (GV, immature) egg is enucleated for the purpose of transferring the patient's own nucleus into that cytoplasm.[68,69] The hope is that nuclear transfer at the GV stage would allow meiosis to complete more successfully with the patient's own chromatin within a younger, healthier egg cytoskeleton, thus reducing the risk of egg-derived aneuploidy in the subsequent embryo. As with partial cytoplasmic transfer, the need for synchrony between the stages of the donating and recipient cytoplasms seems critical.[70] Live births have not been reported for this approach. Further, with both these technologies there has been considerable debate and concern with respect to their premature use in the human without prior extensive investigation in animal models.[71] A significant issue that has arisen with respect to

cytoplasmic donation has been the generation of mitochondrial heteroplasmy and the relevance of this to unwitting mitochondriopathies that may have a possible impact on numerous crucial cellular processes. Recognizing the limitations of subcellular gamete studies and proteomics based on animal experimentation suggests that continued clinical studies in this area may be troublesome and merit only very cautious exploration.[71]

▶ CRYOPRESERVATION

Cryostorage of Female Gamete

The last few years have seen a significant resurgence of interest in the potential benefits of human egg freezing. Essentially, these benefits may be

- Formation of donor egg banks to facilitate and lessen the cost of oocyte donation for women who are unable to produce their own oocytes
- Provision of egg cryostorage for women wishing to delay their reproductive choices
- Convenient cryopreservation of ovarian tissue taken from women about to undergo therapy deleterious to such tissue that may threaten their reproductive health

The technology so far applied clinically has been based directly on traditional human embryo cryopreservation protocols and has produced relatively few offspring (approximately 200 infants). Fortunately, to date, no major abnormalities have been reported from these pregnancies regardless of the persistent concerns that freezing and thawing of mature oocytes may disrupt the meiotic spindle and thus increase the potential for aneuploidy in the embryos arising from thawed oocytes. With respect to cryostorage of donated oocytes, several reports have shown some success with this approach.[72,73] Cryostorage of a woman's own oocytes was reported originally in the case of three births in the 1980s.[74,75] More recently, these results have been reproduced by others.[76–79] All these pregnancies came from frozen-thawed mature oocytes except one notable exception, in which a pregnancy arose from an immature GV-stage oocyte.[77] Interestingly, this stage of egg development may prove to be a more successful approach for cryopreservation because its oolemma is more permeable to cryoprotectant and its chromatin is more conveniently and safely packaged in the nucleus.[80] Such eggs, however, still have to undergo GV breakdown and maturation to the meiosis II stage before fertilization, and therefore, their developmental competency is not so clearly established as with fully mature oocytes that are frozen. Source of the GV eggs and whether they have been exposed to any exogenous gonadotropins may play a key role in the competency of these eggs.[81] Whether mature or not, standard cryopreservation technologies appear to have their ultimate limitations not only in cryosurvival but also more importantly in their lack of consistency. Consequently, radically different types of protocols may provide the answer to more consistent success such that traditional slow-cooling/ rapid-thaw protocols may be replaced with vitrification[82] (Fig. 23-9). This again has been applied successfully in the mouse[83] and bovine[84] models and in humans.[78] While the mouse can be a useful model, it must be remembered that the murine oocyte is only just over one-half the volume of a human oocyte; this can have a major impact on permeability and perfusion of the two types of eggs.[85] ICSI has become the accepted norm for insemination of oocytes after thawing to avoid any reduction in sperm penetration of the zona with premature cortical granule release.[86]

The most plentiful source of oocytes potentially is ovarian tissue itself, containing as it does many thousands of primordial follicles in healthy cortical tissue. Earlier successful work with cryopreservation of rodent ovarian tissue has led the way to successful cryostorage of both sheep and human tissue.[86,87] Up to 80 percent survival of follicles has been reported,

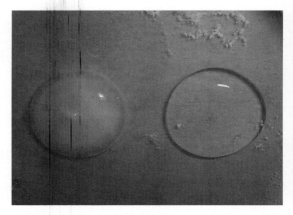

Figure 23-9 Vitrification is the solidification of a solution (glass formation) without ice crystallization. Two droplets of different solutions plunged directly into liquid nitrogen. Left droplet is pure Dulbecco's phosphate-buffered saline (DPBS) with ice crystallization, in contrast to the right droplet containing a mixture of 20% ethylene glycol (EG) and 20% dimethyl sulfoxide (DMSO) plus 0.4 M sucrose in DPBS without ice crystallization (glassy, vitrified state).

but the issue is how to handle this tissue following its thaw. Tissue that has been removed, for example, from a woman about to undergo cancer therapy may contain malignant cells and therefore may not be used safely for autografting. The tissue may be screened before or after thawing for the presence of malignant cells to enable some assessment of the safety of such an approach, or it may be grown in a host animal [e.g., severe combined immune deficient SCID (mouse)] until such time as in vitro maturation could be undertaken more effectively. Extended culture of primordial follicles to full oocyte maturity with subsequent embryonic development and birth has been recorded only in the mouse, and this was not from cryopreserved tissue.[88] Early studies are being undertaken in humans[89] with much to be done. Fertility has been restored in sheep, in a good model for the human ovary, following cryostorage of ovarian cortex and autografting,[87] and this seems the most likely successful clinical model for restoration of fertility in women who are at risk of losing their ovarian function. This may include not only women about to undergo cancer therapy but also women who have a family history of early menopause and those with nonmalignant diseases such as thalassemia or certain autoimmune conditions that may be treated by high-dose chemotherapy. It has been reported that ovarian function can be restored by such means in humans both by orthotopic grafting of thawed ovarian cortical tissue[90] and by heterotopic grafting into the forearm.[91]

The myriad routes for cryostorage of female gamete make for a confusing picture of where clinical applications may occur. However, different clinical needs actually may be met by differing technological approaches, whether they incorporate whole-tissue freezing, separate follicle storage, or cryopreservation of mature oocytes themselves.

Future of Oocyte Cryopreservation

Vitrification protocols are starting to enter the mainstream of human assisted reproductive technology (ART) procedures,[82] and protocols applied successfully to bovine oocytes and embryos have now been used successfully with human oocytes[78,92,93] (Fig. 23-10). Vitrification

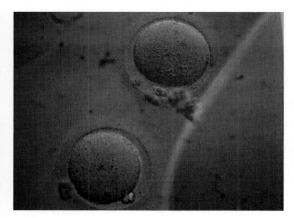

Figure 23-10 Human uninseminated oocytes after vitrifcation and warming.

is very simple, requires no expensive programmable freezing equipment, and relies especially on placement of the oocyte in a very small volume of vitrification medium that must be cooled at extreme rates not obtainable in regular enclosed cryostraws and vials[94] (Fig. 23-11). Oocyte cryopreservation will slowly enter the mainstream of ART techniques, most likely in the area of oocyte donation. Here information, in terms of clinical success of protocols, is generated within months not years, as would be the case with freezing of eggs for single women concerned with their future reproductive choices. Increasingly, couples may choose oocyte cryopreservation over embryo cryopreservation for reasons of an ethical and religious nature. Indeed, a woman may not wish to commit all her gametes to one partner in a single IVF attempt, in which any frozen surplus embryos become the property of the couple, potentially creating litigious complications should the relationship founder. Alternatively, frozen oocytes would remain the sole property of the woman. If these frozen oocytes were not to be used by the woman, then they would make a potentially useful cheap source of "adoptable eggs."

Embryo Cryopreservation

Many of the comments with respect to oocyte cryopreservation may be applied to the allied technology of embryo cryopreservation. That is, there appears a distinct potential for the conventional protocols using slow cooling rates to be replaced by vitrification. The difference, however, is that embryo freezing, regardless of developmental stage, seems more consistent and routinely returns a cryosurvival rate per embryo thawed of over 70 percent. This does mean that there will be greater resistance to effect this change in approach, although ultimately the convenience and rapidity of vitrification that make expensive programmable cell freezers obsolete will sway even the most die-hard cryoembryologist to accept the

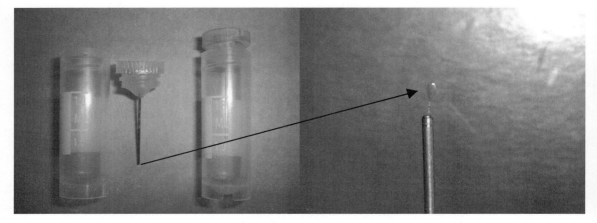

Figure 23-11 Cryoloop system: Cryovial and nylon loop mounted on a stainless steel rod is loaded with the specimen, vitrified and inserted into the lid of the cryovial, and sealed to hold the oocytes or embryos securely. *Inset:* The nylon loop.

cost-effectiveness of rapid cryopreservation (Fig. 23-12). In any event, there will still remain an ongoing debate as to which developmental stage represents the most appropriate stage at which to cryostore embryos. Currently, conventional freezing can be executed successfully at any stage of preimplantation development, although the morula (approximately day 4 to 5) stage may be seen to be the least popular for a variety of organizational reasons.

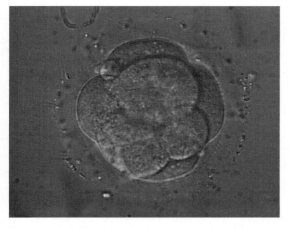

Figure 23-12 Vitrified human day 3 stage embryos 1 hour after warming.

While human embryo cryopreservation has become a well-established technology in ART approaches, it has yet to become fully clear as to which stage preimplantation embryos are best cryostored. Our personal preference is for blastocyst-stage freezing, which has yielded good success rates over recent years (Table 23-4). The superiority of blastocyst-stage freezing over one-cell pronucleate-stage freezing in terms of implantation per thawed embryo transferred is countered by the loss of embryos that lack the wherewithal to grow for up to a week in vitro.[95] Countering the benefits of freezing cleavage-stage embryos is the partial survival of multicellular embryos,[96] where "partial" embryos may give rise to live births even from one surviving cell, but viability is reduced.[97] Nevertheless, given the consistently high rates of cryosurvival of cryopreserved early-stage embryos, there probably will continue to be certain clinical circumstances where early-stage freezing is justified. For example, a woman at risk for ovarian hyperstimulation appropriately may have all her embryos frozen at the one-cell zygote stage prior to any developmental selection, so putting her therapy "on ice." Most embryo cryopreservation protocols currently use a slow-freeze/rapid-thaw approach. Roughly speaking, slow-freeze protocols use lower con-

▶ **TABLE 23-4:** BLASTOCYST CRYOPRESERVATION RESULTS, GEORGIA REPRODUCTIVE SPECIALISTS, 2000–2002

Source of Blastocysts	Nondonor	Donor
Thaws	110	9
Transfers	106	8
No. thawed	312	23
No. FET	263 (84.5%)	17 (75%)
Mean no. at ET	2.5	2.1
Cl.PR/FET	60 (57%)	7 (87.5%)
Viable PR/FET	50 (47%)	6 (75%)
Embryos implanted	59 (22.5%)	6 (35.3%)

centrations of cryoprotectant ($\sim$1.5 M) to avoid the toxicity of such agents during the initial exposure and slow cooling; higher concentrations of cryoprotectant ($\sim$4.0 M) allow shorter exposure times to the cryoprotectant and rapid freezing. Regardless of uncertainties about which protocols for cryopreservation will prevail, the future seems to point to increasing success and consistency with embryo cryopreservation. Preparation of the uterus into which the thawed embryos ultimately will be placed seems to be an area of study that has been better resolved. Both natural and hormone-replacement cycles seem to provide comparable levels of receptivity in naturally cycling women, although they differ in level of convenience.[97] Indeed, artificially prepared cycles may even effectively dispense with the use of gonadotropin-releasing hormone agonists to lessen cost and improve convenience without loss of success.[98]

▶ EMBRYO DONATION

The concept of using donated oocytes and embryos within the context of IVF therapy first became a practical reality during the mid-1980s with the establishment of pregnancies in women without ovarian function[99]; this was a landmark paper. Ultimately, with the honing of human embryo and oocyte cryopreservation,

all the components to allow oocyte and embryo donation have come together to allow us to view these as routine adjuncts of human IVF-ET therapy. As such, newer technologies within the IVF laboratory in general, therefore, apply automatically to donor-oocyte programs specifically. The ability to achieve high success rates in general (see Tables 23-1 and 23-2) allows even higher results to be achieved using donor oocytes.

There exist two different approaches to this therapeutic modality for couples in whom egg donation alone would be insufficient, i.e., couples in need of both donor eggs and sperm. Most clinics, when drawing up consensual agreements for embryo cryopreservation, offer in their options for ultimate disposal of surplus frozen embryos a choice to donate to other recipients or for scientific research. When embryos are donated in such a way, it offers a very cost-effective way to manage a recipient couple's needs, assuming that the quality of the embryos donated is adequate, giving a reasonable chance of pregnancy. Clearly, genetic preselection of the donated embryos by the recipients is very limited and relies on the not easily anticipated generosity of the donor couple. Meanwhile, the recipient couples need to be well screened for commitment to such a therapeutic approach, or even apparently positive outcomes may prove unbearable to that couple.[100]

While this use of "surplus" embryos may seem to be a very ethically easy course to take, nevertheless, such tissue should still be subject to some level of screening with respect to the donating couple. That is, the rescreening of the donors for transmissible diseases is warranted, thus potentially causing significant inconvenience and possible cost to the donors, unaware that their decision to donate might require such actions. From the IVF laboratory perspective, once all the paperwork is in order, then thawing of these donor embryos represents an appealing course, helping as it does to reduce the medicolegal burden of long-term storage of human embryos. In this regard, it would seem increasingly sensible to seek to freeze preimplantation embryos at their most advanced stage, that of the blastocyst. This offers two key advantages over earlier-stage embryo freezing: Blastocysts, if they survive thawing, possess a higher implantation potential and so improve expectation of outcomes per embryo transferred following all thaw/replacement cycles. Additionally, because fewer blastocysts overall are cryopreserved from any one egg collection cycle, it helps to reduce the aforementioned burden of surplus cryostored human embryos.

A second source of donor embryos may be to "purpose-build" them; i.e., by preselecting both donor sperm and oocytes from prearranged donors, "designer" embryos can be generated.[101] While to some minds this may seem inappropriate, willfully creating what seem to be "special" embryos for fastidious clients, it nevertheless does provide better choice and prescreening opportunities than does the donation of "surplus" frozen embryos. The embryos may be generated using thawed donor semen and fresh oocytes for fresh transfer, or all embryos so formed are then cryopreserved to allow complete quarantine of the oocyte donor. Either way the IVF laboratory is very capable of handling the specific techniques required. In cases of donated embryos, as with the more straightforward oocyte donation, where sperm quality is not significantly compromised, it is usually prudent to minimize embryo numbers at transfer. From a clinical perspective, this would best be done with extended in vitro culture to the blastocyst stage allowing routinely two- or even single-embryo transfer.

▶ IN VITRO MATURATION (IVM)

Reports of immature oocyte retrieval from unstimulated ovaries exist.[102,103] These immature oocytes can be cultured successfully to the meiosis II stage in vitro to achieve live births.[104] The overall efficiency of this approach, however, remains in question. Some degree of ovarian stimulation inevitably will increase the potential for recruitment of more competent oocytes, and even if GV oocytes are sought for freezing or nuclear transfer, stimulation protocols tailored to maximize collection of such eggs are to be favored. After retrieval and collection of immature oocytes from unstimulated patients with polycystic ovarian syndrome (PCOS), about 89 percent of them are morphologically normal. After 36 to 48 h of in vitro culture, about 63 to 85 percent of these normal oocytes matured. Development after ICSI to the normal pronuclear stage is about 60 to 75 percent (with or without coculture), and the cleavage rates were about 88 to 95 percent. The pregnancy rate using oocytes from IVM ranged between 18 to 27 percent. Immature oocytes seem to have the same potential after IVM to reach the pronucleate stage and cleavage stage as mature oocytes that were injected on the day of oocyte retrieval.[105–107] Finally, immature oocytes from women whose ovaries have been stimulated can be matured, fertilized by ICSI, and cleave successfully in vitro. Moreover, the IVF rate can be increased with the use of ICSI. Therefore, successful maturation in vitro of oocytes from stimulated cycles coupled with ICSI after maturation ensures a larger population of fertilized, potentially competent oocytes and embryos that increase the opportunity for ensuring a pregnancy.

Oocytes are not the only gamete that may require some degree of IVM prior to use in ART procedures. Testicular biopsy may yield only immature sperm that may need further time in appropriate culture conditions for up to 72 h to allow adequate maturation of the spermatozoon to occur. This enables the male gamete to develop the competency to participate competently in both fertilization and embryonic development to enhance the potential of generating a viable pregnancy. When specific maturation arrest exists in certain men, it seems that pharmacologic concentrations of follicle-stimulating hormone (FSH; 500 IU/L) and testosterone (10 μM) improve in vitro germ cell differentiation and maturation rates from certain men.[108]

► CONCLUSION

The current state of the art in human IVF is the evolution of over a quarter of a century of clinical experience. Although this makes human IVF a relatively recent therapy to have been developed, nonetheless it is clear that while success rates have improved dramatically during this time, it is the case that the way forward becomes increasingly cautiously taken. The consequences of our developments in this field, if not appropriately screened in preclinical trials, may lead to unwitting complications for the offspring that we generate. Additionally, the high rates of multiple births that have become a hallmark of ART techniques obviously must be reduced significantly, and the ability to undertake routine single human embryo transfer may take some time to be achieved. Nevertheless, single-embryo transfer should remain our ultimate goal, with good-prognosis patients and donor-oocyte programs leading the way in this regard.

KEY POINTS

1. With over 1 million offspring now born from IVF-ET procedures, this has provided a reasonable comfort level with the general safety of the therapy. Vigilance nevertheless is warranted with the ever-increasing technology applied in this area.

2. If performed with minimal impact thermally, chemically, and physically, then ICSI should provide normal fertilization rates at least comparable with conventional insemination technologies. In cases of severe male factor infertility, ICSI is clearly essential and the only form of insemination available.

3. Assisted hatching continues to be a controversially applied technique in that there are no fully definitive studies establishing its efficacy in specific IVF patient groups. Nevertheless, certain in vitro studies strongly suggest a continued benefit of this procedure for women of advanced reproductive age and for slowly and poorly developing embryos. Use of the noncontact 1.48-μm infrared laser is allowing assisted hatching to be undertaken increasingly swiftly with minimal impact on or disruption to the preimplantation embryo.

4. Use of the noncontact laser is seen to be of great benefit for the rapid, atraumatic biopsy of the human embryo, with both delivered offspring and improved embryo development after laser biopsy indicating the worth of this somewhat costly technology within the IVF laboratory. Embryo biopsy for aneuploidy, translocation, and specific gene defect screening is being applied increasingly, with approximately 3000 offspring now born following such early-stage diagnostic procedures. DNA microarray chip technology offers the hope on the technological horizon of a broader screen analysis per cell biopsied, possibly diagnosing not only potential disease and abnormal states but also fundamental markers of embryo viability.

5. Routine growth of all human preimplantation embryos in vitro to the blastocyst stage is a central feature of the push toward ultimately single-embryo transfers for all IVF couples. Culture conditions need continued study, and this in particular will include the move away from static culture systems

to those which incorporate a more dynamic (possibly) microfluidic nature. This would allow continuous alteration and manipulation of the culture environment, changing culture components to meet changing metabolic needs while removing metabolic waste products on a constant basis.

6. Cryopreservation of all stages of human embryos will take an increasing role in human IVF therapy. Currently, offspring arising from embryo cryopreservation approaches in the United States constitute approximately one-fifth of all babies born on an annual basis. Improved consistency with human oocyte cryopreservation (especially in the area of oocyte donation), plus the move toward fewer embryos transferred fresh, will see these numbers rise proportionally on an annual basis. Cryopreservation of limited-availability spermatozoa, e.g., from men with certain extreme forms of male factor infertility, will occur more, in particular with improved handling of such gametes after thawing when maturation or reactivation of the spermatozoon is necessary. Throughout the field of human gamete and embryo cryopreservation, the penetration of vitrification technologies will increase with their promise of low-cost, high-speed application with the possible benefit of improved consistency in survival after cryopreservation.

REFERENCES

1. Palermo G, Joris H, Devroey P, et al. Pregnancies after intracytoplasmic single sperm injection into an oocyte. *Lancet* 1992;340:17–18.
2. Tucker MJ, Wright G, Morton PC, et al. Practical evolution and application of direct intracytoplasmic sperm injection for male factor and idiopathic fertilization failure infertilities. *Fertil Steril* 1995;63:820–827.
3. Miller KF, Falcone T, Goldberg JM, et al. Previous fertilization failure with conventional in vitro fertilization is associated with poor outcome of intracytoplasmic sperm injection. *Fertil Steril* 1998;69:242–245.
4. Oehninger S, Gosden RG. Should ICSI be the treatment of choice for all cases of in-vitro conception? *Hum Reprod* 2002;17:2237–2242.
5. Rienzi L, Greco E, Ubaldi F, et al. Laser-assisted intracytoplasmic sperm injection. *Fertil Steril* 2001;76:1045–1047.
6. Witt MA, Elsner C, Kort HI, et al. A live birth from intracytoplasmic injection of a spermatozoon retrieved from testicular parenchyma. *J Urol* 1995;154:1136–1137.
7. Bhattacharya S, Hamilton MP, Shaaban M, et al. Conventional in vitro fertilisation versus intracytoplasmic sperm injection for treatment of non-male-factor infertility: A randomised controlled trial. *Lancet* 2001;357:2075–2079.
8. Tucker M, Graham J, Han T, et al. Conventional insemination versus intracytoplasmic sperm injection. *Lancet* 2001;358:1645–1646.
9. Hansen M, Kurinczuk JJ, Bower C, et al. The risk of major birth defects after intracytoplasmic sperm injection and in vitro fertilization. *N Engl J Med* 2002;346:769–770.
10. Bonduelle M, Van Assche E, Joris H, et al. Prenatal testing in ICSI pregnancies: Incidence of chromosomal anomalies in 1586 karyotypes and relation to sperm parameters. *Hum Reprod* 2002;17:2600–2614.
11. Cox GF, Burger J, Lip V, et al. Intracytoplasmic sperm injection may increase the risk of imprinting defects. *Am J Hum Genet* 2002;71:162–164.
12. Edwards RG. Aspects of the molecular regulation of early mammalian development. *Reprod Biomed Online* 2003;6:97–113.
13. Yanagimachi R. Gamete manipulation for development: New methods for conception. *Reprod Fertil Dev* 2001;13:3–14.
14. Tesarik J. Reproductive semicloning respecting biparental embryo origin: Embryos from syngamy between a gamete and a haploidized somatic cell. *Hum Reprod* 2002;17:1933–1937.
15. Eichenlaub-Ritter U. Reproductive semicloning respecting biparental origin: Reconstitution of gametes for assisted reproduction. *Hum Reprod* 2003;18:473–475.
16. Schoolcraft WB, Schlenker T, Gee M, et al. Assisted hatching in the treatment of poor prognosis in vitro fertilization candidates. *Fertil Steril* 1994;62:551–554.

17. Lanzendorf SE, Nehchiri F, Mayer J, et al. A prospective, randomized, double-blind study for the evaluation of assisted hatching in patients with advanced maternal age. *Hum Reprod* 1998;13:409–413.

18. Alikani M, Cohen J, Tomkin G, et al. Human embryo fragmentation in vitro and its implications for pregnancy and implantation. *Fertil Steril* 1999;71:836–842.

19. Antinori S, Selman HA, Caffa B, et al. Zona opening of human embryos using a noncontact UV laser for assisted hatching in patients with poor prognosis of pregnancy. *Hum Reprod* 1996;11:2488–2492.

20. Malter HE, Cohen J. Blastocyst formation and hatching in vitro following zona drilling of mouse and human embryos. *Gamete Res* 1989;24:67–80.

21. Jones GM, Trounson AO, Lolatgis N, et al. Factors affecting the success of human blastocyst development and pregnancy following in vitro fertilization and embryo transfer. *Fertil Steril* 1998;70:1022–1029.

22. Porter RN, Tucker MJ, Graham J, et al. Advanced embryo development during extended in vitro culture: Observations of formation and hatching patterns in non-transferred human blastocysts. *Hum Fertil* 2002;5:215–220.

23. Tucker M. Relevance of assisted hatching with blastocyst stage transfer, in *Proceedings of the 1st World Congress on Controversies in Obstetrics/Gynecology and Infertility, Prague, Czech Republic, October 28–31, 1999*. Bologna, Italy: Monduzzi Publishing, 2000:49–52.

24. Strohmer H, Feichtinger W. Successful clinical application of laser for micromanipulation in an in vitro fertilization program. *Fertil Steril* 1992;58:212–214.

25. Boada M, Carrera M, De La Iglesias C, et al. Successful use of a laser for human embryo biopsy in preimplantation genetic diagnosis: Report of two cases. *J Assist Reprod Genet* 1998;15:79–84.

26. Germond M, Nocera D, Senn A, et al. Microdissection of mouse and human zona pellucida using a 1.48-μm diode laser beam: Efficacy and safety of the procedure. *Fertil Steril* 1995;64:604–611.

27. Malter H, Schimmel T, Cohen J. Zona dissection by infrared laser: Developmental consequences in the mouse, technical considerations

and controlled clinical trial. *Reprod Biomed Online* 2001;3:117–123.

28. Neev J, Schiewe MC, Sung VW, et al. Assisted hatching in mouse embryos using a non contact Ho:YSGG laser system. *J Assist Reprod Genet* 1995;12:288–293.

29. Antinori S, Panci C, Selman HA, et al. Zona thinning with the use of laser: A new approach to assisted hatching in humans. *Hum Reprod* 1996;11:590–594.

30. Blake DA, Forsberg AS, Johansson BR, et al. Laser zona pellucida thinning: An alternative approach to assisted hatching. *Hum Reprod* 2001;16:1959–1964.

31. Entezami F, Olivennes F, Volante M, et al. Comparison of two procedures for assisted hatching of human embryo: Acidified tyrode versus noncontact laser. *Fertil Steril* 2001;76:3(suppl 1):S248.

32. Graham J, Han T, Greenhouse SJ, et al. Acid Tyrode's or laser: Are they equivalent for assisted hatching? *Fertil Steril* 2001;76:3(suppl 1):S248.

33. Han TS, Sagoskin AW, Graham JR, et al. Laser-assisted human embryo biopsy on the third day of development for preimplantation genetic diagnosis: Two successful case reports. *Fertil Steril* 2003;80:453–455.

34. Verlinsky Y, Cieslak J, Ivakhnenko V, et al. Chromosomal abnormalities in the first and second polar bodies. *Mol Cell Endocrinol* 2001;183:S47–49.

35. Munne S. Preimplantation genetic diagnosis of structural abnormalities. *Mol Cell Endocrinol* 2001;183:S55–58.

36. Munne S, Magli C, Cohen J, et al. Positive outcome after preimplantation diagnosis of human embryos. *Hum Reprod* 1999;14:2191–199.

37. Rechitsky S, Verlinsky O, Amet T, et al. Reliability of preimplantation diagnosis for single-gene disorders. *Mol Cell Endocrinol* 2001;183:S65–68.

38. Montag M, van der Ven K, Delacretaz G, et al. Laser-assisted microdissection of the zona pellucida facilitates polar body biopsy. *Fertil Steril* 1998;69:539–542.

39. Veiga A, Sandalinas M, Benkhalifa M, et al. Laser blastocyst biopsy for preimplantation genetic diagnosis in the human. *Zygote* 1997;5:351–354.

40. Braude P, Pickering S, Flinter F, et al. Preimplantation genetic diagnosis. *Nature Rev Genet* 2002;3:941–953.

41. ESHRE PGD Consortium. Data collection III (May 2001). *Hum Reprod* 2002;17:233–246.

42. Shenfield F, Pennings G, Devroey P, et al. Task-force 5: Preimplantation genetic diagnosis. *Hum Reprod* 2003;18:649–651.

43. Charo RA. Children by choice: Reproductive technologies and the boundaries of personal autonomy. *Nature Cell Biol Med* 2002 Oct; 4 suppl:S23–28.

44. Robertson JA. Extending preimplantation genetic diagnosis: The ethical debate. *Hum Reprod* 2003;18:465–471.

45. Weier HG, Munne S, Lersch RA, et al. Toward a full karyotype screening of interphase cells: "FISH and chip" technology. *Mol Cell Endocrinol* 2001;183:S41–45.

46. Houghton FD, Hawkhead JA, Humpherson PG, et al.Non-invasive amino acid turnover predicts human embryo developmental capacity. *Hum Reprod* 2002;17:999–1007.

47. Carter MG, Hamatani T, Sharov AA, et al. In situ–synthesized novel microarray optimized for mouse stem cell and early developmental expression profiling. *Genome Res* 2003;13: 1011–1021.

48. Jenkins RE, Pennington SR. Arrays for protein expression profiling: Toward a viable alternative to two-dimensional gel electrophoresis? *Proteomics* 2001;1:13–29.

49. Sjoblom C, Wikland M, Robertson SA. Granulocyte-macrophage colony-stimulating factor promotes human blastocyst development in vitro. *Hum Reprod* 1999;14:3069–3076.

50. Khorram O, Shapiro SS, Jones JM. Transfer of non-assisted hatched and hatching human blastocysts after in vitro fertilization. *Fertil Steril* 2000;74:163–165.

51. Sagoskin AW, Han T, Graham JR, et al. Healthy twin delivery after day 7 blastocyst transfer coupled with assisted hatching. *Fertil Steril* 2002;77:615–617.

52. Sills ES, Sweitzer CL, Morton PC, et al. Dizygotic twin delivery following in vitro fertilization and transfer of thawed blastocysts cryopreserved at day 6 and 7. *Fertil Steril* 2003;79: 424–427.

53. Graham J, Han T, Porter R, et al. Day-three morphology is a poor predictor of blastocyst quality in extended culture. *Fertil Steril* 2000; 74:495–497.

54. Alper MM, Brinsden P, Fischer R, et al. To blastocyst or not to blastocyst? That is the question. *Hum Reprod* 2001;16:617–619.

55. Richter KS, Harris DC, Daneshmand ST, et al. Quantitative grading of a human blastocyst: Optimal inner cell mass size and shape. *Fertil Steril* 2001;76:1157–1167.

56. Hardy K, Stark J, Winston RML. Maintenance of the inner cell mass in human blastocysts from fragmented embryos. *Biol Reprod* 2003;68: 1165–1169.

57. Janny L, Menezo YJR. Maternal age effect on early human embryonic development and blastocyst formation. *Mol Reprod Dev* 1996;45: 31–37.

58. Janny L, Menezo YJR. Evidence for a strong paternal effect on human preimplantation embryo development and blastocyst formation. *Mol Reprod Dev* 1994;38:36–42.

59. Dokras A, Sargent I, Barlow DI. Human blastocyst grading: An indicator of developmental potential? *Hum Reprod* 1993;8:2119–2127.

60. Gardner DK, Lane M. Embryo culture systems, in Trounson AO, Gardner DK (eds), *Handbook of in Vitro Fertilization,* 2d ed. Boca Raton, FL: CRC Press, 2000:205–264.

61. Menezo YJ, Kauffman R, Veiga A, et al. A mini-atlas of the human blastocyst in vitro. *Zygote* 1999;7:61–65.

62. Beebe D, Wheeler M, Zeringue H, et al. Microfluidic technology for assisted reproduction. *Theriogenology* 2002;57:125–135.

63. Cohen J, Scott R, Alikani M, et al. Ooplasmic transfer in mature human oocytes. *Mol Hum Reprod* 1998;4:269–280.

64. Barritt J, Willadsen S, Brenner C, et al. Cytoplasmic transfer in assisted reproduction. *Hum Reprod Update* 2001;7:428–435.

65. Levron J, Willadsen S, Bertoli M, et al. The development of mouse zygotes after fusion with synchronous and asynchronous cytoplasm. *Hum Reprod* 1996;11:1287–1292.

66. Huang CC, Cheng TC, Chang HH, et al. Birth after the injection of sperm and the cytoplasm of tripronucleate zygotes into metaphase II oocytes in patients with repeated implantation failure after assisted fertilization procedures. *Fertil Steril* 1999;74:702–706.

67. Lanzendorf SE, Mayer JF, Toner J, et al. Pregnancy following transfer of ooplasm from

cryopreserved-thawed donor oocytes into recipient oocytes. *Fertil Steril* 1999;71:575–577.

68. Zhang J, Wang CW, Krey L, et al. In vitro maturation of human preovulatory oocytes reconstructed by germinal vesicle transfer. *Fertil Steril* 1999;71:726–731.

69. Takeuchi T, Gong J, Veeck LL, et al. Preliminary findings in germinal vesicle transplantation of immature human oocytes. *Hum Reprod* 2001;16:730–736.

70. Liu H, Wang CW, Grifo JA, et al. Reconstruction of mouse oocytes by germinal vesicle transfer: Maturity of host oocyte cytoplasm determines meiosis. *Hum Reprod* 1999;14:2357–2361.

71. Sills ES, Takeuchi T, Tucker MJ, et al. Genetic and epigenetic modifications associated with human ooplasm donation and mitochondrial heteroplasmy: Considerations for interpreting studies of heritability and reproductive outcome. *Med Hypotheses* 2004;62:612–617.

72. Polak de Fried E, Notrica J, Rubinstein M, et al. Pregnancy after human donor oocyte cryopreservation and thawing in association with intracytoplasmic sperm injection in a patient with ovarian failure. *Fertil Steril* 1998;69:555–557.

73. Tucker MJ, Morton PC, Wright G, et al. Clinical application of human egg cryopreservation. *Hum Reprod* 1998;13:3156–3159.

74. Chen C. Pregnancies after human oocyte cryopreservation. *Ann NY Acad Sci* 1988;541:541–549.

75. Van Uem JFHM, Siebzehnrubl ER, Schuh B, et al. Birth after cryopreservation of unfertilized oocytes. *Lancet* 1987;1:752–753.

76. Porcu E, Fabbri R, Damiano G, et al. Clinical experience and applications of oocyte cryopreservation. *Mol Cell Endocrinol* 2000;169:33–37.

77. Tucker MJ, Wright G, Morton PC, et al. Birth after cryopreservation of immature oocytes with subsequent in vitro maturation. *Fertil Steril* 1998;70:578–579.

78. Kuleshova L, Gianaroli L, Magli C, et al. Birth following vitrification of a small number of human oocytes. *Hum Reprod* 1999;14:3077–3079.

79. Young E, Kenny A, Puigdomenech E, et al. Triplet pregnancy after intracytoplasmic sperm injection of cryopreserved oocytes: Case report. *Fertil Steril* 1998;70:360–361.

80. Van Blerkom J, Davis P. Cytogenetic, cellular and developmental consequences of cryopreservation of immature and mature mouse and human oocytes. *Microsc Res Tech* 1994;27:165–193.

81. Cortvrindt RG, Hu Y, Liu J, et al. Timed analysis of the nuclear maturation of oocytes in early preantral mouse follicle culture supplemented with recombinant gonadotropin. *Fertil Steril* 1998;70:1114–1125.

82. Liebermann J, Nawroth F, Isachenko V, et al. The potential importance of vitrification in reproductive medicine. *Biol Reprod* 2002;67:1671–1680.

83. O'Neil L, Paynter SJ, Fuller BJ. Vitrification of mature mouse oocytes: Improved results following addition of polyethylene glycol to a dimethyl sulfoxide solution. *Cryobiology* 1997;34:295–301.

84. Vajta G, Holm P, Kuwayama M, et al. Open pulled straw (OPS) vitrification: A new way to reduce cryoinjuries of bovine ova and embryos. *Mol Reprod Dev* 1998;51:53–58.

85. Paynter SJ, Cooper A, Gregory L, et al. Permeability characteristics of human oocytes in the presence of the cryoprotectant dimethyl-sulphoxide. *Hum Reprod* 1999;14:2338–2342.

86. Gook DA, Edgar DH. Cryopreservation of the human female gamete: Current and future issues. *Hum Reprod* 1999;14:2938–2940.

87. Gosden RG, Baird DT, Wade JC, et al. Restoration of fertility to oophorectomised sheep by ovarian autografts stored at −196°C. *Hum Reprod* 1994;9:597–603.

88. Eppig JJ, O'Brien MJ. Development in mouse oocytes from primordial follicles. *Biol Reprod* 1996;54:197–201.

89. Abir R, Roizman P, Fisch B, et al.: Pilot study of isolated early human follicles cultured in collagen gels for 24 hours. *Human Reproduction* 1999;14:1299–1301.

90. Oktay K, Yih M. Preliminary experience with orthotopic and heterotopic transplantation of ovarian cortical strips. *Semin Reprod Med* 2002;20:63–74.

91. Oktay K, Economos K, Kan M, et al. Endocrine function and oocyte retrieval after autologous transplantation of ovarian cortical strips to the forearm. *JAMA* 2001;286:1490–1493.

92. Yoon TK, Chung HM, Lim JM, et al. Pregnancy and delivery of healthy infants developed

from vitrified oocytes in a stimulated in vitro fertilization–embryo transfer program. *Fertil Steril* 2000;74:180–181.

93. Liebermann J, Tucker MJ, Sills ES. Cryoloop vitrification in assisted reproduction: Analysis of survival rates in >1000 human oocytes after ultrarapid cooling with polymer augmented cryoprotectant. *Clin Exp Obstet Gynecol* 2003;30: 125–129.

94. Liebermann J, Tucker MJ. Effect of carrier system on the yield of human oocytes and embryos as assessed by survival and developmental potential after vitrification. *Reproduction* 2002;124:483–489.

95. Mandelbaum J, Belaish-Allart J, Junca A. Cryopreservation in human assisted reproduction is now routine for embryos but remains a research procedure for oocytes. *Hum Reprod* 1998;13(suppl 3):161–177.

96. Van den Abbeel E, Van Steirteghem A. Zona pellucida damage to human embryos after cryopreservation and the consequences for their blastomere survival and in vitro viability. *Hum Reprod* 2000;15:373–378.

97. Tucker MJ, Morton PC, Sweitzer CL, et al. Cryopreservation of human embryos and oocytes. *Curr Opin Obstet Gynecol* 1995;7:188–192.

98. Simon A, Hurwitz A, Zentner BS, et al. Transfer of frozen-thawed embryos in artificially prepared cycles with and without prior gonadotropin-releasing hormone agonist suppression: A prospective, randomized study. *Hum Reprod* 1998; 13:2712–2717.

99. Lutjen P, Trounson A, Leeton J, et al. The establishment and maintenance of pregnancy using in vitro fertilization and embryo donation in a patient with primary ovarian failure. *Nature* 1984;307:174–175.

100. Marcus SF, Brinsden PR. Termination of pregnancy after conception with donor oocytes and donor spermatozoa. *Hum Reprod* 2001;15: 719–722.

101. Lindheim SR, Sauer MV. Embryo donation: A programmed approach. *Fertil Steril* 1999;72: 940–941.

102. Barnes FL, Crombie A, Gardner DK, et al. Blastocyst development and birth after in vitro maturation of human primary oocytes, intracytoplasmic sperm injection and assisted hatching. *Hum Reprod* 1995;10:3243–3247.

103. Cha KY, Han SY, Chung HM, et al. Pregnancies and deliveries after in vitro maturation culture followed by in vitro fertilization and embryo transfer without stimulation in women with polycystic ovary syndrome. *Fertil Steril* 2000; 73:978–983.

104. Yoon HG, Yoon SH, Son WY, et al. Pregnancies resulting from in vitro matured oocytes collected from women with regular menstrual cycle. *J Assist Reprod Genet* 2001;18:325–329.

105. Child TJ, Abdul–Jalil AK, Gulekli B, et al. In vitro maturation and fertilization of oocytes from unstimulated normal ovaries, polycystic ovaries, and women with polycystic ovary syndrome. *Fertil Steril* 2001;76:936–942.

106. Kim BK, Lee SC, Kim KJ, et al. In vitro maturation, fertilization, and development of human germinal vesicle oocytes collected from stimulated cycles. *Fertil Steril* 2000;74:1153– 1158.

107. Son WY, Yoon SH, Lee SW, et al. Blastocyst development and pregnancies after IVF of mature oocytes retrieved from unstimulated patients with PCOS after in vivo HCG priming: Case report. *Hum Reprod* 2002;17:134–136.

108. Tesarik J, Nagy P, Abdelmassih R, et al. Pharmacological concentrations of follicle-stimulating hormone and testosterone improve the efficacy of in vitro germ cell differentiation in men with maturation arrest. *Fertil Steril* 2002;77:245–251.

CHAPTER 24

Recurrent Pregnancy Loss

WILLIAM H. KUTTEH

Recurrent pregnancy loss is a profound personal tragedy to couples seeking parenthood and a formidable clinical challenge to their physicians. While spontaneous abortion occurs in approximately 15 percent of clinically diagnosed pregnancies of reproductive-age women, recurrent pregnancy loss occurs in about 1 to 2 percent of this same population.[1] Great strides have been made in characterizing the incidence and diversity of this heterogeneous disorder, and a definite cause of pregnancy loss can be established in approximately two-thirds of couples after a thorough evaluation.[2] A complete evaluation includes investigations into genetic, endocrinologic, anatomic, immunologic, microbiologic, thrombophilic, and iatrogenic causes. In cases of idiopathic recurrent miscarriage, intense supportive care is indicated, and successful outcomes will occur in over two-thirds of all couples.[3]

▶ DEFINITION OF PREGNANCY LOSS

The traditional definition of recurrent pregnancy loss included couples with three or more spontaneous, consecutive pregnancy losses. However, several recent studies have indicated that the risk of recurrent miscarriage after two successive losses is similar to the risk of miscarriage in women after three successive losses;

thus couples with two or more consecutive spontaneous miscarriages warrant an evaluation to determine the etiology of their pregnancy loss.[4,5] Miscarriages are considered any loss before 20 gestational weeks and can be further divided into embryonic losses, which occur before the ninth gestational week, and fetal losses, which occur at or after the ninth gestational week to 20 weeks. Couples with primary recurrent loss have never had a previous viable infant, whereas couples with secondary recurrent loss have previously delivered a pregnancy beyond 20 weeks and then suffered subsequent losses.

▶ RECURRENCE RISK

The risk of recurrence depends on several factors, including maternal age, the number of previous miscarriages, and the history of previous term deliveries. Studies that evaluated the frequency of pregnancy loss based on highly sensitive tests for quantitative human chorionic gonadotropin (hCG) indicated that the total clinical and preclinical losses in women ages 20 to 30 is approximately 25 percent, whereas the loss rate in women age 40 or more is at least double that figure.[6,7] Similarly, a greater number of prior losses is associated with an increased risk of recurrence in most studies. A patient with two prior losses has a recurrence risk of at least 25 percent, and after four losses, that figure is at least doubled. Most studies have indicated a more favorable prognosis in women with secondary recurrent pregnancy loss.

▶ ETIOLOGIES OF RECURRENT PREGNANCY LOSS

Genetic Factors

Structural abnormalities in parental chromosomes occur in 3 to 5 percent of couples with recurrent pregnancy loss. The most common chromosomal abnormality is a balanced translocation, an event that occurs at meiosis with an abnormal genetic complement in the germ cells. In recurrent pregnancy loss, this abnormality is found more frequently in the female partner at a ratio of 2:1 and up to 3:1 (female to male). Other parental chromosome abnormalities occur less frequently, such as robertsonian translocations, inversions, sex chromosome aneuploidies, and supernumerary chromosomes. Treatment includes genetic counseling, prenatal diagnoses by amniocentesis or chorionic villus sampling, donor gametes, or preimplantation genetic diagnosis.

Endocrinologic Factors

Luteal-Phase Deficiency

Progesterone produced from the corpus luteum is necessary for successful implantation and maintenance of early pregnancy until progesterone production by the placenta takes over. Luteal-phase deficiency has been described as a cause of pregnancy loss. Classically, diagnosis was obtained after an endometrial biopsy on day 26 or day 27 of the cycle that was more than 2 days out of phase, and more recently, the use of a midluteal progesterone concentration of <10 ng/mL has been suggested to be diagnostic. Women with out-of-phase endometrial biopsies are unable to maintain endometrial progesterone receptors and have abnormal expression of the $\alpha_V\beta_3$ integrin, a biomarker of uterine receptivity.[8] The $\alpha_V\beta_3$ integrin normally appears in the endometrial glands on cycle days 20 to 21 during the "window of implantation." Most of these patients, when treated with supplemental progesterone or low-dose clomiphene citrate, will have restoration of normal histologic endometrium and normal $\alpha_V\beta_3$ expression. Late implantation of the embryo also has been associated with an increased miscarriage rate.[9]

Untreated Hypothyroidism

Untreated hypothyroidism may increase the risk of miscarriage. A recent study of over 700 patients with recurrent pregnancy loss identified 7.6 percent with hypothyroidism.[10] Hypothyroidism is easily diagnosed with a sensitive thyroid-stimulating hormone (TSH) test, and patients should be treated to become euthyroid before attempting a next pregnancy.

Insulin Resistance

Patients with poorly controlled diabetes are known to have an increased risk of spontaneous miscarriage, which is reduced to normal spontaneous loss rates when women are euglycemic preconceptually.[6] It is known that women with polycystic ovarian syndrome have an increased risk of miscarriage. The high prevalence of insulin resistance in women with polycystic ovarian syndrome may account for the increased risk of miscarriage in this group.[11] Testing for fasting insulin and glucose is simple, and treatment with insulin-sensitizing agents can reduce the risk of recurrent miscarriage.[12]

Elevated Day 3 Follicle-Stimulating Hormone (FSH)

Elevated day 3 FSH levels have been associated with decreased pregnancy rates in women undergoing in vitro fertilization. Although the frequency of elevated day 3 FSH levels in women with recurrent miscarriage is similar to the frequency in the infertile population, the prognosis for recurrent miscarriage is decreased with increased day 3 FSH levels.[13] Although no treatment is available, testing should be performed in women over age 35 with recurrent pregnancy loss, and appropriate counseling should follow.

Anatomic Factors

Congenital Uterine Anomalies

Congenital uterine anomalies associated with müllerian fusion defects have been associated with an increased risk of pregnancy loss.[14] The most common abnormality associated with pregnancy loss is the septate uterus. Uncontrolled studies suggest that resection of the uterine septum results in higher delivery rates than in women without treatment. Other congenital abnormalities, such as bicornuate and unicornuate uterus, are associated more frequently with later-trimester losses or preterm delivery.

Acquired Uterine Abnormalities

Intrauterine synechiae (Asherman's syndrome) have been associated with recurrent miscarriage. The most common causes of intrauterine adhesions are curettages occurring after abortion or postpartum. The adhesions are thought to interfere with normal placentation and are treated with hysteroscopic resection. Intrauterine cavity abnormalities, such as leiomyomas

and polyps, can contribute to pregnancy loss by interfering with implantation. Until recently, it was felt that only submucous leiomyomas should be removed surgically prior to subsequent attempts at pregnancy. However, several recent studies investigating the implantation rate in women undergoing in vitro fertilization clearly have demonstrated decreased implantation with intramural myomas in the range of 30 mm.[15] When smaller myomas are identified, it is unclear if myomectomy is beneficial.[16]

Immunologic Factors

Autoimmune Factors
ANTIPHOSPHOLIPID ANTIBODIES

Autoantibodies to phospholipids, thyroid antigens, nuclear antigens, and others have been investigated as possible causes for pregnancy loss.[10] Antiphospholipid antibodies include both the lupus anticoagulant and anticardiolipin antibodies. The occurrence of recurrent pregnancy loss, fetal death, and/or thrombosis in conjunction with antiphospholipid antibodies is termed the *antiphospholipid antibody syndrome*[17] (Table 24-1). There is still controversy concerning testing for other phospholipids, but an increasing number of studies suggest that antibodies to phosphatidyl serine are also associated with pregnancy loss.[18] In the

▶ **TABLE 24-1:** CLINICAL AND LABORATORY CHARACTERISTICS OF ANTIPHOSPHOLIPID ANTIBODY SYNROME

Clinical	Laboratory
Pregnancy morbidity	IgG aCL (≥20 GPL)
≥1 unexplained death at ≥10 weeks or	IgM aCL (≥20 MPL)
delivery at ≤34 weeks with severe PIH or	
three or more losses before 10 weeks	Positive lupus anticoagulant test
Thrombosis	
Venous	
Arterial, including stroke	

Patients should have at least one clinical and one laboratory feature at some time in the course of their disease. Laboratory tests should be positive on at least two occasions more than 6 weeks apart. GPL = IgG phospholipid units; MPL = IgM phospholipid units; PIH = pregnancy-induced hypertension.
Modified from Wilson et al.[17]

past, treatment with low-dose steroids was advocated; however, recent studies indicate that this treatment significantly increases maternal and fetal complications without enhancing live birth rate.[19,20] Independent prospective investigations have indicated the efficacy of subcutaneous heparin and aspirin for the treatment of antiphospholipid antibody syndrome.[21–23]

ANTITHYROID ANTIBODIES

Antithyroid antibodies (antithyroid peroxidase, antithyroglobulin) have been reported in an increased frequency in women with recurrent pregnancy loss. However, if the patient is euthyroid, the presence of antithyroid antibodies does not affect pregnancy outcome.[24] Women who have positive antithyroid antibodies and are euthyroid are at an increased risk for hypothyroidism during and after pregnancy. These women should have their TSH tested during each trimester and postpartum for thyroiditis.[25]

ANTINUCLEAR ANTIBODIES

Approximately 10 to 15 percent of all women will have detectable antinuclear antibodies regardless of their history of pregnancy loss. Their chance of successful pregnancy outcome does not depend on the presence or absence of antinuclear antibodies. Treatments such as steroids have been shown to increase the maternal and fetal complications without benefiting live births[20]; thus routine testing and treatment for antinuclear antibodies are not indicated.

Alloimmune Factors

Alloimmune factors have been suggested to be associated with recurrent pregnancy loss. Human leukocyte antigen (HLA) sharing was thought to be associated with recurrent pregnancy loss based on a decreased maternal immune response and thus decreased production of blocking antibodies. Recent large studies, however, reveal no association between HLA (and HLA-DQα), homozygosity, and recurrent pregnancy loss.[26] Other investigators have im-

plicated certain embryotoxic factors, such as tumor necrosis factor α (TNF-α) and interferon-δ, identified in the supernatants of peripheral blood lymphocytes from women with pregnancy loss; however, this has not been confirmed by independent studies. Immunophenotypes of endometrial cells from women with recurrent pregnancy loss demonstrate altered natural killer cell (CD56+) populations. Some practitioners have suggested that *increased* natural killer cells are associated with pregnancy loss, whereas others have indicated that *decreased* natural killer cells are associated with pregnancy loss. None of these tests has been clearly associated with pregnancy loss; thus there are no recommended tests or treatments at this time.[27] Therapies such as leukocyte immunotherapy and intravenous immunoglobulin have not been shown to be efficacious.[28,29]

Microbiologic Factors

Certain infectious agents have been identified more frequently in cultures from women who have had spontaneous pregnancy losses.[30] These include *Ureaplasma urealyticum, Mycoplasma hominis, Chlamydia,* and other less frequent pathogens. Although no studies have associated any infectious agent with recurrent pregnancy loss, it is unthinkable that a clinician would leave a patient untreated to determine this association. Because of the clear association with sporadic pregnancy losses and the ease of diagnosis, women with recurrent pregnancy loss should be cultured for these organisms, and both partners should be treated if positive.

Thrombophilic Factors

Recent attention has focused on certain inherited disorders that may predispose to arterial and/or venous thrombosis and their possible association with pregnancy complications.[31,32]

These include the group of mutations leading to a hypercoagulable state, such as factor V Leiden *(G1691A),* factor II–prothrombin mutation *(G20210A),* and hyperhomocysteinemia (thermolabile *MTHFR C677T*). Other possible abnormalities leading to hypercoagulable states that may be associated with recurrent miscarriage include the antithrombin III deficiency, protein C deficiency, protein S deficiency, and elevated factor VIII (Table 24-2). It has been recommended that when these thrombophilias are found in association with unexplained recurrent pregnancy loss, women should be treated with prophylactic or therapeutic heparin.[32] It is clear that some of these hypercoagulable states are found more commonly in women with early pregnancy losses.[31,33] Hyperhomocysteinemia has been reported in early pregnancy losses and is treated with folic acid supplementation.[34]

▶ LIFESTYLE ISSUES

Tobacco use of more than 15 cigarettes a day has been associated with an increased risk of pregnancy loss by 1.5- to 2-fold, as well as alcohol consumption of greater than five drinks per week. When both personal habits are used in the same individual, the risk of pregnancy loss may increase fourfold. Couples should be counseled concerning these habits and strongly encouraged to discontinue them prior to attempting subsequent conception.[35]

▶ EVALUATION FOR PREGNANCY LOSS

When the clinician makes the decision to initiate an evaluation for recurrent pregnancy loss, it is recommended that complete diagnostic testing be performed. This obviously includes a complete history, including documentation of prior pregnancies, any pathologic tests that were performed on prior miscarriages, any evidence of chronic or acute infections or diseases, any recent physical or emotional trauma, a history of cramping or bleeding with a previous miscarriage, any family history of pregnancy loss, and any previous gynecologic surgery or complicating factor. A summary of the diagnosis and management of recurrent pregnancy loss includes an investigation of genetic, endocrinologic, anatomic, immunologic, microbiologic, iatrogenic, and thrombophilic causes (Table 24-3).

▶ **TABLE 24-2:** COMMON THROMBOPHILIAS POSSIBLY ASSOCIATED WITH RECURRENT PREGNANCY LOSS

Thrombophilia	Inheritance	Prevalence	Risk of DVT
Factor V Leiden G1691A mutation (activated protein C resistance)	Autosomal dominant	2–15%	3–8×
Factor II G20210A mutation (prothrombin mutation)	Autosomal dominant	2–3%	3×
MTHFR C677T mutation (hyperhomocysteinemia)	Autosomal recessive	11%	2.5–4×
Antithrombin deficiency	Autosomal dominant	0.02%	25–50×
Protein C deficiency	Autosomal dominant	0.2–0.3%	10–15×
Protein S deficiency	Autosomal dominant	0.1–0.2%	2×
Elevated factor VIII	X-linked	5–15%	5×

Prevalence is in the general population; however, significant ethnic differences are known. Risk of deep vein thrombosis (DVT) in the nonpregnant individual with the listed thrombophilia compared with a nonpregnant individual without the thrombophilia.

▶ **TABLE 24-3:** DIAGNOSIS AND MANAGEMENT OF RECURRENT PREGNANCY LOSS

Etiology	Diagnostic Evaluation	Abnormal Result	Therapy
Genetic	Karyotype partners	3–5%	Genetic counseling Donor gametes
Anatomic	Hysterosalpingogram Hysteroscopy Sonohysterography	15–20%	Septum transection Myomectomy Lysis of adhesions
Endocrinologic	Midluteal progesterone TSH Prolactin Fasting insulin:glucose Day 3 FSH, estradiol	8–12%	Progesterone Levothyroxine Bromocriptine, Dostinex Metformin Counseling
Immunologic	Lupus anticoagulant Antiphospholipid antibodies ? Embryotoxicity assay ? Immunophenotypes	15–20%	Aspirin Heparin + aspirin ? IV Gamma globulin
Microbiologic	Cervical cultures	5–10%	Antibiotics
Thrombophilic	Antithrombin III Protein C, protein S Factor V Leiden mutation Factor II (prothrombin) mutation Hyperhomocysteinemia	8–12%	 Heparin + aspirin LMW heparin Folic acid
Psychological	Interview Questionnaire	Varies	Support groups Counseling
Iatrogenic	Tobacco, alcohol use Exposure to toxins, chemicals	5%	Eliminate consumption Eliminate exposure

▶ **OUTCOME**

In approximately 70 percent of all cases of recurrent pregnancy loss, a complete evaluation will reveal a possible etiology.[2] If no cause can be found, most couples eventually will have a successful pregnancy outcome with supportive therapy alone.[3] Couples who have experienced recurrent pregnancy loss want to know what caused the miscarriage. Unexplained reproductive failure can lead to anger, guilt, and depression. Anger may be directed toward the physician for not being able to solve the reproductive problems. Feelings of grief and guilt following an early loss are often as intense as those following a stillbirth, and parents experience a grief reaction similar to those associated with the death of an adult. The couple should be assured that exercise, intercourse, and dietary indiscretions do not cause miscarriage. Any questions or concerns that the couple may have about personal habits should be discussed.

Women who suffer recurrent pregnancy loss already have begun to prepare for their baby, both emotionally and physically, as compared with couples with infertility who have never conceived. When a miscarriage occurs, a couple may have great difficulty informing friends or family about the loss. Feelings of hopelessness may continue long after the loss. Patients may continue to grieve and have episodes of depression on the expected due date or the date of the pregnancy loss. Participation in support groups or referral for grief counseling may be beneficial in many cases.[36]

KEY POINTS

1. A complete evaluation for recurrent pregnancy loss will reveal a possible cause in 70 percent of cases.

2. The complete evaluation (genetic, endocrinologic, anatomic, immunologic, microbiologic, and thrombophilic) should be initiated when the decision to evaluate a couple is made.

3. Couples with primary pregnancy loss have identifiable causes just as frequently as couples with secondary recurrent pregnancy loss; therefore, both couples should be evaluated.

4. Women with two losses have identifiable problems just as frequently as women with three or more losses; thus an evaluation for causes can be initiated after two losses.

5. If no cause is identified after a complete evaluation, 65 percent of couples will have a successful subsequent pregnancy.

REFERENCES

1. Kutteh WH. Recurrent pregnancy loss, in Precis, *An Update in Obstetrics and Gynecology, Reproductive Endocrinology,* 2nd edition. American College of Obstetrics and Gynecology, Washington. 2002; pp 151–161.

2. Stephenson M. Frequency of factors associated with habitual abortion in 197 couples. *Fertil Steril* 1996;66:24–29.

3. Brigham SA, Conlon C, Farguharson RG. A longitudinal study of pregnancy outcome following idiopathic recurrent miscarriage. *Hum Reprod* 1999;14:2868–2871.

4. Branch DW, Silver RM. Antiphospholipid syndrome. *ACOG Educ Bull* 1998;244:302–211.

5. Carson SA, Branch DW. Management of recurrent early pregnancy loss. *ACOG Pract Bull* 2001;24:1–12.

6. Mills JL, Simpson JL, Driscoll SG, et al. Incidence of spontaneous abortion among normal women and insulin-dependent diabetic women whose pregnancies were identified within 21 days of conception. *N Engl J Med* 1988;319:1617–1623.

7. Clifford K, Rai R, Regan L. Future pregnancy outcome in unexplained recurrent first trimester miscarriage. *Hum Reprod* 1997;12:387–389.

8. Castelbaum AJ, Lessy BA. Infertility and implantation defects. *Infertil Reprod Med Clin North Am* 2001;12:427–446.

9. Wilcox AJ, Baird DD, Weinberg CR. Time of implantation of the conception and loss of a pregnancy. *N Engl J Med* 1999;340:1796–1799.

10. Ghazeeri GS, Clark DA, Kutteh WH. Immunologic factors in implantation. *Infertil Reprod Med Clinics North Am* 2001;12:315–337.

11. Craig LB, Ke RW, Kutteh WH. Increased prevalence of insulin resistance in women with a history of recurrent pregnancy loss. *Fertil Steril* 2002;78:487–490.

12. Sills ES, Perloe M, Palermo GD. Correction of hyperinsulinemia in oligoovulatory women with clomiphene-resistant polycystic ovary syndrome: A review of therapeutic rationale and reproductive outcomes. *Eur J Obstet Gynecol Reprod Biol* 2000;91:135–141.

13. Hoffman GE, Khoury J, Thie J. Recurrent pregnancy loss and diminished ovarian reserve. *Fertil Steril* 2000;74:1192–1195.

14. Lin PC. Reproductive outcomes in women with uterine anomalies. J Women's Health 2004;13:33–39.

15. Stovall DW, Parrish SB, Van Voorhis BJ, et al. Uterine leiomyomas reduce the efficacy of assisted reproduction cycles: Results of a matched follow-up study. *Hum Reprod* 1998;13:192–197.

16. Surrey ES, Lietz AK, Schoolcraft WB. Impact of intramural leiomyomata in patients with a normal endometrial cavity on in vitro fertilization-embryo transfer cycle outcome. *Fertil Steril* 2001;75:405–410.

17. Wilson WA, Ghavari AK, Piette JC. International classification criteria for antiphospholipid syndrome: Synopsis of a postconference workshop held at the Ninth International (Tours) APL Symposium. *Lupus* 2001;10:457–460.

18. Franklin RD, Kutteh WH. Antiphospholipid antibodies and recurrent pregnancy loss: treating a unique APA positive population. *Hum Reprod* 20092;17:2981–2985.

19. Cowchock FS, Reece EA, Balaban D. Repeated fetal losses associated with antiphospholipid antibodies: A collaborative randomized trial comparing prednisone with low-dose aspirin treatment. *Am J Obstet Gynecol* 1992;166: 1318–1323.

20. Laskin CA, Bombardier C, Hanna ME, et al. Prednisone and aspirin in women with autoantibodies and unexplained recurrent fetal loss. *N Engl J Med* 1997;337:148–153.

21. Kutteh WH: Antiphospholipid antibody–associated recurrent pregnancy loss: treatment with heparin and low-dose aspirin is superior to low dose aspirin alone. *Am J Obstet Gynecol* 1996;174:1584–1589.

22. Rai R, Cohen H, Dave M, et al. Randomized, controlled trial of aspirin and aspirin plus heparin in pregnant women with recurrent miscarriage associated with phospholipid antibodies. *BMJ* 1997;314:253–257.

23. Empson M, Lassere M, Craig JC, et al. Recurrent pregnancy loss with antiphospholipid antibody: A systematic review of therapeutic trials. *Obstet Gynecol* 2002;99:135–144.

24. Rushworth FH, Bakos M, Rai R, et al. Prospective pregnancy outcome in untreated recurrent miscarriers with thyroid antibodies. *Hum Reprod* 2000;15:1637–1639.

25. Esplin MS, Branch DW, Silver R, et al. Thyroid antibodies are not associated with recurrent pregnancy loss. *Am J Obstet Gynecol* 1998;179: 1583–1586.

26. Ober C, Karrison T, Odem RR, et al. Mononuclear-cell immunisation in prevention of recurrent miscarriages: A randomised trial. *Lancet* 1999;354:365–369.

27. Laird SM, Tuckerman EM, Cork BA, Linjawi S, Blakemore AI, Li TC. A reviw of immune cells and molecules in women with recurrent miscarriage. *Hum Reprod Update* 2003;9:163–174.

28. Daya S, Gunby J, Porter F, et al. Critical analysis of intravenous immunoglobulin therapy for recurrent miscarriage. *Hum Reprod Update* 1999;5:475–482.

29. Scott JR. Immunotherapy for recurrent miscarriage. *Cochrane Database Syst* Rev 2003;(1): CD000112.

30. Penta M, Lukic A, Conte MP, et al. Infectious agents in tissues from spontaneous abortions in the first trimester of pregnancy. *New Microbiol* 2003;26:329–337.

31. Kovalevsky G, Garcia CR, Berlin JA, et al. Evaluation of the association between hereditary thrombophilias and recurrent pregnancy loss: A metaanalysis. *Arch Intern Med* 2004;164:558–563.

32. Regan L, Rai R. Thrombophilia and pregnancy loss. *J Reprod Immunol* 2002;55:163–180.

33. Rey E, Kahn SR, David M, et al. Thrombophilic disorders and fetal loss: A metaanalysis. *Lancet* 2003;361:901–908.

34. Quéré I, Mercier E, Bellet H, et al. Vitamin supplementation and pregnancy outcome in women with recurrent early pregnancy loss and hyperhomocysteinemia. *Fertil Steril* 2002;75:823–825.

35. Ness RB, Grisso JA, Hirschinger N, et al. Cocaine and tobacco use and the risk of spontaneous abortion. *N Engl J Med* 1999;340: 333–339.

36. SHARE, Pregnancy and Infant Loss Support, Inc., St. Joseph Health Center, 300 First Capitol Drive, St. Charles, MO 63301, 1-800-821-6819, *www.nationalshareoffice.com.*

CHAPTER 25

Clinical Trials in Reproductive Medicine

DALE W. STOVALL

Results from clinical investigation provide health care providers with the best information available to make daily practice decisions. Never before has this been more palpable than over the past few years with the publication of the results of the Heart and Estrogen/progesterone Replacement Study (HERS) and the Women's Health Initiative (WHI).[1,2] New medical therapies and surgical instruments are becoming available on the world market at an increasing pace. To continue to practice evidence-based medicine, clinicians must be capable of assessing the data regarding the efficacy, safety, and cost-effectiveness of multiple clinical interventions. Therefore, it is important for all health care providers to understand the various study designs, hierarchy of data quality, and most commonly used biostatistical terms from scientific reports. Armed with this information, the clinician can assess the evidence for causation and make appropriate evidence-based recommendations in their clinical practice.

The role of the clinical investigator includes the generation of important clinical questions, the completion of properly designed clinical trials, data analysis, and the reporting of study results using the highest scientific standards. With the appropriate study design, execution, and analysis, an investigator can evaluate the causal relationship between a therapy or exposure and a given outcome(s). Although it is clear that the gold standard in clinical research is the randomized clinical trial, randomized trials are not the most common study design used in clinical research. This chapter will discuss the different study designs used in clinical research and provide a detailed discussion of the many issues encountered in the design, execution, and analysis of randomized clinical trials. Ethical issues in clinical research also will be addressed, and a glossary of frequently used statistical terms is included for quick reference.

▶ STUDY DESIGNS

To assess the cause-and-effect relationship between an intervention or exposure and one or more outcomes, the investigator may choose either an observational or interventional study design. As compared with any observational study, an intervention study provides the best evidence of causation. However, each of the observational and interventional study types contain their own inherent flaws. Although there are various interventional study designs,

► **TABLE 25-1:** STUDY DESIGNS

Descriptive (case series)
Cross sectional
Case-control
Cohort
Uncontrolled investigational
Nonrandomized, controlled trials
Randomized, controlled trials

all interventional studies are prospective in nature. In contrast, observational studies can be either prospective or retrospective. In a retrospective study, information regarding the exposure or outcome status is known at initiation of the study, and the investigator must go back to determine the unknown variable. Interventional studies have the advantage of investigator-directed assignment of treatment or exposure. The gold standard of the interventional study is the randomized clinical trial. The prediction of causation from a retrospective study is less reliable as compared with the prediction of causation from a prospective study. The various clinical study designs are listed in Table 25-1.

► OBSERVATIONAL STUDIES

One of the simplest types of clinical investigation is the *descriptive study*. The most common descriptive study is the case study or case series. Although their usefulness in determining causation is modest, case series can be very useful in the assessment of rare events. A prime example is the reporting of the occurrence of adverse events that are seen as a result of administration of a new pharmaceutical agent after its release into the marketplace. No clinical trial can be expected to identify all the safety and tolerability factors associated with a new compound, especially drugs that subsequently will be taken for many years. Therefore, as a new drug becomes widely prescribed in patients with various clinical conditions, it is possible that new safety, efficacy, and tolerability

issues will arise. Through case series, clinicians can identify and report these adverse experiences. Depending on the severity and frequency of the events, one of several actions may be taken by the drug's manufacturer. Further clinical investigation may be initiated, changes can be made with regard to prescribing information, or labeling changes may be indicated. Recently, the insulin-sensitizing agent troglitazone was removed from the market after case reports of severe hepatic toxicity.

The *cross-sectional study* is another type of observational study. In cross-sectional studies, individuals are assessed for the presence or absence of both exposure to the independent variable of interest and the outcome(s) of interest at a given time point. For example, if one is trying to determine if estrogen therapy prevents coronary artery atherosclerosis, women would be identified from a population and asked about their use of estrogen. At the same time, these women would be evaluated for coronary atherosclerosis using an accepted methodology. Then some measure of estrogen consumption in women who do and do not have atherosclerosis is compared. The strengths of cross-sectional studies are their ability to yield correlations and disease prevalence. Their weakness is their inability to determine temporal relationships between exposure and outcome status. Furthermore, other factors that may contribute to the outcome of interest are not taken into account. The cross-sectional study, therefore, has limited utility in determining cause and effect.

Case-control studies are a type of retrospective observational study in which a group of participants with a particular disease state (cases) is compared with a group of participants who are not affected by that same disease or outcome (controls). In other words, in case-control studies, the outcome of interest is known at initiation of the study. After identifying cases and controls, the investigator looks back to determine if the cases or controls were exposed to the intervention or risk factor of interest. Data from case-control studies are used to calculate one of the estimates of the actual risk of disease associated with exposure to a risk factor. That estimate is called an *odds ratio*. Odds ratios are calculated by dividing the proportion of participants who received a given intervention or were exposed to a risk factor and developed the outcome of interest by the proportion of individuals who underwent the same intervention and yet did not develop the outcome of interest. Case-control studies have several flaws. First, the case or control group may include or exclude participants with a particular exposure or disease status that may bias the results. For example, if the outcome of interest is pregnancy, and the exposure is intracytoplasmic sperm injection (ICSI), couples who did not conceive (controls) may have included a greater proportion of women with poor ovarian response to follicle-stimulating hormone (FSH) stimulation as compared with the cases. Second, cases and controls may differ in their recall of their exposure status. This is known as *recall bias*. This is likely to occur in cancer survivors who may have spent time thinking about the exposures or therapies that may have caused their disease. Finally, in case-control studies, there is the possibility that unknown confounding factors exist that are related to exposure status. These factors are more likely to be equally distributed among cases and controls if the treatment allocation is randomized.

The last of the observational study types is the *cohort study*. Cohort studies may be prospective or retrospective. Unlike case-control studies, where the disease or outcome of interest is known at the onset of the study, with prospective cohort studies it is the exposure status that is known at the beginning of the study. After participants are identified by their exposure to a risk factor or therapy, they are followed for a specified interval of time to determine the occurrence of the outcome or disease of interest. For example, if one wants to determine if estrogen therapy reduces the risk for Alzheimer's disease, participants who were (study group) and were not (control group) given estrogen would be followed to determine whether the study or control group developed Alzheimer's disease. In a retrospective cohort study, both exposure and outcome status are known at initiation of the study. Cohort studies have several flaws. First, assessment of the exposure status itself may be flawed. In our preceding example, women who simply received a prescription for estrogen from their primary care provider may have been included in the study group when in fact many of these women may not actually have taken estrogen. Second, the method of assessment for Alzheimer's disease may differ in the study and control groups. And finally, women who did not receive a prescription for estrogen based on their primary care provider's own risk-benefit assessment may not represent an appropriate comparison group.

▶ THE RANDOMIZED CLINICAL TRIAL

A *randomized clinical trial* is a prospective comparative study between an intervention group and a control group that uses a method of assignment of participants such that all participants are equally likely to be assigned to either the intervention or control group. Randomized clinical trials are accepted as the standard by which investigators can best evaluate the efficacy, efficiency, and effectiveness of clinical therapies. Although a properly planned and executed clinical trial is a powerful experimental tool, the development and completion of a clinical trial often require significant time, effort, and monies, as well as collaboration and cooperation from a mixture of statisticians, epidemiologists, and clinical scientists.

The evolution of the clinical trial dates back beyond the eighteenth century.[3] In the twentieth century, substantial advancements in the design of clinical trials were introduced by several investigators. Most of the early foundations for the design of controlled experiments were established in the agricultural field. R. A. Fisher is credited with introducing the principle of randomization to clinical trials,[4] and J. B. Amberson's manuscript, published in 1931, regarding the use of sanocrysin in pulmonary tuberculosis was the first to introduce the concept of blindness or masking in clinical trials.[5] In that same decade, H. S. Diehl was the first to use the term *placebo* in reference to a saline solution given to participants of a trial evaluating the efficacy of a cold vaccine.[6] It was not until the early 1950s that the need for a control group in clinical trials was widely accepted.[7] In 1964, clinical trials received unequivocal federal support in the form of legislation requiring the Food and Drug Administration (FDA) to obtain proof of efficacy through randomized trials before approving any new drug for the U.S. market. This decision came on the heels of reports that thalidomide was responsible for producing phocomelia in infants of exposed mothers in Europe.[8] The irony of this turn of events is that the FDA does not currently require clinical trials of new drugs to include pregnant women, and therefore, if thalidomide were developed today, it could very well gain FDA approval without any knowledge of its teratogenic effects. Of course, its pregnancy class would be so designated.

In the past there had been some concern that women were underrepresented in clinical trials. Significant progress has been made in this area with the completion of the HERS trial[1] and initiation of the WHI.[2] Furthermore, there are now requirements stating that minority populations must be included in appropriate numbers in clinical trials.[9] Few randomized clinical trials were reported in the infertility literature until the 1980s. Of those reported, many lacked sufficient statistical power. Although multicenter trials would address this problem, funding for multicenter trials remains limited. The need for clinical trials in reproductive medicine has been addressed initially by development of the Reproductive Medicine Network, which is funded by the National Institutes of Health. This section will review the phases of the clinical trial, including its uses, development, design, execution, closeout, data analysis, and interpretation, and will discuss some of the ethical concerns surrounding implementation of a clinical trial.

Uses

Clinical trials have three primary uses. First, they can be used to evaluate the efficacy, efficiency, and effectiveness of pharmaceutical agents. For example, clinical trials may be used to assess the effectiveness of a new contraceptive agent or the efficacy of a new drug in the treatment of obesity. The FDA requirements for approval of new drug applications into the U.S. market has had a significant impact on the number of trials being conducted by pharmaceutical companies. Assisting in the conduct of these pharmaceutical trials are investigators in both the academic and private-practice sectors.

In addition to testing the efficacy of pharmacologic agents, clinical trials can be used to evaluate the therapeutic value of new technologies. Such trials might evaluate procedures performed in the laboratory, such as intracytoplasmic sperm injection (ICSI) or assisted hatching of embryos, or procedures performed in the operating room, such as endometrial ablation or metroplasty.

Finally, clinical trials can be used to evaluate the effectiveness of screening tests. In this regard, the clinical trial is designed to evaluate the sensitivity, specificity, and predictive value of a test at given cut points and to determine if the beneficial information provided by the test offsets its costs. Randomized trials might be used to evaluate the use of serum free testosterone levels in the evaluation of hirsutism, the utility of assessing insulin sensitivity in the evaluation of polycystic ovary syndrome, and the usefulness of ultrasound for pelvic pain.

Clinical trials are not appropriate or cost-effective in the evaluation of small variations in a clinical procedure or to assess the impact of therapeutic agents on rare events. For example, if a previously approved drug is made available as a depot form, and the depot form has been shown to have acceptable bioavailability, a new clinical trial evaluating the depot formulation is not warranted. Likewise, the effects of pharmaceutical agents on rare events such as the effect of ovarian stimulation on the incidence of ovarian cancer should be evaluated by case-control studies instead of clinical trials. Once an unproven pharmaceutical agent or procedure has become part of accepted clinical practice, carrying out a clinical trial is much more difficult.

Design

The ideal clinical trial is one that is randomized, double-blinded, and placebo-controlled. The design is the key to success of a clinical trial. The basic components of a clinical trial are outlined in Table 25-2.

Developing a Hypothesis
The planning of a clinical trial depends on the development of a testable hypothesis. The hypothesis should be clearly defined and stated as specifically as possible. The hypothesis should contain the primary question the investigator(s) is interested in answering. The investigator may wish to evaluate changes in

▶ **TABLE 25-2:** COMPONENTS
OF A CLINICAL TRIAL

Central research hypothesis
Concurrent comparison of interventions
Placebo control
Masking
Randomized allocation of interventions
Homogeneous study population
Power analysis
Clearly defined and measurable outcome events
Analysis method(s) defined before data collection

severity of a disease or functional changes in various biologic parameters. Usually, the study or null hypothesis states that no difference in outcome exists between two given therapies. For example, in patients with chronic anovulation, treatment with clomiphene citrate at daily doses of 100 mg for 5 days is no better at treating infertility over a 6-month period than treatment with metformin at daily doses of 2000 mg. The clinical trial is designed to determine whether or not the null hypothesis can be rejected. When selecting a hypothesis, the investigator must take several issues into account: Has the question been sufficiently addressed by other investigators? Does the question have significant clinical importance and interest, and are the results of the trial likely to change clinical management? Can the response to therapy be precisely and reliably measured? Given the resources available, can the trial be completed in a reasonable time at a finite cost? And finally, is the trial ethical?

Besides the primary question(s) to be addressed by the trial, there also may be several secondary hypotheses to be addressed. For example, in a trial evaluating intravenous immunoglobulin for treatment of recurrent pregnancy loss, one primary question might be whether a subject's live birth rate is altered after therapy. A secondary question might address the incidence of preterm labor, premature rupture of membranes, and fetal anomalies. Secondary hypotheses may address the analysis of certain subgroups. In the recurrent pregnancy loss example, the investigator may want to determine if the presence of a prior live birth alters outcome. Whenever subgroup analyses are to be performed, they should be specified before the trial is begun. The same is not the case with regard to the assessment of adverse events.

Choosing a Baseline State
During development of the hypothesis, the investigator takes the first step in selecting a study population, which is to identify a group of patients with an important therapeutic need.

The subjects that actually will be included in the clinical trial are further defined by a set of eligibility and exclusion criteria that constitute the *admission criteria*. A set of clearly defined admission criteria needs to be established to avoid the enrollment of ineligible participants. The *eligibility criteria* are used to define the disease state to be studied. The eligibility criteria, as well as the reason for the selection of each criterion, should be precisely defined. For example, when studying a new therapy for the treatment of unexplained infertility, it is important to define what history and diagnostic tests will be used to identify patients with unexplained infertility. Furthermore, it should be specified when, with what instruments, how often, and by whom the tests are to be performed. With tests such as semen analyses that have more than one parameter, it should be determined whether a single abnormal parameter on one occasion is evidence of abnormality. It should be made clear whether or not inclusion is based on previously measured parameters, on measurements obtained during screening of participants, or on investigator judgment. An example of the latter might occur in a trial evaluating a new treatment for endometriosis-associated infertility. With regard to the diagnosis of endometriosis, one needs to specify whether or not all participants have biopsy-proven disease or if the diagnosis is based on the surgeon's judgment that a participant has endometriosis. This approach is advantageous because of its simplicity and cost savings, yet not all the scientific community may agree with this definition.

The eligibility criteria not only define the disease to be studied, but they also attempt to select participants who will benefit from the study and who have a high probability of having the hypothesized result. For example, in a trial of a new selective estrogen receptor modulator for the treatment of osteoporosis, choosing a group of women with a suspected high rate of fracture, such as women in their seventies with low T scores, will reduce the number of subjects needed to detect an effect. Commonly, an investigator uses what is known about the mechanism of action of a new intervention to select which participants have the greatest potential to benefit from therapy. For example, women with a history of thromboembolic disease with menopausal symptoms are appropriate to enroll in a study of a new selective estrogen receptor modulator that has been demonstrated to act as an agonist in the brain and bone but as an antagonist in the liver and uterus. If the mechanism of action of a new drug is unknown, or if it has more than one potential mechanism of action, it may be difficult to select a specific group of participants that is most likely to respond to the new therapy.

Once the eligibility criteria have been selected, the *exclusion criteria* are defined. The exclusion criteria contain those criteria but for which a participant would have been eligible for the study. One common example is an age restriction. When age restrictions are used, it should be made clear when the age limit applies. For example, in a trial on assisted reproduction therapy in which 41 years is used as an exclusionary age, it should be made clear whether a patient is eligible who is 40 on the day of screening but will be 41 before the day of oocyte retrieval. Exclusionary criteria are used often to eliminate participants at high risk for a particular adverse event. In a trial involving a new oral contraceptive therapy, a history of hypertension or deep venous thrombosis might be used as an exclusion criterion. In this case, the investigator should define how the thrombosis is to be diagnosed. Is the participant's history sufficient, or is documentation from one or more diagnostic tests required. Often these decisions are based on the severity of the adverse event. Exclusion criteria are also used to exclude subjects who have medical conditions that might obscure assessment of the outcome of interest. For example, in a trial on a new therapy in the treatment of endometriosis-associated pelvic pain, women with a history of gastrointestinal diseases that may cause pelvic pain, such as Crohn's disease, might be excluded from enrollment because their intestinal disease might preclude assessment of their response to the therapy being investigated. Pregnancy is often used as an exclusion criterion. Whether or not pregnant women should be excluded from drug trials in which pregnancy is not the focus of the intervention is controversial.[10]

In the development of the ideal admission criteria, one must maintain an appropriate balance between practicality and fastidiousness. On the one hand, it is desirable for the criteria to allow enrollment of a *heterogeneous population* of patients. This has three major advantages. First, recruitment will benefit. By including a heterogeneous population of patients, one will increase the percentage of subjects screened who are eligible for the study, making the performance of the study more feasible. Second, if a heterogeneous population is studied, the results of the study are more likely to be generalizable to a broader population of patients with the disease. Furthermore, studying a diverse population provides a greater opportunity to evaluate the effectiveness of the intervention in several subgroups or stages of a disease. On the other hand, however, enrollment of a *homogeneous population* has its advantages. Strict admission criteria simplify the conduct of the study and sharpen the statistical precision of the results. Moreover, if the study population is too diverse, a less susceptible study group may be selected, diluting the effect and decreasing the probability of finding a significant benefit. Clearly, there are instances when selecting a homogeneous study population is not feasible because the technology to do so is not available. Examples include clinical trials evaluating the treatment of a new therapy for premenstrual syndrome or pelvic pain. In this case, the mechanisms that cause premenstrual syndrome and pelvic pain often are unclear, making it difficult to identify a homogeneous population based on the etiology of the disease.

Issues regarding homogeneity and heterogeneity of study populations extend beyond the influences of the admission criteria. There is some evidence to suggest that subjects who agree to sign an informed consent to participate in a study are different from those who do not volunteer.[11,12] Volunteers tend to be healthier and are more likely to be compliant with the study protocol. The influence of these observations on those who participate in clinical trials and how to account for these influences are still unclear. By no means should this undermine the importance of selecting the baseline state because one cannot claim that a therapy is or is not effective unless one can clearly define the population in which the intervention was tested. This level of detail not only allows the reader to identify which patients in his or her practice are appropriate for therapy but also allows other investigators to analyze the appropriateness of the study and to perform confirmatory trials, if necessary. In general, the admission criteria should exclude individuals who are not likely to benefit from the therapy, might be harmed by the therapy, and/or are not likely to comply with the study protocol. A qualification period should be considered before the treatments are imposed to demonstrate that the admission criteria have been fulfilled. Exclusion criteria only apply to subjects who have not been enrolled in the trial. If a participant who has been enrolled in a trial develops a condition that would have excluded him or her from enrollment, the participant may be removed from the trial but should be included in the final analysis of the trial. Table 25-3 includes a brief checklist of the important components of the admission criteria.

Selection of Interventions and Comparisons

Because the natural history of most diseases is still unclear, and because a broad variability of individual responses to medical intervention is common, the need for a defined control or comparison group rarely can be disputed. The choice of the comparative treatment depends on whether the comparison is intended to show

► **TABLE 25-3:** CHECKLIST FOR ADMISSION
CRITERIA

Eligibility Criteria
- Define the basic disease process
- Select the most susceptible participants
- Select participants with a high event rate
- Select participants most likely to adhere to the protocol

Exclusion Criteria
- Subjects with competing disease processes
- Subjects with insufficient prognostic susceptibility
- Subjects with a high risk of therapeutic vulnerability
- The presence of confounding therapies
- Referral bias

the treatment's efficacy, efficiency, or effectiveness.[13] If a clinical trial is to evaluate a new therapy's *efficacy* (i.e., whether it is better than nothing), the appropriate comparison is against a placebo.

There has been considerable debate regarding the ethics of using placebos in clinical trials.[14] Placebo-controlled trials can best be supported under two specific conditions.[15] First, there should be no standard intervention that is clearly superior to placebo. If such a standard therapy does exist, it could be used in combination with the new intervention and placebo. Second, the informed consent for participation in the clinical trial should state clearly that the participant may receive a placebo and what the chances are of receiving either the placebo or alternative.

If a trial is to determine a new treatment's *efficiency,* the decision that the treatment works better than a previously proven standard therapy, the comparison is against the standard therapy. In this case, the new therapy would be used as an alternative to the previously proven therapy.

Finally, a trial may be developed to determine a new therapy's effectiveness. *Effectiveness* refers to the impact of a therapeutic agent on a population and is not necessarily the result of a comparison. Although a new therapy may be proven to be efficacious or efficient, it may be ineffective if it is so expensive, uncomfortable to administer, or inconvenient to take that patients refuse to use it. A new therapy also may be ineffective if participants simply are not motivated to sustain its use. If a new therapy is to be used as a supplement, then the combination of the new and existing treatment should be compared with the existing treatment alone.

When selecting an intervention for investigation, the investigator must consider several issues. First, the intervention's potential for benefit should be maximized while keeping adverse events to a minimum. In the case of a new hormone-replacement regimen, this would mean determining the best dose, route, and frequency of administration. Second, the intervention should be standardized and made stable over the course of the trial so that variations in the intervention will not affect the outcome(s). This is especially true when new procedures are being tested and when multicenter trials are being performed. Furthermore, the duration of intervention needs to be determined. This may be affected by potential side effects of the therapy, such as the problems with loss of bone density found with gonadotropin-releasing hormone agonist (GnRH-a) therapy, or by the length of time needed to obtain the outcome of interest, such as in infertility therapies. The investigator also must determine if multiple drug doses are to be evaluated. If a procedure or new device is being evaluated, the investigator must determine who will perform the procedure or will operate the device. The total number and types of treatments to be evaluated should be kept to a minimum because increasing the number of treatment arms will decrease the feasibility of the study.

Allocation of Treatments

RANDOMIZATION

Historical control studies compare a group of participants on a new therapy or intervention with a previous group of participants on standard or control therapy. Clinical trials compare a group of participants being administered a new therapy to a group of participants who are concurrently being administered a standard or control therapy. Although there is little debate that concurrent controls are the most appropriate with regard to drug evaluation, there is still some controversy and debate regarding the evaluation of new procedures and devices.[16]

The preferred method of assigning participants to intervention and control groups is by randomization. *Randomization* is a process of assignment that gives each participant the same chance of being assigned to either the intervention or control group. Normally, study participants are not chosen for participation in a study in a random manner. However, once an individual has decided to participate in a clinical trial, placement into the control or treatment group should be a random event. Although sometimes used as a randomization surrogate, an alternating assignment of participants to the intervention and control groups is not a form of randomization. The two most common mechanisms from which randomized assignments are obtained are from a *random digit table* and a *computer-generated random-number algorithm*.

Randomized treatment allocations have several advantages. First, randomization tends to create *comparable study groups*. If participants are assigned to two study groups by chance, the distribution of both known and unknown diagnostic variables will tend to be evenly balanced between the two groups. This is probably more important for unknown prognostic variables because the distribution of known prognostic variables can be evaluated and controlled for when the data are analyzed. In large

studies involving several hundred or more participants, the chance that randomization will fail to achieve a balance of prognostic factors is negligible; however, small clinical trials involving less than 100 subjects are much more likely to contain an unbalanced distribution of prognostic factors.[18] Another advantage of a randomized allocation schedule is the potential for the *removal of allocation bias*. If participants are assigned randomly, neither the participant nor the investigator can influence the choice of intervention. For example, in a trial evaluating the efficacy of preoperative therapy with a GnRH-a in the treatment of leiomyoma-associated anemia, if referring physicians would only refer their patients with large leiomyomas to the study if they would be guaranteed allocation of the agonist, the allocation would be biased. Again, neither the participant nor the investigator should know what the intervention assignment will be before the participant's decision to enter the study. Otherwise, the potential for bias will not be affected by the randomization procedure. The third and probably most often overlooked advantage of a randomized allocation schedule is for the *validation of statistical tests*.[19] The validity of statistical tests (e.g., chi-square test and Student's t test) can be justified on the basis of randomization alone. Otherwise, further assumptions regarding the comparability of the study groups, such as equal variances, must be established to validate these statistical comparisons. If this is not done, the p values obtained may not be valid.

Randomization protocols can be either equal or proportional. In an *equal randomization schedule,* the allocations are constrained so that the same numbers of subjects are assigned to each of the maneuvers under investigation. *Proportional assignments* are used to create an unbalanced yet proportional assignment of the comparative agents. For example, a randomization schedule may be arranged so that two-thirds of subjects receive a new hormone therapy for oligospermia and one-third of the subjects receive a placebo. There are two potential advantages to this 2:1 intervention-to-control allocation schedule. First, more information regarding participant responses to the new intervention, such as adverse events, will be gained. Second, if the therapy was found to be beneficial, more subjects will have benefited from the new therapy. Of course, the therapy may be found to be nonefficacious. Allocations proportionally can be tilted toward the control group. If a new intervention is expensive or believed to have a significant chance for one or more toxic side effects, a 1:2 or 1:3 intervention-to-control allocation could be selected. The disadvantages of any proportional allocation schedule are substantial. Most important, proportional allocations are less sensitive and have less statistical power as compared with equal allocation methods,[20] and a proportional allocation schedule may suggest a bias for or against a new intervention, especially in the eyes of the referring physician.

Besides simply randomizing participants into different study groups, participants can be randomized by blocks or strata.[21–23] One disadvantage to a simple stratification procedure is that at any one time during the study, and potentially at the end of the study, a significant imbalance in the number of participants in each group may exist. For example, in a trial of 20 participants with a simple stratification method, there is a 50 percent chance that at the end of the study there will be a 12:8 unbalanced distribution of participants or worse. The advantage of a blocked randomization is that balance between the number of participants in each group is ensured during the course of the study. An example of a *blocked randomization* would be in the assignment of 100 participants to a new procedure (T) for embryo transfer and to a conventional method of transfer (C). A schedule could be devised so that participants are randomized in 25 blocks each with four assignments. In this example, there are six different combinations of group assignments (e.g., TTCC, TCTC, etc.). In this example, one of the six assignments is selected at random for the

purpose of group assignment, and this is repeated 25 times until all participants have been randomized.

In contrast, a *stratified randomization* schedule is used to randomized participants not over time but with regard to one or more prognostic characteristics. Stratification will help to evenly distribute prognostic variables that are strongly associated. If only one prognostic factor is used, it is divided into several subgroups or strata. Otherwise, more than one prognostic factor can be used. For example, in a study comparing two different ovarian stimulation protocols, one might want to stratify subjects based on their cycle day 3 FSH level (e.g., 0 to 10, 11 to 20, or 21 mIU/mL) and smoking history (e.g., never smoker, ever smoker, or current smoker). When two or more variables are used, the total number of strata is the product of the number of subgroups in each factor; therefore, the number of prognostic factors should be kept to a minimum. In this example, the total number of strata is 9. Once a subject has been placed in one of the nine strata, she can then be randomized to receive one of the two stimulation protocols using either a simple or blocked stratification method. Using a blocked randomization method as opposed to a simple randomization method does have important statistical implications.[24] If the appropriate analysis is performed, a blocked randomization scheme will increase the power of the study. Stratified randomizations usually are reserved for smaller studies (e.g., <100 participants). An alternative to stratifying participants at the time of randomization is to stratify participants during analysis. Evaluation by subgroups may help to elucidate the mechanism(s) of action of the intervention.

CROSSOVER DESIGNS

The *crossover study design* is a variation of the randomized clinical trial. In the beginning of a crossover study, each participant is randomly assigned to either the intervention or control group. After a defined period, the control group is "crossed over" and begins receiving treatment and vice versa with the treatment group. Both single and double crossover periods have been described, known as *two-period* and *three-period crossover studies,* respectively. Crossover study designs have several advantages. First, because the measured effect of the intervention is the difference in an individual's response to intervention and control, the statistical variance is reduced. Therefore, fewer participants are required to detect a specific difference in response. Some evidence suggests that parallel study designs require as many as 2.5 to 3 times as many participants as three-period crossover designs.[25] This could result in significant cost savings, especially with regard to recruitment. However, crossover designs have one significant disadvantage. To use a crossover design, a very important assumption must be made; that is, the effects of the therapy in the first or second period must not carry over to the second or third period. This carry-over effect can be avoided if a sufficiently long washout or no treatment period is used before crossing over. Washout periods lengthen the trial and therefore increase costs and reduce participant retention. Furthermore, outcome events may occur during the washout period, such as pregnancies in an infertility therapy trial, making the results difficult to interpret. A statistical test to assess period-treatment interaction has been described, but it has limited power.[26] The most appropriate use for crossover study designs is in conditions that are not cured by therapy, such as diabetes mellitus and hypertension; otherwise, the participant cannot return to the initial state. Finally, crossover designs are only recommended if there is clear evidence that no carry-over effect exists.

MASKING THE STUDY

Masking or *blinding* refers to the process of concealing the identity of the assigned intervention. The principal function of blinding is to avoid problems of bias during data collection and analysis that might lead to false conclusions. A study is particularly susceptible if the response variables are subjective. There are three separate groups that can be masked: the participants, the investigators and staff, and committees that monitor response variables or adverse events. In a *double-masked study,* both the participants and the investigators and staff are kept unaware of the identity of the intervention assignment. If participants are masked, their reporting of symptoms and side effects are less likely to be biased. Participants' preconceived notions regarding a particular therapy or placebo might yield biased reporting of subjective outcome variables. Masking participants can help to prevent study withdrawal that occurs when participants learn that they have been placed on what they think is an undesirable treatment arm. Masking the investigators and staff can help to prevent bias in both data collection and analysis and the unequal administration of concomitant nonstudy treatment that is likely to influence the outcome variables. For example, in a trial of hormone-replacement therapy versus placebo in which quality-of-life parameters are being evaluated, if an investigator is not masked to the intervention assignment, he or she might tend to unequally prescribe concomitant hormonal therapy to the treatment group in cases of vaginal bleeding or other known side effects of hormone-replacement therapy. Furthermore, if the investigator's bias is that hormone-replacement therapy does improve the quality of life, he or she may subconsciously counsel the placebo group regarding lifestyle changes to improve their quality of life or vice versa if he or she wants the study results to be positive. To bias the outcome of a trial, concomitant therapy must be effective, and it must be prescribed to a significant proportion of the participants.

In a *single-masked study,* only the participants are unaware of the identity of the intervention. These studies are easier to carry out. However, the preconceived ideas of the investigator may lead to bias in data collection and concomitant therapy. If a trial is not double-masked, the outcome of response variables should be assessed by investigators who are not involved in follow-up of the participants and are blinded to the treatment group. Some investigators prefer single-masked study designs because this design allows investigators to use their judgment to do what is best for a participant's health and safety should an adverse event occur. Some trials are very difficult to single or double blind. *Unmasked* or *open studies* are used most commonly when a medical therapy is compared against a surgical therapy or laparotomy is compared against laparoscopy. It is possible to design a masked study comparing two surgical procedures if only the surgeon and not the investigator knows the type of surgery being performed. Clearly, initiating and maintaining a masked study design can be very difficult.[27] In pharmaceutical trials, if a drug has one or more identifying characteristics such as its shape, color, or taste, the blind can be broken.[28] In a study involving hormone-replacement therapy, certain side effects, including telltale changes on mammography, may tip off the staff to the participants who are on the study drug. Included in the protocol of any masked trial should be the reason(s) why and the mechanisms for breaking the mask.

Choosing Outcome Events

Anything that happens after the initiation of therapy can be regarded as an *outcome event,* also called a *response variable.* Certain outcomes will be chosen carefully and will represent the specific focus of the study, such as the primary and secondary outcome events, and these events should be stated clearly as such before the trial begins. Other outcomes may be unanticipated yet also may be of critical importance to the conclusions or completion of the study. These outcomes are known as *adverse experiences* or *events* and are discussed in the next section. Because decisions regarding sample size will depend in large part on the primary outcome event, careful consideration should be made when choosing the outcomes that relate to the principal hypothesis of

the study. It is important to have only objective, unambiguous response variables that are not too costly to measure and can be measured accurately. Ascertainment of all outcomes must be complete and honest. The investigator must be capable of measuring the primary response variable(s) in all study participants. By the same accord, all response variables must be measured by the same mechanism in all participants and, if possible, by the same investigator. In a study evaluating a new therapy in the treatment of luteal-phase deficiency in a group of women with infertility, pregnancy rates would be a preferred outcome over correction of an abnormal endometrial biopsy, and delivery rates would be a preferred outcome over pregnancy rates.

In general, a single response variable should be chosen to answer the primary question. In some situations, combining response variables may be considered. For example, in a hormone-replacement study involving women with cardiovascular disease, combined events might include death from coronary heart disease and nonfatal myocardial infarction. Here, both events measure a similar outcome, a cardiac event, so it may be acceptable to use this combined response variable if it is defined as such before the trial begins. When combined responses are used, only one response event is counted per participant. If a single or combined response variable cannot be chosen, the feasibility of conducting the trial should be reconsidered. Response variables are categorized as either continuous or noncontinuous and may change from one *noncontinuous variable* (not pregnant) to another (pregnant) or from one noncontinuous variable (stage I endometriosis) to anyone of a number of others (stage II or III endometriosis). Response variables also may change from one level of a *continuous variable* (e.g., a serum estradiol level) to another. Both the type and quantity of the response variable has implications for sample size. For example, if the primary response is continuous (e.g., serum estradiol levels), change is easier to detect when the initial level is extreme.

Adverse Experiences

Any event or outcome that occurs after the beginning of the study can be categorized as desirable, undesirable, or neutral. Adverse experiences or events are the undesirable signs, symptoms, and clinical events that occur during the clinical trial. Unlike the events that define the primary and secondary outcome variables, adverse experiences are not always well defined or anticipated. The assessment and reporting of adverse events are important for development of the risk-benefit ratio that is considered when a new treatment is appraised. For example, if a new treatment is being compared against a known efficacious therapy and no difference in the primary outcome variable(s) is found between the two groups, the therapy of choice might be decided on based on the frequency of adverse experiences. Before beginning a clinical trial, the investigators should make a list of the adverse events that have been associated with the intervention and are clinically important. A clear definition of each event, based on history, physical examination, and laboratory criteria, should be denoted in the procedure manual. This allows the investigators to record important adverse experiences in a consistent manner. There is some controversy as to whether or not the investigator or staff should elicit specific adverse events from participants or if adverse events should be volunteered by participants.[29–31] I prefer a combination of these two approaches. A limited checklist of what are considered the most important adverse events should be reviewed with the participant, followed by a general question regarding any health-related problems encountered by the participant. This allows for accurate and consistent assessment of what are considered to be the most important adverse events.

Another alternative is to use an *event diary*. The advantage of this technique is a potential reduction in recall bias. One clear disadvantage is the exorbitant amount of time required to review the diaries. No matter which technique is used, the frequency of each experience in each participant during the duration of the trial should be recorded. Clear step-by-step instructions should be developed that define what evaluation, therapy, and follow-up will be performed for certain adverse experiences. An example would be in a clinical trial assessing hormone-replacement therapy in which clear guidelines for vaginal bleeding would need to be developed. Several points should be considered when reporting adverse experiences. Besides reporting the frequency of specific events, it should be clear whether or not a particular adverse experience was defined before the study, how the event was diagnosed, and whether or not its presence was elicited by the investigator or volunteered by the participant. The impact of the event should be reported, e.g., whether it required hospitalization, surgery, additional medical therapy, discontinuation of the study drug, or a reduced drug dosage.

The Operations Manual

All large or complex clinical trials, especially multicenter trials, require the development of an operations manual. Contained within the operations manual is a definitive description of all aspects of the trial, including the study protocol. An example of the contents of a *study protocol* is given in Table 25-4. Besides the study protocol, the operations manual will contain the standard operating procedures, including protocol amendments, a timetable for initiation and completion of the trial, recruitment information, a description of clinical and laboratory procedures, protocols on early termination, protocols on how and when to inform participants about the identity of their study intervention, quality control procedures, algorithms for the evaluation and treatment of specific adverse events, and all clinical research forms. Research forms are developed to record the data that will be collected during the study. Forms need to be developed to record the results of the preliminary screening procedures

▶ **TABLE 25-4:** THE STUDY PROTOCOL

1. Title of the study
2. Specific aims
   a. Primary aim
   b. Secondary aims
3. Background and significance
4. Investigators
5. Experimental design and methods
   a. Study population
   b. Recruitment plan
   c. Schedule and description of visits
   d. Treatment regimen
   e. Randomization
   f. Blinding
   g. Compliance
   h. Adverse events
   i. Sample size calculations
6. Statistical analysis
7. Appendices
   a. Admission criteria
   b. Definition of outcome variables
   c. Definition of adverse events

and information from follow-up visits, concomitant therapies, and adverse experiences. The list of standard operating procedures most likely will grow as the study progresses and new clinical issues arise. Completion dates are especially helpful to inform both participants and coinvestigators as to when the results of the study will become available.

Budget

Making a budget for the clinical trial may be one of the most difficult duties for the investigator. It is helpful to use the resources available from the hospital or university, including personnel, when compiling a budget. A clinical trial contains numerous direct and indirect costs. Table 25-5 lists the potential costs of a clinical trial. Since clinical trials involve screening procedures, there are likely to be positive tests that require further follow-up or therapy. It should be clear in the consent form whether or not tests or procedures not included in the initial screening will be covered by the investigators or trial; this is usually not the case. An example would be a positive Pap smear or mammogram that requires more than an annual follow-up.

Calculating the Sample Size (Power Analysis)

Analysis of the sample size needed for a trial is one of the most important and commonly overlooked components of the clinical trial. Several good reviews of the basic concepts used in sample size calculations are available.[32,33] Sample size calculations should be

▶ **TABLE 25-5:** THE STUDY BUDGET

1. Personnel
   a. Investigator(s)
   b. Study coordinator
   c. Recruitment staff
   d. Data entry staff
   e. Secretary or clerk
2. Equipment
   a. Mammography, ECG machine
   b. Centrifuge, autoclave, freezer
   c. Computer hardware/software
3. Supplies
   a. Clinical supplies for Pap smear, blood draws, endometrial biopsies
   b. Medications/placebos
   c. Postage/shipping of materials
4. Travel for investigators and staff for off-site training and national meetings
5. Other expenses
   a. Travel reimbursement for study participants
   b. Participant parkinig
   c. Recruitment mailings
   d. Recruitment advertising (newspaper, radio, television)
   e. Long-distance phone calls
   f. Rent
6. Indirect costs

performed before any study is begun to address the feasibility of testing the null hypothesis. In other words, sample size calculations are important to ensure that a clinical trial will have sufficient statistical power to detect differences between treatment and control groups that would be considered clinically important. Sample size calculations are based on the primary outcome defined in the null hypothesis. The admission criteria are also important in sample size calculations because these criteria define a specific baseline state with a specific, although not always known, therapeutic susceptibility. Regarding sample size calculations, it is desirable to study participants with a high probability of an anticipated outcome event. Of course, sample size calculations are only estimates of the true sample size required for a study, and therefore, the investigator should considering being conservative and err on overestimating the sample size.

The components of a power analysis are listed in Table 25-6. A sample size is chosen that will adequately test the null hypothesis. When stating a null hypothesis, investigators generally state that no difference exists regarding the primary outcome between the two study groups. The study is then conducted to determine whether this hypothesis is true and should be accepted or is false and should be rejected. Because differences in outcomes can occur by chance alone, the investigator may falsely reject the null hypothesis when in fact it is true. When an investigator falsely rejects the null hypothesis, he or she is said to have made a *type I error*. The probability that a type I error will occur is denoted by α and is called the *significance level*. On the other hand, if the investigator fails to find a difference between the outcome variable of interest when in fact a difference does exist, this is called a *type II error*. The probability of a type II error is denoted by β. The *power* of a study is a quantification of its ability to correctly reject the null hypothesis and is denoted by $1 - \beta$. Traditionally, investigators have set α at 0.01 or 0.05, making the probability of a type I error low (1 to 5 percent). Investigators have accepted a greater probability for a type II error. For example, β is often set at 0.20, making the power of the study 80 percent.

The total sample size (control plus treatment group) is a function of α, β, and the effect size. The *effect size* is the difference in the primary outcome variable that the investigator would consider clinically important. With a fixed sample size, the power of a study depends on the size of the difference of the primary outcome, as shown in the power curve in Figure 25-1. Since α and β generally are fixed at 0.05 and 0.20, the only variable needed to calculate the sample size is the effect size. Therefore, the investigator is forced to define what difference in outcomes he or she thinks would be considered successful treatment. For example, in a study of a fertility-enhancing

▶ **TABLE 25-6:** COMPONENTS
OF A POWER ANALYSIS

Significance level or probability of a type I
  error (α)
Probability of a type II error (β)
Power ($1 - \beta$)
Effect size
Sample size
One-sided versus two-sided hypothesis
Variable type (categorical versus
  continuous)

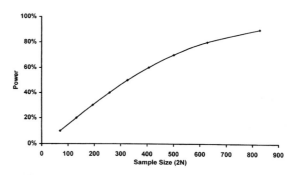

Figure 25-1 Power curve for increasing sample size with baseline pregnancy rate 20 percent, effect size 50 percent, and $\alpha = 0.05$.

procedure, does the intervention need to increase the chance for conception by 10, 25, or 50 percent or more before it can be recommended for general use? As the magnitude of the difference in response is decreased, the sample size must increase at a given α and β. If the calculated sample size is larger than can be obtained realistically, then one of the parameters could be modified. For example, one may relax α if a therapy is being tested that has no side effects and is inexpensive but may provide benefit for an illness with significant morbidity and cost. In this scenario, it would be unfortunate to discard such a therapy without further consideration because a type II error was made. However, if no compromise in α, β, or the effect size can be agreed on and the sample size is still unattainable, serious consideration should be given to abandoning the trial.

Once an α, β, and effect size have been chosen, power can be calculated from standard tables once three additional pieces of information are known.[34,35] First, the investigator must categorize the outcome variables as *categorical (dichotomous),* such as pregnant or not pregnant; or *continuous,* such as mean serum androgen levels, because power calculations are different for different types of variables. Second, it must be determined if the treatment allocation method will result in an equal or unequal proportion of participants in each group. If the variability in the responses for the two groups is approximately the same, equal allocation of interventions will provide a more powerful design. If the variability in the treatment groups is significantly different, an uneven allocation may be more powerful. Third, the investigator must decide if he or she is interested in differences that are in one direction only—a *one-sided test*—or if differences in either direction are important—a *two-sided test*. In general, a two-sided test is recommended unless it is clear that the only changes to be expected are in one direction. In other words, it is clear that a given therapy can only be better and not worse than another. If a one-sided test is used, in most circumstances the signifi-

cance level should be reduced by one-half of what would have been used for a two-sided test. Both methods require the same documentation to declare a treatment effective. This methodology in effect provides two one-sided (e.g., 0.025) hypothesis tests, for an overall 0.05 significance level.

► UNIQUE CLINICAL TRIAL DESIGNS

Pharmaceutical Trials and the FDA Approval Process

The administration of pharmaceutical agents that are proven to be both safe and effective is a cornerstone of clinical care. One function of the U.S. Food and Drug Administration (FDA) is to review data regarding the safety and efficacy of pharmaceutical agents and approve their use before they are available for marketing. Every health care professional depends on the FDA to conduct this process in a critical and comprehensive manner to ensure the efficacy of new agents and to reduce the risks of those individuals who are prescribed a new therapy. Likewise, every health care provider should have a working knowledge of the FDA approval process.

Even before the first clinical trial is conducted, preclinical research is required to synthesize, purify, and test the new pharmaceutical agent in a nonhuman model. If the preliminary results are positive, information from the preclinical studies can be submitted to the FDA as part of an Investigational New Drug (IND) application. The FDA review includes an assessment of the pharmacology and toxicology of the new agent, as well as an assessment of the study design of any preclinical trials and a review of the data analysis. The highest data quality standards are used. If the IND is approved, clinical trials in humans can be initiated.

Pharmaceutical clinical trials are divided into three or four phases. *Phase I studies* are designed to determine the metabolic and pharmacologic actions of a new drug and to determine how well the drug is tolerated.[36] Phase I studies are not true clinical trials in that the proposed intervention is not compared against a control. In contrast, during phase I trials, a relatively small group of participants, often in groups of three, are administered a drug in a step-up manner to determine the pharmacologic actions and maximally tolerated dose (MTD) of the drug. Usually, the MTD is the dosage at which approximately one-third of the participants experience significant toxicity.

If the phase I study reveals that a new drug is sufficiently well tolerated, a phase II study can be initiated. *Phase II studies* involve small numbers of participants and are designed to evaluate the adverse experiences of a new drug and to provide preliminary evidence of efficacy.[37] Phase II studies often involve less than 50 participants and therefore are usually not sufficient to obtain a precise estimate of the true percentage of patients who would respond to therapy (i.e., the response rate). Furthermore, the eligibility criteria of phase II trials are often more restrictive than those of phase III trials, and the primary outcome(s) of a phase II trial may be more short-term-oriented as compared with those used in phase III trials.

Phase III studies are true clinical trials performed to evaluate the effectiveness and safety of a new pharmacologic agent and thus determine its role in clinical practice. Phase III studies usually include several hundred to several thousand subjects and can precisely estimate the true response rate to a given therapy. There are some shortcomings of the phase III trial. Their size makes both cost and quality control significant problems, especially since they are almost always multicenter trials and may involve as many as 80 different centers. In addition to the problems associated with their size, phase III studies often are designed with short follow-up intervals. This is particularly problematic when evaluating treatments in chronic disease states such as osteoporosis. For this reason, trials with long-term follow-up, known as *phase IV studies,* are sometimes performed in subjects with chronic illnesses. Phase IV studies do not include a control group. From the initial animal testing to final approval of a new therapy takes approximately 8.5 years, on average, and costs millions of dollars.

Surgical Trials

The reproductive endocrinology literature contains few appropriately conducted clinical trials evaluating new surgical procedures or instruments. The difficulty in the timing of the performance of a clinical trial that evaluates a new surgical procedure may be one reason why. When deciding when to initiate a trial evaluating a new surgical procedure, one must consider the evolution of the procedure. Enough time must have passed since introduction of the new technique to allow for its optimization before it is appropriate to conduct a trial. On the other hand, if one waits too long, a new procedure may become an integrated part of general medical practice, and the opportunity to conduct a new study may no longer exist because of a loss of clinical equipoise. The medical community may be unwilling to refer patients for randomization once a bias toward the benefit(s) of a procedure has been established. If this occurs, a clinical trial with sufficient power might never be conducted to determine if a given procedure is better than any other therapy or if only a selected group of patients will benefit from the procedure. Furthermore, if various methods of performing a procedure exist, the best method may never be established.

Surgical trials have specific outcomes of interest. Which outcomes are the most important depends on one's perspective. Outcomes that are most important to the surgeon might not be as important to the patient, third-party payor, or an employer. Because of the expense of surgical procedures and new surgical instruments, cost is commonly one of the primary outcomes of interest. There are many costs associated with any surgical procedure, and calculating these costs can be laborious. Surgical procedures harbor both direct and indirect costs. The direct costs include the surgeon's fee, the anesthesiologist's fee, operating room costs, the cost of a hospital room, laboratory fees, the cost of postoperative pain control, and the cost of the surgical instruments. The cost of surgical instruments can be calculated from two perspectives, the cost to the hospital and the cost (price) to the consumer. Thus, when performing a cost analysis, one must differentiate between the cost of acquisition of materials and the cost to the patient. The indirect costs of surgical procedures include the cost of time off from work, which may be difficult to measure, and the cost of diagnosing and treating complications from the procedure. Besides costs, another outcome of particular interest in surgical trials is *patient satisfaction* and the effects of a surgical procedure on the patient's quality of life. One article used a patient satisfaction scale to evaluate the differences in satisfaction between patients undergoing either endometrial ablation or hysterectomy.[38] A patient's satisfaction with a procedure may include the procedure's impact on the patient's physical, psychological, and social functioning.[39] Additionally, the procedure may influence the patient's personal productivity, pain perception, sexual functioning, and sleep habits.

There are several potential risks for bias in surgical trials. Like other clinical trials, the study population may be affected by the selective referral of the most difficult surgical cases, and the participants may be self-selected based on their beliefs. Unlike some pharmaceutical trials, it is especially difficult to blind surgical trials. It is possible to design a study in which the surgeon performing the procedure is the only one that knows the type of surgical procedure, but neither the participant nor the study investigators do. However, this is not possible when a laparoscopic procedure is being compared with a laparotomy procedure or when either of these two procedures is being com-

pared with a hysteroscopic or other transvaginal procedure. Therefore, it is especially important to use objective outcomes, such as delivery rates, whenever possible. Still, the selection of objective outcomes will not alleviate the bias that occurs with regard to the level of skill of the surgeon. For example, if several surgeons are performing the procedures in a trial comparing laparoscopic fimbrioplasty with fimbrioplasty via laparotomy, if the laparoscopic skills of one of the surgeons are particularly good or poor, the results of the trial may be positively or negatively biased toward laparoscopy. Further, if there are only a small number of surgeons participating in a trial, the skill of one surgeon will have an even greater impact on the outcome. One way to overcome this problem is to randomize patients to a few selected surgeons who only perform one of the two procedures being evaluated and who do not assess the outcome variables. Failing to mask a surgical trial will tend to decrease the effect seen, not unlike failing to randomize participants tends to increase the effect seen.[40]

Multicenter Trials

As discussed in the section on sample size, studies evaluating infrequent events and those attempting to detect small differences between study groups require large sample sizes. Recruitment of the necessary number of participants (e.g., hundreds to several thousand) within an acceptable length of time by a single center would not be possible; therefore, multicenter trials were developed. A *multicenter trial* is a collaborative trial in which several university and/or non-university-based investigators contribute subjects to a common protocol.[40] In addition to making a large trial feasible, multicenter trials have several other advantages. First, multicenter trials enable numerous investigators with similar interests to work together to answer a particularly difficult or important clinical question. Second, recruitment of participants from several geographic areas allows for evaluation of a study population that may be more representative of the general population, making the results of the trial more generalizable. The multicenter study design has been used in several recently completed and ongoing studies in women's health, including the Postmenopausal Estrogen/Progestin Intervention (PEPI) study, the HERS trial, and the WHI.

Developing a multicenter trial requires the establishment of an *organizing group.* Members of the organizing group may be primarily investigators from academic institutions but also may be from governmental agencies or private industry. The organizing group has the task to organize and oversee all phases of the trial, including whether or not a particular trial is worth pursuing, the timeliness of the trial, the feasibility of the study, planning of the study, sample size analysis, cost of the trial, participant follow-up, and data analysis. Occasionally, a pilot study is needed to answer some of these questions. The organizing group will select at least some of the clinical centers that will participate in the trial. Out of these centers, a *coordinating center* will be selected. The coordinating center will help with the design, management, and analysis of the trial, including implementation of the randomization process, evaluation of data quality from the various clinical centers, and the day-to-day running of the trial. Therefore, the coordinating center must have particular expertise in clinical, epidemiologic, and biostatistical issues and must be readily accessible and free of any overriding interest in the outcome of the trial. Once the coordinating center and some of the clinical centers have been selected, the final work on the organizational structure, including establishing lines of authority and the final protocol, may begin.

A *steering committee,* made up of a subset of investigators in the trial, is formed to oversee development of the protocol and study forms, approve all scientific publications, select members of subcommittees, and make final decisions regarding safety issues. Some multicenter trials will elect an *executive committee* from the members of the steering committee.

The executive committee may help set the agenda for the steering committee by setting the priorities of the trial and make quick operational decisions when necessary. A *data-monitoring committee,* independent of the investigators and the study sponsor, is charged with periodic monitoring of response-variable data and assessment of intervention toxicity and center performance.[42] *Subcommittees* often are developed to carry out numerous important functions, including patient recruitment, quality control, publication functions, and protocol adherence. Furthermore, specialized centers may need to be selected to prepare medications and perform specialized laboratory assays. During the initial meeting of the investigators, the final and usually most difficult protocol decisions are made. All investigators must agree to follow a common protocol. To expedite some of these decisions, a small group of investigators may be assembled with particular expertise in a given area. Continued communication between the coordinating center and the clinical centers is important through all stages of the trial. Because of the complexity of a multicenter trial, successful monitoring of the trial can be difficult.[43,44] Periodic meetings of the steering committee and the investigators is necessary to maintain the quality of the data and address problems that arise. Training workshops are useful for the investigators and clinical coordinators of multicenter studies and can improve the quality of a clinical trial significantly. Finally, issues regarding publications, presentations, and authorship should be addressed before the trial is begun. A diagram of the structure of a hypothetical three-site trial is presented in Figure 25-2.

▶ CONDUCTING THE CLINICAL TRIAL

Standards for the ethical conduct of clinical research are contained within federal guidelines. In 1974, Congress passed the National Research Act. The National Research Act required regulations for the protection of human subjects

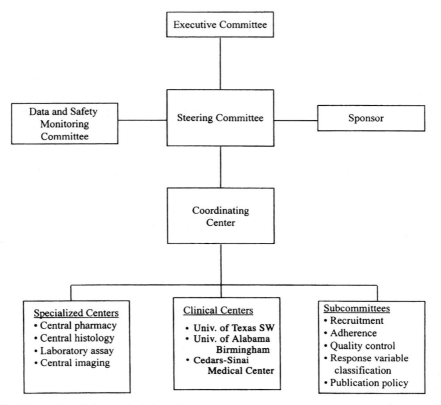

Figure 25-2 Example of the administrative structure in a multicenter trial.

that included requirements for informed consent and review of research by institutional review boards (IRBs). The National Research Act also created the National Commission for the Protection of Human Subjects of Biomedical and Behavioral Research. This commission wrote the Ethical Principles and Guidelines for the Protection of Human Subjects of Research, which now serves as the cornerstone for all federal regulations regarding the protection of subjects in clinical trials. The basic principals of these guidelines include treatment of individuals as autonomous agents, a requirement to protect those with diminished autonomy, a requirement for maximization of benefits with reduction of risks, and fairness in the selection of subjects for clinical trials. In 1981, the Department of Health and Human Services and the FDA published convergent regulations that

were based on the Ethical Principals and Guidelines for the Protection of Human Subjects of Research. These regulations mandated a role on the IRB for persons with broad backgrounds and members who could represent community attitudes. In 1991, 17 federal departments and agencies adopted a set of basic human subject protections that are commonly referred to as the *Common Rule*. Whereas the Common Rule governs research that is conducted or supported by a federal agency, the FDA governs research involving drugs, biologicals, and devices regardless of sponsorship.

Informed Consent

Within the ethical guidelines of clinical research is the concept that subjects should be able to choose what will or will not happen to them. The essential elements contained within the consent form are listed in Table 25-7. Informed consent; however, is not merely a form or witnessed signature but a process of information exchange that takes place between the prospective study participant and the investigator. The *process of informed consent* takes place throughout the conduct of the study and often continues after the study results are obtained. The exchange of information includes subject recruitment materials, verbal instructions, and written materials. Although the original consent should be signed, dated, and kept in the investigator's records, a copy should be given to the study participant for review during the trial.

There are several components of the informed consent process. First, the process must be voluntary. Therefore, the participant's consent must be free from coercion and undue influence. Second, sufficient information must be made available to the subject. The information provided should included the research procedures, the purpose of the study, the risks and anticipated benefits, alternative therapies or actions, and a statement that allows the partici-

▶ **TABLE 25-7:** ESSENTIAL ELEMENTS OF THE INFORMED CONSENT

Statement of voluntary participation in a research study
Purpose of the study
Description of the study procedures
Duration of involvement
Potential risks
Unforeseen risks statement
Potential benefits
Alternative therapies
Reasons for involuntary termination of the participant
Additional costs to participate
Potential consequences for withdrawal
New findings statement
Payments
Statement of confidentiality of records
Statement of compensation for injury

pant to withdraw from the study at any time. Finally, the individual who is giving consent must be capable of comprehending the information that he or she is provided. Thus the information within the consent document must be presented in a clear manner with ample time for questions and discussion so that the prospective subject can clearly understand the information. Technical language should be eliminated from the consent form or explained in lay terms. Overly optimistic language should be avoided.

IRB Approval

Peer review and ethical review are both key elements of the research monitoring system. Scientific merit and methods are reviewed under a system of peer review at major research institutions. The purpose of the IRB is to review research and determine if the rights and welfare of human subjects involved in research are adequately protected. Institutions establish policies that ensure that peer review and IRB review are properly conducted. By institutional policy, even studies that may otherwise be exempt form federal regulations may require review or verification of exempt status. Documents provided to peer-review committees and IRBs by investigators must contain enough information to allow valid judgments about the science and ethics of the research.

The IRB has the authority to approve, require modification in, or disapprove of all research activities, including proposed changes in previously approved human subject research. Based on factors including risks to subjects, IRBs determine which activities require continuing review more frequently than once a year and which need verification that no changes have occurred since previous review and approval. Before a research proposal is approved, the IRB must consider the risks to the subjects, the anticipated benefits, the importance of the knowledge that may result from the study, and the informed-consent process to be employed.

The IRB has an obligation to report any injuries, serious or continuing noncompliance, and suspension or termination of IRB approval for research to the appropriate institutional officials, Office of Protection from Research Risks (OPRR), FDA, and any sponsoring agency of the federal government. Both initial and continuing review and approvals must be in compliance with federal regulations. It is the responsibility of the research investigators to promptly report proposed changes in previously approved research activities. The proposed changes may not be initiated without IRB review and approval, except where necessary to protect subjects from immediate harm.

Recruitment

A common mistake in the planning of a clinical trial is underestimation of the time and effort needed to recruit study participants. The investigator must ensure that an adequate amount of time, funds, and energy will be appropriated to the recruitment of study participants. A well-thought-out plan for recruitment is essential. Obtaining the institutional review board's approval of the study is part of the planning process. Several recruitment strategies should be devised,[45] and the necessary staff, facilities, and equipment for recruitment and screening of participants need to be secured. An experienced and organized coordinator in charge of recruitment is helpful.

Several recruitment strategies are available. No one strategy will work in all geographic locations, and some strategies may not work in any geographic location. The success of recruitment will depend on the recruitment strategies used, the prevalence of the disease being studied, the study design, the admission criteria, and the population base of the clinical center. No matter what recruitment strategy is used, potential participants should undergo a screening evaluation, in person or by phone, before the baseline assessment is initiated to eliminate participants who do not meet the admission criteria. Most clinical trials in reproductive endocrinology require a community-based screening program. One way to identify eligible study participants is by reviewing office records. Once eligible participants are identified, the appropriate channels should be followed before subjects are contacted. Another recruitment strategy is to advertise the study through various media, including mass mailings, various newspapers, and radio and television stations. All advertisements must be approved through the IRB. A combination of approaches will tend to yield the best results. Records should be kept of recruiting activities, including which activities yield the most participants for a given cost. Regular meetings should be held to keep the investigators and staff up to date on how recruitment is progressing. A timetable for recruitment of all participants should be set, as well as short-term (monthly) recruitment goals.

Problems that may occur in recruitment include inadequate funding for the screening process, unwillingness of physicians to refer patients,[46,47] overestimation of the prevalence of the disease, and strenuous requirements of the admission criteria.[48] When recruitment lags, there are several possible solutions. First, if the trial is a multicenter study, investigators can solicit solutions from centers that have had success with their recruitment strategies. Second, depending on costs, the length of recruitment can be extended. This might be particularly attractive if recruitment was initiated during a holiday season, when recruitment might be expected to lag. Another idea is to determine if there were potential participants who failed their screening process because of self-limiting problems, such as a washout period that was not completed or lack of transportation for a given period of time. These participants could be given a second opportunity to be screened. Attention to detail is important during the recruitment phase in order to avoid enrolling ineligible patients. When recruitment lags, the investigator and staff should avoid any temptation to begin to loosely interpret or alter the inclusion criteria. Changes in the admission criteria are appropriate only after a thorough analysis has determined that the design of the study will not suffer. Recently, Congress has directed the National Institutes of Health (NHI) to establish guidelines for the recruitment and inclusion of women and minorities in clinical research.[49]

Executing the Study

Once participants pass the *initial screening evaluation,* a baseline assessment is performed. Depending on the admission criteria, the baseline assessment may measure variables by history, physical examination, blood tests, tissue samples, and imaging studies. Because of cost concerns, only factors that are pertinent to the study and admission criteria should be evaluated. One prerequisite for inclusion into a study is the participant's willingness to comply with the study protocol. For example, in a study that requires an endometrial biopsy to be performed at the baseline visit and at an additional follow-up visits, a participant who does not tolerate the baseline endometrial biopsy may not be a good candidate for the study. Occasionally, when evaluating continuous variables such as prolactin levels, the serum level obtained in an office setting may have met the inclusion criteria, but the evaluation at the baseline visit, with no interim therapy, may not meet the inclusion criteria. This is particularly problematic when the inclusion criteria include an extreme cut point, such as >150 ng/mL in this example. One possible reason for this occurrence is that successive samples of continuous variables tend to yield values that are closer to the mean of the population. This is known as *regression toward the mean.*[50] This problem can be decreased by using a higher cut point in the screening visit or using a mean of two or three samples during the screening visit. The later technique may not be cost-effective or tolerable depending on the variable being evaluated. With either technique, to ensure that the baseline data reflect the true condition of the participants, some time limit should be set for the interval between the baseline evaluation and the allocation of interventions.

Monitoring and maintaining *participant compliance* to the study protocol are critical to the success of the study. Usually, minimal compliance guidelines are established. For example, in studies involving pharmaceutical agents, a 90 percent minimum compliance rate per individual may be reasonable. If the compliance rate is as low as 80 percent, a significant increase in the sample size ($\geq$50 percent) may be necessary to maintain the power of the study.[51] Study protocols that are short and contain simple (e.g., single dose) interventions yield higher compliance rates.[52,53] Better-informed participants and those with a higher level of education are more likely to comply with the study protocol.[54,55] Further, participant compliance is improved if participants think that their health will be improved by the intervention.[56] Therefore, it is important for the staff to stay in close contact with study participants, especially after randomization, and to spend time answering participants' questions and reminding them of upcoming visits and making each clinic visit a pleasant experience by decreasing waiting times and increasing the accessibility of the clinic. In trials that include elderly participants, involving family and friends can help improve compliance. Pill dispensers help keep track of medications taken.[57] Monitoring compliance can be difficult. Frequent follow-up visits can ease the task of compliance monitoring. In pharmaceutical trials, pill counts and diaries can be useful in monitoring compliance. In a study of insulin administration for the treatment of diabetes mellitus, assessment of hemoglobin A1c levels could be useful to assess compliance. Both noncompliance and *losses to follow-up* need to be monitored. Noncompliance is the better of these two evils because one still has the data and may be able to adjust one's analysis appropriately. Usually with losses to follow-up, information bias is lost to the treatment arm at a greater rate than the control arm.

Proper execution of the study is required to maintain data quality and therefore reduce bias. Special attention should be given to controlling the quality of the assessment and recording of important information such as baseline characteristics and outcome measures. To help maintain high-quality data, all investigators and staff should be well versed in the study protocol and have a clear understanding of how all variables are defined and assessed. The operations manual should be constantly updated, made available to all staff, and consulted anytime there is a question regarding the definition or assessment of any variable. Maintaining the quality of data includes assessing all variables in a similar manner in all participants, consistently and completely filling out all data forms, properly labeling tissue specimens, asking questions in a consistent manner, calibrating instruments on a regularly scheduled basis, and using technology instead of technicians to assess variables whenever possible. Histology slides should be evaluated by a single pathologist, if possible. Imaging procedures should be assessed by a single radiologist. Whenever possible, repetitive measures should be performed. For example, in a study using ultrasonography to evaluate the endometrial effects of a new hormone-replacement regimen, the mean of three endometrial stripe measurements should be used for analysis instead of the results from a single measurement. Data forms should be easy to follow and complete and be devoid of any essay-type questions.[58,59] During the study, data forms should be reviewed for completeness. *Extreme values,* such as an FSH concentration of 0.5 mlU/mL or an estradiol level of 3000 pg/mL, should be checked. Finally, computers and data-entry programs should be used to assess data quality when available.

During the execution phase of the trial, an *ongoing statistical evaluation* of the differences in response variables between the intervention groups is important to determine if early termination of the trial is necessary in cases of unanticipated toxicity, greater-than-expected benefit, or high likelihood of indifferent results. If any of these suspicions are confirmed, the trial may be terminated before its scheduled completion. It is preferred that this analysis be performed by a person or group that has no formal involvement with the participants or the investigators[60] but that has experience in clinical trials, epidemiology, and statistical analysis.[61,62] There is no best formula to determine how often the data should be reevaluated. One possibility is to use discrete intervals of time (e.g., every other month); another possibility is to reanalyze the data when a given percentage of the total number of participants has received therapy (e.g., 20, 40, or 60 percent).[63] Repetitive testing is not without its problems. For example, if one reevaluates the data 100 times, five of these evaluations, on average, will show a significant difference based on chance alone if a 0.05 level of significance is used. More specifically, if a hypothesis is tested twice, first when half the data are known and again at the end of the trial, the probability of a type I error increases from 5 to 8 percent.[64]

The solution to this problem is to adjust the critical value used in each analysis so that the overall probability of a type I error remains at the level desired. One method that is commonly used to monitor the accumulating data in a clinical trial is known as the *group sequential method.*[65,66] In this procedure, the number of repeat analyses that will be performed is specified before the trial is begun, and the analysis is performed only with equal numbers of participants or after an equal number of events have occurred between analyses. In a multicenter trial, monitoring committees may not be able to meet at prespecified intervals, making this method less useful for multicenter trials. Another method known as a *flexible group sequential procedure* does not require an equal number of participants or events to have occurred between analyses or a prespecified number of analyses.[67] Comparisons of life-table analysis curves, means, proportions, and linear regression slopes, as well as linear and nonlinear random effects models for continuous data and repeated measure methods for discrete data; can be monitored using the group sequential approach.[68–72] Computer programs are available for statistical calculations using these various procedures.[73] *Confidence intervals* also can be used to monitor data using the group sequential approach.[74] Before deciding to terminate a trial early, several factors must be evaluated, including the distribution of prognostic factors, data quality of all intervention groups, consistency of results across subgroups, presence of concomitant therapy, and whether or not randomization errors have occurred. A trial should not be terminated without definitively resolving whether or not the intervention effects are harmful. Otherwise, an intervention may continue to be used in practice even though its harmful effects were deemed significant enough to terminate a clinical trial.

Closing Out the Study

The closeout of a clinical trial begins with the last follow-up visit of the first participant randomized and ends with the archiving of study material. During the closeout phase of the trial, every effort is made to ensure that the final data regarding the outcome variables are as complete as possible. This process involves both verification of incomplete data and assessment of missing data when possible. All efforts should focus on obtaining data with regard to the primary outcome(s) of interest. To minimize the delay in the final data analysis, a reasonable time is allotted for data cleanup before the data are locked. Most clinical trials close out participants after a defined period of follow-up per participant. Other trials follow all participants to a preselected month or year, during which the closeout process is completed in all participants. Depending on the size of the study and the closeout interval, the latter method may not be feasible. After the data are finalized, they should be stored in an easily re-

trievable form. The investigator may have to choose if all biologic specimens and seemingly less important data not related directly to the outcomes of interest should be stored. Archiving of data will allow investigators and other interested groups to audit the results of the trial and may be important for future metaanalyses.

Several additional points are important to consider at the conclusion of a clinical trial. First, when should the participants be told which intervention they received? Second, how does the investigator advise the participant regarding future therapy? Third, should a participant wish to continue therapy, how will treatment and follow-up be performed? Fourth, how will the results of the study be disseminated to referring physicians and other health care providers? And finally, is a poststudy follow-up warranted for ascertainment of additional data?

The investigator has several obligations during the closeout phase of the study. One of these obligations is to inform each participant which intervention he or she received. As soon as all the data from an individual have been collected, the participant can be unmasked. In some studies, to determine if the study was truly masked, participants and study coordinators may be asked, before being unmasked, if they can guess which intervention they had received. Participants should be advised regarding future therapy at closeout. This may be difficult because the final results of the study may not be known for many months or longer. In any case, the participant needs to be referred to a local physician for continued medical care. Both participants and referring physicians may have to be contacted at a later date when the results of the study are known. It is best if participants and referring physicians can be informed of the study results before the data are made public.[75] The NIH has issued guidelines for informing the public and physicians regarding the benefit or harm of therapies of significant importance to public health.[76] In the case of a trial that is investigating a new drug or device, specific regulatory agencies may need to be informed of the study conclusions.

Because the actions and mechanisms of action of a new therapy are rarely understood, and because the beneficial or adverse effects of an intervention may last long after the intervention has been discontinued, some investigators have designed follow-up visits to evaluate poststudy events. The optimal interval of the *poststudy follow-up* depends on the intervention under investigation and the outcomes of interest. In a trial involving hormone-replacement therapy, if a positive cardiovascular effect was obtained, an investigator may want to determine if the cardiovascular benefit continues for a period of 5 or 10 years after therapy has been discontinued. In the same trial, women with vaginal bleeding or other adverse events could be followed to determine how long these events persist or if other adverse events, such as breast disease, occur 1 or 2 years after discontinuation of therapy. Poststudy follow-up has been used to determine whether participants changed their lifestyles based on results from a clinical trial or if participants comply with the therapeutic recommendations given to them by the study coordinator or investigator.[77,78] Clearly, it may be very difficult to maintain contact with participants over an extended period, making poststudy follow-up complex and expensive.

▶ ANALYSIS OF THE DATA

Analysis and interpretation of data collected during a clinical trial are affected by decisions made during development of the protocol, the performance and modification of the protocol during the trial, the compliance of study participants, and the quality of the data.[79] In addition to the outcomes of interest, several other parameters must be evaluated. Included are the admission eligibility, evaluation for randomization, participant compliance, and placebo response. Follow-up of control groups allows investigators to learn about the natural history of a disease. Just as the hypotheses to be tested are stated a priori, so too are the statistical tests that will be used to evaluate these hypotheses. Otherwise, numerous statistical tests may be performed on the data, increasing the probability of a type I error and potentially allowing a false conclusion that a difference in outcomes exists. Stated another way, data analysis should be used for formal hypothesis testing and not as a method to determine how one can manipulate the data so that a significant difference can be found.[80]

Who Should Be Included?

The first question to be answered in the data analysis is which participants and which events will be included in the analyses. An investigator may want to exclude participants who dropped out of the study, were noncompliant with their intervention, took competing interventions, or had incomplete data. A policy regarding withdrawal of participants should be stated in the study protocol before initiation of the study. Any withdrawals should be done early in the study, preferably before any outcomes have occurred. Participants should never be excluded from analysis based on their outcome status because this will tend to bias the study.[81] In general, an *intention-to-treat analysis* is recommended for all clinical trials. In other words, all participants who were randomized to an intervention should be included in the initial analysis. The reason for adopting this strategy is that the reason a participant may have dropped out of a study or been noncompliant with therapy may be related to the adverse effects or complexity of the intervention. This type of analysis will give the investigator a better understanding of the impact an intervention will have on the population—its effectiveness. Likewise, all events should be included in the initial analysis. One might argue that including noncompliant participants in the analysis will not allow the investigator to evaluate the true efficacy of an intervention. For this reason, it is also recommended that the data be analyzed without including participants who were determined to be noncompliant based on a pretrial definition of noncompliance.

No matter how good an effort is made to have participants come in for all follow-up visits, subjects may be lost to follow-up, yielding missing data. The participants lost to follow-up in one group may be very different in terms of their prognosis or susceptibility to therapy compared with the subjects lost to follow-up in the comparison group. Life-table analysis, which assumes that losses to follow-up are random, can be used to assess differences in dichotomous response variables, such as pregnant or not pregnant, in situations in which the length of follow-up is variable.[82–84] Many methods for imputation of missing values have been described. Included is the method of *end-point analysis,* or carrying the last observation forward.[85] Others use the derivation of a regression equation employed for the basis of the input of missing data.[86] One potential problem with these methods of imputation of missing data is that each model assumes that the reason for missing data is simply a random event.[87] In any case, if more than one method is used to assess outcomes in cases of missing data, the results of all analyses should be presented.

Stratification and Subgroup Analysis

Even if randomization is used in a trial, all the baseline prognostic factors may not be perfectly balanced. If this is the case, and if the baseline variables are highly correlated with outcome, the analysis may require that the data be adjusted for this imbalance. If stratification was used in the randomization, the analysis should be stratified. The type of adjustment used depends on the type of baseline variable being adjusted and the type of outcome variables being analyzed. If the baseline variables are not discrete, these variables can be redefined into strata and made discrete. If the outcome variable is discrete, then a Mantel-Haenszel statistic can be used.[88] If the outcome variable is continuous and there is a

linear relationship between the two variables, then the stratified analysis is called an *analysis of covariance.*[89,90]

If the overall comparison between the intervention and the outcome(s) is significant for beneficial or harmful effects, then the investigator may want to determine which subgroup of participants is most susceptible to therapy.[91] Subgroup analysis is only appropriate if the subgroups were specified in the study protocol.[92] Only baseline variables are used to define subgroups; outcome variables should never be used to define subgroups. In a subgroup analysis, the investigator is only concerned about intervention and control comparisons within one or more subgroups. Because of reductions in sample size per group, the probability of finding a significant difference is reduced. Post hoc analysis of subgroups that are not predefined but are suggested by the data has less credibility. This type of retrospective subgroup analysis should be used to generate new hypotheses for future study.

▶ BIOSTATISTICAL METHODS

Biostatistics concerns the application of the discipline of statistics to problems of biology, including human biology, medicine, and public health. Statistics is a branch of applied mathematics with roots in a part of mathematics called *probability theory.* More specifically, *statistics* is the study of methods and procedures for collecting, classifying, summarizing, and analyzing data and for making scientific inferences from such data. The decision as to which statistical test to use to assess differences between two or more groups of participants depends on several factors. First, the type of variable being evaluated must be categorized. Variables are either discrete (i.e., categorical) or continuous. *Discrete variables* are intrinsically "gappy," in the sense that between two potentially attainable values lies at least one unattainable value. The simplest example in reproductive endocrinology is in counting the number of pregnancies after a given therapy. One can have one, two, three, or more pregnancies but 2.5 pregnancies is impossible. On the other hand, if a variable potentially can take any value within a range, it is called a *continuous variable*. Examples of continuous variables include mean serum blood levels, height, and temperature. In addition to defining the type of variable under investigation, several assumptions must be accepted before the appropriate statistical test is selected. Certain assumptions involve how the data were collected, whereas other assumptions involve the distribution of the data. Appropriate questions about a set of data would include: Are the treatment groups a random sample of the population? Are the study groups independent? Were the interventions randomly assigned? Are the variances of the study groups equal? and Are the distributions of the variable of interest normal? If these assumptions are not considered, the wrong statistical test may be applied. Tests are available to evaluate most of these assumptions. Furthermore, data can be transformed so that one might work with a variable's logarithm instead of its original value.

In general terms, statistical tests can be categorized into parametric and nonparametric tests. *Parametric tests* are used when the distribution of the data is known or can be assumed to be normal. *Nonparametric tests* are distribution-free methods of hypothesis testing. Nonparametric tests are much easier to calculate but are often less sensitive and lack statistical power as compared with parametric tests. In general, when the appropriate assumptions are met, if the variables being evaluated are both discrete, a chi-square test should be performed. If one variable is discrete and one is continuous, either a Student's *t* test or analysis of variance is appropriate. If both variables are continuous, either a correlation or regression analysis is appropriate. An annotated list follows of some of the most commonly used statistical tests in reproductive endocrinology.

Statistical Tests

The methods used to calculate the statistics that describe the utility of a test designed to screen for a particular disease are detailed in Table 25-8. The *chi-square* (χ^2) *test* is used to evaluate associations between two variables. It is particularly useful for noncontinuous covariates such as proportions. A χ^2 test is not appropriate if any expected frequency is less than 1 or if over 20 percent of the expected frequencies are less than 5. The χ^2 test is not normally distributed and therefore is a nonparametric test. The exact distribution of χ^2 depends on the number of degrees of freedom.

The *Fisher's exact test* is one form of "correction" of the χ^2 test and can be used with small sample sizes when expected frequencies are less than 1. Another example of a correction of the χ^2 test is *Yates-corrected χ^2 statistic*.

The *Mantel-Haenszel statistic* has a χ^2 distribution with one degree of freedom.[93] This test is used for covariates that are noncontinuous or for continuous covariates that have been classified into intervals, such as age. Any value for the Mantel-Haenszel statistic >3.84 is significant at the 0.05 level.

The *Student's t test*, discovered by W. S. Gosset, is used to evaluate group mean differences in continuous variables (e.g., the differences in mean androgen levels before and after treatment with an oral contraceptive). As described earlier, this design has the advantage of controlling for many extraneous sources of variation in the data. The *t* distribution is normal.

Both the *Wilcoxon signed-rank test* and the *Spearman's rank correlation* are examples of nonparametric tests. The Wilcoxon signed-rank test is used to compare mean differences for paired data, whereas the Spearman's test is used when the assumptions for a parametric test cannot be met but one wishes to investigate the correlation between two random variables.

An *analysis of variance* (ANOVA) is used when one is comparing differences between three or more means. If a difference is found between the means, the investigator can then

▶ **TABLE 25-8:** PREVALENCE, SENSITIVITY, SPECIFICITY AND PREDICTIVE VALUE

	With Disease	Without Disease	Total
Screened positive	a	b	a + b
Screened negative	c	d	c + d
Total	a + c	b + d	n
Prevalence rate	$\dfrac{a + c}{n}$		
Sensitivity	$\dfrac{a}{a + c}$		
Specificity	$\dfrac{d}{b + d}$		
False-positive rate	$\dfrac{b}{b + d}$		
False-negative rate	$\dfrac{c}{a + c}$		
Positive predictive value	$\dfrac{a}{a + b}$		

make comparisons between specific pairs or combinations of groups. *Multivariate analysis of variance* (MANOVA) is used when both multiple dependent variables and multiple independent variables are being evaluated. Conceptually, MANOVA is an extension of ANOVA.

Receiver operating curves (ROC) are used to assess differences between screening tests. The sensitivity of a test is plotted on the x axis against 1 minus specificity on the y axis. Receiver operating curves are advantageous because they do not require the investigator to split continuous variables into two categories, e.g., by an arbitrary cut point, which otherwise must be done to assess sensitivity and specificity. The area under the curve or the equation of the lines can be used to assess differences between two ROC curves.

Life-table analysis is used in trials in which participants are entered into intervention over an extended period of time and followed after therapy for various lengths of time. This type of analysis could be used to evaluate pregnancy rates after myomectomy or metroplasty in infertile women as compared with pregnancy rates in participants who do not undergo surgical intervention. In this situation, participants may have varying intervals between surgery and pregnancy and may be lost to follow-up at various lengths of time. With life-table analysis, every month of follow-up can be used to calculate a cumulative pregnancy rate. Life-table analysis curves are generated for each intervention, and comparisons can be made between two survival curves to determine if the pregnancy rates are significantly different. There are both parametric and nonparametric tests available to assess the significance of differences between life-table analysis curves. Regression models for the analysis of life-table data that allow for the variation of covariates over time are also available.[94]

Metaanalysis

When data from several clinical trials performed at different research centers, often over a period of several years, are pooled and analyzed together to answer one or more preselected questions, the overview is known as a *metaanalysis*.[95,96] Metaanalyses are performed to obtain sufficient power to detect small yet clinically significant and generalizable intervention effects.[97] Ideally, a metaanalysis should only be performed on randomized clinical trials that study the same type of participant, use precisely the same intervention, measure the same outcome variables, have similar lengths of follow-up, and have similar quality of data. One problem with metaanalyses is that some of the data regarding the question to be answered may not be available. A MEDLINE search may find only 30 to 60 percent of published trials.[98] Furthermore, trials that demonstrated a negative effect may not be available because of publication bias.[99] The results of a metaanalysis are usually summarized by calculating a *relative risk* or *odds ratio* with a *95 percent confidence interval*. Both the relative risk and odds ratios are a product of the intervention success rate divided by the control success rate. A relative risk is calculated from prospective data and is a better estimate of the true risk than an odds ratio, which is inherently retrospective. The method used for calculation of the relative risk depends on whether or not the effects of therapy are similar (homogeneous) among trials or heterogeneous. If the effects are homogeneous, then a *Mantel-Haenszel method* is appropriate; if the effects are found to be heterogeneous, a *random-effects model* is used.[100] Table 25-9 compares three predictors of risk in clinical studies.

►**TABLE 25-9:** PREDICTORS OF RISK

Type	Study Design	Censored Observation
Odds ratio	Case-Control	No
Hazards ratio	Clinical trial or cohort study	Yes
Relative risk	Clinical trial or cohort study	No

*Study participants may not have experienced the outcome of interest for the period of time they are evaluated because of a short length of follow-up.

Often data are combined from several observational studies and are reported as a metaanalysis. Such combined analyses suffer from the lack of reliability that flows from aggregating data across studies with widely varying entry criteria, methods of intervention, definitions of outcome variables, and methods of data management and analysis.

► PRESENTATION AND PUBLICATION

A policy for presentation and publication of the data from the clinical trial should be agreed on before initiation of the trial. This may seem trivial and premature, but it can be extremely beneficial in the long run to clarify responsibilities and expectations. Each investigator has an obligation to critically review his or her study and its findings and to present sufficient information so that readers can properly evaluate the trial. Ideally, the manuscript should be completely prepared before the data are presented in a scientific setting to decrease the delay between the presentation and publication of the data.[101] In any presentation or publication, the hypotheses should be clearly stated, a clear but brief description of the randomization procedure should be included,[102] the selection of the study population should be clearly defined, and the methods used to assess the outcome variables should be described. All presentations and publications should state how the sample size was determined (e.g., a sample size of 200 was required to detect a 25 percent relative increase in pregnancy rates after intervention, with a two-sided significance level of 5 percent and a power of 90 percent). The method(s) of analysis should be stated and the results of all analyses should be reported. Finally, the investigator should report all major outcome categories, such as total mortality, cause-specific mortality, and morbid events. This information will help other investigators to assess the appropriateness of the methods and conclusions of the study.

► ETHICS OF CLINICAL TRIALS

Questions regarding the participant's best interest surround most clinical trials. Ethical issues regarding clinical trials commonly center around the process of randomizing participants to interventions[103,104] and whether investigators are fully truthful when seeking informed consent. All investigators would agree that patients should receive the best therapy available and that it is unethical to treat a patient with a therapy that is known to be inferior. Presumably, the reason a clinical trial is being conducted is because there is uncertainty about which therapy is best with regard to health benefits, adverse effects, and costs. Investigators should only recruit participants for a clinical trial if they believe that there is insufficient evidence to suggest that the intervention should be favored over a control. One could argue that clinical trials are a much more ethical method of approach to clinical problems than routinely prescribing medications or performing procedures that have never been proven to be beneficial and that might be harmful.

► CONCLUSIONS

Designing and completing a clinical trial are challenging undertakings. However, when performed appropriately, clinical trials allow one to compare the outcome in a treatment group with the outcome in a control group that is comparable with the treatment group in every way except for the treatment being studied. Clinical trials also can assist in determining the incidence of adverse events, cost implications of an intervention, and if the benefits of therapy outweigh the risks. The influence of the results of a clinical trial depends on the direction of the findings, the means used to disseminate the results, and any confirmatory evidence regarding the efficacy of the therapy in question. While well-designed clinical trials can provide sound rationale for the use of a given intervention, clinical trials that are poorly designed or executed can yield misleading data.

Well-run clinical trials with sufficient statistical power are costly and should be performed only after a given treatment has evolved completely and after preliminary data regarding efficacy look promising. On the other hand, the consequences of delaying clinical trials can have a serious impact on health care because new procedures of unproven clinical benefit are allowed to become part of general medical practice.

Clinical trials do have limitations. Occasionally, the prevalence of a disease is so rare that a large enough population cannot be readily obtained, making a case-control study, not a clinical trial, the most appropriate method of evaluating the disease. Although a randomized trial could be developed to determine if cessation of an allegedly noxious agent, such as cigarette smoke, would prevent disease, one cannot ethically assign participants to begin using noxious agents. In the final analysis, no single study is definitive. Instead, each trial should be interpreted in regard to its consistency with known biologic and epidemiologic information.

KEY POINTS

1. In a retrospective study, information regarding the exposure or outcome status is known at the initiation of the study, and the investigator must go back to determine the unknown variable(s). Interventional studies have the advantage of investigator-directed assignment of treatment or exposure. The gold standard of the interventional study is the randomized clinical trial. The prediction of causation from a retrospective study is less reliable as compared with the prediction of causation from a prospective study.

2. A randomized clinical trial is a prospective comparative study between an intervention group and a control group that uses a method of assignment of participants such that all participants are equally likely to be

assigned to either the intervention group or the control group. Randomized clinical trials are used to evaluate the efficacy, efficiency, and effectiveness of clinical therapies.

3. During development of the hypothesis, the investigator takes the first step in selecting a study population, which is to identify a group of patients with an important therapeutic need. The subjects who actually will be included in the clinical trial are further defined by a set of eligibility and exclusion criteria that constitute the admission criteria. One cannot claim that a therapy is or is not effective unless one can clearly define the population in which the intervention was tested.

4. The choice of the comparative treatment group in a clinical trial depends on whether the comparison is intended to show the treatment's efficacy, efficiency, or effectiveness.

5. The three advantages of a randomized treatment allocation scheme are the creation of comparable study groups, the removal of allocation bias, and the validation of statistical analysis of the data generated from the trial.

6. Any event or outcome that occurs after the initiation of a clinical trial can be categorized as desirable, undesirable, or neutral. Adverse experiences or events are the undesirable signs, symptoms, and clinical events that occur during the clinical trial. Unlike the events that define the primary and secondary outcome variables, adverse experiences are not always well defined or anticipated.

7. When making decisions regarding data analysis, the investigator must decide if he or she is interested in therapeutic differences that are in one direction only—a one-sided test—or if differences in either direction are important—a two-sided test. In general, a two-sided test is recommended unless it is clear that the only changes to be expected are in one direction.

8. Because of the expense of surgical procedures and new surgical instruments, cost is commonly one of the primary outcomes of interest in a surgical procedure trial. Besides costs, another outcome of particular interest in surgical trials is patient satisfaction and the effects of a surgical procedure on the patient's quality of life.

9. A common mistake in the planning of a clinical trial is the underestimation of the time and effort needed to recruit study participants. The investigator must ensure that an adequate amount of time, funds, and energy will be appropriated to the recruitment of study participants.

10. A policy regarding withdrawal of participants should be clearly stated in the protocol before initiation of the study. Any withdrawals should be done early in the study, preferably before any outcomes have occurred. Participants should never be excluded from analysis based on their outcome status because this will tend to bias the study.

11. A policy for presentation and publication of the results of a clinical trial should be agreed on before initiation of the study. This may seem premature, but it can be extremely beneficial in the long run to clarify responsibilities and expectations.

REFERENCES

1. Hulley S, Grady D, Bush T, et al. Randomized trial of estrogen plus progestin for secondary prevention of coronary heart disease in postmenopausal women. *JAMA* 1998;280:605.

2. Writing Group for the Women's Health Initiative Investigators. Risks and benefits of estro-

gen plus progestin in healthy postmenopausal women: principal results from the Women's Health Initiative randomized, controlled trial. *JAMA* 2002;288:321.

3. Lilienfeld AM. Ceteris paribus: The evolution of the clinical trial. *Bull Hist Med* 1982;56:1.

4. Box JF. RA Fisher and the design of experiments, 1922–1926. *Am Stat* 1980;34:1.

5. Amberson JB Jr, McMahon BT, Pinner M. A clinical trial of sanocrysin in pulmonary tuberculosis. *Am Rev Tuberc* 1931;24:401.

6. Diehl HS, Baker AB, Cowan DW. Cold vaccines: An evaluation based on a controlled study. *JAMA* 1938;111:1168.

7. Hill AB. Observation and experiment. *N Engl J Med* 1953;248:995.

8. McBride WG. Thalidomide and congenital abnormalities (letter). *Lancet* 1962;2:1358.

9. NIH Revitalization Act of 1993, Public Law 103-43.

10. Committee on the Ethical Issues Relating to the Inclusion of Women in Clinical Studies, Institute of Medicine, Mastroianni AC, Faden R, Federman D, eds. *Women and Health Research: Ethical and Legal Issues of Including Women in Clinical Studies*. Washington: National Academy Press, 1994.

11. Wilhelmsen L, Ljungberg S, Wedel H, et al. A comparison between participants and nonparticipants in a primary preventive trial. *J Chron Dis* 1976;29:331.

12. Smith P, Arnesen H. Mortality in nonconsenters in a postmyocardial infarction trial. *J Intern Med* 1990;228:253.

13. Cochrane AL. *Effectiveness and Efficiency: Random Reflections on Health Services*. London: Nuffield Provincial Hospitals Trust, 1972.

14. Bok S. The ethics of giving placebos. *Sci Am* 1974;231:17.

15. Rothman KJ, Michels KB. The continuing unethical use of placebo controls. *N Engl J Med* 1994;331:394.

16. Sapirstein W, Alpert S, Callahan TJ. The role of clinical trials in the Food and Drug Administration approval process for cardiovascular devices. *Circulation* 1994;89:1900.

17. Byar DP, Simon RM, Friedewald WT, et al. Randomized clinical trials: Perspectives on some recent ideas. *N Engl J Med* 1976;295:74.

18. Lachin JM. Statistical properties of randomization in clinical trials. *Control Clin Trials* 1988;9:289.

19. Armitage P. The role of randomization in clinical trials. *Stat Med* 1982;1:345.

20. Brittain E, Schlesselman JJ. Optimal allocation for the comparison of proportions. *Biometrics* 1982;38:1003.

21. Kalish LA, Begg CB. Treatment allocation methods in clinical trials: A review. *Stat Med* 1985; 4:129.

22. Lachin JM. Properties of simple randomization in clinical trials. *Control Clin Trials* 1988;9: 312.

23. Zelen M. The randomization and stratification of patients to clinical trials. *J Chron Dis.* 27:365, 1974

24. Matts JP, Lachin JM. Properties of permutated-blocked randomization in clinical trials. *Control Clin Trials* 1988;9:327.

25. Carriere KC. Crossover designs for clinical trials. *Stat Med* 1994;3:1063.

26. Grizzle JE. The two period change-over design and its use in clinical trials. *Biometrics* 1986; 21:467.

27. Moscucci M, Byrne L, Weintraub M, et al. Blinding, unblinding, and the placebo effect: An analysis of patients' guesses of treatment assignment in a double-blind clinical trial. *Clin Pharmacol Ther* 1987;41:256.

28. Farr BM, Gwaltney JM Jr. The problems of taste in placebo matching: An evaluation of zinc gluconate for the common cold. *J Chron Dis* 19897; 40:875.

29. Avery CW, Ibelle BP, Allison B, et al. Systematic errors in the evaluation of side effects. *Am J Psychiatry* 1967;123:875.

30. Huskisson EC, Wojtulewski JA. Measurement of side effects of drugs. *Br Med J* 1974;2:698.

31. Simpson RJ, Tiplady B, Skegg DCG. Event recording in a clinical trial of a new medicine. *Br Med J* 1988;280:1133.

32. Lachin JM. Introduction to sample size determination and power analysis for clinical trials. *Control Clin Trials* 1981;2:93.

33. Donner A. Approaches to sample size estimation in the design of clinical trials: A review. *Stat Med* 1984;3:199.

34. Kraemer HC, Thiemann S. *How Many Subjects? Statistical Power Analysis in Research*. Newburgh Park, CA: Sage Publications, 1987.

35. Brittain E, Schlesselman JJ. Optimal allocation for the comparison of proportions. *Biometrics* 1982;38:1003.

36. Storer BE. Design and analysis of phase I clinical trials. *Biometrics* 1989;45:925.

37. Chang MN, Therneau TM, Wieand HS, et al. Designs for group sequential phase II clinical trials. *Biometrics* 1987;43:865.

38. Sculpher MJ, Dwyer N, Byford S, et al. Randomized trial comparing hysterectomy and transcervical endometrial resection: Effects on health related quality of life and costs two years after surgery. *Br J Obstet Gynecol* 1996;103:142.

39. Berzon R, Hays RD, Shumaker SA. International use, application and performance of health-related quality of life instruments. *Qual Life Res* 1993;2:367.

40. Miller JN, Colditz GA, Mosteller F. How study design affects outcomes in comparison of therapy: II. Surgical. *Stat Med* 1989;8:455.

41. Meinert CL. *Clinical Trials: Design, Conduct and Analysis*. New York: Oxford University Press, 1986.

42. Friedman L, DeMets DL. The data monitoring committee: How it operates and why. *IRB* 1981;3:6.

43. Fleming TR, DeMets DL. Monitoring of clinical trials: Issues and recommendations. *Control Clin Trials* 1993;14:183.

44. Cohen J. Clinical trial monitoring: Hit or miss? *Science* 1994;264:1534.

45. Hunninghake DB. Summary conclusions. *Control Clin Trials* 1987;8:1S.

46. Tognoni G, Alli C, Avanzini F, et al. Randomised clinical trials in general practice: Lessons from a failure. *Br Med J* 1991;303:969.

47. Peto V, Coulter A, Bond A. Factors affecting general practitioners' recruitment of patients into a prospective study. *Fam Pract* 1993; 10:207.

48. Tilley BC, Shorek MA. Designing clinical trials of treatment for osteoporosis: Recruitment and follow-up. *Calcif Tissue Int* 1990;47:327.

49. Freedman LS, Simon R, Foulkes MA, et al. Inclusion of women and minorities in clinical trials and the NIH Revitalization Act of 1993: The perspective of NIH clinical trial lists. *Control Clin Trials* 1995;16:277.

50. James KE. Regression toward the mean in uncontrolled clinical studies. *Biometrics* 1973;29:121.

51. Davis CE. Prerandomization compliance screening: A statistician's view, in Shumaker SA, Schron EB, Ockene JK (eds), *Health Behavior Changes*. New York: Springer, 1990.

52. Sackett DL, Snow JC. The magnitude of compliance and noncompliance, in Hayes RB, Taylor DW, Sackett DL (eds), *Compliance in Health Care*. Baltimore: Johns Hopkins University Press, 1979.

53. Pullar T, Kumar S, Feely M. Compliance in clinical trials. *Ann Rheum Dis* 1989;48:871.

54. Shulman N, Cutter G, Daugherty R, et al. Correlates of attendance and compliance in the Hypertension Detection and Follow-up Program. *Control Clin Trials* 1982;3:13.

55. Green LW. Educational strategies to improve compliance with therapeutic and preventive regimens: The recent evidence, in Haynes RB, Taylor OW, Sackett DL (eds), *Compliance in Health Care*. Baltimore: Johns Hopkins University Press, 1979.

56. Dunbar J. Predictors of patient adherence: Patient characteristics, in Schumaker SA, Schron EB, Ockene JK (eds), *Health Behavior Changes*. New York: Springer, 1990.

57. Moulding TS. The unrealized potential of the medication monitor. *Clin Pharmacol Ther* 1979;25:131.

58. Knatterud GL, Forman SA, Canner PL. Design of data forms. *Control Clin Trials* 1983;4:429.

59. Wright P, Haybittle J. Design of forms for clinical trials. *Br Med J* 1979;2:529.

60. Fleming T, DeMets DL. Monitoring of clinical trials: Issues and recommendations. *Control Clin Trials* 1993;14:183.

61. Fleming TR. Data monitoring committees and capturing relevant information of high quality. *Stat Med* 1993;12:565.

62. Walters L. Data monitoring committees: The moral case for maximum feasible independence. *Stat Med* 1993;12:575.

63. Li Z, Geller NL. On the choice of times for data analysis in group sequential trials. *Biometrics* 1991;47:745.

64. Armitage P, McPherson CK, Rowe BC. Repeated significance tests on accumulating data. *J R Stat Soc* 1969;132A:235.

65. Popock SJ. Interim analyses for randomized clinical trials: The group sequential approach. *Biometrics* 1982;38:153.

66. O'Brien PC, Fleming TR. A multiple testing procedure for clinical trials. *Biometrics* 1979;35:549.

67. DeMets DL, Lan KKG. Interim analyses: The alpha spending function approach. *Stat Med* 1994;13:1341.

68. Lan KKG, Lachin J. Implementation of group sequential log rank tests in a maximum duration trial. *Biometrics* 1990;46:759.

69. Kim K, DeMets DL. Sample size determination for group sequential clinical trials with immediate response. *Stat Med* 1992;11:1391.

70. Lee JW. Group sequential testing in clinical trials with multivariate observations: A review. *Stat Med* 1994;13:101.

71. Su JQ, Lachin JU. Group sequential distribution-free methods for the analysis of multivariate observations. *Biometrics* 1992;48:1033.

72. Gange SJ, DeMets DL. Sequential monitoring of clinical trials with correlated categorical responses. University of Wisconsin Department of Biostatistics, Madison, technical report no. 86, July 1994.

73. Reboussin DM, DeMets DL, Kim K, et al. Programs for computing group sequential bounds using the Lan-Demets method. University of Wisconsin Department of Biostatistics, Madison, technical report no. 60, June 1992.

74. Tsiatis AA, Rosnar GL, Mehta CR. Exact confidence intervals following a group sequential test. *Biometrics* 1984;40:797.

75. Klimt CR, Canner PL. Terminating a long-term clinical trial. *Clin Pharmacol Ther* 1979;25:641.

76. Healy B. From the National Institutes of Health. *JAMA* 1993;269:3069.

77. Cutler JA, Grandits GA, Grimm RH, et al. Risk factor changes after cessation of intervention in the Multiple Risk Factor Intervention Trial. *Prev Med* 1991;20:183.

78. Hypertension Detection and Follow-up Program Cooperative Group. Persistence of reduction in blood pressure and mortality of participants in the Hypertension Detection and Follow-up Program. *JAMA* 1988;259:2113.

79. Sackett DL, Gent M. Controversy in counting and attributing of ends in clinical trials. *N Engl J Med* 1979;301:1410.

80. Byars DB. Assessing apparent treatment: Covariant interactions in randomized clinical trials. *Stat Med* 1985;4:255.

81. May GS, DeMets DL, Friedman LM, et al. The randomized clinical trial: Bias in analysis. *Circulation* 1981;64:669.

82. Crowly J, Breslow N. Statistical analysis of survival data. *Annu Rev Public Health* 1984;5:385.

83. Cox DR, Oakes D. *The Analysis of Survival Data*. New York: Chapman & Hall, 1984.

84. Fleming T, Harrington D. *Counting Processes and Survival Analysis*. New York: Wiley, 1991.

85. Pledger GW. Basic statistics: Importance of adherence. *J Clin Res Pharmacoepidemiol* 1992; 6:77.

86. Espeland MA, Byington RP, Hire D, et al. Analysis strategies for serial multivariate ultrasonographic data that are incomplete. *Stat Med* 1992;11:1041.

87. Laird NM. Missing data in longitudinal studies. *Stat Med* 1988;7:305.

88. Bishop YM, Fienberg SE, Holland PW. *Discrete Multivariate Analysis: Theory and Practice*. Cambridge, MA: MIT Press, 1975.

89. Egger MJ, Coleman ML, Ward JR, et al. Uses and abuses of analysis of covariance in clinical trials. *Control Clin Trials* 1985;6:12.

90. Thall PF, Lachin JM. Assessment of stratum-covariate interaction in Cox's proportional hazards regression model. *Stat Med* 1986;5:73.

91. Simon R. Patient subsets and variation in therapeutic efficacy. *Br J Clin Pharmacol* 1982;14: 473.

92. Ingelfinger JA, Mosteller F, Thibodeau LA, et al. *Biostatistics in Clinical Medicine*. New York, Macmillan, 1983.

93. Mantel N, Haenszel W. Statistical aspects of the analysis of data from retrospective studies of disease. *J Natl Cancer Inst* 1959;22:719.

94. Cox DR. Regression models and lifetables. *J R Stat Soc* 1972;34B:187.

95. Meinert CL. Meta-analysis: Science or religion? *Control Clin Trials* 1989;10:257S.

96. Sacks HS, Berrier J, Reitman D, et al. Meta-analyses of randomized, controlled trials. *N Engl J Med* 1987;316:450.

97. Peto R. Why do we need systematic overviews of randomized trials? *Stat Med* 1987;6:233.

98. Chalmers TC, Frank CS, Reitman D. Minimizing the three stages of publication bias. *JAMA* 1990;263:1392.

99. Berlin JA, Begg CB, Louis TA. An assessment of publication bias using a sample of published clinical trials. *J Am Stat Assoc* 1989;84:381.

100. DerSimonian R, Laird N. Meta-analysis in clinical trials. *Control Clin Trials* 1986;7:177.

101. Editorial. Reporting clinical trials: Message and medium. *Lancet* 1994;344:347.

102. Williams OS, Davis CE. Reporting of assignment methods in clinical trials. *Control Clin Trials* 1994;15:294.

103. Byar DP, Simon RM, Friedewald WT, et al. Randomized clinical trials: Perspectives on some recent ideas. *N Engl J Med* 1976;295:74.

104. Levine RJ, Lebacqz K. Some ethical considerations in clinical trials. *Clin Pharmacol Ther* 1979;25:728.

APPENDIX 25A

Glossary of Terms

Association When two variables are associated with each other, certain values of one variable tend to occur more often with certain values of the second variable. Two variables are positively associated when larger values of one tend to be accompanied by larger values of the other. Association may be due to causation, common response, or confounding.

Attributable risk The increase or decrease in the actual number of cases in a population that is attributed to a given risk factor. For example, if the baseline risk of a given disease is 1 percent and the relative risk is 1.3, the new absolute risk is 1.3 percent, and the attributable risk of the exposure is 0.3 percent.

Bias A type of error associated with collection of the data that is a consistent, repeated divergence of the sample statistic from the population parameter in the same direction.

Confounding variable The effects of two independent variables on a dependent variable are said to be confounded when they cannot be distinguished from one another.

Continuous variable A variable that potentially can take any value within a range. Examples are body temperature, blood pressure, and serum estradiol level.

Dependent variable A variable whose changes one wishes to study; a response variable.

Discrete variable A variable that is intrinsically gappy, in the sense that between any two potentially attainable values is at least one unattainable value. Counts take values of 1, 2, 3, ... A count of 2.5 is not possible. The opposite of a discrete variable is a *continuous variable*.

Distribution The sampling distribution of a statistic describes the frequency or relative frequency with which the statistic takes each possible value in repeated sampling. A distribution is symmetric if its two sides are approximately mirror images of each other about a center line.

Incidence The number of individuals newly diagnosed with a disease in a given time period.

Independent variable A variable whose effect on the dependent variable one wishes to study.

Lack of precision Means that in repeated sampling the values of the sample statistic are spread out or scattered (i.e., the results of the sampling is not repeatable).

Mean The arithmetic average, calculated by dividing the sum of observations by the number of observations.

Median The typical value; it is the midpoint of the observations when they are arranged in increasing order.

Mode The most frequent value; it is any value having the highest frequency among the observations.

95 Percent confidence interval An interval of a sample statistic that one can be 95 percent confident contains the population parameter. This does not mean that the probability is 95 percent that the true parameter falls between the limits of the interval. One way to reduce the confidence interval is to increase the sample size.

Parameter A summary descriptive characteristic of a population.

Prevalence The number of individuals in a population with a given disease at a specific point in time.

p Value The level of significance at which the observed value of the test would just be significant.

Quantiles Division points of a set of observations that includes percentiles, tertiles, quartiles, quintiles, and deciles that divide the total frequency of an observation into hundredths, thirds, fourths, fifths, or tenths, respectively. The first quartile is the same as the 25th percentile.

Random sample A subset of units drawn from a population of units in such a way that every unit in the population has the same probability of selection.

Relative risk The relative increase or decrease in the risk of developing a disease or outcome as a result of a given risk factor or exposure. A relative risk of 1.3 means a 30 percent relative increase in the chance of a disease or outcome, and a relative risk of 0.7 means a 30 percent relative decrease in the risk of a disease. Relative risk is the ratio of risk of disease of those who are exposed to the risk factor over those who were not exposed to the same risk factor.

Standard deviation The positive square root of the variance. A standard variation of zero means no spread at all; otherwise, the standard deviation is always positive and increases as the spread of the data increases.

Statistic A summary descriptive characteristic of a sample, used for making inferences about a parameter.

Type I error The error made when one rejects the tested hypothesis when it is true. The probability of a type I error is denoted by α, also called the *level of significance*.

Type II error The error made when one accepts the tested hypothesis when it is false. The probability of a type II error is denoted by β. β is equal to $1 - $ power.

Unit The smallest object or individual that can be investigated.

Variable A characteristic observable on the units, e.g., pregnancy rates. The characteristic is called a *variable* because it can vary. Different women have different pregnancy rates. Characteristics that do not vary are called *constants*.

Variance A measure of the spread or variability of values about the mean. It is the mean of the squares of the deviations of the observations from the mean.

SECTION IV

Contraception

CHAPTER 26

Hormonal Contraception

BRUCE R. CARR

The world population grew rather slowly until the nineteenth century. Since then, there has been a drastic increase from less than 1 billion to approximately 5.5 billion by the year 2000. It has been projected that the world population will be near 10 billion by 2050 and that 90 percent of people will live in developing countries[1] (Fig. 26-1). The implication of these predictions on food supply, energy resources, pollution, and political stability support a strong interest in developing reliable and safe methods of birth control.

The discovery of estrogen and progesterone and their potential contraceptive effects stimulated research on the regulation of fertility in women. The effectiveness and safety of oral contraceptive agents in controlling ovulation and fertility are a result of these efforts. Consequently, most research and application of fertility control techniques continue to be directed toward the control of female fertility, and unfortunately, there is no readily reversible

and effective pharmacologic contraceptive for men. Some believe that this inequity is due to societal prejudice as to which gender should bear the primary responsibility for contraception and that this bias has influenced investigators and granted agencies controlling monies for such research.[2] An alternative explanation is that there was not so much a lag in research in the field of male contraception as there was a large positive stimulus for research directed toward a female contraceptive device. Thus the moral support and financial aid that the birth control advocates Margaret Sanger and Mrs. Stanley McCormack provided for a pioneering investigator of reproduction and endocrinology, Gregory Pincus, may explain to a certain extent the rapid early development of the oral contraceptive for women and the continued present efforts.

The failure during the succeeding decades of the development of better means of fertility control in men probably has several causes.

631

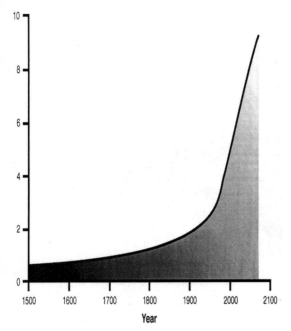

Figure 26-1 Past and future estimated world population. *(Adapted, with permission, from Trussell in Hatcher RA et al.* Contraceptive Technology, 17th ed. *1998; p 745.)*

One is that it has proved to be easier to prevent the production of only one ovum per month in the female than to prevent the production of millions of sperm each day in the male. In addition, the processes of sperm migration from the vagina to the fallopian tubes, the development of the ability of sperm to fertilize an ovum, capacitation, fertilization, and implantation of the fertilized ovum all take place in women. Thus even some measures designed to affect the sperm, such as inhibition of capacitation and implantation, are effective in women but not in men.

This chapter summarizes the present status of hormonal methods of fertility control in women. The methods of fertility control that are used in the United States are compiled in Figure 26-2. A discussion of failure rates of contraception is provided in Chapter 27.[3,4]

▶ ORAL CONTRACEPTIVES

The development of hormonal forms of contraception represents one of the greatest advances of modern gynecology. The concept of pregnancy prevention from administration of hormones originated with the realization that ovulation was inhibited by the presence of the corpus luteum. Ludwig Haberlandt, a professor of physiology in Innsbruck, Austria, demonstrated in 1919 that fertile adult rabbits became sterile after receiving subcutaneous transplants of ovaries from pregnant does.[5] A number of investigators showed that extracts of ovaries, and later progesterone or estrogen, inhibited ovarian function. Progestins were shown to inhibit ovulation; the addition of estrogen was found both to regulate menstrual bleeding and increase contraceptive effectiveness.[5] The first clinical trials of oral contraceptives were described in 1958 by Pincus, Rock, and Garcia, with approval for marketing in the United States obtained in 1960.[6] Within 5 years of their introduction, more than 30 million prescriptions for oral contraceptives were being prescribed annually, making them one of the most common medications in use.

Current Formulations of Hormonal Contraceptives

While both estrogens and progestins affect many different organs, producing a broad range of clinical effects, comparisons of these compounds frequently have been based on isolated hormonal or biochemical effects. However, the clinical effects of these compounds given in combination are markedly different from their effects when they are administered alone. The high steroid doses in early oral contraceptives were chosen because of the effects of the isolated components to prevent pregnancy in laboratory animals, with the synergistic effects of combined estrogen-progestin formulations recognized only some years later.

Percentage of Women Ages 15-50

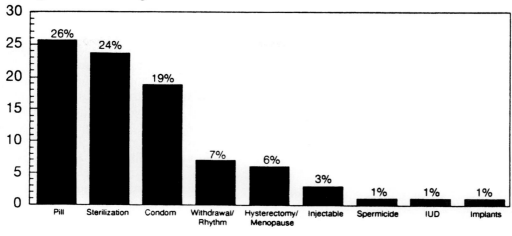

Figure 26-2 Contraceptive use in the United States, 1995 *(Reproduced, with permission, from Ortho Pharmaceuticals, Annual Birth Control Study, 1995.)*

Thus the rational approach to the evaluation of contraceptive steroids relies more on the results of comparative clinical trials than on studies of isolated effects in animals or humans.

The two estrogens in oral contraceptive agents are ethinyl estradiol and mestranol. Eight different synthetic progestagens are used in oral contraceptives in the United States: norethindrone, norethynodrel, norethindrone acetate, ethynodiol diacetate, norgestrel (D,L-norgestrel or D-levonorgestrel), desogestrel, norgestimate, and drospirenone (Fig. 26-3). Additional progestagens (gestodene, lynestrenol, and cyproterone acetate) are used in oral contraceptives marketed in western Europe.

Combined Oral Contraceptives

Orally active contraceptives contain either a combination of estrogen and a progestin or a progestin alone. As discussed previously, two types of estrogen are currently used: ethinyl estradiol and its 3-methyl ether, mestranol. These compounds share an ethinyl group in the 17α position that inhibits hepatic metabolism of the molecule, thus enhancing oral potency. Mestranol does not bind to estrogen receptors and must undergo conversion to ethinyl estradiol to become biologically active. Oral contraceptives containing 50 µg mestranol produce plasma ethinyl estradiol concentrations approximately equivalent to those containing 35 µg ethinyl estradiol.[7] No oral contraceptive containing <50 µg mestranol has been marketed in the United States, whereas the dose of ethinyl estradiol in currently available pills ranges from 20 to 50 µg. In the future, even lower doses will be available.

Removal of the C-19 from testosterone converts the major hormonal effect from androgenic to progestational, with the addition of a 17α ethinyl group producing an orally active compound. Of the eight progestins currently marketed for contraceptive use in the United States, six are 17α ethinyl analogues of 19-nortestosterone (see Fig. 26-3). Concomitant with the hormonal effects associated with progesterone, synthetic progestins exhibit varying degrees of estrogenic and androgenic side

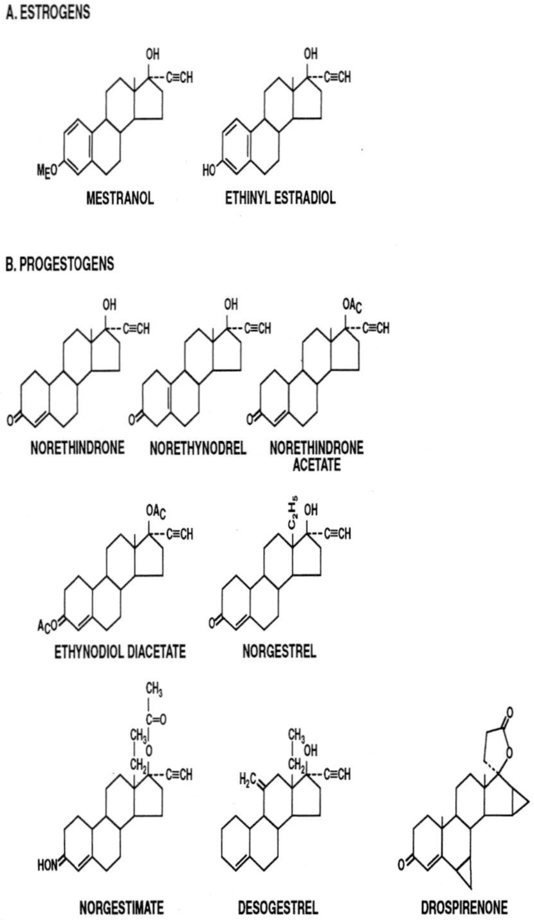

Figure 26-3 Structural formulas of estrogens (A) and progestins (B) in hormonal contraceptive pills approved for use in the United States.

effects. Levonorgestrel, the most potent contraceptive progestin currently available, is the biologically active stereoisomer of norgestrel and is thus about twice as potent as the racemic mixture. Norgestrel generally is considered the most androgenic progestin, whereas norgestimate has been shown to have fewer androgenic side effects than other derivatives of 19-nortestosterone.[8] This effect may be of importance because many of the adverse effects of steroid contraceptives are thought to be mediated by the androgenic actions of progestins. Desogestrel

has clinical profiles similar to those of norgestimate.[9] Drospirenone is similar in structure to spironolactone and has some antimineralocoid activity and is also considered a low androgenic progestin.[10] Ethynodiol diacetate is also considered a low androgenic progestin.

Currently, multiple formulations of combined oral contraceptives are available. Most contain ethinyl estradiol in combination with a progestin. Most oral contraceptives are combined with a constant daily dose of progestin and estrogen given for 21 consecutive days, usually followed by a placebo. Recently, an extended-use contraceptive, Seasonale, has been approved for use in the United States consisting of daily tablets of levonorgestrel 0.15 mg and ethinyl estradiol 30 μg for 84 days followed by 7 days of placebo, reducing the number of withdrawal periods to 4 per year. Other methods include phasic formulations in which the estrogen and progestin dose varies during the cycle, attempting to match the normal menstrual cycle. The advantages of the phasic pills include a slightly lower total progestin dose. The products available today are mostly generic and appear to vary little among the types with respect to efficacy and side effects.

Progestin-Only Contraceptives

Current oral progestin-only formulations available in the United States contain either norethindrone or norgestrel. These drugs have found limited acceptance due to problems with irregular vaginal bleeding and the fact that the efficacy is slightly less than that of combined oral contraceptives. They may be useful for lactating women or for patients intolerant of estrogen.

▶ MECHANISM OF ACTION

Current formulation of hormonal contraceptives rely on the effects of both the progestin and the estrogen, if included. These hormones have both

► **TABLE 26-1:** MECHANISM OF ACTION OF ESTROGEN/PROGESTIN CONTRACEPTIVES

Inhibition of ovulation by suppression of follicle-stimulating hormone (FSH) and luteinizing hormone (LH)
Alteration of cervical mucus to inhibit sperm transport
Interference with ovum transport
Inhibition of implantation by suppression of normal endometrial development

direct and indirect actions on the reproductive tract (Table 26-1). Both estrogen and progestin prevent ovulation by suppression of follicle-stimulating hormone (FSH) and luteinizing hormone (LH) secretion. This occurs through inhibition of hypothalamic gonadotropin-releasing hormone (GnRH) release and possibly through a direct effect on the pituitary.[11] In users of combination estrogen-progestin contraceptives, levels of LH, FSH, progesterone, and estradiol are suppressed.[12] The progestin induces the formation of thick, viscid cervical mucus, which limits the penetrability of sperm. Both estrogen and progestin alter motility of the fallopian tube, but the contraceptive importance of this effect in women is not known.[13] Normal endometrial development is interrupted by estrogen and progestin; this effect may be more important in progestin-only contraceptives or when estrogen-progestin combinations are used for postcoital contraception.[14]

► **NONCONTRACEPTIVE HEALTH BENEFITS OF HORMONAL CONTRACEPTION**

Hormonal contraceptives have other salutary effects on the reproductive system besides prevention of pregnancy. In particular, oral contraceptives have been used widely therapeutically in a variety of gynecologic conditions, even though noncontraceptive uses are not specifically approved by the Food and Drug Administration (FDA). It has been estimated

that as many as 50,000 hospital admissions are prevented annually because of the noncontraceptive benefits of these drugs. While many of these health benefits were described among users of higher-dose oral contraceptives, it is likely that women taking progestin-only agents that inhibit ovulation will derive similar advantages[15] (Table 26-2).

Reproductive Tract Tumors

Perhaps the most important noncontraceptive benefit of hormonal birth control is the prevention of genital tract neoplasms. Data from the Oxford Family Planning Clinic Study observed a 30 percent decrease in the incidence of uterine leiomyomas in oral contraceptive users.[16] The risk for developing endometrial or ovarian cancer is decreased by about half with oral contraceptive use. This protective effect seems to be more profound in nulliparas and appears to persist long after pills are discontinued.[17,18] In the United States, about 1700 cases of ovarian cancer are averted every year by the use of oral contraceptives.[19] Recent data suggest that oral contraceptives can provide primary prevention for women at risk for hereditary ovarian cancer such as $BRCA_1$ and $BRAC_2$.[20] Current users of oral contraceptives have a 50 percent reduction in the incidence of chronic breast cysts and an 85 percent decrease in the incidence of breast fibroadenomas.[15]

Pelvic Inflammatory Disease

The risk of hospitalization for pelvic inflammatory disease (PID) is reduced by 50 percent in users of oral contraceptives.[21] The mechanism for this effect is not clear but is most likely the result of progestin-induced changes in cervical mucus and decreased menstrual blood flow. Whether the effect of oral contraceptives on the incidence of PID involves gonococcal or chlamydial infections or both has not been resolved.

► **TABLE 26-2:** NONCONTRACEPTIVE HEALTH BENEFITS OF ORAL CONTRACEPTIVES

	Percent Reduction/ Protection (%)	Minimum Use Required	Duration of Effect	OCP Formulation*	Comments
Definitive evidence					
Ovarian cancer	40	3–6 months	At least 15 years	>20 μg EE	Also protective against hereditary ovarian cancer
Endometrial cancer	50	12 months	15 years	All monophasic	No data on multiphasic or progestin-only forms
Benign breast disease	30	12–24 months	1 year	>20 μg EE	Effect consistent across all age groups
Pelvic inflammatory disease	50	12 months	Current use	>20 μg EE	? Effect on outpatient cases of PID
Ectopic pregnancy	90	Current use	Current use	>20 μg EE	No increased risk for ectopic pregnancy in women who become pregnant with OCP use
Iron-deficiency anemia	50†	Current use	Current use	>20 μg EE	Amount of reduction unknown but 15% increase in hematocrit
Conflicting evidence, favor beneficial effect					
Bone mineral density	60	Unknown	Unknown	>35 μg EE	Decreased incidence of hip fractures with higher doses
Colorectal cancer	40	96 months	Unknown	>50 μg EE	Increasing protection with increased duration

(Continued)

▶ **TABLE 26-2:** NONCONTRACEPTIVE HEALTH BENEFITS OF ORAL CONTRACEPTIVES (*Continued*)

	Percent Reduction/ Protection (%)	Minimum Use Required	Duration of Effect	OCP Formulation*	Comments
Uterine leiomyomas	30, 50	10 years; 7 years	Unknown	Unclear	If used in setting of fibroids, no clinically significant uterine growth
Toxic shock syndrome	50	Current use	Current use	Unclear	May be influenced by change in tampon composition/absorbency
Conflicting evidence, favor no effect					
Functional ovarian cysts	80, 48, 8	Current use	Current use	Monophasic >35 μg EE; monophasic <35 mcg EE; triphasic all types	No statistically significant effect
Rheumatoid arthritis	40	Current use	Current use	Unclear	May alter severity and clinical course rather development

*Effect of 20 μg EE pills is unknown.

†Exact amount of reduction unknown.

Abbreviations; OCP = oral contraceptive pill; EE = ethinyl estradiol; PID = pelvic inflammatory disease.

Adapted from Dayal M, Barnhart KT. Noncontraceptive benefits and therapeutic uses of the oral contraceptive pill. Semin Reprod Med 2001;19:295, with permission.

Functional Ovarian Cysts

In a study of 17,000 women enrolled in a family planning program, Vessey and colleagues noted a 78 percent reduction in corpus luteum cysts and a 49 percent reduction in follicular cysts among monophasic combination oral contraceptive users.[22] While it has been suggested that multiphasic pills may not be as effective as higher-dose formulations in the prevention of cyst formation, this has not been established with certainty. Oral contraceptives have been advocated to hasten the resolution of functional ovarian cysts. However, the efficacy of such therapy was not confirmed in a recent randomized clinical trial, and estrogen-progestin treatment appears to have little effect on the course of such cysts once they have developed.[23]

Other Benefits

The decreased blood flow associated with hormonal contraceptive use diminishes the risk of iron-deficiency anemia. Oral contraceptives also appear to stimulate bone mass and prevent osteoporosis, particularly in premenopausal women with estrogen deficiency such as amenorrhea due to excessive exercise or anorexia. In addition to noncontraceptive benefits, oral contraceptives are useful for the therapeutic treatment of menstrual disorders, endometriosis, and androgen excess.[24]

Regulation of Menstrual Dysfunction

Oral contraceptives are useful for the management of irregular bleeding associated with anovulatory states such as polycystic ovary syndrome, in which unopposed estrogen exposure results in prolonged endometrial proliferation.[25] Patients with menorrhagia not associated with a demonstrable organic cause have been shown to respond to oral contraceptive treatment with a reduction in menstrual blood loss.

Menstrual pain is also decreased significantly in women with primary dysmenorrhea treated with oral contraceptives, and some women also report lessening in premenstrual discomfort. Because ovulation is blocked with combined oral contraceptives, periovulatory discomfort (mittelschmerz) is relieved. The effect is of considerable importance in women with coagulopathies, in whom normal ovulation may result in shock from intraabdominal bleeding.[24]

Endometriosis

Progestins have long been used for the treatment of symptoms associated with endometriosis, either alone or combined with estrogens as part of a "pseudopregnancy" regimen. Although this approach to therapy has been superseded by the development of danazol and GnRH analogues, progestins or estrogen-progestin combinations are still useful for the long-term treatment of patients with symptomatic endometriosis who wish to preserve fertility but are not actively attempting pregnancy.[26]

Androgen Excess

Estrogen treatment increases hepatic synthesis of sex hormone–binding globulin (SHGB), and both estrogen and progestin limit ovarian androgen production by suppression of pituitary LH release. These effects result in decreased free (and hence biologically active) testosterone levels, which can limit symptoms such as acne and hirsutism caused by androgen excess.[27] Patients treated with oral contraceptives specifically for this problem benefit most from pills containing at least 35 μg ethinyl estradiol and a progestin with limited androgenic activity such as norethindrone, norgestimate, ethynodiol diacetate, or drosperinone.[24]

▶ POTENTIAL RISKS OF ORAL CONTRACEPTIVES

No contraceptive is 100 percent effective, and none is without risk. In women who are at increased risk, i.e., smokers over age 35, the risks are increased so that their use is contraindicated[28] (Fig. 26-4). However, it needs to be emphasized that the potential lethal side effects of hormonal contraceptives are significantly less than the mortality associated with pregnancy. Death rates from surgical procedures such as tubal sterilization (8 to 10 per 100,000 procedures) are higher than the death rate in young, nonsmoking women using low-dose contraceptives.[29,30]

Pregnancy

Hormonal contraceptives are among the most effective methods for preventing pregnancy. While the theoretical risk of pregnancy is lowest with combined oral contraceptives, long-acting injections and contraceptive implants achieve higher efficacy in actual use because compliance is ensured. Progestin-only contraceptives are more effective in preventing intrauterine than ectopic pregnancies; thus, among progestin-only contraceptive failures, the ratio of ectopic to intrauterine pregnancies is higher than in women who are not receiving oral contraceptives.

Early retrospective studies suggested that oral contraceptive use during pregnancy was associated with an increased risk of fetal limb-reduction defects and cardiovascular anomalies. Prospective surveys have failed to confirm these initial observations; warnings about possible birth defects with oral contraceptive use in pregnancy were ordered removed from package inserts by the FDA in 1989.[31]

Norethindrone in high doses (10 to 40 mg/d) in early pregnancy can cause labioscrotal fusion, urethral displacement, and clitoral hypertrophy in female fetuses. Less is known about the virilization potential of other 19-nortestosterone derivatives, although similar effects can be expected at high doses.[32] Masculinization of female fetuses has not been reported as a result of modern hormonal contraceptive use most likely because of the small amounts of progestins in the formulations.[33]

A temporary delay in pregnancy after discontinuation of oral contraceptives has been

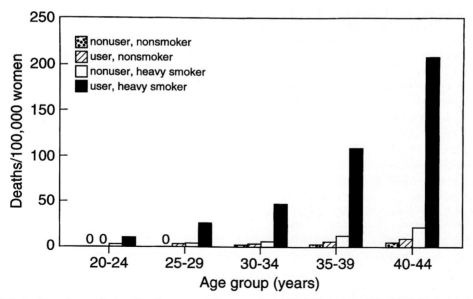

Figure 26-4 Number of deaths from cardiovascular diseases per 100,000 women by smoking status or nonuse of oral contraceptives. *(Reproduced, with permission, from Kost et al. Fam Plan Perspect 1991;23:54.)*

observed; one recent study found that the chance of conception was decreased significantly for the first six cycles after pill discontinuation and that the delay in conception was longer in users of higher-dose (≥50 μg) estrogen pills.[34]

Circulatory System

Oral contraceptive pills have been reported to cause an increase in the incidence of stroke, myocardial infarction, and venous thromboembolism (VTE).[35] Because the actual incidence of these serious adverse events in women prior to the menopause is low, large changes in relative risk compared with nonusers result from small changes in the attributable risk. These need to be discussed with the patient to put the proper risk in perspective.

Stroke

The association of oral contraceptive pills and stroke was first described in the literature in the 1960s and 1970s when high dose oral contraceptives were in use (e.g., 150 μg ethinyl estradiol).[36] By the year 2000, most women were using low-dose contraceptive pills containing 20 to 35 μg ethinyl estradiol. Thus data generated in older studies do not pertain to the present. More recently, numerous studies in western developed countries have shown minimal or no increased risks of stroke in women taking low-dose oral contraceptives.[35] In a study by Thorogood conducted in England and Wales, there was a slight increased risk in subarachnoid hemorrhage, but the study did not report estrogen dose.[37] When the adjusted death rate for this disorder was evaluated, the differences were not statistically significant. One of the largest studies of hemorrhagic and ischemic stroke was conducted by the World Health Organization (WHO).[38] The investigators reported no statistically significant increased risk of stroke in nonsmoking women using <50-μg pills. However, smoking appeared to increase the risk of hemorrhagic and

ischemic stroke in women using low-dose pills. In two U.S. studies with low dose-oral contraceptives (<50 μg ethinyl estradiol), the risk of stroke was not increased significantly except in smokers and women with hypertension.[35]

In summary, stroke is a rare event in reproductive-age women (approximately 10 per 100,000 women over 1 year). Women with a history of hypertension and smoking are at higher risk.

Myocardial Infarction

Studies performed between 1960 and 1980 suggested that women who smoke and are over 35 are at increased risk for myocardial infarction (see Fig. 26-4). These studies were conducted in women using oral contraceptives of at least 50 μg ethinyl estradiol.[39] A number of recent studies have not confirmed a relationship between smoking, low-dose contraceptive use, and myocardial infarction.[35,40] A recent review of low-dose oral contraceptives using the third-generation oral contraceptive desogestrel, gestodene, and norgestimate were not associated with an increased risk of myocardial infarction.[41] Low-dose oral contraceptives have minor effects on lipoproteins but increase triglycerides. Consequently, oral contraceptives are contraindicated in women with significantly elevated triglycerides.

In summary, healthy women do not appear to be at increased risk of myocardial infarction even up to age 50. However, it is still prudent to continue to avoid using estrogen-containing pills in women over 35 who smoke.

Venous Thromboembolism (VTE)

The use of oral contraceptives has been known to be associated with an increased risk of VTE in a dose-related fashion.[35] There is some debate as to whether the type of progestin is associated with increased risk. The risk of VTE in the general population is low (1 per 10,000 people), and it is estimated that the use of oral contraceptives causes a small but significant increase to 3 per 10,000 women.[35] Recent studies suggest that women carrying defects in hereditary thromboembolism such as factor V Leiden mutation are at significantly increased risk of VTE compared with normal women.[41] Even low-dose hormone therapy is associated with a small but significant increase in VTE.[42] Thus it is important to prescribe low-dose oral contraceptives when possible.

In women who have a history of thromboembolism, oral contraceptives are contraindicated. If a patient has a family history of VTE or stroke, it may be helpful to screen for factor V Leiden and other thrombophilias, and if a defect is noted, nonhormonal methods of contraception should be used.

Neoplasms

Given the responsiveness of some malignancies to sex steroids and the association between reproductive status and tumor development, the potential neoplastic effect of steroidal contraception has been a continuing concern to health professionals. As noted previously, current formulations of hormonal contraceptives appear to be protective against the development of endometrial and ovarian cancer. Twelve studies have been performed regarding oral contraceptives and colorectal cancer, and a metaanalysis of these reports suggests a significant decrease in the rate of cancer.[24,43] The effects on the incidence of other tumors are less certain. There is no current consensus as to whether cancers of the breast, cervix, colon, and skin are influenced by oral contraceptive use.[44,45]

Early studies suggesting a protective effect of oral contraceptive use on breast cancer development have not been confirmed, and further analyses indicated that certain subgroups of women might be at increased risk. However, the findings from a number of investigations have been inconsistent and contradictory.[46–48] Retrospective studies, in general, have not shown a difference in the breast cancer incidence in women who have used oral contraceptives. In a comprehensive survey of research dealing with breast cancer and oral contraceptives, oral contraceptive use did not appear to increase the risk of breast cancer in women over age 45.[49] A recent report concluded that among women ages 35 to 64 years, current or former use of oral contraceptives was not associated with an increased risk of breast cancer.[50]

Controversy still exists as to the risk of breast cancer in younger women using or having used oral contraception, but the lack of consistency among investigations argues against a causal relationship between oral contraceptive use and the development of breast cancer. Little can be said with confidence about the risk of breast cancer with other hormonal contraceptive formulations due to limited patient experience; although depot medroxyprogesterone acetate (DMPA) has been shown to increase the development of breast nodules in beagle dogs. However, this was not confirmed in case-control studies in humans.[51]

The results of several studies have suggested an increase in the development of cervical cancer in users of oral contraceptives.[52,53] Vessey and colleagues found the risk of cervical neoplasia (including dysplasia and cancer) to be about 70 percent higher among oral contraceptive users as compared with intrauterine device (IUD) users.[52] However, potential confounding factors such as age at first intercourse, number of sexual partners, and frequency of Pap smear screening have not been fully controlled for in these investigations. The use of control patients who employ barrier methods that prevent the transmission of papillomavirus, thought to be a precursor of cervical neoplasia, is another potential source of bias in these surveys. It is likely that hormonal contraception does not in itself induce the development of cervical neoplasia.

A strong association exists between oral contraceptive use and the development of benign hepatic adenomas. An increased incidence of 3.3 cases per 100,000 uses has been estimated, with the risk further increasing after 4 or more years of use, especially with higher-dose oral contraceptives.[54] Data from Great Britain have indicated an increased risk of hepatocellular carcinoma with oral contraceptive use, but a large multicenter study was unable to confirm these observations.[55] Due to the rarity of these tumors, the attributable risk (if it exists) has been estimated to be less than 1 case per 1 million users.

Gallbladder Disease

Early studies of oral contraceptive users reported a twofold increase in gallstones and cholecystitis. More recent data indicate only a minimal effect, probably due to the low hormone doses in newer formulation.[56] The risk of gallbladder disease with progestin-only formulations is not known precisely but is probably less than that seen with combined oral contraceptive use.

Other Potential Adverse Effects

A number of minor side effects have been ascribed to oral contraceptive use, including nausea, amenorrhea, edema, facial hyperpigmentation (chloasma), breast tenderness and enlargement, lactation, migraine, mental depression, and change in corneal curvature. The precise mechanisms of these changes have not been elucidated. Galactorrhea develops in up to 10 percent of combined oral contraceptive users, and it has been suggested that combination oral contraceptives may promote the growth or development of prolactinomas; however, this was not confirmed in a multicenter case-control study.[57]

Combined oral contraceptive use in the postpartum period can decrease milk production and may affect infant growth if feedings are not supplemented, but progestin-only formulations have no significant effect on lactation.[58] The amount transferred to infants of mothers taking currently available formulations is clinically negligible, the equivalent of about one pill for every 4 years of full lactation.[59]

Accelerated metabolism of steroidal contraceptives has been reported with concurrent use of drugs such as rifampin and anticonvulsants that induce microsomal liver enzymes or increase SHBG levels.[60] Breakthrough bleeding and contraceptive failure are more likely to occur in hormonal contraceptive users who take these drugs, and it has been suggested that such patients be placed on oral contraceptives containing at least 50 μg ethinyl estradiol to ensure contraceptive efficacy. Disturbance of the enterohepatic circulation by steroids through alteration of gut flora has been suggested as a cause for contraceptive pill failure among users of antibiotics, but controlled trials have failed to document a consistent effect on contraceptive steroid serum levels.[61,62] Physicians who care for patients on hormonal contraceptives also should be aware of changes in clinical laboratory values induced by sex steroid use (Table 26-3).

Carbohydrate Intolerance

Impaired glucose tolerance has been observed with the use of combined or progestin-only oral contraceptives.[63] Progestins induce a decrease in insulin receptors on the cell membrane. Orally administered norgestrel seems to have the most pronounced effect, whereas injectable levonorgestel and medroxyprogesterone acetate (MPA) induce little or no alteration in carbohydrate metabolism.[64,65] Thus patients with diabetes who desire hormonal contraception may benefit from a parenteral formulation.

▶ INJECTABLE CONTRACEPTIVE STEROIDS

Currently, two injectable forms of hormonal contraception are available in the United States. These include depot medroxyprogesterone acetate (DMPA, Depo-Provera) and medroxyprogesterone acetate–estradiol cypionate

▶**TABLE 26-3:** POTENTIAL EFFECTS OF COMBINED ORAL CONTRACEPTIVES ON LABORATORY TEST RESULTS

	Specific Tests and Potential Alteration of Lab Value	
Group	Increased	Decreased
Carbohydrate Metabolism	FBS and 2 h pp Insulin level	Glucose tolerance
Hematologic/coagulation	Coagulation factor II, VII, XIII, IX, time; plasma volume, plasmin, and plasminogen; platelet count, platelet aggregation, and platelet adhesiveness; prothrombin time	Antithrombin III; erythrocyte count (total); hematocrit; prothrombin time
Lipid metabolism	Cholesterol; lipoproteins (pre-β, β, and α); phospholipids, total; total lipids; triglycerides	
Liver function/ gastrointestinal tests	Alkaline phosphatase; bilirubin, SGOT, SGPT; cephalin flocculation; formiminoglutamic acid excretion after histidine (urine); γ-glutamyl *trans*-peptidase; leucine aminopeptidase; protoporphyrin, coproporphyrin excretion (urine); uroporphyrin excretion (urine); sulfobromophthalein retention	Alkaline phosphatase; etiocholanolone excretion (urine); haptoglobin (serum); urobilinogen excretion (urine)
Metals	Copper and ceruloplasmin; iron, iron binding capacity, and transferrin	Magnesium; zinc
Thyroid function	Butanole extractable iodine; protein bound iodine; thyroid-binding globulin; triiodothyronine (serum)	Triiodothyronine resin (serum); free thyroxine
Vitamins	Vitamin A (blood and plasma)	Folate (serum); vitamin B_2 (red blood cell and urine excretion); vitamin B_6; vitamin B_{12}; vitamin C
Other hormones/enzyme measurements	Aldosterone (blood and urine); angiotensinogen; angiotensin I and II; cortisol (blood and urine); growth hormone; prolactin; testosterone (serum); total estrogens	Estradiol and estriol; FSH (urine), LH (blood and urine); gonadotropin excretion (urine); 17-hydroxycorticosteroid excretion (urine); 17-ketosteroid excretion (urine); pregnanediol excretion (urine); renin (serum); tetrahydrocortisone
Miscellaneous laboratory	α_1-Antitrypsin; antinuclear antibody; bilirubin; complement-reactive protein; globulins a-1, a-2; lactate; lupus erythematosus cell preparation; pyruvate; sodium	Albumin; α-amino nitrogen; calcium (serum) and calcium excretion (urine); complement reactive protein; immuno-globulin A, G, and M

Adapted, with permission, from Hatcher et al. Contraceptive Technology, *16th ed. New York:Irvington, 1994.*

(MPA/E$_2$C, Lunelle).[66] Both these formulations have demonstrated a high degree of efficacy, safety, and ease of use in international and U.S. trials.

DMPA has been available for a number of years as a contraceptive in the United States. It consists of 150 mg DMPA and is given intramuscularly every 3 months. The mechanisms of DMPA includes inhibition of ovulation, production of a thick cervical mucus, induction of a decidual reaction that results in a thin endometrium, and possibly delayed ovum transport.[67] The benefits of DMPA include reduced vaginal bleeding, induction of amenorrhea, and reduction in the risk of endometrial cancer.[68] On the other hand, side effects include irregular uterine bleeding and spotting, weight gain, depression, and a decrease in high-density lipoprotein (HDL) cholesterol. In addition, when DMPA is discontinued, there is a significant delay in time to conception.[66]

MPA/E$_2$C became available in the United States in the year 2000 and is given as a monthly injection containing 25 mg MPA and 5 mg E$_2$C.[69] The mechanism of action appears to be similar to that of DMPA and includes decreased cervical mucus and inhibition of ovulation. The addition of estradiol to MPA regulates vaginal bleeding, so instead of experiencing amenorrhea, women who choose this form of contraception generally experience cyclic withdrawal bleeding.[66] The noncontraceptive benefits have not yet been determined but are probably similar to those of DMPA. Regarding potential risks, the findings appear to be similar to those of DMPA. However, the return to fertility is much more rapid than for DMPA.[70] See Table 26-4 for a comparison of DMPA and MPA/E$_2$C injectable contraception.

▶ SUBDERMAL IMPLANTS

Currently, one method of steroidal hormonal implant is approved for use in the United States.[71] This is Norplant, which contains levonorgestrel in six Silastic capsules and has a duration of effectiveness ranging from 5 to 10 years. Recently, the manufacture of Norplant was discontinued, and it is no longer available in the United States. A new implant containing etonogestrel has been under study. If and when it is approved, it will consist of one Silastic rod and will have a length of contraception effectiveness of up to 3 years.[72]

Progestin-containing rods have multiple modes of action that include inhibition of ovulation, changes in cervical mucus, and a thinning of the endometrial lining. These methods are highly effective, and fertility improves rapidly on removal. Implants have minimal metabolic effect. The principal problem with implants includes the need for surgical insertion and removal and potential problems with

▶ **TABLE 26-4:** COMPARISON OF DMPA AND MPA/E$_2$C CONTRACEPTIVE INJECTIONS

Parameter	DMPA	MPA/E$_2$C
Formulation	Progestin only	Combined progestin-estrogen
Administration site	Gluteus, deltoid	Gluteus, deltoid, or anterior thigh
Dosage	150 mg medroxyprogesterone acetate	25 mg medroxyprogesterone acetate/ 5 mg estradiol cypionate
Injection schedule	Every 12–13 weeks	Every 28–33 days
Failure rate	0.3%	0.1%
Typical return to fertility after discontinuation	7–15 months	35–84 days

From Kaunitz AM. *Current options for injectable contraception in the United States.* Semin Reprod Med 2001;19:331, with permission.

removal of the implant, requiring hospitalization and removal under anesthesia. This appears to be less of a problem with the single implant containing etonorgestrel that is being studied at present.

▶ TRANSDERMAL PATCHES

A new series of hormonal methods of contraception has been marketed recently[73] (Table 26-5). The transdermal contraception patch contains once-a-week dosing of 150 μg norelgestromin and 20 μg ethinyl estradiol each day,[74] and it is applied for 3 weeks followed by a 1-week rest, when the patient experiences withdrawal bleeding. The mechanism of action of the hormonal patch is similar to that of oral contraceptive pills, primarily by preventing ovulation. The advantage of the patch is that it may increase compliance in women who have a problem taking a daily oral pill. The risks appear to be the same as those of the oral contraceptive pills, and thus contraindications are also similar to those for oral contraceptive pills, including in women who smoke over age 35 (see Fig. 26-4). The only other side effect is skin reactions or allergies.

▶ CONTRACEPTIVE VAGINAL RING

The most recent contraceptive device available consists of a vaginal ring that contains the progestin etonogestrel and ethinyl estradiol.[75] The ring is a combined hormonal contraceptive method that the woman inserts in the vagina herself. The ring is inserted for a 3-week period, after which it is removed, followed by a 1-week hormone-free period in which withdrawal bleeding is anticipated. Once it is inserted, the ring releases continuous doses of hormones into blood, and the mechanisms of action are similar to those of the contraceptive patch. Cycle control appears to be similar to that of the patch and oral contraceptive pills.[76] The efficacy and other aspects of safety are similar to that of oral contraceptive pills, and the contraindications are also the same. Benefits include improved compliance because the patient only has to remember to change this device every 3 weeks. The downside is that in some patients a vaginal ring is not well tolerated by the patient or her partner.[77]

▶ HORMONE-CONTAINING INTRAUTERINE DEVICE (IUD)

The second IUD available in the U.S. market in addition to the copper IUD, which is discussed in Chapter 27, is the levonorgestrel intrauterine system (Mirena).[78] The levonorgestrel IUD is a small plastic T-shaped IUD that releases 20 μg levonorgestrel per day. This progestin is contained in many oral contraceptive pills. Once in place, the IUD provides contraception for up to 5 years.[79] Its mechanism of action includes cervical mucous thickening, reduced sperm motility, endometrial suppression, and a weak foreign-body reaction in the uterine cavity and, in a small percentage of patients, the inhibition of ovulation. Its safety has been well established and is similar to that of the copper IUD. Although infections are rare with IUDs if used in monogamous couples, the risk of infection is further reduced if cervical cultures ruling out gonorrhea and chlamydia are obtained prior to insertion.

One of the principal advantages of this device is that it often induces amenorrhea, and patients generally do not experience menstrual

▶ TABLE 26-5: NEW METHODS OF CONTRACEPTION

Progestin IUD
Vaginal ring
Transdermal patch
Daily injectable
Subdermal implant

▶ **TABLE 26-6:** POSSIBLE CONTRAINDICATIONS TO USE OF COMBINED ORAL
CONTRACEPTIVE PILLS

Absolute Contraindications
1. Thrombophlebitis or thromboembolic disorder
2. Past history of deep vein thrombophlebitis or thromboembolic disorders
3. Cerebrovascular or coronary artery disease
4. Known or suspected breast carcinoma
5. Known or suspected estrogen-dependent neoplasia
6. Pregnancy
7. Benign or malignant liver tumor
8. Known impaired liver function
9. Previous cholestasis during pregnancy or with prior pill use

Strong Relative Contraindications
10. Severe headaches, particularly vascular or migraine headaches, that start after initiation of oral contraceptives
11. Hypertension with resting diastolic BP of 140 mmHg or greater on three or more separate visits or an accurate measurement of 110 mmHg diastolic or more on a single visit
12. Mononucleosis, acute phase
13. Elective major surgery or major surgery requiring immobilization planned in next 4 weeks
14. Long-leg cast or major injury to lower leg
15. Over 40 years old, accompanied by a second risk factor for the development of cardiovascular disease (such as diabetes or hypertension)
16. Over 35 years old and currently a heavy smoker (15 or more cigarettes/day)
17. Abnormal genital bleeding

Other Considerations
Diabetes, prediabetes, or a strong family history of diabetes
Sickle cell disease or sickle C disease
Active gallbladder disease
Congenital hyperbilirubinemia (Gilbert's disease)
Undiagnosed abnormal genital bleeding
Over 50 years old
Completion of term pregnancy within past 10 to 14 days
Weight gain of 10 lb or more while on the pill
Cardiac renal disease (or history thereof)
Conditions likely to make patient unreliable at following pill instructions (mental retardation, major psychiatric illness, alcoholism or other chemical abuse, history of repeatedly taking oral contraceptives or other medication incorrectly)
Lactation
Family history of death of a parent or sibling due to myocardial infarction before age 50; *myocardial infarction in a mother or sister is especially significant and indicates a need for lipid evaluation*
Family history of hyperlipidemia

Adapted, with permission, from Hatcher et al. Contraceptive Technology, *16th ed. New York:Irvington, 1994.*

bleeding even though they still continue to ovulate and produce estrogen. This occurs because a direct local effect of the progestin reduces the thickness of the endometrium. Other potential future noncontraceptive benefits of this device include use as a primary treatment for abnormal uterine bleeding, possibly in postmenopausal women, for the prevention of endometrial hyperplasia. Once the IUD is removed, fertility returns rapidly.[80]

► EMERGENCY POSTCOITAL CONTRACEPTION

Emergency contraceptive methods that prevent pregnancy are effective when used after unprotected sexual intercourse.[81] In the United States, three different emergency contraceptive methods have been studied widely, including: (1) taking ordinary combined oral contraceptive pills consisting of, for example, ethinyl estradiol and levonorgestrel used at high dose for a short period of time within a few days of unprotected intercourse, (2) taking levonorgestrel-only tablets, or (3) inserting a levonorgestrel IUD within 1 week of unprotected intercourse. Emergency contraception is best known for its use in women who have been raped. Emergency contraception methods are also appropriate for women who have experienced condom breaks, women who did not use any method because they were not planning on having sexual intercourse, or women who have unprotected intercourse for other reasons.

One of the problems with emergency contraception is that it is used infrequently, and many patients and physicians are unaware of its availability and effectiveness. The most experience available is with the use of combined contraceptive pills, also known as the "morning-after pill." To be effective, the first dose of medication must be administered within 72 hours of unprotected intercourse and a second dose within 12 hours of the

first.[81] Other options include a product known as Plan B that contains 75 mg levonorgestrel given in two doses within 72 hours of exposure. Most studies have shown that the risk of pregnancy is reduced by approximately 75 percent. Side effects of emergency oral contraceptive pills are upper gastrointestinal symptoms, including nausea and vomiting.[81] It may be helpful to take nonprescription antinausea medicine to reduce this. Safety is very good because the medication is used for only a short period of time. The mechanism of action of combined contraceptive pills used as emergency contraception appears to be inhibition or delay of ovulation. A direct effect on the endometrium and implantation is also possible.

► PRESCRIBING HORMONAL CONTRACEPTIVES: A PRACTICAL APPROACH

The benefits of hormonal contraceptives outweigh the risks for most women. A thorough history and physical examination should be performed and testing of cholesterol and fasting blood sugar may be appropriate, especially in older women. Contraindications for hormonal contraceptive use should be considered and reviewed periodically (Table 26-6). All patients should be encouraged to stop smoking and achieve their ideal body weight. Many clinicians feel that the initial choice of an oral contraceptive for most women should be one containing 35 μg ethinyl estradiol or less. Patients should be reassured that mortality among healthy nonsmokers who use oral contraceptives is decreased relative to women who use no contraception. Consideration should be given to longer-acting formulations in women who have difficulty complying with daily pill use. Patients with multiple sexual partners should be encouraged to use condoms to minimize the transmission of sexually transmitted diseases.

KEY POINTS

1. The world population will be 10 billion by the year 2050.

2. The estrogen contained in modern contraceptive pills except for one pill is ethinyl estradiol.

3. The progestins in todays' oral contraceptive products include norethindrone, norethynodrel, norethindrone acetate, ethynodiol diacetate, norgestrel, desogestrel, norgestimate, and drospirenone.

4. The estrogen component of the oral contraceptive controls bleeding, and the progestin component inhibits ovulation.

5. Oral contraceptives decrease the risk of ovarian, uterine, and colon cancer. They do not increase breast cancer risk. There is a slight increase in cervical cancer and hepatic adenomas.

6. Oral contraceptives at all doses increase the risk of VTE, but the risk is reduced with low-dose estrogen-containing oral contraceptives.

7. Injectable contraceptives can be given in monthly injections (Lunelle) or every 3 months (Depo-Provera).

8. Subdermal implants are currently not available but have minimal metabolic effects.

9. Transdermal patches are changed weekly for 3 weeks followed by a rest of 1 week. The patch releases the equivalent of 20 μg ethinyl estradiol per day.

10. Vaginal contraceptive rings contain ethinyl estradiol and etonorgestrel and are effective for 3 weeks.

REFERENCES

1. Trussell J. Dynamics of reproductive behavior and population change, in Hatcher RA, Trussel J, Stewart F, et al (eds), *Contraceptive Technology,* 17th ed. New York: Ardent Media, 1998:745.

2. Segal AJ. Contraceptive research: A male chauvinist plot? *Fam Plan Perspect* 1972;4:21.

3. Cunningham FA, MacDonald PC, Gant NF, et al. *Williams Obstetrics,* 19th ed. Norwalk, CT: Appleton & Lange, 1993:1321.

4. Trussell J, Hatcher RA, Cates W, et al. Contraceptive failure in the United States: An update. *Stud Fam Plan* 1990;21:51.

5. Goldzieher JW, Rudel HW. How the oral contraceptives came to be developed. *JAMA* 1982; 274:3210.

6. Pincus G, Rock J, Garcia CR. Effects of certain 19-nor steroids upon the reproductive process. *Ann NY Acad Sci* 1958;71:677.

7. Goldzieher JW. Pharmocokinetics and metabolism of ethynol estrogens, in Goldzieher JW, Fotherby K (eds), *Pharmacology of the Contraceptive Steroids.* New York: Raven Press, 1994; p 127.

8. Hatcher RA, Trussel J, Stewart F, et al. *Contraceptive Technology,* 16th ed. New York: Irvington, 1994.

9. Fotherby K. Pharmocokinetics and metabolism of progestins in humans, in Goldzieher JW, Fotherby K (eds), *Pharmacology of the Contraceptive Steroids.* New York: Raven Press, 1994; p 99.

10. Borenstein J, Yu HT, Wade S,et al. Effect of an oral contraceptive containing ethinyl estradiol and drospirenone on premenstrual symptomatology and health-related quality of life. *J Reprod Med* 2003;48(2):79.

11. Spellacy WN, Kalra PS, Buhi WR, et al. Pituitary and ovarian responsiveness to a graded gonadotropin-releasing factor stimulation test in women using a low estrogen on a regular type of oral contraceptive. *Am J Obstet Gynecol* 1980;137:109.

12. Carr BR, Parker CR Jr, Madden JD, et al. Plasma levels of adrenocorticotropin and cortisol in women receiving oral contraceptive steroid treatment. *J Clin Endocrinol Metab* 1979;49: 346.

13. Greenwald GS. In vivo recording of intraluminal pressure changes in the rabbit oviduct. *Fertil Steril* 1963;14:666.

14. Rowlands D, Kubba AA, Guillebaud J, et al. A possible mechanism of action of danazol and an ethinyl estradiol/norgestrel combination

used as postcoital contraceptive agents. *Contraception* 1986;33:539.

15. Baird DT, Glasier AF. Hormonal contraception. *N Engl J Med* 1993;328:1543.

16. Vessey MP, McPherson K, Johnson B. Mortality among women participating in the Oxford/Family Planning Association Contraceptive Study. *Lancet* 1977;2:731.

17. Cancer and Steroid Hormone Study of the Centers for Disease Control and the National Institute of Child Health and Human Development. Combined oral contraceptive use and the risk of endometrial cancer. *JAMA* 1987;257:796.

18. Rossenberg L, Shapiro S, Stone D, et al. Epithelial ovarian cancer and combination oral contraceptives. *JAMA* 1982;274:3210.

19. Brinton LA, Vessey MP, Flavel R, et al. Risk factors for benign breast disease. *Am J Epidemiol* 1981;113:203.

20. Narod SA, Risch H, Moslehi R, et al. Oral contraceptives and the risk of hereditary ovarian cancer. *N Engl J Med* 1998;339:424.

21. Grimes DA, Cates W Jr. Family planning and sexually transmitted diseases, in Holmes KK, Mardh P-A, Sparling PF, et al. (eds), *Sexually Transmitted Diseases,* 2d ed. New York: McGraw-Hill, 1990.

22. Vessey M, Metcalfe A, Wells C, et al. Ovarian neoplasms, functional ovarian cysts, and oral contraceptives. *Br Med J* 1987;294:1518.

23. Steinkampf MP, Hammond KR, Blackwell RE. Hormonal treatment of functional ovarian cysts: A randomized, prospective study. *Fertil Steril* 1990;54:775.

24. Dayal M, Barnhart KT. Noncontraceptive benefits and therapeutic uses of the oral contraceptive pill. *Semin Reprod Med* 2001;19:295.

25. Mishell DR Jr. Noncontraceptive benefits of oral contraceptives. *J Reprod Med* 1993;38:1021.

26. Moore J, Kennedy S, Prentice A. Modern combined oral contraceptives for pain associated with endometriosis (Cochrane Review). *Cochrane Library Syst Rev* 1999;2.

27. Carr BR, Breslau NA, Givens C, et al. Oral contraceptive pills, gonadotropin-releasing hormone agonists, or use in combination for treatment of hirsutism: A clinical research center Study. *J Clin Endocrinol Metab* 1995;80:1169.

28. Kost K, Forrest JD, Harlap S. Comparing the health risks and benefits of contraceptive choices. *Fam Plan Perspect* 1991;23:54.

29. Gray MJ, Grimes DA. Birth control, abortion and sterilization, in Romney SC, Gray MJ, Little AB, et al (eds), *Gynecology and Obstetrics: The Health Care of Women.* New York: McGraw-Hill, 1981:817.

30. Peterson HB, DeStefano F, Greenspan JR, et al. Mortality risk associated with tubal sterilization in Unites States hospitals. *Am J Obstet Gynecol* 1982;142:125.

31. Bracken MB. Oral contraception and congenital malformations in offspring: A review and meta-analysis of the prospective studies. *Obstet Gynecol* 1990;76:552.

32. Wilkins L. Masculinizations of female fetuses due to the use of orally given progestins. *JAMA* 1960;172:1028.

33. Carson SA, Simpson JL. Virilization of female fetuses following maternal ingestion for progestational and androgenic steroids, in Mahesh VB, Greenblatt RB (eds), *Hirsutism and Virilism.* Boston: John Wright-PSG, 1983:177.

34. Bracken MB, Hellenbrand KG, Holford TG. Conception delay after oral contraceptive use: The effect of estrogen dose. *Fertil Steril* 1990;53:21.

35. Pymar HC, Creinin MD. The risks of oral contraceptive pills. *Semin Reprod Med* 2001;19:305.

36. Inman W, Vessey M. Investigation of deaths from pulmonary, coronary, and cerebral thrombosis and embolism in women of child-bearing age. *Br J Med* 1968;2:193.

37. Thorogood M, Mann J, Murphy M, et al. Fatal stroke and use of oral contraceptives: Findings from a case-control study. *Am J Epidemiol* 1992;136:35.

38. World Health Organization Collaborative Study of Cardiovascular Disease and Steroid Hormone Contraception. Hemorrhagic stroke, overall stroke risk, and combined oral contraceptive: Results of an international, multicenter, case control study. *Lancet* 1996;348:505.

39. Rosenberg L, Kaufman D, Helmrich S, et al. Myocardial infarction and cigarette smoking in women younger than 50 years of age. *JAMA* 1969;253:2965.

40. Spitzer WO, Faith JM, MacRae KD. Myocardial infarction and third generation oral contraceptives: Aggregation of recent studies. *Hum Reprod* 2002;17:2307.

41. Vandenbroucke J, Koster T, Briet E, et al. Increased risk of venous thrombosis in oral con-

traceptive users who are carriers of factor V leiden mutation. *Lancet* 1994;344:1453.

42. Rossouw JE, Anderson GL, Prentice RL, et al, for Writing Group for the Women's Health Initiative. Risks and benefits of estrogen plus progestin in healthy post-menopausal women: principle results from the Women's Health Initiative. *JAMA* 2002;288:321.

43. Fernandez E, La Vecchia C, Balducci A, et al. Oral contraceptives and colorectal cancer risk: a meta-analysis. *Br J Cancer* 2001;84:722.

44. Sartrwell PE, Arthea FG, Tonascia JA. Exogenous hormones, reproductive history and breast cancer. *J Natl Cancer Inst* 1979;59:1589.

45. Ravnihar B, Seigel DB, Lindtner J. An epidemiologic study of breast cancer and benign breast neoplasias in relation to the oral contraceptive and estrogen use. *Int J Cancer* 1979; 15:395.

46. Lipnick RJ, Buring JE, Hennekins CH, et al. Oral contraceptives and breast cancer: A prospective cohort study. *JAMA* 1986;255:58.

47. Kay CR, Hannaford PC. Breast cancer and the pill: A further report from the Royal College of General Practitioners Oral Contraception Study. *Br J Cancer* 1988;58:675.

48. Vessey MP, McPherson K, Villard-Mackintosh L, et al. Oral contraceptives and breast cancer: Latest findings in a large cohort study. *Br J Cancer* 1989;59:613.

49. Harlap S. Oral contraceptives and breast cancer: Cause and effect? *J Reprod Med* 1991;36:374.

50. Marchbanks PA, McDonald JA, Wilson HG, et al. Oral contraceptives and the risk of breast cancer. *N Engl J Med* 2002;346:2025.

51. World Health Organization. Depot-medroxyprogesterone acetate (DMPA) and cancer: Memorandum from a WHO meeting. *Bull WHO* 1986;64:375.

52. Vessey MP, Lawless M, McPherson K, Yeates D. Neoplasia of the cervix uteri and contraception: A possible adverse effect of the pill. *Lancet* 1983;2:930.

53. WHO Collaborative Study of Neoplasia and Steroid Contraceptives. Invasive cervical cancer and combined oral contraceptives. *Br Med J* 1985;290:961.

54. Rooks JB, Ory HW, Ishak KG, et al. Epidemiology of hepatocellular adenoma: The role of oral contraceptive use. *JAMA* 1979;242:644.

55. Forman D, Vincent TJ, Doll R. Cancer of the liver and oral contraceptives. *Br J Med* 1986;292:1357.

56. Storm BL, Tamragouri RT, Morse ML, et al. Oral contraceptives and other risk factors for gallbladder disease. *Clin Pharmacol Ther* 1986;39:335.

57. Pituitary Adenoma Study Group. Pituitary adenomas and oral contraceptives: A multicenter case-control study. *Fertil Steril* 1983;39:753.

58. Koetsawang S. The effects of contraceptive methods on the quality and quantity of breast milk. *Int J Gynaecol Obstet* 1987;258:115.

59. Labbock MH. Consequences of breastfeeding for mother and child. *J Biosoc Sci* 1985;9(suppl):43.

60. Guengerich FP. Oxidation of 27-α-ethinyl estradiol by human liver cytochrome P-450. *Mol Pharmacol* 1988;33:500.

61. Friedman CI, Humeke AL, Kim NH, Powell J. The effect of ampicillin on oral contraceptive effectiveness. *Obstet Gynecol* 1980;55:33.

62. Neely JL, Abate M, Swinder M, et al. The effect of doxycycline on serum levels of ethinyl estradiol, norethindrone, and endogenous progesterone. *Obstet Gynecol* 1991;77:416.

63. Spellacy WN, Buhi WC, Birk SA, et al. Metabolic studies in women taking norethindrone for 6 months' time (measurements of blood glucose, insulin, triglyceride concentrations). *Fertil Steril* 1973;24:419.

64. Spellacy WN, Buhi WE, Birk SA. Prospective studies of carbohydrate metabolism in "normal" women using norgestrel for eighteen months. *Fertil Steril* 1981;35:167.

65. Liew DF, Ng CS, Young YM, et al. Long-term effects of Depo-Provera on carbohydrate and lipid metabolism. *Contraception* 1985;31:51.

66. Kaunitz AM. Current options for injectable contraception in the United States. *Semin Reprod Med* 2001;19:331.

67. Mishell DR Jr. Pharmacokinetics of depot medroxyprogesterone acetate contraception. *J Reprod Med* 1991;41(suppl):191.

68. Cullins VE. Noncontraceptive benefits and therapeutic uses of depot medroxyprogesterone acetate. *J Reprod Med* 1996;41(suppl 5):428.

69. Kaunitz AM, Garceau RJ, Cromie MA. Comparative safety, efficacy, and cycle control of Lunelle monthly contraceptive injection (medroxyprogesterone acetate and estradiol cypionate injectable suspension) and Ortho-Novum 7/7/7

oral contraceptive (norethindrone/ethinyl estradiol triphasic). *Contraception* 1999;60:179.

70. Rahimy MH, Ryan KK. Lunelle monthly contraceptive injection (medroxyprogesterone acetate and estradiol cypionate injectable suspension): assessment of return of ovulation after three monthly injections in surgically sterile females. *Contraception* 1999;60:189.

71. Meckstroth KR, Darney PD. Implant contraception. *Semin Reprod Med* 2001;19:339.

72. Bennink HJ. The pharmacokinetics and pharmacodynamics of Implanon, a single-rod etonogestrel contraceptive implant. *Eur J Contracept Reprod Health Care* 2000;5(suppl 2):12.

73. Creasy GW, Abrams LS, Fisher AC. Transdermal contraception. *Semin Reprod Med* 2001;19:373.

74. Abrams L, Skee D, Natarajan J, et al. An overview of the pharmacokinetics of a contraceptive patch. *Int J Gynaecol Obstet* 2000; 70(suppl 1):78.

75. Mulders TMT, Dieben TO. Use of the novel combined contraceptive vaginal ring NuvaRing for ovulation inhibition. *Fertil Steril* 2001;75: 865.

76. Roumen FJME, Apter D, Mulders TMT, et al. Efficacy, tolerability and acceptability of a novel contraceptive vaginal ring releasing etonogestrel and ethinyl oestradiol. *Hum Reprod* 2001;16:469.

77. Harwood B, Mishell DR. Contraceptive vaginal rings. *Semin Reprod Med* 2001;19:381.

78. Luukkainen T, Pakarinen P, Toivonen J. Progestin-releasing intrauterine systems. *Semin Reprod Med* 2001;19:355.

79. Luukkainen T, Toivonen J. Levonorgestrel-releasing IUD as method of contraception with therapeutic properties. *Contraception* 1995; 52:269.

80. Pakarinen P, Toivonen J, Luukainen T. Therapeutic use of the LNG IUS, and counseling. *Semin Reprod Med* 2001;19:365.

81. Ellertson C, Trussell J, Stewart F, et al. Emergency contraception. *Semin Reprod Med* 2001;19:323.

CHAPTER 27

Nonhormonal Contraception

RICHARD E. BLACKWELL

It is difficult to use population demographics to estimate the use of contraception and its failure. In the United States it is estimated that there are 466 births per hour, 249 deaths, 101 net immigration, 318 net population growth, 268 marriages, and 136 divorces. Approximately 35 percent of the births in this country are out of wedlock; however, this reflects a worldwide trend, with countries such as Iceland having nearly 60 percent of their children born out of wedlock. Further, the demand for single-woman insemination in this country is rising rapidly as many women who have put off child-bearing are approaching the end of their reproductive lifespan. *Time* Magazine recently pointed out the subject of babies versus careers, indicating that nearly one-half the women in corporate America were childless and unmarried. At the opposite end of the spectrum, the percentage of births to mothers younger than 12 years of age was the highest in Los Angeles at 45.3 percent, and the percentage of births to teenagers who were already mothers was highest in the District of Columbia at 28 percent. Teenage motherhood was lowest in the state of Massachusetts at 7.2 percent and highest in Mississippi at 20 percent. Louisiana, Mississippi, Alabama, Georgia, South Carolina, and North Carolina had the highest rates of gonorrhea in the country. Despite the fact that we spend more of our gross national product on health care than any other country, contra-

ception is covered in the United States in Maine, New Hampshire, Vermont, Connecticut, Maryland, Virginia, Kentucky, North Carolina, Georgia, Texas, Iowa, Minnesota, Idaho, Nevada, California, and Hawaii. There are active bills before the legislature to provide coverage in Illinois and New York.

▶ HISTORY

Contraception has been used for 3000 years. The forerunner of modern contraception includes sea sponges, medicated steams and douches to instill anti–human seed medicates, cervical caps and diaphragms made in China and Japan, disks of oil silk paper placed against the cervix, and wax wafers and linen cloths as diaphragms in Europe. Other methods included honey and crocodile dung, rock salt, alum, quinoquin, fried quicksilver and oil, swallowing fourteen live tadpoles, and eating mule uteri. Tubes of cat liver have been tied to the left foot, and potions of willow leaves, slag, iron rust, clay, and mule kidneys have been used, European brides were taught to sit on their fingers while riding in a coach, and walnuts placed in the bosom have been used for every barren year desired.[1]

Until recently, among women ages 15 to 50 years, the following methods were used for contraception[2] (Table 27-1): 26 percent used

▶ **TABLE 27-1:** CONTRACEPTIVE USE

Birth control pills (BCPs)	26%
Sterilization	24%
Condoms	19%
Withdrawal and rhythm	7%
Hysterectomy	6%
Injectable	3%
Spermicide	1%
Intrauterine devices (IUDs)	1%
Implants	1%

the birth control pill, 24 percent used sterilization, 19 percent used condoms, 7 percent used withdrawal and rhythm, 6 percent used hysterectomy and menopause, 3 percent used injectable contraceptives, 1 percent used spermicide, 1 percent used intrauterine devices (IUDs), and 1 percent used implants. The failure rate of these techniques is quoted as 26 percent for spermicides, about 24 percent for withdrawal and rhythm, 21 percent for periodic abstinence, 14 percent for male condoms, 13 percent for diaphragms and cervical caps, 7 percent for oral contraceptive agents (although recent studies have suggested that this may be as high as 9 percent), 3 percent for injectable contraceptives, and 2 percent for contraceptive implants[3,4] (Table 27-2). There was a change in contraceptive use by married couples between 1973 and 1988. Female sterilization has increased, as has male sterilization. The use of oral contraceptive agents has decreased, and the use of IUDs has decreased. As expected, the use of contraception varies markedly by age, with women ages 35 to 44 being much

▶ **TABLE 27-2:** FAILURE RATE OF VARIOUS CONTRACEPTIVE AGENTS

Spermicide	26%
Withdrawal and rhythm	24%
Condoms	14%
Diaphragms	13%
Birth control pills (BCPs)	7-9%
Injectable	3%
Implants	2%
Sterilization	0.4%

more likely to undergo sterilization than their younger counterparts; the same is true for males. Women in the 15- to 24-year age group are much more likely to use birth control pills as well as condoms for contraception. Women in the 25- to 34-year age group are more likely to use a diaphragm or the rhythm method, and IUDs seem to be used more frequently in the 35- to 44-year age group. However, with the advent of newer contraceptive technologies, such as the Ortho Evra skin patch, the Nuva intrauterine ring, the Lunelle injection, and the Mirena progesterone-secreting IUD, these statistics are very likely to change (see Chapter 26).

Ninety-five percent of the 54 million U.S. women between the ages of 15 and 44 use contraception. It is of interest that female physicians use contraceptive agents at different rates than their patients.[5] For instance, 4501 physicians were studied between 1993 and 1994 as part of the women's physician health study. They range in age between 30 and 44 years, and it was found that physicians used more contraception than the general population; they used greater numbers of IUDs, diaphragms, and condoms; and they used far fewer sterilizations of all types. The younger physicians were less likely to be sterilized than the general population; one in five physicians used more than one type of contraception; Caucasian physicians did not tend to use tubal ligations; Asian and black physicians did not use vasectomy; black and Caucasian physicians used a great deal more birth control pills; Asian and Hispanic physicians used condoms; and Caucasians but not Asians used diaphragms. Female physicians have 1.55 children versus 2.04 for the general population.

▶ TYPES OF CONTRACEPTION

Condoms have been used since antiquity. The Romans used animal bladders for this purpose; Egyptians dyed sheaths various colors. Fallopius devised the linen sheath in the sixteenth century; in 1838, rubber was vulcanized. Casanova described the condom as "the armor against enjoyment and a spiderweb against danger." The latex condom is typically between 0.3 and 0.8 mm thick, whereas sperm is 0.003 mm in diameter (Fig. 27-1). The condom excludes virus and bacteria and is made of lambskin, latex, polyurethane, and neoprene.[6,7] An issue that has been raised with latex condom use has to do with type I and type II allergic reactions. There are significant numbers of reactions to latex condoms, and deaths have been reported. There is a movement toward making nonlatex condoms from polyurethane; however, these devices, while quite sturdy, are hard to fit and frequently slip off during intercourse.

Dr. Frederick Wilde invented the diaphragm in 1858. Diaphragms ranged between 50 and 105 mm, although 60- to 70-mm diaphragms are worn by most women. The diaphragm must be fitted and seems to be most effective when used with a spermicide generally containing nonoxynol-9. Cervical caps are a smaller version of the diaphragm and fit over the cervix. Two prototypes are available, the Fem Cap and the Leah shield. The latter was not approved by the Food and Drug Administration (FDA) for use[8–10] (see Fig. 27-1).

The female condom, sold under the trade name Reality, is a polyurethane device with an

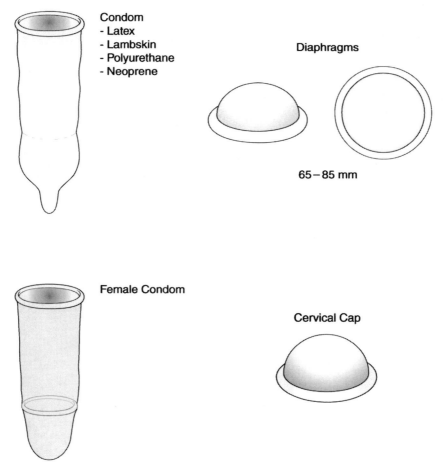

Figure 27-1 Barrier contraceptive devices.

internal ring that fits behind the symphysis pubis and an external ring that lies on the labia. The female condom has a failure rate of about 26 percent per year and in preference studies was one of the least appealing contraceptive devices evaluated[11,12] (see Fig. 27-1).

The intrauterine device (IUD) was developed by Jack Lippes. It is said that the Lippes loop was prepared originally using a cookie cutter and that the IUDs were baked in an oven on a cookie sheet. It is also said that "the IUDs turned out perfectly but Mrs. Lippes' cookie sheet was ruined." The IUD, while not enjoying wide use in the United States, with

sales in 1988 of 0.7 million, is the most widely used form of contraception in the world. Seventy-nine million IUDs were placed in China, and the world use of IUDs is 83 million units. Lack of popularity in the United States stems from the experience with the Dalkon shield, which had a braided tail and appeared to enhance pelvic infection rates among certain social classes of users. All of today's IUDs have monofilament strings; most contemporary IUDs are either copper wound or release a progestogen over time, although there are rings used in China that have no string and are designed not be removed (Fig. 27-2). Contraindications to

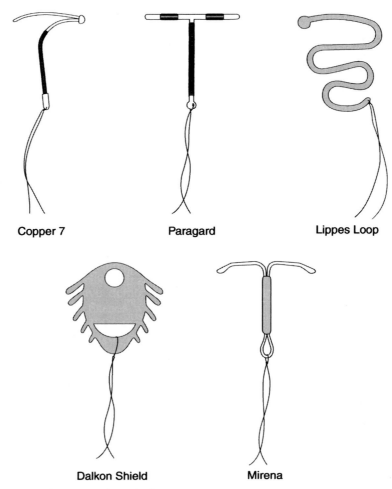

Copper 7   Paragard   Lippes Loop

Dalkon Shield   Mirena

Figure 27-2 Types of intrauterine devices.

IUD use include pelvic infection, abnormal uterine bleeding, and obviously, pregnancy.[13–15]

Spermicides, primarily the detergent nonoxynol-9, have been used for many years as contraceptive agents either with condoms or diaphragms or alone. This observation suggests that the failure rate alone is approximately 26 percent, and some recent evidence suggests that rather than retard the transmission of human immunodeficiency virus (HIV), perhaps the rate of transmission is enhanced at least in sex providers in Subsaharan Africa.[16–18] Since these gels or foams contain detergents, irritation of the urethra may occur in men or in women. Nevertheless, they are relatively inexpensive, easy to use, and do not require a prescription. A number of other agents are being examined for spermicidal activities; for instance, AZT derivatives have both spermicide and anti-HIV properties, and phenethyl-5-bromopyridyl, thiourea (PBT), and venatium-4 metalasine complexes have been described as having spermicidal properties.[19] None of these are available commercially; however, the National Institutes of Health (NIH) are very interested in providing a new spermicidal preparation and are currently testing the biogel product in clinical trials.

▶ SURGERY

The surgical approach to sterilization consists of vasectomy in men, and tubal ligation, hysterectomy, possibly endometrial ablation, and hysteroscopic tubal occlusion in women. The vasectomy can be performed as an outpatient procedure under local anesthesia and has been adopted widely in third-world countries such as India. The process is potentially reversible, but the highest pregnancy rates tend to occur within 2 years of the original procedure, with 6 to 10 years being the maximum time that should elapse between the initial procedure and reversal. It is said that approximately 50 percent of men who have vasectomies will have sperm antibodies involving either the head, midpiece, or tail of the spermatozoa. In

the event that the male is antibody-positive, intrauterine insemination (ISI), in vitro fertilization (IVF), or IVF with intracytoplasmic injection may well produce pregnancy.[20,21]

There are numerous types of tubal ligations, the most widely used being the postpartum type, which involves making a small incision in the umbilicus either at the time of delivery or the morning after (Fig. 27-3). The fallopian tubes generally are delivered through the incision, grasped at the isthmic ampullary junction. A knuckle of tube is ligated twice with no. 3 plain gut suture, and the tubal segment is resected and sent to pathology for evaluation. Alternative techniques include fimbriectomy with resection of the distal end of the fallopian tubes, bringing the proximal end of the fallopian tube into the uterus (the Irving procedure) or burying the fallopian tubes in the mesosalpinx (the Uchida procedure). A popular technique used some years back was a vaginal tubal ligation, in which a posterior colpotomy incision was made, the tubes were delivered into the vagina, and either a Pomeroy-type technique or fimbriectomy was performed. These procedures are quick and straightforward; however, the couple must avoid intercourse long enough to allow the colpotomy incision to heal. The advent of the laparoscope allowed for the fallopian tube to be occluded in a number of manners, with a clip such as the Hulka or Bealer clip, the tube may be occluded by placing a plastic grommet over a Pomeroy-type knuckle using the Fallope ring, or the tube may be cauterized at the isthmic ampullary junction and allowed to occlude thermally, or the tube can be transected. The failure rate with all these techniques is about 2 women per 1000 per lifetime.[22,23]

Endometrial ablation, either using a rollerball, rollerbar, deep resection, or thermal ablation, will essentially destroy the endometrium and render a patient amenorrheic. None of these techniques has FDA approval for use as a contraceptive agent, and there is some concern that pregnancy possibly may be able to occur after such a procedure. Nevertheless, the

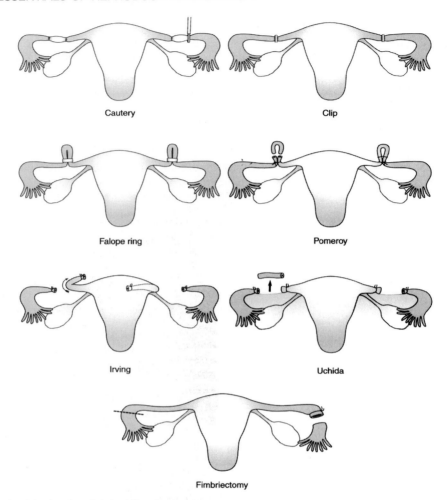

Figure 27-3 Methods of tubal ligation.

likelihood of a pregnancy following such a technique is slight.

Hysterectomy historically was used for sterilization, particularly when performed in Catholic hospitals, which banned tubal ligations. Given the large array of contraceptive means available today, there seems to be little indication for performing such an invasive procedure unless the patient had other pathology such as extensive endometriosis, cancer, large fibroids, or significant prolapse.

Transcervical tubal occlusion has been investigated for many years. A number of agents

have been injected into the fallopian tube, including silicon, methrylates, quinocrine, and other sclerosing agents. The failure rate with these techniques was as high as 26 percent. Recently, a springlike device has been approved by the FDA for transcervical sterilization. Essure was developed by Conceptus, Inc. It involves the hysteroscopic placement of a microinsert into the fallopian tubes that causes tissue ingrowth and occlusion. It has been shown to be 99.8 percent effective in 2 years of follow-up in hundreds of women who participated in the Stop Prehysterectomy Investigation Group Trial carried out worldwide.[24] The acceptability of this method remains to be seen. While reversal appears to be unlikely due to the inflammation and fibrosis produced from the tubal ostia into the isthmic portion of the tube, the effect of this technique on the outcome of IVF is unknown. One question that would have to be answered is whether the device would have to be removed from the fallopian tube because it is made of inert metal, which might prove to be embryotoxic. The other question is how to removed it. It would seem that the extensive fibrosis produced by the device may make it exceedingly difficult to remove transcervically, and obviously, cutting into the cornual area of the tube endoscopically or with open abdominal surgery may well weaken the uterus and result in cornual rupture during an intrauterine pregnancy.

▶ FUTURE

While a number of new contraceptive devices have been introduced into the market, they are by and large redesigns of old products. There is a dearth of contraceptive research, which is of great concern to the NIH. This shortage of investigation is due to the fact that these are difficult trials to perform; the obvious outcome of a trial failure is pregnancy with the possibility of a teratogenic effect on the offspring. Further, the legal climate is not conducive for contraceptive research, and many products are sold on the international market at a highly discounted price. Nevertheless, several areas of investigation have been suggested. There is interest in developing a vaccine to the beta chain of human chorionic gonadotropin (hCG), gonadotropin-releasing hormone (GnRH), follicle-stimulating hormone (FSH), luteinizing hormone (LH), zona pellucida (ZP) antigen, acrosome-associated protein, and low-density lipoprotein (LDH). There is also considerable interest in a male contraceptive device that would involve a combination of treatment with a GnRH antagonist combined with replacement testosterone. Further, several medications such as calcium channel blockers, Azulfidine, and other medications have been shown to decrease male fertility, as have herbal therapies such as echinacea, St. John's Wort, and gingko. This would seem to leave open many possible avenues for the development of the next generation of contraceptive devices.

Despite the negative financial, economic, and legal pressures on contraceptive development, developed countries such as those in Europe have entered a critical phase of their demographic evolution. Somewhere around the year 2000 the population began to generate *negative momentum*. This event occurred because of the low fertility rate over the last 30 years. It is estimated that for each additional decade that fertility remains at its current level, the European union will decline by 20 to 40 million people. The fertility rate is falling because European couples are delaying reproduction until later ages presumably because of social and economic advantages. This has resulted in a population decline of about 88 million people. This fuels a deeply rooted fear of population decline being linked with a possible weakening of national identity and loss of international policy and economic standing. Some have said that childbearing should come to be considered a social act rather than purely a private decision. In 1976, East Germany implemented a policy of improved child care facilities, financial benefits, and government-supported housing for women who became pregnant. Consequently, fertility, which had paralleled that of West Germany, increased from 1.5 to 1.9. This would suggest that current contraceptive practices are highly effective in bringing about these population declines and that this process can be readily reversed given favorable social, economic, and political circumstances.

These types of population declines are being seen in all developed countries. It is estimated that the population in Japan will shrink by 40 to 50 percent over the next 30 to 40 years, and couples in the United States are reproducing at below-replacement rates with the exception of the Hispanic population. These population shifts have profound implications in terms of support ratio, with the number of working-age persons declining significantly against the number of increasing retirees. It has been estimated that by 2065 there could be as few as 0.5 workers per elderly person in developed populations. Add to these trends the use of therapeutic abortions, population control, and interceptive abortive agents such as RU486, and one could easily see that the whole topic of contraception and contraception development exists in an economic, social, political, and religious cauldron. All these factors come into play when the public chooses to reward or punish government agencies and corporations for manipulating the human reproductive process.[25]

KEY POINTS

1. The populations of underdeveloped countries are declining due to the success of currently available contraceptive agents and social, economic, and political motivating factors.

2. The three most popular contraceptive techniques used in the United States are birth control pills (26 percent), sterilization (24 percent), and condoms (19 percent).

3. The most popular means of contraception worldwide is the IUD.

4. Ninety-five percent of U.S. women between the ages of 15 and 45 use contraception.

5. While most condoms are made of latex, the increasing rate of type I and type II allergic reactions has brought about the development of polyurethane- and neoprene-based condoms.

6. The estimated use of IUDs worldwide is 83 million units.

7. Tubal ligation enjoys a failure rate of 2 women per 1000 per lifetime.

8. The newest form of sterilization is transcervical occlusion of fallopian tubes using the Essure system, which claims a 99.8 percent efficacy rate in a 2-year follow-up period.

REFERENCES

1. Tatum HJ, Connell-Tatum EB. Barrier contraception: A comprehensive overview, in Wallach EE, Kempers RD (eds), *Modern Trends in Infertility and Conception Control*, Vol 2. Chicago: Year Book medical, 1982:437–447.

2. Forrest JD. Has she or hasn't she? U.S. women's experience with contraception. *Fam Plan Perspect* 1987;19:133.

3. Forrest JD, Fordyee RR. U.S. women's contraceptive attitudes and practice: How have they changed in the 1980s? *Fam Plan Perspect* 1988;20:112–118.

4. Trussell J, Hatcher RA, Cates W, et al. Contraceptive failure in the United States: An update. *Stud Fam Plan* 1990;21:51–54.

5. Frank A. Contraceptive use by female physicians in the USA. *Obstet Gynecol* 1999;99:66.

6. Rietmeijer CA, Krebs JW, Feorino PM, et al. Condoms as physical and chemical barriers against human immunonondeficiency virus. *JAMA* 1988;259:1851–1853.

7. Connell EB. Barrier methods of contraception: A reappraisal. *Int J Gynaecol Obstet* 1979;16:479.

8. Bounds W, Guillebaud J, Dominik R, Dalberth B. The diaphragm with and without spermicide: A randomized comparative efficacy trail. *J Reprod Med* 1995;40:764–774

9. Cook L, Nanda K, Grimes D. The diaphragm with and without spermicide for contraception: A Cochrane review. *Eur Soc Hum Reprod Embryol* 2002;1.4:867–869.

10. Archer D, Mauck C, Viniegra-Sibal A, Anderson FD. Lea shield: A phase I postcoital study of a new contraceptive study barrier device. *Contraception* 1995;52:162–173.

11. Trussell J, Sturgen K, Strickler J, et al. Comparative contraceptive efficacy of the female condom and other barrier methods. *Fam Plan Perspect* 1994;26:66–72.

12. Shihata A, Trussell J. New female intervaginal barrier contraceptive device. *Contraception* 1991;44:11–19.

13. Population Reports. *IUDs: A New Look,* Series B, No 5: *Intrauterine Devices.* Baltimore: Johns Hopkins University Press, 1988:1–31.

14. American College of Obstetricians and Gynecologists. The intrauterine devices and pelvic inflammatory disease: An international perspective. *Lancet* 1992;339:785.

15. Grimes DA. The intrauterine device, pelvic inflammatory disease and infertility: The confusion between hypothesis and knowledge. *Fertil Steril* 1992;58:670.

16. Curtis KM, Chrisman CE, Peterson HB. Contraception for women in selected circumstances. *Obstet Gynecol* 2002;99:1100–1112.

17. Roddy RE, Zekeng L, Ryan KA, et al. Effect of nonoxynol-9 gel on urogenital gonorrhea and chlamydial infection: A randomized, controlled trial. *JAMA* 2002;287:1117–1122.

18. Richardson BA. Nonoxynol-9 as a vaginal microbicide for prevention of sexually transmitted infections. *JAMA* 2002;287:1171–1172.

19. D'Cruz OJ, Uckun FM. Contraceptive activity of a spermicidal aryl phosphate derivative of bromo-methoxy-zidovudine (compound WHI-07) in rabbits. *Fertil Steril* 2003;79:864–872.

20. Alexander NJ, Anderson DJ. Vasectomy: Consequences of autoimmunity to sperm antigens, in Wallach EE, Kempers RD (eds), *Modern Trends in Infertility and Conception Control,* Vol 2. Chicago: Year Book Medical, 1982:448–455.

21. Li S, Golten M, Zhu J, Huber D. The no scalpel vasectomy. *Gen Urol* 1991;145:341.

22. Trussell J, Guilbert E, Hedley A. Sterilization reversal, and pregnancy after sterilization reversal in Quebec. *Am Coll Obstet Gynecol* 2003;101:677–684.

23. Jamieson DJ, Kaufman SC, Costello C, et al. A comparison of women's regret after vasectomy versus tubal sterilization. *Am Coll Obstet Gynecol* 2002;99:1073–1069.

24. Valle RF, Carignan CS, Wright TC. The Stop Prehysterectomy Investigation Group. *Fertil Steril* 2001;76:574–980.

25. Lutz W, O'Neill BC, Scherbov S. Europe's population at a turning point. *Science* 2003;299:1991–1992.

Menopause

CHAPTER 28

Physiology of the Perimenopause and Menopause

Nora R. Miller and Nanette F. Santoro

As preventative and interventional medicine continue to improve, the average American life expectancy is predicted to lengthen[1] (Fig. 28-1). Many women today are living up to a third of their lives postmenopausally. These trends are resulting in an enormous increase in the population of postreproductive-age women. In the year 2020, population projections estimate that almost 52 million women will be ages 55 and older.[2] Women's health issues during the transition from perimenopause through the postmenopausal years are becoming increasingly prevalent and are important to address. In this chapter we will discuss the physiology of the perimenopause and menopause. We will attempt to differentiate the consequences of aging per se from the effects of menopause.

▶ CLINICAL FEATURES

Definitions

Menopause refers to the time period that begins 1 year after the cessation of menstruation.[3] The definition of menopause is based on the low likelihood (<10 percent) that a woman age 45 or older will have another menstrual period after 1 year of amenorrhea.[4] Menopause can occur at any age, with a median age of 51.5 years. A woman is considered to have *premature ovarian failure* if menses stop for at least 6 months before age 40 and is accompanied by an elevated follicle-stimulating hormone (FSH) level, usually >40 IU/mL.[5] The term *premature menopause* is considered

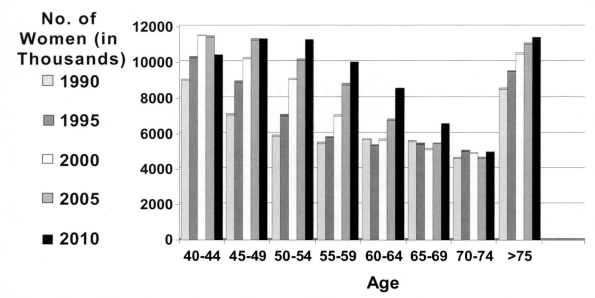

Figure 28-1 Women by age group. Women are living longer. The most substantial increase in populations are in women ages 55 to 59 and greater than 75 years old. *(Adapted from projections by the U.S. Census Bureau.[1,2])*

inappropriate because these women often will have evidence of estrogen or progesterone production and, although rare, can conceive. Women who undergo menopause between the ages of 40 and 45 are considered to have *early menopause* and comprise about 5 percent of the population.[6]

A woman's age at menopause can be affected by several variables. A mother's age at menopause is predictive of the age at which her daughter will stop menstruating.[7] Nulliparity or unopposed ovulation is associated with an earlier menopause, whereas multiparity and oral contraceptive use are predictive of a later age at menopause.[8] Environmental conditions can accelerate the age at which a woman will become menopausal. Tobacco use advances menopause by an average of 1.5 years.[7,8] Chemotherapy and radiation treatment can cause menopause to occur sooner.[9] Pelvic surgery, including uterine artery embolization, can cause ovarian failure to occur earlier by compromising ovarian blood flow.[10] A vegetarian diet was shown to advance the age at

menopause by 2 years in one study.[7] Conversely, a woman's age at menarche is the only reproductive factor that does not affect when menopause will happen. The age at which menopause occurs has not changed over the past century.[11]

Perimenopause defines the interval in the late reproductive years when menstrual cycles become irregular[12] (Fig. 28-2). Perimenopause usually begins when women are in their midforties, and the average duration is 4 years. Intermenstrual lengths can vary greatly because some cycles are anovulatory, whereas others still remain normal. During this time, FSH is elevated compared with younger women, and serum estrogen may be increased at first and then declines more precipitously as cycles get longer. Perimenopause has been divided into an early and a late phase. Early perimenopause starts when a woman's menstrual cycles begin to change from the regular pattern of her reproductive years. Late perimenopause is characterized by lengthened intermenstrual cycles. After a woman experiences 3 to 11 months of

				Final Menstrual Period (FMP)			
Stages:	**-5**	**-4**	**-3**	**-2**	**-1** **0**	**+1**	**+2**
Terminology:	Reproductive			Menopausal Transition		Postmenopause	
	Early	Peak	Late	Early	Late*	Early*	Late
				Perimenopause			
Duration of Stage:	variable			variable		(a) 1 yr (b) 4 yrs	until demise
Menstrual Cycles:	variable to regular	regular		variable cycle length (*>7 days different from normal*)	≥2 skipped cycles and an interval of amenorrhea (*≥60 days*)	Amen x 12 mos none	
Endocrine:	normal FSH		↑ FSH	↑ FSH		↑ FSH	

Stages most likely to be characterized by vasomotor symptoms   ↑ = elevated

Figure 28-2 Stages of menopause transition. This diagram demonstrates a staging system for the menopausal transition. The early perimenopause begins at stage −2 when menstrual cycle irregularity starts. Stage −1 correlates with the late perimenopause when episodes of amenorrhea are prevalent and vasomotor symptoms typically begin. One year after the FMP *(a)*, the patient is menopausal and has entered stage +1, the early menopause. Five years after the FMP, the patient is in the late postmenopause, stage +2, which is the final stage and continues until death.

amenorrhea, she has entered the late phase.[13] Perimenopause ends 1 year after the final menstrual period (FMP).

Symptoms

Hot Flashes

Most women will experience vasomotor instability (i.e., hot flashes) as they traverse the menopause. The prevalence varies from 60 to 82 percent among women who undergo a natural menopause.[14] However, women who undergo a surgical menopause have a 90 percent prevalence of hot flashes.[15] The probability of experiencing vasomotor symptoms is related to

socioeconomic status, body mass index (BMI), cultural factors, geographic location, and diet.[16]

Symptomatic women describe a hot flash as lasting 1 to 5 minutes. Forty percent have a premonition before the flash occurs. The median duration of hot flashes is 4 years, with 87 percent of women having them daily and, among those, 33 percent having more than 10 per day.[17] The actual hot flash has been described as sweating of the face, head, neck, and chest with the sensation traveling from a cranial to caudal direction. Other frequent symptoms include a sense of heat and flushing, followed by clamminess, chills, and sometimes anxiety.[14] Sweating can be profuse following the episode.

Studies of symptomatic women have identified peripheral vasodilatation of the forehead, cheek, chest, upper arm, back, and thigh. Skin conductance, a means of measuring sweating, increased in 90 percent of recorded hot flashes and concurred with actual sweating. However, core body temperature measurements using esophageal and tympanic temperatures do not identify a precipitating rise. It is possible that the lag time using these measurements is too long to identify a temperature change. Freedman and colleagues used an ingested telemetry pill to monitor rapid changes in core body temperature in real time and found 60 percent of hot flashes to be preceded by a small but significant temperature rise—with no change in rectal temperature. Heart rate also increases during hot flashes by 7 to 15 beats per minute. Peripheral warming can be used to reproduce hot flashes. Water pads set at 42°C and applied to the torso can cause hot flashes in symptomatic but not in asymptomatic women.[14]

What causes one woman to be symptomatic and another not to be? Plasma and urinary estrogens, as well as vaginal maturation index, do not differ between women who experience hot flashes and those who do not. No differences in FSH or luteinizing hormone (LH) have been determined,[14] although the hot flash itself is associated with an acute rise in LH[18] in some, but not all, women. Women who have pituitary insufficiency, are hypophysectomized, or have been administered a gonadotropin-releasing hormone (GnRH) agonist have no LH release but still may experience hot flashes.[14] This finding rules out a causal relationship between the LH pulse and the hot flash.

There is evidence that central norepinephrine may be responsible for triggering hot flashes. Peripheral norepinephrine is not elevated prior to or after a hot flash. The main metabolite of brain norepinephrine is 3-methoxy-4-hydroxyphenylglycol (MHPG), of which 50 percent is metabolized to vanillylmandelic acid (VMA). Freedman found a significant increase in MHPG but not VMA after a hot flash.[19] Consistent with these data, administration of α_2-adrenergic antagonist yohimbine reproduced hot flashes in symptomatic but not in asymptomatic women. The converse is also true. By treating symptomatic women with the α_2-adrenergic agonist clonidine, the frequency of hot flashes was decreased. The length of time required to reproduce hot flashes in clonidine-pretreated patients using heated water pads also was increased.[20] Systemic estrogen therapy appears to decrease the frequency and even suppress hot flashes in women. Estrogen regulates adrenergic receptors in numerous tissues. Therefore, the withdrawal of estrogen may affect the hypothalamic adrenergic receptors, causing increased central norepinephrine levels.[14]

Current understanding of the pathophysiology of hot flashes centers on the brain's thermoregulatory system, which seems to be altered in women susceptible to hot flashes. Women with hot flashes begin sweating at a lower temperature than asymptomatic females (37.2 versus 37.6°C). Symptomatic women also begin shivering at a higher temperature than women without hot flashes (36.4 versus 36.1°C).[14] In other words, the shivering threshold is raised, and the sweating threshold is lowered. As a result, women who experience hot flashes have a narrower temperature range in which they feel comfortable when compared with asymptomatic women. Current investigation is focused on treatments that may widen or restore the thermal "comfort zone" for symptomatic women. In the meantime, simple measures such as layering of clothing and maintaining the ambient temperature several degrees lower than is customary may help to reduce the frequency and severity of hot flashes in susceptible women by avoiding or reducing the environmental triggers.

Menstrual Irregularities

Perimenopause begins when menstrual cycle irregularity starts.[12] While there is no specific pattern that definitively describes the onset of perimenopause, it is best characterized by a deviation from a woman's previously regular cycling pattern. Virtually nothing is known about women with chronically irregular menstrual cycles in their midreproductive years. These menstrual-based definitions, though crude, appear to have relevance to hormonal patterns and to the timing of the transition stages (see Fig. 28-2).

Metcalf and colleagues were the first to investigate urinary hormones during the perimenopause. They described cycle shortening at the onset of the perimenopause.[21] Shideler and collaborators also studied hormones of perimenopausal women. They identified elevations in estrogen that rose two- to threefold higher than in normal cycles.[22] Santoro and colleagues studied perimenopausal women prospectively by measuring daily urinary hormones in six regularly cycling women age 47 and older for 1 year. For controls, midreproductive-age women and postmenopausal women were compared with the perimenopausal patients. By analyzing the urinary

hormones of the perimenopausal women, follicular-phase shortening and decreased cycle length were identified when compared with the younger patients. FSH, LH, and estrone excretion were significantly higher when compared with the younger women. However, peak estrone concentrations in the perimenopausal patients were not different from those of reproductive-age women.[23] Pregnanediol excretion and serum progesterone concentration have been reported to be significantly lower in some[24,25] but not other[26] studies of perimenopausal women (Fig. 28-3).

Investigators have divided the perimenopause into early and late phases to more accurately describe menstrual pattern alterations. In the early perimenopause, menstrual cycle irregularity has started (usually defined as either a "skipped" cycle or a change in intermenstrual interval of 7 or more days) from the normal 21 to 35 days.[27] The transition to

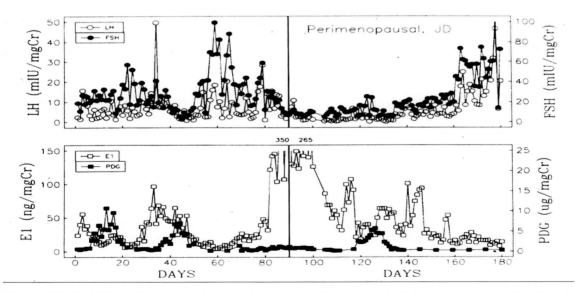

Figure 28-3 Urinary hormones in a perimenopausal woman. In this figure, one patient's urinary FSH, LH, estrone (E$_1$), and pregnanediol (PDG) levels are recorded. Both FSH and LH elevations are demonstrated in the follicular phase. Estrone clearly is elevated, particularly between days 60 and 110, when no ovulation occurred. Three ovulatory cycles are shown with a rise in PDG, but there are also prolonged intervals of anovulation demonstrated by no rise in PDG. This is an example of the erratic menstrual cycles of the perimenopause. *(Reprinted, with permission, from the Endocrine Society.[23])*

late perimenopause occurs after a woman begins having episodes of amenorrhea from 3 to 11 months in duration.[13] In Taffe's study, patients in the late perimenopause had long intermenstrual intervals. When the mean cycle length was greater than 42 days, the final menstrual period was likely to occur within the next 18 months.[27] After the FMP, for the first year serum estrone levels can vary. However, there is no progesterone secretion.[28]

Urogenital Atrophy

Late perimenopausal and menopausal women complain of urogenital atrophy. The most common symptoms include dryness, burning, irritation, dyspareunia, and pruritus.[29] Due to the loss of endogenous estrogen, all the tissues that have estrogen receptors are affected by the hormonal changes of menopause. The vaginal epithelium may become dry and atrophied, which causes vaginal itching, discomfort, and dyspareunia for some women. Dysuria, frequency, and urgency may follow. The increase in vaginal pH also may predispose some women to develop urinary tract infections.[30]

▶ MENOPAUSE EFFECTS BY ORGAN SYSTEM

The Endocrine System

The Hypothalamus

The medial basal hypothalamus releases GnRH in a pulsatile manner to stimulate pituitary gonadotropin secretion. During the reproductive years, ovarian steroids cause negative feedback on GnRH burst quantity (amplitude) and frequency. With the menopause-associated removal of ovarian steroids, the negative-feedback loop is opened, and GnRH is released at a maximal frequency and amplitude. Circulating FSH and LH rise up to fourfold higher after menopause than during the reproductive years.

There is no evidence in humans that hypothalamic changes contribute to the onset of menopause. Hall and colleagues have described some changes in GnRH secretion with age. They studied postmenopausal women, some of whom were recently menopausal and some of whom were about 20 years postmenopausal (mean ages 52 and 72 years, respectively). They measured free α subunit, FSH, and LH to track GnRH activity. GnRH pulsatility was detectably slower in older women compared with younger postmenopausal women, implying that aging is associated with a decrease in hypothalamic GnRH secretion.[31] There is also evidence that pulsatile LH and, by inference, GnRH secretion is less organized in its pattern with advancing age.[32]

The Pituitary

The pituitary is responsible for stimulating the ovary by secreting FSH and LH. However, after menopause, the ovary is no longer able to provide feedback and inhibit pituitary output. As a result, FSH and LH levels are tonically and maximally elevated. In a study by Hall and colleagues, 11 postmenopausal women who were an average of 52 years old had an FSH level of 172 IU/L and LH level of 86 IU/L. When compared with 11 women who were an average of 72 years old, a 27 to 40 percent decrease in circulating gonadotropins with advancing age was demonstrated in the face of similarly low estradiol concentrations.[31] These findings suggest that aging causes a decrease in the release of GnRH from the hypothalamus or of gonadotropins from the pituitary.

The Ovary

During perimenopause, the ovarian response to gonadotropin stimulation is variable. Some cycles are normal, with FSH and LH inducing ovulation. Other cycles may be anovulatory because no dominant follicle arises. The perimenopause is a result of the decreased number of remaining ovarian follicles. O'Connor has proposed a means of understanding how the diminished ovarian pool affects the menstrual cycle. Perimenopause begins when there are approximately 100 to 1000 remaining follicles per ovary. The reason that menstrual periods become variable in length is because there are cycles in which the ovary does not respond to gonadotropins. O'Connor describes this as an "inactive phase" in which there is no cohort of growing follicles. This probably occurs by chance, but because there are few remaining follicles, it becomes more common when a woman is older. Since there is no dominant follicle during the inactive phase, no feedback inhibition of gonadotropins occurs. FSH rises and eventually recruits follicles to grow. However, because the cycle had an inactive phase initially, it lasts longer than the usual 28 days.[33] In some cycles of perimenopausal women, this pattern clearly occurs. However, other cycles in which there is a normal-appearing follicle but no ovulation, with or without an LH surge, have been reported.[34,35] Park and associates hypothesized that perimenopausal women had a change in their mechanism for an LH surge. To test this hypothesis, they performed an estrogen challenge test using mid-reproductive-age women as controls. In response to the high dose of estrogen, all the younger patients had an LH surge, whereas only 1 of 8 of the perimenopausal women did.[35] The pathophysiologic basis of these types of cycles is at present less clear.

After menopause, there are few to no remaining ovarian follicles. As a result, the ovary is no longer able to respond to FSH and LH. Estradiol levels decrease to <20 pg/mL and do not decrease further after oophorectomy.[36] It has been proposed that the postmenopausal ovary is a source of androgens, even in the absence of functioning. However, there is now evidence that steroidogenic enzymes are not present in the postmenopausal ovarian stroma or hilum.[37]

Couzinet and colleagues studied 10 postmenopausal women with complete adrenal insufficiency and another 3 patients who also were ovariectomized. These investigators compared those women with 15 postmenopausal women and 15 women who were ovariectomized. Both these groups had normal adrenal function. Women with adrenal insufficiency had similarly low levels of testosterone, androstenedione, and dehydroepiandrosterone sulfate (DHEAS) whether they were ovariectomized or just postmenopausal. The authors then treated the postmenopausal women who had adrenal insufficiency with human chorionic gonadotropin (hCG) and observed no increase in androgens. Dexamethasone administration resulted in significant decreases in testosterone, androstenedione, and DHEAS in all the patients with normal adrenal function. In vitro analysis of tissue homogenates from postmenopausal ovaries lacked four key steroidogenic enzymes. FSH and LH receptors also were absent.[37] An independent laboratory has found similar results.[38]

The Adrenal Gland

The primary hormone secreted by the adrenal is DHEAS. Labrie and colleagues studied adrenal hormone levels in women from age 20 to 80 to determine the effects of aging. DHEAS concentrations peaked in women aged 20 to 30, with an average of 6.2 μM, and then decreased steadily. At ages 70 to 80, DHEAS levels were diminished by 74 percent to 1.6 μM, in agreement with others.[39,40] Other adrenal hormones also decrease with aging. Androstenedione peaks at ages 20 to 30 and then decreases to 62 percent in women 50 to 60 years old. Pregnenolone diminishes by 45 percent, and dehydroepiandrosterone (DHEA) drops by 69.7 percent between women in their twenties to those in their seventies. The ovary contributes to the production of these hormones during the reproductive years, but after menopause, it is only the adrenal gland that continues hormone production.[40]

The age-related decrease in DHEAS and its relationship to menopause are controversial. As a part of the Melbourne Women's Midlife Health Project, Burger and colleagues prospectively studied 172 women during the menopausal transition. By analyzing hormone levels longitudinally in these patients, these investigators observed no relationship between

DHEAS and a woman's FMP. DHEAS declined 1.5 percent with each year of advancing age, modified in an inverse fashion by BMI.[39] In a prospective, longitudinal study of the menopausal transition in the United States—the Study of Women's Health Across the Nation (SWAN)—Lasley and colleagues had different findings. DHEAS was noted to be elevated in some women in the latter stages of their menopausal transition. DHEAS also was shown to differ by ethnicity. Chinese and Japanese women had the highest DHEAS levels (168 and 142 μg/mL, respectively), whereas Hispanic and African-American women had the lowest (116 and 109 μg/mL, respectively).[41]

The Thyroid Gland

The secretion of thyroxine is the main endocrine function of the thyroid. Menopausal symptoms can be very similar to those of hypothyroidism. Fatigue, malaise, weight gain, cold intolerance, and dry skin can be presenting complaints for either menopause or a thyroid disorder. TSH testing has been recommended as a part of routine screening for women over age 60.[42] Thyroid function remains stable overall through menopause and beyond, but hypothyroidism is a relatively common disease, and screening should be ongoing throughout a woman's life. As a part of the National Health and Nutrition Examination Survey III, thyroid function testing was performed in 16,533 participants without known thyroid disease. Ten percent of the participants had antithyroperoxidase antibodies, with a higher prevalence seen in women and an increased rate with advancing age. The presence of antithyroperoxidase antibodies was significantly associated with thyroid dysfunction.[43]

Body Composition

Menopause may cause alterations in body composition and fat mass. In a study by Douchi and associates, 365 premenopausal and 201 postmenopausal women were analyzed for lean body and fat mass. With advancing age and postmenopausal status, lean mass significantly decreased, whereas the percentage of body and trunk fat increased. These investigators have suggested that menopause is responsible for the decrease in the trunk and total-body lean mass.[44]

Another study by Ferrara and colleagues analyzed adipose tissues of perimenopausal and postmenopausal women to determine if there are differences in metabolism. Using an in vitro model, these investigators compared adipose tissue in the abdominal and gluteal subcutaneous regions in women who were matched for race, BMI, and percentage of body fat. The two groups of women had similar fat cell sizes. The postmenopausal women had significantly lower lipolysis in the gluteal fat cells and significantly higher lipoprotein lipase activity in both the abdominal and gluteal regions, indicating slower adipose tissue metabolism when compared with younger women.[45] This could explain the increase in body fat and its distribution after menopause.

However, other studies have demonstrated that advancing age is responsible for the weight increases in women, not the menopausal transition. In a longitudinal study of 271 premenopausal women over 5 years, all the participants gained weight. There was no difference in weight accumulation between the patients who experienced menopause during the study and those who remained premenopausal.[45] Similarly, Davies investigated two cohorts of women through the menopausal transition. Weight rose linearly as a function of age in both patient groups, and menopausal status did not have any effect on weight gain.[47]

Physical activity is a powerful modifier of weight gain. BMIs were compared among premenopausal, perimenopausal, and menopausal women in a cross-sectional study of the participants of SWAN. The perimenopausal and surgically menopausal women had higher BMIs than the premenopausal women. However, the participants who underwent a natural menopause did not have higher BMIs than the premenopausal patients when corrected for age. After statistical analysis, the investigators determined that physical activity was the most accurate predictor of BMI, whereas menopausal status and age were the least predictive.[48]

The Cardiovascular System

Maintaining Cardiovascular Health

Before menopause, women have a much lower risk for cardiovascular events when compared with men their age. However, after menopause, this benefit slowly disappears over time such that a woman of 70 begins to have a risk identical to that of a male of the same age. Cardiovascular events are the leading cause of death in adult women[49] (Fig. 28-4). Perhaps the most important single intervention that a physician can make for his or her postmenopausal patients is to help prevent or delay the onset of this devastating disease. Since

recent data do not support the widespread prescription of hormones to avert this common problem, other strategies must be considered.

As a part of the Women's Health Initiative, an observational study of women's activity levels was conducted. Manson and colleagues identified the cardiovascular benefits of physical activity. They determined that walking—as well as vigorous exercise—prevented cardiovascular events in postmenopausal women regardless of their age, BMI, or ethnic background. On the other hand, a sedentary lifestyle correlated directly with an increase in the risk for a coronary event.[50]

Intermediate markers of the effects of exercise on the cardiovascular system have been studied. Healthy postmenopausal women who self-reported their activity levels were evaluated for vasoreactivity in response to cold pressor testing. There was a statistically significant

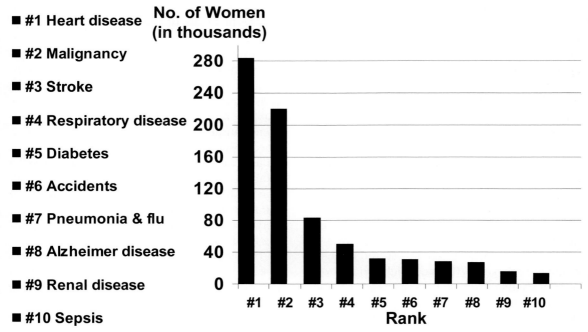

Figure 28-4   Most common causes of death in women in 2000. This figure demonstrates the 10 most common causes of death in women in 2000. Heart disease is by far the most common cause, accounting for the death of 284,304 women.   *(Used, with permission, from Minino et al.[23])*

increase in the percentage change for the patients who reported moderately demanding daily activities when compared with less active women.[51] Patients with preexisting coronary artery disease also were studied to determine the effects of exercise on endothelial function. Women who participated in a cardiac rehabilitation of leg exercises three times weekly over 10 weeks were compared with patients who did not exercise. The group that exercised had significant improvements in endothelial-dependent flow dilatation of the lower extremity and a 29 percent increase in their functional capacity at the end of the study.[52] Physical activity appears to be cardioprotective and should be recommended to menopausal patients.

Lipids

Physiologic levels of estrogen are known to help maintain a favorable lipoprotein profile. Therefore, after menopause and the subsequent decrease in estrogen, this favorable effect is lost. As a result, high-density lipoprotein (HDL) levels decrease and total cholesterol levels increase. Low HDL and increased low-density lipoproteins (LDL) are two independent risk factors for coronary heart disease.[53]

Diet and exercise can be used to improve cholesterol levels. Stefanick and colleagues studied lipoprotein levels in 180 postmenopausal women who had moderately elevated LDL or low HDL levels but were otherwise healthy. The patients were randomized to exercise, National Cholesterol Education Program (NCEP) step 2 diet, or both for 1 year. Substantial decreases in LDL and total cholesterol levels, diastolic blood pressure, resting heart rate, and weight were observed in women who followed the combined diet and exercise regimen for 1 year. HDL and triglyceride levels did not change.[53] These patients were at higher risk for heart disease and were still able to reduce their risk by modifying their diet and exercising regularly.

Coagulation

Changes in clotting parameters occur with aging. Fibrinogen, plasminogen activator inhibitor 1, and factor VII increase and cause a relative hypercoagulable state. This is thought to be a contributor to the increase in cardiovascular disease and cerebrovascular disease in older women.[42]

The Skeleton

Bone Architecture

Bone is constantly undergoing remodeling. A balance exists between the osteoblasts, cells that produce new bone, and osteoclasts, multinucleated giant cells that resorb bone. Bone is accrued during childhood, adolescence, and until age 30 by maintaining a positive balance between osteoblasts and osteoclasts.[54] Then, during adulthood, after peak bone mass has been achieved, there is a slow but steady decrease in bone mass of about 0.4 percent per year. There is a dramatic increase in bone loss beginning in the late perimenopause. Women lose 2 to 5 percent of their bone mass per year for the first 5 to 10 years from the FMP.[55]

Osteoporosis

Osteoporosis is characterized by a deterioration of the microarchitecture of the skeleton causing increased fragility of bones.[56] Osteoporosis is a major health problem in postmenopausal women and is the most common bone disease. Currently, it is estimated that 4 million to 6 million postmenopausal Caucasian women have osteoporosis, and another 13 million to 17 million women have osteopenia at the hip. One of two Caucasian females will experience an osteoporosis-related fracture during her lifetime. The most serious consequence of osteoporosis is a hip fracture. A woman's risk of hip fracture equals her combined risk of developing breast, ovarian, and uterine cancers.[57]

Women can be screened and those at risk identified before they develop osteoporosis (Table 28-1). Osteoporosis is both a preventable and a treatable disease. Screening is recommended for (1) all women over age 65, (2) postmenopausal women with a fracture

▶ **TABLE 28-1:** RISK FACTORS FOR OSTEOPOROSIS

Unmodifiable Risks	Diseases	Medications	Diet	Lifestyle
Female	Hyperthyroid	Corticosteroids	Low in calcium	Tobacco use
Caucasian or Asian	Hyperparathyroid	Heparin	Low in vitamin D	High in alcohol
Advancing age	Anorexia nervosa	Anticonvulsants	Poor nutrition	Sedentary
Family history in first-degree relative	Amenorrhea or hypoestrogenism	GnRH agonists	Excess caffeine	Thin or underweight
Prior fracture at age <50	Malabsorption syndromes	Lithium	Aluminum	
Early menopause	Multiple myeloma	Depo Provera		

From National Osteoporosis Foundation.[5]

(so that the diagnosis of osteoporosis can be confirmed), (3) women who are considering therapy for osteoporosis if knowing their bone mineral density (BMD) would assist in their decision making, (4) women who have been on prolonged hormone-replacement therapy (HRT) in order to monitor the effectiveness of their treatment, and (5) postmenopausal women younger than age 65 who have more than one risk factor for the development of osteoporosis.[57]

There are many tests that can be done to measure BMD. The most widely available and most reproducible clinical test for screening and measuring response to treatment is a dual-energy x-ray absorptiometry (DEXA).[57] When using DEXA to measure BMD, the hip (the femoral neck, trochanter, and total hip—a combination of trabecular and cortical bone), lumbar spine (L_1–L_4, primarily trabecular bone), and sometimes the wrist are analyzed. Measurements are compared with those in age- and race-matched women. The Z score is based on a comparison of the patient with women her own age, and the T score is a comparison between the patient and women with peak BMDs. The T score is used to define osteoporosis and osteopenia. If a patient's T score is within 1 standard deviation (SD), she has a normal BMD. *Osteopenia,* which means "thin

bone," is defined as a T score of less than −1 SD but greater than −2.5 SD. Osteoporosis is diagnosed by BMD when a woman has a T score of −2.5 SD or less.[56] A woman has severe or established osteoporosis if she has a T score of less than −2.5 SD with a fracture. Common fracture sites for patients with osteoporosis include vertebral compression fracture, distal radial (Colle's) fracture, and hip fracture. Secondary osteoporosis is diagnosed when osteoporosis is the result of other conditions, diseases, or medications.[57]

Women who have a normal DEXA test result should be encouraged to take steps to maintain skeletal health and prevent the development of osteoporosis. Preventative treatment strategies should be initiated during the perimenopause. Calcium supplementation and regular weight-bearing exercise can slow bone loss but usually will not prevent it entirely in postmenopausal women. For postmenopausal women, the recommended daily allowance for calcium is 1200 mg, along with 400 to 800 IU of vitamin D. Exercise that exerts stress on the patient's bones helps to maintain BMD. This can be achieved by walking or running (to maintain the spine and hips) and weight lifting (to keep the upper extremities strong). An added benefit of exercise is that patients develop stronger muscles, making it less likely that they will fall.[57] Behavior modification also should be encouraged. Women should abstain from or decrease the amount of alcohol they consume, tobacco smoking should be halted, and medication that adversely affects BMD, such as corticosteroids, should be avoided.

Therapy for Osteoporosis

After a patient is appropriately screened for osteoporosis, treatment can be started. It is recommended that therapy be instituted in all women with a T score of less than -2 SD. If a woman has other risk factors for the development of osteoporosis and a T score of less than -1.5, treatment also should be initiated.[57] The diagnosis of osteoporosis is based on the lowest T score of either the hip or the spine.[58] Women with osteopenia and osteoporosis can be counseled similarly as a first step but also should begin treatment to prevent further bone loss. The Food and Drug Administration (FDA) has approved several medications for osteoporosis treatment (Table 28-2). Although estrogen-replacement therapy prevents bone loss and fractures, it is no longer recommended for osteoporosis treatment because its benefit in reducing fractures is offset by increased risks of breast cancer, venous thromboembolism, and cardiovascular events.[59] The newest medication available for the treatment of osteoporosis is human parathyroid hormone 1-34 [hPTH(1-34)], which is the only anabolic treatment available. Tibolone is another promising drug for the prevention of osteoporosis. Although tibolone has been used in Europe for almost 20 years, it is not yet approved by the FDA in the United States.[60]

After initiating therapy, response should be monitored to ensure patient compliance and the effectiveness of the treatment. Urinary and serum markers of bone formation and resorption can be used for this purpose (Table 28-3). Treatment response can be measured over an interval of days to months. However, these markers do not predict fracture risk, are only weakly associated with bone mass changes, and are expensive.[57] While DEXA also can be used to monitor treatment efficacy, frequent measurements can provide misleading results.[61]

The Genitourinary System

The Female Reproductive Tract

There are estrogen and progesterone receptors in most of the muscles and ligaments of the pelvic floor. These include the levator ani muscles, uterus, cervix, round ligaments, vagina, urethra, and bladder. Treatment for vaginal symptoms includes estrogen therapy (local or systemic) and vaginal moisturizers. Both these medications relieve symptoms by decreasing the vaginal pH and altering the fluid content of the endothelium.[62] Lubricants can help to restore moisture, and regular sexual activity may maintain epithelial health.[63]

The Bladder

Urinary tract infections (UTIs) become more common with advancing age. According to

▶ **TABLE 28-2:** THERAPY FOR OSTEOPOROSIS

Medication	Type	Dose	Indications
Alendronate	Bisphosphonate	10 mg qd	Prevention and treatment
Calcitonin	Salmon calcitonin	200 IU/spray qd	Treatment
hPTH(1-34)	Parathyroid hormone	400 U	Treatment
Raloxifene	SERM	60 mg qd	Prevention and treatment
Risedronate	Bisphosphonate	5 mg qd	Prevention and treatment
Tibolone	Synthetic steroid	2.5 mg qd	Prevention (not FDA approved)

From ref. 55.

▶ **TABLE 28-3:** MARKERS OF BONE FORMATION AND RESORPTION

Bone Formation	Bone Resorption
Bone-specific alkaline phosphatase	C-telopeptides (urinary or serum)
Osteocalcin	N-telopeptides (urinary or serum)
Protein breakdown products of procollagen	Urinary pyridinolines
	Urinary deoxypyridinolines

From ref. 55.

some investigators, this is a direct effect of menopause,[64] whereas others interpret these changes as a result of aging.[65] Postmenopausal women who suffered from recurrent and symptomatic UTIs were randomized to local estrogen treatment or no therapy. Patients who were prescribed estrogen had a significant decrease in their incidence of another UTI. After 36 weeks of therapy, 45 percent of the women receiving estrogen had no recurrence, whereas only 20 percent of the control group remained infection-free. Local estrogen therapy significantly reduced the vaginal pH after 12 weeks of treatment when compared with the baseline level. Subjectively also, estrogen-treated patients had significant improvements in their symptoms when compared with the control group.[66]

Some studies have found incontinence to be related to menopausal status,[62] whereas others have not.[67] Sherburn and colleagues performed a cross-sectional study of Australian women between the ages of 45 and 55. In this population they identified a 15 percent prevalence of incontinence. Associated risk factors included gynecologic surgery, higher BMI, UTIs, constipation, and multiparity. Next, these investigators studied a subset of 373 premenopausal females over 7 years to determine if the menopause transition itself was associated with an increased incidence of incontinence. In this group of women the overall incidence of incontinence was 35 percent, with no increase associated with menopause. Incontinence was most closely related to hysterectomy during the course of the study.[67]

The Central Nervous System

Memory, Cognition

Memory decreases with advancing age. Although no direct effect on memory and cognition has been determined, many investigators suspect that there is a relationship to or an acceleration at menopause. In a cohort study of reproductive-age and postmenopausal women (not using HRT), cognitive functioning was assessed. In the postmenopausal patients, performance declined with advancing age. This was not the case for reproductive-age women. Premenopausal women in their forties were then compared with postmenopausal patients in the same decade of life. The premenopausal patients did substantially better in one aspect of testing—simulated driving reaction time. All other test results were similar between the two groups. These investigators concluded that there is an acceleration in the deterioration of some forms of cognitive function after menopause.[68]

Nappi and colleagues took another approach to identify whether menopause affects memory by comparing patients with natural and surgically induced menopause. The number of years since surgical menopause was inversely related to short-term memory, independent of age. There was a significant decrease in the short-term memory of the surgically menopausal women when compared with the naturally menopausal patients. There were no differences between the two groups with respect to long-term memory, selective and divided attention, or psychomotor functioning.[69]

Sherwin studied premenopausal women treated with GnRH analogues for 12 weeks, thereby creating a menopausal state. All the patients had a significant decline in their verbal memory testing when compared with baseline. Then one-half the patients were randomly prescribed add-back HRT in addition to the GnRH analogue for an additional 8 weeks. The patients taking estrogen replacement improved their verbal memory testing, whereas the patients who were taking the GnRH analogue alone had no change in their performance.[70] Some aspects of memory appear to be affected by menopause. However, women suffering from hot flashes have impaired sleep, which may have an impact on their short-term memory. Further studies are necessary before menopause can be definitively blamed for causing a decline in memory.

Libido

Although there has been a great deal of investigation of the relationship of circulating hormones to libido, definitive data are lacking. Many studies demonstrate that other factors besides menopause can account for changes in libido. Avis and colleagues studied sexual function in a subgroup of 200 women in the Massachusetts Women's Health Study II who underwent natural menopause. None took HRT, and all had sexual partners. Menopausal status was observed to be significantly related to decreased sexual interest. However, after adjustment for physical and mental health, smoking, and marital status, menopause status no longer had a significant relationship to libido.[71] Dennerstein prospectively evaluated 438 Australian women over 6 years during the menopausal transition. Menopause was significantly associated with dyspareunia and indirectly with sexual response. Psychological factors of feelings for one's partner, stress, and other social factors also indirectly affected sexual functioning.[72] These findings demonstrate that psychological as well as physical issues affect libido.

Other investigators have demonstrated that sexual problems are more prevalent after menopause. A longitudinal study of women during the perimenopause until at least 1 year after the FMP demonstrated a significant decrease in the rate of weekly coitus. Patients reported a significant decrease in the number sexual thoughts, sexual satisfaction, and vaginal lubrication after becoming menopausal.[73] In a study of 100 naturally menopausal women, both sexual desire and activity decreased when compared with the premenopausal period. Patients reported loss of libido, dyspareunia, and orgasmic dysfunction, with 86 percent reporting no orgasms after menopause.[74]

Clinical trial evidence suggests that estrogen and/or testosterone can help to restore sexual interest in surgically induced menopausal women.[75,76] DHEA supplementation also may acutely improve sexual interest and arousal in postmenopausal females, as well as in women with adrenal insufficiency.[77,78] However, to achieve normal libido in women, the levels of androgens need to be sufficiently high, which may lead to unwanted virilizing side effects.

The Breast

Breast Changes with Menopause

The breast undergoes change after menopause mainly as a result of hormonal withdrawal. Estrogen and progesterone bind to their respective receptors in the breast and exert proliferative effects on the ductal and glandular structures, respectively. Unlike in the uterus, there is chronic proliferative input to the breast. One therefore would expect that withdrawal of estrogen and progesterone accompanying menopause would lead to a relative reduction in breast proliferation. A significant reduction in the area and percentage of dense tissue on mammography was noted in a longitudinal study of peri- to postmenopausal patients. The areas of dense breast tissue were replaced with nondense (i.e., adipose) tissue. This was not the case for those women who were age-matched but remained premenopausal throughout the course of the study. These results imply that menopause has a greater effect on mammographic density than age.[79]

Further proof that breast tissue changes are a direct result of hormonal withdrawal comes from studies of women taking HRT. Greendale and colleagues studied radiographic changes in breast tissue in a subset of 307 women who were part of the Postmenopausal Estrogen/Progestin Intervention Trial. None of the participants had taken hormones within 5 years of their baseline mammogram. A comparison of breast density changes from baseline in women who took estrogen, HRT, or placebo was made. Women who initiated estrogen alone had a 3.5 percent increase in breast density, those who took estrogen with cyclic medroxyprogesterone acetate had a 23.5 percent increase, and women taking placebo had no increase in breast density after 1 year.[80]

Breast Cancer

The greatest risk factor for the development of breast cancer is advancing age. The probability of developing breast cancer in a woman's lifetime is 1 in 8. Risk factors for the development of breast cancer include being female, early menarche and late menopause, and nulliparity or age greater than 30 at the time of a first live birth. A history of atypical hyperplasia on a breast biopsy, lobular or ductal carcinoma in situ, hereditary breast cancer, and prior breast cancer constitute other risk factors. There are also several environmental conditions that can increase a woman's risk for developing breast cancer. HRT, radiation therapy, a high-fat diet, adult weight gain, alcohol consumption, and sedentary lifestyle also increase the likelihood for a woman to develop breast cancer.[81]

A patient's individual breast cancer risk may be estimated using the Gail or the Claus model. The Gail model, which is used more commonly, allows the clinician to estimate the likelihood of developing breast cancer over the subsequent 5 years and over a woman's remaining lifetime. The model uses (1) the number of first-degree relatives with breast cancer, (2) age at menarche, (3) age at first live birth, and (4) number of breast biopsies to determine the risk for developing breast cancer. The Claus model is based only on family history. The number of first- and second-degree relatives with breast cancer and their age at diagnosis are used to determine the patient's 10-year risk of developing breast cancer. However, the best method for determining a woman's risk if she is genetically predisposed to develop breast cancer from a familial hereditary syndrome (e.g., *BRCA1* or *BRCA2*) is to have genetic testing performed.[81]

▶ CONCLUSION

In this chapter we have discussed the pathophysiology of the perimenopause and menopause. Many patients will present complaining of hot flashes, irregular menses, and urogenital atrophy. Understanding the changes that happen to women as they enter the menopausal transition will help clinicians to take better care of their patients. Besides treating a woman's symptoms, this is an opportunity to screen the patient for potential diseases. Evaluation of lipoprotein levels and encouragement of physical activity and dietary modification can help to prevent cardiovascular disease. In addition, risk factors for the development of osteoporosis need to be considered, and appropriate diagnosis and therapy should be instituted. Breast cancer prevalence increases with advancing age. Therefore, the importance of routine screening should be emphasized.

KEY POINTS

1. The perimenopausal woman has unique issues. Hot flashes, urogenital atrophy, and irregular menses are troublesome problems for many women during this time.

2. The incidence of hypothyroidism increases with advancing age. Regular thyroid screening is recommended.

3. Cardiovascular disease is the leading cause of death in menopausal women. Efforts should be made to screen patients regularly for risk factors of cardiovascular disease, treat contributing conditions (i.e., hypertension, high LDL), and employ preventive strategies such as exercise.

4. Osteoporosis is a common disease for postmenopausal women. It is important to screen patients and institute preventive therapy or treatment to avoid the consequences of fractures.

5. The prevalence of breast cancer increases with advancing age for a lifetime risk of 1 of 8. When making treatment decisions, a woman's individualized risk for breast cancer should be taken into account.

REFERENCES

1. US Bureau of Census; *eire.census.gov/popest/archives/national/nation2/intfile2-1.txt,* pp 2, 5.
2. US Bureau of Census; *www.census.gov/population/projections/nation/detail,* pp. 6,11.
3. Soules MR, Sherman S, Parrott E, et al. Executive summary: stages of reproductive aging workshop (STRAW). *Fertil Steril* 2001;76(5):874–878.
4. Wallace RB, Sherman BM, Bean JA. Probability of menopause with increasing duration of amenorrhea in middle-aged women. *Am J Obstet Gynecol* 1979;135(8):1021–1024.
5. Adashi EY, Rock JA, Rosenwaks Z, eds. *Reproductive Endocrinology, Surgery, and Technology,* Vol 2. Philadelphia: Lippincott Raven, 1996; p 1394.
6. Cramer DW, Xu H. Predicting age at menopause. *Maturitas* 1996;23:319–326.
7. Biela U. Determinants of the age at natural menopause. *Przegl Lek* 2002;59(3):165–169.
8. Harlow BL, Signorello LB. Factors associated with early menopause. *Maturitas* 2000;35(1): 3–9.
9. Meirow D, Nugent D. The effects of radiotherapy and chemotherapy on female reproduction. *Hum Reprod Update* 2001;7(6):535–543.
10. Chrisman HB, Saker MB, Ryu RK, et al. The impact of uterine fibroid embolization on resumption of menses and ovarian function. *J Vasc Intervent Radiol* 2000;11(6):699–703.
11. Bromberger JT, Matthews KA, Kuller LH, et al. Prospective study of the determinants of age at menopause. *Am J Epidemiol* 1997;145(2):124–133.
12. Weiss G. Menstrual irregularities and the perimenopause. *J Soc Gynecol Invest* 2001;8(suppl 1):S65–66.
13. Dudley EC, Hopper JL, Taffe J, et al. Using longitudinal data to define the perimenopause by menstrual cycle characteristics. *Climacteric* 1998;1(1):18–25.
14. Freedman RR. Physiology of hot flashes. *Am J Human Biol* 2001;13(4):453–464.
15. Feldman BM, Voda A, Gronseth E. The prevalence of hot flash and associated variables among perimenopausal women. *Res Nurs Health* 1985;8:261–268.
16. Grisso JA, Freeman EW, Maurin E, et al. Racial differences in menopause information and the experience of hot flashes. *J Gen Intern Med* 1999;14(2):98–103.
17. Kronenberg F. Hot flashes: Epidemiology and physiology. *Ann NY Acad Sci* 1990;592:52–86.
18. Tataryn IV, Meldrum DR, Lu KH, et al. LH, FSH and skin temperature during the menopausal hot flash. *J Clin Endocrinol Metab* 1979;49(1):152–154.
19. Freedman RR. Biochemical, metabolic, and vascular mechanisms in menopausal hot flushes. *Fertil Steril* 1998;70:1–6.
20. Freedman RR, Woodward S, Sabharwal SC. α_2-Adrenergic mechanism in menopausal hot flushes. *Obstet Gynecol* 1990;76:573–578.
21. Metcalf MG, Donald RA, Livesey JH. Pituitary-ovarian function in normal women during the menopausal transition. *Clin Endocrinol* 1981;14(3):245–255.
22. Shideler SE, DeVane GW, Kalra PS, et al. Ovarian-pituitary hormone interactions during the perimenopause. *Maturitas* 1989;11(4):331–339.
23. Santoro N, Rosenberg Brown J, Adel T, et al. Characterization of reproductive hormonal dynamics in the perimenopause. *J Clin Endocrinol Metab* 1996;81(4):1495–1501.
24. Reyes FI, Winter JS, Faiman C. Pituitary-ovarian relationships preceding the menopause. *Am J Obstet Gynecol* 1977;129:557–564.

25. The SWAN Daily Hormone Study Writing Group. Validation of urinary hormone assays. The Endocrine Society's 84th Annual Meeting, San Francisco, 2002 (abstract P-103).

26. Batista MC, Cartledge TP, Zellmer AW, et al. Effects of aging on menstrual cycle hormones and endometrial maturation. *Fertil Steril* 1995;64(3):492–499.

27. Taffe JR, Dennerstein L. Menstrual patterns leading to the final menstrual period. *Menopause* 2002;9(1):32–40.

28. Metcalf MG, Donald RA, Livesey JH. Pituitary-ovarian function before, during and after the menopause: A longitudinal study. *Clin Endocrinol* 1982;17(5):489–494.

29. Willhite LA, O'Connell MB. Urogenital atrophy: prevention and treatment. *Pharmacotherapy* 2001;21(4):464–480.

30. Pandit L, Ouslander JG. Postmenopausal vaginal atrophy and atrophic vaginitis. *Am J Med Sci* 1997;314(4):228–231.

31. Hall JE, Lavoie HB, Marsh EE, et al. Decrease in gonadotropin-releasing hormone (GnRH) pulse frequency with aging in postmenopausal women. *J Clin Endocrinol Metab* 2000;85:1794–1800.

32. Santoro N, Banwell T, Tortoriello D, et al. Effects of aging and gonadal failure on the hypothalamic-pituitary axis in women. *Am J Obstet Gynecol* 1998;178(4):732–741.

33. O'Connor KA, Holman DJ, Wood JW. Menstrual cycle variability and the perimenopause. *J Hum Biol* 2001;13:465–478.

34. Santoro N, Isaac B, Adel G, et al. Increased variability in follicle growth in older reproductive aged women. The Society of Gynecologic Investigators 49th Annual Meeting, Los Angeles, 2002 (abstract 833).

35. Park SJ, Goldsmith LT, Reinert A, et al. Perimenopausal women are deficient in an estrogen positive feedback on LH secretion mechanism. The Endocrine Society's 82d Annual Meeting, Toronto, Canada. 2000 (abstract 248).

36. Shifren JL, Schiff I. The aging ovary. *J Womens Health Gend Based Med* 2000;9(suppl 1):S3–7.

37. Couzinet B, Meduri G, Lecce MG, et al. The postmenopausal ovary is not a major androgen-producing gland. *J Clin Endocrinol Metab* 2001;(10):5060–5066.

38. Jabara S, Christenson LK, Wang CY, et al. Stromal cells of the human postmenopausal ovary displays a distinctive biochemical and molecular phenotype. *J Clin Endocrinol Metab* 2003;88(1):484–492.

39. Burger HG, Dudley EC, Cui J, et al. A prospective longitudinal study of serum testosterone, dehydroepiandrosterone sulfate, and sex hormone–binding globulin levels through the menopause transition. *J Clin Endocrinol Metab* 2000;85(8):2832–2838.

40. Labrie F, Belanger A, Cusan L, et al. Marked decline in serum concentrations of adrenal C_{19} sex steroid precursors and conjugated androgen metabolites during aging. *J Clin Endocrinol Metab* 1997;82(8):2396–2402.

41. Lasley BL, Santoro N, Randolf JF et al. The relationship of circulating dehydroepiandrosterone sulfate, testosterone, and estradiol to stages of the menopausal transition and ethnicity. *J Clin Endocrinol Metab* 2002;87(8):3760–3467.

42. Speroff, L, Glass RH, Kase NG, eds. *Clinical Gynecologic Endocrinology and Infertility,* 6th ed. Baltimore: Lippincott Williams & Wilkins, 1999; pp 654–707.

43. Hollowell JG, Staehling NW, Flanders WD. Serum TSH, T_4, and thyroid antibodies in the United States population (1998 to 1994): National Health and Nutrition Examination survey (NHANES III). *J Clin Endocrinol Metab* 2002;87(2):489–498.

44. Douchi T, Yamamoto S, Yoshimitsu N, et al. Relative contribution of aging and menopause to changes in lean and fat mass in segmental regions. *Maturitas* 2002;42(4):301–306.

45. Ferrara CM, Lynch NA, Nicklas BJ, et al. Differences in adipose tissue metabolism between postmenopausal and perimenopausal women. *J Clin Endocrinol Metab* 2002;87(9):4166–4170.

46. Blumel JE, Castelo-Branco C, Rocangliolo ME, et al. Changes in body mass index around menopause: A population study of Chilean women. *Menopause* 2001;8(4):239–244.

47. Davies KM, Heaney RP, Recker RR, et al. Hormones, weight change and menopause. *Int J Obes Relat Metab Disord* 2001;25(6):874–879.

48. Matthews KA, Abrams B, Crawford S, et al. Body mass index in midlife women: Relative influence of menopause, hormone use, and ethnicity. *Int J Obes Relat Metab Disord* 2001;25(6):863–873.

49. Minino AM, Arias E, Kochanek KD, et al. Deaths: Final data for 2000. *Natl Vital Stat Rep* 2002;50(15):1–120.

50. Manson JE, Greenland P, LaCroix AZ, et al. Walking compared with vigorous exercise for the prevention of cardiovascular events in women. *New Engl J Med* 2002;347(10):716–725.

51. McKechnie R, Rubenfire M, Mosca L. Association between self-reported physical activity and vascular reactivity in postmenopausal women. *Atherosclerosis* 2001;159(2):483–490.

52. Gokce N, Vita JA, Bader DS, et al. Effect of exercise on upper and lower extremity endothelial function in patients with coronary artery disease. *Am J Cardiol* 2002;90(2):124–127.

53. Stefanick ML, Mackey S, Sheehan M, et al. Effects of diet and exercise in men and postmenopausal women with low levels of HDL cholesterol and high levels of LDL cholesterol. *N Engl J Med* 1998;339(1):12–20.

54. Shoback D, Marcus R, Bikle D, et al.: Mineral metabolism and metabolic bone disease, in Greenspan FS, Gardner DG (eds), *Basic and Clinical Endocrinology,* 6th ed. New York: McGraw-Hill, 2001:306–318.

55. Prevention and management of osteoporosis in women. *ASRM Committee Opinion,* 2001.

56. World Health Organization. Assessment of fracture risk and its application to screening for postmenopausal osteoporosis: report of a WHO study group. Technical report series 843. Geneva: WHO, 1994.

57. National Osteoporosis Foundation; *http://nof. org/physguide/diagnosis.htm.*

58. Hamdy RC, Petak SM, Lenchik L. Which central dual x-ray absorptiometry skeletal sites and regions of interest should be used to determine the diagnosis of osteoporosis? *J Clin Densitom* 2002;5(suppl):S11–18.

59. Roussouw JE, Anderson GL, Prentice RL, et al. Risks and benefits of estrogen plus progestin in healthy postmenopausal women. *JAMA* 2002;288(3):321–333.

60. Modelska K, Cummings S. Tibolone for postmenopausal women: Systematic review of randomized trials. *J Clin Endocrinol Metab* 2002;87(1):16–23.

61. Cummings SR, Palermo L, Browner W, et al. Monitoring osteoporosis therapy with bone densitometry: Misleading changes and regression to the mean. *JAMA* 2000;283(10):1318–1321.

62. Smith P. Estrogens and the urogenital tract: Studies on steroid hormone receptors and a clinical study on a new estradiol-releasing vaginal ring. *Acta Obstet Gynaecol Scand* 1993;157:1–26.

63. Leiblum S, Bachmann G, Kemmann E, et al. Vaginal atrophy in the postmenopausal woman: The importance of sexual activity and hormones. *JAMA* 1983;249(16):2195–2198.

64. Hextall A. Oestrogens and lower urinary tract function. *Maturitas* 2000;36(2):83–92.

65. Hextall A, Hooper R, Cardozo L, et al. Does the menopause influence the risk of bacteriuria? *Int Urogynecol J Pelvic Floor Dysfunct* 2001;12(5):332–336.

66. Eriksen B. A randomized, open, parallel-group study on the preventative effect of an estradiol-releasing vaginal ring (Estring) on recurrent urinary tract infections in postmenopausal women. *Am J Obstet Gynecol* 1999;180(5):1072–1079.

67. Sherburn M, Guthrie JR, Dudley EC, et al. Is incontinence associated with menopause? *Obstet Gynecol* 2001;98(4):628–633.

68. Halbreich U, Lumley LA, Palter S, et al. Possible acceleration of age effects on cognition following menopause. *J Psychiatr Res* 1995;29(3):153–163.

69. Nappi RE, Sinforiani E, Mauri M, et al. Memory functioning at menopause: Impact of age in ovariectomized women. *Gynecol Obstet Invest* 1999;47(1):29–36.

70. Sherwin BB, Tulandi T. "Add-back" estrogen reverses cognitive deficits induced by a gonadotropin-releasing hormone agonist in women with leiomyomata uteri. *J Clin Endocrinol Metab* 1996;81(7):2545–2549.

71. Avis NE, Stellato R, Crawford S, et al. Is there an association between menopause status and sexual functioning? *Menopause* 2000;7(5):297–309.

72. Dennerstein L, Lehert P, Burger H, et al. Factors affecting sexual functioning of women in the midlife years. *Climacteric* 1999;2(4):254–262.

73. McCoy NL, Davidson JM. A longitudinal study of the effects of menopause. *Maturitas* 1985;7(3):203–210.

74. Tungphaisal S, Chandeying V, Sutthijumroon S, et al. postmenopausal sexuality in Thai women.

Asia Oceania J Obstet Gyencol 1991;17(2): 143–146.

75. Barrett-Connor E, Young R, Notelovitz M, et al. Two-year, double-blind comparison of estrogen-androgen and conjugated estrogens in surgically menopausal women. *J Reprod Med* 1999; 44(12):1012–1020.

76. Shifren JL, Braunstein GD, Simon JA, et al. Transdermal testosterone treatment in women with impaired sexual function after oophorectomy. *N Engl J Med* 2000;343(10):682–688.

77. Hackbert L, Heiman JR. Acute dehydroepiandrosterone (DHEA) effects on sexual arousal in postmenopausal women. *J Womens Health Gend Based Med* 2002;11(2):155–162.

78. Arlt WA, Callies F, van Vlijmen JC, et al. Dehydroepiandrosterone replacement in women with adrenal insufficiency. *N Engl J Med* 1000; 341(14):1013–1020.

79. Boyd N, Martin L, Stone J, et al. A longitudinal study of the effects of menopause on mammographic features. *Cancer Epidemiol Biomarkers Prev* 2002;11(10 pt 1):1048–1053.

80. Greendale GA, Rebousin BA, Sie A, et al. Effects of estrogen and estrogen-progestin on mammographic parenchymal density. *Ann Intern Med* 1999;130:262–269.

81. Sakorafas GH, Krespis E, Pavlakis G. Risk estimation for breast cancer development: A clinical perspective. *Surg Oncol* 2002;10:183–192.

CHAPTER 29

Androgen Deficiency in Women

GLENN D. BRAUNSTEIN

► ANDROGEN PRODUCTION IN WOMEN

Androgen production in women derives from direct secretion by the ovaries and adrenals and from conversion of androgen precursors of ovarian and adrenal origin in various peripheral tissues, including the skin, muscles, and adipose tissue. The circulating concentrations of the androgens depend on their production rate and metabolic clearance rate. The latter, in turn, is influenced by the metabolism of the androgen and the degree and affinity of binding to serum proteins, especially sex hormone–binding globulin (SHBG; low capacity, high affinity) and albumin (high capacity, low affinity).

The major androgens and androgen precursors are testosterone, dihydrotestosterone (DHT), androstenedione, and dehydroepiandrosterone (DHEA) and its sulfate (DHEAS). Figure 29-1 depicts the approximate contribution of the ovaries, adrenals, and peripheral conversion sources of these androgens based on a number of studies.[1–5] The contribution of each of these steroids to the androgenic biologic activity in blood depends on the quantitative level in the circulation; the amount that is free or weakly bound to serum proteins, which determines how much is bioavailable to the target tissues; the relative biologic potency of the androgen; and the rapidity and degree of interconversion to other androgens of greater or lesser biologic activity or aromatization to estrogens. Table 29-1 summarizes the relative potency, degree of protein binding, and serum concentrations of these steroids in premenopausal and postmenopausal women.[5–10] Because of these factors, testosterone best reflects the overall androgen status of women, with mild to moderately elevated levels being found in women with acne and hirsutism, marked elevations in women with virilization, and low levels in women with hypopituitarism and adrenal insufficiency or following oophorectomy.[5,11–13]

One of the major determinants of the amount of free or bioavailable testosterone is the concentration of SHBG in the circulation. This protein strongly binds testosterone and DHT, weakly binds androstenedione and DHEA, and does not bind DHEAS.[1,2,10,14] SHBG concentrations are increased by endogenous or exogenous estrogens, hyperthyroidism, and cirrhosis, as well as with some antiepileptic drugs. The levels are decreased in hyperandrogenic states, obesity, hypothyroidism, acromegaly, and during growth hormone therapy, Cushing

PREMENOPAUSE

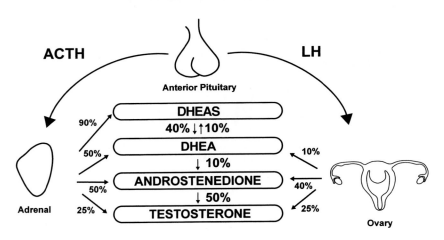

POSTMENOPAUSE

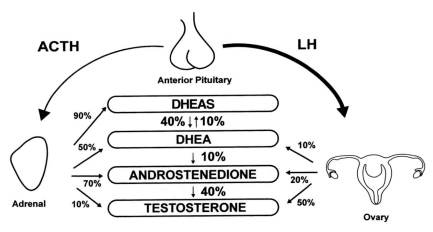

Figure 29-1 Sources of androgens in premenopausal *(upper panel)* and postmenopausal *(lower panel)* women with approximations of the quantitative amounts derived from the ovaries, adrenals, and peripheral tissues.

syndrome, and hyperinsulinemic states (e.g., polycystic ovary syndrome or metabolic syndrome). Unlike the situation in males, the testosterone concentrations in women are not tightly controlled by a feedback loop. An elevated testosterone concentration may be the result of increased production or decreased clearance due to elevations of SHBG. There-fore, the free testosterone concentration, or bioavailable testosterone (the sum of free and the freely dissociable fraction from albumin) concentration, is a better reflection of the androgen status of a woman than is the total testosterone level. The free testosterone level can be estimated from measurements of total testosterone and SHBG and calculation of the

► **TABLE 29-1:** RELATIVE POTENCY, MEAN SERUM CONCENTRATIONS, AND PROTEIN BINDING OF MAJOR ANDROGENS OR ANDROGEN PRECURSORS IN WOMEN

Androgen	Relative Potency	Percent Unbound	Percent Bound to Albumin	Percent Bound to SHBG	Premenopausal Serum Concentrations, ng/dL	Postmenopausal Serum Concentrations, ng/dL
DHT	5	0.5	21	78	20	11
Testosterone	1	1.4	30.4	66	32	22
Androstenedione	0.1	7.5	84.5	6.6	140	77
DHEA	0.01	3.9	88.1	7.9	415	186
DHEAS	0.001	5.0	95.0	—	188,500	106,000

From refs. 5–10.

free testosterone index (FTI), also referred to as the *free androgen index* (FAI).

The most potent androgen, DHT, is secreted in small amounts by the adrenal and ovary but is produced primarily in androgen target tissues through 5α-reduction of testosterone, and therefore, the circulating concentrations correlate with testosterone levels but may not reflect the local tissue concentrations. Since the androgen prohormones DHEA and DHEAS are converted to androstenedione and testosterone and then to DHT or estrone and estradiol, an assessment of the overall androgen activity actually may be best reflected by measurements of the conjugated metabolites of DHT, namely, androsterone-glucuronide (ADT-G), androstane-3α,17β- diol-glucuronide (3α-diol-G), androstane-3β,17β-diol-glucuronide (3β-diol-G), and androsterone sulfate (ADT-S).[15]

► EFFECT OF AGE AND NATURAL MENOPAUSE

Testosterone and Androstenedione

Serum testosterone and androstenedione concentrations exhibit a circadian rhythm, with peak levels at 8 A.M. and lowest levels in the evening, undoubtedly reflecting the effect of adrenocorticotropic hormone (ACTH) stimulation of the adrenal zona reticularis.[5,16] During most of the reproductive years, there is a midcycle peak of total and free testosterone and androstenedione concentrations that coincides with the luteinizing hormone (LH) preovulatory surge.[16,17] Older premenopausal women (>43 years of age) with regular menstrual cycles lose the midcycle rise in free testosterone and androstenedione.[17]

Serum testosterone concentrations in women decline before the menopausal transition, beginning before age 30.[15,18] In one study, the levels at age 40 were approximately one-half those at age 21.[18] Since the calculated percentage of free testosterone did not vary with age, the FTI also decreased. A recent analysis of data from over 3000 women participating in the Study of Women's Health Across the Nation (SWAN) found about a 20 percent drop in mean testosterone levels between the ages of 42 and 50 years.[19] Androstenedione levels also have been found to decrease before the menopause.[15,20]

Studies that have examined the changes in androgens across the menopausal transition have shown conflicting results. Some studies indicate that there is an approximately 15 percent or more decline in testosterone and androstenedione during this period.[1,2,21,22] However, there are relationships between these steroids and smoking, body mass index (BMI), and aging that are confounding variables in the cross-sectional studies independent of the menopause.[22] In a carefully conducted longitudinal study of women from 5 years before to 7 years after the menopause, there was no change in serum total testosterone concentrations, and the SHBG levels decreased, reflecting the decline in serum estrogens and resulting in an actual rise in the free androgen index.[23] In a study of 438 postmenopausal women with intact ovaries who were not taking estrogens, the BMI–adjusted mean testosterone levels actually rose from the youngest cohort of 50 to 59 years of age to the oldest group of 80 to 89 years of age, with most of the increase occurring after age 59.[24] In the same study, androstenedione levels decreased 27 percent from the 50- 59-year age group to the 80- to 89-year age group. Taken together, these studies indicate that menopausal women have lower testosterone and androstenedione levels than young reproductive-age women but that the decrease precedes the menopausal transition.

Whether the ovaries in a postmenopausal woman actually secrete androgens also is a controversial topic. Support for active androgen secretion includes several lines of evidence. First, there is a higher concentration of testosterone in ovarian venous effluent than in the peripheral blood.[25,26] Second, in women whose adrenal androgen production has been suppressed by dexamethasone, injections of human chorionic gonadotropin (hCG) results in a significant rise in testosterone.[27] Third, the administration a gonadotropin-releasing hormone (GnRH) agonist or antagonist, which lowers LH, results in a decrease in testosterone and androstenedione concentrations in both peripheral serum and ovarian venous effluent.[28–31] Fourth, one study actually has shown a rise in testosterone with age following a nadir around the time of the menopause, a time when adrenal androgen secretion is decreasing, suggesting an increase in the ovarian contribution.[24] Finally, as will be discussed below, oophrectomy in postmenopausal women significantly reduces the peripheral serum concentrations of testosterone and androstenedione.[12,32,33] These findings support the proposition that the ovarian interstitial and hilar cells in menopausal women are steroidogenically active and respond to the high concentrations of LH by continuing to secrete androgens.

Several longitudinal studies have documented an approximately 50 percent decrease in circulating concentrations of testosterone following oophorectomy in both premenopausal and postmenopausal women[12,32,33] (Fig. 29-2). In addition, serum androstenedione levels also decrease by 40 to 50 percent following removal of the postmenopausal ovaries.[12,33] A cross-sectional comparison of women with and without oophorectomy residing in a southern California community (Rancho Bernardo) demonstrated that postmenopausal women without ovaries had total and bioavailable testosterone levels that were 40 percent lower and androstenedione concentrations that were 10 percent lower than postmenopausal women with ovaries.[24] These findings clearly support the importance of the postmenopausal ovary as an androgen-producing organ.

However, a contrary view has been expressed based on a reassessment of the steroidogenic potential and gonadotropin responsiveness of the postmenopausal ovary. In postmenopausal women with adrenal insufficiency, plasma testosterone, bioavailable testosterone, free testosterone, and androstenedione concentrations were below or close to the limit of the assays, and no increases were observed following the administration of hCG.[34] Dexamethasone dramatically decreased all the steroids in postmenopausal women with intact adrenals. In addition, there were negligible quantities of testosterone and androstenedione in homogenates of ovarian tissue from postmenopausal women, absent or very low amounts of the androgen steroidogenic enzymes in the ovarian tissue, and no gonadotropin receptors detected by immunocytochemistry.[34] These findings suggest that postmenopausal ovaries are not a major source of circulating androgens. Rather,

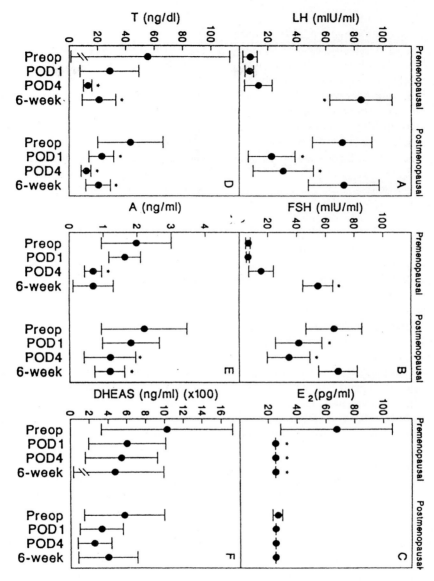

Figure 29-2   Hormone levels (mean ± SD) in premenopausal or postmenopausal women before (Preop), 1 day (POD1), 4 days (POD4), and 6 weeks following oophorectomy. Statistically significant differences between preoperative and postoperative values for each hormone within each group are indicated with asterisks for $p < 0.05$. (LH = luteinizing hormone; T = testosterone; FSH = follicle-stimulating hormone; A = androstenedione; E_2 = estradiol; DHEAS = dehydroepiandrosterone sulfate.)   *(Used, with permission, from Hughes et al.[12])*

adrenal androgen and androgen precursor production may be responsible for maintaining the androgen levels found in postmenopausal women. It is difficult to reconcile these findings, as well as the data demonstrating a continued age-related reduction of adrenal DHEA and DHEAS secretion, with the information supporting the continued androgen production by the postmenopausal ovaries summarized above.

DHEA and DHEAS

DHEA is secreted primarily by the zona reticularis and to a lesser extent by the ovaries, whereas DHEAS is secreted exclusively by the adrenals, as well as being formed peripherally from DHEA.[35] DHEAS serves as a major prohormone for tissue production of androgens and estrogens in women, which is controlled by the degree of expression and activity of the various steroidogenic and metabolizing enzymes in tissues.[15] This concept of local tissue regulation has been termed *intracrinology*.[36] Both DHEA and DHEAS peak in the third decade and then decline such that a 70-year-old woman has DHEA and DHEAS levels that are approximately one-fifth to one-third those found at the time of peak production.[15,23,35,37,38] This decline has been termed the *andropause*.[39] The sharpest decline in adrenal androgen precursors is found between the ages of 20 and 30 years and 50 and 60 years, with smaller changes after age 60.[15] Thus the decline in DHEA and DHEAS primarily reflects an aging phenomenom and is not specifically temporally related to the menopause.[23,40]

DHT and Conjugated Metabolites

DHT is primarily an intracellular product of testosterone and is the most potent of the endogenous androgens. In women, there is a progressive 44 percent decrease in serum DHT levels between the age ranges of 20 and 30 and 70 and 80 years.[15] This reduction is also reflected in marked age-related decreases in the serum concentrations of the conjugated metabolites of DHT. Between the ages of 20 and 80 years, there are decreases of approximately 62 percent in ADT-G, 72 percent in 3α-diol-G, 48 percent in 3β-diol-G, and 66 percent in ADT-S.[15] As with the other steroids, the reductions begin during the reproductive years, well before the menopause, and continue after the menopausal transition, reflecting age-related changes in steroid production rather than menopausal changes.

▶ ANDROGEN MEASUREMENTS

Total serum testosterone levels are measured by immunoassay. Commercial assays generally have been optimized for the testosterone concentrations found in men, whose values are 10 to 20 times higher than those found in reproductive-age women and 20 to 40 times those found in women who have undergone menopause. Therefore, unless meticulous attention is paid to assay performance, the results of the assays run on sera from women may be relatively imprecise. Since the free testosterone concentration more closely reflects the biologically active fraction, and the relationship between the total testosterone concentration and the free concentration is highly dependent on the concentration of SHBG and the SHBG binding sites available, measurements of free testosterone are preferred to those of total testosterone.

Nonetheless, measurements of free testosterone are fraught with a number of technological issues. The most accurate method is equilibrium dialysis in which labeled testosterone is incubated with serum followed by dialysis. The percentage of the labeled testosterone that is dialyzable and therefore free is multiplied by the total testosterone concentration measured by immunoassay to arrive at the free testosterone concentration. This method is time-consuming and requires both a highly purified testosterone tracer and a reliable total testosterone immunoassay. The percentage of free testosterone also may be measured accurately using a sensitive ultrafiltration method that yields similar values to those obtained by equilibrium dialysis.[41] Since the levels of free testosterone are generally low in women who have undergone oophorectomy, often below the limits of the standard assays, methods have been devised to measure levels down to 2 pmol/L (0.6 pg/mL), which is important for the biochemical diagnosis of androgen insufficiency in women.[42] Direct measurement of free testosterone by radioimmunoassay using an analogue ligand is a rapid method that has been developed as an alternative to equilibrium dialysis.[43] However, this method underestimates the free testosterone concentration in both men and women, with the fraction of free testosterone varying as a function of SHBG levels, and there are discrepancies in results on the same serum samples with kits from different manufacturers.[41,44,45]

The free testosterone concentration can be estimated by three other techniques. The first is a calculation of free testosterone based on measurements of total testosterone, SHBG, and in some instances albumin using the known association constants for testosterone binding to SHBG and albumin. SHBG levels are measured by immunoassay[46] or by competitive binding.[46a] The calculated free testosterone correlates well with free testosterone measured by equilibrium dialysis, except with pregnancy samples, in which the calculated levels are lower because of the high amount of estradiol binding to SHBG.[45,47] The second method is calculation of the FTI or FAI, which is: 100 × (total testosterone concentration/SHBG concentration). Although the ratio of the FAI to free testosterone measured by equilibrium dialysis varies as a function of the SHBG level, rendering it less useful for measurements over a wide range of SHBG concentrations, it has been used widely in population studies of women going through the menopausal transition.[23,45] A third method measures all bioavailable testosterone, i.e., both free testosterone and the testosterone weakly bound to albumin,

both of which are able to diffuse into target tissues. The non-SHBG-bound testosterone is determined after precipitation of SHBG-bound hormone by the addition of 50% ammonium sulfate to the sample.[48] The value obtained is approximately 20 times the free testosterone concentration and correlates well over a wide range of SHBG concentrations.[45]

The assays used to measure androstenedione and DHT also suffer from similar problems as the measurement of total and free testosterone. Since these steroids also bind to SHBG, the total serum concentration may not reflect the free or bioavailable concentrations. Alternatively, the assays available for DHEA and DHEAS generally are accurate and do not suffer from some of the methodologic issues that plague testosterone assays in women.

In addition to the methodologic issues with each of these assays, there exist other problems in interpretation of the assay results. First, because of the diurnal variation in androgen levels, the samples generally should be obtained during the morning. Second, if samples are to be collected in premenopausal women with normal menstrual cycles, they should be obtained during the early follicular phase to avoid the midcycle rise in testosterone and androstenedione. Third, and most important, there is a paucity of normative data over the adult lifespan in women with carefully characterized sexual function, ovulatory function, or the absence of dermatologic signs of androgen excess (e.g., hirsutism). In addition, because of the above-described age-related changes in adrenal androgen production, the normative data must be age-adjusted.

▶ RELATIONSHIP OF ANDROGENS AND SEXUAL DYSFUNCTION

Studies that have attempted to correlate various parameters of female sexual function with hormone levels have provided conflicting results. Significant correlations between FTI, androstenedione, and DHEAS and sexual thoughts and masturbation in ninth and tenth grade Caucasian girls have been found.[50] The midmenstrual cycle increase in testosterone has been correlated with an increase in masturbation frequency and, in some studies, libido, arousability, and frequency of sexual activity with their partners.[51–55] Of course, there also are increases in estradiol, gonadotropins, and cervical mucus, as well as other changes that occur at periovulatory time, that confound interpretation of the data. In a study of testosterone levels across the menstrual cycle, women who had high-normal testosterone levels exhibited less depressed mood, had a greater capacity to form interpersonal relationships, and experienced more sexual gratification than women with low-normal levels.[52]

Positive correlations also have been found in premenopausal women over 40 years of age between testosterone concentrations and sexual desire and arousal.[56] In a study that examined two groups of women (21 to 31 and 50 to 60 years of age), plasma androstenedione and testosterone concentrations were each negatively associated with sexual avoidance ($r = -0.41$), whereas testosterone correlated with sexual initiation ($r = 0.53$) and responsivity ($r = 0.47$).[57] Frequency of intercourse and sexual gratification, but not orgasmic frequency, were significantly correlated with testosterone, androstenedione, DHT, and DHEA concentrations.[57] All these findings were derived from cross-sectional studies. A longitudinal study of women from 2 years before menopause to 2 years after demonstrated a decline in sexual interest and frequency of sexual intercourse beginning before the menopause. The frequency of sexual intercourse over the 4-year period significantly correlated with the plasma testosterone levels.[58]

In contrast to these positive reports, several other cross-sectional studies have failed to find an association between circulating androgens and sexual function in pre- and post-menopausal women.[52,59–62,64,65] This is not surprising because even in the reports showing positive associations between androgens and sexual function, the correlations generally were modest, indicating that factors other than androgen concentrations are of importance in determining sexual function. Clearly, the individual's overall health and that of her partner, the use of medications or drugs that potentially can alter sexual function (e.g., serotonin reuptake inhibitors, antihypertensives, alcohol), strength of the relationship, attitudes toward sexual activity, and other factors are important determinants of libido, sexual responsiveness, and overall sexual function. Thus testosterone appears to be an important, but not sufficient, component in maintaining normal female sexual function.

▶ EFFECTS OF ANDROGEN THERAPY ON SEXUAL FUNCTION

Several trials of physiologic or pharmacologic testosterone-replacement therapy have been performed on women who developed low libido following oophorectomy or natural menopause. Most have studied women who were receiving estrogens concomitantly, an important feature because estrogen deficiency per se results in decreased vaginal secretions and lubrication that can lead to dyspareunia. If a woman repeatedly experiences pain during intercourse, avoidance of sexual activity generally occurs. Vaginal dryness and dyspareunia readily respond to estrogen-replacement therapy.[66] The randomized, controlled trials that have examined the effect of testosterone on sexual function generally have shown an increase in libido, desire, arousal, sexual fantasies, enjoyment of sex, initiation of sexual activity, pleasure, sensation, and in some studies, orgasm in women receiving testosterone.[67–75] A double-blind, placebo-controlled trial with DHEA supplementation in women who were androgen deficient from primary adrenal insufficiency showed that along with an increase in serum levels of DHEA, DHEAS, androstenedione, and testosterone, libido and sexual function also improved.[13] Similar effects with DHEA supplementation have been reported in hypopituitary androgen-deficient women.[76]

Although the androgen treatment trials generally have shown similar positive effects on various parameters of sexual function, it should be noted that several trials included women with both natural and surgical menopause, who, as previously noted, often exhibit different baseline androgen levels, and that the doses of testosterone often resulted in supraphysiologic blood testosterone concentrations. Only two studies were randomized, double-blind, and placebo-controlled, an important feature because there is a very large placebo effect in studies of sexual response to medications.[66,73,77] Also, the duration of the studies appears to be important because the full effects of testosterone on sexual function may not be apparent for several months.[67–70,75,78] This factor may account for the lack of an effect seen in some studies.[79]

In addition to the effects on sexual function, several of the androgen therapy studies have examined their effects on mood and other psychological parameters. Those studies have shown that androgens improve overall energy and sense of well-being, decrease depression and somatization, but increase hostility.[69,73,78,80,81]

▶ ANDROGEN INSUFFICIENCY SYNDROME

Evaluation of women with conditions known to be associated with low testosterone levels has led to an empirical definition of a female *androgen insufficiency syndrome* based on a constellation of symptoms, signs, and historic features[82–85] (Table 29-2). The major presenting symptoms often include fatigue, lack of energy, problems "getting started," absent or greatly diminished sexual motivation (libido), lack of desire to be intimate, and a generalized decrease in a sense of well-being. These symptoms often are the cause of considerable personal distress. Thus the androgen insufficiency syndrome fulfills the definition of the *hypoac-*

▶ **TABLE 29-2:** COMPONENTS OF FEMALE ANDROGEN INSUFFICIENCY SYNDROME

Symptoms
- Low libido with global decrease in sexual desire, fantasy, or arousability
- Persistent unexplained fatigue
- Decreased sense of well-being
- Blunted motivation
- Flattened mood

Signs
- Thinning or loss of public hair
- Decreased lean body mass
- Osteopenia or osteoporosis

Other Indications
- Onset following an event associated with decreased androgen production
- Other causes of symptoms have been evaluated and ruled out
- Symptoms persist despite having normal estrogen production if premenopausal or being on adequate estrogen replacement if hypogonadal

From refs. 81–84.

tive sexual desire disorder as defined by a recent consensus group.[86] The women may exhibit thinning or sparsity of pubic hair, a decrease in muscle mass, and bone loss detected by bone mineral density measurements. A decrease in vaginal vasocongestion in response to erotic stimuli and decreased sensitivity to sexual stimulation of the nipples and clitoris also have been included as manifestations of androgen insufficiency.[84,87]

An important operative part of the definition is that the onset of the symptoms begins with an event that is known to be associated with androgen deficiency, such as oophorectomy or the administration glucocorticoids. In addition, other conditions, including primary depression, hypothyroidism, anemia, iron deficiency, and drug or medication use, first must be considered, investigated, and eliminated as a cause of the symptoms. It is important that these women not be estrogen-deficient because estrogen deficiency may lead to dyspareunia and a loss of libido.[66,72] Therefore, a post-menopausal woman should receive adequate estrogen-replacement therapy for several months before being evaluated for the androgen insufficiency syndrome.

► CONDITIONS ASSOCIATED WITH ANDROGEN INSUFFICIENCY

Reduced production of androgens has been found in a variety of conditions (Table 29-3). Structural abnormalities in the hypothalamus such as tumors, infiltrative diseases, or vascular injury may result in a reduction in the synthesis, secretion, or transmission of anterior pituitary releasing or inhibitory factors. A decrease in GnRH results in a reduction in LH secretion and thus a reduction in ovarian androgen production, whereas the loss of corticotropin-releasing hormone leads to insufficient ACTH secretion and decreased adrenal androgen production. Hypothalamic lesions also frequently are associated with loss of normal dopamine release and inhibition of lac-

► **TABLE 29-3:** CONDITIONS ASSOCIATED WITH ANDROGEN INSUFFICIENCY IN WOMEN

Hypothalamic-Pituitary Abnormalities
- Structural
- Functional

Ovarian Insufficiency
- Oophorectomy
- Premature ovarian failure
- Gonadal dysgenesis
- ? Natural menopause

Adrenal Insufficiency

Drug-Induced
- Glucocorticoids
- Estrogen-replacement therapy
- Oral contraceptives
- Antiandrogens
- GnRH agonists or antagonists

Adapted from refs. 81 and 82.

totroph production and secretion of prolactin. In males, the resulting hyperprolactinemia interferes with the action of testosterone, and it is likely, but not shown, that women also would experience symptoms of androgen deficiency. Thus hypothalamic-pituitary structural abnormalities may cause androgen insufficiency through a combination of factors.[11] Functional abnormalities of the hypothalamic-pituitary-gonadal axis (hypothalamic hypogonadotropic hypogonadism), as occurs with anorexia nervosa and systemic illnesses, are associated with low androgen levels.[88,89] Hypogonadotropic hypogonadism with or without secondary adrenal insufficiency is found in patients with destruction of the anterior pituitary from tumors, vascular accidents, or trauma.

Dysgenesis, removal, or destruction of ovarian tissue leads to loss of androgen-producing theca-interstitial cells and both androgen and estrogen insufficiency. As noted previously, cross-sectional studies have suggested no fall or even an increase in free androgen levels during the menopausal transition, although the androgen levels decrease prior to the transition, suggesting an age-related phenomenon. Symptomatic androgen insufficiency can be precipitated in some menopausal women by the administration of oral estrogen-replacement therapy, which increases the production of SHBG by the liver, resulting in more protein binding of testosterone and a reduction in free testosterone concentrations.[7,10,90,91] Estrogen-replacement therapy may decrease pituitary LH production, which may contribute to decreased ovarian androgen production, a phenomenon that also may occur in premenopausal women who receive combined hormone contraceptive pills.[92,93] Of interest, high doses of oral estrogens (e.g., 1.25 mg esterified estrogens orally per day) are associated with reduced concentrations of androstenedione and DHEA, possibly due to direct inhibition of the adrenal 17-hydroxylase/17,20-lyase enzyme system, a reduction in the sensitivity of the adrenal zona reticularis to ACTH stimulation, or an alteration in ACTH or prolactin bioactivity.[90,94–96]

Reduced adrenal androgen production is found with primary or secondary adrenal insufficiency.[13,89] Therapeutic glucocorticoid administration lowers ACTH secretion and hence adrenal androgen production and may be associated with symptomatic androgen insufficiency.[32]

In addition to oral contraceptives, menopausal estrogen-replacement therapy, and glucocorticoids, GnRH agonists[29] and antagonists, and antiandrogens (e.g., spironolactone) can lower androgen production or action, resulting in androgen insufficiency.

► EVALUATION OF PATIENTS SUSPECTED OF HAVING ANDROGEN INSUFFICIENCY SYNDROME

Androgen insufficiency should be suspected in a women presenting with decreased libido, sexual receptivity, and/or pleasure; persistent unexplained fatigue; and a diminished sense of well-being or dysphoric mood[82,83,97] (see Table 29-2). Suspicion should be heightened if the onset began in a close temporal relationship to an event known to be associated with decreased androgen production (see Table 29-3). The evaluation should proceed along the algorithm shown in Figure 29-3.[82]

It is important to consider the possibility of alternative causes of the symptoms. These include medical illnesses such as thyroid, metabolic, and nutritional disorders; iron deficiency; major life stresses; relationship conflicts or other psychosocial issues; and depression.[83,97,98] These should be evaluated through an appropriate history, physical examination, and laboratory studies. Since decreased vaginal lubrication and dyspareunia can be a consequence of estrogen deficiency, and estrogen deficiency may have effects on mood, the estrogen state of the woman should be optimized with adequate estrogen-replacement therapy. Failure of estrogen replacement to improve the symptoms increases the likelihood that androgen insufficiency is present.

The diagnosis of androgen deficiency should be confirmed with measurements of a free testosterone concentration by equilibrium dialysis in an assay optimized for the low levels found in women who have undergone oophorectomy or measurements of total testosterone and SHBG with calculation of the FAI or free androgen concentration. Although there is a dearth of normative data established in age-matched women with and without sexual dysfunction to accurately define androgen insufficiency biochemically, a recent consensus conference of international experts suggested that the diagnosis is supported by the finding of serum androgen levels in the lowest quartile of the normal range for reproductive-age women.[97] Measurement of serum DHEAS concentration provides a good index of adrenal androgen production and is especially important in women with pituitary or adrenal abnormalities or in individuals in whom DHEA replacement therapy is contemplated.

If the measured or calculated free testosterone concentration, or FAI, is in the upper portion of the normal range, then it is unlikely that androgen insufficiency is the cause of the woman's symptoms. If the free androgen levels are low, then it is useful to know if the SHBG level is elevated. Since oral estrogens usually elevate SHBG concentrations, an attempt should be made to switch to a transdermal preparation because these are associated with little or no elevation of the SHBG levels. If the symptoms fail to improve with this change, a trial of androgen-replacement therapy is then reasonable.

► ANDROGEN-REPLACEMENT THERAPY

Preparations

There are no androgen preparations that are approved by the Food and Drug Administration (FDA) for the treatment of androgen insufficiency symptoms in women as of press time,

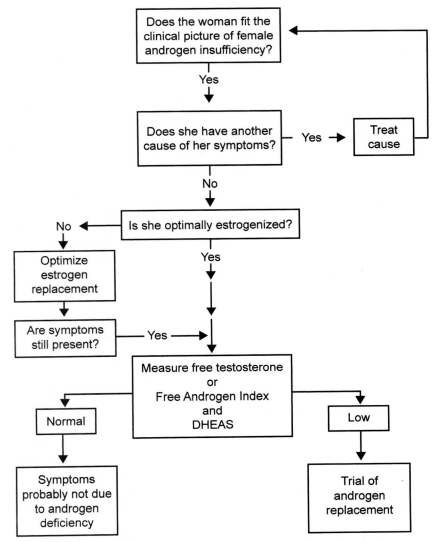

Figure 29-3 Algorithm for the diagnosis and treatment of female androgen insufficiency syndrome. *(Adapted from Braunstein.[82])*

although a number are available (Table 29-4). An oral preparation of esterified estrogens and methyltestosterone is available for the treatment of menopausal vasomotor symptoms not responsive to estrogen therapy alone. This combination is available as 0.625 mg esterified estrogens plus 1.25 mg methyltestosterone (Estratest HS, Solvay Pharmaceuticals, Marietta, GA) or 1.25 mg esterified estrogens and 2.5 mg methyltesterone (Estratest, Solvay Pharmaceuticals, Marietta, GA). Methyltestosterone is a 17α-alkylated compound of testosterone that resists the first-pass hepatic detoxification that inactivates unsubstituted, micronized testosterone. Other 17α-alkylated androgen preparations that are available for the oral treatment of male hy-

▶ **TABLE 29-4:** ANDROGEN PREPARATIONS AND DOSAGES THAT HAVE BEEN USED FOR ANDROGEN REPLACEMENT IN WOMEN

Route	Medication	Dose/Range	Frequency
Oral	Methyltestosterone	1.25–2.5 mg	Daily
	Testosterone undecanoate	40–80 mg	2–4 ×/d
	Micronized testosterone	2.5–5 mg	Daily
	DHEA	25–50 mg	Daily
	Androstenedione	50–100 mg	Daily
IM	Mixed testosterone esters	50–100 mg	4–6 weeks
	Testosterone enanthate	50–100 mg	4–6 weeks
	Testosterone cypionate	50–100 mg	4–6 weeks
	Testosterone undecanoate	1000 mg	6 weeks
	Nandrolone decanoate	25–50 mg	4–6 weeks
Subcutaneous	Cystalline testosterone pellets	50–100 mg	3–6 months
Transdermal	Gel	1 mg	Daily
	Patch	300 µg/d	Twice a week
Sublingual	Testosterone cyclodextrin	tbd	tbd
	Testosterone propionate lozenges	1 mg	2–4 ×/day

Adapted from refs. 99–111.

pogonadism include mesterolone, methenolone acetate, methandrostenolone, and stanozolol. None of these is optimal for the treatment of androgen insufficiency symptoms in women. In addition to androgenic side effects, combination esterified estrogens and methyltestosterone treatment in women lowers total cholesterol and high-density lipoprotein (HDL) cholesterol without altering low-density lipoprotein (LDL) cholesterol through its action on the liver.[75,99–101] Triglyceride levels may be unaltered or reduced with this therapy.[75,99–101]

Testosterone undecanoate is an orally active 17β-ester of testosterone that is lipophilic and is absorbed through intestinal lymphatics and thus enters the circulation without passing through the liver. This preparation must be given two to four times a day and has variable absorption with wide individual variation in testosterone levels and therefore is not optimal for replacement therapy.[102]

Intramuscular administration of testosterone esters has been used in some of the randomized, controlled trials of estrogen-androgen therapy for sexual dysfunction but results in pharmacologic levels of testosterone that may

persist for months following the injections.[71,78,103,104] Despite the supraphysiologic levels of testosterone, the lipid profiles generally remain normal.

Another parenteral form of testosterone replacement that is popular in Europe and Australia involves the subcutaneous insertion of crystalline testosterone pellets that contain 50 or 100 mg testosterone. These are replaced every 3 to 6 months and also result in supraphysiologic concentrations of testosterone without significantly altering lipid levels.[67–69]

Testosterone also can be administered percutaneously either by patches,[73,102] by a micronized testosterone gel,[105] or via a testosterone spray.[106] These preparations have the capacity to provide physiologic (i.e., for a woman age 20 to 30 years) steady-state concentrations of free testosterone, bioavailable testosterone, and DHT without adverse effects on lipids, carbohydrate metabolism, liver or renal function, or hemoglobin.[73,105]

Absorption of testosterone across the oral mucous membranes is being studied in women using testosterone cyclodextrin for sublingual administration and testosterone propionate lozenges.[103,105] These must be administered multiple times during the day and lead to rapid supraphysiologic increases in testosterone, followed by rapid falls. Therefore, it is unlikely that this will become a viable alternative to the transdermal methods currently undergoing clinical trials.

Oral DHEA has been used to provide androgen substitution for women with primary and secondary adrenal insufficiency.[13,76,107] In both these populations, testosterone and androstenedione concentrations rose, and there was marked improvement in mood and sexual function. Doses above 30 mg/d were required to see an effect on sexual function because a dose of 25 mg/d did not alter sexuality.[108] The salutory effects of DHEA replacement in women without adrenal or pituitary insufficiency have been a controversial topic, with some studies showing an increase in libido, increased intercourse and masturbation frequency, and increased sexual satisfaction in women over 70 years of age, whereas others have demonstrated a mood-enhancing effect without a change in libido.[109,110] Oral androstenedione also has been found to increase testosterone concentrations in postmenopausal women, but no studies have examined the effectiveness of this type of substitution therapy on quality of life or sexual function parameters.[111]

Safety

Acne and hirsutism are the major androgenic cutaneous side effects found with androgen-replacement therapy. Acne has been found in 3 to 38 percent of patients receiving esterified estrogens and methyltestosterone, about 4 percent of those receiving testosterone pellets (100 mg), and up to a third of women receiving 50 mg DHEA.[75,99–101,112,113] Hirsutism is reported in 6 to 36 percent of women taking methyltestosterone with esterified estrogens, 15 to 20 percent of women receiving pharmacologic doses of testosterone esters intramuscularly, 6 to 21 percent of women with subcuta-

neous testosterone pellets containing 100 mg crystalline testosterone but not with 50 mg, and 6 to 8 percent of women taking 50 mg oral DHEA.[67,70,81,99,101,112–114] In a double-blind, placebo-controlled trial of transdermal testosterone patches, the incidence of acne or hirsutism was not increased above that of women receiving placebo patches.[73] Other signs of virilization are seen rarely with the doses of androgens used to treat androgen insufficiency in women, with only anecdotal reports of deepening of the voice and clitoromegaly.[115]

As noted earlier, an adverse lipid profile has been noted primarily with methyltestosterone administered with esterified estrogens. In prospective, randomized, double-blind studies, total cholesterol, HDL cholesterol, apolipoprotein A_1, and triglycerides were significantly lower in the women receiving the estrogen-testosterone combination in comparison with the women taking only the esterified estrogens.[99–101] Although the androgens may create a more athrogenic profile than in women receiving estrogens alone, there is a great deal of individual variability, and to date there has not been an increase in cardiovascular disease found in women taking this combination.[116]

Androgen therapy does increase lean body mass and reduce fat free mass.[114,117] Weight gain has been noted in some studies but not others.[73,112,114] The addition of androgens to estrogen therapy increases bone mineral density in multiple sites over and above that found with estrogen therapy alone.[118]

With the exception of the 17α-alkylated and C_{11} fluorinated (e.g., fluoxymesterone) androgens, hepatic toxicity is rare with the use of androgen preparations. Both oral and parenteral 17α-alkylated androgens have been associated with hepatic enzyme elevations, cholestatic hepatitis, peliosis hepatitis, jaundice, and hepatocellular adenoma and carcinoma formation.[115] These adverse effects generally are found in women receiving supraphysiologic doses of androgens taken for athletic performance enhancement or for medical conditions but not for androgen-replacement therapy.

Other potential concerns that have not been borne out with androgen therapy given to women include excessive endometrial stimulation, breast cancer, sleep apnea, polycythemia, and insulin resistance.

Monitoring Therapy

Since the most common androgenic side effects are acne and hirsutism, a careful baseline assessment with semiquantification of both with instruments such as modifications of the Ferriman-Gallwey Hirsutism Scoring Method,[119] the Lorenzo Hirsutism Scale,[120] or the Palatsi and colleagues acne assessment scale[121] should be performed. Acne and hirsutism should be assessed after 1 month of therapy and then every 3 months for the next year. Following 1 to 2 months of therapy, hemoglobin, serum lipids, and liver enzymes should be assessed and, if normal, should be repeated after 6 months of therapy. Ideally, the effectiveness of therapy should be assessed through validated measurement tools to examine sexual-parameter response and quality of life.[122]

KEY POINTS

1. Androgens are produced by the adrenals, ovaries, and peripheral tissues. Hence hypopituitarism, adrenal insufficiency, and oophorectomy result in lowered androgen production.

2. Serum androgen levels decrease with age prior to the menopause.

3. Estrogen-replacement therapy may precipitate androgen insufficiency in menopausal women by increasing SHBG levels, resulting in a lowering of the free testosterone concentration.

4. At present, most serum free testosterone measurement methods lack sensitivity for measuring low levels in women suspected of having androgen insufficiency. Normal ranges of total and free testosterone in serum at different ages have not been well established for women.

5. Some, but not all, studies have demonstrated a relationship between basal serum androgen levels and sexual desire, arousal, and frequency of sexual activity.

6. Symptoms of androgen insufficiency include fatigue, decreased libido, and a generalized decrease in the sense of well-being.

7. Androgen therapy in women with androgen insufficiency improves sexual function.

8. Acne and hirsutism are the major side effects with current androgen-replacement therapy in women with androgen insufficiency.

REFERENCES

1. Vermeulen A. Plasma androgens in women. *J Reprod Med* 1998;43:725–733.
2. Longcope C. Androgen metabolism and the menopause. *Semin Reprod Endocrinol.* 1998;16:111–115.
3. Judd HL, Fournet N. Changes of ovarian hormonal function with aging. *Exp Gerontol* 1994;29:285–298.
4. Adashi EY. The climacteric ovary as a functional gonadotropin-driven androgen-producing gland (comment; erratum appears in *Fertil Steril* 1995;63:684). *Fertil Steril* 1994;62:20–27.
5. Buster JE, Casson PR. Where androgens come from, what controls them, and whether to replace them, in Lobo RA (ed), *Treatment of the Postmenopausal Woman: Basic and Clinical Aspects,* 2d ed. Philadelphia: Lippincott Williams & Wilkins, 1999.
6. Plouffe LJ. Ovaries, androgens and the menopause: Practical applications. *Semin Reprod Endocrinol* 16:117–120, 1998.
7. Simon JA. Estrogen replacement therapy: Effects on the endogenous androgen milieu. *Fertil Steril Suppl* 2002;4:S77–S82.
8. Longcope C. Androgen metabolism and the menopause. *Semin Reprod Endocrinol* 1998;16:111–115.

9. Simpson ER. Aromatization of androgens in women: Current concepts and findings. *Fertil Steril Suppl* 2002;44:S6–S10.

10. Dunn JF, Nisula BC, Rodbard D. Transport of steroid hormones: Binding of 21 endogenous steroids to both testosterone-binding globulin and corticosteroid-binding globulin in human plasma. *J Clin Endocrinol Metab* 1981;53:58–68.

11. Miller K, Sesmilo G, Schiller A, et al. Androgen deficiency in women with hypopituitarism. *J Clin Endocrinol Metab* 2001;86:561–567.

12. Hughes CL Jr, Wall LL, Creasman WT. Reproductive hormone levels in gynecologic oncology patients undergoing surgical castration after spontaneous menopause. *Gynecol Oncol* 1991;40:42–45.

13. Arlt W, Callies F, van Vlijmen JC, et al. Dehydroepiandrosterone replacement in women with adrenal insufficiency. *N Engl J Med* 1999; 341:1013–1020.

14. Lobo RA. Androgens in postmenopausal women: Production, possible role, and replacement options. *Obstet Gynecol Surv* 2001; 56:361–376.

15. Labrie F, Belanger A, Cusan L, et al. Marked decline in serum concentrations of adrenal C_{19} sex steroid precursors and conjugated androgen metabolites during aging. *J Clin Endocrinol Metab* 1997;82:2396–2402.

16. Vermeulen A, Verdonck L. Plasma androgen levels during the menstrual cycle. *Am J Obstet Gynecol* 1976;125:491–494.

17. Mushayandebvu T, Castracane VD, Gimpel T, et al. Evidence for diminished midcycle ovarian androgen production in older reproductive aged women. *Fertil Steril* 1996;65:721–723.

18. Zumoff B, Strain GW, Miller LK, Rosner W. Twenty-four-hour mean plasma testosterone concentration declines with age in normal premenopausal women. *J Clin Endocrinol Metab* 1995;80:1429–1430.

19. Lasley BL, Santoro N, Randolf JF, et al. The relationship of circulating dehydroepiandrosterone, testosterone, and estradiol to stages of the menopausal transition and ethnicity. *J Clin Endocrinol Metab* 2002;87:3760–3767.

20. Longcope C, Franz C, Morello C, et al. Steroid and gonadotropin levels in women during the perimenopausal years. *Maturitas* 1986;8:189–196.

21. Rannevik G, Carlstrom K, Jeppsson S, et al. A prospective long-term study in women from premenopause to postmenopause: Changing profiles of gonadotrophins, oestrogens and androgens. *Maturitas* 1986;8:297–307.

22. Bancroft J, Cawood EH. Androgens and the menopause: A study of 40- to 60-year-old women. *Clin Endocrinol* 1996;45:577–587.

23. Burger HG, Dudley EC, Cui J, et al. A prospective longitudinal study of serum testosterone, dehydroepiandrosterone sulfate, and sex hormone–binding globulin levels through the menopause transition. *J Clin Endocrinol Metab* 2000;85:2832–2838.

24. Laughlin GA, Barrett-Connor E, Kritz-Silverstein D, von Muhlen D. Hysterectomy, oophorectomy, and endogenous sex hormone levels in older women: The Rancho Bernardo Study (comment). *J Clin Endocrinol Metab* 2000;85:645–651.

25. Judd HL, Judd GE, Lucas WE, Yen SS. Endocrine function of the postmenopausal ovary: Concentration of androgens and estrogens in ovarian and peripheral vein blood. *J Clin Endocrinol Metab* 1974;39:1020–1024.

26. Lucisano A, Acampora MG, Russo N, et al. Ovarian and peripheral plasma levels of progestogens, androgens and oestrogens in postmenopausal women. *Maturitas* 1984;6:45–53.

27. Vermeulen A. The hormonal activity of the postmenopausal ovary. *J Clin Endocrinol Metab* 1976;42:247–253.

28. Sluijmer AV, Heineman MJ, De Jong FH, Evers JL. Endocrine activity of the postmenopausal ovary: The effects of pituitary downregulation and oophorectomy. *J Clin Endocrinol Metab* 1995;80:2163–2167.

29. Andreyko JL, Monroe SE, Marshall LA, et al. Concordant suppression of serum immunoreactive luteinizing hormone (LH), follicle-stimulating hormone, alpha subunit, bioactive LH, and testosterone in postmenopausal women by a potent gonadotropin releasing hormone antagonist (Detirelix). *J Clin Endocrinol Metab* 1992;74:399–405.

30. Rabinovici J, Rothman P, Monroe SE, et al. Endocrine effects and pharmacokinetic characteristics of a potent new gonadotropin-releasing hormone antagonist (Ganirelix) with minimal histamine-releasing properties: Studies in postmenopausal women. *J Clin Endocrinol Metab* 1992;75:1220–1225.

31. Dowsett M, Cantwell B, Lal A, et al. Suppression of postmenopausal ovarian steroidogene-

sis with the luteinizing hormone–releasing hormone agonist goserelin. *J Clin Endocrinol Metab* 1988;66:672–677.

32. Judd HL, Lucas WE, Yen SS. Effect of oophorectomy on circulating testosterone and androstenedione levels in patients with endometrial cancer. *Am J Obstet Gynecol* 1974;118: 793–798.

33. Heinonen PK, Koivula T, Rajaniemi H, Pystynen P. Peripheral and ovarian venous concentrations of steroid and gonadotropin hormones in postmenopausal women with epithelial ovarian tumors. *Gynecol Oncol* 1986;25:1–10.

34. Couzinet B, Meduri G, Lecce MG, et al. The postmenopausal ovary is not a major androgen-producing gland. *J Clin Endocrinol Metab* 2001; 86:5060–5066.

35. Hornsby PJ. Biosynthesis of DHEAS by the human adrenal cortex and its age-related decline. *Ann NY Acad Sci* 1995;774:29–46.

36. Labrie F, Luu-The V, Labrie C, et al. Endocrine and intracrine sources of androgens in women: Inhibition of breast cancer and other roles of androgens and their precursor dehydroepiandrosterone. *Endocr Rev* 2003;24:152–182.

37. Orentreich N, Brind JL, Rizer RL, Vogelman JH. Age changes and sex differences in serum dehydroepiandrosterone sulfate concentrations throughout adulthood. *J Clin Endocrinol Metab* 1984;59:551–555.

38. Ravaglia G, Forti P, Maioli F, et al. The relationship of dehydroepiandrosterone sulfate (DHEAS) to endocrine-metabolic parameters and functional status in the oldest-old: Results from an Italian study on healthy free-living over-ninety-year-olds. *J Clin Endocrinol Metab* 1996;81:1173–1178.

39. Alesci S, Bornstein R. Intra-adrenal mechanisms of DHEA regulation: A hypothesis for andropause. *Exp Clin Endocrinol Diabetes* 2001; 109:75–82.

40. Lasley BL, Santoro N, Randolf JF, et al. The relationship of circulating dehydroepiandrosterone, testosterone, and estradiol to stages of the menopausal transition and ethnicity. *J Clin Endocrinol Metab* 2002;87:3760–3767.

41. Gruschke A, Kuhl H. Validity of radioimmunological methods for determining free testosterone in serum. *Fertil Steril* 2001;76:576–582.

42. Sinha-Hikim I, Arver S, Beall G, et al. The use of a sensitive equilibrium dialysis method for the measurement of free testosterone levels in healthy, cycling women and in human immunodeficiency virus-infected women [comment; erratum appears in *J Clin Endocrinol Metab* 1998;83(8):2959]. *J Clin Endocrinol Metab* 1998;83:1312–1318.

43. Wilke TJ, Utley DJ. Total testosterone, free androgen index, calculated free testosterone and free testosterone by analog RIA compared in hirsute women and in otherwise normal women with altered binding of sex hormone binding globulin. *Clin Chem* 1987;33:1372–1375.

44. Rosner W. An extraordinarily inaccurate assay for free testosterone is still with us. *J Clin Endocrinol Metab* 2001;86:2903.

45. Vermeulen A, Verdonck L, Kaufman JM. A critical evaluation of simple methods for the estimation of free testosterone in serum (comment). *J Clin Endocrinol Metab* 1999;84:3666–3672.

46. Guay AT. Screening for androgen deficiency in women: Methodological and interpretive issues. *Fertil Steril* 2002;4:83–88.

46a. Pearlman WII, Crepy O. Steroid-protein interaction with particular reference to testosterone binding by human serum. *J Biol Chem* 1967;242: 182–189.

47. Buch AB, Destefano AJ, Skuster J, et al. Accuracy of free testosterone measurements in women: Comparison to calculated values. 85th Annual Meeting of the Endocrine Society, Philadelphia, 2003 (abstract P2-219).

48. Cumming DC, Wall SR. Non-sex hormone-binding globulin-bound testosterone as a marker for hyperandrogenism. *J Clin Endocrinol Metab* 1985;61:873–876.

49. Laumann EO, Paik A, Rosen RC. Sexual dysfunction in the United States: Prevalence and predictors. *JAMA* 1999;281:537–544.

50. Udry JR, Talbert LM, Morris NM. Biosocial foundations for adolescent female sexuality. *Demography* 1986;23:217–230.

51. Bancroft J, Sanders D, Davidson D, Warner P. Mood, sexuality hormones, and the menstrual cycle: III. Sexuality and the role of androgens. *Psychosom Med* 1983;45:509–516.

52. Persky H, Lief AI. Plasma testosterone levels and sexual behavior of couples. *Arch Sex Behav* 1978;7:157–173.

53. Morris NM, Udry JD, Khan-Dawood F, Dawood MY. Marital sex frequency and midcycle female testosterone. *Arch Sex Behav* 1987;16:27–38.

54. Van Goozen SH, Wiegant VM, Endert E, et al. Psychoendocrinological assessment of the menstrual cycle: The relationship between hormones, sexuality, and mood. *Arch Sex Behav* 1997;26:359–382.

55. Riley A, Riley E. Controlled studies on women presenting with sexual drive disorder: I. Endocrine status. *J Sex Marital Ther* 2000;26: 269–283.

56. Floter JA, Nathorst-Boos J, Carlstrom BK, von Schoultz B. Androgen status and sexual life in perimenopausal women. *Menopause* 1997;4: 95–100.

57. Persky H, Dreisbach L, Miller WR, et al. The relation of plasma androgen levels to sexual behaviors and attitudes of women. *Psychosom Med* 1982;44:305–319.

58. McCoy NL, Davidson JM. A longitudinal study of the effects of menopause on sexuality. *Maturitas* 1985;7:203–210.

59. Studd JWW, Collins WP, Chakravarti S, et al. Oestradiol and testosterone implants in the treatment of psychosexual problems in the post-menopausal woman. *Br J Obstet Gynaecol* 1977;84:314–316.

60. Bachmann GA, Leiblum SR, Colburn DW, et al. Sexual expression and its determinants in the post-meonpausal woman. *Maturitas* 1984;6: 19–29.

61. Dennerstein L, Randolph J, Taffe J, et al. Hormones, mood, sexuality, and the menopausal transition. *Fertil Steril* 2002;4:42–48.

62. Dennerstein L, Dudley EC, Hopper JL, Burger H. Sexuality, hormones and the menopausal transition. *Maturitas* 1997;26:83–93.

63. Cutler WB, Garcia CR, Huggins GR, Preti G. Sexual behavior and steroid levels among gynecologically mature premenopausal women. *Fertil Steril* 1986;45:496–502.

64. Schreiner-Engel P, Schiavi RC, White D, Ghizzani A. Low sexual desire in women: the role of reproductive hormones. *Horm Behav* 1989; 23:221–234.

65. Bancroft J, Sherwin BB, Alexander GM, et al. Oral contraceptives, androgens, and the sexuality of young women: II. The role of androgens. *Arch Sex Behav* 1991;20:121–135.

66. Sarrel PM. Broadened spectrum of menopausal symptom relief. *J Reprod Med* 1998;43:734–740.

67. Burger HG, Hailes J, Menelaus M, et al. The management of persistent menopausal symptoms with oestradiol-testosterone implants: Clinical, lipid and hormonal results. *Maturitas* 1984;6:351–358.

68. Burger H, Hailes J, Nelson J, Menelaus M. Effect of combined implants of oestradiol and testosterone on libido in postmenopausal women. *Br Med J Clin Res Ed* 1987;294:936–937.

69. Davis SR, McCloud P, Strauss BJ, Burger H. Testosterone enhances estradiol's effects on postmenopausal bone density and sexuality. *Maturitas* 1995;21:227–236.

70. Sherwin BB, Gelfand MM, Brender W. Androgen enhances sexual motivation in females: A prospective, crossover study of sex steroid administration in the surgical menopause. *Psychosom Med* 1985;47:339–351.

71. Sherwin BB, Gelfand MM. The role of androgen in the maintenance of sexual functioning in oophorectomized women. *Psychosom Med* 1987;49:397–409.

72. Sarrel P, Dobay B, Wiita B. Estrogen and estrogen-androgen replacement in postmenopausal women dissatisfied with estrogen-only therapy: Sexual behavior and neuroendocrine responses. *J Reprod Med* 1998;43:847–856.

73. Shifren JL, Braunstein GD, Simon JA, et al. Transdermal testosterone treatment in women with impaired sexual function after oophorectomy (comment). *N Engl J Med* 2000;343: 682–688.

74. Brincat M, Magos A, Studd JW, et al. Subcutaneous hormone implants for the control of climacteric symptoms:. A prospective study. *Lancet* 1984;1:16–18.

75. Lobo RA, Rosen RC, Yang HM, et al. Comparative effects of oral esterified estrogens with and without methyltestosterone on endocrine profiles and dimensions of sexual function in postmenopausal women with hypoactive sexual desire. *Fertil Steril* 2003;79:1341–1352.

76. Johannsson G, Burman P, Wiren L, et al. Low-dose dehydroepiandrosterone affects behavior in hypopituitary androgen-deficient women: A placebo-controlled trial. *J Clin Endocrinol Metab* 2002;87:2046–2052.

77. Modelska K, Cummings S. Female sexual dysfunction in postmenopausal women: Systematic review of placebo-controlled trials. *Am J Obstet Gynecol* 2003;188:286–293.

78. Sherwin BB, Gelfand MM. Sex steroids and affect in the surgical menopause: A double-blind,

cross-over study. *Psychoneuroendocrinology* 1985;10:325–335.

79. Myers LS, Dixen J, Morrissette D, et al. Effects of estrogen, androgen, and progestin on sexual psychophysiology and behavior in postmenopausal women. *J Clin Endocrinol Metab* 1990;70:1124–1131.

80. Sherwin BB. Affective changes with estrogen and androgen replacement therapy in surgically menopausal women. *J Affect Disord* 1988;14:177–187.

81. Davis SR, Tran J. Testosterone influences libido and well being in women. *Trends Endocrinol Metab* 2001;12:33–37.

82. Braunstein GD. Androgen insufficiency in women: Summary of critical issues. *Fertil Steril Suppl* 2002;4:S94–99.

83. Davis SR. When to suspect androgen deficiency other than at menopause. *Fertil Steril Suppl* 2002;4:S68–71.

84. Bachmann GA. The hypoandrogenic woman: Pathophysiologic overview. *Fertil Steril Suppl* 2002;4:S72–76.

85. Kaplan HS, Owett T. The female androgen deficiency syndrome. *J Sex Marital Ther* 1993;19:3–24.

86. Basson R, Berman J, Burnett A, et al. Report of the international consensus development conference on female sexual dysfunction: Definitions and classifications. *J Urol* 2000;163:888–893.

87. Rako S. Female hypoactive sexual desire disorder due to androgen deficiency: Clinical and psychometric issues. *Psycopharmacol Bull* 1997;33:761–766.

88. Masi AT, Feiggenbaum SL. Hormonal and pregnancy relationships to rheumatoid arthritis: Convergent effects with immunological and microvascular systems. *Semin Arthritis Rheum* 1995;25:1–27.

89. Miller K, Corcoran C, Armstrong C, et al. Transdermal testosterone administration in women with acquired immunodeficiency syndrome wasting: A pilot study. *J Clin Endocrinol Metab* 1998;83:2717–2725.

90. Simon J, Klaiber E, Wiita B, et al. Differential effects of estrogen-androgen and estrogen-only therapy on vasomotor symptoms, gonadotropin secretion, and endogenous androgen bioavailability in postmenopausal women. *Menopause* 1999;6:138–146.

91. Casson PR, Elkind-Hirsch KE, Buster JE, et al. Effect of postmenopausal estrogen replacement on circulating androgens. *Obstet Gynecol* 1997; 90:995–998.

92. Mathur RS. The effect of estrogen treatment on plasma concentrations of steroid hormones, gonadotropins, prolactin and sex hormone–binding globulin in post-menopausal women. *Maturitas* 1985;7:129–133.

93. Krug R, Pietrowsky R, Fehm HL, Born J. Selective influence of menstrual cycle on perception of stimuli with reproductive significance. *Psychosom Med* 1994;56:410–417.

94. Albrecht ED, Pepe GJ. Suppression of maternal adrenal dehydroepiandrosterone and dehydroepiandrosterone sulfate production by estrogen during baboon pregnancy. *J Clin Endocrinol Metab* 1995;80:3201–3208.

95. Madden JD, Milewich L, Parker CR Jr, et al. The effect of oral contraceptive treatment on the serum concentration of dehydroisoandrosterone sulfate. *Am J Obstet Gynecol* 1978;132: 380–384.

96. Tazuke S, Khaw KT, Barrett-Connor E. Exogenous estrogen and endogenous sex hormones. *Medicine* 1992;71:44–51.

97. Bachmann G, Bancroft J, Braunstein G, et al. Female androgen insufficiency: The Princeton consensus statement on definition, classification, and assessment. *Fertil Steril* 2002;77: 660–665.

98. Verdon F, Burnand B, Stubi CL, et al. Iron supplementation for unexplained fatigue in non-anaemic women: Double blind randomized placebo controlled trial. *Br Med J* 2003;326: 1124.

99. Hickok LR, Toomey C, Speroff L. A comparison of esterified estrogens with and without methyltestosterone: Effects on endometrial histology and serum lipoproteins in postmenopausal women. *Obstet Gynecol* 1993;82:919–924.

100. Watts NB, Notelovitz M, Timmons MC, et al. Comparison of oral estrogens and estrogens plus androgen on bone mineral density, menopausal symptoms, and lipid-lipoprotein profiles in surgical menopause [erratum appears in *Obstet Gynecol* 1995;85:668]. *Obstet Gynecol* 1995;85:529–537.

101. Barrett-Connor E, Timmons C, Young R, et al. Interim safety analysis of a two-year study comparing oral estrogen-androgen and conjugated estrogens in surgically menopausal women. *J Womens Health* 1996;5:93–101.

102. Buckler HM, Robertson WR, Wu FC. Which androgen replacement therapy for women? *J Clin Endocrinol Metab* 1998;83:3920–3924.

103. Casson PR, Carson SA, Buster JE. Testosterone delivery systems for women: present status and future promise. *Semin Reprod Endocrinol* 1998;16:153–159.

104. Urman B, Pride SM, Yuen BH. Elevated serum testosterone, hirsutism, and virilism associated with combined androgen-estrogen hormone replacement therapy (comment). *Obstet Gynecol* 1991;77:595–598.

105. Slater CC, Souter I, Zhang C, et al. Pharmacokinetics of testosterone after percutaneous gel or buccal administration. *Fertil Steril* 2001;76:32–37.

106. Davis SR, Humberstone AJ, Wilne RW, Evans AM. Measurement of serum total testosterone levels after administration of testosterone can underestimate the amount of testosterone that has been absorbed. 85th Annual Meeting of the Endocrine Society, Philadelphia, 2003 (abstract P2-220).

107. Arlt W, Allolio B. Dehydroepiandrosterone replacement therapy. *Curr Opin Endocrinol Diabetes* 2001;8:130–139.

108. Lovas K, Gebre-Medhin G, Trovik TS, et al. Replacement of dehydroepiandrosterone in adrenal failure: No benefit for subjective health status and sexuality in a 9-month, randomized, parallel group clinical trial. *J Clin Endocrinol Metab* 2003;88:1112–1118.

109. Baulieu EE, Thomas G, Legrain S, et al. Dehydroepiandrosterone (DHEA), DHEA sulfate, and aging: Contribution of the DHEAge Study to a sociobiomedical issue. *Proc Natl Acad Sci USA* 2000;97:4279–4284.

110. Morales AJ, Nolan JJ, Nelson JC, Yen SS. Effects of replacement dose of dehydroepiandrosterone in men and women of advancing age.[erratum appears in *J Clin Endocrinol Metab* 1995;80(9):2799]. *J Clin Endocrinol Metab* 1994;78:1360–1367.

111. Leder BZ, Leblanc KM, Longcope C, et al. Effects of oral androstenedione administration on serum testosterone and estradiol levels in postmenopausal women. *J Clin Endocrinol Metab* 2002;87:5449–5454.

112. Hunt PJ, Gurnell EM, Huppert FA, et al. Improvement in mood and fatigue after dehydroepiandrosterone replacement in Addison's disease in a randomized, double-blind trial. *J Clin Endocrinol Metab* 2000;85:4650–4656.

113. Cardozo L, Gibb DM, Tuck SM, et al. The effects of subcutaneous hormone implants during climacteric. *Maturitas* 1984;5:177–184.

114. Dobs AS, Nguyen T, Pace C, Roberts CP. Differential effects of oral estrogen versus oral estrogen-androgen replacement therapy on body composition in postmenopausal women. *J Clin Endocrinol Metab* 2002;87:1509–1516.

115. Slayden SM. Risks of menopausal androgen supplementation. *Semin Reprod Endocrinol* 1998;16:145–152.

116. Sarrel PM. Cardiovascular aspects of androgens in women. *Semin Reprod Endocrinol* 1998;16:121–128.

117. Gower BA, Nyman L. Associations among oral estrogen use, free testosterone concentration, and lean body mass among postmenopausal women. *J Clin Endocrinol Metab* 2000;85:4476–4480.

118. Notelovitz M. Androgen effects on bone and muscle. *Fertil Steril Suppl* 2002;77(4):S34–41.

119. Ferriman D, Gallwey JD. Clinical assessment of body hair growth in women. *J Clin Endocrinol Metab* 1961;21:1440–1447.

120. Lorenzo E. Familial study of hirsutism. *J Clin Endocrinol Metab* 1970;31:556–564.

121. Palatsi R, Hirvensalo E, Liukko P, et al. Serum total and unbound testosterone and sex hormone–binding globulin (SHBG) in female acne patients treated with two different oral contraceptives. *Acta Derm Venereol* 1984;64:517–523.

122. Rosen RC. Assessment of female sexual dysfunction: Review of validated methods. *Fertil Steril Suppl* 2000;77:S89–93.

CHAPTER 30

Benefits of Hormone-Replacement Therapy

ELLEN E. WILSON AND BRUCE R. CARR

An average woman can expect to spend more than one-third of her life in a postmenopausal state.[1] According to data from the Massachusetts Women's Health Study, the average age of natural menopause is 51.3 years.[2] Whereas approximately 95 percent of women will go through menopause somewhere between the ages of 44 and 56,[3] about 1 percent of women will undergo premature menopause before the age of 40.[4] Over 40 million women in the United States are postmenopausal, and about 16 million of these women are over the age of 65. The question remains: What happens to women physically and psychologically when they become postmenopausal, and how might hormone therapy be of benefit to some?

► MENOPAUSE AND THE ADVERSE EFFECTS OF HORMONE LOSS

After menopause, there is a marked decline in estrogen levels due to loss of ovarian follicular competence. Postmenopausal women will have some estrogen production, but this is from the extraglandular conversion of androstenedione and testosterone. The blood production rate of estrogen in the premenopausal years is approximately 0.35 mg/d, whereas the rate is re-

duced to 0.045 mg/d in women in the post-menopausal years and in those who have been oophorectomized.[5] Short-term adverse effects of estrogen loss in the climacteric years are reflected in vasomotor symptoms of hot flashes and night sweats. These symptoms can affect quality of life by causing sleep and mood disturbances and irritability. Intermediate adverse effects of estrogen loss include atrophic conditions of the genitourinary tract, which can result in vaginal atrophy with resulting sexual dysfunction and an increase in stress urinary incontinence. Skin collagen loss also occurs. Long-term consequences of estrogen loss include osteoporosis with increased risk of fracture and potentially an increased rate for cardiovascular disease and dementia.

► BENEFITS OF POSTMENOPAUSAL ESTROGEN THERAPY

Vasomotor Symptoms

Hot flushes sometimes are described as the hallmark of menopause. A hot flush is described as a sudden intense feeling of heat beginning in the face and neck and extending to the chest and body and lasting, on average, several minutes. It is often followed by sweating and a chill. It may recur infrequently, such as once a month, or as often as every 30 minutes and occurs more often at night and at times of stress or warmer weather.[6]

As many as 25 percent of postmenopausal women will not experience hot flashes, another 50 percent will experience minor flushing occasionally, and almost 25 percent will report severe frequent flushing that interferes with normal daily professional and social activities. In fact, as many as 20 percent of premenopausal women will report some hot flashing usually in their middle to late forties.[2,7] Hot flashes generally diminish over time. On average, women will experience hot flashes for a period lasting from 6 months to 2 years; however, some women will report having them for several decades.[8,9] The etiology of the hot flash is not completely understood but is believed to be due to a decline in estrogen level. Specifically, the degree of the drop in estrogen levels is more crucial than the actual estrogen level itself. Premenopausal bilateral oophorectomy and administration of gonadotropin-releasing hormone (GnRH) analogues are two situations where hot flashes are prominent.[10–13] Patients with Turner syndrome and low estrogen levels from birth will not have hot flashes unless prescribed estrogen replacement is later withdrawn.[14,15] Estrogen is the most effective known treatment for hot flashes. Several placebo-controlled studies have demonstrated a significant decrease in hot flashes with oral estrogen therapy.[16–20] The Postmenopausal Estrogen/Progestin Interventions (PEPI) Trial, which enrolled 875 postmenopausal women on either estrogen alone or three estrogen-progestin combinations, found a reduced severity of vasomotor symptoms in all therapeutic groups.[21] Transdermal estrogen can offer some advantages over oral regimens, including a sustained release of hormone, increased absorption, and fewer gastrointestinal side effects. The once- or twice-weekly application of transdermal estrogen may improve therapy compli-

ance issues.[22,23] A practical approach is to prescribe a low-dose estrogen initially when hot flashes become bothersome. Some women will experience an immediate effect, whereas others may not experience a therapeutic effect for months. (Others will benefit from the addition of other nonestrogenic treatment options.) For women whose primary concern is hot flashes, taking estrogen-alone treatment (ET) or estrogen plus progestin, known as *hormone treatment* (HT), is a good strategy on a short-term basis. However, in some women, longer-term therapy may be indicated if, after discontinuing ET or HT, hot flashes recur and are moderate to severe. A very slow taper of hormone over a 3- to 6-month period is advised to decrease the recurrence of vasomotor symptoms. Recent studies have reported a reduction in the frequency and severity of hot flashes even when using a very low dose of ET or HT[24] (Fig. 30-1).

Vulvovaginal Atrophy

It is well known that estrogen deprivation often will lead to atrophy of the genitourinary system. Atrophy of the vulvar and vaginal mucosa may precipitate symptoms of pruritus, dyspareunia, and stenosis.[25] Atrophy of the urethra and bladder mucosa may lead to symptoms of dysuria, urge incontinence, and frequency.[26] Whereas hot flashes and night sweats usually will diminish in time without any therapy, vulvovaginal disturbances are progressive in nature. As the vaginal epithelium thins, dryness is a frequent complaint, along with irritation, which can lead to sexual dysfunction and/or incontinence.[27] Women who are smokers can expect an exacerbation of their urogenital symptoms.[28] Intravaginal estrogen application provides a direct, immediate, and effective therapy to relieve atrophic effects. Various modalities include creams, rings, tablets, and pessaries.[29] Intravaginal estrogen has been shown to moisten the vagina and decrease dyspareunia, as well as urinary tract infections.[30] Very

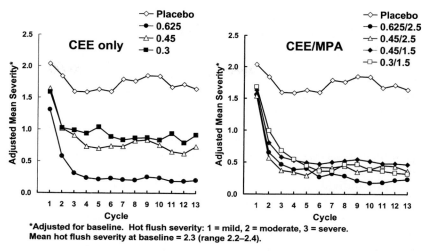

Figure 30-1 Reduction in the mean severity of hot flushes in women on placebo and standard-dose and low-dose ET and HT. *(Data from the Heart, Osteoporosis, Progestin, Estrogen Study. Utian WH, et al.* Fertil Steril *2001;75:1065; used with permission.)*

little systemic absorption occurs with intravaginal estrogen application, and therefore, such products may be used in women who have a uterus without progesterone supplementation because the risk of endometrial hyperplasia is low. However, a new estrogen ring is available that provides higher levels of estrogen and reduces hot flushes, and in women with a uterus, a progestin is indicated. Over-the-counter vaginal lubricants and moisturizers can ease vaginal dryness, as can regular sexual intercourse, which serves to maintain vaginal elasticity.

Skin Changes

Skin is our largest body organ and has significant collagen content, particularly in the deep dermis layer. The peri- and postmenopausal years are marked by a decrease in skin collagen and thickness. Research has shown the amount of collagen in the skin to drop sharply after menopause.[31] As the skin becomes dryer and thinner, an increase in the amount of wrinkling occurs, especially on the face and hands. Billions of dollars each year are spent on cosmetic products and procedures to diminish fine

lines and wrinkles in women.[32] Postmenopausal estrogen therapy has been shown to decrease collagen turnover. Skin wrinkling and dry skin were improved with estrogen use, as shown in data from the U.S. First National Health and Nutrition Examination Survey.[33] Another study showed an increase in skin thickness (11.5 percent) and dermis thickness (30 percent) in a group of 60 women who were taking oral estrogen over that of women taking a placebo.[34] Several studies have shown an increase in skin thickness with estrogen-replacement therapy, as well as an association between osteoporosis and thinning of the skin.[35,36] Vascularization of the skin may improve with estrogen use.[37] Finally, estrogen-replacement therapy has a beneficial effect on several mechanical properties of the skin, such as distensibility and elasticity.[38]

Osteoporosis

Osteoporosis is a major public health concern. Of the 25 million Americans who have osteoporosis, 80 percent are women. It is the most common skeletal disorder, characterized by microarchitectural deterioration of bone tissue with resulting fragility. Low bone mass results in thin, porous bones that fracture more easily. By definition, osteoporosis is low bone mineral density that is more than 2.5 standard deviation below the mean normal peak bone mass. In the United States, osteoporotic fractures of the vertebrae, hip, and wrist total 1.5 million cases a year. The total annual cost of the associated complications of osteoporosis is estimated at over $14 billion. It is termed a "silent disorder" because an individual will remain asymptomatic for many years until a fracture occurs. Bone mass is greater in the hip than in the spine; therefore, osteoporotic fractures of the hip occur later in life. Approximately 16 percent of those who suffer a hip fracture will die within a 3-month period because of complications related to the fracture, including pulmonary embolism and myocardial infarction.[39]

Bone mass growth results from a constant remodeling process when new bone formation by osteoblasts exceeds resorption by osteoclasts until approximately the age of 35. After that, both men and women lose a small amount of bone mass each year because the remodeling process favors osteoclastic resorption over osteoblastic building of bone. Estrogen deficiency at menopause is thought to accelerate bone loss due to stimulation of osteoclastic bone resorption through the activation of various lymphokines including interleukin 1 (IL-1), IL-6, and tumor necrosis factor.[40] Estrogen is also a modulator of calcium regulatory hormones such as parathyroid hormone and 1,25-dihydroxyvitamin D, as well as of intestinal calcium absorption. Numerous investigators have shown an increase in bone mineral density (BMD) with postmenopausal estrogen therapy. The PEPI trial, which specifically examined the spine and hip in postmenopausal women who were, on average, 52 years of age, compared placebo to estrogen alone, estrogen plus medroxyprogesterone acetate (MPA), and estrogen plus micronized progesterone. Investigators, over the 3-year time span of the study, demonstrated a loss of BMD in the placebo

group and a gain in BMD in all the hormone-treated groups.[41]

Lindsay demonstrated the benefit of starting estrogen replacement soon after menopause in a 16-year placebo-controlled trial of oophorectomized women. Estrogen therapy retarded bone loss, whereas those who did not take estrogen lost 20 percent of their bone mineral content over the course of the study.[42] The Swedish Hip Fracture Study was an observational study of 1327 women ages 50 to 81 years with hip fracture and 3262 controls. Women using estrogens had an odds ratio of 0.35 (0.24–0.53) for hip fracture compared with never-users.[43] One study of 36 patients with gonadal dysgenesis ages 16 to 35 years demonstrated a marked decrease in the BMD of the lumbar spine and femoral neck. Ninety percent of these women presented with osteopenia or osteoporosis of the lumbar spine. The duration of estrogen therapy had a positive association with the BMD at the lumbar spine in those participating.[44] Therefore, early diagnosis and medical intervention with HT are important to ensure adequate bone mass development in patients with hypogonadal amenorrhea. Finally, the Women's Health Initiative (WHI) study is a randomized, multicenter, double-blind, placebo-controlled set of three clinical trials studying the effect of HT on the prevention of heart disease, breast and colon cancer, and osteoporosis in postmenopausal women.[45a] One arm of the study consisted of 16,608 healthy women with an intact uterus who received estrogen and progestin between the ages of 50 and 79 (average age was 63.3 years). This study was to be conducted for 8 years yet was halted at 5.2 years due to the observation that the risks of the intervention outweighed its benefits. The investigators initially hypothesized a significant reduction in the risk of coronary heart disease and stroke and some increase in the risk of breast cancer. The study was halted due to the finding of a small increase in the risk of breast cancer and cardiovascular events (myocardial infarction, stroke, pulmonary embolism, and deep-vein thrombosis) but a statistically significant reduction in the risk of both hip and vertebral fracture in women treated with estrogen and progestin compared with placebo. Specifically, the WHI study showed one-third fewer hip and vertebral fractures and a 24 percent decreased risk for total fractures (Fig. 30-2). This report is the first definitive data supporting the ability of postmenopausal estrogen therapy to prevent fractures at the hip, vertebrae, and other sites. As a result of this study, the North American Menopause Society (NAMS) Advisory Panel considered individual circumstances for which *extended* (i.e., greater than 5 years) use of hormonal therapy would be appropriate. Even though a consensus was not reached, these circumstances include women with increase risk of osteoporosis who may not tolerate other therapeutic options. Importantly, a separate arm of the WHI study, initiated at the same time was designed to examine women without a uterus and on estrogen alone. This arm of the study was halted after 6–8 years due to a lack of prevention of cardiovascular disease, and a small increase in the risk of stroke. Hip and vertebral fractures were 39 percent and 38 percent lower in the estrogen-treated group than in the placebo group. These differences were statistically significant.[45b]. It appears appropriate to advise women who are taking HT for the first few years after menopause that they do not need the addition of another antiresorptive agent for the prevention of osteoporosis. Finally, the use of lower doses of ET and HT appears to maintain bone density at or near that for standard doses[46] (Fig. 30-3)

Osteoarthritis

There is some evidence that estrogen may protect older women against osteoarthritis, which is an inflammatory and degenerative disorder of the hip. One study of 4366 women older than 65 years of age showed a significant reduction in the risk of hip osteoarthritis [odds ratio (OR) 0.62; 95 percent confidence interval (CI) 0.49–0.86]. There was a greater reduction with current use over 10 years in duration (OR 0.57; 95 percent CI 0.40–0.82).[47]

Periodontal Disease

Evidence of HT's dental benefits comes from the Nurses' Health Study of 14,171 women. The relative risk for tooth loss among current HT users was 0.76 (0.72–0.80) compared with nonusers.[48] Two other studies also noted that

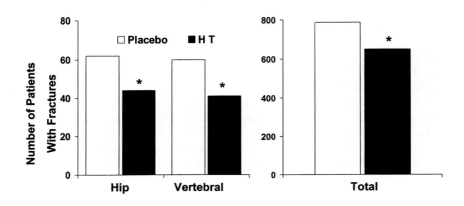

*P < .05 vs placebo.

Figure 30-2 The number of hip, vertebral, and total fractures in women treated with placebo or hormone therapy (HT). *(From Women's Health Initiative. JAMA 2003;288: 321–333.)*

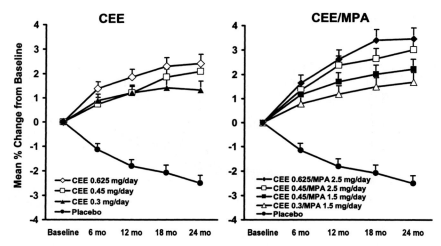

Figure 30-3 Bone mineral density of the spine (percentage change from baseline). *(Data from the Heart, Osteoporosis, Progestin, Estrogen Study. Lindsay R, et al. JAMA 2002;287:2668–2676; used with permission.)*

both past and current use of ET is associated with a decreased risk of tooth loss.[49,50]

Alzheimer Disease

The prevalence of Alzheimer disease increases dramatically with aging, and the disease is observed in approximately 15 percent of individuals who are 80 years of age or older. It now affects 4.5 million Americans. Several studies have provided a link between ET and a reduced risk of Alzheimer disease.[51–54] Two studies have demonstrated a decrease in the incidence of Alzheimer disease with increased duration of estrogen use.[52,53] The Cache County Study reported an effect of treatment duration with a decrease in the incidence of Alzheimer's disease in HT users versus nonusers. The risk of Alzheimer disease in former HT users (>10 years) was reduced 67 percent [hazard ratio (HR) 0.33; 95 percent CI 0.15–0.16][55] (Fig. 30-4). However, the use of ET or HT in established Alzheimer disease does not appear beneficial.[56] Also in the Women's Health Initiative Memory Study (WHIMS), the initiation of HT in women over 65 years of age did not improve and slightly increased the risk for dementia.[57]

Clearly, there is a need for further prospective studies on HT in postmenopausal women prior to the onset of Alzheimer disease. Thus routine therapeutic use of estrogen in women who are at risk for Alzheimer disease is not as yet justified.

Colorectal Cancer

Among U.S. women, colorectal cancer is the third most common malignancy. Colon cancer is more common in women than in men, and the incidence peaks at 60 to 75 years of age. Many epidemiologic studies have examined the relationship between estrogen use and colorectal cancer. Several studies have reported as much as a 50 percent reduction in the incidence of this cancer among current or recent users of ET.[58–67] The WHI study, as mentioned earlier under "Osteoporosis," found a reduced risk of colon cancer in estrogen-progestin users with an overall hazard ratio of 0.63, suggesting a 37 percent reduction in risk.[45a] These data are consistent with previously published observational data and data from clinical trials[58–67] (Fig. 30-5). A precise mechanism of action for estrogen's role in the reduction of colon can-

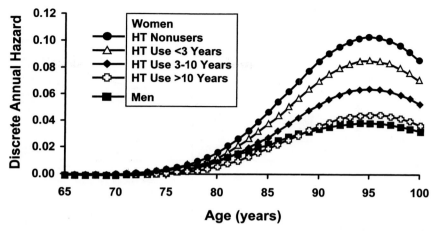

Figure 30-4   The effect of HT on the risk of developing Alzheimer's disease.   *(Data from the Cache County Study. Zandi PP, et al. JAMA 2003;288:2123–2129; used with permission.)*

cer is not known. One theory suggests that hormone use decreases bile acids that are carcinogenic.[68] Another theory involves the fact that decreased levels of estrogen receptor β (ER-β) is associated with colon tumors in women. ET increases ER-β, which is the prominent subtype in the human colon.[69] Finally, one study suggests that tumor growth suppression results from estrogen receptor activity

by preventing a "methylation imbalance" that leads to tumor progression.[70]

Cardiovascular Disease

Until recently, data have suggested that ET and HT were beneficial in reducing the risk of cardiovascular disease (CVD) in women. Beginning

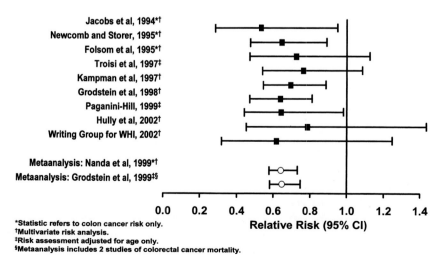

*Statistic refers to colon cancer risk only.
†Multivariate risk analysis.
‡Risk assessment adjusted for age only.
§Metaanalysis includes 2 studies of colorectal cancer mortality.

Figure 30-5   A summary of studies reporting reduction in the risk of developing colorectal cancer in women who take HT.

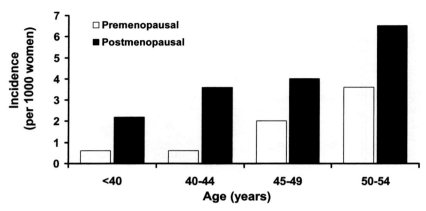

Figure 30-6 The incidence of cardiovascular events in women related to their menstrual status. *(Data adapted, with permission, from Kannel WB, et al. Ann Intern Med 1976;85: 447–452.)*

with the report of the Framingham Study in 1976, which reported that women who experienced premature menopause had an increased risk of heart disease compared with women at the same age who were still having menstrual cycles[71] (Fig. 30-6), observational studies have shown overwhelmingly a reduction in CVD risk in patients who used estrogen therapy or combined hormone therapy with progestin.[72] The largest observation trial is the Nurse's Health Study, which demonstrated a reduction in relative risk of around 50 percent in both ET and HT users compared with nonusers[73] (Table 30-1). ET and HT could prevent CVD by two mechanisms. A primary prevention mechanism would reduce the risk of developing CVD. Secondary prevention would reduce coronary occlusion in women with established CVD. There

are a number of studies that have demonstrated that ET in particular decreased the subsequent or second cardiac event or death rates in women who previously have had a myocardial infarction. A marked reduction was found in both reinfarction and death rates in current ET users and past users.[74] These results led investigators to develop the HERS I and HERS II trials, which evaluated the ability of a combination of hormone therapy and estrogen and progestin treatment to reduce the risk of recurrent events in women with previously established heart disease. These women were an average of 65 years of age. In the HERS I trial, there appeared to be more cardiac events in the first year of use in HT users, and thereafter they declined.[75] The conclusions of the HERS I and II trials were that there is no significant

▶ **TABLE 30-1:** EFFECT OF ESTROGEN DOSE ON RISK OF COROINARY HEART DISEASE (NURSES' HEALTH STUDY, 1980–1996)

Hormone Use	Person-Years of Follow-up	Cases (*n*)	Multivariate-Adjusted RR (95% CI)
Never	313,661	609	1.0
0.3 mg	19,964	19	0.58 (0.37–0.92)
0.625 mg	116,150	99	0.54 (0.44–0.67)
≥1.25 mg	39,026	41	0.70 (0.51–0.97)

RR = relative risk for current versus never-users.

From Grodstein et al.,[73] with permission.

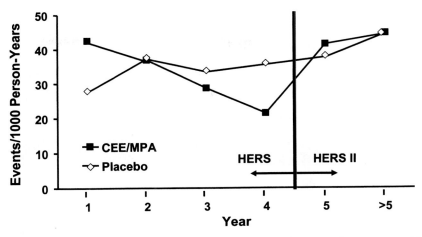

Figure 30-7   The effect of HT on the risk of coronary heart decease in women with established heart disease.   *(Data from HERS I and HERS II. Grady D, et al. JAMA 2002;88: 49–57.)*

difference in rates of coronary heart disease or second cardiovascular outcomes among women assigned to conjugated equine estrogens plus MPA compared with those assigned to a placebo[75,76] (Fig. 30-7). The conclusion of the Hodus study and the ERA also support the view that women with established heart disease appear not to have any benefit from HT use.[77,78]

In contrast, there are significant data supporting that estrogens are protective in healthy vessels both in vitro and in animal models. Particularly in a primate model, Clarkson has demonstrated that estrogens, as well as estrogens plus MPA, prevented the occurrence of coronary occlusion in oophorectomized monkeys subsequently given an unhealthy high-fat diet.[79] Again, the WHI evaluated the use of

▶ **TABLE 30-2:** WHI RESULTS: ABSOLUTE AND RELATIVE RISK OR BENEFIT OF HRT

Health Event	Relative Risk versus Placebo at 5.2 Years	Confidence Interval		Increased Absolute Risk per 10,000 Women/Year	Increased Absolute Benefit per 10,000 Women/Year
		Nominal 95%	Adjusted 95%		
Coronary heart disease (CHD)	1.29	1.02–1.63	0.85–1.97	7	
Strokes	1.41	1.07–1.85	0.86–2.31	8	
Breast cancer	1.26	1.00–1.59	0.83–1.92	8	
VTEs	2.11	1.58–2.82	1.26–3.55	18	
Colorectal cancer	0.63	0.43–0.92	0.32–1.24		6
Hip fractures	0.66	0.45–0.98	0.33–1.33		5
Total fractures	0.76	0.69–0.85	0.63–0.92		44

Nominal = variability based on simple trial for single outcome; adjusted = corrects variability for multiple analyses over time.
From Writing Group for the Women's Health Initiative Investigators,[45] with permission.

▶ **TABLE 30-3A:** ORAL PRODUCTS (ESTROGEN-ONLY)

Product	Estrogen	Common Daily Dose (mg)	Available Doses (mg)
Cenestin (Duramed)	Oral synthetic conjugated estrogens	0.625	0.3 0.625 0.9 1.25
Gynodiol (Novavax)	Oral ethinyl estradiol	1.0	0.05 1.0 1.5 2.0
Estrace (Warner Chilcott) Estradiol (Watson Labs)	Oral micronized estradiol	1.0 mg	0.5 1.0 2.0
Menest (Monarch)	Oral esterfied estrogen	0.625	0.3 0.625 1.25 2.5
Ogen (Abbot)	Oral estropipate	0.625	0.625 1.25 2.5
Premarin (Wyeth)	Oral conjugated equine estrogen	0.625 mg	0.3 0.45 0.625 0.9 1.25 2.5

▶ **TABLE 30-3B:** TRANSDERMAL PRODUCTS (ESTROGEN-ONLY)

Product	Estrogen	Common Doses	Available Dosages (mg)
Alora (Watson) Climara (Berlex) Esclim (Women First Healthcare) Estraderm (Ciba Geigy)	Transdermal Estradiol-17β	Estraderm, Alora, Vivelle, Vivelle-Dot, Esclim (change patch twice weekly)	Alora: 0.025, 0.05, 0.075, 0.1 Climara: 0.025, 0.0375, 0.05, 0.06, 0.075, 0.1 Fempatch: 0.025
FemPatch (Parke-Davis) Vivelle (Novartis) Vivelle-Dot (Novartis)		Climara and FemPatch (change patch weekly)	Esclim: 0.025, 0.0375, 0.05, 0.075, 0.1 Estraderm: 0.05, 0.1 Vivelle: 0.025, 0.05, 0.075, 0.1 Vivelle-Dot: 0.025, 0.05, 0.075, 0.1

▶ **TABLE 30-3C:** VAGINAL PRODUCTS (ESTROGEN-ONLY)

Product	Estrogen	Dosage
Estrace Vaginal (Warner Chilcott)	Estradiol vaginal cream 0.1 mg/g	2–4 g/day for 1–2 weeks. Gradually reduce to ½ initial dosage. Maintenance dose 1 g 1 to 3 times/week.
Estring (Pharmacia & Upjohn)	Estradiol vaginal ring 2.0 mg	Change q3 months
Premarin (Wyeth)	Conjugated equine estrogen vaginal cream 0.625 mg/g	2–4 g/day for 1–2 weeks. Gradually reduce to ½ initial dosage. Maintenance dose 1 g 1 to 3 times/week.
Femring (Warner Chilcott)	Estradiol vagina ring 0.05 mg/d 0.10 mg/d	Change q 3 months
Ortho Dienestrol Vaginal Cream (Ortho Pharm.)	0.01% dienstrol cream	Administer cyclically. 1 or 2 applicators/day for 1 or 2 weeks, then reduce to ½ initial dosage. Maintenance dose of one applicator 1 to 3 times/week
Vagifem (Novo Nordisk)	Estradiol vaginal tablet 0.025 mg (with applicator)	Initial: 1 tab qd × 2 weeks Maintenance: twice weekly

▶ **TABLE 30-3D:** INTRAMUSCULAR PRODUCT (ESTROGEN-ONLY)

Product	Estrogen	Strengths	Dosage
Delestrogen (Monarch)	Estradiol valerate	10 mg/ml (5 ml) 20 mg/ml (5 ml) 40 mg/ml (5 ml)	10–20 mg IM every few weeks

▶ **TABLE 30-3E:** COMBINATION HRT

Product	Estrogen	Progestin
Activella (Novo Nordisk)	Oral estradiol, 1.0 mg	Norethindrone acetate, 0.5 mg
Climara Pro	Transdermal estradiol, 0.045 mg/d	Levonorgestrel 0.015 mg/d
Combipatch (Novartis)	Transdermal estradiol, 0.05 mg	Norethindrone acetate, 0.14 mg/d
(Apply patch twice weekly)	Transdermal estradiol, 0.05 mg	Norethindrone acetate, 0.25 mg/d
Femhrt (Phizer)	Oral ethinyl estradiol, 0.05 mg	Norethindrone acetate, 1.0 mg
Premphase (Wyeth)	Oral conjugated equine estrogen 0.625 mg	Medroxyprogesterone, 5 mg (14 days/28-day cycle)
Prempro (Wyeth)	Oral conjugated equine estrogen 0.625 mg	Medroxyprogesterone, 2.5 mg or 5.0 mg
Prempro (Wyeth)	Oral conjugated equine estrogen 0.45 mg	Medroxyprogesterone, 1.5 mg
Prempro (Wyeth)	Oral conjugated equine estrogen 0.3 mg	Medroxyprogesterone, 1.5 mg
Prefest (Monarch)	Oral estradiol, 1.0 mg	Norgestimate, 0.09 mg (on 3 days and off 3 days cycling)

▶ **TABLE 30-3F:** PROGESTIN-ONLY HRT

Product	Progestin	Cyclic Regimen 10–14 days/mo (mg)	Continuous Regimen (daily) (mg)
Amen (Carnrick)	Oral MPA*	10 mg	
Provera (Pharmacia & Upjohn)	Oral MPA*	5 or 10	2.5
Crinone (Serono)	Progesterone gel 4%, 8%	Every other day for up to 6 doses	
Prometrium (Solvay)	Oral micronized progesterone	200	100–200
Micronor (Ortho) .35 mg	Oral norethindrone	0.7–1.0	0.35
Nor-QD (Watson) .35 mg	Oral norethindrone	0.7–1.0	0.35

*MPA, medroxyprogesterone acetate.

▶ **TABLE 30-3G:** ESTROGEN-ANDROGEN HRT

Product	Estrogen	Methyltestosterone (mg)
Estratest (Solvay)	Oral 1.25 mg esterfied estrogen	2.5
Estratest HS (Solvay)	Oral 0.625 mg esterfied estrogen	1.25

combination conjugated equine estrogens plus progestin used continuously compared with placebo in 10,608 women with an average age of 63.3 years. Although most of these women were healthy, their body weight, incidence of smoking, and history of previous myocardial infarction or coronary bypass procedure was greater than that observed in the Nurse's Health Study. The conclusions of the WHI demonstrate a slight increased risk of coronary heart disease [relative risk (RR) 1.29; 95 percent CI 1.02–1.63)[45a] (Table 30-2). The estrogen-alone arm of the WHI in hysterectomized women after a following of 6.8 years revealed no effect (either positive or negative) on the risk of CHD.[45b] This is the first study that suggested that HT might slightly increase the risk of heart disease. However, a reevaluation of these data was published recently, and the overall risk of CVD was not statistically significant in users of HT versus nonusers (RR 1.24; 95 percent CI 1.00–1.50).[80] The WHI also reported a small increased risk of strokes and venous throm-

boembolism in hormone users. Based on these studies, the current belief is that hormone therapy is no longer indicated for a secondary prevention of cardiac disease and probably not for primary prevention, at least in patients who fit the parameters of the WHI, i.e., women who are not having hot flashes or symptoms and were distant from the onset of menopause. The question of whether ET/HT is beneficial to women in the early premeno-pausal years as a primary prevention of heart disease is currently unanswered.

▶ ESTROGEN-PROGESTIN METHODS OF DELIVERY

Estrogen Only

Methods of hormone delivery of estrogen include oral preparations, transdermal products and vaginal creams, tablets, and rings (Table 30-3). Vaginal preparations typically have had a local estrogenizing effect on the mucosal lining without significant systemic effects. However, recently, a new vaginal estrogen-containing ring product has been introduced that does have systemic effects to the extent of a reduction in hot flashes.

Estrogen-Progestin Combination Products

Products containing both estrogen and progestin preparations include oral preparations as well as a transdermal patch.

KEY POINTS

1. The mean or average age of menopause is 51 years.

2. The early or short-term effects of estrogen deficiency are vasomotor symptoms. The intermediate effect of estrogen deficiency is vaginal atrophy. The long-term consequences of estrogen deficiency are osteoporosis and, possibly, cardiovascular disease and dementia.

3. Hormone therapy (HT) is very effective in relieving hot flushes and vaginal dryness and in preventing osteoporosis.

4. Skin changes that improve with HT include thickness, wrinkling, and dryness.

5. HT increases bone density and prevents fractures of the spine and femur in postmenopausal women.

6. HT *may* reduce the risk of dementia if initiated early in the perimenopause.

7. HT significantly reduces the risk of colorectal cancer.

8. HT does not reduce the risk of secondary coronary events in women with cardiovascular disease. The effect on primary cardiac prevention is unclear.

REFERENCES

1. US Bureau of the Census. *Statistical abstract of the United States: 1991,* 3d ed. Washington: US Government Printing Office, 1991:16.

2. McKinlay SM, Brambilla DJ, Posner JG. The normal menopause transition. *Maturitas* 1992; 14:103.

3. Treolar AE. Menarche, menopause, and intervening fecundability. *Hum Biol* 1974;46:89.

4. Coulam CB, Adamsen SC, Annegers JF. Incidence of premature ovarian failure. *Obstet Gynecol* 1986;67:604.

5. Longcope C, Jaffe W, Griffing G. Production rates of androgens and oestrogens in postmenopausal women. *Maturitas* 1981;3:215.

6. Kronnenberg F, Barnard RM. Modulation of menopausal hot flashes by ambient temperature. *J Therm Biol* 1992;17:43.

7. Oldenhave A, Jaszmann LJB, Haspels AA, Everaerd WTAM. Impact of climacteric on well-being. *Am J Obstet Gynecol* 1993;168:772.

8. Kronnenberg F. Hot flashes: Epidemiology and physiology. *Ann NY Acad Sci* 1990; 592:52.

9. Feldman BM, Voda AM, Gronseth E. The prevalence of hot flash and associated variables among perimenopausal women. *Res Nurse Health* 1985;8:261.

10. Aksel S, Schomberg DW, Iyrey L, Hammond CB. Vasomotor symptoms, serum estrogens and gonadotropins levels in surgical menopause. *Am J Obstet Gynecol* 1976;12:165..

11. Utian WH. The true clinical features of postmenopause and oophorectomy, and their response to estrogen therapy. *S Afr Med J* 1972;46:732.

12. DeFazio J, Meldrum DR, Laufer L, et al. Induction of hot flashes in premenopausal women treated with a long-acting GnRH agonist. *J Clin Endocrinol Metab* 1983;56:445.

13. Lemay A, Maheux R, Faure N, et al. Reversible hyperestrogenism induced by repetitive LHRH agonist administration in the treatment of endometriosis. Presented at the 17th International Congress of Endocrinology, 1984.

14. Casper RJ, Yen SSC, Wilkes MM. Menopausal flushes: A neuroendocrine link with pulsatile luteinizing hormone secretion. *Science* 1979; 205:823.

15. Yen SSC. The biology of menopause. *J Reprod Med* 1977;18:287.

16. Coope J, Thomson JM, Poller L. Effects of natural oestrogen replacement therapy on menopausal symptoms and blood clotting. *BMJ* 1975;4:139.

17. Campbell S, Whitehead M. Oestrogen therapy and the menopausal syndrome. *Clin Obstet Gynecol* 1977;4:31.

18. Derman RJ, Dawood MY, Stone S. Quality of life during sequential hormone replacement therapy: A placebo-controlled study. *Int J Fertil Menopaus Stud* 1995;40:73.

19. Steingold KA. Treatment of hot flashes with transdermal estradiol administration. *J Clin Endocrinol Metab* 1985;61:627.

20. Haas S, Walsh B, Evans S, et al.. The effect of transdermal estradiol on hormone and metabolic dynamics over a six-week period. *Obstet Gynecol* 1988;71:671.

21. Greendale GA, Reboussin BA, Hogan P, et al. Symptom relief and side effects of postmenopausal hormones: Results from the Postmenopausal Estrogen/Progestin Interventions Trial. *Obstet Gynecol* 1998;92:982.

22. Notelovitz M, Cassel D, Hille D, et al. Efficacy of continuous sequential transdermal estradiol and norethindrone acetate in relieving vasomotor symptoms associated with menopause. *Am J Obstet Gynecol* 2000;182:7.

23. Ellerington MC, Whitcroft SI, Whitehead MI. HRT: Developments in therapy. *Br Med Bull* 1991;48:401.

24. Utian WH, Shoupe D, Bachman G, et al. Relief of vasomotor symptoms and vaginal atrophy with lower doses of conjugated equine estrogens and medroxyprogesterone acetate. *Fertil Steril* 2001;75:1065.

25. Pandit L, Ouslander JG. Postmenopausal vaginal atrophy and atrophic vaginitis. *Am J Med Sci* 1997;314:228.

26. Speroff L. Menopause and the perimenopausal transition, in *Clinical Gynecologic Endocrinology and Infertility,* 6th ed. Philadelphia: Lippincott Williams & Wilkins, 1999; p 643.

27. McKenna SP, Whalley D, Renck-Hooper U, et al. The development of a quality of life instrument for use with postmenopausal women with urogenital atrophy in the UK and Sweden. *Qual Life Res* 1999;8:393.

28. Kalogeraki A, Tamiolakis D, Relakis K, et al. Cigarette smoking and vaginal atrophy in postmenopausal women. *In Vivo* 1996;10:597.

29. Notelovitz M. Urogenital aging: Solutions in clinical practice. *Int J Gynaecol Obstet* 1997;59:S35.

30. Raz R, Stamm WE. A controlled trial of intravaginal estriol in postmenopausal women with recurrent urinary tract infections. *N Engl J Med* 1993;329:753.

31. Castello-Branco C, Duran M, Gonzalez-Merlo J. Skin collagen changes related to age and hormone replacement therapy. *Maturitas* 1992;15:113.

32. Holland EFN, Studd JWW, Mansell JP, et al. Changes in collagen composition and cross-links in bone and skin of osteoporotic postmenopausal women treated with percutaneous estradiol implants. *Obstet Gynecol* 1994;83:180.

33. Dunn LB, Damesyn M, Moore AA, et al. Does estrogen prevent skin aging? Results from the First National Health and Nutrition Examination Survey (NHANES I). *Arch Dermatol* 1997;133:339.

34. Maheux R, Naud F, Rioux M, et al. A randomized, double-blind, placebo-controlled study on the effect of conjugated estrogens on skin thickness. *Am J Obstet Gynecol* 1994;170:642.

35. Brincat M, Moniz CF, Kabalan S, et al. Decline in skin collagen content and metacarpal index after the menopause and its prevention with sex hormone replacement. *Br J Obstet Gynaecol* 1987;94:126.

36. Brincat M, Kabalan S, Studd JWW, et al. A study of the relationship of skin collagen content, skin thickness and bone mass in the postmenopausal woman. *Obstet Gynecol* 1987;70:840.

37. Goodrich SM, Wood JE. The effect of estradiol-17β on peripheral venous distensibility and velocity of venous blood flow. *Am J Obstet Gynecol* 1966;96:407.

38. Pierard GE, Letawe L, Dowlati A, Pierard-Franchimant C. Effect of hormone replacement therapy for menopause on the mechanical properties of skin. *J Am Geriatr Soc* 1995;43:662.

39. Gallagher JC, Melton LJ, Riggs BL, et al. Epidemiology of fractures of the proximal femur in Rochester, Minnesota. *Clin Orthop* 1980;150:163.

40. Jilka RL. Cytokines, bone remodeling, and estrogen deficiency: A 1998 update. *Bone* 1998;23:75.

41. Writing Group for the PEPI Trial. Effects of hormone therapy on bone mineral density: Results from the Postmenopausal Estrogen/Progestin Interventions Trial. *JAMA* 1996;276:389.

42. Lindsay R. The menopause: Sex steroids and osteoporosis. *Clin Obstet Gynecol* 1987;30:847.

43. Michaelsson K, Baron JA, Farahmand BY, et al for the Swedish Hip Fracture Study Group. Hormone replacement therapy and risk of hip fracture: Population based case-control study. *Br Med J* 1998;316:1858.

44. Benetti-Pinto CL, Bedone A, Magna LA, et al. Factors associated with the reduction of bone density in patients with gonadal dysgenesis. *Fertil Steril* 2002;77: 571.

45a. Writing Group for the Women's Health Initiative Investigators. Risks and benefits of estrogen plus progestin in healthy postmenopausal women: Principal results from the Women's Health Initiative randomized controlled trial. *JAMA* 2002;288:321.

45b. Effects of conjugated equine estrogens in postmenopausal women with hysterectomy. The Women's Health Initiative randomized controlled trial. *JAMA* 2004;291:1701.

46. Lindsay R, Gallagher JC, Kleerekoper M, et al. Effect of lower doses of conjugated equine estrogens with and without medroxyprogesterone acetate on bone in early post-menopausal women. *JAMA* 2002;287:2668.

47. Nevitt MC, Cummings SR, Lane NE, et al. Association of estrogen replacement therapy with the risk of osteoarthritis of the hip in elderly white women. Study of Osteoporotic Fractures Research Group. *Arch Intern Med.* 1996;156: 2073.

48. Grodstein F, Colditz GA, Stampfer MJ. Postmenopausal hormone use and tooth loss: a prospective study. *J Am Dent Assoc* 1996;127:370.

49. Pagagnini-Hill A. The benefits of estrogen replacement therapy on oral health. *Arch Intern Med* 1995;155:2325.

50. Krall EA, Dawson-Hughes B, Hannan MT, et al. Postmenopausal estrogen replacement and tooth retention. *Am J Med* 1997;102:536.

51. Paganini-Hill A, Henderson VW. Estrogen deficiency and risk of Alzheimer's disease in women. *Am J Epidemiol* 1994;140:256.

52. Paganini-Hill A, Henderson VW. Estrogen replacement therapy and risk of Alzheimer's disease. *Arch Intern Med* 1996;156:2213.

53. Tang M-X, Jacobs D, Stern Y, et al. Effect of oestrogen during menopause on risk and age at onset of Alzheimer's disease. *Lancet* 1996; 348:429.

54. Kawas C, Resnick S, Morrison A, et al. A prospective study of estrogen replacement therapy and the risk of developing Alzheimer's disease: The Baltimore Longitudinal Study of Aging. *Neurology* 1997;48:1517.

55. Zandi PP, Carlson MC, Plassman BL, et al. Cache County Memory Study Investigators. Hormone replacement therapy and incidence of Alzheimer disease in older women: The Cache County Study. *JAMA* 2002;288:2123.

56. Mulnard RA, Cotman CW, Kawas C, et al. Estrogen replacement therapy for treatment of mild to moderate Alzheimer disease: A randomized, controlled trial. *JAMA* 2000;283:1007.

57. Shumaker SA, Legault C, Rapp SR, et al. Estrogen plus progestin and the incidence of dementia and mild cognitive impairment in postmenopausal women. The Women's Health Initiative Memory Study: A randomized controlled trial. *JAMA* 2003;289:2651.

58. Jacobs EJ, White E, Weiss NS. Exogenous hormones, reproductive history, and colon cancer (Seattle, Washington, USA). *Cancer Causes Control* 1994;5:359–366.

59. Newcomb PA, Storer BE. Postemenopausal hormone use and risk of large-bowel cancer. *J Natl Cancer Inst* 1995;87:1067.

60. Folsom AR, Mink PJ, Sellers TA, et al. Hormonal replacement therapy and morbidity and mortality in a prospective study of postmenopausal women. *Am J Public Health* 1995;85: 1128–1132.

61. Troisi R, Schairer C, Chow WH, et al. A prospective study of menopausal hormones and risk of colorectal cancer (United States). *Cancer Causes Control* 1997;8:130.

62. Kampman E, Potter JD, Slattery ML, et al. Hormone replacement therapy, reproductive history, and colon cancer: A multicenter, case-control study in the United States. *Cancer Causes Control* 1997;8:146.

63. Grodstein F, Martinez ME, Platz EA, et al. Postmenopausal hormone use and risk for colorectal cancer and adenoma. *Ann Intern Med* 1998;128:705.

64. Paganini-Hill A. Estrogen replacement therapy and colorectal cancer risk in elderly women. *Dis Colon Rectum* 1999;42:1300.

65. Hulley S, Furberg C, Barett-Conner E, et al. Noncardiovascular disease outcomes during 6.8 years of hormone therapy: Heart and Estrogen/progestin Replacement Study follow-up (HERS II). *JAMA* 2002;288:58.

66. Nanda K, Bastian LA, Hasselblad V, Simel DL. Hormone replacement therapy and the risk of colorectal cancer: A meta-analysis. *Obstet Gynecol* 1999;93:880.

67. Grodstein F, Newcomb PA, Stampfer MJ. Postmenopausal hormone therapy and the risk of colorectal cancer: A review and meta-analysis. *Am J Med* 1999;106:574.

68. Kamano T, Mikami Y, Kurasawa T, et al. Ratio of primary and secondary bile acids in feces: Possible marker for colorectal cancer? *Dis Colon Rectum* 1999;42:668.

69. Campbell-Thompson M, Lynch IJ, Bhardwaj B. Expression of estrogen receptor (ER) subtypes and ER-(isoforms in colon cancer. *Cancer Res* 2001;61:632.

70. Al-Azzawi F, Wahab M. Estrogen and colon cancer: current issues. *Climacteric* 2002;5:3.

71. Kannel WB, Hjortland MC, McNamara PM, et al. Menopause and risk of cardiovascular disease: The Framingham Study. *Ann Intern Med* 1976;85:447.

72. Grodstein F, Stampfer MH, Falkeborn M, et al. Postmenopausal hormone therapy and risk of cardiovascular disease and hip fracture in a cohort of Swedish women. *Epidemiology* 1999; 10:476.

73. Grodstein F, Manson JE, Coditz GA, et al. A prospective observational study of postmenopausal hormone therapy and primary prevention of cardiovascular disease. *Ann Intern Med* 2000;133:933.

74. Newton KM, LaCroix AZ, McKnight B. Estrogen replacement therapy and prognosis after first myocardial infarction. *Am J Epidemiol* 1997; 145:269.

75. Hulley S, Grady D, Bush T, et al. Randomized trial of estrogen plus progestin for secondary prevention of coronary heart disease in postmenopausal women. Heart and Estrogen/progestin Replacement Study (HERS) Research Group. *JAMA* 1998;280:605.

76. Grady D, Herrington D, Bittner V, et al. Cardiovascular disease outcomes during 6.8 years of hormone therapy: Heart and Extrogen/progestin Replacement Study follow-up (HERSII). *JAMA* 2002;288:49.

77. Hodis HN, Mack WJ, Azen SP, et al. Hormone therapy and the progression of coronary-artery atherosclerosis in postmenopausal women. *N Engl J Med* 2003;349:535.

78. Herrington DM, Reboussin DM, Brosnihan KB, et al. Effects of estrogen replacement on the progression of coronary-artery atherosclerosis. *N Engl J Med* 2000;343:522.

79. Clarkson TB, Anthony MS, Wagner JD. A comparison of tibolone and conjugated equine estrogens effects on coronary artery atherosclerosis and bone density of postmenopausal monkeys. *J Clin Endorinol Metab* 2001;86: 5396.

80. Manson JE, Johnson KC, Rossouw JE, et al. Women's Health Initiative Investigators: Estrogen plus progestin and the risk of coronary heart disease. *N Engl J Med* 2003;349:523.

CHAPTER 31

Risks of Hormone-Replacement Therapy

DAVID F. ARCHER

Hormone-replacement therapy has been used for over 60 years in the United States. A recent recommendation is to change the term from *hormone-replacement therapy* to use *hormone therapy* (HT) as the descriptor for estrogen or estrogen plus progestin use in postmenopausal women. Hormone-replacement therapy has been studied intensively since it was introduced as a means to increase low estrogen levels in postmenopausal women or following a surgical menopause with removal of one or both functioning ovaries.

Until 1998, hormone therapy was felt to be a significant, positive intervention to control symptoms and prevent cardiovascular disease for postmenopausal women.[1-3] The reasons for this have been described for the control of symptoms in postmenopausal women (see Chap. 30). Observational data strongly supported a reduction in the risk of coronary heart disease, maintenance of bone mineral density, and a reduced incidence of Alzheimer's disease.[4-7]

There has been a recent series of publications based on two prospective, randomized clinical trials that have questioned the utility and efficacy of HT (estrogen plus progestin therapy) in reducing cardiovascular risk. These studies, the Heart and Estrogen Progestin Replacement Study (HERS) and the Women's Health Initiative (WHI), have had a significant amount of media attention and have resulted in a reassessment of the role of HT in postmenopausal women.[8,9]

This chapter provides the background evidence and balance between opposing viewpoints in the ongoing discussion as to the risks of HT.

▶ CARDIOVASCULAR DISEASE

Cardiovascular disease, specifically coronary artery disease, increases as individuals age. This statement is true for both men and women. The overwhelming cause of death in older individuals is heart disease. Although many women feel that neoplasia is the principal cause of death in the United States, this is a fallacy because the most common cause of death is myocardial infarction.

The arterial side of the circulation is involved in coronary heart disease and ischemic stroke, and the venous side of the circulation is involved in venous thrombosis and pulmonary emboli. Whether or not these morphologically distinct blood vessels have different etiologies with the use of hormone therapy (HT) is a matter of conjecture and debate.

Coronary Heart Disease

Beginning in the late 1980s, a series of reports appeared based on observational data of older women in a variety of clinical settings. It appeared that women who used HT enjoyed a privileged position for reduction in the risk of coronary heart disease compared with women who were not using HT. That is to say that there appeared to be a reduction in the incidence of coronary heart disease by approximately 30 percent in women using HT compared with nonusers.[2,10] Studies reported from the National Lipid Research database presented compelling evidence that women on HT had higher high-density lipoprotein (HDL) cholesterol and lower low-density lipoprotein (LDL) cholesterol, and their overall total cholesterol was less than nonusers of HT.[11–13] There is pervasive biology strongly supporting estrogen and estrogen plus progestin as having a significant positive impact in terms of reduction in atherosclerosis, changes in endothelial cell function, and vasodilatation of arteries.[14] It should be appreciated that all these positive outcomes supported a conclusion that HT was efficacious in reducing the incidence of coronary heart disease.

Beginning in the 1990s, questions were raised as to the true efficacy of HT in coronary heart disease. Specifically, it was debated whether or not there were biases in the observational studies that identified a group of women who were at low risk for heart disease.[15,16] These low-risk women represented a subset of postmenopausal women who, through self-imposed diet, exercise, and other positive lifestyles, including HT, improved their general health. Therefore, they were at less risk of developing coronary heart disease than their non-HT-using contemporaries. The impact of exercise on coronary heart disease was confirmed from the observational arm of the WHI, which found a 30 percent reduction in the risk of coronary heart disease in women who exercised three times a week for 30 minutes.[17]

The HERS was a prospective, randomized trial of women whose average age was 67 years. These women had evidence of preexisting coronary artery disease, as demonstrated by a previous myocardial infarction, previous coronary artery bypass graft, or a percutaneous coronary artery angioplastic procedure.[8,18,19] The use of conjugated estrogens 0.625 mg and medroxyprogesterone acetate 2.5 mg as continuous combined HT had no effect on reducing the recurrence rate for coronary heart disease events and/or mortality. There appeared to be an increase in the incidence of coronary heart disease events in the first year after starting HT in this study.[8] There was a trend for the reduction in the number of coronary heart disease events in the HT group compared with placebo with time. An extension of this trial was carried out for an additional 2.5 years on a voluntary basis.[19] The overall outcome in terms of HT and the incidence of coronary heart disease events was null throughout the course of the 6.5 years of treatment and follow-up.[19] That is to say there was no increased or decreased incidence of recurrent cardiac events between the two groups. These data resulted in a significant discussion within the medical/scientific community as to why there was no benefit of HT. A variety of hypotheses were put forward to try to explain the fact that HT was not found to be efficacious in reducing the incidence of heart disease in established coronary heart disease patients.[20–28]

Some of the hypotheses argued that there was a subset of women at increased risk due to an unsuspected hypercoagulable state. Alternatively, it was felt that perhaps there were changes in the capillary endothelium in established atherosclerosis that resulted in increasing thrombosis. Third was the concern that the progestin, medroxyprogesterone acetate was the culprit by altering vascular responsivity.[29–31]

A unique finding was that the use of statin therapy provided protection from increased risk of coronary heart disease events during the first year in the HT user.[28] It was considered that the use of statins may have introduced a bias into the placebo population. Statins were prescribed more frequently in the placebo group compared with the HT group. Subgroup analysis failed to show that there was a difference in the use of statins that could account for the first-year discrepancy in the coronary heart disease events in the HERS trial.

The overall relative risk was 0.99 [95 percent confidence interval (CI) 0.84–1.17] for coronary heart disease in the individuals using HT versus placebo in the HERS trial over the 6.8 years of the study.[32]

These data from a prospective, randomized clinical trial were contrasted to the observational studies published at the same time. The observational study (Nurses Health Study) continued to show a protective effect with the use of estrogens or estrogen plus progestin in women with established heart disease who had been hospitalized for myocardial infarction or who had evidence of atherosclerosis.[33] The multivariate-adjusted relative risk for major coronary heart disease in HT users was 1.25 (95 percent CI, 0.78–2.00) compared with never-users. The relative risk of a coronary heart disease event with increasing time of HT use was 0.61 (95 percent CI 0.52–0.71).[33]

The use of statins, aspirin, and other therapies has been shown to significantly reduce the risk of coronary heart disease events.[34] Recommendations and guidelines from national organizations do not support the use of HT for the primary or secondary prevention of coronary heart disease.[35–37]

Primary Prevention of Coronary Heart Disease

There are meta-analyses that, based on observational data, suggest that women who used HT have a 40 percent reduction in the incidence of coronary heart disease compared with nonusers.[1,38] The WHI is a prospective, randomized, double-blind study supported by the National Institutes of Health (NIH) to investigate whether or not estrogen or estrogen plus progestin would prevent coronary heart disease in postmenopausal women. The estrogen plus progestin (HT) trial enrolled 18,600 women whose average age was 63 years and who were "healthy." This statement really meant that these women were currently asymptomatic at the time of enrollment in the clinical trial. The reason for saying asymptomatic is that approximately 3 percent of the women had had previous myocardial infarction or coronary artery procedures prior to enrollment. Thirty-six percent of the women had hypertension, and 4 percent were diabetic. The incidence of these coronary heart disease risks was equally divided between the HT and placebo groups. The HT in this study was 0.625 mg conjugated estrogen and 2.5 mg medroxyprogesterone acetate as a continuous combined daily therapy versus placebo.[9]

The primary outcome of the WHI was the occurrence of coronary heart disease events, either myocardial infarction diagnosed on clinical evidence following admission to a hospital, changes in electrocardiogram (ECG) suggesting myocardial infarction at 3 and 6 years after entry, or a death that on review of the records was felt to be a myocardial infarction. The final outcome of this trial was similar to that found in HERS. There was neither a statistically significant increase nor a decrease in the occurrence of coronary heart disease in this group of women over the 5 years of the clinical trial.[39] The overall relative risk was 1.24 (nominal 95 percent CI 1.00–1.54). There was an increase in the occurrence of coronary heart disease events in the first year of HT with a relative risk of 1.81 (95 percent CI 1.09–3.01). There was a trend down in the subsequent years with a z score of -2.36 ($p = 0.02$).[39]

These data have been used to indicate that there is no primary prevention of coronary heart disease with the use of HT. The debate has centered around the fact that two-thirds of the women who were enrolled in the WHI had never before used HT, and that the average age of the WHI participants was 63 years. The opposing point is that it is possible that these women already had established coronary heart disease.[31] A subset of these women could be at greater risk with the use of HT, and therefore, the increased risk in the first year identified susceptible individuals. These data from WHI are similar to those from the HERS trial that of an increased incidence of disease in the first year with a subsequent decline in the occurrence of coronary heart disease. The long-standing Nurses Health Study, an observational trial, found that women using HT had a reduced incidence of coronary heart disease with a relative risk of 0.61.[10]

The data from the WHI have been debated in the scientific community with a variety of arguments as to the potential biases that were present in this study and the statistics used to document whether or not there was indeed an increase in the incidence of coronary heart disease.[31,40,41] It should be pointed out that in the WHI interim report in 2002 there was a statistically significant increase in the incidence of coronary heart disease in the group using HT.[9] The final WHI report in 2003 stated that there was no statistically significant increase in the incidence of coronary heart disease between the HT group and the placebo group.[39]

Hypothesis to Explain the Discrepancy in Findings

The persistent problem is that observational trials showed coronary heart disease protection and prospective, randomized clinical trials failed to show protection.[31] To explain this discrepancy, a hypothesis has been put forward. This hypothesis has been promulgated mainly by those who support the efficacy of HT in preventing coronary heart disease. The hypothesis supports a concept of a window of opportunity for intervention to retard the development of atherosclerosis.[31,42]

The discussion regarding primary prevention of atherosclerosis hinges on findings from the cynomolgus monkey, in which surgical menopause (bilateral oophorectomy) in the presence of an atherogenic diet increases the size of the atherosclerotic plaque found in the coronary arteries of these female monkeys on necropsy.[42] The monkeys who were initially maintained on a normal diet and then oophorectomized and placed on an atherosclerotic diet with estrogen replacement had a significant reduction in the occurrence of atherosclerotic plaque. If the animals were first maintained on an atherosclerotic diet but then were given estrogen or estrogen plus progestin plus the atherogenic diet after oophorectomy, there was less reduction in the size of the atherosclerotic plaque. Lastly, if the primate had a surgical menopause and then after 1 year of an atherogenic diet was placed on HT, there was no reduction in plaque size.

It is difficult to emulate this type of controlled investigation in the human. There have been several studies that suggest that the use of estrogen in young women will retard the progressive development of the intimal medial thickness of the carotid artery.[43] Intimal medial thickness is a surrogate marker for coronary atherosclerosis.[43] Using conjugated estrogen with medroxyprogesterone acetate did not retard or improve the extent of the atherosclerotic plaque in the Estrogen Replacement and Atherosclerosis (ERA) trial.[44] These data have been interpreted to indicate that in order to prevent the development of atherosclerosis, intervention should be at an early stage in the atherosclerotic process. Intervention with HT may be beneficial, but of course there are other positive things that the consumer could do. Diet modification and/or exercise have been found to significantly reduce the occurrence of coronary heart disease and type 2 diabetes mellitus.[39]

This hypothesis takes into consideration that atherosclerosis is a pervasive disease in the U.S. population. We should be intervening at 30 or 40 years of age, not 50 plus, to prevent the development of coronary heart disease in women. Positive changes occur in total cholesterol, HDL cholesterol, and LDL cholesterol with HT.[45–49] The increase in HDL cholesterol and decrease in LDL cholesterol are changes that one would anticipate with using statin therapy. These findings suggest that there should be improvement in atherosclerotic progression if HT were started early. The HERS trial, in which similar positive lipid changes were found without evidence of protection from coronary heart disease, would suggest that as in the ERA study, established atherosclerosis cannot be reversed with HT.[8,27]

There are also several other potential mechanisms that may effect the interaction between hormones and cardiovascular disease. A genetic alteration in a gene coding for thrombin has been suggested. Postmenopausal women with hypertension, who have the prothrombin 20210G→A variant of the thrombin gene, are at greater risk for myocardial infarction when using HT as compared with nonusers.[50]

Second, there has been evidence of polymorphic differences in the estrogen receptor that result in significant lipid changes. Women who have a specific polymorphism of estrogen receptor 401A have a significant increase in their HDL cholesterol when using HT.[51] This increase in HDL cholesterol theoretically could lower the incidence of cardiovascular disease based on changes in HDL cholesterol from other clinical interventions.[51]

Other Hormonal Preparations

Most clinical data and the randomized, double-blind clinical trials in the United States are based on using a combination of conjugated estrogen 0.625 mg with medroxyprogesterone acetate 2.5 mg in a continuous combined fashion. There has been speculation that this is perhaps the wrong type of estrogen and/or progestin that should be used for postmenopausal women. There is one prospective, randomized trial of estradiol for the prevention of reinfarction in postmenopausal women who had survived a myocardial infarction. This trial did not find any difference between estradiol valerate (2.0 mg/d) compared with placebo for reinfarction or cardiac death. The odds ratio was 0.99 (95 percent CI 0.70–1.41) for reinfarction over the 2 years of the study.[52]

There was a small randomized, placebo-controlled trial of transdermal estradiol in women with preexisting ischemic heart disease.[53] This trial randomized 255 women, and in the intention-to-treat analysis, the odds ratio of 1.29 (95 percent CI 0.84–1.95) was not significantly different between the transdermal estrogen and placebo arms.[53]

Stroke

Ischemic Stroke

As individuals age and develop other medical problems such as hypertension and diabetes, there is an increasing occurrence of arterial thrombotic events leading to cerebral ischemia or stroke.[54] It has been well documented that hypertension and smoking are two independent risk factors for stroke in older women.[55,56] A review of the literature was unable to arrive at a definite conclusion confirming a relationship between estrogen therapy and estrogen plus progestin therapy and stroke.[57,58]

An increase in the incidence of ischemic stroke was found in the WHI study.[9,59] This increased incidence occurred in a group of older women whether or not they had identified risk factors such as diabetes mellitus or hypertension.

The WHI found the hazard ratio for ischemic stroke to be 1.44 (95 percent CI 1.09–1.90) in women using estrogen plus progestin.[59] These data are similar to those found in the Nurses Health Study, with a relative risk of 1.45 (95 percent CI 1.10–1.92) for any type of stroke.[10] There was no increase in the incidence of stroke in HERS, but this study was not powered for this end point.[54] The WHI did not find an increase in hemorrhagic stroke relative risk, namely, 0.82 (95 percent CI 0.43–1.56).[59]

The use of estrogen alone in the Nurses Health Study was not associated with an increased incidence of ischemic stroke [relative risk (RR) 1.18; 95 percent CI 0.95–1.46].[10]

In women who had had a stroke (the Women's Estrogen for Stroke Trial) it was found that the immediate intervention of estradiol

1 mg/day neither increased nor decreased the recurrence rate for ischemic stroke.[60] These data again support the contention that with established arterial disease, estrogen or HT does not appear to add any efficacy in reducing the incidence of subsequent events.

Hemorrhagic Stroke

Hemorrhagic stroke is different than ischemic or thrombotic stroke. The underlying pathophysiology appears to be different, and there is, at the present time, no large enough study that supports the fact that estrogen or estrogen plus progestin increases the incidence of hemorrhagic stroke.[58,61,62] The WHI did not find an increase in hemorrhagic stroke (RR 0.82; 95 percent CI 0.43–1.56).[59]

Venous Thromboembolism/ Pulmonary Embolism

Based on the WHI results, as well as published observational studies, there is an increase in the occurrence of deep vein thrombosis (DVT)/pulmonary emboli (PE) in postmenopausal women who are receiving HT.[39,63–67] This risk is approximately doubled (RR 2) in all the published studies. There does appear to be a predilection for an increasing incidence of venous thromboembolism (VTE) in women who have underlying coagulation disorders and specifically factor V Leiden.[68,69]

VTE incidence increases with age in both men and women, and estrogen itself appears to be a significant risk factor. Data from the HERS trial indicated that the use of aspirin in this population of women negated the increased incidence of VTE in those women on estrogen plus progestin.[63]

The pathophysiology of the occurrence of VTE/PE in these women is unknown. There is no evidence of coagulation changes induced by estrogen that correlate at all with the occurrence of VTE/PE.

A recent observational study has indicated that transdermal estradiol use is associated with a significant reduction in the occurrence of VTE compared with nonusers. This trial is the first to show any effect with the use of transdermal estrogen on VTE.[70]

Both factor V Leiden and prothrombin gene mutations have been associated with an increased risk for DVT in women who are on HT.[68,69,71,72] However, the incidence of these two abnormalities in the general population is low enough to preclude screening as a worthwhile endeavor.[68]

Anticoagulant Therapy

In individuals who are receiving anticoagulant therapy for either DVT or PE, there is no contraindication to the use of HT. HT appears to act via the coagulation cascade, and in the presence of active therapeutic anticoagulation, there does not appear to be an increased risk of thrombosis.[73]

Previous VTE or PE

The WHI unequivocally shows that individuals who have had a prior VTE or PE emboli are at significantly increased risk for recurrence with the use of HT. The relative risk for recurrent thrombotic events was 5.0.[9] These data highlight the fact that in the presence of a prior history of VTE/PE, the use of estrogen or estrogen plus progestin as replacement therapy is contraindicated.

Hypertension

Most clinical trials of the use of estrogen or estrogen plus progestin have reported no or an insignificant change in blood pressure.[45,74–78] In the current clinical trials that have been reported, the systolic blood pressure has changed approximately 1 to 2 mmHg, and the diastolic pressure has not changed significantly at all. There are reports of idiosyncratic reactions with increase in blood pressure in women on HT. At the present time, the occurrence of hypertension per se is not a contraindication to HT if the hypertension is controlled. The subgroup analysis from the WHI did not find any significant interaction between HT and hypertension.[9]

Neoplasia

Breast Cancer

The medical literature is replete with a variety of observational studies that have shown an increase, a decrease, and no significant change in the incidence of breast cancer in postmenopausal women receiving estrogen or estrogen plus progestin therapy.[79] The most compelling aspect of this argument is that estrogen or estrogen plus progestin could increase the incidence or growth of a neoplasia in postmenopausal women. One aspect of the hypothesis argues that the use of exogenous estrogen or estrogen plus progestin does not cause breast cancer; rather, it increases the growth of the breast cancer, resulting in an increase in the size of the tumor that leads to its clinical detection.

Estrogen and progestins can stimulate the growth of breast cancer cells in animal models and in vitro.[80] There is no direct evidence that HT can cause neoplasia.[80] One of the most compelling pieces of information is that after stopping HT, the risk of breast cancer rapidly returns to that observed in never-users of HT.[81–84]

Epidemiologic studies that have shown an increase in the incidence of breast cancer may be interpreted to demonstrate an overall increase in breast cancer detection in a population of women who are using HT. Over 80 percent of breast cancers in postmenopausal women occur in women who have never received HT. Age is positively correlated with the occurrence of breast cancer.[84] That is to say that as an individual ages, the incidence of breast cancer increases.[83]

The two randomized clinical trials of conjugated estrogen and medroxyprogesterone acetate (MPA) show different outcomes. The HERS trial in a group of women (average age 67 years) did not find an increase in the incidence of breast cancer with a relative risk of 1.38 (95 percent CI 0.82–2.31).[18] The HERS trial certainly was not powered to detect any effect and only lasted for 3 years.

The WHI did show an increase in the occurrence of breast cancer with an unweighted hazard ratio of 1.24 (95 percent CI 1.01–1.54).[85] It should be stressed that the hazard ratio for those women who had never before used HT was not increased.[85] This finding is in agreement with the collaborative group report of a relative risk of 1.05 (95 percent CI 0.99–1.12) in women who used HT for less than 5 years.[83] The overall risk of breast cancer in the WHI trial being elevated may reflect previous use of HT in these women. Prior HT use was associated with an increased incidence of breast cancer.[9,85] These data would argue that it takes 5 or more years before the effects of the HT are apparent in terms of the detection of breast cancers.

It is important to understand that none of the women, on entry into the WHI, had evidence of breast cancer. During the first 4 years of the study, breast cancers were detected both in the placebo and the HT groups. These findings would support the contention that these were preexisting tumors. The subsequent increase in the incidence of invasive breast cancer in the HT group of the WHI could be related to the fact that they grew to a size that was detectable. Therefore, the WHI has a hazard ratio for the detection of breast cancer rather than a hazard ratio that is increased due to HT causing breast cancer.

In support of this latter hypothesis is the fact that the tumor size in the HT group was slightly larger than in the placebo group (1.7 versus 1.5 cm; $p = 0.4$).[85] The HT group had a higher rate of positive lymph nodes (25.9 versus 15.8 percent). There were no differences in the histology or grade of the tumors between the two groups.[85]

The Million Women's Study also has found that duration of HT is related to the incidence or occurrence of breast cancer.[81] Both estrogen alone and estrogen plus progestin users have an increase in the relative risk for breast cancer in current users. The most important aspect of the Million Women's Study is the fact that on stopping HT, the increased incidence of breast cancer dissipates rapidly. The reduction in the risk of breast cancer with stopping HT also was present in the collaborative group analysis.[83] These data would support the hypothesis that the neoplastic change in the breast cancer cell may not be caused by estrogen but that existing breast cancer is grown secondary to increased mitotic activity by the use of either estrogen or estrogen plus progestin.

There is concern over the fact that the progestogen may be a more significant issue than estrogen in the risk of breast cancer. These data are based on biologic finding that there is a stimulation of mitotic activity in female breast tissue by progestins.[86,87] Continued use of a progestin or increase in the concentration of the progestin often results in an increase in apoptosis and cessation of cell growth.[88,89] Progestins also have been found to increase the mitotic activity in normal human breast tissue from postmenopausal women.[87,90]

Observational studies, case-controlled trials, and even prospective, randomized trials generally have shown a relatively small and borderline statistically significant increase in the occurrence of breast cancer in postmenopausal women using HT. The relative risk or hazard usually has been about 1.2, a point estimate found in the WHI.[85] The absolute increase was approximately 7 more cases of breast cancer per 10,000 women per year. The overall incidence of breast cancer in a 50-year-old woman not on HT is 20 per 1000 based on data from the collaborative group analysis. This figure rises to approximately 20 cases per 1000 at age 60.[83]

In terms of causality, the basic and clinical literature is very mixed as to whether or not there is an ability of estrogen to cause breast cancer.[79,91] At the present time, my opinion is that mitotic activity or growth in the breast cancer is stimulated by both estrogen and progestin. There was no compelling evidence at the time that either estrogen or progestin is a carcinogen causing breast cancer.[91]

Neither the Gail model used to estimate the risk of breast cancer nor a family history of breast cancer was found to correlate with the occurrence of breast cancer in the WHI study.[9] The Gail model, although useful for clinical trial work, is not particularly suited to the individual patient because a major factor in the model is the age of the individual. As a woman ages, she has an increasing incidence of breast cancer that results in a significant risk factor for breast cancer in women over the age of 62. The Gail model, therefore, is not useful for counseling individual patients.

RADIOGRAPHIC BREAST DENSITY

Data from both the Postmenopausal Estrogen/Progestin Intervention (PEPI) and WHI indicate that women using HT have an increase in breast density on their mammograms.[85,92] Published studies have reported an association between increased mammographic density and breast cancer.[92–94] The link between HT increased mammographic density and breast cancer is not known.[95] The WHI investigators have pointed out that increased mammographic density may impede the detection of breast cancers in women on HT.[85]

Endometrial Cancer

All epidemiologic studies to date have shown an increase in the occurrence of endometrial cancer in women who have received unopposed estrogen.[96] The incidence of endometrial cancer is negated or reduced with the addition of a progestational agent.[96] The WHI, a prospective, randomized clinical trial found that the incidence of endometrial cancer was not increased in women using both an estrogen and a progestin with an overall relative risk of 0.83 (95 percent CI 0.29–2.32).[97] There were cases of endometrial cancer in both the placebo and control group during the course of the trial. None of the women on entry into the trial had evidence of an endometrial cancer based on medical history and physical examination.

There is an increase in the occurrence of endometrial cancer at year 4 in the trial that probably reflects an observational bias because 42 percent of the women in the HT arm of the study experienced irregular endometrial bleeding versus 7.0 percent in the placebo group, resulting in active investigation by their gynecologists.

There was not an estrogen-only randomized clinical trial in women who have an intact uterus because of the results of the PEPI.[98] This study found that the use of unopposed conjugated estrogen increased the incidence of endometrial hyperplasia by approximately 20 percent each year over the 3 years of this trial.[98] Postmenopausal women who had an intact uterus and used unopposed estrogen had a reported incidence of endometrial hyperplasia similar to the type and dose of the estrogen between 8 to 20 percent.[49,98–103]

Ovarian Cancer

The occurrence of ovarian cancer in women who are postmenopausal and using HT has been reported to be increased. There appears to be an increase in the occurrence of ovarian neoplasia in long-term users of estrogen but not estrogen plus progestin users. The Breast Cancer Detection Project found a relative risk of 1.6 (95 percent CI 1.2–2.0) in women who only used estrogen.[104] The women in this trial using estrogen plus progestin had a relative risk of 1.1 (95 percent CI 0.64–1.7).[104] Other smaller studies and a meta-analysis have shown a variable occurrence of ovarian cancer in women using HT.[104–107]

One study suggests that there is an increase in mortality in women with ovarian cancer who have used HT.[108] At present, the strength of the evidence is not sufficient to document that there is an increase in the occurrence of ovarian cancer in women using HT.

Uterine/Cervical Cancer

The incidence of carcinoma of the cervix uteri increases with age, and therefore, postmenopausal women are at an increased risk for developing cervical cancer. To date, there has been no evidence that suggests that estrogen or estrogen plus progestin increases the incidence of cervical cancer.[109–112]

REFERENCES

1. Barrett-Connor E, Grady D. Hormone replacement therapy, heart disease, and other considerations. *Annu Rev Public Health* 1998;19: 55–72.
2. Grady D, Rubin SM, Petitti DB, et al. Hormone therapy to prevent disease and prolong life in postmenopausal women. *Ann Intern Med* 1992;117:1016–1037.
3. Grady D. Exercise, hormone therapy, and lipoproteins in women. *J Am Geriatr Soc* 1996; 44:331–332.
4. Hammond CB. Women's concerns with hormone replacement therapy: Compliance issues. *Fertil Steril* 1994;62:157S–160S.
5. Genant HK, Cooper C, Poor G, et al. Interim report and recommendations of the World Health Organization Task Force for Osteoporosis. *Osteoporos Int* 1999;10:259–264.
6. Lindsay R. The role of estrogen in the prevention of osteoporosis. *Endocrinol Metab Clin North Am* 1998;27:399–409.
7. Zandi PP, Carlson MC, Plassman BL, et al. Hormone replacement therapy and incidence of Alzheimer disease in older women: The Cache County Study. *JAMA* 2002;288:2123–2129.
8. Hulley S, Grady D, Bush T, et al. Randomized trial of estrogen plus progestin for secondary prevention of coronary heart disease in postmenopausal women. Heart and Estrogen/progestin Replacement Study (HERS) Research Group. *JAMA* 1998;280:605–613.
9. Rossouw JE, Anderson GL, Prentice RL, et al. Risks and benefits of estrogen plus progestin in healthy postmenopausal women: Principal results From the Women's Health Initiative randomized controlled trial. *JAMA* 2002;288: 321–333.
10. Grodstein F, Manson JE, Colditz GA, et al. A prospective, observational study of postmenopausal hormone therapy and primary prevention of cardiovascular disease. *Ann Intern Med* 2000;133:933–941.
11. Bush TL. Evidence for primary and secondary prevention of coronary artery disease in women

taking oestrogen replacement therapy. *Eur Heart J* 1996;17(suppl D):9–14.

12. Barrett-Connor E, Bush TL. Estrogen and coronary heart disease in women. *JAMA* 1991;265: 1861–1867.

13. Bush TL, Cowan LD, Barrett-Connor E, et al. Estrogen use and all-cause mortality: Preliminary results from the Lipid Research Clinics Program Follow-Up Study. *JAMA* 1983;249: 903–906.

14. Mendelsohn ME, Karas RH. The protective effects of estrogen on the cardiovascular system. *N Engl J Med* 1999;340:1801–1811.

15. Barrett-Connor E. Heart disease in women. *Fertil Steril* 1994;62:127S–132S.

16. Barrett-Connor E. The menopause, hormone replacement, and cardiovascular disease: The epidemiologic evidence. *Maturitas* 1996;23:227–234.

17. Manson JE, Greenland P, LaCroix AZ, et al. Walking compared with vigorous exercise for the prevention of cardiovascular events in women. *N Engl J Med* 2002;347:716–725.

18. Grady D, Applegate W, Bush T, et al. Heart and Estrogen/progestin Replacement Study (HERS): Design, methods, and baseline characteristics. *Control Clin Trials* 1998;19:314–335.

19. Hulley S, Furberg C, Barrett-Connor E, et al. Noncardiovascular disease outcomes during 6.8 years of hormone therapy: Heart and Estrogen/progestin Replacement Study follow-up (HERS II). *JAMA* 2002;288:58–66.

20. Bush TL. Lessons from HERS: The null and beyond. *J Womens Health* 1998;7:781–783.

21. Wells G, Herrington DM. The Heart and Estrogen/Progestin Replacement Study: What have we learned and what questions remain? *Drugs Aging* 1999;15:419–422.

22. Blumenthal RS, Zacur HA, Reis SE, Post WS. Beyond the null hypothesis: Do the HERS results disprove the estrogen/coronary heart disease hypothesis? *Am J Cardiol* 2000;85: 1015–1017.

23. Skouby SO. The rationale for a wider range of progestogens. *Climacteric* 2000;3(suppl 2): 14–20.

24. Bush T. Beyond HERS: Some (not so) random thoughts on randomized clinical trials. *Int J Fertil Womens Med* 2001;46:55–59.

25. Mendelsohn ME, Karas RH. The time has come to stop letting the HERS tale wag the dogma. *Circulation* 2001;104:2256–2259.

26. Rosano GM, Fini M. Comparative cardiovascular effects of different progestins in menopause. *Int J Fertil Womens Med* 2001;46:248–256.

27. Furberg CD, Vittinghoff E, Davidson M, et al. Subgroup interactions in the Heart and Estrogen/progestin Replacement Study: Lessons learned. *Circulation* 2002;105:917–922.

28. Herrington DM, Vittinghoff E, Lin F, et al. Statin therapy, cardiovascular events, and total mortality in the Heart and Estrogen/progestin Replacement Study (HERS). *Circulation* 2002;105: 2962–2967.

29. Clarkson TB. Progestogens and cardiovascular disease: A critical review. *J Reprod Med* 1999;44: 180–184.

30. Clarkson TB. The new conundrum: Do estrogens have any cardiovascular benefits? *Int J Fertil Womens Med* 2002;47:61–68.

31. Grodstein F, Clarkson TB, Manson JE. Understanding the divergent data on postmenopausal hormone therapy. *N Engl J Med* 2003;348:645–650.

32. Grady D, Herrington D, Bittner V, et al. Cardiovascular disease outcomes during 6.8 years of hormone therapy: Heart and Estrogen/progestin Replacement Study follow-up (HERS II). *JAMA* 2002;288:49–57.

33. Grodstein F, Manson JE, Stampfer MJ. Postmenopausal hormone use and secondary prevention of coronary events in the nurses' health study: A prospective, observational study. *Ann Intern Med* 2001;135:1–8.

34. Lenfant C, Chobanian AV, Jones DW, Roccella EJ. Seventh report of the Joint National Committee on the Prevention, Detection, Evaluation, and Treatment of High Blood Pressure (JNC 7): Resetting the hypertension sails. *Hypertension* 2003;41:1178–1179.

35. Mosca L, Grundy SM, Judelson D, et al. Guide to preventive cardiology for Women's. AHA/ACC Scientific Statement Consensus Panel statement. *Circulation* 1999;99:2480–2484.

36. Mora S, Kershner DW, Vigilance CP, Blumenthal RS. Coronary artery disease in postmenopausal women. *Curr Treat Options Cardiovasc Med* 2001;3:67–79.

37. Estrogen and progestogen use in peri- and postmenopausal women. September 2003 position statement of the North American Menopause Society. *Menopause* 2003;10: 497–506.

38. Research on the menopause in the 1990s: Report of a WHO Scientific Group. *WHO Tech Rep Ser* 1996;866:1–107.

39. Manson JE, Hsia J, Johnson KC, et al. Estrogen plus progestin and the risk of coronary heart disease. *N Engl J Med* 2003;349:523–534.

40. McDonough PG. The randomized world is not without its imperfections: Reflections on the Women's Health Initiative Study. *Fertil Steril* 2002;78:951–956.

41. Grimes DA, Lobo RA. Perspectives on the Women's Health Initiative trial of hormone replacement therapy. *Obstet Gynecol* 2002;100:1344–1353.

42. Mikkola TS, Clarkson TB. Estrogen replacement therapy, atherosclerosis, and vascular function. *Cardiovasc Res* 2002;53:605–619.

43. Hodis HN, Mack WJ, Lobo RA, et al. Estrogen in the prevention of atherosclerosis: A randomized, double-blind, placebo-controlled trial. *Ann Intern Med* 2001;135:939–953.

44. Herrington DM, Reboussin DM, Brosnihan KB, et al. Effects of estrogen replacement on the progression of coronary-artery atherosclerosis. *N Engl J Med* 2000;343:522–529.

45. Pickar JH, Wild RA, Walsh B, et al. Effects of different hormone replacement regimens on postmenopausal women with abnormal lipid levels. Menopause Study Group. *Climacteric* 1998;1:26–32.

46. Lobo RA, Pickar JH, Wild RA, et al.. Metabolic impact of adding medroxyprogesterone acetate to conjugated estrogen therapy in postmenopausal women. The Menopause Study Group. *Obstet Gynecol* 1994;84:987–995.

47. Lobo RA, Bush T, Carr BR, Pickar JH. Effects of lower doses of conjugated equine estrogens and medroxyprogesterone acetate on plasma lipids and lipoproteins, coagulation factors, and carbohydrate metabolism. *Fertil Steril* 2001;76:13–24.

48. Davidson MH, Maki KC, Marx P, et al. Effects of continuous estrogen and estrogen-progestin replacement regimens on cardiovascular risk markers in postmenopausal women. *Arch Intern Med* 2000;160:3315–3325.

49. Speroff L, Rowan J, Symons J, et al. The comparative effect on bone density, endometrium, and lipids of continuous hormones as replacement therapy (CHART study): A randomized, controlled trial. *JAMA* 1996;276:1397–1403.

50. Psaty BM, Smith NL, Lemaitre RN, et al. Hormone replacement therapy, prothrombotic mutations, and the risk of incident nonfatal myocardial infarction in postmenopausal women. *JAMA* 2001;285:906–913.

51. Herrington DM, Howard TD, Hawkins GA, et al. Estrogen-receptor polymorphisms and effects of estrogen replacement on high-density lipoprotein cholesterol in women with coronary disease. *N Engl J Med* 2002;346:967–974.

52. Cherry N, Gilmour K, Hannaford P, et al. Oestrogen therapy for prevention of reinfarction in postmenopausal women: A randomised, placebo-controlled trial. *Lancet* 2002;360:2001–2008.

53. Clarke SC, Kelleher J, Lloyd-Jones H, et al. A study of hormone replacement therapy in postmenopausal women with ischaemic heart disease: The Papworth HRT atherosclerosis study. *Br J Obstet Gynaecil* 2002;109:1056–1062.

54. Simon JA, Hsia J, Cauley JA, et al. Postmenopausal hormone therapy and risk of stroke: The Heart and Estrogen/progestin Replacement Study (HERS). *Circulation* 2001;103:638–642.

55. Sacco RL, Wolf PA, Gorelick PB. Risk factors and their management for stroke prevention: Outlook for 1999 and beyond. *Neurology* 1999;53:S15–24.

56. Boden-Albala B, Sacco RL. Lifestyle factors and stroke risk: Exercise, alcohol, diet, obesity, smoking, drug use, and stress. *Curr Atheroscler Rep* 2000;2:160–166.

57. Paganini-Hill A. Hormone replacement therapy and stroke: risk, protection or no effect? *Maturitas* 2001;38:243–261.

58. Hu FB, Grodstein F. Postmenopausal hormone therapy and the risk of cardiovascular disease: The epidemiologic evidence. *Am J Cardiol* 2002;90:26F–29F.

59. Wassertheil-Smoller S, Hendrix SL, Limacher M, et al. Effect of estrogen plus progestin on stroke in postmenopausal women: the Women's Health Initiative: A randomized trial. *JAMA* 2003;289:2673–2684.

60. Viscoli CM, Brass LM, Kernan WN, et al. A clinical trial of estrogen-replacement therapy after ischemic stroke. *N Engl J Med* 2001;345:1243–1249.

61. Lemaitre RN, Heckbert SR, Psaty BM, et al. Hormone replacement therapy and associated risk of stroke in postmenopausal women. *Arch Intern Med* 2002;162:1954–1960.

62. Angeja BG, Shlipak MG, Go AS, et al. Hormone therapy and the risk of stroke after acute myocardial infarction in postmenopausal women. *J Am Coll Cardiol* 2001;38:1297–1301.

63. Grady D, Wenger NK, Herrington D, et al. Postmenopausal hormone therapy increases risk for venous thromboembolic disease. The Heart and Estrogen/progestin Replacement Study. *Ann Intern Med* 2000;132:689–696.

64. Jick H, Derby LE, Myers MW, et al. Risk of hospital admission for idiopathic venous thromboembolism among users of postmenopausal oestrogens. *Lancet* 1996;348:981–983.

65. Daly E, Vessey MP, Hawkins MM, et al. Risk of venous thromboembolism in users of hormone replacement therapy. *Lancet* 1996;348:977–980.

66. Miller J, Chan BK, Nelson HD. Postmenopausal estrogen replacement and risk for venous thromboembolism: A systematic review and meta-analysis for the U.S. Preventive Services Task Force. *Ann Intern Med* 2002;136:680–690.

67. Grodstein F, Stampfer MJ, Goldhaber SZ, et al. Prospective study of exogenous hormones and risk of pulmonary embolism in women. *Lancet* 1996;348:983–987.

68. Herrington DM, Vittinghoff E, Howard TD, et al. Factor V Leiden, hormone replacement therapy, and risk of venous thromboembolic events in women with coronary disease. *Arterioscler Thromb Vasc Biol* 2002;22:1012–1017.

69. Bloemenkamp KW, Helmerhorst FM, Rosendaal FR, Vandenbroucke JP. Thrombophilias and gynaecology. *Best Pract Res Clin Obstet Gynaecol* 2003;17:509–528.

70. Scarabin PY, Oger E, Plu-Bureau G. Differential association of oral and transdermal oestrogen-replacement therapy with venous thromboembolism risk. *Lancet* 2003;362:428–432.

71. Cano A, Van Baal WM. The mechanisms of thrombotic risk induced by hormone replacement therapy. *Maturitas* 2001;40:17–38.

72. Rosendaal FR, Vessey M, Rumley A, et al. Hormonal replacement therapy, prothrombotic mutations and the risk of venous thrombosis. *Br J Haematol* 2002;116:851–854.

73. Chandramouli NB, Rodgers GM. Management of thrombosis in women with antiphospholipid syndrome. *Clin Obstet Gynecol* 2001;44:36–47.

74. Barrett-Connor E, Slone S, Greendale G, et al. The Postmenopausal Estrogen/Progestin Interventions study: Primary outcomes in adherent women. *Maturitas* 1997;27:261–274.

75. Harvey PJ, Molloy D, Upton J, Wing LM. Dose response effect of conjugated equine oestrogen on blood pressure in postmenopausal women with hypertension. *Blood Press* 2000;9:275–282.

76. Harvey PJ, Molloy D, Upton J, Wing LM. Dose-response effect of cyclical medroxyprogesterone on blood pressure in postmenopausal women. *J Hum Hypertens* 2001;15:313–321.

77. Harvey PJ, Wing LM, Savage J, Molloy D. The effects of different types and doses of oestrogen replacement therapy on clinic and ambulatory blood pressure and the renin-angiotensin system in normotensive postmenopausal women. *J Hypertens* 1999;17:405–411.

78. Zacharieva S, Atanassova I, Kirilov G, et al. Effect of transdermal estrogen therapy on some vasoactive humoral factors and 24-h ambulatory blood pressure in normotensive postmenopausal women. *Climacteric* 2002;5:293–299.

79. Bush TL, Whiteman M, Flaws JA. Hormone replacement therapy and breast cancer: A qualitative review. *Obstet Gynecol* 2001;98:498–508.

80. Goss PE, Ingle JN, Martino S, et al. A randomized trial of letrozole in postmenopausal women after 5 years of tamoxifen therapy for early-stage breast cancer. *N Engl J Med* 2003;349:1793–1802.

81. Beral V. Breast cancer and hormone-replacement therapy in the Million Women Study. *Lancet* 2003;362:419–427.

82. Beral V, Banks E, Reeves G, Appleby P. Use of HRT and the subsequent risk of cancer. *J Epidemiol Biostat* 1999;4:191–210; discussion: 210–215.

83. Breast cancer and hormone replacement therapy: Collaborative reanalysis of data from 51 epidemiological studies of 52,705 women with breast cancer and 108,411 women without breast cancer. Collaborative Group on Hormonal Factors in Breast Cancer. *Lancet* 1997;350:1047–1059.

84. Breast cancer and hormone replacement therapy: Collaborative reanalysis of data from 51 epidemiological studies of 52,705 women with breast cancer and 108,411 women without breast cancer. Collaborative Group on Hormonal Factors in Breast Cancer. *Lancet* 1997;350:1047–1059.

85. Chlebowski RT, Hendrix SL, Langer RD, et al. Influence of estrogen plus progestin on breast cancer and mammography in healthy post-menopausal women: the Women's Health Initiative randomized trial. *JAMA* 2003;289: 3243–3253.

86. Cline JM, Soderqvist G, von Schoultz E, et al. Effects of conjugated estrogens, medroxyprogesterone acetate, and tamoxifen on the mammary glands of macaques. *Breast Cancer Res Treat* 1998;48:221–229.

87. Conner P, Soderqvist G, Skoog L, et al. Breast cell proliferation in postmenopausal women during HRT evaluated through fine needle aspiration cytology. *Breast Cancer Res Treat* 2003;78:159–165.

88. Sitruk-Ware R, Plu-Bureau G. Progestins and cancer. *Gynecol Endocrinol* 1999;13(suppl 4): 3–9.

89. Speroff L. Role of progesterone in normal breast physiology. *J Reprod Med* 1999;44:172–179.

90. Conner P, Skoog L, Soderqvist G. Breast epithelial proliferation in postmenopausal women evaluated through fine-needle-aspiration cytology. *Climacteric* 2001;4:7–12.

91. Clemons M, Goss P. Estrogen and the risk of breast cancer. *N Engl J Med* 2001;344: 276– 285.

92. Greendale GA, Reboussin BA, Sie A, et al. Effects of estrogen and estrogen-progestin on mammographic parenchymal density: Postmenopausal Estrogen/Progestin Interventions (PEPI) Investigators. *Ann Intern Med* 1999;130: 262–269.

93. Boyd NF, Martin LJ, Stone J, et al. Mammographic densities as a marker of human breast cancer risk and their use in chemoprevention. *Curr Oncol Rep* 2001;3:314–321.

94. Greendale GA, Reboussin BA, Slone S, et al. Postmenopausal hormone therapy and change in mammographic density. *J Natl Cancer Inst* 2003;95:30–37.

95. Boyd NF, Stone J, Martin LJ, et al. The association of breast mitogens with mammographic densities. *Br J Cancer* 2002;87:876–882.

96. Archer DF. The effect of the duration of progestin use on the occurrence of endometrial cancer in postmenopausal women. *Menopause* 2001;8:245–251.

97. Rousseau ME. Hormone replacement therapy: Short-term versus long-term use. *J Midwifery Womens Health* 2002;47:461–470.

98. Effects of estrogen or estrogen/progestin regimens on heart disease risk factors in postmenopausal women. The Postmenopausal Estrogen/Progestin Interventions (PEPI) Trial. The Writing Group for the PEPI Trial. *JAMA* 1995;273:199–208.

99. Woodruff JD, Pickar JH. Incidence of endometrial hyperplasia in postmenopausal women taking conjugated estrogens (Premarin) with medroxyprogesterone acetate or conjugated estrogens alone. The Menopause Study Group. *Am J Obstet Gynecol* 1994;170:1213–1223.

100. Kurman RJ, Felix JC, Archer DF, et al. Norethindrone acetate and estradiol-induced endometrial hyperplasia. *Obstet Gynecol* 2000;96: 373–379.

101. Pickar JH, Thorneycroft I, Whitehead M. Effects of hormone replacement therapy on the endometrium and lipid parameters: A review of randomized clinical trials, 1985 to 1995. *Am J Obstet Gynecol* 1998;178:1087–1099.

102. Pickar JH, Yeh I, Wheeler JE, Cunnane MF, Speroff L. Endometrial effects of lower doses of conjugated equine estrogens and medroxyprogesterone acetate. *Fertil Steril* 2001;76: 25–31.

103. Pickar JH, Yeh IT, Wheeler JE, et al. Endometrial effects of lower doses of conjugated equine estrogens and medroxyprogesterone acetate: Two-year substudy results. *Fertil Steril* 2003;80: 1234–1240.

104. Lacey JV Jr, Mink PJ, Lubin JH, et al. Menopausal hormone replacement therapy and risk of ovarian cancer. *JAMA* 2002;288:334–341.

105. Sit AS, Modugno F, Weissfeld JL, et al. Hormone replacement therapy formulations and risk of epithelial ovarian carcinoma. *Gynecol Oncol* 2002;86:118–123.

106. Garg PP, Kerlikowske K, Subak L, Grady D. Hormone replacement therapy and the risk of epithelial ovarian carcinoma: A meta-analysis. *Obstet Gynecol* 1998;92:472–479.

107. Coughlin SS, Giustozzi A, Smith SJ, Lee NC. A meta-analysis of estrogen replacement therapy and risk of epithelial ovarian cancer. *J Clin Epidemiol* 2000;53:367–375.

108. Rodriguez C, Patel AV, Calle EE, et al. Estrogen replacement therapy and ovarian cancer mortality in a large prospective study of US women. *JAMA* 2001;285:1460–1465.

109. Persson I. Estrogens in the causation of breast, endometrial and ovarian cancers: Evidence and hypotheses from epidemiological findings. *J Steroid Biochem Mol Biol* 2000;74:357–3564.

110. Parazzini F, La Vecchia C, Negri E, et al. Case-control study of oestrogen replacement therapy and risk of cervical cancer. *Br Med J* 1997; 315:85–88.

111. Lacey JV Jr, Brinton LA, et al. Use of hormone replacement therapy and adenocarcinomas and squamous cell carcinomas of the uterine cervix. *Gynecol Oncol* 2000;77:149–154.

112. Anderson GL, Judd HL, Kaunitz AM, et al. Effects of estrogen plus progestin on gynecologic cancers and associated diagnostic procedures: The Women's Health Initiative randomized trial. *JAMA* 2003;290:1739–1748.

CHAPTER 32

Alternative Treatment for the Aging Woman: Phytoestrogens and Herbs

RICHARD E. BLACKWELL

Management of menopause really translates into management of aging. On October 12, 1999, the world population reached 6 billion. The projection as of 1992 was for 11.5 billion by 2150, yet revision of those projections done in 1999 suggests that the world population will be about 9.8 billion. The most populous countries will be India, China, and the United States. Each of these countries views menopausal symptoms differently, and obviously, the first two have long traditions of alternative and complementary medicine.

The United States will have large population concentrations along the eastern seaboard and throughout Florida, central Texas, and the southwest, and extending up to the pacific northwest. Different racial groups will be clustered in different areas, African-Americans being concentrated in the south, Hispanics in Florida and the southwest, American Indians in the northwest and the central plains, Pacific Islanders in the Hawaiian Islands, and Eskimos in Alaska. The U.S. labor force will become increasingly heterogeneous, with the primary inflow in immigrants coming from Latin America, followed by Asia.

These population shifts are reflected across the world, with Europe having an increasingly older population and a smaller, younger labor force. The pattern is similar in the United States except our younger labor force will represent this heterogeneous population. Most European nations today fall below the two-children replacement rate, and in the United States, only the Hispanic population is growing.

These changes in population and age bring about altered social dynamics. In the United States, families tend to be disbursed, with few support systems in place. In other countries, notably Asia, two and three generations often live under the same roof.

In 1900, menopause was not a social issue for this country. The average lifespan of women was approximately 42 years of age, and 1 in 4 died in childbirth. These statistics are reflected in third-world countries, such as those found in central Africa today. As of 2003, women could expect to live into the mid-80s, and by 2050, it will not be unreasonable to expect to find women living beyond 100 years. It is projected that the longevity of men will not equal that of women given our propensity for violence, homicide, and dangerous activities; and in fact, in subhuman primates it is felt that reproduction alone decreases male lifespan.

Different societies value the human body and its age differently. For instance, Upanisadic St. Matiri described the human body "as an ill-smelling mess of skin, marrow, blood, and mucus," "a bag filled with phlegm, feces, urine, wind, and bile—what good is the enjoyment of desires in this?" Joshua Blank, author of *Arrows of the Blue Skin God,* raised the question, "Should the flesh be glorified or mortified? Is the human frame a temple or a prison?" Most Americans feel that a good life should be a long one filled with good health, yet when one reaches the end, both mind and body should be prepared to leave. Therefore, it would seem that the goal of menopausal management is to help smooth the passage through this journey.

Until recently, estrogen was considered to be a menopausal cure-all, a virtual pharmacologic fountain of youth. Recent studies such as the Heart and Estrogen/progestin Replacement Study (HERS) I and II and the Women's Health Initiative (WHI) have cast doubt on the wisdom of prescribing estrogen replacement therapy or hormone replacement therapy for all women.[1–5] In fact, some proponents would suggest that these agents carry too high a general health risk and that alternative therapies should be used to treat various menopausally associated conditions. Combined with this therapeutic turn of events, there is a developing skepticism among the public with regard to allopathic medicine. Mind you, this is the same public that has become the most obese population in the world, has terrible dietary habits, continues to smoke and abuse alcohol, continues to use recreational drugs, produces the highest homicide rate in the world, is one of the most sedentary populations in the world, refuses to wear seatbelts, and is reluctant to undergo medical screening procedures that prolong not only the length but improve the quality of their life.[6–8] Alternative and complementary therapies have been embraced so widely that in 2000 the sales of herbal and botanical supplements exceeded $5 billion, and the current projection is that the amount of money spent on all alternative and complementary therapies equals that spent on prescription pharmaceuticals. The question that must be raised is: Why would individuals gravitate to nutraceuticals that are classified as food supplements with no Food and Drug Administration (FDA) regulation, limited manufacturer oversight, and no quality control or control of uses? For the answer, perhaps we should go back and examine the personality of the traditional healer. Healers are interested in others, have a sense of humor, need to help others, tend to be spiritual, often have little formal education, and are more interested in others than in themselves. "They do not take themselves, disease, healing, life, or death too seriously and believe that humor is an integral part of the healing process." Don Julio Ponte, the Shaman of Belize, feels that "most people think too much. Get them to laugh, and half their troubles and sickness will go away and the blessed herbs will do the rest." Perhaps we as allopathic practitioners should reflect on some of these traits and comments.

▶ ROLE OF SOY IN THE TREATMENT OF MENOPAUSAL SYMPTOMS

Since the intensity of menopausal symptoms increases in the 12 months prior to menopause and decreases within 6 months afterward, 9 of 10 women who seek either hormonal or nontraditional therapy do so for relief of psychomotor symptoms. However, accompanying the psychomotor symptoms frequently will be fatigue, unexplained depression, decreased libido, insomnia, decreased cognitive function, and memory loss. All these have been attributed to either hypoestrogenism and/or hypoandrogenism. One of the most common therapies to combat psychomotor symptoms would be the use of phytoestrogens (isoflavones). There are approximately 20 phytoestrogens, the most widely known being Genistein.(Table 32-1) The phytoestrogens generally are found in high concentrations in soy and in red clover. They function like selective estrogen receptor modulators, bind weakly to the estrogen receptor α, and have an 87 percent affinity for the estrogen receptor β. Phytoestrogens have both agonists and antagonist properties, free isoflavones are absorbed in the gut, and the rest are metabolized to aglycones. Isoflavinoids are metabolized to dihydrodiadzein, Equal, *O*-desmethylangolasin. There is great variability in metabolism within individuals that produces a large mix of agonists and antagonists. These agents have great biologic activity: They have antioxidant effects, they inhibit the enzymes involved in estrogen metabolism, they inhibit protein kinases, they affect both ion and glucose transport, they alter protein synthesis, they alter cell proliferation, and they alter angiogenesis and growth factor action. They have been demonstrated to inhibit bone loss in animals, although this is limited to the spine, and no fracture data are available. They are thought to have a positive effect on the brain, to increase high-density lipoprotein (HDL) cholesterol and decrease low-density lipoprotein (LDL) cholesterol, have a positive effect on coronary artery dilatation, inhibit the breast, and inhibit the uterus. An epidemiologic observation has suggested that soy decreases the incidence of breast and prostate cancer and decreases mastalgia. Japanese women consume 45 mg daily and have 75 percent less breast cancer than their U.S. counterparts, and soy re-duces proliferation of breast cancer cells 28 to 30 percent in vitro, the same as tamoxifen or raloxifene. It is recommended that 50 mg soy be consumed in the diet; however, for the prevention of osteoporosis, a dose of 80 mg has been recommended. High consumption of phytoestrogens has no known adverse effect.[9,10]

Flaxseed is a food source rich in lignans, one of the major groups of phytoestrogens. Lignans have been implicated as having antitumorigenic activity, estrogenic and antiestrogenic activity, and antioxidant properties. In animal models it has been reported that the major lignan of flaxseed produces little change in cholesterol or LDL concentrations. When women consumed 40 g ground flaxseed daily for 3 months compared with controls, the flaxseed supplementation lowered total cholesterol and non-HDL cholesterol by 6 percent. The flaxseed regimen also reduced serum levels of LDL and HDL cholesterol by 4.7 percent and triglycerides by 12.8 percent. Serum apolipoprotein A_1 and apolipoprotein B concentrations were reduced significantly by 6 and 7.5 percent, respectively. It should be noted that there was no change in bone formation or resorption with this therapy.[11]

▶ CNS ALTERNATIVE AGENTS

Other agents that have been used to treat menopausal symptoms include dong quai. This is an aromatic herb that contains 12 coumarin-like derivatives. It is vasodilatory and antispasmodic, and doses up to 4.5 g have no effect on hot flashes. Side effects include photosensitization and dermatitis.[12] Black cohosh (Remifemin, Glaxo at Zomg BD) is used for menstrual control and contains isoflavinoids and trteperpenses. Uncontrolled trials show some effect on hirsutism. It has been approved by the German FDA for the treatment of hot flashes and menstrual cramps, but it is contraindicated in pregnancy.[13,14]

Extract of red clover (Promensil), in small studies including 48 patients treated for 6

▶ **TABLE 32-1:** ETHANOBOTANICALS

- Soy
- Red clover
- Snake root
- Hops
- Vitamin E
- Dong quai
- Primitive dill
- Flaxseed dill

months, showed an increase in HDL cholesterol, a decrease in apoprotein B, and an increase in cortical bone in the proximal radius and ulna at doses of 28.5 mg.[15]

Wild yam creams contain saponins, which can be converted to progesterone in vitro. This conversion cannot occur in vivo because the human body lacks the effective enzymes for the last conversion step. Discoria, an intermediate, cannot be converted to either progesterone or dehydroepiandrosterone (DHEA) in vitro. Therefore, these therapies are essentially worthless with the exception of the placebo effect.

St. John's Wort affects the uptake of serotonin, epinephrine, and norepinephrine. It inhibits monoamine oxidase and increases γ-aminobutyric acid (GABA) turnover. It is thought to be effective for the treatment of mild depression, but it has been shown not to be effective for major depressive disorders. Its side effects include gastrointestinal upset and photosensitivity.[16]

▶ COMPOUNDED PREPARATIONS

Often confused with natural hormonal products are the tri- and biestrogens. These are mixtures of estriol, estrone, and estradiol, all of which obviously have to be synthesized by a pharmaceutical house before they can be placed into compound preparations. Patients often are told that these preparations do not cause breast cancer; no data exist either refuting this statement or supporting it. Since estriol is produced in high quantities only during pregnancy, it seems that this type of therapy would be nonphysiologic.

Progesterone creams often are presented in a similar manner, and patients frequently are upset to find that these agents are made by a major pharmaceutical house and sold to compounding pharmacists. Topical progesterones usually come in 3% to 6% formulations; preparations show tremendous variability of absorption ranging from 0 to 100 percent. When used in a perimenopausal patient, these preparations do not convert the endometrium appropriately. Many of these patients are transiently amenorrheic, and when bleeding occurs, they are found to have adenocarcinomas. In general, use of these preparations by a perimenopausal patient should be discouraged. Further, lay books portray menopause and perimenopause as a progesterone-deficiency state. Proponents of progesterone-only therapy fail to recognize the physiology of normal folliculogenesis and the relationship of estrogen to progesterone in maintaining homeostasis. In general, the only use of topical progesterone seems to be the application of its sedative effect to the induction of sleep.

▶ PSYCHOPHARMACEUTICALS

While not generally considered part of complementary and alternative medicine, central nervous system (CNS)–affecting agents can be used to control psychomotor symptoms. These include selective serotonin reuptake inhibitors (SSRIs), gabapentin, clonidine, beralipride, tibolone, propranolol, bellergal, and α-methyldopa.

SSRIs

The SSRIs paroxetine (Paxil), sertraline (Zoloft), fluoxetine (Prozac/Sarafem), and venlafaxine (Effexor) have all been used to inhibit hot flashes (Table 32-2). The paroxetines have been

▶ **TABLE 32-2:** CNS-ALTERING PHARMACEUTICALS

• Selective serotonin reuptake inhibitors (SSRIs)
• Clonidine
• α-Methyldopa
• Gabapentin
• Veraliprid

involved in two pilot trials involving 43 patients being treated with 20 mg/d for 4 to 5 weeks. This resulted in a decrease in hot flashes by about 75 percent. Paroxetine 20 mg/d for 4 weeks in 81 patients was reported to decrease hot flashes by about 50 percent. This has been controlled in crossover trials. Effexor has been shown in three studies to decrease symptoms up to 61 percent.[17–20]

Clonidine

Clonidine is a central α_2-adrenergic agonist that inhibits catecholamine release. A dose of 0.1 mg/d produces an appreciable reduction in hot flashes, but side effects include sleep disturbance, constipation, drowsiness, and dry mouth.[21,22]

Neurontin

Neurontin at 300 to 600 mg/d decreases hot flashes up to 70 percent. Veraliprid (Agreal) is a European nonhormonal agent used to treat hot flashes. It has antidopaminergic activity and enhances opioid activity. At a dose of 100 mg/d it has some beneficial effects on hot flashes.[23]

α-Methyldopa

α-Methyldopa at doses of 250 to 500 mg used at bedtime seems to have a positive effect on hot flashes in about 80 percent of patients, but fatigue is a significant side effect.[24]

Tibilone

Tibilone is a synthetic steroid prodrug with estrogenic, progestogenic, and androgenic activity. The product has been used in Europe at 2.5 mg/d. It has been shown to reduce hot flashes and is currently under FDA review.[25]

Vitamin E

One vitamin E has been evaluated in 105 patients for 4 weeks at 80 IU/d and has a marginal effect on decreasing hot flashes.

▶ WELL WOMEN'S CARE

It is my feeling that patients experiment with complementary and alternative therapies hoping to receive all the benefits of hormone replacement but with none of the hypothetical risks. It is my goal to ensure that patients get all the benefits promised by these therapies and also ensure that they have minimal risks. I would suggest that the practitioner be very aggressive in patients using these therapies. Individuals should have mammograms, periodic DEXA scans, ultrasounds of the ovaries and uterine lining, measurement of CA-125 antigen, measurement of lipids and a vascular assessment profile, assessment of C reactive protein levels, measurement of thyroid-stimulating hormone (TSH), assessment for insulin resistance, dietary counseling, and appropriate gastrointestinal screening (Table 32-3).

▶ TABLE 32-3: PREVENTIVE MEDICINE IN ADULT WOMEN

- H & P, each year
- Mammogram, each year
- Lipids, each year
- C-reactive protein, each year
- Thyroid stimulating hormone (TSH), every 2 years
- DEXA scan, baseline
- Pelvic ultrasound, each year
- Diet coverage, each year
- Fasting blood sugar (FBS) and insulin, as needed
- Stool guaiac, each year
- Colon screen, every 5 to 8 years

► **TABLE 32-4:** ALTERNATIVE MENOPAUSAL SYMPTOMS

1. Lifestyle changes
   - Proper diet (vegetables, grain, fiber, fruits)
   - Soy, 60–80 mg/day
   - Exercise (aerobic, weight bearing)
   - Adequate sleep
   - Discontinue alcohol, smoking, caffeine
   - Maintain healthy weight [body mass index (BMI) 25]
2. Yoga for relaxation
3. Ethanobotanicals for psychomotor symptoms
   - Black cohosh
   - Flax seed oil
   - Red clover extract
   - Ginseng ($\pm$)

The role of complementary and alternative medicine and how it will relate to allopathic medicine in the future remains unclear. A recent cover of Newsweek had a title that said, "The Science of Alternate Medicine." There certainly appears to be a role for such therapies as acupuncture in the management of pain and the use of Botox injections in the treatment of migraines; soy has a place in the healthy diet; Tai massage appears to be an alternate form of physical therapy; moxibustin seems similar in many regards to the therapeutic use of various vapors; yoga and other forms of relaxation clearly can help to relieve stress; and ethnobotanicals include such well-known agents as digitalis and curare. It is likely that the future will lead to an incorporation of complementary and alternative medical practices into allopathic medicine guided by evidence[26] (Table 32-4).

KEY POINTS

1. The U.S. population is becoming more diverse as a result of immigration from Central and South America and Asia, parts of the world that have a strong tradition in alternative and complementary medicine.

2. Studies such as HERS I, HERS II, and the WHI have cast doubt on the wisdom of using traditional hormone replacement therapy.

3. Most women seek treatment for psychomotor symptoms, and nonhormonal alternatives such as herbal medications and neuropharmaceuticals have proven useful in treating these conditions.

4. Menopausal symptoms usually increase in the first 12 months prior to the cessation of menses and decrease within the next 6 months.

5. Approximately 80 percent of women are symptom-free within 8 months to 1 year after the cessation of menstruation.

6. Soy is a widely used food product that contains ethanobotanical agents such as isoflavones. The isoflavones have some modest effect on reducing psychomotor symptoms and seem to produce favorable lipid profiles, although they have minimal effect on bone stability.

7. SSRIs such as fluoxetine reduce hot flashes.

REFERENCES

1. Grady D, Herrington D, Bittner V, et al, for the HERS Research Group. Cardiovascular disease outcome during 6.8 years hormone therapy. Heart and Estrogen/progestin Replacement Study follow-up study (HERS II). *JAMA* 2002; 288:49–57.

2. Simon JA, Hsia J, Cauley JA, et al. Postmenopausal hormone therapy and risk of stroke: The Heart and Estrogen/progestin Replacement Study (HERS). *Circulation* 2001;103: 638–642.

3. Hulley S, Furberg C, Barrett-Connon E, et al, for the HERS Research Group. Noncardiovascular disease outcome during 6.8 years of hormone therapy. Heart and Estrogen/progestin Replacement Study follow-up (HERS II). *JAMA* 2002;288:58–66.

4. Grady D, Wenger NK, Herrington D, et al. Post-menopausal hormone therapy increases risk for venous thromboembolic disease: The Heart and Estrogen/progestin Replacement Study. *Ann Intern Med* 2000;1997:389–396.
5. Writing Group for the Women's Health Initiative Investigators. Risks and benefits of estrogen plus progestin in healthy postmenopausal women. *JAMA* 2002;288:321–333.
6. Strauss RS, Pollack HA. Epidemic increase in childhood overweight, 1986–1998. *JAMA* 2001;286:2845–2848.
7. Ford ES, Giles WH, Dietz WH. Prevalence of the metabolic syndrome among US adults. *JAMA* 2002; 287:356–376.
8. Irwin MI, Yasui Y, Ulrich CM, et al. Effect of exercise on total and intra-abdominal body fat in postmenopausal women: A randomized, controlled trial. *JAMA* 2003;289:323–330.
9. Naftolin F, Guadelupe SM. Phytoestrogens: Are they really estrogen mimics? *Fertil Steril* 2002; 68:981–986.
10. Han KK, Soares JM Jr, Haidar MA, et al. Benefits of soy isoflavone therapeutic regimen on menopausal symptoms. *Obstet Gynecol* 2002;99:289–293.
11. Lucas EA, Wild RD, Hammond LJ, et al. Flaxseed improves lipid profile without altering biomarkers of bone metabolism in postmenopausal women. *J Clin Endocrinol Metab* 2002;87(4): 1527–1532.
12. Hirata JD, Swiersz LM, Zell B. Does dong quai have estrogenic effects of postmenopausal women. *Fertil Steril* 1996;68:981–986.
13. Blumenthal M, Goldberg A, Gruenwald J. *Black Cohash*. German Commission E Monograph (translated). Austin, TX: American Botanical Council, 1998.
14. Jacobson JS, Troxel AB, Evans J. Randomized trial of black cohost for treatment of hot flashes among women with a history of breast cancer. *J Clin Oncol* 2001;19(10):2739–2745.
15. Van de Weijer, Baremtsen R. Isoflavones from red clover (Promentsil) significantly reduces menopausal hot flush symptoms compared with placebo. *Maturitas* 2002;42(3):187.
16. Hypericum Depression Trial Study Group. Effect of *Hypericum perforatum* (St. John's Wort) in major depressive disorder: A randomized, controlled trial. *JAMA* 2002;287:1807–1814.
17. Loprinzi CL, Pisansky TM, Fonseca R. Pilot evaluation of venlafaxine for therapy of hot flashes in cancer survivors. *J Clin Oncol* 1998;16:2377.
18. Weitzner MA, Moncello J, Jacobson PB. A pilot trial of paroxetine for treatment of hot flashes and associated symptoms in women with breast cancer. *J Pain Symptom Manage* 1001;23(4):337.
19. Loprinzi CL, Sloan JA, Perez EA. Phase III evaluation of fluoxetine for treatment of hot flashes. *J Clin Oncol* 2001;20(6):1578.
20. Roth AJ, Scher HI. Sertraline relieves hot flushes secondary to medical castration. *Psychiatr Oncol* 1998;7(2):129.
21. Pandya KJ, Raubertas RF, Flynn PJ. Oral clonidine in postmenopausal patients with breast cancer experiencing tamoxifen-induced hot flashes. *Ann Intern Med* 2000;132(10):788.
22. Nagamani M, Kelver ME, Smith ER. Treatment of menopausal hot flushes with transdermal administration of clonidine *Am J Obstet Gynecol* 1987;156(3):561.
23. Guttuso TJ. Gabapentins effect on hot flashes and hypothermia. *Neurology* 2000;54:2161–2163.
24. Hammond MC, Hatley L, Talbert LM. A double-blind study to evaluate the effect of methyldopa on menopausal vasomotor flushes. *J Clin Endocrinol Metab* 1984;56:1158–1160.
25. Barton DL, Loprinzi CL, Quella SK. Prospective evaluation of vitamin E for hot flashes in breast cancer survivors. *Fertil Steril* 1996;495:500.
26. Renckens CNM. Alternative treatments in reproductive medicine: Much ado about nothing. *Eur Soc Hum Reprod* 2002;3:528–533.

Index

Page numbers followed by *f* indicate figures, by *t* indicate tables.